Textbook of
BIOCHEMISTRY
for
Dental/Nursing/Pharmacy Students

Other Publications by the Same Author

- Textbook of Medical Biochemistry, 4th Edn, 2000
- Clinical Chemistry: Organ Function Tests and Laboratory Investigations, 1st Edn, 1999
- Viva in Biochemistry, 1st Edn, 1999

Textbook of BIOCHEMISTRY *for* *Dental/Nursing/Pharmacy Students*

(Also for Medical Science/Life Science/Agriculture/DMLT and Homeopathy/Ayurvedic Colleges, etc.)

Third Edition

Dr (Brig) MN Chatterjea
BSc MBBS DCP MD (Biochemistry)

Formerly
Professor and Head
Department of Biochemistry
Armed Forces Medical College, Pune

Professor and Head
Department of Biochemistry
Christian Medical College, Ludhiana

Professor and Head
Department of Biochemistry
MGM's Medical College, Aurangabad

Specialist in Pathology and Biochemistry and
Reader in Pathology
Armed Forces Medical College
Pune, India

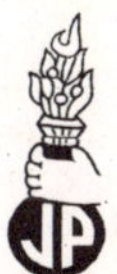

JAYPEE BROTHERS MEDICAL PUBLISHERS (P) LTD

New Delhi • Ahmedabad • Bengaluru • Chennai
Hyderabad • Kochi • Kolkata • Lucknow • Mumbai • Nagpur • St Louis (USA)

Published by
Jitendar P Vij
Jaypee Brothers Medical Publishers (P) Ltd
Corporate Office
4838/24 Ansari Road, Daryaganj, **New Delhi** - 110002, India, Phone: +91-11-43574357
Registered Office
B-3 EMCA House, 23/23B Ansari Road, Daryaganj, **New Delhi** - 110 002, India
Phones: +91-11-23272143, +91-11-23272703, +91-11-23282021
+91-11-23245672, Rel: +91-11-32558559, Fax: +91-11-23276490, +91-11-23245683
e-mail: jaypee@jaypeebrothers.com, Visit our website: www.jaypeebrothers.com

Branches

- 2/B, Akruti Society, Jodhpur Gam Road Satellite
Ahmedabad 380 015, Phones: +91-79-26926233, Rel: +91-79-32988717
Fax: +91-79-26927094, e-mail: ahmedabad@jaypeebrothers.com
- 202 Batavia Chambers, 8 Kumara Krupa Road, Kumara Park East
Bengaluru 560 001, Phones: +91-80-22285971, +91-80-22382956, 91-80-22372664
Rel: +91-80-32714073, Fax: +91-80-22281761 e-mail: bangalore@jaypeebrothers.com
- 282 IIIrd Floor, Khaleel Shirazi Estate, Fountain Plaza, Pantheon Road
Chennai 600 008, Phones: +91-44-28193265, +91-44-28194897, Rel: +91-44-32972089
Fax: +91-44-28193231 e-mail: chennai@jaypeebrothers.com
- 4-2-1067/1-3, 1st Floor, Balaji Building, Ramkote Cross Road,
Hyderabad 500 095, Phones: +91-40-66610020, +91-40-24758498
Rel:+91-40-32940929, Fax:+91-40-24758499 e-mail: hyderabad@jaypeebrothers.com
- No. 41/3098, B & B1, Kuruvi Building, St. Vincent Road
Kochi 682 018, Kerala, Phones: +91-484-4036109, +91-484-2395739
+91-484-2395740 e-mail: kochi@jaypeebrothers.com
- 1-A Indian Mirror Street, Wellington Square
Kolkata 700 013, Phones: +91-33-22651926, +91-33-22276404
+91-33-22276415, Rel: +91-33-32901926, Fax: +91-33-22656075
e-mail: kolkata@jaypeebrothers.com
- Lekhraj Market III, B-2, Sector-4, Faizabad Road, Indira Nagar
Lucknow 226 016 Phones: +91-522-3040553, +91-522-3040554
e-mail: lucknow@jaypeebrothers.com
- 106 Amit Industrial Estate, 61 Dr SS Rao Road, Near MGM Hospital, Parel
Mumbai 400 012, Phones: +91-22-24124863, +91-22-24104532,
Rel: +91-22-32926896, Fax: +91-22-24160828
e-mail: mumbai@jaypeebrothers.com
- "KAMALPUSHPA" 38, Reshimbag, Opp. Mohota Science College, Umred Road
Nagpur 440 009 (MS), Phone: Rel: +91-712-3245220, Fax: +91-712-2704275
e-mail: nagpur@jaypeebrothers.com

USA Office
1745, Pheasant Run Drive, Maryland Heights (Missouri), MO 63043, USA, Ph: 001-636-6279734
e-mail: jaypee@jaypeebrothers.com, anjulav@jaypeebrothers.com

Textbook of Biochemistry for Dental/Nursing/Pharmacy Students

First Edition: 1997
Second Edition: 2004
Third Edition: 2009

ISBN 978-81-8448-531-8

Typeset at JPBMP typesetting unit
Printed at Replika Press Pvt. Ltd.

To
the memory
of my
late parents

CHRISTIAN DENTAL COLLEGE

POST BOX NO. 109

C.M.C., LUDHIANA-141008, PUNJAB

(REGISTERED SOCIETY UNDER ACT NO. XXI OF 1860 AS A CHARITABLE MINORITY INSTITUTION)

Dr. J.L. Joshi
B.Sc., B.D.S., M.D.S.,
F.O.S. (U.S.A), F.A.D.I., F.P.F.A
PRINCIPAL

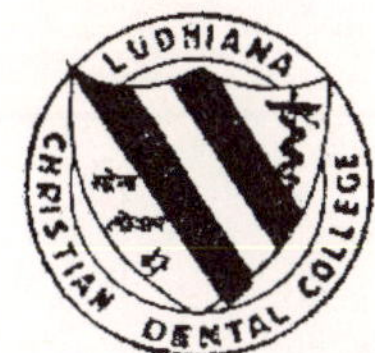

Phones : Office 665659
Residence 609641
Fax : (91) (0161) 665958
Cables Grams : CHRISMED

Foreword

I consider this a privilege to be associated with this publication of the *Textbook of Biochemistry* by Dr (Brig) MN Chatterjea which is a book specially for Dental/Nursing and Pharmacy students.

Biochemistry is one of the basic sciences on which the Medical Science is built upon. This subject needs special talent to make it attractive, enjoyable and understandable to students. The discipline of biochemistry has expanded in recent years and accordingly, a good knowledge is essential for all students related with allied basic sciences. The book is written in simple and lucid language, easily understandable and clinically oriented.

I am sure that this book will prove handy and will be welcomed by undergraduate dental and other students.

Dr JL Joshi BSc BDS MDS FOS (USA) FADI FPFA
Principal, Professor and Head
Christian Dental College
Ludhiana

Preface to the Third Edition

I feel great pleasure and satisfaction to present the third edition of the book *Textbook of Biochemistry for Dental/Nursing/Pharmacy Students* to my beloved students and esteemed teachers. As already pointed out the book can be useful for students of Ayurveda, Homeopathy, DMLT Course and Home Sciences. The book can be of immense value to MBBS students also, who can use the book as a concise companion for rapid revision.

Though, the main framework has been retained, extensive revisions of certain portions have been made. Topics like 'Protein Synthesis' have been rewritten keeping in view of the recent advances. New chapters like 'Recombinant DNA Technology' and 'Biochemistry of AIDS' hot topics have been incorporated.

The overall objective has been to provide concise yet authoritative coverage of the "Basics of Biochemistry" to the Dental/Nursing/Pharmacy students, for applying the knowledge gained for understanding the disease processes.

I have highlighted the important points to be remembered by the students by bold/italic prints. I have tried my utmost to ensure that the language used is simple, lucid and easily understandable by the students. My aim has been to make the book clinically oriented and I have given clinical significance and biomedical importance wherever necessary.

I hope the new edition of the book will fulfil the needs and expectations of the students and teachers of Dental/Nursing/Pharmacy and allied disciplines. I shall look forward for valuable comments and fruitful suggestions, if any, for further inclusions/corrections for improving the quality of the book.

I extend my appreciation and sincere thanks to Shri Jitendar P Vij (Chairman and Managing Director), Mr PG Bandhu (Director-Sales) and Mr Tarun Duneja (Director-Publishing) for their untiring work and keen efforts to bring out the new revised edition of the book.

Dr (Brig) MN Chatterjea

Preface to the First Edition

It gives me immense pleasure and satisfaction in introducing a *Textbook of Biochemistry for Dental/Nursing/Pharmacy Students.*

The discipline of biochemistry, in recent years has expanded by leaps and bounds. The current efflorescence in the knowledge in this subject has necessitated that it should be learnt separately from physiology.

A sound and comprehensive knowledge in biochemistry has now become essential for the students of dental and allied basic sciences. At present there is paucity of a comprehensive standard clinically oriented biochemistry textbook for these students.

My *Textbook of Medical Biochemistry* is being used in certain Dental and Homeopathy Colleges. The book is rather voluminous for them and contains a few topics which are not required by them. Hence, I have attempted to extract the essential elements from the parent book and put in the present concise form.

An attempt has been made in this book to present the subject pointwise, clinically oriented in simple and lucid language avoiding complicated chemical formulae so that it becomes comprehensive, and an average student of dental and basic science can easily understand the subject.

No one can claim to be perfect and even with best of my efforts, there may be some flaws and shortcomings in the book. I shall be highly delighted to welcome constructive criticisms and comments, if any, along with fruitful suggestions to improve the quality of the book in its future editions.

In writing a textbook, one has to take help from others and this book is no exception. I am highly indebted to all my colleagues, friends and authors consulted and referred in compiling the book.

I am grateful to Mr JP Vij, CMD and Mr RK Yadav, Director (Publishing) and the staff of Jaypee Brothers Medical Publishers (P) Ltd. for giving a proper shape in bringing out the first edition of the book successfully.

Dr (Brig) MN Chatterjea

Contents

Chemistry of Carbohydrates

CARBOHYDRATES

DEFINITION

Carbohydrates are defined chemically as aldehyde or ketone derivatives of the higher polyhydric alcohols, or compounds which yield these derivatives on hydrolysis.

CLASSIFICATION

Carbohydrates are divided into *four* major groups—monosaccharides, disaccharides, oligosaccharides and polysaccharides.

1. ***Monosaccharides*** (also called "simple" sugars) are those which cannot be hydrolyzed further into simpler forms.

General formula—$C_nH_{2n}O_n$

They can be subdivided further:

- ***depending upon the number of carbon atoms*** they possess, as trioses, pentoses, hexoses, etc.
- ***depending upon whether aldehyde (–CHO) or ketone (–CO) groups are present*** as aldoses or ketoses.

General formula	*Aldosugars*	*Ketosugars*
• ***Trioses*** ($C_3H_6O_3$)	Glyceraldehyde	Dihydroxyacetone
• ***Tetroses*** ($C_4H_8O_4$)	Erythrose	Erythrulose
• ***Pentoses*** ($C_5H_{10}O_5$)	Ribose	Ribulose
• ***Hexoses*** ($C_6H_{12}O_6$)	Glucose	Fructose

2. ***Disaccharides*:** are those sugars which yield two molecules of the same or different molecules of monosaccharide on hydrolysis.

General formula—$C_n (H_2O)_{n-1}$

Examples

- **Maltose** yields 2 molecules of glucose on hydrolysis.
- **Lactose** yields one molecule of glucose and one molecule of galactose on hydrolysis.
- **Sucrose** yields one molecule of glucose and one molecule of fructose on hydrolysis.

3. ***Oligosaccharides:*** are those which yield 3 to 10 monosaccharide units on hydrolysis.

4. ***Polysaccharides (Glycans):*** are those which yield more than ten molecules of monosaccharides on hydrolysis.

General formula—$(C_6H_{10}O_5)_n$

Polysaccharides are further divided into **two groups:**

- ***Homopolysaccharides (Homoglycans):*** Polymer of same monosaccharide units.

  Examples: Starch, glycogen, inulin, cellulose, dextrins, dextrans.

- ***Heteropolysaccharides (Heteroglycans):*** Polymer of different monosaccharide units or their derivatives.

  Example: Mucopolysaccharides (glycosaminoglycans "GAG").

BIOMEDICAL IMPORTANCE

- Chief source of energy.
- Constituents of compound lipids and conjugated proteins.
- Degradation products act as "promoters" or "catalysts".
- Certain carbohydrate derivatives are used as drugs like cardiac glycosides/antibiotics.
- Lactose: principal sugar of milk, in lactating mammary gland.
- Degradation products utilized for synthesis of other substances such as fatty acid, cholesterol, amino acid, etc.
- Constituents of mucopolysaccharides which form the ground substance of mesenchymal tissues.
- Inherited deficiency of certain enzymes in metabolic pathways of different carbohydrates can cause diseases. ***Derangement of glucose metabolism is seen in diabetes mellitus.***

GENERAL PROPERTIES IN REFERENCE TO GLUCOSE

Asymmetric carbon: A carbon atom to which ***four different atoms or groups of atoms*** are attached is said to be asymmetric ***(Fig. 1.1)***.

Vant Hoff's rule of 'n': The number of possible isomers of any given compound depends upon the number of asymmetric carbon atoms the molecule possesses.

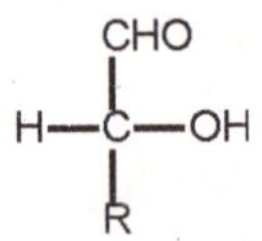

```
     CHO
      |
  H — C — OH
      |
      R
```

Fig. 1.1: Asymmetric carbon

According to Vant Hoff's rule of '*n*', 2^n equals the possible isomers of that compound, where, '*n*' represents the number of asymmetric carbon atoms in a compound.

Stereoisomerism: The presence of asymmetric carbon atoms in a compound gives rise to the formation of isomers of that compound. Such compounds which are identical in composition and differ only in spatial configuration are called ***"stereoisomers".***

Two such isomers of glucose—D-Glucose and L-Glucose are "mirror" image of each other ***(Fig. 1.2)***.

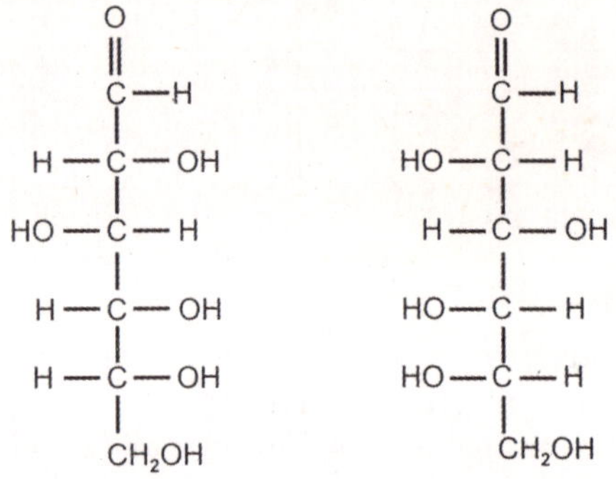

```
        O                     O
        ‖                     ‖
        C — H                 C — H
        |                     |
  H  —  C — OH          HO —  C — H
        |                     |
  HO —  C — H            H —  C — OH
        |                     |
  H  —  C — OH          HO —  C — H
        |                     |
  H  —  C — OH          HO —  C — H
        |                     |
       CH2OH                 CH2OH

    D-Glucose             L-Glucose
```

Fig. 1.2: Stereoisomers of glucose

D-series and L-series: The orientation of H and OH groups around the carbon atom just adjacent to the terminal primary alcohol carbon, e.g. C-atom 5 in glucose determines the series.

When the –OH group on this carbon is on the **right,** it belongs to **D-series,** when the **–OH** group is on the **left,** it is a member of **L-series** ***(Fig. 1.3)***.

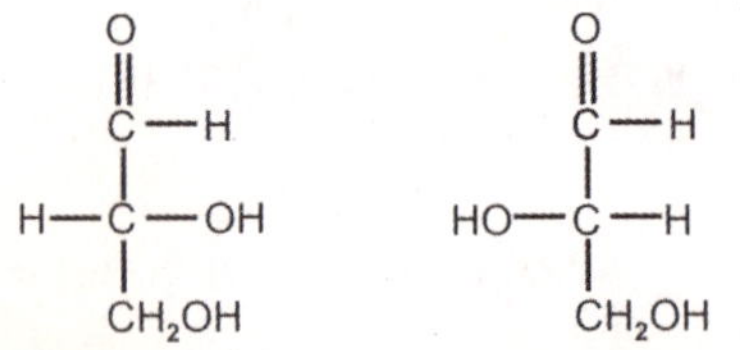

```
        O                       O
        ‖                       ‖
        C — H                   C — H
        |                       |
   H —  C — OH            HO —  C — H
        |                       |
       CH2OH                   CH2OH

     D-Glycerose             L-Glycerose
 (D-Glyceraldehyde)      (L-Glyceraldehyde)
```

Fig. 1.3: D- and L-series

Optical Activity: Presence of asymmetric carbon atoms also confers optical activity on the compound. When a beam of ***plane-polarized*** light is passed through a solution exhibiting optical activity, it will be rotated to the right or left in accordance with the type of compound, i.e. the *"optical isomers"* or *"enantiomorphs"*; when it is rotated to right, the compound is called **"dextrorotatory" (d or + sign),** but when rotated to left, the compound is called **"laevorotatory"** *(l or –sign).*

Racemic: When equal amounts of dextrorotatory and laevorotatory isomers are present, the resulting mixture has no optical activity, since the activities of each isomer cancels the other. Such a mixture is said to be *"racemic".*

Resolution: The separation of optically active isomers from a racemic mixture is called **'resolution'.**

Cyclic structures: As the two reacting groups aldehyde and alcoholic group belong to the same molecule, a cyclic structure takes place. If the open-chain form of D-glucose, which may be called as *"aldehydo-D-glucose"* is taken, and condense the aldehyde group on carbon-1 with the alcoholic-OH group on carbon-5, two different forms of glucose are formed. **When the OH group extends to right,** it is *"α-D-glucose"* and **if it extends to left,** it is *"β-D-glucose" (Fig. 1.4).*

Anomers and anomeric carbon: Carbon 1, after cyclization has four different groups attached to it, and thus it becomes now *asymmetric.*

The two cyclic compounds, **α and β** have different optical rotation, but they will not be same because the compounds as a whole are not mirror-images of each other. Compounds related in this way are called ***anomer*** and ***carbon-1, after cyclization becomes asymmetric is now called anomeric carbon atom (Fig. 1.4).***

MUTAROTATION

Definition: When an aldo sugar is first dissolved in water and the solution is put in optical path so that plane polarized light is passed, the initial optical rotation shown by the sugar gradually changes until a constant ***fixed rotation*** characteristic of the sugar is reached. ***This phenomenon of change of rotation is called as "mutarotation".***

Explanation: ***Ordinary crystalline glucose happens to be in the α-form.*** The above change in optical rotation represents a conversion from α-glucose to an equilibrium mixture of α- and β-forms. The mechanisms of mutarotation probably involves opening of the hemiacetal ring to form traces of the aldehyde form, and then recondensation to the cyclic forms. ***The aldehyde form is extremely unstable and exists only as a transient intermediate.*** In **glucose solutions—approx 2/3 of the sugar exists as the β-form and 1/3 as α-form, at equilibrium** *(Fig. 1.5).*

Epimers and Epimerisation

Two sugars which differ from one another only in configuration around a single carbon atom are termed as ***epimers.***

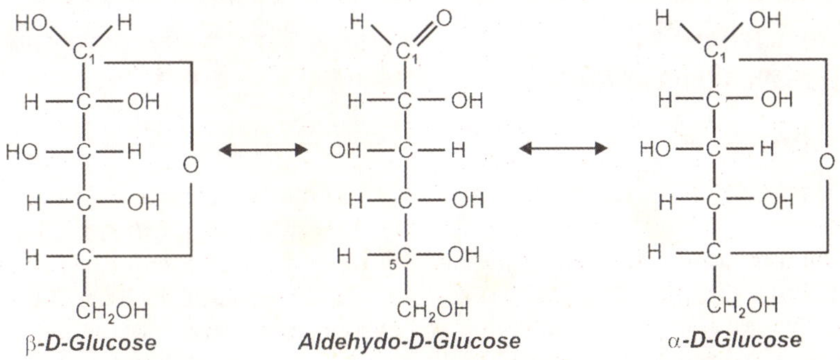

Fig. 1.4: C_1 after cyclization becomes asymmetric—it is called "anomeric" carbon and α-D glucose and β-D-glucose are "anomers"

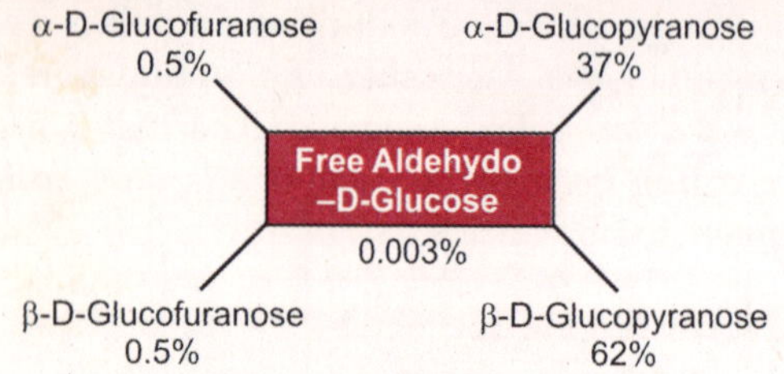

Fig. 1.5: Pyranose and furanose forms of glucose in solution

Examples: **Glucose and galactose are examples of an epimeric pairs** which differ only with respect to C_4 *(Fig. 1.6)*.

Similarly, mannose and glucose are epimers in respect of C_2.

Epimerisation: The process by which one epimer is converted to another is called ***epimerisation*** and it requires the enzyme ***epimerase***, e.g. conversion of galactose to glucose in liver.

D-Glucose *D-Galactose* *D-Mannose*

Fig. 1.6: Epimers

MONOSACCHARIDES

MONOSACCHARIDES OF BIOLOGICAL IMPORTANCE

1. Trioses

- Both D-glyceraldehyde and dihydroxyacetone occur in the form of phosphate *esters*, as intermediates in glycolysis.
- They are also the precursors of glycerol, which the organism synthesizes and incorporates into various types of lipids.

2. Tetroses

- Erythrose-4-P occurs as an intermediate in hexosemonophosphate shunt which is an alternative pathway for glucose oxidation.

3. Pentoses

- ***D-ribose*** is a constituent of nucleic acid RNA; also as constituent of certain coenzymes, e.g.
  - FAD (flavin adenine dinucleotides),
  - NAD (nicotinamide adenine dinucleotide)
  - Coenzyme A.
- ***D-2 deoxyribose*** is a constituent of DNA. ***L-xylulose*** is a metabolite of D-glucuronic acid and is excreted in urine of humans afflicted with a hereditary abnormality in metabolism called pentosuria.
- ***L-fructose*** (methylpentose): occurs in glycoproteins.

4. Hexoses

i. ***D-glucose:*** (Synonyms of D-glucose are dextrose, grape sugar).

- It is the chief physiological sugar present in normal blood continually and at fairly constant level, i.e. about 0.1 percent.
- All tissues utilise glucose for energy. ***Erythrocytes and brain cells utilise glucose solely for energy purposes.***
- It occurs as a constituent of disaccharide and polysaccharides.
- It is stored as glycogen in liver and muscles mainly.
- **It shows mutarotation.**

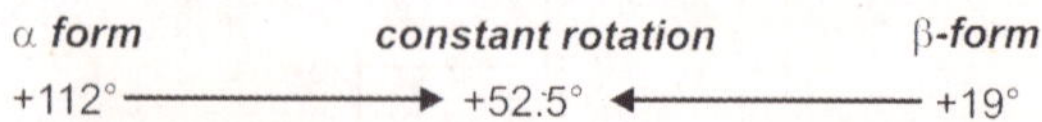

ii. ***D-galactose:*** D-galactose is seldom found free in nature. In combination, it occurs both in plants and animals.

- It ***occurs as constituent of milk sugar lactose*** and also in tissues as a constituent of galactolipid and glycoproteins.
- It is **an epimer of glucose** and differs in orientation of H and OH **on carbon-4**. It is formed in body from glucose by epimerization by the enzyme *epimerase* in liver.

- It is less sweet than glucose and less soluble in water
- It is *dextrorotatory* and **shows mutarotation.**

α form	specific rotation	β-form
+150.7° ⟶	+80°	⟵ +43°

- On oxidation with hot HNO_3, it yields dicarboxylic acid, ***mucic acid*** which helps in its identification, since the crystals of mucic acid are not difficult to produce and have characteristic shape.

iii. D-Fructose: It is a **keto-hexose** and commonly called **"fruit sugar"** as it occurs free in fruits.

- It is very sweet sugar, much sweeter than sucrose and more reactive than glucose.
- It occurs as a constituent of sucrose and also of the polysaccharide inulin.
- It is ***laevorotatory*** and hence is called ***"laevulose"***.
- It ***exhibits mutarotation***

α form	specific rotation	β-form
−21° ⟶	−92°	⟵ −133.5°

BIOMEDICAL IMPORTANCE

Seminal fluid is rich in fructose and sperms utilise fructose for energy. Fructose is formed in the seminiferous tubular epithelial cells from glucose.

iv. D-mannose: does not occur free in nature but is widely distributed in combination as the polysaccharide mannan, e.g. in ivory nut.

- In the body, it is found as a constituent of glycoproteins.

IMPORTANT PROPERTIES OF MONOSACCHARIDES

1. OSAZONE FORMATION

It is useful means of preparing crystalline derivatives of sugars.

Osazones have characteristic:

- ***Melting points***
- ***Crystal structures,*** and
- ***Precipitation time,*** and thus are valuable in identification of sugars.

Preparation: They are obtained by adding a mixture of phenyl hydrazine hydrochloride and sodium acetate to the sugar solution and heating in a boiling water bath for 30 to 45 minutes. The solution is allowed to cool slowly **(not under tap)** by itself. Crystals are formed. A coverslip preparation is made on a clean slide and seen under the microscope.

Basis of reaction: The reaction ***involves only the carbonyl carbon (i.e. aldehyde or ketone group) and the next adjacent carbon.*** First phenyl hydrazone is formed and then the hydrazone reacts with two additional molecules of phenyl hydrazine to form the osazones. The reaction with ketose is similar.

Types of crystals are given in ***Fig. 1.7.***

- ***Glucosazone crystals***: are fine, yellow needles in fan-shaped aggregates or sheaves or crosses, typically described as ***"bundle of hay"*** whose melting point is 204° to 205°C.

Why fructose and mannose form same osazones and galactose forms different osazones? Glucose, mannose and fructose due to similarities of structures form the same osazones. But since the structure of galactose differs on C-4, that part of the molecule unaffected in osazone formation, it would form a different osazone.

- ***Lactosazone crystals:*** are irregular clusters of fine needles and look like a **"powder puff"**.
- ***Maltosazone***: are starshaped and compared to ***"Sunflower"*** petals.

2. INTERCONVERSION OF SUGARS

Glucose, fructose and mannose are interconvertible in solutions of ***weak alkalinity*** such as $Ba(OH)_2$ or $Ca(OH)_2$ ***(Fig. 1.8).*** These interconversions are due to the fact that all give the same ***"Enediol"*** form, which tautomerises to all three sugars.

Physiological Significance

- Enediol formation in weak alkali is necessary for reducing action.
- It has been used for synthesis of certain sugars.

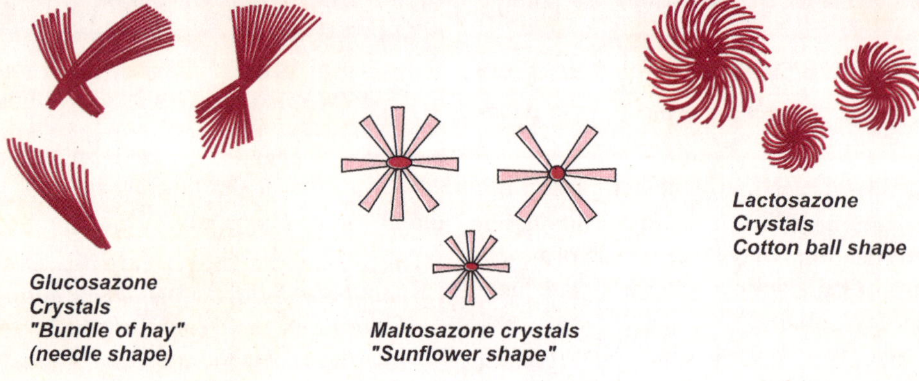

Fig 1.7: Osazone crystals

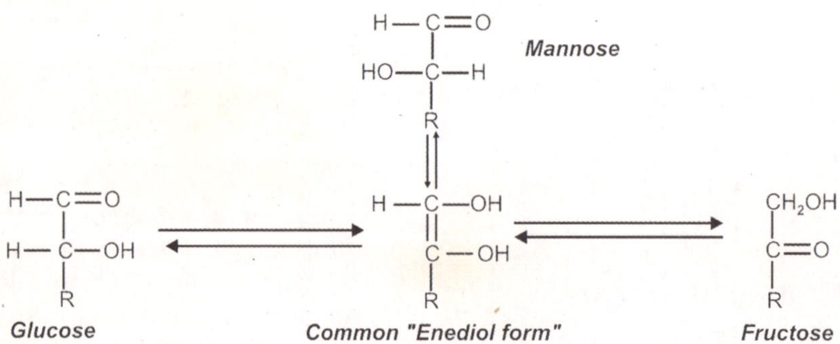

Fig 1.8: Interconversions of sugars in weak alkalinity

3. OXIDATION TO PRODUCE SUGAR ACIDS

When oxidized under different conditions, the aldoses may form

- ***Monobasic aldonic acids***, e.g. D-Glucose → D-Gluconic acid
- ***Dibasic saccharic acids***, e.g.
  D-Glucose → D-Glucaric acid
  D-Galactose → Mucic acid
- ***Monobasic uronic acids*** containing aldehyde groups thus possessing reducing properties, e.g. D-Glucose→D-Glucuronic acid

BIOMEDICAL IMPORTANCE OF D-GLUCURONIC ACID

In the body D-Glucuronic acid is formed from glucose in liver by uronic acid pathway, an alternative pathway for glucose oxidation. It occurs as a constituent of certain muco-polysaccharides. In addition, it is of importance in that it conjugates toxic substances, drugs, hormones and even bilirubin (a breakdown product of Hb) and converts them to nontoxic substance, a glucuronide, which is excreted in urine.

4. REDUCTION OF SUGARS TO FORM SUGAR ALCOHOLS

The monosaccharides may be reduced to their corresponding alcohols by reducing agents such as Na-amalgam. Similarly, ketoses may also be reduced to form keto-alcohol.

Examples:

- *D-Glucose yields D-Sorbitol*
- *D-Galactose yields D-Dulcitol*

- *D-Mannose yields D-Mannitol*
- *Ketosugar D-fructose yields D-mannitol and D-sorbitol.*

5. ACTION OF ACIDS ON CARBOHYDRATES

- Polysaccharides and the compound carbohydrates in general are hydrolyzed into their constituent monosaccharides by boiling with dilute mineral acids (0.5-1.0N) such as HCl or H_2SO_4.
- With conc. mineral acids the monosaccharides are decomposed.
- ***Pentoses*** yield the cyclic aldehyde ***furfural.*** 12% HCl has been found most satisfactory for decomposition.

Practical application
The reaction is used for the quantitative determination of pentoses and compound carbohydrates containing pentoses. Furfural can combine with phloroglucinol to form a relatively insoluble compound, ***furfural phloroglucide,*** which may be used in estimating the furfural formed in the reaction as a measure of the pentose present.

- ***Hexoses*** are decomposed by hot strong mineral acids to give ***hydroxy methyl furfural,*** which decomposes further to produce laevulinic acid, formic acid, CO and CO_2.

Practical application
The furfural products thus formed by decomposition with strong mineral acid can condense with certain organic phenols to form compounds having characteristic colours. ***Thus, it forms basis for certain tests used for detection of sugars.***

Examples:

- ***Molishch's test:*** With α-naphthol (in alcoholic solution) gives ***red-violet ring***. A sensitive but non-specific reaction is given by all sugars.
- ***Seliwanoff's test:*** With resorcinol, a cherry-red color is produced. It is characteristic of D-fructose.

  Other tests are anthrone test, Bial-orcinol test.

6. ACTION WITH ALKALIES

With alkalies, monosaccharides react in various ways.

a. ***In dilute alkali:***
   - The sugar will change to the cyclic **α** and **β** forms with an equilibrium between the two isomeric form (see mutarotation).
   - ***On standing:*** A rearrangement will occur which produces an equilibrated mixture of glucose, fructose and mannose through the common **"enediol"** form (see interconversion).
   - If it is heated to 37°C, the acidity increases, and a series of "enols" are formed in which double bond shifts from the oxygen-carbon atoms.

b. ***In conc. alkali:*** The ***sugar caramelizes*** and produces a series of decomposition products. Yellow and brown pigments develops, salts may form, many double bonds between C-atoms are formed, and C-to-C-bonds may rupture.

7. REDUCING ACTION OF SUGARS IN ALKALINE SOLUTION

All the sugars that contain free sugar group undergo enolization and various other changes when placed in alkaline solution. The ***"enediol" forms of the sugars are highly reactive*** and are easily oxidized by O_2 and other oxidizing agents and form sugar acids. As a consequence, they readily reduce oxidizing ions such as Ag^+, Hg^+, Bi^{+++}, Cu^{++} (cupric) and $Fe(CN)_6^{---}$.

Practical application
This reducing action of sugars in alkaline solution is utilised for both qualitative and quantitative determinations of sugars.

Reagents: Reagents containing Cu^{++} (ic) ions are most commonly used. These are generally alkaline solution of cupric sulphate containing

- Sodium potassium tartarate ***(Rochelle salt)*** and strong alkali NaOH/KOH as in Fehling's solution (not used now).
- Sodium citrate and weak alkali sodium carbonate as in Benedict's qualitative reagent.

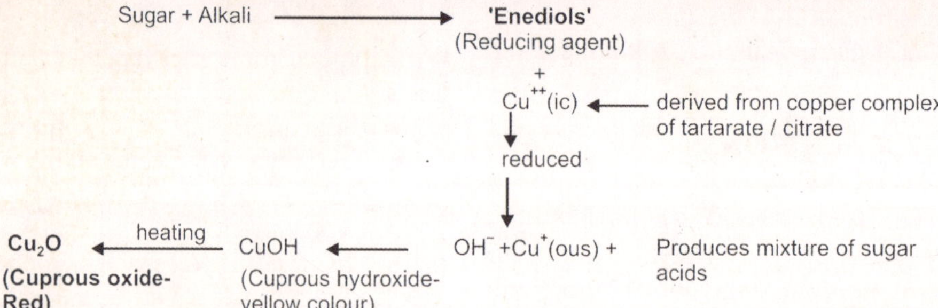

Function of Ingredients:

- Sodium citrate/Rochelle salt in the reagents prevent precipitation of cupric hydroxide or cupric carbonate by forming soluble, slightly dissociable complexes which dissociate sufficiently to provide supply of readily available Cu^{++} (cupric) ions for oxidation.
- The alkali of the reagents enolizes the sugars and thereby causes them to be strong reducing agents. ***Enolization is better in weak alkali than strong alkali.***

Reaction: When a solution of reducing sugar is heated with one of the alkaline copper reagents, the abovementioned reactions occur (as shown above). ***The appearance of a yellow to red precipitate indicates reduction, and the quantity of sugar present can be roughly estimated from colour and amount of precipitate.***

OTHER SUGAR DERIVATIVES OF BIOCHEMICAL IMPORTANCE

1. DEOXY SUGARS

Deoxy sugars represent sugars in which the oxygen of an *-OH group* has been removed, leaving the hydrogen. Thus,—CHOH or $-CH_2OH$ becomes – CH_2 or $-CH_3$.

Deoxy sugars of biological importance are:

- 2-deoxy-D-ribose is found in nucleic acid (DNA).
- 6-deoxy –L-galactose is found as a constituent of glycoproteins, blood group substances and bacterial polysaccharides.

2. AMINO SUGARS (HEXOSAMINES)

Sugars containing an $-NH_2$ group in their structure are called "amino sugars".

Two naturally occurring members are derived from glucose and galactose, in which – ***OH group on carbon 2 is replaced by—NH_2*** group, and forms respectively glucosamine and galactosamine ***(see Fig. 1.9).***

Properties: Generally, they give chemical reactions characteristic of sugars.

D–Glucosamine **D–Galactosamine**

Fig. 1.9: Hexosamines of biomedical importance

- They form hydrazones but not osazones.
- Aminosugars occur combined as N-acetyl derivatives (amino group is acetylated) in a number of important biological substances.

BIOMEDICAL IMPORTANCE

- N-acetyl derivative of D-glucosamine occur as a constituent of certain mucopolysaccharides (MPS) such as hyaluronic acid and heparin and also in blood group substances.
- It is also a constituent of shells of *crustaceae* (crabs, lobsters, etc.) where it occurs as **"chitin"** which is made of repeating units of N-acetylated glucosamine. Hence, Glucosamine is often called as ***Chitosamine.***
- Galactosamine occurs as N-acetyl-galactosamine in a group of complex sulphated mucopolysaccharides (MPS) as chondroitin

sulphates which are present in cartilages, bones, tendons and heart valves. Hence galactosamine is also known as ***Chondrosamine.***

- ***Antibiotics:*** Certain antibiotics such as **erythromycin, carbomycin** contain amino sugars. Erythromycin contains dimethyl amino sugar and carbomycin 3-amino-D-ribose. It is believed that amino sugars are related to the antibiotic activity of these drugs.

3. AMINO SUGAR ACIDS

- ***Neuraminic acid:*** It is an amino sugar acid and structurally an aldol condensation product of pyruvic acid and D-mannosamine.
  Neuraminic acid is unstable and found in nature in the form of acylated derivatives known as ***sialic acids*** (N-acetyl neuraminic acid-NANA).
- ***Muramic acid:*** Another amino sugar acid which is structurally a condensation product of D-glucosamine and lactic acid.

BIOMEDICAL IMPORTANCE

- Neuraminic acid and sialic acids occur in a number of ***mucopolysaccharides*** and in glycolipids like ***gangliosides.***
- A number of nitrogenous oligosaccharides which contain neuraminic acid are found in human milk.
- Certain bacterial cell walls contain "muramic acid"
- ***Neuraminidase*** is the enzyme which hydrolyzes to split NANA from compound.

4. GLYCOSIDES

Definition: Glycosides are compounds containing a ***carbohydrate and a non-carbohydrate residue in the same molecule.*** In these compounds, the carbohydrate residue is attached by an ***acetal linkage*** of carbon-I to the non-carbohydrate residue. ***The non-carbohydrate residue present in the glycoside is called as Aglycone***. The aglycones present in glycosides vary in complexity from simple substances as methyl alcohol, glycerol, phenol, hydroquinones to complex substances like sterols and anthraquinones. The glycosides are named according to the carbohydrate it contain. If they contain glucose it forms ***glucoside.*** If galactose, it forms ***galactoside*** and so on.

BIOMEDICAL IMPORTANCE

Glycosides are found in many drugs, spices and in the constituents of animal tissues. They are widely distributed in plant kingdom,

- ***Cardiac glycosides:*** Cardiac glycosides are important in medicine because of their action on heart and thus used in cardiac insufficiency. They are derivatives of ***Digitalis, Strophanthus*** and squill plants.
- ***Ouabain:*** A glycoside obtained from ***Strophanthus* spp.** is of interest as it **inhibits active transport of Na^+** in cardiac muscle *in vivo* (**"sodium pump" inhibitor**).
- ***Phlorhizin:*** A glycoside obtained from the root and bark of apple tree. It blocks the transport of sugar across the mucosal cells of small intestine and also renal tubular epithelium; it ***displaces Na^+ from the binding site of "carrier protein" and prevents the binding of sugar molecule,*** and ***produces glycosuria.***
- Other glycosides include antibiotics such as streptomycin.

DISACCHARIDES

Three most common disaccharides of biological importance are: ***maltose, lactose*** and ***sucrose.*** Their general molecular formula is $C_{12}H_{22}O_{11}$ and they are hydrolyzed by hot acids or corresponding enzymes as follows:

$$C_{12}H_{22}O_{11} + H_2O \rightarrow C_6H_{12}O_6 + C_6H_{12}O_6$$

Thus, on hydrolysis

- **Maltose** $\xrightarrow{H_2O}$ D-Glucose + D-Glucose
- **Lactose** $\xrightarrow{H_2O}$ D-Glucose + D-Galactose
- **Sucrose** $\xrightarrow{H_2O}$ D-Glucose + D-Fructose

The disaccharides are formed by the union of two constituent monosaccharides with the elimination of one molecule of water. The points of linkage, the **glycosidic linkage** varies as does the manner of linking, and ***the properties of the disaccharides depend to a great extent on the type of the linkage***. If both of the two potential aldehyde/or ketone groups are involved in the linkage the sugar will not exhibit reducing properties and will not be able to form osazones, e.g. ***sucrose.*** But if one of them is not bound in this way, it will permit reduction and osazone formation by the sugars, e.g. ***lactose*** and ***maltose.***

PROPERTIES OF DISACCHARIDES

1. MALTOSE

- Maltose or malt sugar is an intermediary in acid hydrolysis of starch and can also be obtained by enzyme hydrolysis of starch. In the body, dietary starch digestion by *amylase* in gut yields maltose, which requires a specific enzyme *maltase* to form glucose.
- It is a rather sweet sugar and is much soluble in water. Since it has one aldehyde "free" or potentially free ***(see structure-Fig. 1.10)***, it has reducing properties, and forms characteristic osazones which has a characteristic **"sun-flower"** like appearance. As anomeric carbon of one glucose is free, it can form α and β forms and **exhibit mutarotation.**

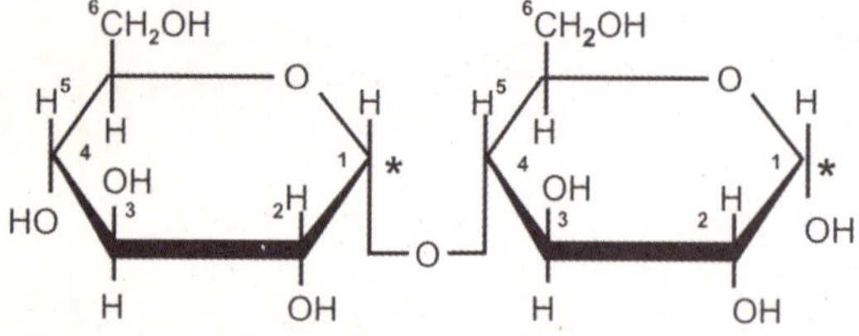

o-α-D-Glucopyranosyl-(1→4)-α-D-Glucopyranoside

Fig. 1.10: Maltose (α-form)

- ***On hydrolysis*** maltose yields two molecules of glucose.

2. LACTOSE

- It is **"milk sugar"** and found in appreciable quantities in milk to the extent of about 5% and occurs at body temperature as an equilibrium mixture of the α and β in 2:3 ratio.
- It is not very soluble and is not so sweet. It is **dextrorotatory.** Specific enzyme which hydrolyzes is ***lactase*** present in intestinal juice. On hydrolysis, it yield one molecule of D-glucose and one molecule of D-galactose.
- Because it contains galactose as one of its constituents, it yields ***"mucic acid"*** on being treated with conc. HNO_3 after hydrolysis.
- As one of the aldehyde group is free or potentially free ***(see structure-Fig. 1.11)***, it has reducing properties and can form osazones. Lactosazone crystals have typical ***hedge-hog*** shape or ***powder-puff*** appearance. As anomeric carbon of glucose is free, it can form **α** and **β** forms and exhibits mutarotation.

o-β-D-Galactopyranosyl-(1→4)-β-Glucopyranoside

Fig. 1.11: Lactose (β-form)

3. SUCROSE

- ***Ordinary "table sugar" is sucrose.*** It is also called as "cane sugar", as it can be obtained from sugarcane. It can also be obtained from sugar beet, and to lesser extent the sugar maple. It occurs free in most fruits and vegetables, e.g. pineapple and carrots.
- It is very soluble and sweet and ***on hydrolysis yields one molecule of D-glucose and one molecule of D-fructose.*** The specific enzyme which hydrolyses sucrose is ***sucrase*** present in intestinal juice.
- ***As both aldehyde and ketone groups are linked together (α 1→2)***, it does not have reducing properties, and cannot form osazones. As both anomeric carbons are involved in "linkage", ***it does not exhibit mutarotation (Fig. 1.12).***

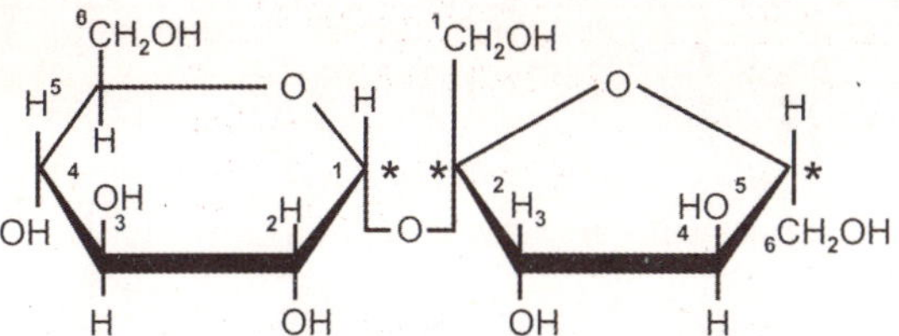

o-α-D-Glucopyranosyl-(1→2)-β-D-Fructofuranoside

Fig. 1.12: Sucrose

- **Invert sugars and 'inversion':** *Sucrose is dextrorotatory* (+62.5°) **but its hydrolytic products are laevorotatory** because fructose has a greater specific laevorotation than the dextrorotation of glucose. As the hydrolytic products invert the rotation, the ***resulting mixtures of glucose and fructose (hydrolytic products) is called as Invert sugar*** and the process is called ***inversion.*** Honey is largely "Invert sugar" and the presence of fructose accounts for the greater sweetness of honey.

Differences between Sucrose and Lactose

Detailed differentiation of lactose from sucrose has been given in *Table 1.1.*

OLIGOSACCHARIDES

BIOMEDICAL IMPORTANCE

- Integral membrane proteins contain covalently attached carbohydrate units, oligosaccharides, on their extracellular face. Such glycoproteins act as **"receptors"**.
- Many secreted proteins, such as antibodies and coagulation factors also contain oligosaccharide units.

POLYSACCHARIDES

Polysaccharides are more complex substances. Some are polymers of a single monosaccharide and are termed as ***homopolysaccharides (homoglycans)***, e.g. starch, glycogen, etc. Some contain other groups apart from carbohydrates such as hexuronic acid and are called as ***heteropolysaccharides (heteroglycans)***, e.g. mucopolysaccharides (GAG).

HOMOPOLYSACCHARIDES (HOMOGLYCANS)

1. STARCH

- Starch is a polymer of glucose, and occurs in many plants as storage foods. It may be found in the leaves, and stem, as well as in roots, fruits and seeds where it is usually present in greater concentration.
- *Starch granules* appear under microscope as particles made up of the concentric layers of material. They differ in shape, size and markings according to the source *(Fig. 1.13)*.
- Starchy foods are the mainstay of diet. Large amounts are present in cereals such as wheat, rye, rice, corn and barley, in potatoes, in legumes and in nuts.

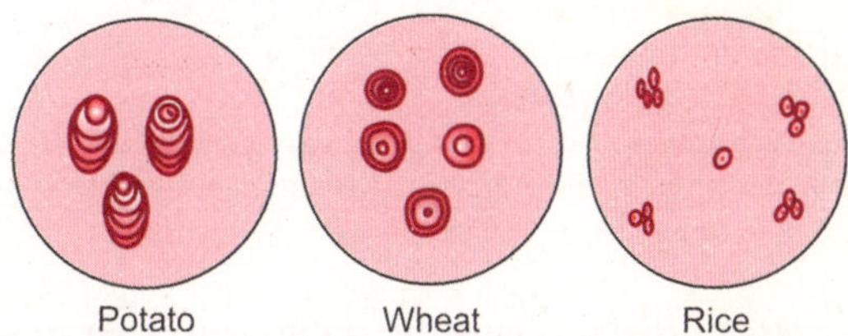

Fig. 1.13: Starch grains under microscope

- *Composition:* Starch granule consists of **two polymeric units of glucose** called *amylose* and *amylopectin*, but they differ in molecular architecture and in certain properties *(Table 1.2)*.
- Starch granules are insoluble in cold water, but when their suspension is heated, water is taken up and swelling occurs at first to a slight degree but later to several hundred times to their original volume, viscosity increases and **starch "gels" or "pastes" are formed.**
- *Reaction with I_2:* Both the granules and the colloidal solutions react with iodine to give a blue colour. This is chiefly due to amylose which forms a deep-blue complex, which dissociates on heating. Amylopectin solutions are coloured blue-violet or purple.

Table 1.1: Differentiation of Lactose from Sucrose

Lactose	*Sucrose*
• Also known as "milk sugar"	• Common table sugar (cane sugar)
• Structurally one molecule of D-glucose and one molecule of D-galactose are joined together by glycosidic linkage (β 1 → 4)	• Structurally one molecule of D-glucose and one molecule of D-fructose joined together (α 1→ 2)
• Hydrolyzed to give one molecule of glucose and one molecule of galactose	• Hydrolyzed to give one molecule of glucose and one molecule of fructose
• Specific enzyme which hydrolyzes is called *lactase*, which is present in intestinal juice	• Specific enzyme which hydrolyzes is called *sucrase* (invertase) which is present in intestinal juice
• Dextrorotatory disaccharide	• Also dextrorotatory (+66.5°), but hydrolytic products are laevorotatory (–19.5°) Hydrolytic products are called **"invert sugars"** and process is called **"inversion"**.
• As anomeric carbon is free, it can form α and β forms and exhibits mutarotation	• As both anomeric carbons are involved in linkage, cannot form α and β forms and does not exhibit mutarotation.
• Specific rotation of the solution is, +55.2°	• Does not exhibit mutarotation.
• Can reduce alkaline copper sulphate solution like Benedict's qualitative reagent, Fehling's solution	• Does not reduce alkaline copper sulphate solution
• Does not reduce Berfoed's solution	• Does not reduce Berfoed's solution
• Forms osazone. Lactosazone crystals have typical "hedge-hog" or powder puff shape".	• Cannot form osazones
• Hydrolytic products on treatment with conc HNO_3 can "form mucic acid".	• Cannot form mucic acid
• Fearon's test is positive	• Fearon's test is negative
• Can be synthesized in lactating mammary gland from glucose	• Not so
• In lactating mother lactose may appear in urine, producing "lactosuria"	• Not so

- ***Hydrolysis of starch:*** Yield succession of polysaccharides of gradually diminishing molecular size.

Course of Hydrolysis	*Reaction with Iodine*
Starch	Blue
↓	
Soluble starch	Blue
↓	
Amylodextrin	Purple
↓	
Erythrodextrin	Red
↓	
Achroodextrin	Colourless
↓	
Maltose	

Enzyme (amylase) hydrolysis ends at maltose. For formation of glucose, it requires the enzyme maltase.

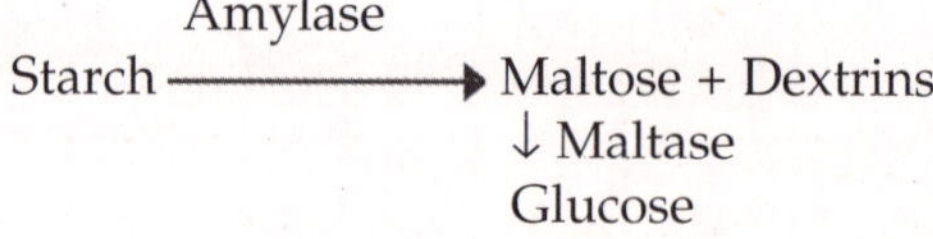

But if the hydrolysis is accomplished by acids, much of the starch will be converted into glucose.

$$\text{Starch} \xrightarrow{\text{Acid}} \text{Glucose}$$

2. GLYCOGEN

- Glycogen is the reserve carbohydrate of the animal, hence it is called as ***"animal starch"***.
- In higher animals, it is ***deposited in the liver and muscle as storage material*** which are readily available as immediate source of energy.
- Formation of glycogen from glucose is called as ***glycogenesis*** and breakdown of glycogen to form glucose is called as ***glycogenolysis.***

Table 1.2: Differentiation of Amylose and Amylopectin

Amylose	*Amylopectin*
• Occurs to the extent 15 to 20%	• Occurs 80 to 85%
• Low molecular weight—approx 60,000	• High molecular weight—approx 500,000
• ***Soluble in water***	• ***Insoluble in water,*** can absorb water and swells up
• Gives blue colour with dilute iodine solution	• Gives reddish-violet colour with I_2 solution
• ***Structure:***	• Highly branched structure
• Unbranched	• More D-Glucose
• Straight chain	• Structure similar to glycogen
• 250 to 300 D-glucose units linked by α 1 → 4 linkages	• Main stem α-1→4 glycoside bonds
• Twist into a helix, with six glucose units perturn	• At branch point α 1 → 6 linkage, approx 80 branches. One branch after every 24 to 30 D-Glucose units

- The molecular weight of glycogen is variable, the size of the molecule depending upon the nutritional status of the animal. The molecular weight varies from 1,000,000 to 4,000,000.
- It is ***dextrorotatory*** with an [α] D 20° = + 196° to +197°.
- ***Solubility:*** Glycogen is not readily soluble in water and it ***forms an opalescent solution.*** It can be precipitated from opalescent solution by ethyl alcohol, and on drying, it forms a pure white powder.
- ***Action of alkali:*** Glycogen is not destroyed by a hot strong KOH or NaOH solution. ***This property is made use of in the method for determining it quantitatively in tissues.***
- ***Action with iodine:*** Glycogen gives a deep red colour. In this respect it resembles erythrodextrin.
- ***Structure:*** Glycogens have a complex structure of **highly branched chains**. It is a polymer of D-glucose units and resemble amylopectin. ***Glucose units in main stem are joined by α1→4 glucosidic linkages*** and ***branching occurs at branch points by α1→6 glucosidic linkage.*** A branch point occurs for every 12 to 18 glucose units ***(Fig. 1.14).***

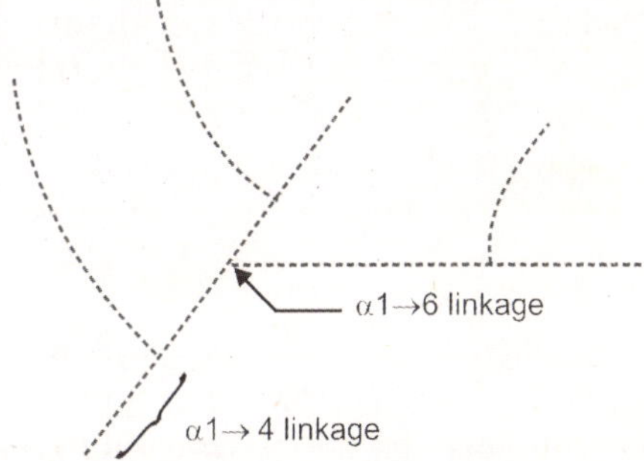

Fig. 1.14: Branched structure of glycogen

3. INULIN

- Inulin is a **polymer of D-fructose** and has a low molecular weight (MW=5000). It occurs in tubers of the Dahlia, in the root of the Jerusalem artichoke, dandelion and in the bulbs of onion and garlic.
- It is a white, tasteless powder. It is ***laevorotatory*** and gives no colour with iodine.
- Acids hydrolyze it to D-fructose; similarly it is also hydrolyzed by the enzyme ***inulinase***, which accompanies it in plants.
- ***It has no dietary importance in human beings.***

BIOMEDICAL IMPORTANCE

- It is used in physiological investigation for determination of the rate of glomerular filtration rate (GFR).
- It has been also used for estimation of body water (ECF) volume.

4. CELLULOSE

- Cellulose is a **polymer of glucose**. It is not hydrolyzed readily by dilute acids, but heating with fairly high concentrations of acids yields, the disaccharide ***cellobiose*** and D-glucose.

- Cellobiose is made up of two molecules of D-glucose linked together by β-***glucosidic-linkage*** between C_1 and C_4 of adjacent glucose units.

BIOMEDICAL IMPORTANCE

Cellulose is a very stable insoluble compound. Since it is the main constituent of the supporting tissues of plants, it forms a considerable part of our vegetable food. ***In human beings no cellulose splitting enzyme is secreted by GI mucosa***, hence it is not of any nutritional value. ***But it is of considerable human dietetic value that it adds bulk to the intestinal contents*** **(roughage)** thereby stimulating peristalsis and elimination of indigestible food residues.

5. DEXTRINS

- When starch is partially hydrolyzed by the action of acids or enzymes, it is broken down into a number of products of lower molecular weight known as ***"dextrins"***.
- The dextrins are water soluble and react with iodine (see hydrolysis of starch). They resemble starch by being precipitable by alcohol, forming sticky, gummy masses.

6. DEXTRANS

- It is a **polymer of D-glucose**. It is synthesized by the action of ***Leuconostoc mesenteroides***, a non-pathogenic gram positive cocci in a sucrose medium. Exocellular enzyme produced by the organisms bring about polymerization of glucose moiety of sucrose molecule, and forms the polysaccharide known as ***dextrans.***

BIOMEDICAL IMPORTANCE

- Dextran solution, having molecular wt approx. 75,000 have been used as ***plasma expander.*** When given IV in cases of blood loss (haemorrhage), it ***increases the blood volume.***
- Because of their high viscosity, low osmotic pressure, slow disintegration and utilization, and slow elimination from the body they remain in blood for many hours to exert its effect.

Disadvantage: The ***only disadvantage is that it can interfere with grouping and crossmatching, as it forms false agglutination*** **(Rouleux formation)**. Hence blood sample for grouping and cross-matching should be collected before administration of dextran in a case of haemorrhage and blood loss, where blood transfusion may be required.

7. AGAR

- It is a homopolysaccharide.
- Made up of **repeating units of galactose** which is sulphated.
- Present in seaweed. It is obtained from them.

BIOMEDICAL IMPORTANCE

- ***In humans: Used as laxative in constipation.*** Like cellulose it is not digested, hence adds bulk to the feces ("roughage" value) and helps in its propulsion.
- ***In microbiology***: Agar is available in purified form. It dissolves in hot water and on cooling it sets like gel. It is **used as agar plate for culture of bacteria.**

Heteropolysaccharides (Heteroglycans)-Mucopolysaccharides (MPS)

Jeanloz has suggested the name ***Glycosamino glycans (GAG)*** to describe this group of substances. They are usually composed of ***amino sugar*** and ***uronic acid*** units as the principal components, though some are chiefly made up of amino sugar and monosaccharides units without the presence of uronic acid. ***The hexosamine present is generally acetylated.*** These are essential components of tissues where they are generally present either in free form or in combination with proteins. Carbohydrates content varies. When carbohydrates content is >4%, they are called ***mucoproteins*** and when <4% they are called as ***glycoproteins.***

Classification

Although there is no agreement on classification, the nitrogenous heteropolysaccharides (mucopolysaccharides) are classified as follows:

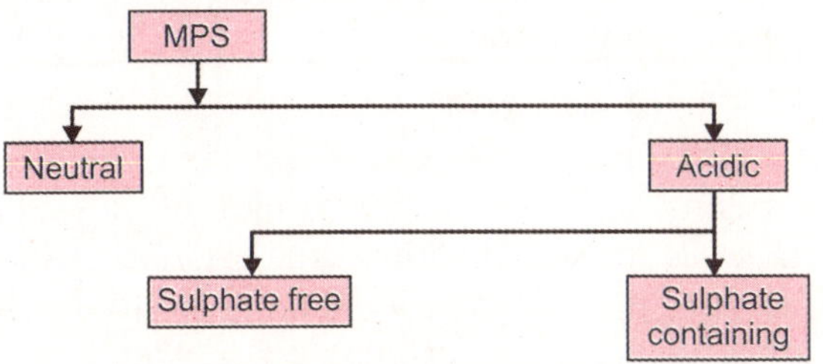

A. ACIDIC SULPHATE FREE MPS

1. HYALURONIC ACID

- A ***sulphate free mucopolysaccharide***. It was first isolated from vitreous humour of eye. Later, it was found to be present in synovial fluid, skin, umbilical cord, haemolytic streptococci and in rheumatic nodule.
- It occurs in both free and salt-like combination with **proteins** and forms so-called ***"ground substance"*** of mesenchyme, an integral part of the gel-like ground substance of connective and other tissues.

Composition: Hyaluronic acid is composed of ***repeating units of N-acetylglucosamine and D-glucuronic acid.***

On hydrolysis: It yields equimolecular quantities of D-glucosamine, D-glucuronic acid and acetic acid ***(Fig.1.15).***

FUNCTIONS

- Hyaluronic acid in ***tissues acts as cementing substance*** and contribution to tissue barriers which permit metabolites to pass through but resist penetration by bacteria and other infective agents.
- In ***joints***, it ***acts as lubricant*** and ***shock absorbant.***

Hyaluronidase

Hyaluronidase is an enzyme present in certain tissues notably testicular tissue and spleen, as well as in several types of pneumococci and haemolytic streptococci. The enzyme catalyzes the depolymerization of hyaluronic acid and by reducing its viscosity facilitate diffusion of materials into tissue spaces. Hence the enzyme, sometime, is designated as ***spreading factor***.

BIOMEDICAL IMPORTANCE

- The invasive power of some pathogenic organisms may be increased because they secrete *hyaluronidase.*
- In the testicular secretions, it may dissolve the viscid substances surrounding the ova to permit penetration of spermatozoa.
- Clinically the enzyme is used to increase the efficiency of absorption of solution administered by clysis.

2. CHONDROITIN

- Chondroitin is another **sulphate free acid mucopolysaccharide**. It is found in ***cornea*** and has been isolated from cranial cartilages.
- Chondroitin differs from hyaluronic acid only in that it contains N-acetyl galactosamine instead of N-acetyl glucosamine.

B. SULPHATE CONTAINING ACID MPS

1. ***Keratan Sulphate (Kerato Sulphate):*** A sulphate acid MPS is found in costal cartilage, and cornea. It has been isolated from bovine cornea. It has been reported to be present in *nucleus pulposus* and the wall of aorta.

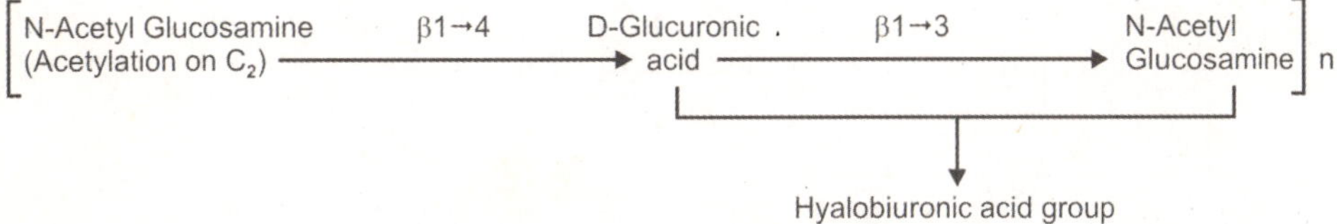

Fig. 1.15: Structure of hyaluronic acid

Composition

- Kerato sulphate is composed of ***repeating disaccharides unit consisting of N-acetyl glucosamine and galactose.***

[N-acetyl Glucosamine → Galactose → N-Acetyl Glucosamine]n

There are no uronic acids in the molecule.

2. ***Chondroitin sulphates:*** Chondroitin sulphates are principal MPS in the ground substance of mammalian tissues and cartilage. They occur in combination with proteins and are called as chondroproteins.

Types

Four Chondroitin sulphates have been isolated so far. They are named as chondroitin SO_4 A,B,C and D.

a. Chondroitin SO_4A

- Chondroitin SO_4A is present mainly in cartilage, adult bone and cornea.
- ***Structure:*** It consists of ***repeating units of N-acetyl-D-galactosamine and D-glucuronic acid.*** N-Acetyl galactosamine is esterified with SO_4 in position 4 of galactosamine.

b. Chondroitin SO_4 B

- Chondroitin SO_4 B is present in skin, cardiac valves and tendons. It is also isolated from aortic wall and lung parenchyma.
- It has ***L-iduronic acid in place of glucuronic acid*** which is found in other chondroitin sulphates.
- It has a weak anticoagulant property, hence sometimes it is called β-***heparin***
- As it is found in skin, it is also known as ***dermatan sulphate.***

Structure: It consists of ***repeating units of L-iduronic acid and N-acetyl galactosamine.*** Sulphate moiety is present at C_4 of N-acetyl galactosamine molecule.

c. Chondroitin SO_4C

Chondroitin SO_4C found in cartilage and tendons. Structure of Chondroitin SO_4C is the same as that of Chondroitin SO_4A, except that the SO_4 group is at position 6 of galactosamine molecule instead of position 4.

d. Chondroitin SO_4D

Chondroitin SO_4D has been isolated from the cartilage of shark. It resembles in structure to chondroitin SO_4C, except that it has a second SO_4 attached probably at carbon 2 or 3 of uronic acid moiety.

3. HEPARIN

- Heparin is called as ***α-heparin***. It is an ***anticoagulant*** present in the liver, produced mainly by ***mast cells* of liver** (originally isolated from liver).
- In addition, it is also found in lungs, thymus, spleen, walls of large arteries and in small quantity in blood.
  Structure: It is a polymer of ***repeating units of L-iduronic acid and D-glucosamine (Fig. 1.16).***
- The $-NH_2$ group at C_2 and OH group at C_6 of glucosamine molecule are sulphated, in addition OH group at C_2 of L-Iduronic acid is also sulphated.

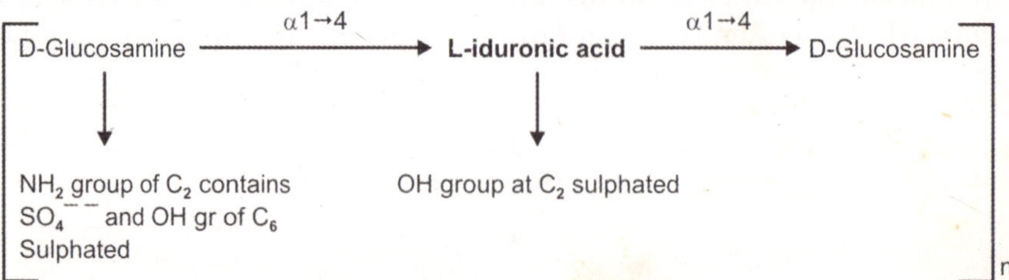

Fig. 1.16: Structure of heparin

Properties

- It is **strongly acidic** due to sulphuric acid groups and readily forms salts.
- The molecular weight of heparin appears to be in the range of 17,000 to 20,000.

BIOMEDICAL IMPORTANCE

- Heparin acts in body to increase the activity of ***lipoprotein lipase*** and hence called **"clearing factor".**
- Heparin ***inhibits formations of thrombin from prothrombin.*** Most satisfactory anticoagulant, it does not produce a change in red cell volume or interfere with subsequent determinations. In clinical practice, 2 mg/10 ml of blood is used.

C. NEUTRAL MPS

- Many of the neutral nitrogenous polysaccharides of various types are found in pneumococci capsule.
- ***Blood Group Substances:*** These contain peptides or amino acids as well as carbohydrates. **Four monosaccharides are found in all types of blood group substances** regardless of source—***galactose, fucose, galactosamine (acetylated) and acetylated glucosamine***. Non-reducing end groups of acetyl glucosamine, galactose and fucose are associated with blood group specificities of A, B and H respectively. The amino acid composition of blood group substances is peculiar in that S-containing and aromatic amino acids are absent.
- Nitrogenous neutral MPS firmly bound-proteins, e.g. ovalbumin (contains mannose and glucosamine).

BIOMEDICAL IMPORTANCE

Mucopolysaccharidosis: The mucopolysaccharidosis are a group of related disorders due to ***inherited enzyme defect***, in which skeletal changes, mental retardation, visceral involvement and corneal clouding are manifested to varying degrees.

Defect/defects in these disorders result in

i. widespread deposits in tissues of a particular MPS and
ii. in excessive excretion of MPS in urine.

At least ***six types*** of mucopolysaccharidosis have been described.

Detection of MPS in urine: cetyl trimethyl ammonium bromide test: Take 5 ml of fresh urine from the suspected case in a test tube. Add 1.0 ml of 5% cetyl trimethyl ammonium bromide (cetavion) in 1 M citrate buffer (pH—6.0). Mix and allow to stand at room temperature for ½ hour. A heavy precipitate is given in gargoylism.

☞ SALIENT POINTS TO REMEMBER

- Carbohydrates are defined chemically as aldehyde or ketone derivatives of the higher polyhydric alcohols or compounds which yield these derivatives on hydrolysis.
- Classified into 4 groups, viz. monosaccharides, disaccharides, oligosaccharides and polysaccharides.
- D-Glucose is the principal monosaccharide present in circulating blood and utilized by tissues to provide energy.
- D-Glucose is converted to Glycogen for storage in liver and muscles.
- D-Glucose is also converted to other carbohydrates, e.g. ribose for nucleic acid, D-Galactose for lacose of milk.
- Seminal fluid is rich in D-fructose which is utilized by the spermatozoa for energy.
- Sucrose is dextrorotatory but hydrolytic products are laevorotatory. Hence the hydrolytic products of sucrose are called invert sugars and the process is called inversion.
- Glycosides are compounds containing a carbohydrate and a non-carbohydrate residue called aglycone, in the same molecule.
- Chief glycosides of biomedical importance are cardiac glycosides, phloridzin, ouabain, antibiotic streptomycin.
- The homoglycans, starch and glycogen are the carbohydrate reserves of plants and

animals respectively. Glycogen is called animal starch.

- Acid hydrolysis of starch ends in glucose but enzyme hydrolysis produces maltose which requires maltase for conversion to glucose.
- Inulin, a polymer of D-fructose, used for determination of rate of glomerular filtration (GFR) and for estimation of body water (ECF volume).
- Dextran, a polymer of D-Glucose is used as a plasma expander to increase blood volume in a case of haemorrhage and shock.
- Cellulose a homoglycan, nondigestable by humans, increases bulk of faeces (roughage) avoiding constipation.
- Mucopolysaccharides (Glycosaminoglycans) are heteroglycans and are essential components of mesenchymal tissues.
- Heparin, a heteroglycan acts as an anticoagulant *"in vitro"* and *"in vivo"*.
- Mucopolysaccharidoses, a group of disorders due to inherited enzyme defect of metabolism of MPS.

MULTIPLE CHOICE QUESTIONS

Give one correct answer:

1. **Cane sugar is:**
   (a) Glucose (b) Fructose
   (c) Maltose (d) Sucrose
   (e) Galactose
2. **Table sugar which is used in making morning tea is:**
   (a) Glucose (b) Lactose
   (c) Sucrose (d) Maltose
   (e) Mannose
3. **Which of the following are reducing sugars?:**
   (a) Sucrose (b) Lactose
   (c) Xylose (d) Dextrin
   (e) Ribose
4. **Glucose and galactose are epimers and they differ structurally in orientation of H and OH on:**
   (a) C_1 (b) C_3
   (c) C_5 (d) C_4 (e) C_2
5. **Starch and glycogen are polymers of:**
   (a) Galactose (b) β-D-Glucose
   (c) α-D-Glucose (d) Fructose
   (e) Mannose
6. **Which of the following is not a polymer of glucose?:**
   (a) Amylose (b) Glycogen
   (c) Dextrins (d) Inulin
   (e) Amylopectin
7. **The repeating disaccharide unit in cellulose is:**
   (a) Dextrin (b) Sucrose
   (c) Maltose (d) Dextrose
   (e) Cellobiose
8. **Inversion is related to which sugar?:**
   (a) Dextrose (b) Sucrose
   (c) Maltose (d) Lactose
   (e) Fructose
9. **Seliwanoff's test is answered by:**
   (a) Glucose
   (b) Galactose
   (c) Mannose
   (d) Fructose
   (e) Lactose
10. **All of the following are pentoses, *except:***
    (a) Xylose
    (b) Ribose
    (c) Mannose
    (d) Arabinose
    (e) Ribulose
11. **The glycosaminoglycans which does not contain uronic acid is:**
    (a) Heparin (b) Karatan sulphate
    (c) Chondroitin sulphate (d) Chondroitin
    (e) Hyaluronic acid
12. **All of the following are homoglycans, *except:***
    (a) Inulin (b) Heparin
    (c) Glycogen (d) Dextran
    (e) Dextrins

13. **Milk sugar is:**
    (a) Maltose (b) Glucose
    (c) Mannose (d) Lactose
    (e) Sucrose

14. **Mucic acid is produced by oxidation of:**
    (a) Galactose (b) Glucose
    (c) Fructose (d) Sedoheptulose
    (e) Mannose

ANSWERS

1. (d)	2. (c)	3. (e)	4. (d)
5. (c)	6. (d)	7. (e)	8. (b)
9. (d)	10. (c)	11. (b)	12. (b)
13. (d)	14. (a)		

Chemistry of Lipids

LIPIDS

INTRODUCTION

The lipids constitute a very important heterogenous group of organic substances in plant and animal tissues and ***related either actually or potentially to the fatty acids.*** Chemically they are various types of esters of different alcohols. In addition to alcohol and fatty acids, some of the lipids may contain phosphoric acid, nitrogenous base and carbohydrates.

Bloor's Criteria: According to ***Bloor,*** lipids are compounds having the following characteristics.

- These are ***insoluble in water.***
- Solubility in one or more organic solvents, such as ether, chloroform, benzene, acetone, etc— so called 'fat solvents'.
- Some relationship to the fatty acids as esters either actual or potential.
- Possibility of utilization by living organisms.

Thus, lipids include fats, oils, waxes and related compound. An ***oil*** is a lipid which is liquid at ordinary temperature. Distinction between fats and oil is a purely physical one. Chemically these are all esters of glycerol with higher fatty acids.

BIOMEDICAL IMPORTANCE

- Lipids are important dietary constituents and ***act as fuel in the body.*** In some respects lipids is even superior to carbohydrates as a raw material for combustion, since,
  - It ***yields more energy per gm (9.5 C/gm*** as compared to carbohydrates 4.0 C/gm).
  - Can be stored in the body in almost unlimited amount in contrast to carbohydrates.
- Some deposits of lipids may exert an ***insulating effect*** in the body, while lipids around internal organs like kidney, etc. may provide padding and protect the organs.
- ***Building materials:*** Breakdown products of fats can be utilized for building biological active materials.
- Lipids supply so-called ***essential fatty acids*** (EFA), which cannot be synthesized in the body and are essential in the diet for normal health and growth.
- The nervous system, is particularly rich in lipids of certain types and are essential for proper functioning.
- Some vitamins like, A,D,E and K are fat soluble, hence lipid is necessary for these vitamins.
- Lipoproteins and phospholipids (PL) are important constituents of many natural membranes such as walls and cell organelles like mitochondrion, etc.
- Lipoproteins are also 'carriers' of triglycerides, cholesterol and PL in the body.

CLASSIFICATION OF LIPIDS

Bloor's classification is generally adopted with a few modifications.

1. Simple lipids: These are esters of fatty acids with various alcohols.

- ***Neutral fats (Triacylglycerol, TG):*** are triesters of fatty acids with glycerol.

- *Waxes:* are esters of fatty acids with monohydroxy aliphatic alcohols other than glycerol.
  - True waxes are esters of higher fatty acids with cetyl alcohol ($C_{16}H_{33}OH$) or other higher straight chain alcohols.
  - Cholesterol esters are esters of fatty acid with cholesterol.
  - Vit A and vit D esters are palmitic or stearic acid esters of vit A (retinol) or vit D respectively.

2. **Compound lipids:** These are esters of fatty acids containing groups, other than, and in addition, to an alcohol and fatty acids.

- ***Phospholipids:*** They are substituted fats containing in addition to fatty acid and glycerol, a phosphoric acid residue, a nitrogenous base and other substituents.
  Examples: Phosphatidyl choline (Lecithin), phosphatidyl ethanolamine (Cephalin), phosphatidyl inositols (Lipositols), phosphatidyl serine, plasmalogens, sphingomyelins, etc.
- ***Glycolipids:*** Lipids containing carbohydrates moiety are called glycolipids. They contain a ***special alcohol called sphingosine or sphingol*** and nitrogenous base in addition to fatty acids ***but does not contain phosphoric acid or glycerol.*** These are of **two types:**
  - ***Cerebrosides***
  - ***Gangliosides***
- ***Sulpholipids:*** Lipids characterized by possessing sulphate groups.
- ***Aminolipids*** (Proteolipids)
- ***Lipoproteins:*** Lipids as prosthetic group to proteins.

3. **Derived lipids:** Derivatives obtained by hydrolysis of those given in groups I and II, still possess the general characteristic of lipids.

- ***Fatty Acids:*** may be saturated, unsaturated or cyclic.
- ***Monoglycerides*** (Monoacylglycerol) and ***Diglycerides*** (Diacylglycerol)
- ***Alcohols:***
  - Straight chain alcohols are water insoluble alcohols of higher molecular weight obtained on hydrolysis of waxes.
  - Cholesterol and other steroids including vit D.
  - Alcohols containing the β-ionone ring—include vit A and certain carotenoids.
  - Glycerol.

DERIVED LIPIDS

FATTY ACIDS

Definition

- A fatty acid (FA) may be defined as an organic acid that occurs in a natural triglyceride and is a **monocarboxylic acid** ranging in chain length from C4 to about 24 carbon atoms.
- FA are obtained from hydrolysis of fats. Fatty acids which occur in natural fats usually contain an even number of carbon atoms (because they are synthesized from two carbon units) and are straight chain derivatives.

TYPES OF FATTY ACIDS

Straight Chain FA

These are divided into **two groups.**

- ***Saturated FA:*** Those which contain no double bonds
- ***Unsaturated FA:*** Those which contain one or more double bonds.

A. ***Saturated FA:*** Their general formula is $C_nH_{2n+1}COOH$.

Examples

- Acetic acid CH_3COOH
- Propionic acid C_2H_5COOH
- Butyric acid C_3H_7COOH
- Caproic acid $C_5H_{11}COOH$
- Palmitic acid $C_{15}H_{31}COOH$
- Stearic acid $C_{17}H_{35}COOH$ and so on.

Saturated fatty acids having 10 carbon or less number of carbon atoms are known ***lower fatty acids***, e.g. acetic acid, butyric acid, etc. Saturated fatty acids having more than 10 carbon atoms are called ***higher fatty acids,*** e.g. palmitic acid, stearic acid, etc. Milk contains significant amount of lower fatty acids.

B. *Unsaturated FA:* These are classified further ***according to the degree of unsaturation.***

1. *Monounsaturated (mono-ethenoid)* fatty acids are those which **contain one double bond.** Their general formula is $C_nH_{2n-1}COOH$

Example: ***Oleic acid*** $C_{17}H_{33}COOH$ is found in nearly all fats **(18:1;9).**

2. *Polyunsaturated (Polyethenoid) fatty acids:* There are ***three polyunsaturated fatty acids of biological importance.***

- ***Linoleic acid series (18:2;9,12):*** It contains **two double bonds** between C9 and C10; and between C12 and C13. Their general formula is $C_nH_{2n-3}COOH$
  Dietary sources: Linoleic acid is present in sufficient amounts in peanut oil, corn oil, cotton seed oil, soybean oil, egg yolk.
- ***Linolenic acid series (18:3;9,12,15):*** It contains **three double bonds** between 9 and 10, 12 and 13 and, 15 and 16. Their general formula is $C_nH_{2n-5}COOH$.
  Dietary sources: It is found frequently with linoleic acid, but particularly present in linseed oil, rapeseed oil, soybean oil, fish visceras and liver oil (cod liver oil).
- ***Arachidonic acid series (20:4;5,8,11,14):*** It contains **four double bonds.** Their general formula is $C_nH_{2n-7}COOH$.
  Dietary sources: Arachidonic acid is found in small quantities with linoleic acid but particularly present in peanut oil. It is found in animal fats including liver fats.

C. *Cyclic FA:* Fatty acids bearing cyclic groups are present in some seeds, e.g.
- **Chaulmoogric acid** obtained from chaulmoogra seeds,
- **Hydnocarpic acid.**

BIOCHEMICAL IMPORTANCE

Both of them have been used earlier since long time for treatment of leprosy.

D. *Eicosanoids:* These are derived from eicosapolyenoic FA.

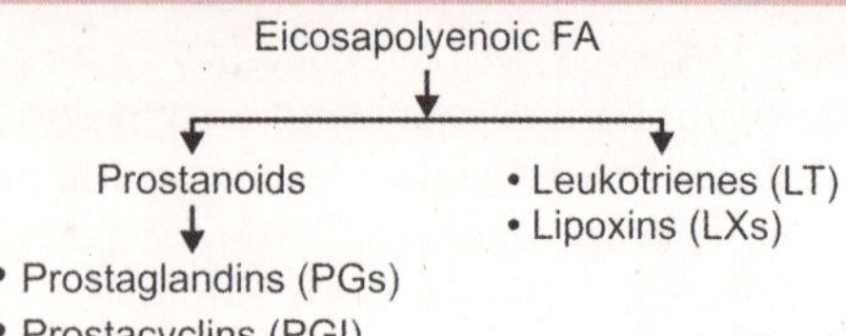

E. Essential Fatty Acids: Three polyunsaturated fatty acids, ***linoleic acid, linolenic acid*** and ***arachidonic acid*** are called ***essential fatty acids (EFA). They cannot be synthesized in the body and must be provided in the diet.*** Lack of EFA in the diet can produce growth retardation and other deficiency manifestation symptoms.

Which EFA is Important?
- Linoleic acid is the most important as arachidonic acid can be formed from linoleic acid by a ***three stage*** reaction by addition of acetyl CoA. ***Pyridoxal phosphate is necessary for this conversion.***
- ***Biologically arachidonic acid is very important*** as it is precursor from which prostaglandins and leukotrienes are synthesized in the body.

Why EFA cannot be Synthesized?
Introduction of additional double bonds in unsaturated fatty acid is limited to the area between –COOH group and the existing double bond and that it is not possible to introduce a double bond between the $-CH_3$ group at the opposite end of the molecule and the first unsaturated linkage. This would explain body's inability to synthesize an EFA from oleic acid.

FUNCTIONS OF EFA

- ***Structural elements of tissues:*** Polyunsaturated fatty acids occur in higher concentration in lipids associated with structural elements of tissues.
- ***Structural element of gonads:*** Lipids of gonads also contain a high concentration of polyunsaturated fatty acids which suggests importance of these compounds in reproductive function.

- ***Synthesis of prostaglandins*** and other compounds: Prostaglandins are synthesized from arachidonic acid by cyclo-oxygenase enzyme system. Leukotrienes are a family of conjugated trienes formed from arachidonic acid in leucocytes by the Lipo-oxygenase pathway.
- ***Structural element of mitochondrial membrane:*** A deficiency of EFA causes swelling of mitochondrial membrane and reduction in efficiency of oxidative phosphorylation. This may explain for increased heat production noted in EFA deficient animals.
- ***Serum level of cholesterol:*** Fats with high content of polyunsaturated fatty acids ***tends to lower serum level of cholesterol.***
- ***Effect on clotting time:*** Prolongation of clotting time is noted in ingestion of fats rich in EFA.
- ***Effect on fibrinolytic activity:*** An increase in fibrinolytic activity follows the ingestion of fats rich in EFA.
- ***Role of EFA in fatty liver:*** Deficiency of EFA produces fatty liver.

Deficiency Manifestations: A deficiency of EFA has not yet been unequivocally demonstrated in humans. In weaning animals, symptoms of EFA deficiency are readily produced. They are:

- *Cessation of growth*
- *Skin lesions:* acanthosis (hypertrophy of prickle cells, and hyperkeratosis (hypertrophy of stratum corneum).
- ***Skin becomes abnormally permeable to water.*** Increased loss of water increases BMR.
- Abnormalities of pregnancy and lactation in adult females.
- *Fatty liver* accompanied by increased rates of fatty acid synthesis.
- Lessened resistance to stress.
- Kidney damage

BIOMEDICAL IMPORTANCE

In human, *deficiency of EFA causes:*

(a) Eczema like dermatitis,
(b) Degenerative change in arterial wall and
(c) Fatty liver in man. There are also some reports that administration of EFA in such cases may produce

- Some improvement of eczema in children kept on skimmed milk.
- Prevent fatty liver (some cases) and
- Lowering of cholesterol levels.

Infants and babies with low fat diet develop typical skin lesion which have shown to be improved with EFA (linoleic acid).

ALCOHOLS

Alcohols contained in the lipid molecule include glycerol, cholesterol and the higher alcohols, e.g. cetylalcohol, $C_{16}H_{33}COOH$ (usually found in waxes).

1. GLYCEROL

Glycerol commonly known as "glycerin" is the simplest trihydric alcohol as it contains three hydroxyl groups in the molecule *(Fig. 2.1)*.

- It is colourless oily fluid with a sweetish taste.
- It is miscible with water and alcohols in all proportions but is almost insoluble in ether.

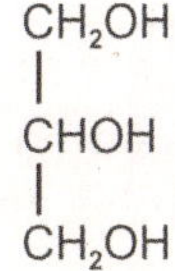

Fig. 2.1: Glycerol

Source

- *Industrial*
  - It is obtained as a by-product of soap manufacture.
- *Physiological*
  - *Endogenous source:* Main source is from lipolysis of fats in adipose tissue.
  - *Exogenous source:* The chief source is from dietary intake. ***Approx. 22% of glycerol directly absorbed to portal blood from the gut.***

Test

- *Acrolein Test:* The presence of glycerol is detected by acrolein test. Glycerol when dehydrated with heat and $KHSO_4$ produces *"acryl aldehyde"* which has pungent or acrid odour.

Uses of Glycerol

- ***Industrial:*** Glycerol has many uses in industry, as a result of its solubility, solvent action and hygroscopic nature. Many pharmaceuticals and cosmetic preparations have glycerol in their formulas.
- ***In Medicine:***
  - **Nitroglycerine** ***is used as a vasodilator.***
  - **Glycerol therapy** ***in cerebrovascular (CV) diseases.*** Glycerol has been used orally as well as IV in cases of CV diseases. It is nontoxic and it reduces cerebral oedema with improvement in CS fluid. Besides, there is no rebound increase in intracranial pressure on discontinuation of therapy as may occur with mannitol or urea.
- ***Physiological:*** In body, glycerol has a ***definite nutritive value. It can be converted to glucose/ and glycogen, the process known as gluconeogenesis.***

STEROIDS AND STEROLS

- The steroids are often found in association with fat.
- They may be separated from the fat, after the fat is saponified, since they occur in **"unsaponifiable residue"**
- All of the steroids have a similar cyclic nucleus resembling **"phenanthrene"** (ring A, B and C) to which a **"cyclopentane"** ring (ring D) is attached. It is designed as ***"cyclopentano perhydrophenanthrene nucleus" (Fig. 2.2).***

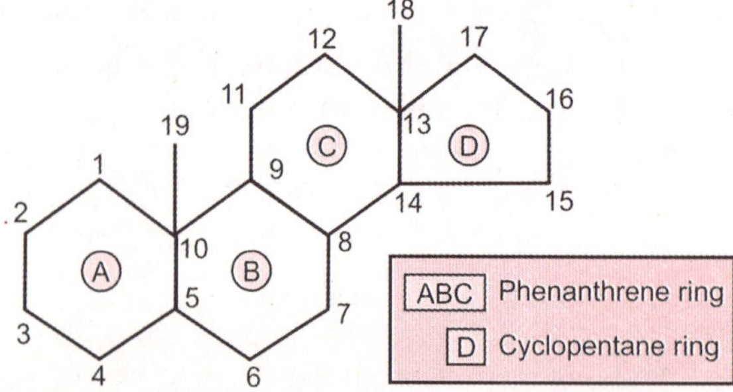

Fig. 2.2: Cyclopentanoperhydrophenanthrene nucleus

- Methyl side chains occur typically at positions 10 and 13 (constituting carbon atoms 19 and 18 respectively).
- A side chain at position 17 is usual. If the compound has one or more –OH groups and no carbonyl or carboxyl groups, it is called a ***'sterol'*** and the name terminates in –ol. ***Most important sterol in human body is cholesterol.***

CHOLESTEROL

Structure: Cholesterol is the most important sterol in human body. Its molecular formula is $C_{27}H_{45}OH$. Its structural formula is given in *Figure 2.3.*

- It possesses ***"Cyclopentanoperhydrophenanthrene nucleus".***
- It has ***an-OH group at C_3***
- It has an ***unsaturated double bond between C_5 and C_6***
- It has an eight carbon side chain attached to C_{17}.

Molecular formula is $C_{27}H_{45}OH$

Fig. 2.3: Cholesterol

Properties: The name cholesterol is derived from the Greek word meaning "solid bile".

- It occurs as a white or faintly yellow, almost odourless, pearly leaflets or granules.
- It is ***insoluble in water,*** sparingly soluble in alcohol and soluble in ether, chloroform, hot alcohol, ethylacetate and vegetable oils.
- It easily crystallizes from such solutions in colourless, rhombic plates with ***one or more characteristic notches in the corner (Fig. 2.4).***

- It is ***not saponifiable.***
- Its melting point is 147° to 150°C.
- Since it has an unsaturated bond, it can take up two halogen atoms.

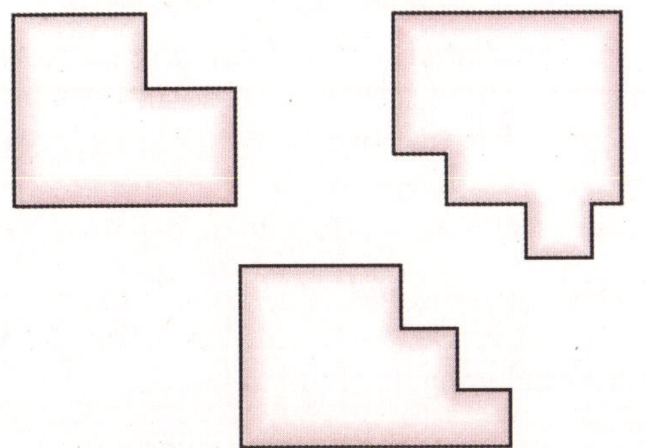

Fig. 2.4: Cholesterol crystals

Source

- ***Exogenous:*** Dietary cholesterol, ***approximately 0.3 gm/day.*** Diet rich in cholesterol are butter, cream, milk, egg yolk, meat, etc. ***A hen's egg weighing 2 oz. gives 250 mg cholesterol.***
- ***Endogenous:*** It is synthesized in the body from acetyl-CoA, ***approximately 1.0 gm/day.***

Occurrence: It is widely present in body tissues. Cholesterol is found in largest amounts in normal human adults.

- **Brain** and nervous tissue 2%
- In the **liver** about 0.3%
- **Skin** 0.3% and **intestinal mucosa** 0.2%, **certain endocrine glands**, viz. adrenal cortex contain some 10% or more. Corpus luteum is also rich cholesterol.
- The relatively high content of cholesterol in skin may be related to vit D formation by UV rays and that in the adrenal gland and gonads to steroid hormone synthesis. Cholesterol is present in blood and bile and is usually a major constituent of gallstones.

FORMS OF CHOLESTEROL

- Cholesterol occurs both in *free* form and in *ester* form, in which it is esterified with fatty acids at –OH group at C_3 position.
- Free cholesterol is equally distributed between plasma and red blood cells, but the latter do not contain esters. In brain and nervous tissue, free from predominates, whereas in adrenal cortex it occurs mainly as esterified form.

Esterification of Cholesterol: Esterification occurs in **two ways:**

- Some cholesterol esters are formed in tissues by the transfer of acyl groups from acyl-CoA to cholesterol by *acyl transferases.*
- But most of the plasma cholesterol esters are produced in the plasma itself by the transfer of an acyl group (mostly unsaturated acyl group) from the β-position of lecithin to cholesterol with the help of the enzyme *lecithincholesterol acyl transferase* (LCAT).

$$\text{Lecithin + Cholesterol} \xrightarrow{\text{LCAT}} \text{Lysolecithin + Cholesterol ester}$$

BIOMEDICAL IMPORTANCE

1. ***Norum's disease:*** A ***genetic deficiency*** of ***LCAT*** produces Norum's disease due to the failure of esterification of cholesterol at the cost of lecithin. The ***disease is characterized by:***
   - Rise in free cholesterol ↑
   - Rise in lecithin in plasma and ↑
   - Fall in cholesterol ester, lysolecithin and α-lipoproteins in plasma. ↓
2. ***Normal level and physiological variations:*** Normal level of serum total cholesterol in an adult varies from 150 to 250 mg%. About 40-50 mg% occurs as "free" cholesterol (approximately 30% of total) and 110-200 mg% as cholesterol "esters" (approximately 70%).
3. ***Variations of cholesterol level:***
   - ***Age:*** Blood cholesterol level is low at birth (50-70% of the values in normal adults) and it gradually increases with age. After 55 years there is a tendency to decrease again.
   - ***Sex and race:*** Sex and race have little effect, but in case of women, the level is increased just before and decreased during the menstrual period.
   - ***Pregnancy:*** The level is also increased during pregnancy, when a progressive rise in free cholesterol and a fall in "ester" fraction are observed.
4. ***Pathological variations:*** See cholesterol metabolism.

COLOUR REACTIONS OF STEROLS

1. *Liebermann-Burchard reaction*

- A chloroform solution of a sterol, when treated with acetic anhydride and conc. H_2SO_4 gives a ***grass-green colour.***
- This reaction forms the basis for a colorimetric estimation of cholesterol by **Sackett's method.**

2. *Salkowski test*

- When a chloroform solution of the sterol is treated with an equal volume of conc H_2SO_4, it develops ***a red to purple colour.***
- The heavier acid, which form a layer below assumes a yellowish colour with a green fluorescence, whereas the upper chloroform layer becomes bluish red first, and gradually turns violet-red.

3. ***Zak's reaction:*** When glacial acetic acid aldehyde free solution of cholesterol is treated with ferric chloride and conc. H_2SO_4 it produces ***a red colour.*** This reaction forms a basis for the colorimetric estimation of cholesterol **(Zak's method).**

OTHER STEROLS OF BIOLOGICAL IMPORTANCE

1. **7-Dehydrocholesterol:** It is an important sterol ***present in the skin.*** This differs from cholesterol only in having a second double bond, between C_7 and C_8.

Source: In man, 7-dehydrocholesterol may be obtained partly by synthesis from cholesterol in skin and/or intestinal wall,

BIOMEDICAL IMPORTANCE

In the epidermis of skin, UV rays of sunshine change 7-dehydrocholesterol (pre-cholecalciferol) to cholecalciferol (vitamin D_3). Hence ***7-dehydrocholesterol is called pro-vitamin-D_3.*** This explain the value of sunshine in preventing rickets, a disease produced from vitamin D deficiency.

2. **Ergosterol:** It is a plant sterol, **first isolated from ergot,** a fungus of *rye* and later from yeast and certain mushrooms. Structurally this sterol has the same nucleus as 7-dehydrocholesterol but differs slightly in its side chain.

BIOMEDICAL IMPORTANCE

When irradiated with UV rays (long wave 265 mμ), ergosterol is changed to vitamin D_2 by the opening of the ring B of the sterol. ***Hence ergosterol is called as pro-vitamin D_2*, Over-irradiation may produce toxic products.**

3. ***Stigmasterol and sitosterol:*** They are plant sterols, occurring in higher plants. They have no nutritional value for human beings.

BIOMEDICAL IMPORTANCE

Sitosterol appears to decrease the intestinal absorption of both exogenous and endogenous cholesterol, thus ***lowering the blood cholesterol level.***

4. **Coprosterol (Coprostanol):** Coprosterol occurs in faeces as a result of the reduction of cholesterol (by hydrogenation of double bond). This is brought about by bacterial action—double bond between C_5 and C_6 is saturated. Rings A and B (between C atoms 5 and 10) is "cis" (cf. Cholesterol—it is "trans").

SIMPLE LIPIDS

NEUTRAL FATS (TRIGLYCERIDES) OR (TRIACYLGLYCEROL)

Neutral fats (triglycerides-TG) are ***all tri-esters of the trihydric alcohol*** with various fatty acids. The type formula for a neutral fat (TG) is given in ***Figure 2.5***, in which R_1, R_2, R_3 represent fatty acids chains which may or may not all be the same.

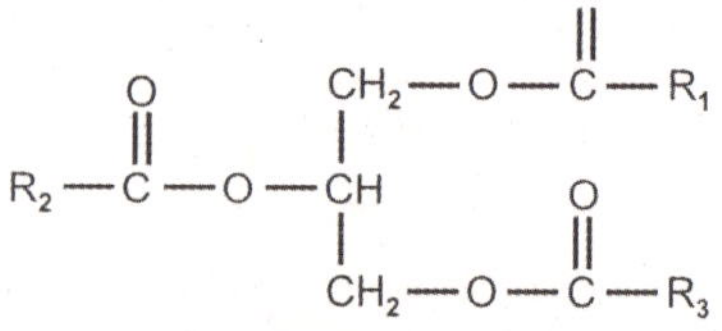

$$
\begin{array}{ccc}
 & CH_2-O-\overset{\overset{\displaystyle O}{\|}}{C}-R_1 \\
 & | \\
R_2-\overset{\overset{\displaystyle O}{\|}}{C}-O- & CH \\
 & | \\
 & CH_2-O-\overset{\overset{\displaystyle O}{\|}}{C}-R_3
\end{array}
$$

Fig. 2.5: Type formula for neutral fat

Physical Properties:

- Neutral fats are colourless, odourless and tasteless substances.
- *Solubility:* They are ***insoluble in water*** but soluble in organic fat solvents.
- *Specific gravity:* The specific gravity of all fats is less than 1.0, consequently all fats float in water.
- *Emulsification:* Emulsions of fat may be made by shaking vigorously in water and by emulsifying agents such as gums, soaps and proteins which produce more stable emulsions.

BIOMEDICAL IMPORTANCE OF EMULSIFICATION

The emulsification of dietary fats in intestinal canal, **brought about by bile salts**, is a prerequisite for digestion and absorption of fats.

Chemical Properties

1. **Hydrolysis:** The fats may be hydrolyzed with:
   - ***Superheated steam.***
   - ***By acids, or alkalies,*** or
   - ***By the specific fat splitting enzymes lipases.***

$$\text{Triolein} \xrightarrow[\text{Hydrolysis}]{H_2O} \text{Glycerol + oleic acid}$$

Lipases: Lipases are enzymes which hydrolyse triglyceride yielding fatty acids and glycerol.

Sites: Lipases are found in human body in following places.

- ***Lingual lipase*** in saliva
- ***Gastric lipase*** in gastric juice
- ***Pancreatic lipase*** in pancreatic juice, ***intestinal lipase*** in intestinal epithelial cell, ***adipolytic lipase*** in adipose tissue and
- ***Serum lipase***

Pancreatic lipase is peculiar in that it can hydrolyze ester bonds in positions 1 and 3 preferentially, than in position 2 of TG molecule.

2. **Saponification:** ***Hydrolysis of a fat by an alkali is called saponification.*** The resultant products are glycerol and the alkali salts of the fatty acids, which are called "soaps".

$$\text{Triolein + 3 NaOH} \xrightarrow{H_2O} \text{Glycerol + 3}D_{17}H_{33}\text{COO Na}$$

(sodium oleate)—soap

3. **Additive reactions:** The unsaturated fatty acids present in neutral fat exhibit all the additive reaction, i.e. hydrogenation, halogenation, etc. Oils which are liquid at ordinary room temperature, on hydrogenation become solidified. This is the basis of vanaspati (Dalda) manufacture, where inedible and cheap oils like cotton seed oil are hydrogenated and converted to edible solid fat.

4. **Oxidation:** Fats very rich in unsaturated fatty acids such as linseed oil undergo spontaneous oxidation at the double bond forming aldehydes, ketones and resins which form transparent coating on the surfaces to which the oil is applied. These are called ***drying oils*** and are used in the manufacture of paints and varnishes.

5. **Rancidity:** The unpleasant odour and taste developed by most natural fats on aging is referred to as rancidity.

Rancidity may be caused by the following methods:

- ***Hydrolysis of fat*** yields free fatty acids and glycerol and/or mono and diglycerides. Process is enhanced by presence of lipolytic enzymes *lipases,* which, in the presence of moisture and warm temperature bring about hydrolysis rapidly.
- ***By various oxidative processes*** oxidation of double bonds of unsaturated glycerides may form ***"peroxides".*** Which then decompose to form aldehydes of objectionable odour and taste. The process is greatly enhanced by exposure to light.

Prevention of rancidity: Vegetable fats contain certain substances like vitamin E, phenols, hydroquinones, tannins and others which are **antioxidants** and prevent development of rancidity. Hence ***vegetable fats preserve for longer periods than animal fats.***

IDENTIFICATION OF FATS AND OILS

Sometimes it becomes necessary to ascertain the following points.

- *To identify a pure fat.*
- *To assess the degree of adulteration.*
- *To determine the proportions of different types of fat in a mixture.*

Besides the characteristic melting point and congealing point several other chemical values ("chemical constants") have been used. Some of them are discussed below:

1. SAPONIFICATION NUMBER

Definition: The number of mgms of KOH required to saponify the free and combined FA in one gram of a given fat is called its saponification number.

Basis: The amount of alkali needed to saponify a given quantity of fat will depend upon the number of –COOH group present. Thus, fats containing short chain fatty acids will have more-COOH groups per gram than long-chain fatty acids and this will take up more alkali and hence will have higher saponification number.

Example: **Butter** containing a large proportion of short-chain fatty acids such as butyric and caproic acids, has relatively high saponification number from 220 to 230. **Oleo-margarine**, with more long chain fatty acids, has a saponification number of 195 or less.

2. REICHERT-MEISSL NUMBER

Definition: It is the number of millilitres of 0.1 (N) alkali required to neutralize the soluble volatile fatty acids distilled from 5 gm of fat.

Significance: The Reichert-Meissl ***measures the amount of volatile soluble fatty acids.*** Butter fat is the only common fat with a high Reichert-Meissl number and this determination, therefore, is of interest in that it aids the food chemist in detecting butter substitutes in food products.

3. IODINE NUMBER

Definition: Iodine number is defined as the number of grams of iodine absorbed by 100 gms of fat.

Significance and Use:

- Iodine number is a ***measure of the degree of unsaturation of a fat.*** The more the iodine number, the greater the degree of unsaturation in the fatty acids part of the fat.
- The determination of iodine number is useful to the chemist in determining the quality of an oil or its freedom from adulteration. *Example:* Iodine number of cottonseed oil varies from 103 to 111, that of olive oil from 79 to 88, and that of linseed oil from 175 to 202. A commercial lot of olive oil which has an iodine number higher than 88 might have been adulterated with cottonseed oil.

4. ACETYL NUMBER

Definition: The number of mgms of KOH required to neutralize the acetic acid obtained by saponification of 1 gm of fat after it has been acetylated.

Example: Castor oil because of its high content of ricinoleic acid has a high acetyl number.

Acetyl numbers of some oils:

- **Castor oil** 146-150
- **Cod liver oil** 1.1
- **Cottonseed oil** 21-25
- **Olive oil** 10.5

It can be used to detect adulteration.

COMPOUND LIPID

PHOSPHOLIPIDS: CHEMISTRY AND FUNCTIONS

Definition: Phospholipids are compound lipids, they contain in addition to fatty acids and glycerol/or other alcohol, a phosphoric acid residue, nitrogen containing base and other substituents.

Classification: Classification given by **Celmer and Carter** is used, which is ***based on the type of alcohol present*** in the phospholipids. Thus, they are classified mainly into following **three groups:**

- *Glycerophosphatides:* In this group, ***glycerol is the alcohol. Examples*** are phosphatidyl ethanolamine (cephalin), phosphatidyl choline (Lecithin), phosphatidyl serine, plasmalogens, phosphatidic acid and cardiolipins, phosphatides.

- *Phospho-inositides:* In this group, ***inositol is the alcohol***, e.g. phosphatidyl inositol (lipositol)
- ***Phospho-sphingosides: Alcohol present is sphingosine*** (also called as sphingol)–an unsaturated amino alcohol, e.g. sphingomyelin.

PROPERTIES OF PHOSPHOLIPIDS IN REFERENCE TO LECITHIN

PHOSPHATIDYL CHOLINE (LECITHIN)

- It is widely distributed in animals in liver, brain, nerve tissues, sperm and egg yolk, having both metabolic and structural functions. In plants, it is particularly abundant in seeds and sprouts.
- Lecithin has also been prepared synthetically.
- Structurally lecithin is considered to be made up of:

```
┌ OH — FA
├ OH — FA
└ OH — Phosphoric acid—choline
Glycerol
```

- ***On hydrolysis,*** lecithin yields – glycerol, fatty acids, phosphoric acid and nitrogenous base choline.

Properties

Physical properties: When purified it is a waxy, white substance.

- It becomes **brown** when exposed to air **(autoxidation).**
- It is hygroscopic, mixes well with water to form cloudy, colloidal solution.
- Lecithin is soluble in ordinary fat solvents except acetone.

Chemical properties:

- When aqueous solution of lecithins is shaken with H_2SO_4, choline is split off, forming **"phosphatidic acid".**
- When lecithin is boiled with alkalies or mineral acids, not only choline is split off, phosphatidic acid is further hydrolyzed to glycerophosphoric acid and two molecules of fatty acids.

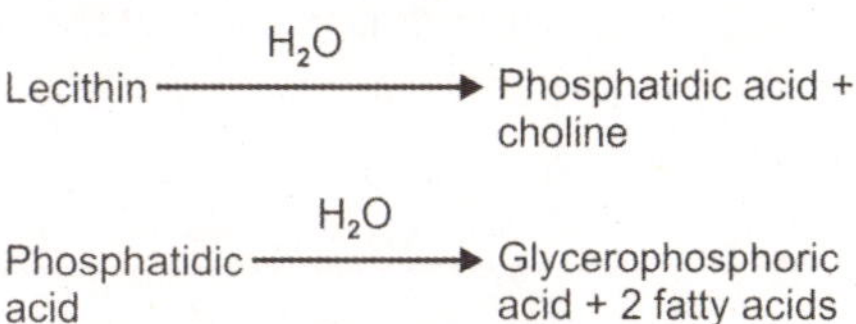

PHOSPHOLIPASES (DAWSON)

Dawson found several types of phospholipases. They hydrolyze phospholipids (lecithin) in a characteristic way. Site of action of different phospholipases are shown in *Figure 2.6.*

OTHER PHOSPHOLIPIDS OF BIOLOGICAL IMPORTANCE

1. Phosphatidyl Ethanolamine (Cephalins):

- Cephalins are structurally identical with lecithins, with the exception that ***the base ethanolamine replaces choline.***

2. Phosphatidyl Inositol (Lipositols):

- Inositol is an alcohol, a cyclic compound hexahydroxycyclohexane with molecular formula $C_6H_{12}O_6$. ***It replaces the base choline of lecithin.***
- Inositol as a constituent of phospholipids was first discovered in acid-fast bacilli. Later, it was found to occur in brain and nervous tissues, moderately in soyabeans, and also occurs in plant phospholipids.

3. Phosphatidyl Serine:

A cephalin like phospholipid ***contains amino acid serine in place of ethanolamine.*** It is found in brain and nervous tissues and in small amounts in other tissues. It is also found in blood.

4. Lysophosphatides:

These are phosphoglycerides containing only one acyl radical in **α** position, e.g. lysolecithin.

Formation Lysophosphatides can be formed in **two ways:**

- ***By the action of phospholipase A_2.***

- Alternatively, it can also be formed by ***interaction of lecithin and cholesterol in presence of the enzyme lecithin cholesterol acyl transferase*** (LCAT), so that cholesterol ester and lysolecithin are formed.

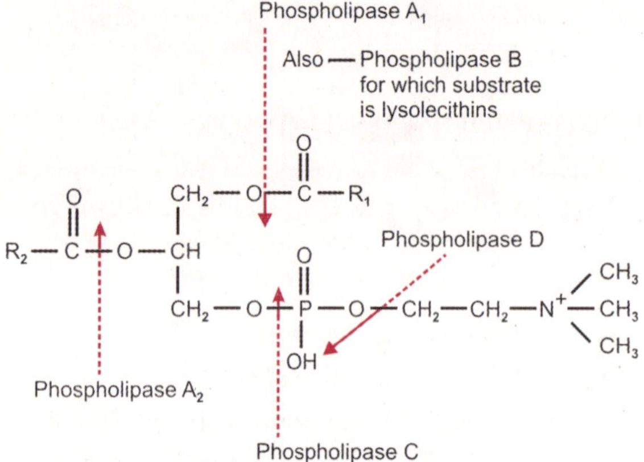

Fig. 2.6: Site of action of phospholipases

Lecithin + Cholesterol

↓ LCAT

Lysolecithin + Cholesterol ester

5. PLASMALOGENS:

- The plasmalogens make up an appreciable amount, about 10 percent of total phospholipids, of brain and nervous tissue, muscle and mitochondria.
- **These compounds yield on hydrolysis**
  - one molecule each of long chain aliphatic aldehyde
  - a FA
  - glycerol-PO_4, and
  - a nitrogenous base which is usually ethanolamine, but may be sometimes choline.

6. SPHINGOMYELINS (PHOSPHATIDYL SPHINGOSIDES)

- Sphingomyelins are found in large quantities in brain and nervous tissues, and in very small amount in other tissues.
- ***It does not contain glycerol.*** In place of glycerol, it contains an 18 carbon unsaturated amino alcohol called ***"sphingosine" (sphingol).***
- A sphingomyelin molecule is built on the following:

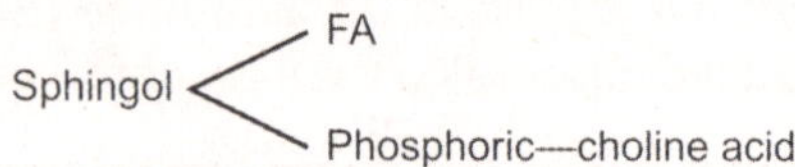

- ***On hydrolysis*, sphingomyelin yields**
  - one molecule of fatty acid +
  - phosphoric acid +
  - nitrogenous base choline +
  - one molecule of complex unsaturated amino alcohol sphingosine (sphingol).
- Sphingosine molecule in which a fatty acyl group is substituted on the $-NH_2$ group is called ***ceramide*** and when a phosphate group is attached to ceramide, it is called ***"ceramide phosphate".*** When choline is split off from sphingomyelin, ceramide phosphate is left.
- *Sphingomylinase* is the enzyme which hydrolyzes sphingomyelin to form ceramide and phosphoryl choline.

Clinical Aspect of Sphingomyelins—Niemann-Pick Disease

- Large accumulations of sphingomyelins may occur in brain, liver and spleen of some persons suffering from **Niemann-Pick disease.**
- Niemann-Pick disease is ***an inherited disorder*** of sphingomyelin metabolism in which sphingomyelin is not degraded, as a result sphingomyelin accumulates.
- It is a lipid-storage disease (lipidoses). Its inheritance is ***autosomal recessive.***
- It is **caused by the deficiency of enzyme sphingomyelinase**, a lysosomal enzyme. It affects children, usually at birth or infancy.
- Abnormal accumulation of sphingomyelins occurs in all organs and tissues of body especially in liver, spleen, and brain.
- Clinically, the child presents with gradual enlargement of abdomen, liver (hepatomegaly),

and spleen (splenomegaly), and manifests progressive mental deterioration (due to accumulation of sphingomyelins in brain).

- Other lipids and cholesterol are usually normal or may be slightly elevated.
- *Prognosis:* It is usually fatal and follows progressive downhill course. Over 80% of infants die within 2 years.

FUNCTIONS OF PHOSPHOLIPIDS

- *Structural:* Phospholipids participate in the lipoprotein complexes which are thought to constitute the matrix of cell walls and membranes, the myelin sheath, and of such structures as mitochondria and microsomes.
- *Role in enzyme action:* Certain enzymes require tightly bound phospholipids for their action, e.g. mitochondrial enzyme system involved in oxidative phosphorylation.
- *Role in blood coagulation:* Phospholipids play an essential part in the blood coagulation process. These are required at two stages.
  - Conversion of prothrombin to thrombin by active factor X
  - Possibly also in the activation of factor VIII by activated factor IX.

  Platelets provide the chief source of PL and that part of total lipid content of the platelets which contribute to intrinsic blood coagulation process is called ***"platelet factor 3"***.
- *Role in lipid absorption in intestine:* Lecithin lowers the surface tension of water and aids in emulsification of lipid water mixtures, a prerequisite in digestion and absorption of lipids from GI tract.
- *Role in transport of lipids from intestines:* Exogenous TG is carried as lipoprotein complex, ***chylomicrons,*** in which PL takes an active part.
- *Role in transport of lipids from liver:* Endogenous TG is carried from liver to various tissues as lipoprotein complex ***"pre-β-lipoprotein" (VLDL),*** PL is required for the formation of the lipoprotein complex.
- *Role in electron transport:* As constituents of mitochondria, endoplasmic reticulum, Golgi apparatus, etc. PL participates in electron transport and oxidative phosphorylation in mitochondria and other functions of these membrane components. Probably PL ***helps to couple oxidation with phosphorylation and maintain electron transport enzymes in active conformation*** and proper relative positions.
- *Lipotropic action of lecithin:* Choline acts as a lipotropic agent as it can prevent formation of fatty liver. ***As lecithin can provide choline it acts as a lipotropic agent.***
- *Ion transport and secretion:* Phospholipids in some way implicated in the mechanism of secretion is suggested by the observation that phospholipids, especially phosphatidic acid and phosphoinositides ***turnover is proportional to the rate of secretion of cells liberating such products as hormones, enzymes, mucins and other proteins.***
- *Membrane phospholipids as source of arachidonic acid:* ***Phospholipids*** of membrane are hydrolyzed by ***phospholipase*** A_2 and provide the unsaturated fatty acid arachidonic acid which is utilized for synthesis of prostaglandins and leukotrienes.
- *Insulation:* Phospholipids of myelin sheaths provide the insulation around the nerve fibres.
- *Cofactor:* Phospholipids are required as a cofactor for the activity of the enzyme *lipoprotein lipase and triacylglycerol lipase.*
- *Role of phosphatidyl inositides metabolite in Ca^{++} dependent hormone action:* Some signal must provide communication between the hormone receptor on the plasma membrane and intracellular Ca^{++} reservoirs. The best candidate appears to be the products of phosphatidyl inositides metabolism.

BIOMEDICAL IMPORTANCE DIPALMITY LECITHIN (DPL)

- DPL acts as a 'surfactant' and lowers the surface tension in lung alveoli.
- Absence of DPL in premature foetus may produce collapse of lung alveoli which produces ***respiratory distress syndrome (hyaline membrane disease).***

GLYCOLIPIDS

CEREBROSIDES (GLYCOSPHINGOSIDES)

Cerebrosides **occurs in large amounts in the white matter of brain and in the myelin sheaths of nerve.** They are not found in embryonic brain, but develop as medullation progresses. In smaller amounts, they appear to be very widely distributed in animal tissues. In medullated nerves, the concentration of cerebrosides are much higher than in nonmedullated nerve fibres.

Structure: A cerebroside is considered to be built on the following:

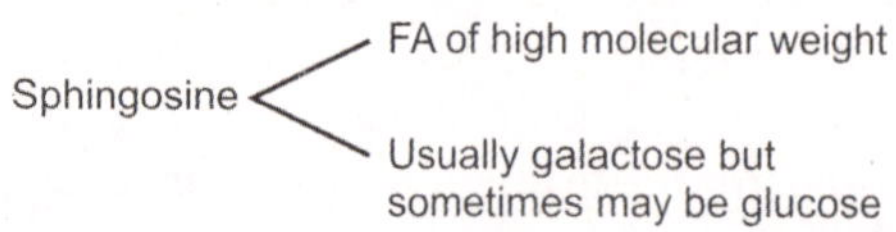

There is no glycerol, no phosphoric acid and no nitrogenous base. On hydrolysis, a cerebroside yields:

- A sugar, **usually galactose, but sometimes glucose**
- A high molecular weight **fatty acid,** and
- The alcohol, **sphingosine** or dihydrosphingosine.

Thus they contain nitrogens though there is no nitrogenous base.

Types of Cerebrosides: Individual cerebrosides are differentiated by the kinds of fatty acids in the molecule. *Four types* of cerebrosides have been isolated and their fatty acids have been identified. They are:

- *Kerasin:* It contains normal lignoceric acid, $C_{23}H_{47}COOH$ as fatty acid.
- *Cerebron (Phrenosin):* It contains hydroxy lignoceric acid, also called *"cerebronic acid".*
- *Nervon:* It contains an unsaturated homologue of lignoceric acid called *"nervonic acid".*
- *Oxynervon:* Oxynervon contains hydroxy derivative of nervonic acid.

Clinical Aspect of Cerebrosides

GAUCHER'S DISEASE

- Gaucher's disease is an *inherited disorder of cerebrosides metabolism* (lipidosis).
- *Inheritance:* It is an autosomal recessive.
- *Enzyme defect:* Deficiency of the enzyme *β-glucocerebrosidase,* a lysosomal enzyme.
- In absence of the enzyme, the cerebrosides cannot be degraded in the body, as a result large amount of glucocerebrosides, (usually) *"kerasin"* accumulate in RE cells, viz. liver, spleen, bone marrow and also brain. Complex lipids appear to collect within mitochondria of the RE cells.
- Biochemically, there is characteristically **elevation in serum *acid phosphatase level.***

Clinical features: Adults as well as infants are affected.

a. *In infancy and childhood:*

- It has fairly acute onset, with rapid course and death in several years. The infant loses weight, fails to grow, progressive mental retardation.
- Initially there is spasticity, later on followed by flaccidity.

b. *In adult:*

- It causes progressive enlargement of spleen (splenomegaly) which may reach to umbilicus or below.
- *Characteristic "bone pain"* due to marrow cells replaced by histiocytes loaded with the lipids. As a result it leads to progressive *anaemia, leucopenia* and *thrombocytopenia*- tendency to get secondary infections and bleeding tendency.

GANGLIOSIDES

- **Klenk,** in 1942, isolated gangliosides from beef brain. It was a new class of carbohydrate rich glycolipid which he called gangliosides.
- Gangliosides have been isolated from ganglion cells, neuronal bodies and dendrites, spleen and RBC stroma. The ***highest concentrations are found in grey matter of brain.***
- Gangliosides are the most complex of the glycosphingolipids. They are large complex lipids, whose molecular weight varies from 180,000 to 250,000.

Structure: Although the exact structures of the gangliosides are not definitely established, ***on hydrolysis,*** gangliosides yield the following products:

- A long chain FA (usually C_{18} to C_{24})
- Alcohol-sphingosine
- A carbohydrate moiety which usually contains:
  - Glucose and/or galactose,
  - One molecule of N-acetyl galactosamine, and
  - At least one molecule of N-acetyl neuraminic acid (NANA) (also called "sialic acid").
- Brain gangliosides are known to be complex and mono-,di-,trisialogangliosides containing 1 to 3 sialic acid residues have been described.

Types of gangliosides: Over 30 types of gangliosides have been isolated from brain tissue. **Four important types are:** GM-1, GM-2, GM-3, and GD-3.

BIOMEDICAL IMPORTANCE

- Gangliosides are mainly components of "membranes".
- The gangliosides, therefore, can serve as specific *membrane binding sites*(receptor sites) for circulating hormones and thereby influence various biochemical processes in the cell.

Clinical Aspect Tay-Sach's Disease (GM_2 Gangliosidosis)

- Accumulation of gangliosides in brain and nervous tissues take place. The affected ganglioside is GM_2
- The enzyme deficiency is ***hexosaminidase*** A.
- **Its Inheritance:** autosomal recessive.
- Normal degradation of GM_2 requires the action of a specific hydrolyzing enzyme *Hexosaminidase A.* In absence of the enzyme *Hexosaminidase A,* GM_2 cannot be degraded and accumulates.

Clinical Features: This rare **inherited disorder** is associated with the following:

- Progressive development of ***idiocy*** and ***blindness*** in infants soon after birth. The above is due to widespread injury to ganglion cells in brain (cerebral cortex) and retina.
- A ***cherry-red spot*** about the macula, seen ophthalmoscopically, is pathognomonic and is caused by destruction of retinal ganglion cells, exposing the underlying vasculature.
- There may be seizures and association of macrocephaly.

Prognosis: is bad, usually death follows.

AMPHIPATHIC LIPIDS

Lipids as such are insoluble in water, since they contain a predominance of "nonpolar" hydrocarbon groups. But fatty acids, phospholipids (PL), bile salts, and to a lesser extent cholesterol contain "Polar" groups. Hence, the part of the molecule is ***hydrophobic*** or water insoluble and part is ***hydrophilic*** or water soluble. Such molecules are called ***amphipathic.***

ORIENTATION OF AMPHIPATHIC LIPIDS

- Amphipathic lipids get oriented at oil-water interfaces with the polar groups in the water phase and non-polar groups in the oil phase ***(Fig. 2.7A).***
- ***Membrane bilayers:*** Orientation of amphipathic lipids as above forms the basic structure of biological membranes ***(Fig. 2.7B).***
- ***Micelles:*** When a critical concentration of these amphipathic lipids is present in an aqueous medium, they form "***micelles***". ***Micelles formation, facilitated by bile salts, is prerequisite for fat digestion*** and absorption from the intestine ***(Fig. 2.7C).***
- ***Liposomes:*** Liposomes are formed by sonicating an amphipathic lipid in an aqueous medium.

  Characteristic of liposomes: They consist of spheres of lipid bilayers that enclose part of the aqueous medium ***(Fig. 2.7D).***

Uses of liposomes

i. They are potential clinical use, particularly when combined with tissue-specific **antibodies**, as carriers of drugs in the circulation, targeted to specific organs, e.g. in cancer therapy,

ii. They are being used for ***gene transfer*** into vascular cells, and

iii. As carriers for topical and transdermal delivery of drugs and cosmetics.

- ***Emulsions:*** They are larger in size and formed usually by non-polar lipids (e.g. T-G) are mixed with water (aqueous medium). They are stabilized by emulsifying agents such as amphipathic lipids (e.g. phosphatidyl choline) which form a surface layer separating the main bulk of non-polar material from the water.

PROSTAGLANDINS

A generic term for a family of closely related biologically "active" lipids, is now called **eicosanoids.**

- Prostaglandins (PGs) have been detected in almost every mammalian tissue and body fluids
- Their production increases or decreases in response to diverse stimuli or drugs
- They are produced in minute amounts
- Broad spectrum and diverse biological effects
- Not stored in body
- They have also been found to modulate cyclic AMP activity in cells either by activating or inhibiting *adenyl cyclase activity*.

CLASSIFICATION

Prostaglandins and related compounds are now classified under the heading eicosanoids as these compounds are derived from "eicosa (20-c) polyenoic FA".

They are classified mainly in ***two groups:***

(i) **Prostanoids** (PGs) and (b) **Leucotrienes** (LTs)

'Prostanoids' are further subdivided into three groups as follows:

CHEMISTRY OF PROSTAGLANDINS

According to structures, PGs can be divided in ***four*** main groups.

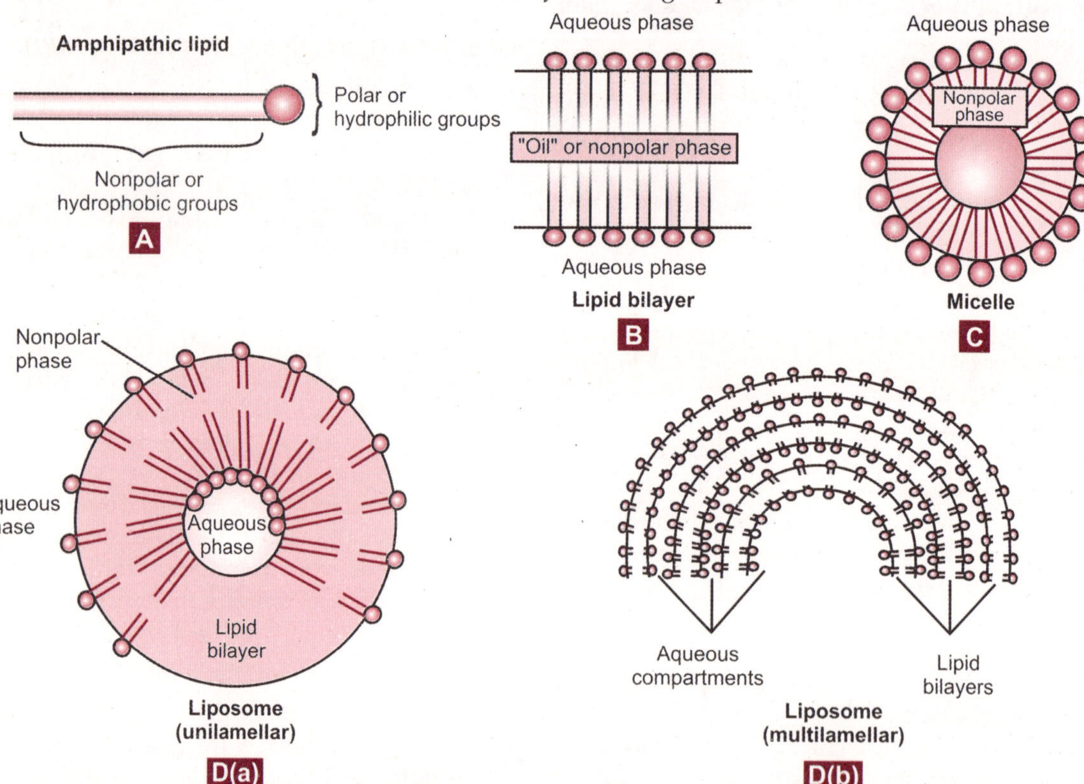

Figs 2.7A to D: Formation of lipid bilayer membrane, micelle, and liposomes from amphipathic lipids

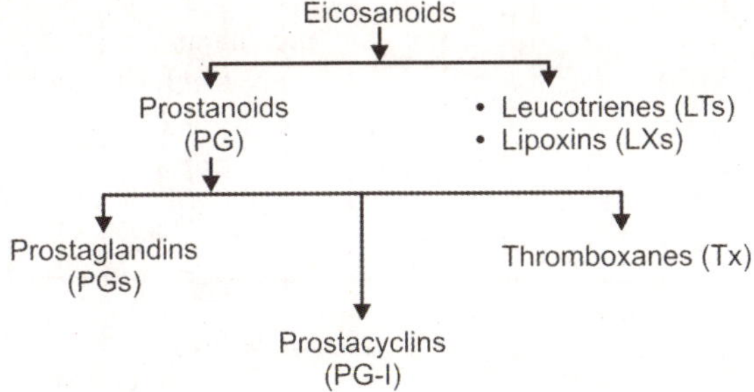

- ***PG-E group***—PGE-1, PGE-2 and PGE-3
- ***PG-F group***—PG-$F_1\alpha$, PG-$F_2\alpha$ and PG-$F_3\alpha$
- ***PG-A group***—PG-A_1, PG-A_2,19-OH PG-A_1, 19-OH PH-A_2
- ***PG-B Group***—PG-B_1, and PG-B_2, 19-OH PG-B_1 and 19-OH PG-B_2

Besides above 14 PGs, PG-C and PG-D group have also been recognised.

CHARACTERISTIC FEATURES OF STRUCTURES

- All naturally occurring PGs are 20C fatty acids containing a ***cyclopentane ring.*** Structures are based on parent saturated acid called ***Prostanoic acid (Fig. 2.8).***

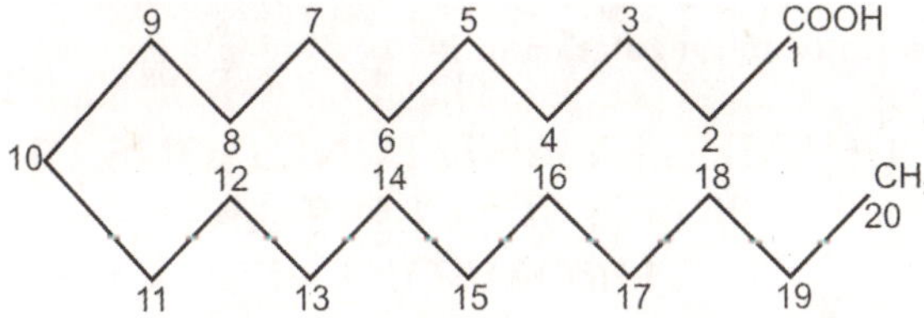

Fig. 2.8: Prostanoic acid

- All PGs have the following salient structural features.
  - ***–OH group at 15 position***
  - ***Trans double bond at 13 position***
- Differences in the four main group is due to difference in structure of cyclopentane ring.

Primary prostaglandins: Six PGs of the E and F series are referred to as primary PGs because none is the precursor of the other. Recently, a new type of prostaglandin has been isolated from human seminal plasma which has been designated as PGx.

Occurrence and distribution: Although PGs were first discovered in seminal plasma and vesicular glands, the distribution of these substances is not restricted to male accessory genital glands and secretions only. They are ***ubiquitous*** in mammalian tissues and have been detected and isolated from pancreas, kidney, brain, thymus, iris, synovial fluid, CS fluid, etc. Recently it has been identified in human amniotic fluid and umbilical cord vessels.

METABOLISM OF PROSTAGLANDINS

Biosynthesis: PGs are synthesized ***aerobically*** from polyunsaturated fatty acid-arachidonic acid (5, 8, 11, 14- eicosa-tetraenoic acid) with the help of a ***multi-enzyme complex*** now called **Prostaglandin H synthase** which consists of two components: (i) ***cyclo-oxygenase* system** and (ii) ***peroxidase system. About 1 mg of PG is normally synthesized in man every day.***

Fig. 2.9 above, shows the biosynthetic pathway and regulation of PGs.

COMMON DRUGS THAT INHIBIT PG

Synthesis

- Aspirin, indomethacin, ibuprofen (brufen), phenyl butazone, fenclozic acid, diclofenac, pyrixocam and other non-steroidal anti-inflammatory agents (NSAIDs): It prevents conversion of arachidonate to PG-G2 (cyclic endoperoxide) by inhibiting cyclooxygenase system and thus stop PG synthesis.

Catabolism: PGs are very rapidly removed from circulation and metabolized in lungs, brain, liver and other tissues. ***Some 80 to 90% or more is destroyed during a single passage through the liver/or the lungs.***

FUNCTIONS OF PROSTAGLANDINS

Prostaglandins have numerous and diverse effects. **Diversity in function is "awesome" and "bewildering".** Not only is the spectrum of action broad, but also different PGs show different activities both qualitatively and quantitatively. Important functions of PGs are as follows:

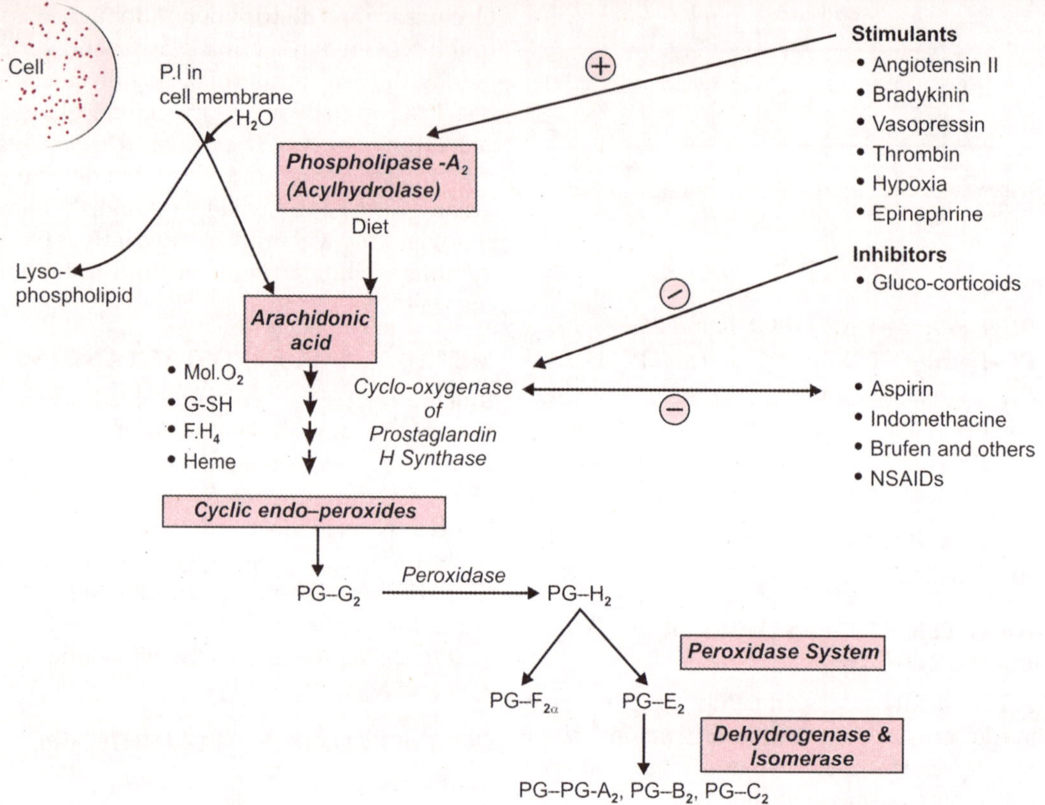

Fig. 2.9: Showing biosynthetic pathway and regulation of PGs

FUNCTIONS OF PGs

- Lowers blood pressure **(antihypertensive)**
- *Inhibition of platelet aggregation*
- Stimulation of smooth muscle of uterus (uterine contraction)
- Inhibition of gastric secretion
- Purgative action
- Mediation of inflammatory response
- Sensitization to pain
- Regulation of steroid synthesis
- Inhibition of hormone sensitive lipases
- Show PTH-like, thyrotropin-like and insulin-like effects.

CHEMISTRY AND FUNCTIONS OF PROSTACYCLINS AND THROMBOXANES

PROSTACYCLINS vs THROMBOXANES

- Both prostacyclins (PG-I_2)and thromboxanes (Tx) are produced from cyclic endoperoxide PG-H_2 ***(Fig. 2.10).***
- Cyclic endoperoxide first formed in PG synthesis is PG-G_2,which is converted to PG-H_2 an immediate precursor of PGI_2, and Tx. ***Both cyclic endoperoxides have a very short half-life (t½ = 5 minute at 37°C) but they are biologically very active,*** and have powerful

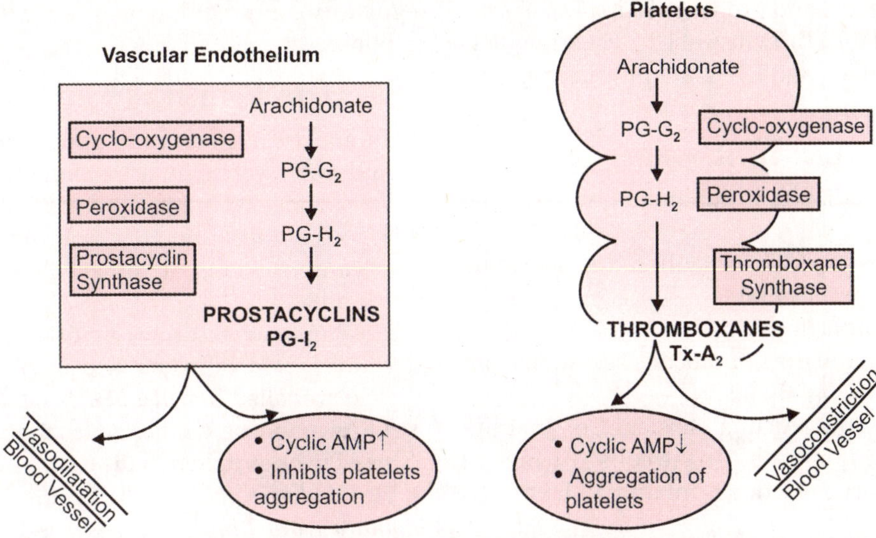

Fig. 2.10: PG-I_2 and Tx-A_2—Formation and actions

effect on contraction of GI smooth muscles, bronchial muscles and umbilical cord vessels. For differentiation of prostacyclins (PG-I_2) from thromboxanes (Tx) is given in *Table 2.1.*

Applied Aspect of PG-I_2 and Tx

Prevention of Thrombus Formation in Health

- Platelets attempting to stick to blood vessels wall release "endoperoxides", which is converted to prostacyclin (PG-I_2) by endothelial cell of blood vessel wall.
- PG-I_2 by its vasodilatation effects and inhibition of platelet aggregation repels the platelets and prevent them from sticking and forming a "nidus" and thus opposes thromboxane activity.
- ***A balance between these two biochemical processes is critical for the thrombus formation.***

Injury to Blood Vessel Wall:

- Injury to blood vessel wall decreases PG-I_2 formation and thus reduces the anti-aggregatory action of PG-I_2. Unopposed action of TX-A_2 in such cases causes platelet aggregation and thrombus formation.

Table 2.1: Differentiation of Prostacyclins and Thromboxanes

Prostacyclins (PGI$_2$)	*Thromboxanes (Tx)*
• Formed in vascular endothelium, heart, kidneys	• Formed in platelets, neutrophils, brain, lungs kidneys
• Synthesized from PG-H_2 by the enzyme *prostacyclin synthase*	• Synthesized from PG-H_2 by the enzyme *thromboxane synthase*
• Acts through cyclic AMP ↑	• Cyclic AMP ↓ can also use Ca^{++} as second messenger
• **Functions:** • Inhibits platelet aggregation • Produces vasodilatation	• **Functions:** • Enhance platelet aggregation • Produces vasoconstriction

LEUCOTRIENES (LTs)

A newly discovered family of conjugated trienes formed from eicosanoic acids in leucocytes, mast cell, and macrophages by the *lipooxygenase* pathway in response to both immunologic and noninflammatory stimuli. LTs possess no ring in its structure but have three characteristic conjugated double bonds.

Synthesis: LTs are synthesized from ***arachidonate*** by the addition of hydroxyperoxy groups to arachidonic acid and produces *hydroperoxy eicosa tetranoates* (HPETE). Different LTs, viz. LT-A_4, LT-B_4, LT-C_4, LT-D_4 and LT-E_4 are produced from 5 HPETE.

FUNCTIONS OF LTs

- Act as mediators in inflammation and anaphylaxis
- Produces capillary dilatation and increases vascular permeability
- Causes bronchospasm
- Potent stimulators of mucous secretion from human airway tissue
- **SRS-A** (slow reacting substance of anaphylaxis) produced by mast cells during an anaphylactic reaction is mixture of LTs.

Applied Aspects

- Lipoxygenase system is not inhibited by aspirin and other anti-inflammatory drugs.
- ***Prolonged use of aspirin:*** Prolonged use of aspirin for certain conditions like arthritis, etc. depresses cyclo-oxygenase system and PG synthesis but enhances lipo-oxygenase system synthesis of LTs, which may lead to bronchospasm and produce ***aspirin-induced (iatrogenic) bronchial asthma.***

LIPOXINS

Lipoxins are a family of conjugated tetraenes recently discovered arising in leucocytes by lipo-oxygenase pathology.

Types

Several lipoxins have been found to be formed Lx-A_4 to Lx-E_4 in a manner similar to the formation of leukotrienes.

Formation

They are formed by the combined action of more than one lipo-oxygenase introducing more oxygen into the molecule from arachidonic acid.

Function

Evidences support a role of lipoxins in vasoactive and immuno-regulatory function, e.g. as counter-regulatory compounds (chalones) of the immune response.

☞ SALIENT POINTS TO REMEMBER

- Lipids are a group of heterogenous organic substances, actually or potentially related to fatty acids and are utilized in the body.
- Lipids are insoluble in water but soluble in organic solvents viz ether, alcohol, chloro form, etc.
- Polyunsaturated fatty acids (PUFAs) like Linoleic acid, Linolenic acid and Arachidonic acid are called ***Essential Fatty acids (EFAs).***
- EFAs cannot be synthesized in the body hence need to be supplied in the diet.
- ***Arachidonic acid can be synthesized in the body from Linoleic acid.*** It is biologically important as prostaglandins (PGs) and Leukotrienes (LTs) are synthesized from it.
- Triacyl glycerol (TG), called simple Lipid, is esters of glycerol with various fatty acids. They are found in adipose tissue and are "Fuel" reserve for animals.
- ***Glycerol can be converted to Glucose*** in the body by a process called Gluconeogenesis. ***Thus it is not a waste product of hydrolysis of fats.***
- Phospholipids (PL) are compound Lipids containing Phosphoric acid. They participate in the Lipoprotein complexes which is the major constituent of cell walls and membrane, the myelin sheaths and mitochondrial/ microsomal membranes.
- Dipalmityl lecithin (DPL) secreted by the epithelial cells of Lung alveoli ***acts as surfactant*** and prevents collapse of Lung alveoli.
- **The absence of DPL leads to "respiratory distress syndrome (RDS)" in infants.**
- Cephalins, a phospholipid, participate in blood clotting, action of certain hormones is mediated through phosphatidyl inositol.
- Absence of the enzyme ***"sphingomyelinase"*** leads to the inherited disorder ***"Niemann-pick disease".***
- Cerebrosides are the simplest form of Glycolipids which occur in membrane of nervous tissue.

- Inherited deficiency of the enzyme *"cerebrosidase"* leads to the disease *"Gaucher's disease"*.
- Gangliosides, a group of complex Glycolipids are found predominantly in ganglions. They differ from cerebrosides in having one or more molecules of N-acetyl neuraminic acids (NANA).
- Inherited deficiency of the enzyme *"Hexoseamidinase A"* leads to the inherited disorder *"Tay-Sach's disease". (GM-2 Gangliosidosis).*
- Cholesterol is the most abundant animal sterol.
- Cholesterol is an important constituent of membrane structure, found in nervous tissues, and is the precursor for formation of bile acids, vitamin D_3, corticosteroids and gonadal hormones.
- 7-dehydrocholesterol is found in skin epidermis. UV rays of sunshine changes 7-dehydro cholesterol to vitamin D_3 (cholecalciferol). Hence called as **provitamin D_3.**
- UV irradiation of Ergosterol (a plant sterol) produces vitamin D_2; hence it is called as **"Provitamin D_2".**
- Prostaglandius (PGs), one of the "Eicosanoids", are synthesized in small amounts in almost all the tissues *(except Erythrocytes)* of the body and act as Local hormones.
- PGs have diverse biochemical functions which include lowering of blood pressure (BP), inhibition of gastric acid secretion (HCl), relaxation of bronchial muscles, increases uterine contractions, decrease in immunological response, and increase in GFR.
- Over production of PGs causes pain, inflammation, fever, nausea/vomiting.
- Aspirin,/NSAIDs like Brufen, Diclofenac etc./ and corticosteroids inhibit PG synthesis and relieve the above symptoms.
- PGs have been used therapeutically for treatment of Gastric ulcers, Bronchial asthma, medical termination of pregnancy, induction of labour, etc.
- Use of PGs as drugs is limited due to-
  (i) Short duration of action, and
  (ii) Lack of tissue specificity.
- Thromboxanes (TX A_2) and PG-E_1 Promote platelet aggregation, while prostacyclins (PG I_2) inhibit platelet aggregation.
- Leukotrienes (LTs) produced by Lipo-oxygenase pathway are implicated in hypersensitivity and asthma.
- SRS-A of anaphylaxis is a mixture of LTs like C_4, D_4 and E_4.

MULTIPLE CHOICE QUESTIONS

Give one correct answer:

1. **Depot fats of mammals comprise mostly of:**
   (a) Phospholipids (b) Triacyl glycerols
   (c) Cerebrosides (d) Gangliosides
   (e) Cholesterol esters
2. **The calorific value of lipid is:**
   (a) 4.0 k cal/gm (b) 6.0 k cal/gm
   (c) 9.0 k cal/gm (d) 12.0 k cal/gm
   (e) 15.0 k cal/gm
3. **Which one of the following is not a phospholipid?**
   (a) Lecithin (b) Plasmalogen
   (c) Cephalin (d) Cerebrosides
   (e) Lysolecithin
4. **In cephalin, choline is replaced by**
   (a) Serine (b) Ethanolamine
   (c) Betaine (d) Inositol
   (e) Sphingosine
5. **Which of the following is not essential fatty acid?**
   (a) Oleic acid (b) Linoleic acid
   (c) Linolenic acid (d) Arachidonic acid
   (e) None of the above
6. **A fatty acid which is not synthesized in human body and need to be supplied in the diet:**
   (a) Palmitic acid (b) Oleic acid
   (c) Linoleic acid (d) Valeric acid
   (e) Stearic acid

7. **The smell of fat turned rancid is due to**
   (a) Presence of vit E
   (b) Presence of phenols
   (c) Presence of quinones
   (d) Volatile fatty acids
   (e) Cholesterol
8. **The ring system of cholesterol is called as**
   (a) Corrin ring
   (b) Phenanthrene ring
   (c) Isoalloxazine ring
   (d) Naphthoquinone ring
   (e) Cyclopentanoperhydrophenanthrene ring
9. **One of the following compound is not derived from cholesterol**
   (a) Cortisol (b) Oestrogen
   (c) Lanosterol (d) Coprosterol
   (e) Bile salt
10. **All of the following are constituents of gangliosides molecule, *except:***
    (a) Glycerol (b) Sialic acid
    (c) Hexose sugar (d) Sphingosine
    (e) Long chain fatty acid
11. **All of the following are useful substances produced from cholesteral *except:***
    (a) Cortisol (b) Bile salts
    (c) Bile pigments (d) Progesterone
    (e) Vitamin D
12. **All PGs have a structure based on prostanoic acid which contains a cyclopentane ring and has carbon atoms.**
    (a) 10 (b) 15
    (c) 18 (d) 20 (e) 25
13. **PG-Es lower cyclic AMP level in:**
    (a) Lungs (b) Adipose tissue
    (c) Thyroids (d) Platelets
    (e) Spleen
14. **All Prostaglandins have in common in addition to cyclopentane ring one double bond between positions:**
    (a) C_5 and C_6 (b) C_7 and C_8
    (c) C_9 and C_{10} (d) C_{11} and C_{12}
    (e) C_{13} and C_{14}

ANSWERS

1. (b)	2. (c)	3. (d)	4. (b)
5. (a)	6. (c)	7. (d)	8. (e)
9. (c)	10. (a)	11. (c)	12. (d)
13. (b)	14. (e)		

Chemistry of Proteins and Amino Acids

INTRODUCTION

In 1839 Dutch chemist ***GJ Mulder*** while investigating substances such as those found in milk, egg found that they could be coagulated on heating and were nitrogenous compounds. Swedish scientist ***JJ Berzelius*** suggested to Mulder that these substances should be called proteins. The term is derived from Greek word ***Proteios*** which means "primary", or "holding first place" or *"preeminent"* because Berzelius thought them to be the most important of biological substances. And now we know that proteins are fundamental structural components of the body. They are ***nitrogenous "macromolecules" composed of many amino acids.***

BIOMEDICAL IMPORTANCE

- Proteins are the main structural components of the cytoskeleton. They are the ***sole source of nitrogen*** of the body.
- Biochemical catalysts known as ***enzymes*** are proteins.
- Proteins known as ***immunoglobulins serve*** as the first line of defence against bacterial and viral infections.
- Several ***hormones*** are protein in nature.
- Structural proteins furnish ***mechanical support*** and some of them like actin and myosin are contractile proteins and help in the movement of muscle fibre, microvilli, etc.
- Some proteins present in cell membrane, cytoplasm and nucleus of the cell act as ***receptors.***
- The ***transport proteins carry*** out the function of transporting specific substances either across the membrane or in the body fluids.
- ***Storage proteins*** bind with specific substances and store them, e.g. iron is stored as ferritin.
- Few proteins are ***constituents of respiratory pigments*** and ***occur in electron transport*** chain or respiratory chain, e.g. cytochromes, haemoglobin, myoglobin.
- Under certain conditions proteins can be catabolized to supply energy.
- Proteins by means of exerting osmotic pressure help in maintenance of electrolyte and water balance in body.

COMPOSITION OF PROTEINS

In addition to C, H, and O which are present in carbohydrates and lipids, proteins also contain N. The nitrogen content is around 16% of the molecular weight of proteins. Small amounts of S and P are also present. Few proteins contain other elements such as I, Cu, Mn, Zn and Fe, etc.

Amino acids: Protein molecules are very large molecules with high molecular weight ranging from 5000 to 25,000,00. Protein can be broken down into smaller units by hydrolysis. ***These small units of the monomers of proteins are called amino acids. Proteins are made up of 20 such standard amino acids in different sequences and numbers.*** So, an indefinite number of protein can be formed and do occur in nature. ***Thus, proteins are the unbranched polymers of L-α amino acids.***

The L-α-amino acid has a general formula as shown below.

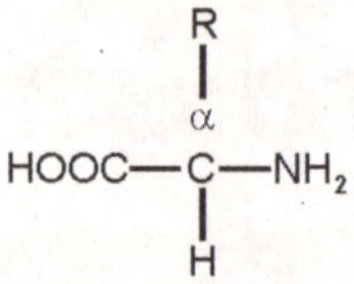

$$HOOC-\overset{\overset{R}{|}\;\alpha}{\underset{\underset{H}{|}}{C}}-NH_2$$

R is called a side chain and can be a hydrogen, aliphatic, aromatic or heterocyclic group. Each amino acid has an amino group-NH_2, a carboxylic acid group –COOH and a hydrogen atom each attached to carbon located next to the –COOH group. Thus, ***the side chain varies from one amino acid to the other.***

AMINO ACIDS

CLASSIFICATION AND STRUCTURE OF AMINO ACIDS

Amino acids can be classified into *three groups* depending on their reaction in solution.

- **Neutral**
- **Acidic**
- **Basic**

A. Neutral Amino Acids: This is the largest group of amino acids and can be further subdivided into aliphatic, aromatic, heterocyclic and S-containing amino acids.

1. *Aliphatic Amino Acids*

- *Glycine (Gly)* or α-amino acetic acid

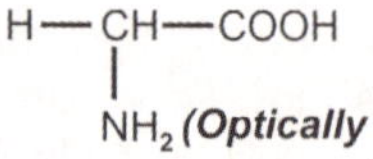

$$H-\underset{\underset{NH_2}{|}}{CH}-COOH$$

NH_2 ***(Optically inactive)***

- *Alanine (Ala)* or α-amino propionic acid

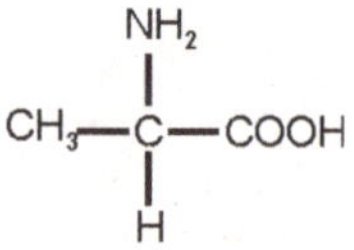

$$CH_3-\overset{\overset{NH_2}{|}}{\underset{\underset{H}{|}}{C}}-COOH$$

- *Valine (Val)* or α-amino-iso-valeric acid

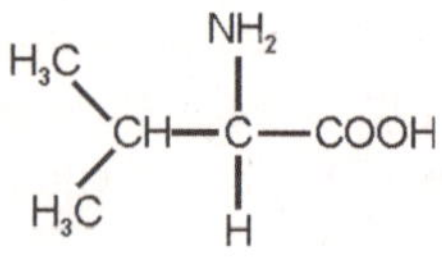

$$(H_3C)(H_3C)CH-\overset{\overset{NH_2}{|}}{\underset{\underset{H}{|}}{C}}-COOH$$

- *Leucine (Leu)* or α-amino-iso-caproic acid

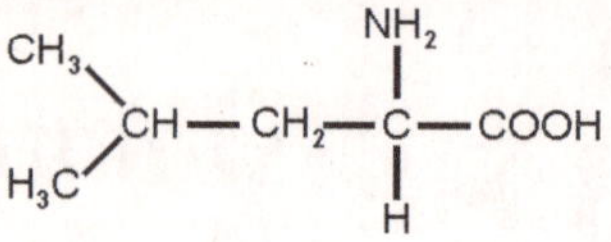

$$(CH_3)(H_3C)CH-CH_2-\overset{\overset{NH_2}{|}}{\underset{\underset{H}{|}}{C}}-COOH$$

- *Isoleucine (Ile)* or α-amino-β-methyl valeric acid

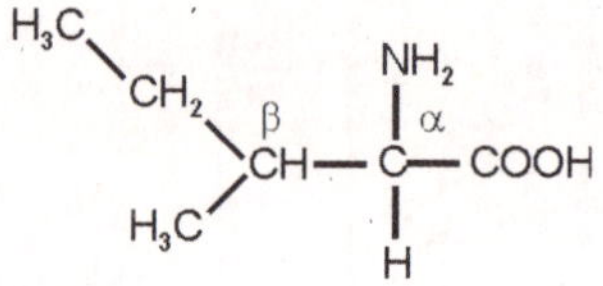

$$(H_3C-CH_2)(H_3C)\overset{\beta}{CH}-\overset{\overset{NH_2}{|}\;\alpha}{\underset{\underset{H}{|}}{C}}-COOH$$

All of the above are simple ***monoamino monocarboxylic acids.***

Hydroxy amino acids:

- *Serine (Ser)* or α amino β-hydroxy propionic acid

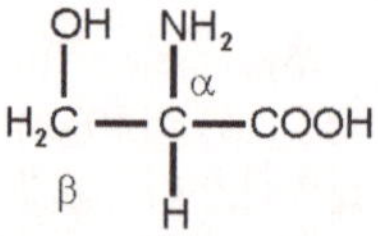

$$\overset{\overset{OH}{|}}{\underset{\beta}{H_2C}}-\overset{\overset{NH_2}{|}\;\alpha}{\underset{\underset{H}{|}}{C}}-COOH$$

- *Threonine (Thr)* or α-amino-β-hydroxy butyric acid

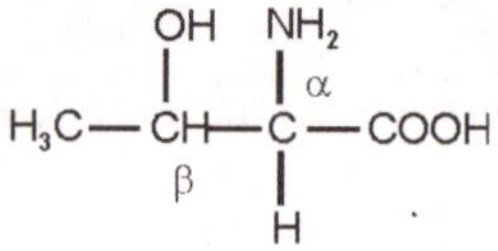

$$H_3C-\overset{\overset{OH}{|}}{\underset{\beta}{CH}}-\overset{\overset{NH_2}{|}\;\alpha}{\underset{\underset{H}{|}}{C}}-COOH$$

2. **Aromatic Amino Acids**

- *Phenylalanine (Phe)* or α-amino β-phenyl propionic acid

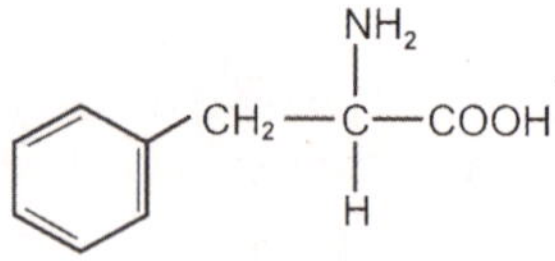

$$C_6H_5-CH_2-\overset{\overset{NH_2}{|}}{\underset{\underset{H}{|}}{C}}-COOH$$

- *Tyrosine (Tyr)* or para-hydroxy phenylalanine or α-amino-β-parahydroxy phenyl propionic acid

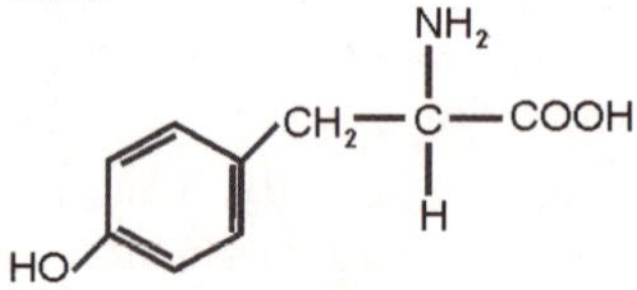

$$HO-C_6H_4-CH_2-\overset{\overset{NH_2}{|}}{\underset{\underset{H}{|}}{C}}-COOH$$

3. **Heterocyclic Amino Acids:**

- ***Tryptophan (Trp)*** or α-amino-β-3-indole propionic acid: This amino acid is often considered as aromatic amino acid since it has aromatic ring in its structure.

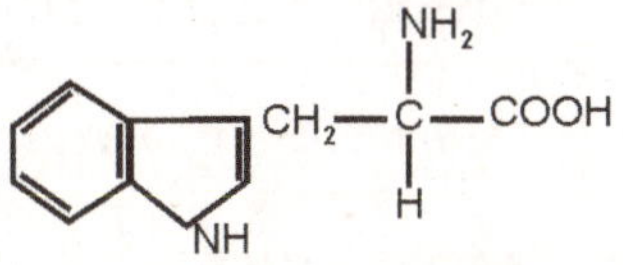

NH_2
CH_2—C—COOH
H
NH

- ***Histidine (His)*** or α-amino-β-imidazole propionic acid. Histidine is ***basic*** in ***solution*** on account of the imidazole ring and often considered as basic amino acid.

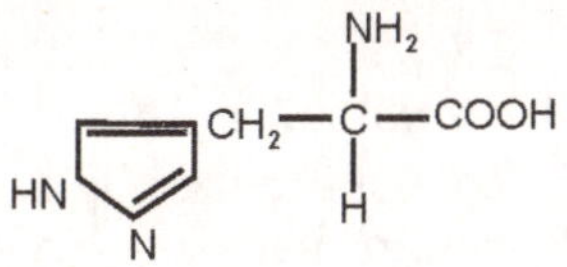

NH_2
CH_2—C—COOH
HN
H
N

4. ***Imino Acids:***

- ***Proline (Pro)*** or Pyrrolidone-2-carboxylic acid

2 COOH
1
NH

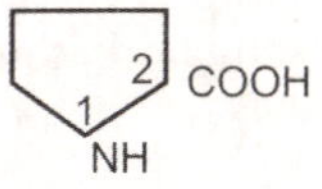

Hydroxyproline (Hyp) or 4 hydroxy pyrrolidone-2 carboxylic acid.

HO 4 3
5 2 COOH
1
NH

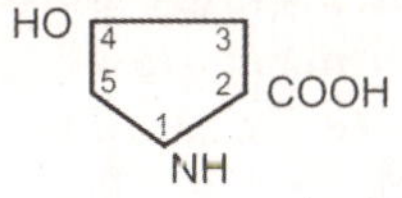

Proline and hydroxyproline do not have a free–NH_2 group but only a ***basic pyrrolidone ring*** in which the nitrogen of the imino group is in a ring but can still function in the formation of peptides. These amino acids are therefore called as ***imino acids.***

5. ***'S' Containing Amino Acids:***

- ***Cysteine (Cys)*** or α-amino-β-mercaptopropionic acid.

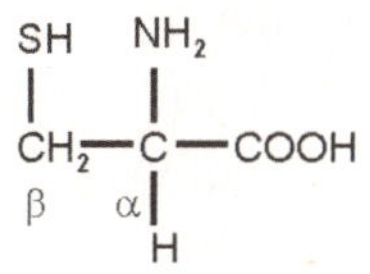

SH NH_2
CH_2—C—COOH
β α
H

Two molecules of cysteine make cystine **(cys-cys)** or dithio-β, β-α-aminopropionic acid. The S—S linkage is called ***disulphide bridge.***

- ***Methionine (Met)*** or α-amino γ-methyl-thio-η-butyric acid

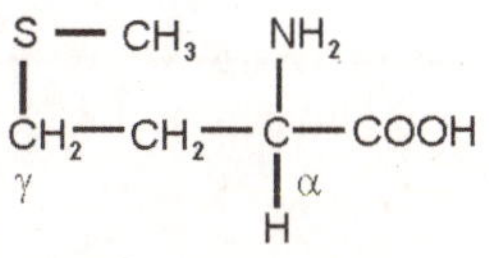

S — CH_3 NH_2
CH_2—CH_2—C—COOH
γ α
H

A. ***Acidic Amino Acids:*** These amino acids have two –COOH groups and one –NH_2 group. They are therefore ***monoaminodicarboxylic acids.***

- ***Aspartic Acid (Asp)*** or α-amino succinic acid

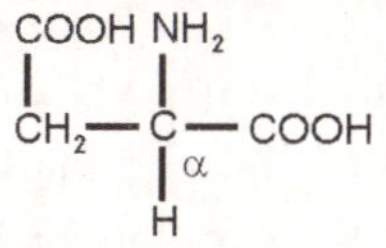

COOH NH_2
CH_2—C— COOH
α
H

Asparagine (Asn) or γ-amide of α-amino succinic acid (Amide of aspartic acid).

- ***Glutamic Acid (Glu)*** or α-aminoglutaric acid.

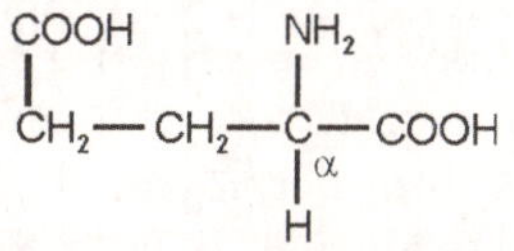

COOH NH_2
CH_2— CH_2—C—COOH
α
H

Glutamine (Gln) or amide of glutamic acid or δ-amide of α-amino glutaric acid.

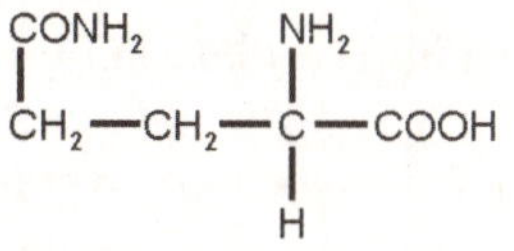

$CONH_2$ NH_2
CH_2—CH_2—C—COOH
H

B. ***Basic Amino Acids:*** This class of amino acids consists of those amino acids which have one –COOH group and two –NH_2 groups. Thus, they are ***diaminomonocarboxylic acids.***

- ***Arginine (Arg)*** or α-amino-δ-guanidino-n-valeric acid

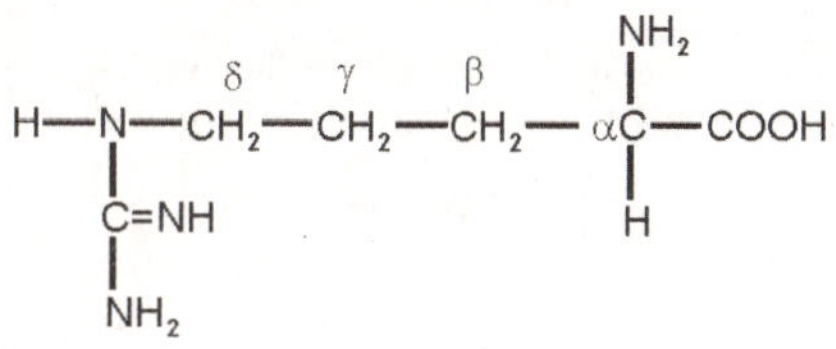

NH_2
δ γ β
H—N—CH_2—CH_2—CH_2— αC—COOH
C=NH H
NH_2

- ***Lysine (Lys)*** or α-ε-diamino caproic acid

$$\underset{NH_2}{\overset{\varepsilon}{CH_2}}-\overset{\delta}{CH_2}-\overset{\gamma}{CH_2}-\overset{\beta}{CH_2}-\underset{H}{\overset{NH_2}{\alpha C}}-COOH$$

- ***Hydroxylysine (Hyl)*** or α, ε-diamino-δ-hydroxy-n-valeric acid

$$\underset{NH_2}{\overset{\varepsilon}{CH_2}}-\underset{OH}{\overset{\delta}{CH}}-\overset{\gamma}{CH_2}-\overset{\beta}{CH_2}-\underset{H}{\overset{NH_2}{\alpha C}}-COOH$$

As already mentioned histidine is also classified as basic amino acid.

FUNCTIONS OF AMINO ACIDS

- Apart from being the monomeric constituents of proteins and peptides, amino acids serve variety of functions.
- Some amino acids are converted to carbohydrates and are called ***glucogenic amino acids.***
- Specific amino acids give rise to specialized products, e.g. Tyrosine forms hormones such as ***thyroid hormones, (T_3,T_4), epinephrine*** and ***norepinephrine*** and a pigment called ***melanin.***
- Tryptophan can synthesize a vitamin called ***niacin.***
- ***Glycine, arginine and methionine synthesize creatine.***
- Glycine and cysteine help in synthesis of bile salts.
- Glutamate, cysteine and glycine synthesize ***glutathione.***
- Histidine changes to *histamine*, by decarboxylation.
- In addition to tripeptides formation, glycine is used for the synthesis of ***heme.***
- Pyrimidines and purines use several amino acids for their synthesis such as asparate and glutamine for pyrimidines and glycine, aspartic acid, glutamine and serine for purine synthesis.
- Some amino acids such as glycine and cysteine, are used as ***detoxicants*** of specific substances.
- Methionine acts as **"active methionine"** ***(S-adenosylmethionine)*** transfers methyl group to various substances by ***trans-methylation.***
- Cystine and *methionine* are ***sources of sulphur.***

ESSENTIAL AMINO ACIDS

Nutritionally, amino acids are of **two types:**

(i) ***Essential*** and
(ii) ***Non-essential***

There is also a third group of ***semi-essential*** amino acids.

- ***Essential amino acids:*** These are the ones which are not synthesized by the body and must be taken in diet. They include ***valine, leucine, isoleucine, phenylalanine, threonine, tryptophan, methionine and lysine.***
- ***Non-essential amino acids:*** These can be synthesized by the body and may not be the requisite components of the diet.
- ***Semi-essential amino acids:*** These are growth promoting factors since they are not synthesized in sufficient quantity during growth. They include ***arginine*** and ***histidine. They become essential in growing children, pregnancy and lactating women.***

Occurrence of Amino Acids

All the standard amino acids mentioned above occur in almost all proteins. Cereals are rich in acidic amino acids Asp and Glu while collagen is rich in basic amino acids and also proline and hydroxyproline.

New Amino Acids

In addition to 20 L-amino acids that take part in protein synthesis, recently two more new amino acids described. They are:

A. Selenocysteine - 21st amino acids

B. Pyrrolysine - 22nd amino acid

PROPERTIES OF AMINO ACIDS

I. Isomerism

Two types of isomerism are shown by amino acids basically due to the presence of asymmetric carbon atom. ***Glycine has no asymmetric carbon atom in its structure hence is optically inactive.***

```
         COOH                 COOH
          |                    |
  NH2 —— C —— H         H —— C —— NH2
          |                    |
          R                    R
   L-Amino Acid          D-Amino Acid
```

Fig. 3.1: L and D forms of amino acid

- ***Stereo-isomerism:*** All amino acids except glycine exist as D and L isomers ***(Fig. 3.1). In D-amino acids–NH_2 group is on the right hand while in L-amino acids it is oriented to the left.*** Natural proteins of animals and plant generally contain L-amino acids. D-amino acids occur in bacteria.
- ***Optical Isomerism:*** All amino acids **except glycine** have asymmetric carbon atom. Few amino acids like isoleucine and threonine have an additional asymmetric carbon in their structures. Consequently, all but glycine exhibit "optical" activities and rotate the plane polarized light and exist as ***dextro-rotatory (d)*** or ***laevorotatory (l) isomers.*** Optical activity depends on the pH and side chain.

II. Amphoteric Nature and Isoelectric pH

The $-NH_2$ and –COOH groups of amino acids are **ionizable groups**. Further, charged polar side chain of few amino acids also ionize. Depending on the pH of the solution ***these groups act as proton donors (acids) or proton acceptors (bases). This property is called amphoteric and therfore amino acids are called ampholytes.*** At a specific pH the amino acid carries both the charges in equal number and exists as dipolar ion or ***Zwitterion. At this point the net charge on it is zero,*** i.e.+ve charges and negative charges on the protein amino acid molecule equalises. The pH at which it occurs without any charge on it is called ***pI or isoelectric pH.*** **On the acidic side of its pI, amino acids exist as a cation by accepting a proton and on alkaline side as anion by donating a proton.**

III. Physical Properties:

- These are colourless, crystalline substances more soluble in water than in polar solvents. Tyrosine is soluble in hot water.
- Amino acids have high melting point usually more than 200°C.
- They have a high dielectric constant.
- They possess a large dipole moment.

IV. Chemical Properties:

1. ***Properties Due to Carboxylic (–COOH) Group***

- ***Formation of esters:*** Amino acids can form esters with alcohols. The COOH group can be esterfied with alcohol.
- ***Reduction to amino alcohol:*** This is achieved in presence of lithium aluminium hydride.
- ***Formation of amines by decarboxylation:*** Action of specific amino acids decarboxylases, dry distillation or heating with $Ba(OH)_2$ or with diphenylamine evolves CO_2 from the – COOH group and changes the amino acid into its ***amine***.
- ***Formation of amides:*** Anhydrous NH_3 may replace alcohol from its combination with an amino acid, in an amino acid ester so that an amide of amino acid and a molecule of free alcohol is produced.

2. ***Properties due to Amino ($-NH_2$) Group***

- ***Salt formation with acids:*** The basic amino group reacts with mineral acids such as HCl to form salts like hydrochlorides.
- ***Reaction with HNO_2:*** Like other primary amines, the amino acids except proline and hydroxy-proline react with HNO_2 (nitrous acid) liberating N_2 from NH_2 group. This forms the basis of Van Slyke method for determining $-NH_2$ group (nitrogen) ***(Fig. 3.2).***
- ***Reaction with formaldehyde:*** Formaldehyde reacts with $-NH_2$ group to form a methylene compound ***(Fig. 3.3).***

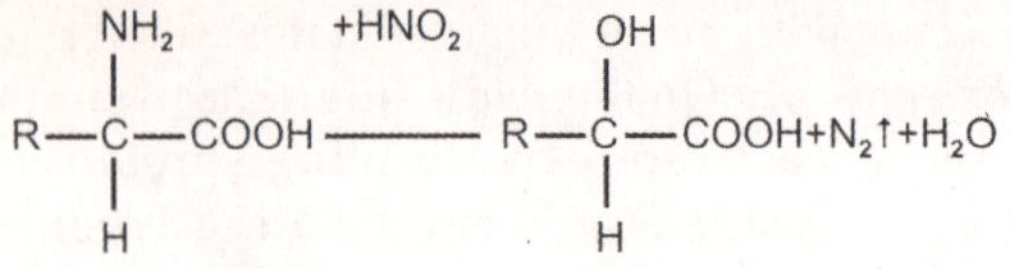

$$R-C(NH_2)(H)-COOH \xrightarrow{+HNO_2} R-C(OH)(H)-COOH + N_2\uparrow + H_2O$$

α-Amino Acid α-Hydroxy Acid

Fig. 3.2: Reaction with HNO_2

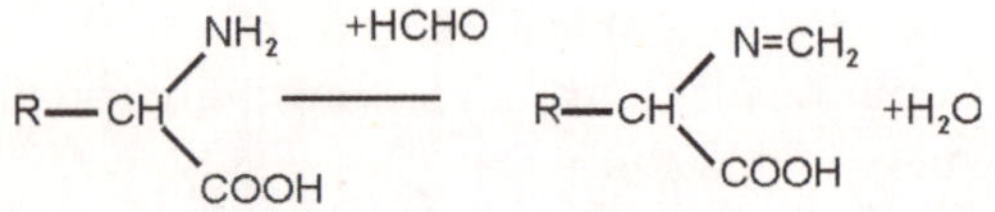

$$R-CH(NH_2)COOH \xrightarrow{+HCHO} R-CH(N{=}CH_2)COOH + H_2O$$

Fig. 3.3: Reaction of glycine with formaldehyde. Basis of Sorensen's formal titration

Application: Because of the presence of free basic amino group in the amino acid molecule, its amount cannot be estimated directly by titration with a standard alkali. On addition of neutral formaldehyde, ***it combines with amino group to form either methylene amino acid or dimethylol amino acid. Both these products are strong acids and may be estimated by titration with a standard alkali.*** This is known as *Sorensen's formol titration method.*

3. *Properties of Amino Acids due to Both NH_2 and COOH Groups:*

In addition to the property of reacting with both cation and anion, the amino acids form chelated, coordination complexes with certain heavy metals and other ions. These include Cu^{++}, CO^{++}, Mn^{++} and Ca^{++}.

Clinical Aspect

Chelates are non-ionic, and therefore amino acids may be used to remove calcium from bones and teeth. It is possible that the amino acids resulting from the breakdown of enamel and dentine could in this way form soluble calcium complexes thereby causing a loss of calcium and the *development of "caries".*

Identification of N-terminal residue

(a) N-terminal residue can be identified by using a reagent that bonds covalently with its α-NH_2 group. Because the bond is stable to hot acid hydrolysis, the derivative of the N-terminal residue can be identified by chromatographic procedures after the protein has been hydrolyzed.

Two Reagents are commonly used:

1. ***Sanger's reagent:*** The reagent contains 1-fluoro-2, 4-dinitro benzene (FDNB). It reacts with free — NH_2 group in an alkaline medium

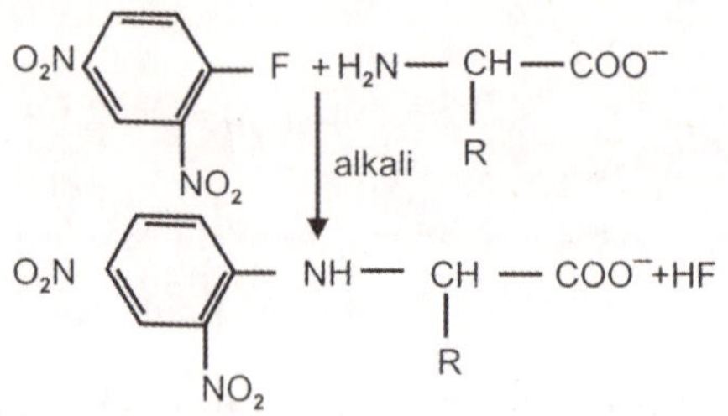

$$O_2N-C_6H_3(NO_2)-F + H_2N-CH(R)-COO^- \xrightarrow{alkali} O_2N-C_6H_3(NO_2)-NH-CH(R)-COO^- + HF$$

The reaction can also take place with the N-terminal—NH_2 group of the polypeptide chain. The compound so formed can be isolated after protein hydrolysis and identified.

2. ***Reaction with Dansyl chloride:*** The N-terminal—NH_2 group can also combine with Dansyl chloride (1-dimethyl amino naphthalene-5-sulphonyl chloride) to ***form a fluorescent dansyl derivative*** which can be isolated and identified.

(b) ***Edman reaction:*** A similar reaction with —NH_2 group can occur with the reagent phenyl isothiocyanate and thus enables the identification of the N-terminal amino acid.

Note:

- The reagent phenyl isothiocyanate was developed for a technique that allow repetitive sequencing of a peptide.

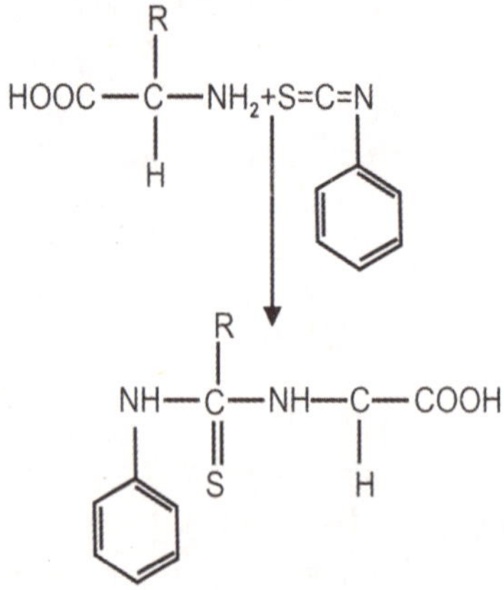

$$HOOC-C(R)(H)-NH_2 + S{=}C{=}N-C_6H_5 \longrightarrow C_6H_5-NH-C(R)(=S)-NH-C(H)-COOH$$

- Under mildly acid conditions, a phenyl thiocarbamyl derivative is formed by the reaction of the reagent with the N-terminal — NH_2 group and is cleaved off the peptide. ***It cyclizes to form a phenyl thiohydantoin derivative that can be identified chromatographically.***
- The remainder of the peptide is left intact with the next residue in the chain bearing a free — NH_2 group. This can inturn be reacted with fresh reagent.
- The procedure has been now automated and can be used to determine the amino acid sequences of peptides having 60 to 70 residues.

Sequenator

Edman and **G. Begg** have perfected an automataed amino acid **"sequenator"** for carrying out sequential degradation of peptides by the phenyl isothiocynate procedure (Edman's reaction).

Automated amino acid sequencers now widely used, which permits very rapid determination of amino acid sequences of polypeptides upto 100 amino acid approximately.

Amino acids are determined sequentially from N-terminal end. **The phenyl thiohydantoin amino acid** liberated is **identified by high performance liquid chromatography (HPLC).**

PROTEINS

CLASSIFICATION OF PROTEINS

Proteins are classified on the basis of their
- **Shape and size**
- **Functional properties**
- **Solubility and physical properties.**

I. On Shape and Size

- *Fibrous proteins:* When the axial ratio of length: width of a protein molecule is **more than 10**, it is called a "fibrous protein".
  Example: α-keratin from hair, collagen.
- *Globular protein:* When the axial ratio of length: width of a protein molecule **is less than 10**, it is called a "globular protein".
  Example: Myoglobin, haemoglobin, ribonuclease, etc.

II. On Functional Properties

The second way of classifying proteins makes use of their ***functional properties.***

- ***Defence proteins:*** Immunoglobulins are involved in defence mechanism.
- ***Contractile proteins:*** Proteins of skeletal muscle are involved in muscle contraction and relaxation.
- ***Respiratory proteins:*** These are involved in the function of respiration, e.g. haemoglobin, myoglobin, cytochromes.
- ***Structural proteins:*** These are the proteins of skin, cartilage, nail.
- ***Enzymes:*** Proteins act as enzymes.
- ***Hormones:*** Proteins act as hormones.

III. On Solubility and Physical Properties

However, both the above classification schemes have many overlapping features. Therefore, a third most acceptable scheme of classification of proteins is adopted. According to this scheme, proteins are ***classified on the basis of their solubility and physical properties*** and divided in to *three* different classes.

- *Simple Proteins:* These are proteins which on complete hydrolysis yield only amino acids.
- *Conjugated Proteins:* These are proteins which in addition to amino acids ***contain a non-protein group called prosthetic group in their structure.***
- *Derived Proteins:* These are the proteins formed from native protein by the action of heat, physical forces or chemical factors.

A. Simple Proteins

These are further subclassified based on their solubilities and heat coagulabilities. These properties depend on the size and shape of the protein molecule. Major subclasses of simple proteins are as given below:

1. *Protamines:* These are small molecules and are soluble in water, dilute acids and alkalies, and dilute ammonia.

- *Non-coagulable by heat*
- They do not contain *cysteine, tryptophan* and *tyrosine*, but are ***rich in arginine***.
- Their isoelectric pH is around 7.4, and they exist as basic proteins in the body.
- They combine with nucleic acids to form nucleoproteins.

  Examples: Salmine, sardinine and cyprinine or fish (sperms) and testes.

2. *Histones:* They are basic proteins with alkaline isoelectric pH and are ***rich in arginine and histidine***.

- They are ***soluble in water***, dilute acids and salt solution but insoluble in ammonia.
- They ***coagulate on heating.***
- They form conjugated proteins with nucleic acids (DNA) and Porphyrins.
- The protein part of haemoglobin, globin is an atypical histone having a predominance of histidine and lysine instead of arginine. *Example:* Nucleohistones, chromosomal nucleoproteins and globin of haemoglobin.

3. *Albumins:* These are proteins which are ***soluble in water*** and in dilute salt solutions and are generally ***deficient in glycine.***

- They are ***coagulable by heat*** and are changed to products that are insoluble in water and solutions of salt.
- The ***"albumins" may be precipitated (salted out) of solution by saturating the solution with ammonium sulphate.***
- Albumins have low isoelectric pH or pI 4.7 and therefore, they are acidic proteins at the pH 7.4.

  Example: **Plant albumins:** legumelin in legumes, leucosin in cereals. **Animal albumins:** ovalbumin in egg, lactoalbumin in milk.

4. *Globulins:* Globulins are ***insoluble in water*** but soluble in dilute neutral salt solutions.

- They also are ***heat coagulable.*** Vegetable globulins coagulate rather completely.
- Globulins are ***precipitated (salted out) by half saturation with ammonium sulphate*** or by full saturation with sodium chloride.
- Globulins bind with haem, e.g. haemopexin, with lipids, e.g. VLDL, with metals, e.g. transferrin, ceruloplasmin and with carbohydrates, e.g. immunoglobulins.

  Examples: In addition to above, ovoglobulin in eggs, lactoglobulin in milk, legumin from legumes.

5. ***Gliadins (Prolamines): Alcohol soluble plant proteins, insoluble in water*** or salt solutions and absolute alcohol, but they dissolve in 50-80% ethanol. ***They are very rich in proline, but poor in lysine.***

Example: ***Gliadin*** of wheat and ***hordein*** of barley.

6. *Glutelins:* These are ***plant proteins insoluble in water*** or neutral salt solutions, but soluble in dilute acids or alkalies.

- They are ***rich in glutamic acid.***
- They are large molecules and can be coagulated by heat.

  Example: *Oryzenin* of rice and *glutelin* of wheat.

7. *Scleroproteins or albuminoids:* These are ***fibrous proteins*** with great stability and very low solubility and form supporting structures of animals. In this group are found ***keratins, collagens*** and ***elastins.***

i. Keratins: These are characteristic constituents of tissues such as horn, hair, nails, wool, hoofs and feathers.

- The outermost layer of skin is keratin and a similar albuminoid keratohyaline is present in the lower layers.
- Human hair has a higher content of cysteine than that of other species, it is called α-keratin.

ii. Collagen: Collagen is a protein found in connective tissues and bone as long, thin, partially crystalline substance.

- These are insoluble in all neutral (salt) solvents.
- This is converted into a tough, hard substance on treatment with tannic acid. This is the basis of tanning process.
- Collagen can be easily converted to gelatin by boiling or by splitting of some amino acids.
- ***Gelatin*** is highly soluble and easily digestible. It forms a gel on cooling and is provided

as diet for invalids and convalescents. ***It is not a complete protein as it lacks an amino acid tryptophan which is an essential amino acid.***

iii. Elastins: These are the proteins present in yellow elastic fibre of the connective tissue, ligaments and tendons.

- Elastins are rich in non-polar amino acids such as alanine, leucine, valine and proline.
- Elastins do not contain cysteine, methionine 5-hydroxylysine and histidine.

B. Conjugated Proteins

Conjugated proteins are simple proteins combined with a non-protein group called ***prosthetic group. Protein part is called apoprotein, and entire molecule is called holoprotein.***

1. *Nucleoproteins:* The nucleoproteins are compounds made up of simple basic proteins such as protamine or histone with nucleic acids as the prosthetic group.

- They are proteins of cell nuclei and apparently are the chief constituents of ***chromatin.***
- ***Deoxyribonucleoproteins*** containing DNA as prosthetic group are found in nuclei, mitochondria and chloroplasts.
- ***Ribonucleoproteins occur*** in nucleoli and ribosome granules. They have *RNA* as prosthetic group.
  Examples: ***Nucleohistone*** **and** ***nucleoprotamine.***

2. *Mucoproteins or Mucoids:* Mucoproteins are the simple proteins combined with ***mucopolysaccharides*** **(MPS)** such as hyaluronic acid, the chondroitin sulphate, etc. They contain large quantities of N-acetylated hexosamine (>4%) and in addition substances such as uronic acid, sialic acid are also present.

- ***Mucoproteins are important constituents of the ground substance of connective tissue,*** and are present as tendomucoid, osseomucoid and chondroproteins in tendons, bones and cartilage respectively.
- These are present in large amounts in umbilical cord, and are also present in all kinds of *mucins* and blood group substances.

3. *Glycoproteins:* Glycoproteins are the proteins with carbohydrate moiety as the prosthetic group. **Karl Meyer** suggested that these proteins carry a small amount of carbohydrates < 4% such as serum albumin and globulin. Carbohydrate is bound much more firmly in the glycoproteins than the mucoprotein. Glycoproteins include mucins, immunoglobulins, complements and many enzymes. They carry mannose, galactose, fucose, xylose, arabinose in their oligosaccharide chains.

4. *Chromoproteins:* These are proteins that contain coloured substance as the prosthetic group.

1. ***Haemoproteins:*** All haemoproteins are chromoproteins which carry haem as the prosthetic group which is a red coloured pigment found in these proteins.

- ***Haemoglobin:*** Haemoglobin is a respiratory protein found in RBC's (See Chapter on Haemoglobin for details).
- ***Cytochromes:*** These are the mitochondrial enzymes of the respiratory chain.
- ***Catalase:*** This is the enzyme that decomposes H_2O_2 to water and O_2.
- ***Peroxidase:*** Is an oxidative enzyme.

2. ***Others:***

- ***Flavoprotein:*** Is a cellular oxidation-reduction protein which has ***riboflavin,*** a constituent of vitamin B complex in its prosthetic group. This is yellow in colour.
- ***Visual purple:*** Is a protein of the retina in which the prosthetic group is a carotenoid pigment which is purple in colour.

5. *Phosphoproteins:* These are the proteins with phosphoric acid as organic phosphate but not the phosphate containing substances such as nucleic acids and phospholipids.

Examples:

- ***Casein*** and ***ovovitellin*** are the two important groups of phosphoproteins found in milk and egg yolk respectively. They contain about 1% of phosphorous.

6. *Lipoproteins:* The lipoproteins are formed in combination with lipids as their prosthetic group. (Refer to Chapter on Metabolism of Lipids).

7. *Metalloproteins:* As the name indicates, they contain a metal ion as their prosthetic group. Several enzymes contain metallic elements such as Fe, CO, Mn, Zn, Cu, Mg, etc.

Examples:
- **Ferritin:** contains Fe
- **Carbonic anhydrase:** contains Zn
- **Caeruloplasmin:** contains Cu
- **Lactate dehydrogenase:** contains Zn, etc.

C. Derived Proteins

This class of proteins includes those protein product formed from the simple and conjugated proteins. It is not a well defined class of proteins. These are produced by various physical and chemical factors and are divided into two major groups.

1. *Primary Derived Proteins: **Denatured*** or ***coagulated proteins*** are placed in this group.
- Their molecular weight is the same as native protein, but ***they differ in solubility, precipitation and crystallization.***
- Heat, X-ray, UV rays, vigorous shaking, acid, alkali cause denaturation and give rise to primary derived proteins.
- There is an intramolecular rearrangement leading to changes in their properties such as solubility.
- ***Primary derived proteins are synonymous with denatured proteins.***
  - i. *Proteans:* These are insoluble products formed by the action of water, very dilute acids and enzymes. They are predominantly formed from certain globulin and differ from globulins being insoluble in dilute salt solution. In general, they are like glutelins.

  Example:
  - *Myosan:* from myosin
  - *Edestan:* from elastin and
  - *Fibrin:* from fibrinogen.
  - ii. *Metaproteins:* These are formed from further action of acids and alkalies on proteins. They are generally soluble in dilute acids and alkalies but insoluble in neutral solvents, e.g. acid and alkali metaproteins such as alkali and acid albuminates.
  - iii. *Coagulated proteins:* The coagulated proteins are insoluble products formed by the action of heat or alcohol on native proteins.

    Example: Cooked meat, cooked egg albumin and alcohol precipitated proteins.

2. *Secondary Derived Proteins:* These are the proteins formed by the ***progressive hydrolysis of proteins at their peptide linkages.*** They represent a great complexity with respect to their size and amino acid composition. They are roughly called as proteoses, peptones and peptides according to relative average molecular size.
- *Proteoses or albumoses:* These are the hydrolytic products of proteins which are soluble in water and are coagulated by heat and are precipitated from their solution by saturation with ammonium sulphate.
- *Peptones:* These are the hydrolytic products of proteoses. They are soluble in water, not coagulated by heat and not precipitated by saturation with ammonium sulphate. They can be precipitated by phosphotungstic acid.

  Example: Protein products obtained by the enzymatic digestion of proteins.
- *Peptides:* Peptides are composed of only a small number of amino acids joined as *"peptide bonds"*. They are named according to the number of amino acids present in them.
- **Dipeptides** are made up of two amino acids,
- **Tripeptides** are made of three amino acids, etc. Peptides are water soluble, uncoagulated by heat and are not salted out of solution, and can be precipitated by phosphotungstic acid.

The complete hydrolytic decomposition of a protein generally follows the stages given below.

Protein → Protean → Metaprotein → Proteose
Amino Acids ← Peptides ← Peptone ←

The products from protein to peptone give a positive Biuret reaction and are relatively large molecules. The **dipeptide and amino acids do not**

give Biuret positive reaction, and, therefore, are called as a biuret products.

Note: In secondary derived proteins the primary structure, i.e. the peptide bond is broken; on the other hand, in ***primary derived Proteins, the peptide bonds remain intact***, the secondary and tertiary structures are broken.

GENERAL PROPERTIES OF PROTEINS

1. **Taste:** Proteins are tasteless. However, the hydrolytic products (derived proteins) are bitter in taste.

2. **Odour:** They are odourless. When heated to dryness they turn brown and give off the odour of burning feather.

3. **Molecular weight:** The protein in general has a large molecular weight. ***Proteins therefore are macromolecules.*** Molecular weight of some common proteins is shown in ***Table 3.1.***

Table 3.1: Molecular Weight of Some Common Proteins

Protein	Molecular weight
• Serum albumin	69,000
• Serum γ-globulin	176,000
• Fibrinogen	330,000
• Haemoglobin	67,000
• Cytochrome-C	15,600
• Pepsin	35,500
• Catalase	250,000

4. **Viscosity of protein solutions:** The viscosity of protein varies widely with the kind of protein and its concentration in solution. ***The viscosity is closely related to molecular shape as long molecules (fibrous proteins) are more viscous than globular proteins.*** Thus, fibrinogen can form a more viscous solution than albumin.

5. **Heat coagulation of proteins:** Several proteins coagulate forming, an insoluble coagulum. ***Coagulation is maximum at the isoelectric pH of the protein.*** During coagulation protein undergoes a change called denaturation. ***Denatured proteins are soluble in extremes of pH, and maximum precipitation occurs at isoelectric pH (pl) of the protein.***

6. **Amphoteric nature of proteins:** In any of the protein molecule, there are amino acids which carry –COOH or NH_2 groups in their side chains. ***These groups can undergo ionization in solution producing both anions and cations.*** In addition to the side chain of polar amino acids, N-terminal $-NH_2$ group, and C-terminal –COOH group may also ionize. Depending on the pH, few groups act as proton donors while few as proton acceptors. Therefore, ***proteins are ampholytes, i.e. act both as acids and bases. At a specific pH called an isoelectric pH (pI), a protein exists as a dipolar ion*** or ***Zwitterion*** or ***"hybrid" ion*** carrying equal number of positive and negative charges on its ionizable groups. ***So, the net charge on protein molecule at its isolectric pH is zero.***

On the acidic side of its isoelectric pH a protein exists as a ***cation*** by accepting a proton and migrates towards anode in an electrical field; while ***on the alkaline side*** of its *pI* a protein exists as ***anion*** by donating a proton and migrates towards cathode. This property is made use of in electrophoresis to separate different proteins depending on the charge present in them at a particular pH.

7. ***Precipitation of proteins:*** Proteins can be precipitated from solutions by a variety of +ve and –ve ions. Such precipitation is of importance in the isolation of protein in the deproteinization of blood and other biological fluids, and extracts for analysis and in the preparation of useful protein derivatives.

a. ***Precipitation by +ve ions:*** The +ve ions most commonly used are those of ***heavy metals*** Zn^{+2}, Ca^{+2}, Hg^{+2}, Fe^{+2}, Cu^{+2}, and Pb^{+2}. These metals precipitate protein at the pH ***alkaline*** to its isoelectric pH. At this pH, protein is dissociated as an anion-proteinate . The metal ions combine with the $-COO^-$ group to give insoluble precipitate of metal proteinate.

BIOMEDICAL APPLICATION

- The use of $AgNO_3$ in cauteries is based on this property. It precipitates the proteins of tissues as Ag-salts.

- Another application of this property is the ***use of proteins as antidotes to metallic poisons***. Egg white, milk and other proteins can be used to precipitate metal ions. The metallic protein precipitate must be removed from the stomach by an emetic or by stomach-tube to prevent the liberation and absorption of the poisonous metal.

b. ***Negative ion precipitation:*** Negative ions combine with proteins when the pH of the medium is on the ***acidic side*** of its isoelectric pH. Acidic pH makes the protein to exist as $protein^+$ and forms precipitate with –ve ions. NH_2 group is the reacting group in this case.

- Among the more common precipitants involving –ve ion precipitation are tungstic acid, phosphotungstic acid, trichloroacetic acid, picric acid, tannic acid, ferrocyanic acid and sulphosalicyclic acid. When these agents are added to protein solution at proper pH, the protein precipitates as its salt. The precipitate is found to be soluble in alkali.

Clinical Application

Trichloroacetic acid, tungstic acid, are commonly used for the preparation of protein-free filtrate of blood (PPF) and other biological materials prior to analysis of few constituents such as sugar and urea by specific methods.

COLOUR REACTIONS OF PROTEINS

Proteins produce colour in certain reactions. These reactions are not quite specific for a protein molecule as such but are ***due to characteristic groups of particular amino acids present in it.***

1. ***Xanthoproteic reaction:*** The aromatic amino acids such as ***phenylalanine, tyrosine*** and ***tryptophan*** present in the protein give ***yellow precipitate*** when heated with conc. HNO_3. On addition of alkali, the ***precipitate turns orange due to nitration of the aromatic ring. Collagen and gelatin do not give a positive reaction.***

2. ***Million's test:*** This is a specific test for ***tyrosine*** of protein. Proteins give a ***white ppt*** with Millon's reagent (10% mercurous chloride in H_2SO_4) on heating. On addition of $NaNO_2$ the ***precipitate turns pink-red.***

3. ***Sakaguchi test:*** This is a specific test for ***arginine*** of the protein. Sakaguchi reagent consists of alcoholic α-naphthol and a drop of sodium hypobromite. ***Guanidine group of arginine ($HN=C-NH_2$) is responsible for the formation of red colour.***

4. ***Hopkins Cole reaction (Glyoxylic acid reaction):*** Reagent containing glyoxylic acid which may be prepared by reduction of oxalic acid with sodium-amalgam. Protein containing ***tryptophan*** gives this test positive. ***The reaction is characteristic of tryptophan.*** **Gelatin, collagen do not contain tryptophan and hence do not give this test positive.** Nitrates, chlorates, nitrites and excess chlorides prevent the reaction. A number of aldehydes other than glyoxylic acid give similar colour reactions with tryptophan.

5. ***Nitroprusside reaction:*** Proteins with free –SH group of ***cysteine*** give ***reddish colour*** with sodium nitroprusside in ammoniacal solution. Many proteins give this test positive after heat coagulation or denaturation indicating the liberation of free-SH groups.

6. ***Sullivan reaction:*** Used for the determination of ***cysteine*** and ***cystine***. ***Red colour*** is produced when cysteine containing protein is heated with sodium 1,2 naphthoquinone-4-sulfonate in the alkaline medium in presence of $Na_2S_2O_4$.

7. ***Lead acetate test (Unoxidized sulfur test):*** This ***test is specific for sulfur containing amino acid.*** The protein containing S-containing amino acids is boiled with strong alkali to split out sulphur as sodium sulphide which reacts with Lead acetate ***to give black precipitate of PbS,***

8. ***Biuret reaction:*** When urea is heated it forms biuret as follows:

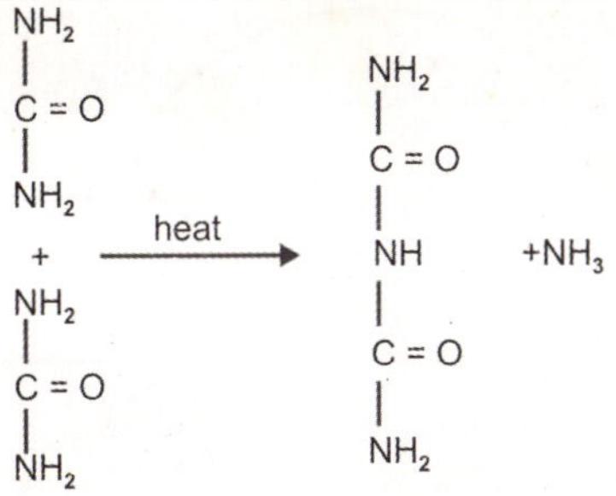

$$H_2N{-}CO{-}NH_2 + H_2N{-}CO{-}NH_2 \xrightarrow{\text{heat}} H_2N{-}CO{-}NH{-}CO{-}NH_2 + NH_3$$

Urea *Biuret*

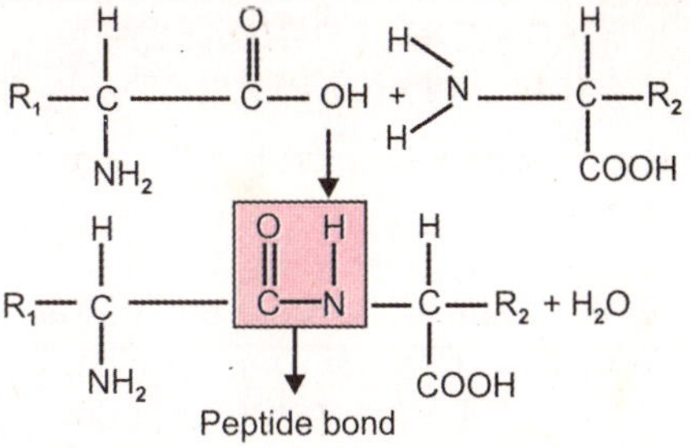

If a strongly alkaline solution of biuret is heated with very dilute copper sulphate ***a purple-violet colour*** is obtained. The ***colour depends upon the presence of 2 or more peptide linkages.***

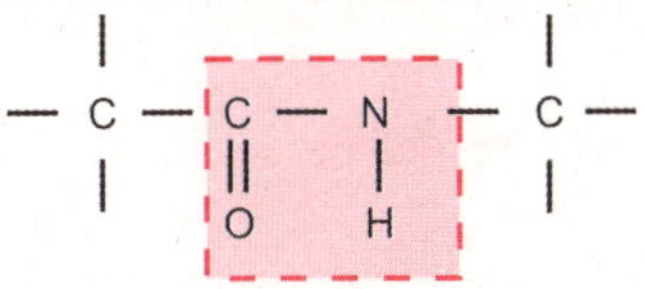

$$-\overset{|}{\underset{|}{C}}-\underset{\|}{\overset{}{C}}-\underset{|}{N}-\overset{|}{\underset{|}{C}}-$$
$$\quad\quad O \quad H$$

Thus dipeptides and free amino acids do not give the biuret test. Only histidine can give a positive reaction. Biuret test is due to co-ordination of cupric ions with the unshared electron pairs of peptide nitrogen and the oxygen of water to form a coloured co-ordination complex.

9. ***Ninhydrin reaction:*** Ninhydrin is a powerful oxidizing agent and causes oxidative decarboxylation of α-amino acids producing an aldehyde with one carbon less than the parent amino acid. The reduced ninhydrin-hydrindantin then reacts with ammonia which has been liberated and one molecule of ninhydrin forming *a* ***blue-coloured compound. A molecule of CO_2 is evolved indicating the presence of α-amino acid.***

PEPTIDE LINKAGE

The –COOH group of one amino acid can be joined to the $-NH_2$ group of another by a covalent bond called ***peptide bond.*** In the process of formation of a peptide bond, a molecule of water is eliminated ***(Fig. 3.4).*** When two amino acids are joined together by one peptide bond, such a structure is called ***dipeptide.*** A third amino acid can form a second peptide bond through its free –COOH end and is called ***tripeptide*** and so on. Thus, it is the peptide linkage which holds various amino acids together in a specific sequence and number. Peptides varying from the simplest dipeptide to very long polypeptides are present in human body and serve specific functions.

$$R_1{-}CH(NH_2){-}CO{-}OH + H{-}NH{-}CH(COOH){-}R_2 \rightarrow R_1{-}CH(NH_2){-}CO{-}NH{-}CH(COOH){-}R_2 + H_2O$$

Peptide bond

Fig. 3.4: **Formation of peptide bond**

Difference between a polypeptide and a protein molecule:

Polypeptides do not contain amino acids more than 100, whereas proteins contain amino acids more than 100.

STRUCTURAL ORGANIZATION OF PROTEINS

Protein structure is normally described at *four levels of organization.*

1. ***Primary structure: Primary structure is the linear sequence of amino acids held together by peptide bonds in its peptide chain.*** The peptide bonds form the backbone, and side chains of amino acid residues project outside the peptide backbone. The free $-NH_2$ group of the terminal amino acids is called ***N-terminal end*** and the free –COOH end is called ***C-terminal end.*** It is a tradition to number the amino acids forming N-terminal end as number 1 towards the C-terminal end. ***Presence of specific amino acids at a specific number is very significant for a particular function of a protein.*** Any change in the sequence is abnormal and may affect the function and properties of protein.

2. ***Secondary structure:*** The peptide chain thus formed assumes a three dimensional secondary structure by way of folding or coiling consisting of a helically coiled, zig-zag linear or mixed form. It results from the steric relationship between amino acids located relatively near each other in the peptide chain. The linkages or bond involved

SOME BIOLOGICALLY IMPORTANT PEPTIDES

1. **Dipeptides:** two dipeptides present in muscle tissues are
- *Carnosine:* β-alanine + histidine
- *Anserine:* β-alanine + methyl histidine
2. **Tripeptides:** ***Glutathione*** is a tripeptide consisting of 3 amino acids—glutamic acid + cysteine + glycine.
   It functions in the body in the oxidation-reduction system.
3. **Angiotensin II:** octapeptide increases BP↑
4. **Brain peptides:** Endorphins
5. **Antibiotics:** Penicillin, chloramphenicol, bacitracin, polymyxin, gramicidin A, actinomycin
6. **Antitumor agent:** Bleomycin.

in the secondary structure formation are hydrogen bonds and disulphide bonds.

- ***Hydrogen bond:*** These are weak, low energy noncovalent bonds sharing a single hydrogen by two electronegative atoms such as O, and N. Hydrogen bonds are formed in secondary structure by sharing H-atoms between oxygen of CO and nitrogen of –NH of different peptide bonds
- ***Disulphide bonds:*** These are ***formed between two cysteine residues.*** They are strong, high energy covalent bonds. The hydrogen bonds in secondary structure may form either an α-helix or β-pleated sheet structure.

a. **α-Helix:**

- A peptide chain forms regular helical coils called **α-helix**. These coils are stabilized by hydrogen bonds between carbonyl O of 1st amino acid and amide N of 4th amino acid residues. ***Thus, in α-helix intrachain hydrogen bonding is present.*** The α-helices can be either right handed or left handed. ***Left handed α-helix is less stable than right handed α-helix*** because of the steric interference between the C = O and the side chains. Only the right handed α-helix has been found in protein structure ***(Fig. 3.5).***

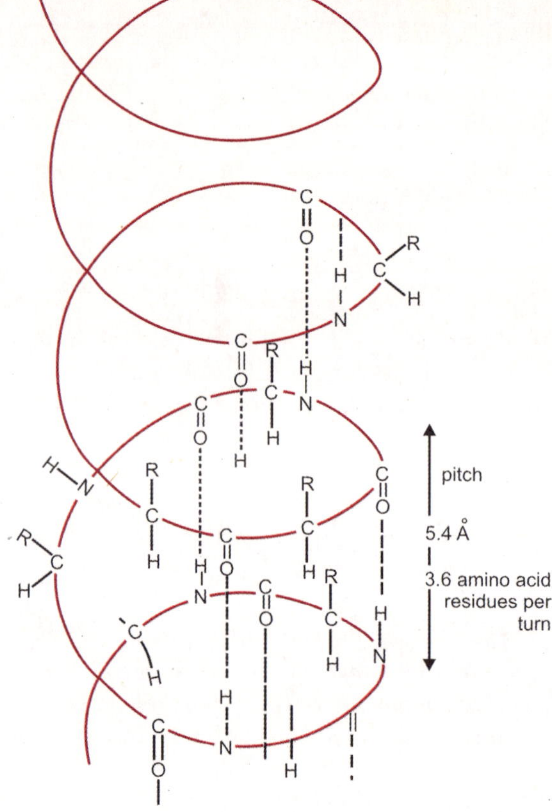

Fig. 3.5: α-helix

- Each amino acid residue advances by 0.15 nm along the helix, and ***3.6 amino acid residues are present in one complete turn.*** The distance between two equivalent points on turn is 0.54 nm and is called ***a pitch.***
- Small or uncharged amino acid residues such as *alanine, leucine and phenylalanine* are often found in α-helix. More polar residues such as arginine, glutamate and serine may repel and destabilize α-helix. **Proline is never found in α-helix.**
- The proteins of hair, nail, skin contain a group of proteins called keratins rich in α-helical structure.

b. ***β-pleated sheet structure:*** β-Keratins present in spider's web, reptilian claw, fibres of silk form almost fully extended chain. A conformation called β-pleated sheet structure is thus formed when hydrogen bonds are formed between the carbonyl oxygens and amide hydrogens of two or more adjacent extended polypeptide chains. ***Thus, the hydrogen bonding in β-pleated sheet structure is interchain.*** The structure is not absolutely planer but is slightly pleated due to the angles of bonds. The ***adjacent chains in β-pleated sheet structure are either parallel or antiparallel***, depending on whether the amino to carbonyl peptide linkage of the chains runs in the same or opposite direction. In both parallel and anti-parallel β-pleated sheet structures, the side chains are on opposite sides of the sheet. Generally glycine, serine and alanine are most common to form β-pleated sheet. Proline occurs in β-pleated sheet although it tends to disrupt the sheets by producing kinks ***(Fig.3.6).*** Silk fibroin, a protein of silkworm is rich in β-pleated sheets.

c. ***Triple helix: Collagen is rich in proline and hydroxyproline, and cannot form α-helix or β-pleated sheet. It forms a triple helix.*** The triple helix is stabilized by both non-covalent as well as covalent bonds. Interchain hydrogen bonds between different peptide chains are formed which are almost perpendicular to the long axis of α-helix. In addition, interchain additional cross links, secondary amide bonds of peptide bonds also are responsible for triple helix.

d. Many globulin proteins have mixed secondary structure of α-helix, β-pleated sheet and non-helical, non-pleated structures called ***random coil.***

3. ***Tertiary Structure:*** The polypeptide chain with secondary structure mentioned above may be ***further folded, superfolded, twisted about itself*** forming many size. Such a structural conformation is called tertiary structure. It is only one such conformation which is biologically active and protein in this conformation is called as native protein. Thus, the tertiary structure is constituted by steric relationship between the amino acids located far apart but brought closer by folding. The bonds responsible for interaction between groups of amino acids are as given below:

- ***Hydrophobic interactions:*** Normally occur between non-polar side chains of amino acids such as alanine, leucine, methionine, isoleucine and phenylalanine. They constitute the major stabilizing forces for tertiary structures forming a compact three-dimensional structure.
- ***Hydrogen bonds:*** Normally formed by the polar side chains of the amino acids.
- ***Ionic or electrostatic interactions:*** These are formed between oppositely charged polar side

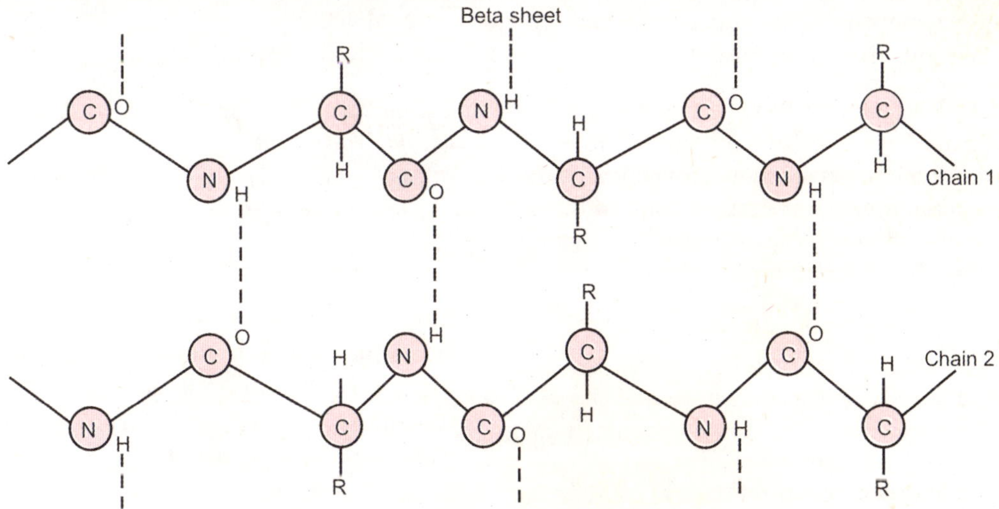

Fig. 3.6: β-pleated sheet

chains of amino acids such as basic and acidic amino acids.

- *van der Waal Forces:* These occur between non-polar side chains.
- *Disulphide bonds:* These are the S-S bonds between –SH groups of distant cysteine residues.

4. ***Quaternary structure:*** Many proteins are made up of only one peptide chain. However, ***when a protein consists of two or more peptide chains held together by non-covalent interaction or by covalent cross-links it is referred to as the quaternary structure.*** The assembly is often called as oligomer and each constituent peptide chain is called monomer or subunit. The monomers of oligomeric protein can be identical or quite different in primary, secondary or tertiary structure.

Example:

- Protein with two monomers (dimer) is an enzyme called creatine phosphokinase (CPK).
- Haemoglobin and lactate dehydrogenase (LDH) are tetramers consisting of four monomers.
- **Apoferritin:** An apoprotein of feritin, an iron binding and storage protein contains 24 identical subunits.
- An enzyme aspartate transcarbamylase has 72 subunits in its structure.

DENATURATION OF PROTEINS

Conformation of a protein molecule is extremely sensitive to changes in their environment. In denaturation, there is a disruption of native or biologically active protein conformation when the environment is altered.

Definition: Denaturation may be defined as a disruption of the secondary, tertiary, and wherever applicable quarternary organization of a protein molecule due to cleavage of non-covalent bonds.

Note: ***Primary structure of protein molecule, i.e. peptide bond is not affected.***

Agents that cause denaturation: Various agents which can disrupt the conformation are given below:

- *Physical agents:* Heat, UV light, ultrasound, and high pressure can cause denaturation. Even violent shaking can denature the protein.
- *Chemical agents:* Organic solvents, acids/alkalies can cause denaturation of proteins.
- *Urea and various detergents:* The disruption/disorganization of the protein molecules results in alteration of the chemical, physical and biological characteristics of the protein.

Alterations in Protein Molecules after Denaturation

1. *Chemical alterations:*
   - Greatly decreased solubility especially at pI of the protein. ***Maximum precipitation as floccules occur at pI of the protein.***
   - Many chemical groups which were rather inactive become exposed, e.g.—SH group.
   - Denaturation can be **reversible.**
2. *Physical alterations:*
   - It ***confers increased viscosity*** of the solution.
   - Rate of diffusion of the protein molecules decreases.
3. *Biological alterations:*
   - Increased digestibility by proteolytic enzymes has been found in the case of certain denatured proteins.
   - Denaturation destroys enzymal and hormonal activity.
   - Biologically becomes inactive.

Relationship of Denaturation, Flocculation and Coagulum Formation

The relationship is explained schematically in case of albumin ***(Fig. 3.7).*** It shows the behaviour of denatured albumin.

- ***Denatured albumin is soluble in extremes of pH.***
- Maximum precipitation occurs at pI of the protein, i.e. albumin as ***floccules (flocculation).***
- ***Denatured protein as floccules, is reversible and soluble in extremes of pH.***
- When the floccules at pI are heated further, they become dense ***coagulum which is irreversible*** and is ***not soluble in extremes of pH.***

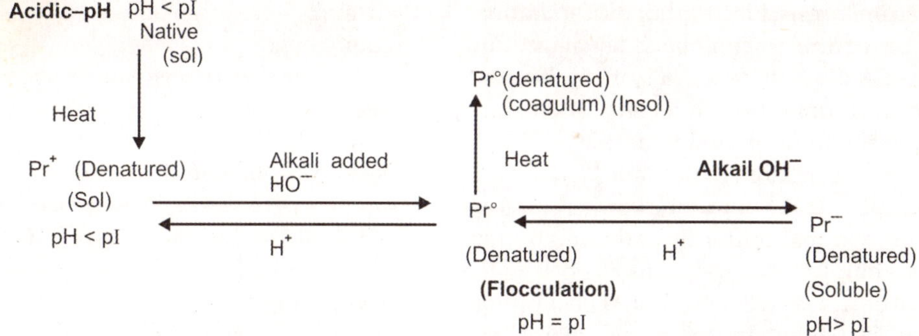

Fig. 3.7: Relationship of denaturation, flocculation and coagulum formation

PURIFICATION OF PROTEINS

Methods of Purification: The **two major** methods employed in purification of protein are (i) **Chromatography** and (ii) **Electrophoresis.**

1. *Chromatography:* There are many different types of chromatography even though the underlying principle is the same for all of them.

- The physicochemical factors involved in chromatography are adsorption, partition, ion exchange and molecular sieving.
- There are ***two phases*** in all types of chromatography (i) ***the stationary phase*** and (ii) the ***other mobile phase***. In paper chromatography, paper is stationary phase and organic solvent is mobile phase. In column chromatography, the glass column filled with appropriate substances is stationary phase while a buffer is mobile phase. The mixture of proteins to be separated is dissolved in smallest possible volume of buffer or solvent and applied on stationary phase. As soon as the solution is soaked into the adsorbent stationary phase, it is followed by a solvent or buffer.

Paper chromatography: Whatmann 1 or Whatmann 3 filter paper is normally used as supporting material for stationary aqueous phase. An organic solvent layer of **mixture of butanol: acetic acid: water in the ratio of 4:1:5** is used as solvent or mobile phase. Normally amino acids are separated by this. When another solvent system in a perpendicular direction in paper is employed, it is a two-dimensional paper chromatography and separates the amino acids more distinctly.

Rf value: The ratio of the distance moved by a compound to the distance moved by the solvent front is known as its Rf value.

For example, if the solvent front has moved 40 cm, and a compound, say an amino acid, has moved 20 cm, then the Rf value of the compound/ amino acid is 20/40 = 0.5.

Importance: Rf values are different for different solvents. For a given solvent, the Rf value is a characteristic of the compound and from this observation, ***it is possible to identify unknown substances by their positions in relation to known substances.***

2. *Electrophoresis:* The second procedure for protein purification or separation is electrophoresis. ***Electrophoresis is the movement of charged particles towards one of the electrodes under the influence of electrical current.*** Depending upon the mode of separation and technique, electrophoresis is divided in three group: (i) boundary, (ii) zone, (iii) immunoelectrophoresis. Moving boundary electrophoresis is now obsolete and immunoelectrophoresis is used only in special cases with a special purpose. Most commonly employed type of electrophoresis is now the zone electrophoresis. Zone electrophoresis can be further divided as *paper electrophoresis,* disc electrophoresis, block electrophoresis and isoelectric focussing, etc.

Paper electrophoresis: Electrophoretic separation depends on various factors such as charge on protein molecules, its size, pH of the buffer, temperature of operation, intensity of current applied and the dilution of the sample.

The papers commonly used are Whatmann filter paper No. 1, 2, 3. For routine work in clinical laboratories, veronal buffer or barbitone buffer of pH 8.6 is employed. Paper is moistened with the veronal buffer, its free end should be dipping in the buffer on both sides in buffer chambers. About 10-20 μl sample of protein mixture is applied as a thin line. A direct current of 0.5 to 10 mA is applied using a suitable power supply unit, and electrophoresis is conducted for 16 hours. The paper is then removed, dried and stained with Amido Black 10B, Bromophenol blue, Azocarmine B, etc. which are protein specific stains.

Ion-exchange papers like **cellulose acetate membrane** (CAM) are employed. In this, the adsorption which occurs to some extent in paper electrophoresis is avoided and there is an added advantage of molecular sieving. Here, the **whole process of electrophoresis is complete in less than one hour.**

Quantitation: The protein bands obtained either in paper or in CAM electrophoresis can be quantified by a ***scanning densitometer*** or by cutting the bands, ***eluting*** and using colorimeters to obtain their absorbance values. The absorbance of each band is added up and individual percentage are calculated.

☞ SALIENT POINTS TO REMEMBER

- Proteins are nitrogen containing most abundant organic macro-molecules widely distributed in animals and plants.
- They perform structural and dynamic functions in the organism. ***They are sole source of nitrogen in the body.***
- Proteins are polymers of monomeric units L-amino acids, joined by peptide bonds.
- L-amino acids are ***twenty in numbers*** and are classified into different groups based on their structure, chemical nature and nutritional requirement.
- Each amino acid possesses two functional groups viz carboxyl (–COOH) and amino-group (–NH_2).
- Depending on the pH of the medium, the amino acid can behave as an acid or a base.
- In the physiological system, they exist as "dipolar ions" commonly referred as **"zwitterions".**
- Nutritionally the amino acids are divided into 3 groups, viz. essential, semiessential and non-essential.
- **Essential amino acids are eight in number** viz. Valine, Leucine, Isoleucine, Phenylalanine, Threonine, Tryptophan, Methionine, and Lysine.
- They must be provided in the diet as they cannot be synthesized in the body. ***All essential amino acids must be taken together in the diet. If one is missing, the others cannot be used for tissue formation.***
- ***Semiessential amino acids are two,*** viz. **Arginine** and **histidine.** They become essential in growing children, pregnancy and lactating women.
- Proteins are classified into three major groups viz. simple proteins, conjugated proteins and derived proteins.
- Simple proteins contain only amino acid residues, e.g. albumin, globulins, prolamines, glutelins, scleroproteins, etc.
- Conjugated proteins contain a ***non-protein moiety*** called as ***prosthetic group*** besides the L-amino acids, e.g. Nucleoproteins, Glycoproteins, Chromoproteins, etc.
- Derived proteins are obtained by degradation/or hydrolysis of simple or conjugated proteins, e.g. primary derived proteins and secondary derived proteins.
- Depending on shape and size, proteins can be of 2 types viz. Fibrous proteins and Globular proteins.
- ***When the axial ratio of length: width is more than 10,*** it is called ***fibrous proteins. Examples:*** α-keratin of hair, collagen.

- ***When the axial ratio of length: width is less than 10,*** it is called as ***globular proteins. Examples:*** Haemoglobin, Myoglobin.
- The -COOH group of one amino acid can be joined to the $-NH_2$ group of another by a covalent bond called **'Peptide bond'** or **'Peptide linkage'**.
- Polypeptides do not contain amino acids more than 100, whereas proteins contain amino acids more than 100.
- Several biologically important peptides are known in the living organisms and serve important functions. Examples:
  - ***Glutathione,*** a tripeptide involved in cellular oxidation-reduction. Required for maintenance of structure and integrity of RB cells and lens of eye.
  - ***Oxytocin,*** an octapeptide causes uterine contraction.
  - ***Vasopressin,*** an octapeptide acts as antidiuretic hormone.
  - ***Encephalins,*** brain peptides—inhibit sense of pain in the brain.
- ***Structure*** of protein is divided into ***four levels of organization:***
  - Primary structure represents the linear sequence of amino acids joined by "Peptide bond". ***The peptide bond is very stable and not affected in denaturation.***
  - Secondary structure is the twisting and coiling of the polypeptide chain. It mainly consists of α-helix and/or β-pleated sheet. α-helix is stabilized by extensive hydrogen bonding. ***Proline is never found in α-helix.***

    β-pleated sheet is composed of two or more segments of fully extended polypeptide chains.
  - Tertiary and quaternary structures of Protein are stabilized by non-covalent bonds such as hydrogen bonds, hydrophobic interactions, ionic bonds, S-S bonds, etc.
  - Collagen is the most abundant protein in mammals. It is rich in OH-proline and OH-lysine, cannot form α-helix or β-pleated sheet. It *forms a triple helix.*
- Proteins can be precipitated by +ve ions or -ve ions.
- +ve ions precipitation take place in presence of heavy metals such as Zn^{+2}, Ca^{+2}, Hg^{+2}, Fe^{+3}, Pb^{+2}, in **an alkaline medium.**
- -ve ions precipitation take place in presence of trichloroacetic acid, tungstic acid, sulphosalicylic acid, picric acid, etc. in **an acidic medium.**
- Protein free filtrate (PFF) of blood is used for biochemical investigations, e.g. estimation of blood sugar, blood urea, etc.
- Denaturation is disruption of secondary, tertiary and wherever applicable quarternary organization of a protein molecule due to cleavage of non-covalent bonds by (i) physical agents like heat, UV light, ultrasound, high pressure, etc. and (ii) chemical agents like acids/alkalis, organic solvents.
- Denaturation brings about physical, chemical and biological alterations in protein molecules.
- In ***denaturation, primary structure, i.e. peptide bond is not affected.***
- Heat coagulation test is most commonly used to detect the presence of albumin in urine. Denatured albumin is soluble in extremes of pH.
- Denatured albumin appears as floccules in pI of albumin. Heating further floccules are converted to congulum which is insoluble and irreversible in extremes of pH.

MULTIPLE CHOICE QUESTIONS

Give one correct answer:

1. **Which bond is present in the primary structure of protein?**
   (a) Hydrogen bond (b) Peptide bond
   (c) Ionic bond (d) Disulfide bond
   (e) Ester bond
2. **Which amino acid listed below is not a basic amino acid?**
   (a) Histidine (b) Lysine
   (c) Glutamine (d) Arginine
   (e) Ornithine

3. **Which of the following amino acid has a hydroxyl group?**
(a) Leucine (b) Valine
(c) Histidine (d) Serine
(e) Lysine

4. **The number of helices present in a collagen molecule is:**
(a) 2 (b) 3 (c) 5
(d) 4 (e) 6

5. **Which of the following amino acid is optically inactive?**
(a) Serine (b) Threonine
(c) Tyrosine (d) Glycine
(e) Proline

6. **Which one is not a fibrous protein?**
(a) Elastin (b) Keratin
(c) Prolamine (d) Collagen
(e) Fibrin

7. **All of the following are sulphur containing amino acids found in proteins *except:***
(a) Cysteine (b) Tyrosine
(c) Cystine (d) Methionine
(e) Homocysteine

8. **In protein structure, the α-helix and β-pleated sheet are examples of:**
(a) Tertiary structure
(b) Primary structure
(c) Secondary structure
(d) Quarternary structure
(e) All of the above

9. **An essential amino acid in man is:**
(a) Tyrosine (b) Threonine
(c) Proline (d) Serine
(e) Aspartate

10. **An amino acid that does not take part in α-helix is:**
(a) Valine (b) Leucine
(c) Lysine (d) Proline
(e) Threonine

11. **Which of the following is a dipeptide?**
(a) Bradykinin (b) Carnosine
(c) Encephalin (d) Glutathione
(e) Prolamine

12. **Pyrrolidine group is present in amino acid stated below:**
(a) Arginine (b) Proline
(c) Tyrosine (d) Histidine
(e) Threonine

13. **In denaturation of proteins, the bond which is not broken:**
(a) Disulfide bond (b) Hydrogen bond
(c) Ionic bond (d) Peptide bond
(e) None of the above

14. **The protein present in hair is**
(a) Elastin (b) Prolamine
(c) Keratin (d) Glutelin
(e) Gliadin

15. **In which category keratin belongs:**
(a) Globulins (b) Albumin
(c) Albuminoids (d) Histone
(e) Protamine

ANSWERS

1. (b)	2. (c)	3. (d)
4. (b)	5. (d)	6. (c)
7. (b)	8. (c)	9. (b)
10. (d)	11. (b)	12. (b)
13. (d)	14. (c)	15. (c)

4 Plasma Proteins—Chemistry and Functions

PLASMA PROTEINS

- The chief solids of plasma are the proteins which are about 7.0 to 9.0 gm percent
- The human plasma proteins are mixture of simple proteins such as
  - **Albumins**
  - **Globulins**
- And **conjugated proteins** such as glycoproteins, lipoproteins, etc.

SEPARATION OF PLASMA PROTEINS

Various methods have been used to separate out the individual proteins in plasma. A brief outline is described here.

1. *Precipitation by salting out:* By this method, different concentrations of salt solutions are used to precipitate the various fractions of proteins which are then separated. **Two types of salt solutions** have been used for this:

- ***Ammonium sulphate solution***
- ***Mixture of sodium sulphate and sodium sulphite solution.***

2. *Fractionation of plasma proteins by ethanol* ***(Cohn's fractionation):*** **Cohn** used varying concentrations of ethanol at low temperature to separate out fractions of proteins which are called fraction I, II, etc. Each fraction is itself a mixture of proteins but contains one of the proteins predominantly. Thus,

- **Fraction I** is rich in fibrinogen
- **Fraction II** is γ globulins
- **Fraction III** contains α and β globulins including iso-agglutinins and prothrombin
- **Fraction IV** contains α and β globulins
- **Fraction V** contains predominantly albumin.

Advantage of this Fractionation

- Solvent used in the procedure can be readily removed by evaporation.
- Mild procedures adopted in fractionation of the proteins do not cause denaturation of the proteins.

> **Clinical Use**
>
> Cohn's method is useful for obtaining purified proteins on a large scale for therapeutic purposes.

3. More recent methods include separation of plasma proteins by:

- Paper electrophoresis (Tselius, 1937)
- Gel electrophoresis
- Immunoelectrophoresis
- Ultracentrifugation
- Column chromatography

Electrophoresis

Original paper electrophoresis was followed by more sensitive agar gel electrophoresis, cellulose acetate membrane electrophoresis, starch gel electrophoresis and immunoelectrophoresis.

By paper electrophoresis, the serum can be separated into a number of fractions, viz albumin, globulins-α_1, α_2, β and γ-globulins *(Fig. 4.1)*. Depending on sensitivity of the method β-globulins can be resolved into β_1 and β_2.

Note: If plasma is used instead of serum, a band of fibrinogen fraction is seen between β and γ-globulins.

Using modern analytical methods, more than 80 proteins have been identified in plasma. Many of them occur only in trace amounts and are either enzymes or transport proteins. Values of different proteins as obtained by standard precipitation methods and by paper electrophoresis are given in ***Table 4.1.***

Table 4.1: Normal Values of Plasma Proteins
Total proteins=7.0 to 7.5 gm%

	By precipitation (gms %)	*By paper electrophoresis (% of total proteins)*
• Albumin	3.7 to 5.3	50 to 70%
• Globulins	1.8 to 3.6	29.5 to 54%
• α_1 globulins	0.1 to 0.4	2.0 to 6.0%
• α_2 globulins	0.4 to 0.8	5.0 to 11.0%
• β-globulins	0.5 to 1.3	7.0 to 16.0%
• γ-globulins	0.6 to 1.5	11.0 to 22.0%
• Fibrinogen	0.2 to 0.4 (200 to 400 mg%)	

A: G ratio = 2.5 to 1.0 to about 1.2 to 1.0, most frequently 2:1

Electrophoretic pattern in some common diseases is shown in the following box.

Electrophoretic Pattern in Different Diseases

Diseases	*Electrophoretic pattern*
• *Nephrosis*	Albumin ↓, α_2-globulin-increased markedly, γ-globulin ↓
• *Chronic liver disease*	γ-globulin ↑ diffuse in nature (polyclonal)
• *Infectious hepatitis*	γ-globulin ↑, α_1 and α_2-globulins ↓
• *Diabetes mellitus*	α_2-globulin-small increase ↑
• *Rheumatoid arthritis*	γ-globulin ↑, slight to moderate α_2 globulin ↑
• *SLE*	γ-globulin ↑, α_2-globulin ↑
• *Sarcoidosis* β-globulin -, α_2- globulin -	γ-globulin ↑
• *Lymphatic leukaemia*	γ-globulin ↓
• *Myelogenous and monocytic leukaemia*	γ-globulin ↑
• *Multiple myeloma*	Sharp paraprotein band in β to γ region (M band-Monoclonal)

CHARACTERISTICS OF INDIVIDUAL PLASMA PROTEINS

A. Albumin

- It is the most abundant and fairly homogeneous protein of plasma with a molecular weight of 69,000.
- Approximately half of the total proteins of plasma is albumin.
- It has a low iso-electric pH (pI = 4.7).
- The protein migrates fastest in electrophoresis at alkaline pH and precipitates last in "salting out" or alcohol precipitation methods.
- It is a simple protein consisting of a single polypeptide chain, having 610 amino acids, having 17 interchain disulphide (S-S) bonds.
- The protein is ***precipitated with full saturation of ammonium sulphate.***
- The molecule is ellipsoidal in shape, measuring 150 Å × 30Å.

Site of Synthesis: Albumin is **mainly synthesized in liver.** Rate of synthesis is approximately 14.0 gm/day.

FUNCTIONS OF ALBUMIN

- It exerts low viscosity.
- Contributes 70 to 80% of osmotic pressure and plays an important role in exchange of water between tissue fluid and blood.
- Also undergoes constant exchange with the albumin present in extracellular spaces of muscles, skin and intestines.
- Helps in transport of several substances, viz. FFA(NEFA/UFA), unconjugated bilirubin, Ca^{++} and steroid hormones.

- Certain drugs also blind to albumin, e.g. sulphonamides, aspirin, penicillin, etc. and are transported to target tissue.
- *Nutritive function:* Albumin in plasma is in a dynamic state with a rapid turnover with a specific half-life. It is delivered to cells where it is hydrolyzed and cellular proteins are synthesized.

The pattern of serum proteins on electrophoresis may be used in the diagnosis of diseases

Normal values	*% of Total Proteins*
Albumin	50-70%
α_1-Globulin	2-6%
α_2- Globulin	5-11%
β-Globulin	7-16%
γ-Globulin	11-22%
	Total Gram/100 ml
Albumin	3.7-5.3
α_1-Globulin	0.1-0.4
α_2- Globulin	0.4-0.8
β-Globulin	0.5-1.3
γ-Globulin	0.6-1.5

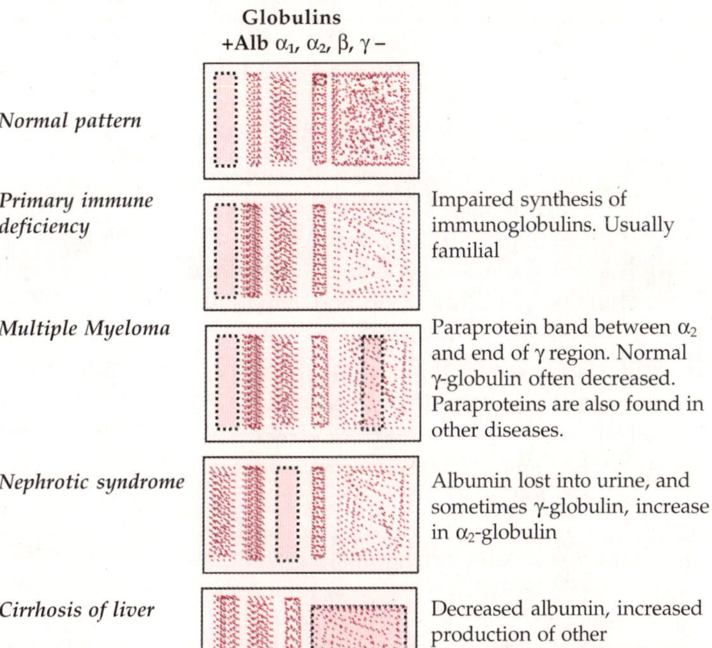

Infection — Elevated α_2 globulin and α_1 globulin, usually decreased albumin.

Chronic lymphatic leukaemia — Quite often accompanied by decreased γ-Globulin

Plasma should not be used — *If plasma is used instead of Serum, fibrinogen band gives the appearance of a paraprotein, leading to misleading diagnosis.*

α_1 antitrypsin deficiency

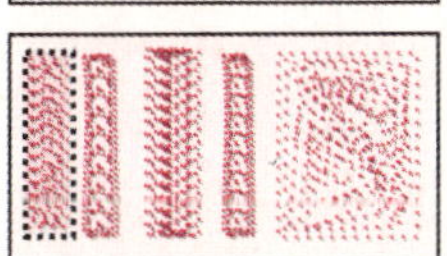

α_1 (antitrypsin) deficiency associated with emphysema of the lung in adults, and Juvenile Cirrhosis.

Fig. 4.1: Electrophoresis pattern of serum proteins

BIOMEDICAL IMPORTANCE

Decrease in albumin concentration: Concentration of albumin decreases in severe protein calorie malnutrition (PCM), liver diseases like cirrhosis liver, (albumin synthesis impaired), nephrotic syndrome (albumin is lost in urine). Decrease in albumin concentration leads to edema formation. ***Oedema occurs when total proteins fall below about 5.0 gm% and albumin level below approx. 2.5 gm%.***

B. *Globulins: Globulins are separated by half saturation with ammonium sulphate,* molecular weight ranges from 90,000 to 13,00,000. By electrophoresis, globulins can be separated into different fractions, viz. α_1-globulins, α_2-globulins, β-globulins and γ-globulins.

Site of synthesis: α-and β-globulins are synthesized in liver. But γ-globulins are synthesized by plasma cells and B-cells of lymphoid tissues (RE system). *Nature and functions of different fractions of globulins alongwith other proteins are given in* ***Table 4.2.***

Some globulins of clinical importance are discussed below:

I. α_1-Globulins

1. *Oroso-mucoid:* It is an α_1- acid glycoprotein. Normal plasma concentration is 0.6 to 1.4 gm per litre (average = 0.9). Its carbohydrate content is approximately 41%.

FUNCTIONS

- Orosomucoid is considered to be a reliable indicator of acute inflammation.
- It binds the hormone progesterone and functions as a transport protein for this hormone.

2. *α_1-fetoglobulin (α_1-feto-protein):* It is present in high concentration in foetal blood during mid-pregnancy. Normal adult blood has less than 1 μg/100 ml. It may increase during pregnancy.

Clinical Importance

Presence of α-fetoprotein is useful diagnostically in determining presence of ***hepato cellular carcinoma or teratoblastomas.*** Hence used as ***"tumor marker".***

3. *α_1-antitrypsin (α_1-AT):* It is α_1-antiprotease, molecular weight approx. 45,000 to 54,000.

- It is synthesized by liver and it is ***principal protease inhibitor (Pi)*** of human plasma. It inhibits trypsin, elastase and certain other proteases by forming complexes with them.

Note: A very low or absent α_1-globulin band in electrophoresis suggests α_1-anti-trypsin deficiency (α_1-AT).

Clinical Significance

a. ***Role in Emphysema:*** A deficiency of α_1-AT has a role to play in approx. 5% of emphysema lung cases.
b. ***Role in cirrhosis liver:*** Juvenile hepatic cirrhosis has also been correlated with α_1-AT deficiency.
c. ***Role as "tumour-marker":*** It is increased in germ cell tumours of testes and ovary.
d. ***Role as an inhibitor of fibrinolysis***

II. α_2-Globulins

1. *Ceruloplasmin:* It is a copper containing α_2-globulin, a glycoprotein with enzyme activities. Molecular weight is $\simeq$ 151,000. It has ***eight sites for binding copper.*** It contains about eight atoms of copper per molecule-½ as cuprous (Cu^+) and ½ as cupric (Cu^{++}). It carries 0.35% Cu by weight. Normal plasma contains approximately 30 mg/ 100 ml and about 75 to 100 μg of Cu may be present in 100 ml of plasma. ***It has enzyme activities,*** e.g. ***copper oxidase, histaminase*** and ***ferrous oxidase.***

Site of Synthesis: It is ***synthesized in liver*** where eight copper atoms are attached to a protein, ***"apoceruloplasmin".***

FUNCTIONS

- Although ceruloplasmin is ***not involved in copper transport,*** 90% or more of total serum copper is contained in ceruloplasmin.
- ***It mainly functions as a ferroxidase*** and helps in oxidation (conversion) of Fe^{++} to Fe^{+++} which can be incorporated into transferrin.

Table 4.2: Various Proteins which have Binding and Transport Functions

Proteins	*Mol. wt.*	*Normal value in adults mg/100 ml*	*Biological functions*
• **Prealbumin**	61,000	10-40 (mean 25)	• Binds and transports thyroxine and retinol
• **Albumin**	69,000	3500-5500 (4400)	• Osmotic, reserve protein, binding and transport of ions, pigments, drugs, etc.
• **α_1-lipoprotein (HDL)**	200,000	290-770 (360)	• Transport of various lipid fractions, fat soluble vitamins, hormones, etc. • ***Removes cholesterol from tissues to liver scavenging action.***
• **Transcortin**	45,000	(~7)	• Binding and transport of cortisol
• **TBG (thyroxine binding globulin)**	~45,000	(1-2)	• Binding and transport of thyroxine
• **Retinol binding protein**	21,000	(~4.5)	• Binding and transport of retinol
• **Ceruloplasmin (α_2 globulin)**	160,000	20-60 (35)	• Binding of copper, ferroxidase activity
• **Haptoglobin (α_2 globulin)**			
phenotypes 1-1		100-220 (170)	• Binding and transport of free Hb
2-1	100,000	160-300 (235)	• Peroxidase activity
2-2		120-260 (190)	
• **β-Lipoprotein (LDL) βLP**	3,200,000	250-800 (500)	• Transport of various fractions of lipids, (rich in cholesterol), hormones, fat soluble vitamins. • ***Carries cholesterol to tissues***
• **Haemopexin, (HPX) (β-B-globulin)**	80,000	70-130 (100)	• Haem binding
• **Transferrin, (Tr) (β globulin) (siderophilin)**	80,000 to 90,000	200-400 (295)	• Binding of Fe and transport
• **Transcobalamine I, II, and III (α_2-β mobility)**		1-20 µg/L II-60 µg/L	• Binding and transport of vit B_{12}

Clinical Importance

Increase: in serum concentration is found in pregnancy, inflammatory processes, malignancies, oral oestrogen therapy and contraceptive pills.

Decrease: Occurs in Wilson's disease and in Menke's disease (Refer Copper Metabolism).

2. ***Haptoglobin* (Hp):** This is another α_2-globulin present in plasma which is of clinical importance. It is composed of two kinds of polypeptide chains, ***two α-chains*** (possibly three) and ***only one form of β-chain.***

Site of formation: It is ***synthesized principally in liver*** by hepatocytes and to a very small extent, in RE cells.

FUNCTIONS

The function of haptoglobin is ***to bind "free Hb"*** by its α-chain and minimises urinary loss of Hb.

- Average binding capacity of Hp, irrespective of phenotype, can be taken approx. as 100 mg/dl.
- After binding, Hp-Hb complex circulates in the blood, which cannot pass through glomerular filter, and ultimately the complex is destroyed by RE cells.

Clinical Importance

Serum Hp concentration is found to be increased in inflammatory conditions.

- Determination of free Hp (or Hp-binding capacity) has been ***used to evaluate the degree of intravascular haemolysis*** which can occur in mismatched blood transfusion reactions and in heamolytic disease of the newborn (HDN).
- It is also used to evaluate the rheumatic diseases.
- ***Methaemalbumin formation:*** Where the degree of intravascular haemolysis is rapid and severe, excess of free Hb in circulation, after binding with Hp, combines with albumin to form ***methaemalbumin,*** which can be detected by sensitive ***Schumm's test.***

When free Hb exceeds 125 mg% or more, it appears in urine and the condition is called ***haemoglobinuria.***

III. β-Globulins

1. ***Transferrin:*** It is non-haem iron-containing protein and formerly used to be called as ***siderophilin.*** It exists in plasma as β-globulin-as a true carrier of Fe (Refer to Iron Metabolism).

Site of Synthesis: The protein is ***synthesized principally*** in liver. There is also evidence of its synthesis in bone marrow, spleen, and lymph nodes perhaps by lymphocytes.

FUNCTIONS

- ***Sole function is the transport of Fe*** between intestine and site of synthesis of Hb and other Fe-containing proteins.
- Recently, it has also been seen that ***unsaturated transferrin has a bacteriostatic function*** which is attributed to sequestration of Fe required by microorganisms.

Clinical Importance

Increase: Serum transferrin levels are seen increased in iron deficiency anaemia and in last months of pregnancy.

Decrease: Serum transferrin decrease parallels albumin decrease in conditions like-protein calorie malnutrition (PCM), cirrhosis liver, nephrotic syndrome, acute illness such as trauma, myocardial infarction and malignancies or other wasting diseases.

IV. γ-Globulins

These are immunoglobulins having antibody activity (see below).

OTHER PROTEINS OF CLINICAL INTEREST

1. Bence-Jones' Protein

- An abnormal protein occurs in blood and urine of people suffering from a disease called ***multiple myeloma*** (a plasma cell tumour). It is defined as "monoclonal" light chains present in the urine of patients with paraproteinaemic states.
- Either monoclonal 'κ' or 'λ' light chains are excreted in significant amount in about 50% cases of multiple myeloma. It has a molecular weight 45000 and has sedimentation co-efficient of 3.5 S. Sometimes the chains excreted may be a "dimer" of L-chains.

Identification

- The protein is identified easily in urine by a simple ***Heat test.*** On heating the urine to 50° to 60°C, Bence-Jones' proteins are precipitated, but when heated further it dissolves again. ***Reverse occurs on cooling.***
- Best detected by zone electrophoresis and immunoelectrophoresis of concentrated urine.

C. Fibrinogen: A soluble glycoprotein, also called as clotting factor I, as it takes part in coagulation of blood, and it is the precursor of fibrin, the substance required for clotting.

Normally, it constitutes 4 to 6% of total proteins of blood. Like globulins, ***it is also precipitated with 1/5th saturation of ammo-nium sulphate.*** Molecular weight ranges between 350,000 and 450,000. It has a ***large asymmetrical molecule,*** which is highly elongated having an axial ratio about 20:1. ***Being asymmetrical and large, it is important for viscosity of blood.***

Site of Synthesis: These are ***formed in liver.*** Concentration in blood decreases rapidly in liver disease where there is extensive destruction of liver tissues.

Structure:

- It is **made of six polypeptide chains,** 2A α, 2Bβ and 2 γ chains (thus, formula is A α_2

B β_2 γ_2) α, β and γ-chains are linked together lengthwise by S-S linkages.

- The terminal portions have helical structures and also *forms two swellings,* one at each end.
- The **head end carries a high –ve charge** ***due to presence of aspartate, glutamate and tyrosine-O-SO_4 residues.***
- These –vely charged termini of the fibrinogen molecules not only contribute to its water solubility, but ***also repulse the termini of other fibrinogen molecules thereby preventing aggregation (clotting).***

FUNCTIONS OF PLASMA PROTEINS

- *Nutritive:* Plasma proteins are simple proteins and a good source of proteins, thus, are largely involved in the nutritive functions. It is useful in hypoproteinaemic states. ***Plasma proteins contribute amino acids for tissue-protein synthesis.***
- *Fluid Exchange:* The colloid osmotic pressure of plasma proteins plays an important role in the distribution of water between the blood and tissues ***(Fig. 4.2).***

  At the ***arterial end*** of capillary, hydrostatic pressure exerted is greater than the osmotic pressure. ***Net filtration pressure is 7 mm Hg which drives the fluid out from vessels to tissue spaces.*** On the other hand, in the ***venous end*** of capillary loop, osmotic pressure is greater than the hydrostatic pressure and ***net absorption pressure is 8 mm Hg which draws fluid from tissue spaces into the vessels.*** This explanation of the mechanism of exchange of fluids and dissolved materials between the blood and tissue spaces is called the ***Starling hypothesis.***
- *Buffering Action:* The serum proteins, like other proteins, are ***amphoteric,*** and thus can combine with acids or bases. ***In acidic pH,*** NH_2 group acts as base and accept a proton and thus converted to $NH^+{}_3$ and ***alkaline pH*** COOH group acts as acid and can donate a "proton" and thus have COO^-.
- ***Binding and Transport Function:*** Already discussed above. See ***Table 4.2*** for important proteins which bind and transport various substances.
- *Viscosity of Blood:* Due to presence of proteins blood is a viscous fluid. ***Globulins and fibrinogen, which are large in size and asymmetrical, accounts for the viscosity of blood.*** The viscosity of blood provides resistance to flow of blood in the blood vessels for maintenance of normal range of blood pressure.
- ***Reserve Proteins:*** The amino acids from plasma proteins can be taken up by tissues

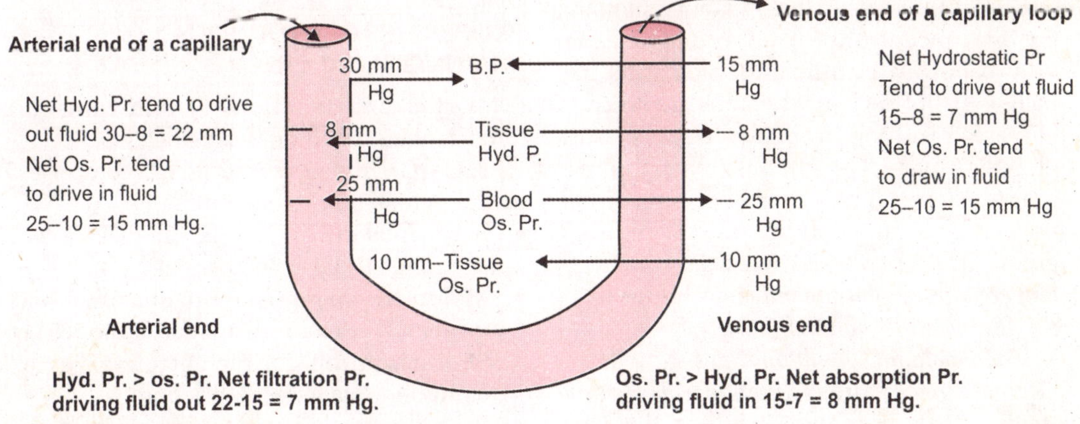

Fig. 4.2: Showing fluid exchange in capillary bed (Hyd. Pr. = Hydrostatic pressure, Os. Pr. = Osmotic pressure, BP = Blood Pressure)

and used for building up new tissue proteins and *vice versa.*

- ***Role in Blood Coagulation and Fibrinolysis:*** In addition to prothrombin and fibrinogen, plasma contains a number of other components, enzymes and clotting factors which participates in the process of coagulation of blood. Intravascular clot known as ***thrombus***, whenever it is formed is digested by the enzymes of fibrinolytic system present in the plasma, which saves from the disastrous effects of thrombosis.
- ***Immunological Function (Body Defence):*** γ-globulins are present in plasma which are antibodies and protect body against microbial infections (refer Immunoglobulins below).
- ***Enzymes: Enzymes are proteins.*** Enzymes like *amylase, transaminases, dehydrogenases, lipases, phosphatases,* etc. are present in small quantities in normal blood. They show quantitative variation, increase/decrease with different disease processes, and thus ***their estimation in blood is of immense help in diagnosis of diseases, and serial estimations help in assessing prognosis.***

Variations in Plasma Proteins

1. *Increase* in total proteins called as ***hyperproteinaemia*** can occur in two situations, they are:

- Haemoconcentration due to dehydration where both albumin and globulins are increased, but A:G ratio remains unaltered.
- Diseases resulting in high levels of plasma globulins-mainly γ-globulins (hypergammaglobulinaemias). Albumin remains either normal or reduced. If albumin is reduced grossly, the A:G ratio is reversed.

  Hypergammaglobulinaemia may be due to:
  - *"Polyclonal" gammopathies*
  - *"Monoclonal" gammopathies*

2. Decrease in total proteins called as ***Hypoproteinaemia*** can occur in two situations, they are:

- ***Haemodilution:*** Where both albumin and globulins are decreased, A:G ratio remains unaltered.
- Conditions resulting in low albumin level is more common accompanied either by no increase in globulin or by an increase which is less than the fall in albumin. **A:G ratio is decreased.** Hypoproteinaemia may also take place due to decrease in γ-globulin (Hypogammaglobulinaemia).

IMMUNOGLOBULINS

Definition: The immunoglobulins constitute a heterogeneous family of serum proteins, which either functions as antibodies or are chemically related to antibodies. On electrophoresis, they mainly occupy the γ-globulin position but also occur in the β- and α_2 regions.

Classification: Immunoglobulins (Igs) are divided into **five** main classes according to their molecular weight, elctrophoretic mobility, ultracentrifugal sedimentation and other properties ***(Table 4.3).***

Table 4.3: WHO Classification

Classes	*Corresponding old Nomenclatures*
• IgG (or γ G)	7S γ, γ_2, γ ss, 6.6s γ
• IgA(or γ A)	γ_1A, β_2A, 7sγ^1
• IgM (or γ M)	19sγ,γ_1M, β_2M
• IgD (or γ D)	—
• IgE(γ E)	—

PROPERTIES OF INDIVIDUAL IMMUNOGLOBULINS

Properties and functions of following three important Igs are discussed below:

1. IgG (γG): In a normal adult, IgG comprises 70 to 80% of total immunoglobulins.

- It amounts to 1200 mg/100 ml plasma (average range = 600 to 1600 mg%).
- Molecular weight is approximately 145,000 (previously determined as 160,000 to 165,000).
- Sedimentation coefficient of IgG is 6.7s (commonly called as 7s fraction).
- It is a glycoprotein, and carbohydrate contents is about 2.5%.
- Electrophoretic mobility in slow $\gamma_2 \rightarrow$ fast γ_1
- ***Transport across placenta*** ++++.

Note: ***IgG is the only class of Igs that can cross the placenta freely and it is responsible for the protection of newborn during the first month of life.***

Several antibodies have been identified which contain IgG. IgG class represents the most of antibacterial and antiviral antibodies thus majority of acquired antibodies are in this fraction.

2. **IgM (γM):** They constitute approximately 7% (3 to 10%) of total Igs in an adult.
   - They amount 100 ± 25 mg/100 ml of plasma (range 60 to 170 mg%)
   - They are the largest Igs molecules. Molecular weight-900,000 to 1,000,000.
   - Sedimentation Co-efficient ranges from 17s to 20s (usually called as 19s globulins).
   - Carbohydrate content of IgM molecule is about 10%. ***They cannot pass through the placenta.***
   - Antigen binding avidity of IgM is greater than that of IgG molecules. ***In early immune response to most antigens, IgM antibodies play a pivotal role.***

Note:
- In **nephrotic syndrome**, IgG and IgA may be lost in urine, but IgM molecules are not lost.
- On the other hand in **protein losing enteropathy**, all Igs are lost equally.

3. **IgA(gA):** IgA accounts for 10-20% of total plasma immunoglobulins in an adult.
   - Normal adult level is approximately 200 ± 50 mg/100 ml (range = 150 to 250 mg%).
   - These are mainly 7s globulins. Sedimentation co-efficient varies from 7 s to 13 s due to the capability to polymerise
   - ***Carbohydrate content:*** They differ from IgG in having 4 times carbohydrates. Carbohydrate content of IgA molecule is about 10%.
   - Molecular weight varies from 150,000 to 500,000.

IgA in secretion (Non-vascular IgA): In addition to its antibody function in serum, IgA is the predominant immunoglobulin class in body secretions. It is found in external secretions such as colostrum, saliva, tears, GI fluids, prostatic secretion, nasal and bronchial secretions.

Secretory IgA: IgA present in these secretions is in the form of
- **Higher polymer:** Molecular weight of secretory IgA is approximately 400,000.
- In addition, antigenically it is slightly different from serum IgA.

This dissimilarity between vascular IgA and non-vascular IgA is due to presence of another small protein, called ***transport piece (T-Protein or secretory protein or transport protein).*** T-piece is a single polypeptide chain of approximately molecular weight of 70,000.

FUNCTIONS OF T-PIECE

This protein is responsible for two important biological properties of nonvascular IgA.
- Its selective transport from serum to secretions or to facilitate the transport of IgA molecule synthesized in lymphoid cells beneath the epithelium.
- Probably, it protects the IgA molecule against digestion by proteolytic enzymes like those found in GI tract.

Antibody Functions of IgA Molecule:
- Secretory IgA provides the primary defence mechanism against some local infections owing to its abundance in saliva, tears, bronchial secretions, the nasal mucosa, prostatic fluid, vaginal secretions and mucous secretions of small intestine. Thus, ***IgA appears to be essential for warding off sino-bronchial infections.***

4. **IgD(γD):** IgD is a class of immunoglobulin discovered by **Rowe** and **Fahey** (1965), who first detected the new protein in serum of a myeloma patient.
   - This Ig is normally present in serum in trace amount, 0.2% of total Igs.
   - It is a monomer and its molecular weight is approximately 180,000.
   - Sedimentation co-efficient is 7 to 8s (slightly higher than that of IgG).

- Mean serum IgD concentration is 3 mg%, but wide variations have been reported.
  Antibody Functions: The main function and the role is not yet determined but following has been reported:
  IgD along with IgM is the predominant immunoglobulin on the surface of human B lymphocytes and it has been suggested that IgD may be involved in the differentiation of these cells.

5. **IgE (γE):** The identification of IgE antibodies as ***reagins*** (or reaginic antibodies) and characterization of this Ig class has marked a major breakthrough in the study of the mechanism involved in allergic disease like hay fever, asthma, etc.

- It is a monomer. Molecular weight approximately 190,000 to 200,000
- Sedimentation coefficient is 8s.
- It comprises only 0.004% of the total serum immunoglobulins.
- Serum level varies from 10 to 70 μg per 100 ml.

Antibody Function of IgE:

- ***Allergic response:*** Combination of IgE ('reagin' or reaginic antibody) with certain specific antigens, called allergens, IgE triggers release from ***mast cells*** of the pharmacologic mediators responsible for the characteristic "wheal" and "flare" skin reactions evoked by the exposure of the skin of allergic individuals to allergens.
- ***Role in Inflammation:*** IgE not only fixes to skin sites, but can also fix to leucocytes and other cells including mast cells. Thus, it can release mediators of inflammation upon exposure to allergens or antigens. These may be important protective mechanisms.
- ***Defence against worm infections:*** IgE defends against worm infections by causing release of enzymes from eosinophils. It does not fix complement. IgE offers main host defense against helminthic infections.

Clinical Aspect

- IgE deficiency has been demonstrated with chronic sino-pulmonary infection.
- IgE deficiency also demonstrated in 11/16 patients with *Ataxia telangiectasia*, a familial disorder of progressive cerebellar ataxia, oculocutaneous telangiectasia and frequent sino-pulmonary infection.

Structure and Chemistry of Immunoglobulins —Model of Ig Molecule (Fig. 4.3)

- The Ig molecule has a V-shape. Each molecule is composed of equal numbers of **two heavy ('H'-chains)** and **two light (L) polypeptide chains** which can be represented by the general formula H_2L_2.
- The chains are held together by non-covalent forces and ***usually covalent interchain disulphide bridges*** to form a bilaterally symmetric structure.
- Each polypeptide chain is made up of a number of loops or ***domains*** of rather constant size (100 to 110 amino acid residues) formed by the intrachain disulphide bonds.
- The N-terminal domain of each chain shows much more variation in amino acid sequence than the others and is designated as ***variable region (v-region)*** to distinguish it from the other relatively constant domains collectively called as ***constant region*** *in* each chain.

Heavy Chain Classes (H-chains): Five classes of H-chains have been identified in human Igs based on structural differences in the constant regions by serologic and chemical methods.

- The different forms of H-chains are designated as-**γ *(gamma)*, α *(alpha)*, μ *(mu)*, δ *(delta)* and ε *(epsilon)*.**
- ***The class of the H-chain determines the class of immunoglobulins.*** Thus, there are ***five classes*** of Igs as discussed above-IgG, IgA, IgM, IgD and IgE, having H-chains γ, α, μ, δ and ε respectively.

Light Chain Types: All L-chains have a molecular weight of approximately 23,000, and are classified into ***two types-"Kappa" (κ) and "lambda" (λ).***

- The proportions of κ to λ chains in Ig molecule varies from species to species, being about 2:1 in humans.

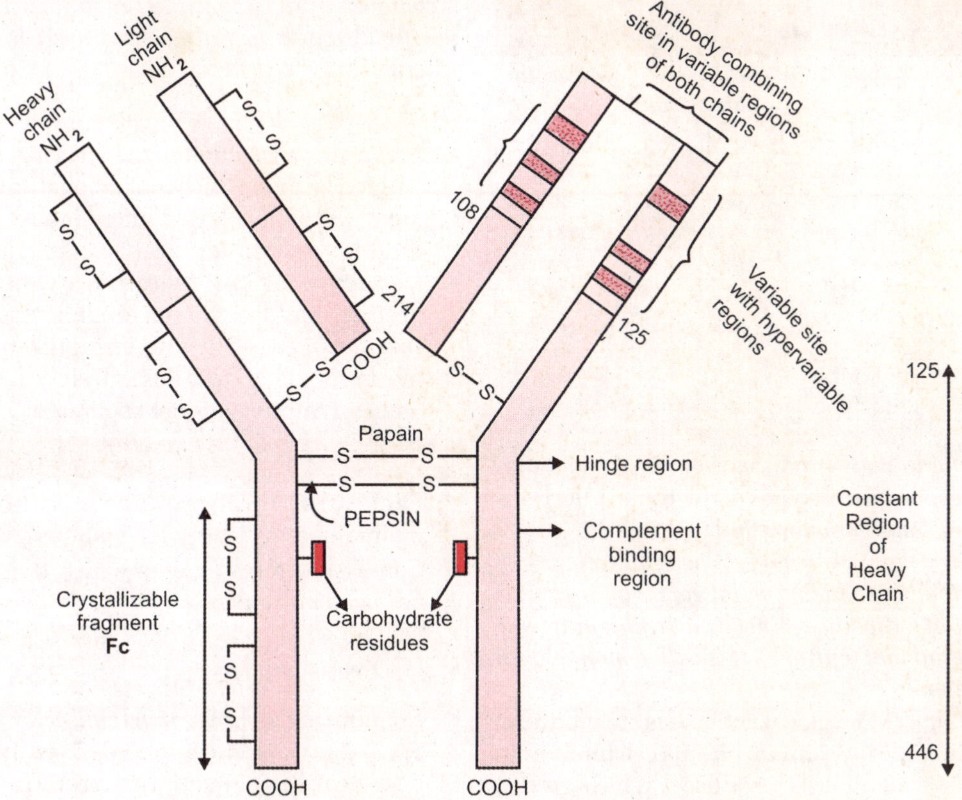

Fig. 4.3: Structure of Immunoglobulin

- ***A given Ig molecule always contains identical κ or λ chains but never both.***

Molecular Formula: Each Ig may be written as formula which expresses both its 'H' and 'L' chains constitutions as in *Table 4.4.*

Degradation of Igs by Proteolytic Enzymes:

- *Papain:* Splits the molecule into **three fragments:**
  - **Two 'Fab' fragments** which include an entire 'L' chain and the VH and CH-1 domains of a heavy chain and,
  - **One 'Fc' fragment**-composed of C-terminal halves of H-chains
- *Pepsin:* Splits the Ig molecule into a large **F (ab)$_2$ fragment** composed of about 2 'Fab' fragments. Fc fragments is extensively degraded.

Antigen Binding Site: Antigen binding activity is associated with the "Fab" fragments or more specifically with V_H and V_L domains (variable regions).

POLYCLONAL vs. MONOCLONAL ANTIBODY: HYBRIDOMA

1. **Polyclonal antibody:** In response to an antigenic challenge the body produces different types of antibodies **against various antigenic determinants (epitopes)** of the antigen. ***The antibodies thus produced are called polyclonal antibodies.*** Under such a situation, the different "clones" of antibody forming cells simultaneously synthesizes the antibody. Different molecules will have different specificities and affinities.

Table 4.4: Type and Molecular Formula of Each Class

Ig Class	*Type*	*H chains*	*L chains*	*Molecular formula*
IgG	IgG K type	γ	κ	$\gamma_2\kappa_2$
	IgG L type	γ	λ	$\gamma_2\lambda_2$
IgA	IgA K type	α	κ	$\alpha_2\kappa_2$
	IgA L type	α	λ	$\alpha_2\lambda_2$
IgM	IgM K type	μ	κ	$\mu_2\kappa_2$
	IgM L type	μ	λ	$\mu_2\lambda_2$
IgD	IgD K type	δ	κ	$\delta_2\kappa_2$
	IgD L type	δ	λ	$\delta_2\lambda_2$
IgE	IgE K type	ε	κ	$\varepsilon_2\kappa_2$
	IgE L type	ε	λ	$\varepsilon_2\lambda_2$

Example: Body produces polyclonal antibodies in response to all types of microbial infections *(polyclonal gammopathy).*

2. **Monoclonal antibody:** ***When one "clone" of antibody producing cells secrete a particular type of antibody against a particular antigenic determinant (epitope), it is called monoclonal antibody.***
   Example: Monoclonal antibodies are produced in multiple myeloma, a plasma cell tumour. In this para protein is produced, which gives a sharp para protein band in β to γ region **(M-band)** in electrophoresis ***(monoclonal gammopathy).***

- ***In vitro*** in the laboratory monoclonal antibodies can be produced by the hybridoma technology.

3. **Hybridoma:** ***Hybridoma is a hybrid cell capable of producing monoclonal antibodies.*** It has been possible to fuse two different types of cultured animal cells, the resulting "hybrid" cell contained the chromosome of both the parent cells. **Kohler** and **Milstein,** in 1975, first produced monoclonal antibodies from hybridoma cells. They showed that cultured splenic cells from mouse immunized with specific antigen can be fused with that of cultured mouse myeloma cells. ***The hybrid cells so produced will remain "immortal in culture" like the myeloma cell and produce monoclonal antibodies like the immunized splenic cells.***

Technique: In principle, the technique of hybridoma cell production is rather simple. It is shown schematically in next page.

Steps

- ***Preparation of immunized spleen cells:*** The antigen against which monoclonal antibodies are required is injected into a mouse, so that the mouse is immunized. Dose, route and frequency of antigen administration for optimal yield of monoclonal antibodies is standardized. After the immunization, the mouse is killed and the spleen is removed. Spleen lymphocytes are separated.

Properties of Splenic Cells

- **Lack proliferation**, hence cannot be maintained in culture for long periods
- Can produce Igs against which the animal has been immunized
- *HGPRTase* +
- HAT resistant

- ***Preparation of mouse myeloma cells:*** Usually Sp 2/0 myeloma cell line derived from Bal b/c mouse is used for preparation of hybridoma cell.

Properties of Myeloma Cells

- ***Proliferation +, cells are self-propagating*** in tissue culture and can be maintained indefinitely.
- Cannot produce Igs (antibody).
- Lacks the enzyme *HGPRTase*, hence they cannot synthesize DNA by salvage pathway.

- ***Preparation of cell mixture:*** Immunized splenic lymphocytes are mixed with mouse myeloma cells in the ratio of $10^8 : 2 \times 10^7$.
- ***Fusion of the two cells:*** Fusion of the splenic cells with myeloma cells is brought about by the addition of **"polyethylene glycol"** (PEG-1500). Fused cell mixture is maintained in tissue culture in "HAT" medium.

HAT medium: contains

- **hypoxanthine,**
- **aminopterin,** and
- **thymidine.**

Aminopterin, a folic acid antagonist will inhibit the *"de Novo"* synthesis of purines.

- ***Hybridization (Hybridoma):*** Result of fusion will be production of hybridoma cells.
- Hybrid of normal + normal cells lack proliferation, hence the ***"normal hybrids"*** die in the culture medium in 5 to 6 days.
- Unfused myeloma cells also die in HAT medium as they lack *HGPRTase*.
- Only cells that survive are the hybrid cells formed by fusion of normal immunized splenic cells and mouse myeloma cells. ***Such hybridoma cells survive in the culture medium because they can use hypoxanthine and thymidine through salvage pathway.***

Properties of Hybridoma Cell

- Can propagate for indefinite period **(Immortal).**
- **Can secrete Igs.**
- Has *HGPRTase* enzyme, hence salvage pathway of purnie synthesis can operate.

- ***Propagation of hybridoma cells:***
  - The monoclonal antibody producing hybrid cells are cloned and subcloned (separated into individual cells) in plates containing small wells.
- Supernatent medium is tested for specific antibody. The cells producing desired antibody are selected.
- These cells are propagated in culture bottles or injected into mice peritoneum where they are grown in ascitic fluid.

USES OF MONOCLONAL ANTIBODIES

(a) ***Diagnostic uses:***

- Monoclonal antibodies have been raised for the diagnosis of many bacterial, viral and parasitic diseases.
- Monoclonal antibodies have been used for blood grouping.
- Also being used for standardization and leucocyte identification through the cluster differentiation (CD antigen).
- Recently used against HLA antigens for phenotype screening purposes.

(b) ***Therapeutic uses:***

Recently, monoclonal antibodies are being used for treatment, viz.

- anti tumour therapy
- immunosuppression in organ transplantation

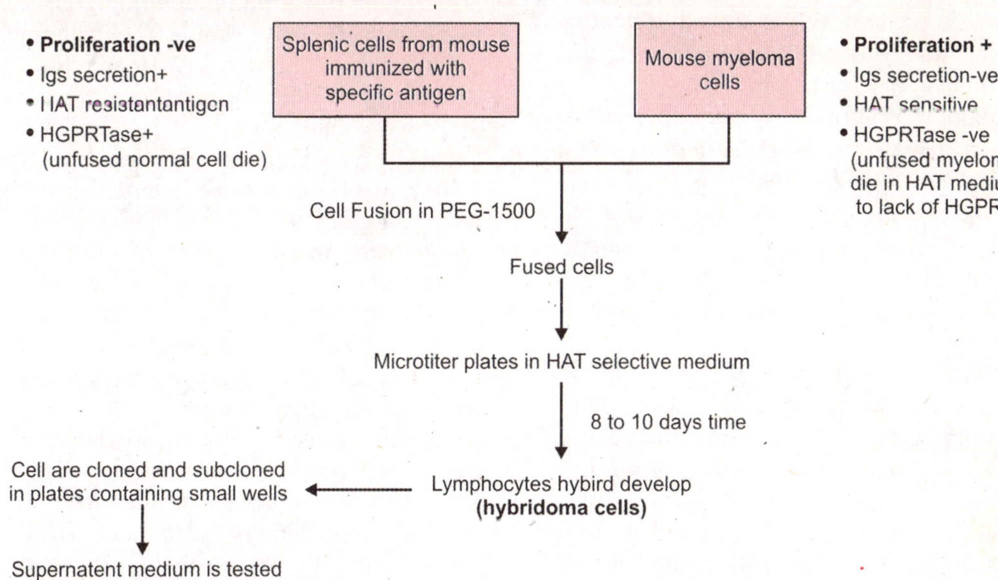

- and in auto-immune diseases, e.g. recently in rheumatoid arthritis monoclonal CD_4 antibody tried.

☞ SALIENT POINTS TO REMEMBER

- The total concentration of plasma proteins is about 7.0 to 7.5 gm percentage.
- Proteins of plasma can be separated into different fractions—albumin, globulins and fibrinogen by salting out technique.
- Albumins are precipitated on full saturation with ammonium sulphate, globulins by half-saturation and fibrinogen by 1/5th saturation of ammonium sulphate.
- Electrophoretically serum proteins are separated into distinct fractions, viz. albumin, α_1 globulin, α_2 globulin, β globulin and γ- globulins.
- Albumin is the major constituent (60%) of plasma proteins with a concentration of 3.7 to 5.2 gm percent.
- Albumin is exclusively synthesized in liver and have nutritive function, exerts low viscosity, and 70 to 80% osmotic pressure, fluid exchange in capillary bed and binding and transport certain proteins and drugs.
- Caeruloplasmin, a Cu-containing α_2 globulin, a glycoprotein is synthesized in liver. It mainly functions as ***"ferro-oxidase"*** and helps in oxidation of Fe^{++} to Fe^{+++}.
- Haptoglobin is another α_2 globulin, synthesized principally in liver and ***mops up free Hb produced by intravascular haemolysis.***
- Average binding capacity of Hp is approximately 100 mg/dl. Hp-Hb complex circulates in the blood. It cannot pass through glomerular filter and ultimately the complex is destroyed by RE cells.
- Transferrin is a β-globulin, synthesized principally in liver. Its main function is to transport Fe between intestine and site of synthesis of Hb and other Fe containing proteins.
- Bence-Jones' protein, an abnormal protein found characteristically in blood and urine of people suffering from a ***disease called multiple myeloma (a plasma cell tumor).***
- This abnormal protein can be identified easily in urine by a ***simple heat test.*** On heating the urine in a test tube to 50° to 60°C, Bence-Jones' proteins get precipitated, but when heated further precipitate dissolves. The reverse occurs on cooling.
- Immunoglobulins (Igs) are specialized proteins to defend the body against foreign substances such as bacteria, viruses and proteins.
- They function as antibodies and are chemically related to antibodies.
- On electrophoresis, they mainly occupy the γ-globulin position but may occur in the β and α_2 regions.
- Five classes of immunoglobulin, viz. IgG, IgA, IgM, IgD and IgE are found in humans.
- IgG is most abundant and is mainly responsible for humoral immunity.
- Both IgG and IgM are involved for humoral immunity. ***IgG seems to have evolved later than IgM***. The sequence in the organism's response to antigenic stimulation usually consists of IgM being produced initially, followed later, and ultimately replaced by IgG.
- IgE is associated with allergic reactions. IgE can fix to mast cells and can release pharmacologic mediators.
- Structurally the immunoglobulins consist of two identical "Heavy chains" (H-chains) and two identical "Light chains" (L-chains) held together by disulfide bridges.
- The heavy chains are γ, α, μ, δ and ε respectively in IgG, IgA, IgM, IgD and IgE.
- The ***type of H-chains in a Ig molecule determines the class of Igs.***
- Light chains are of 2 types: "κ" (kappa) and 'λ' (lambda).
- A given Ig molecule always contains identical 'κ' or 'λ' chains **but never both.**
- Ig molecules can be degraded by proteolytic enzymes like papain or pepsin.
- Antigen binding activity is associated with the "Fab" fragments or more specifically with V_H and V_L domains (variable region).
- ***IgG is the only class of Igs that can cross the placenta*** and it is responsible for the protection of the newborn during the first month of life.

MULTIPLE CHOICE QUESTIONS

Give one correct answer:

1. **The number of amino acids present in one molecule of albumin are:**
(a) 510 (b) 580
(c) 600 (d) 610
(e) 650

2. **Normal level of albumin in blood is:**
(a) 1.5 to 2.5 mg/dl
(b) 2.5 to 3.0 mg/dl
(c) 3.0 to 3.5 mg/dl
(d) 3.5 to 4.0 gm/dl
(e) 3.7 to 5.3 gm/dl

3. **All the following are bound with albumin in blood, *except:***
(a) Unconjugated bilirubin
(b) Sulphonamides
(c) Iron
(d) Non-esterified fatty acid (NEFA)
(e) Aspirin

4. **One caeruloplasmin molecule can bind _____ copper ions:**
(a) 4 (b) 6
(c) 8 (d) 10
(e) 12

5. **Plasma proteins which are precipitated best by 1/5th saturation of ammonium sulphate.**
(a) Albumin (b) Fibrinogen
(c) α_2-globulin (d) β-globulins
(e) Euglobulin

6. **Transferrin can bind ____ atoms of Fe^{++} per molecule:**
(a) 1 (b) 2
(c) 3 (d) 4 (e) 5

7. **β-globulin fraction contains:**
(a) Oroso-mucoid
(b) Transferrin
(c) Haptoglobin
(d) Bence-Jones Protein
(e) TBG (Thyroxine binding globulin)

8. **Haemopexin carries which of the following:**
(a) Free bilirubin
(b) Free copper
(c) Free haemoglobin
(d) Free heme
(e) Free iron

9. **Which of the following immunoglobulin is a pentamer?**
(a) IgG, (b) IgM
(c) IgA (d) IgE
(e) IgD

10. **The serum antibody responsible for fighting gm +ve pyogenic bacteria is:**
(a) IgD (b) IgE
(c) IgG (d) IgA
(e) All of the above

11. **The immunoglobulin that binds to mast cells is:**
(a) IgA (b) IgE
(c) IgG (d) IgM
(e) IgD

12. **Which immunoglobulin possesses the highest molecular weight?**
(a) IgA (b) IgG
(c) IgD (d) IgM
(e) IgE

13. **Which of the following immunoglobulins can cross the placenta?**
(a) IgM (b) IgG
(c) IgA (d) IgD
(e) IgE

14. **Which of the immunoglobulins class has reaginic antibody?**
(a) IgG (b) IgM
(c) IgD (d) IgE
(e) IGA

15. **The antigen binding capacity resides at which site of the immunoglobulin molecule:**
(a) Hinge region (b) Constant region
(c) Variable region (d) Fc fragment
(e) T-Piece

ANSWERS

1. (d)	2. (e)	3. (c)	4. (c)
5. (b)	6. (b)	7. (b)	8. (d)
9. (b)	10. (c)	11. (b)	12. (d)
13. (b)	14. (d)	15. (c)	

Chemistry of Nucleotides

NUCLEOPROTEINS

INTRODUCTION

- A group of *conjugated proteins.*
- Characterized by the *presence of non-protein prosthetic group, nucleic acid,* and are attached to one or more molecules of a simple protein and a basic protein—*histone or protamine.*
- Nucleoproteins are so named because they constitute a large part of nuclear material. Chromatin is largely composed of nucleoproteins, which indicates that these compounds are involved in cell division, and transmission of hereditary factors.

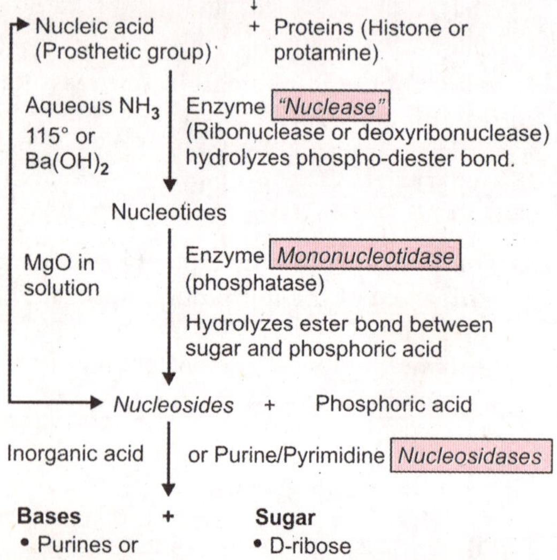

COMPOSITION

When the purified nucleoprotein is hydrolyzed with acid or by the use of enzymes, various components as shown in LHS are obtained.

SUGARS

- **D-ribose** and **D-2 deoxyribose** are the only sugars so far found in the nucleic acids from which the sugars have been isolated and identified, and they are assumed to be the sugars universally present in nucleic acids.

D-ribose *D-2-deoxyribose*

Both sugars are present in nucleic acids as the ***β-Furanoside ring structures*** as depicted below.

β-*D-ribofuranose* β-*D-2-deoxyribofuranose*

PYRIMIDINE BASES

There are mainly **three pyrimidine bases** found in nucleic acids.

- **Cytosine** is found both in DNA and RNA
- **Thymine** is found in DNA only
- **Uracil** is found in RNA only.

A pyrimidine nucleus is represented below:

All the pyrimidine bases can exist in ***lactam*** and ***lactim form***. If the group is –HN-CO-, it is called as *lactam* type *(keto)*, while the same if isomerizes to-N=C-OH, it is called *lactim* form *(enol)*.

At the physiological pH, the *lactam* (keto) forms are predominant.

1. **Cytosine:** Chemically cytosine is a ***"2-deoxy-4 amino pyrimidine"***, which can exist both as *lactam* or *lactim* forms.

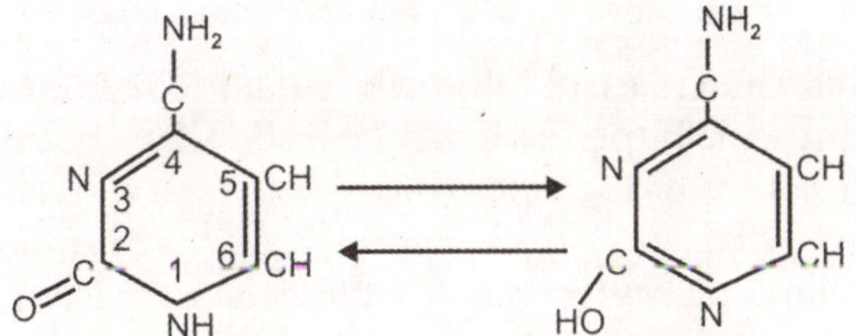

Lactam form of cytosine (Keto) ***Lactim form of cytosine (Enol)***

- Cytosine is found in all nucleic acids except DNA of certain viruses.

2. **Thymine (5-methyl uracil):** Chemically it is **2, *4-deoxy-5-methyl pyrimidine.***

- Thymine ***occurs only in DNA***, which contain deoxyribose as sugar.
- Minor amounts have recently been found in t-RNA.

Lactam form of thymine ***Lactim form of thymine***

3. **Uracil:** Chemically it is **2, *4-dioxy pyrimidine.***

- ***Uracil is confined to RNA only, not found in DNA.***

Lactam form of uracil ***Lactim form of uracil***

- In addition to three major pyrimidine bases, there occurs in small quantities bases like 5-OH-methyl cytosine, methylated derivatives and reduced uracil compounds.

PURINE BASES

The Purine ring is more complex than the pyrimidine ring. It can be considered the product of fusion of a pyrimidine ring with an imidazole ring.

Pyrimidine ***Imidazole***

Purine nucleus

Adenine and guanine are the two principal purines found in both DNA and RNA.

1. **Adenine:** Chemically it is ***6-amino purine.***

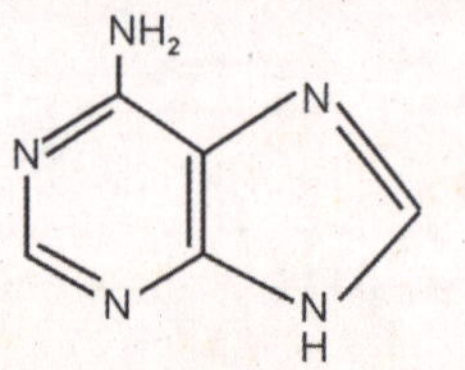

Adenine (6-aminopurine)

2. **Guanine:** Chemically it is ***2-amino-6-oxy purine.***
   - Guanine can be present as lactam and lactim forms.

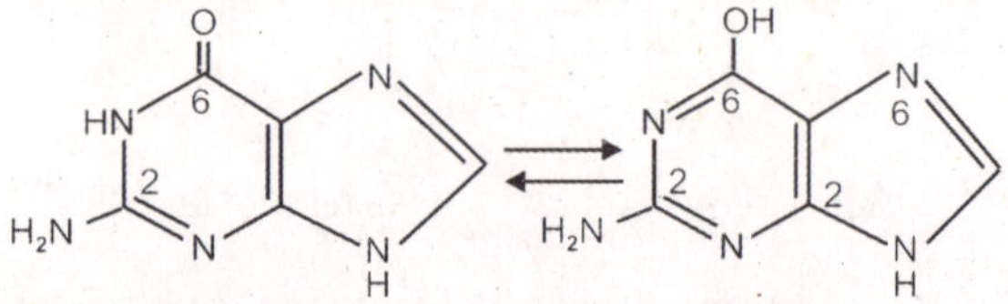

Guanine (lactam form) ⇌ *Guanine (lactim form)*

In human beings, a completely oxidized form of purine base uric acid occurs, which is of great biomedical importance. ***Uric acid is the catabolic end product of purines in human beings.***

BIOMEDICAL IMPORTANCE

Solubility of the Bases:

At neutral pH, guanine is the least soluble of the bases followed in this respect by xanthine.

- Although uric acid as urate is relatively soluble at a neutral pH, it is highly insoluble in solutions with a lower pH such as urine.
- Guanine is not normal constituent of human urine, but xanthine and uric acid occur in human urine. These two purines frequently occur as constituents of urinary tract stones, e.g. xanthine stones/and urate stones.

NUCLEOSIDES

- The nucleosides are composed of purine or pyrimidine base linked to either D-ribose (in RNA) or D-2-deoxyribose (in DNA).
- These are joined by "**β-N-glycosidic linkage**".
  - This linkage in purine nucleosides is at position-9-of the purine base and carbon 1′ of sugar or deoxy sugar.

  Example: Adenosine (adenine-9-riboside)
- In pyrimidine nucleosides, β-N-glycosidic linkage is formed at position-1 of the pyrimidine base linked to carbon-1′ of ribose or deoxyribose sugar.

  Example: Uridine (uracil-1-riboside)
- In cytidine and uridine, ribose is attached to N_1-position of cytosine and uracil respectively.

Adenosine (Adenine-9-riboside)
(Adenine purine base + ribose sugar)

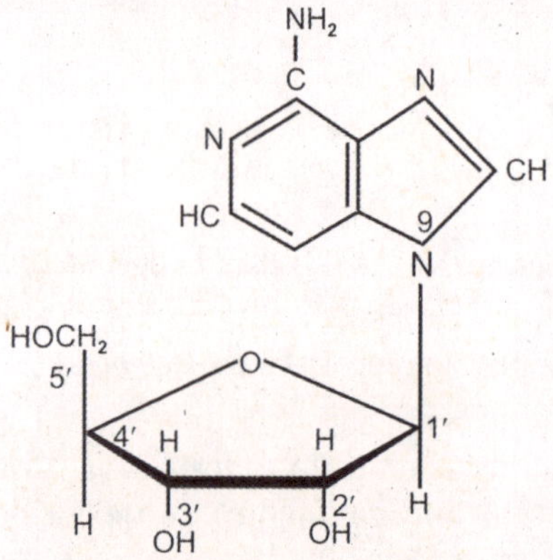

β-N-glycosidic linkage with position 9 of purine base-adenine and 1′ carbon of ribose sugar

Note: If in place of ribose, the sugar deoxyribose is present, the prefix "deoxy" may be added before the name of the nucleoside in all cases ***except thymidine. It is to be remembered that uridine remains present only in RNA but absent in DNA.***

Uridine (Uracil-1-riboside)
(Uracil pyrimidine base + ribose sugar)

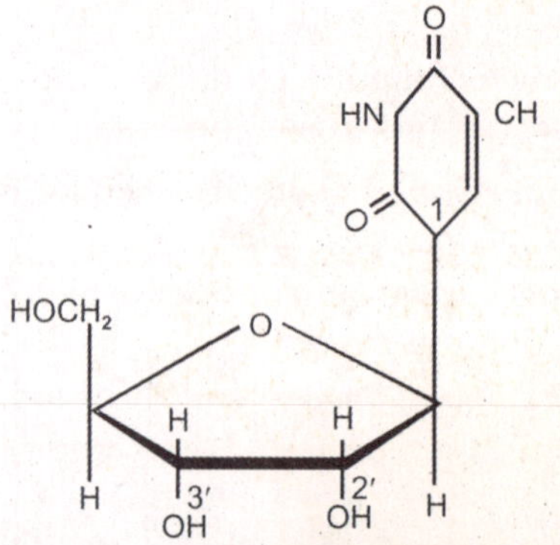

β-N-glycosidic linkage with position 1 of pyrimidine base-Uracil and 1′ carbon of ribose sugar

Table 5.1 shows the different nucleosides and their corresponding base (purine/pyrimidine) and sugar. Though these are the usual types of nucleoside, relatively small amounts of what is called ***"pseudouridine"*** (Ψ) is also present in RNA in which carbon-5-pyrimidine is linked to C-1′ of sugar.

Table 5.1: Nucleosides with their Different Bases and Sugars

Nucleoside	*Base*		*Sugar*
• **Adenosine**	Adenine	+	Ribose
• **Deoxyadenosine**	Adenine	+	Deoxyribose
• **Guanosine**	Guanine	+	Ribose
• **Deoxyguanosine**	Guanine	+	Deoxyribose
• **Uridine**	Uracil	+	Ribose
• **Cytidine**	Cytosine	+	Ribose
• **Deoxycytidine**	Cytosine	+	Deoxyribose
• **Thymidine**	Thymine	+	Deoxyribose

NUCLEOTIDES

A nucleotide is a nucleoside to which a phosphoric acid group has been attached to the sugar molecule by "esterification" at a definite –OH group, and thus has the general composition-**base-sugar-PO_4.** Thus, ***nucleotides are nucleoside-P.***

- In ribose nucleosides, there are three possible positions for phosphate esterification, namely 2′, 3′ and 5′.
- In deoxynucleosides, there are free-OH groups only at the 3′ and 5′ positions in the deoxyribose nucleosides. PO_4 can be attached only at these positions. The name of each nucleotide may be derived from its constituent nitrogenous base.

  Table 5.2 shows the different nucleotides and their corresponding base (purine/pyrimidine) and sugar.

Internucleotide Bonds

- The bond between the nucleotides is the ***"Phosphoric acid di-ester bond".***
- The phosphate di-ester bond between the nucleotides is formed mainly by 3′ OH group of sugar of one nucleotide to 5′-OH group of sugar of another nucleotide. This 3′, 5′-linkage is to be expected in DNA since these are only sugar –OH groups available in deoxyribose for the formation of phosphate di-ester bond.
- In RNA-3′-5′ linkages predominate but 2′, 3′ linkages are also possible.

SYNTHETIC ANALOGUES OF BIOMEDICAL IMPORTANCE

Synthetic analogues of nucleobases, nucleosides and nucleotides are of wide use in medical sciences and clinical medicine. Synthetic analogues have become the chief fighting weapons in the hands of oncologists for cancer chemotherapy.

Basis of Chemotherapy

- The heterocyclic ring structure or the sugar moiety is altered in such a way as to induce toxic effects when the analogues get incorporated in to cellular constituents of the body.
- ***Effects result either due to:***
  - Inhibition by the drug of specific enzyme activities necessary for the nucleic acid synthesis of the cells or,
  - Due to incorporation of metabolites of the drug into the nucleic acids, where they adversely affect the base pairing essential for accurate transferring of information.

Synthetic Derivatives: Some synthetic derivatives are described below.

SYNTHETIC DERIVATIVES

- ***6-thioguanine and 6-mercaptopurine:*** Used in clinical medicine
- ***Azapurine, Aza-cytidine, and 8-Azaguanine:*** Also used in clinical medicine
- ***Allo-purinol:*** Inhibits the enzymes *xanthine oxidase* and thus inhibits uric acid formation. Widely used for treatment of gout
- ***Cytarabine (arabinosyl cytosine, Ara-C) and vidarabine (arabinosyl adenine, Ara-A):*** Used in chemotherapy of cancer and certain viral infections.
- ***Azathioprine:*** It is catabolized to 6-mercaptopurine, used in organ transplantation to prevent immunologic graft rejection
- ***5-iodo-deoxyuridine:*** Found useful in treatment of herpetic keratitis (an infection of cornea of eye by herpes simplex virus).

Table 5.2: Nucleotides with their Corresponding Bases and Sugars

Nucleotide	Base		Sugar		Phosphoric acid
a. Present in RNA					
• Adenylic acid or Adenylate (AMP)	Adenine	+	Ribose	+	Phosphoric acid
• Guanylic acid or Guanylate (GMP)	Guanine	+	Ribose	+	Phosphoric acid
• Cytidylic acid or Cytidylate (CMP)	Cytosine	+	Ribose	+	Phosphoric acid
• Uridylic acid or Uridylate (UMP)	Uracil	+	Ribose	+	Phosphoric acid
b. Present in DNA					
• Deoxy adenylic acid or Deoxy adenylate (dAMP)	Adenine	+	Deoxyribose	+	Phosphoric acid
• Deoxy guanylic acid or Deoxy guanylate (d GMP)	Guanine	+	Deoxyribose	+	Phosphoric acid
• deoxy cytidylic acid or Deoxy cytidylate (d CMP)	Cytosine	+	Deoxyribose	+	Phosphoric acid
• Thymydylic acid or Thymidylate (TMP)	Thymine	+	Deoxyribose	+	Phosphoric acid

Note: 1. Uridylic acid occur in RNA only, hence there will be only ribose. There is no deoxy uridylic acid.
2. There is no thymidylic acid in RNA.

NUCLEOTIDES/NUCLEOSIDES OF BIOLOGICAL IMPORTANCE

Besides the nucleosides which occur as integral part of DNA and RNA, there are many biologically important nucleotides present in tissues and cells, where they have diverse biochemical functions.

CLASSIFICATION

1. *Adenosine nucleotides:* ATP, ADP, AMP and cyclic AMP.
2. *Guanosine nucleotides:* GTP, GDP, GMP and cyclic GMP.
3. *Uridine nucleotides:* UTP, UDP, UMP, UDP-G.
4. *Cytidine nucleotides:* CTP, CDP, CMP and certain deoxy CDP derivatives of glucose, choline, ethanolamine.
5. *Miscellaneous:* PAPS (active sulphate), "active" methionine (S-adenosyl methionine) certain coenzymes like NAD^+ and $NADP^+$, FAD and FMN, cobamide coenzyme, CoA.
6. *Cyclic nucleotides:* c-AMP and cyclic GMP. Only two important nucleotides are discussed here.

ADENOSINE TRI-PHOSPHATE (ATP)

It is called "***storage battery***" of the tissues. It is the storehouse of energy.

Formation of ATP: See the Chapter on Biological Oxidation.

Functions: Two of the three phosphate residues are high energy "phosphates" (~*P*) and on hydrolysis each releases energy (7.6 K cal); energy is utilized for ***"endergonic processes"***.

- Many synthetic reactions require energy, e.g. argininosuccinate synthetase reaction in the urea cycle.
- ATP is also required in the synthesis of phosphocreatine from creatine, synthesis of FA from acetyl CoA, synthesis of peptides and proteins from amino acids, formation of glucose from pyruvic acid, synthesis of glutamine, etc.
- ATP is an important source of energy for muscle contraction, transmission of nerve impulses, transport of nutrients across cell membranes, motility of spermatozoa.
- ATP is required for formation of ***"active methionine"*** which is required for methylation reactions.
- ATP donates phosphate for a variety of *phosphotransferase* reactions, e.g. hexokinase reaction.
- ATP is required for formation of ***"active" sulphate*** which is necessary for incorporation of SO_4 in compounds like formation of chondroitin SO_4 etc.

- *"In vivo"*-ATP is converted to ADP, AMP and cyclic nucleotides like 3′-5′ c-AMP which have important role to play in many biochemical processes.

CYCLIC NUCLEOTIDES

1. c-AMP

Cyclic adenosine monophosphate 3′-5′ c-AMP was first discovered as a mediator in hepatic glycogenolysis. ***Sutherland*** and ***Rall*** discovered this factor in the cell while they were studying the mechanism by which epinephrine and glucagon promoted glucose release in the liver. The structure of c-AMP was first described by the ***Markham*** and by ***Sutherland's group***. Since then work in many laboratories has established the ubiquity of c-AMP in living organisms. c-AMP in the cell is now known to participate in many important endocrinal and physiological functions in the body. Sutherland's brilliant concept of the ***second messenger***, a hypothesis which states that cyclic nucleotides mediate the effect of a variety of hormones and other biologically active agents has found ample confirmation. ***EW Sutherland (Jr) was awarded the Nobel Prize in 1971 in physiology and medicine*** for his outstanding "discoveries" concerning the mechanisms of the action of hormones.

FORMATION AND DEGRADATION OF c-AMP

c-AMP is a cyclic nucleotide and chemically it is 3′5′-adenosine monophosphate ***(Fig. 5.1)***.

c-AMP is synthesized in the tissues from ATP under the influence of an enzyme ***adenyl cyclase*** in the presence of Mg^{++} ion ***(Fig. 5.2)***. The activity of the enzyme is regulated by a series of complex interactions many of which involve hormone receptors.

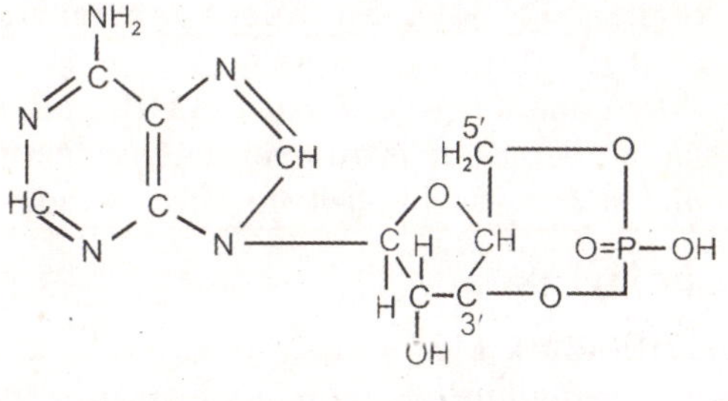

Fig. 5.1: Structure of c-AMP

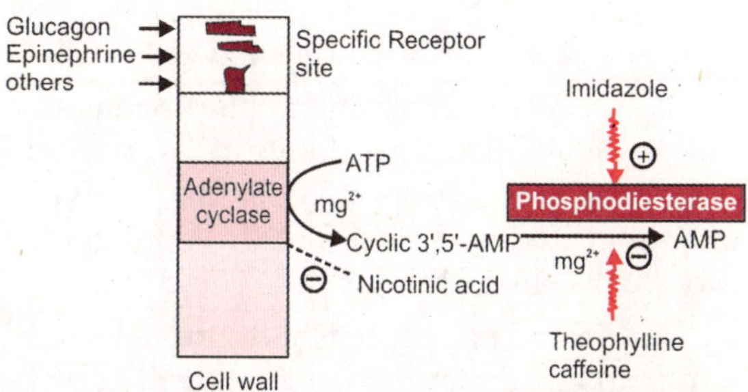

Fig. 5.2: Formation and degradation of cyclic AMP

c-AMP is degraded in the tissues by its conversion to 5′-AMP in a reaction catalyzed by the enzyme ***phosphodiesterase.***

Adenyl cyclase: The enzyme is widely distributed in nature and has been identified in every mammalian tissue studied with the ***exception of nature mammalian erythrocytes***. Adenyl cyclase has been found to be associated with either the cytoplasmic, mitochondrial or endoplasmic membrane. The profound physiological and metabolic importance of adenyl cyclase resides in the fact that its activity responds to a wide variety of hormones and other pharmacologically active agents, viz. histamine, 5-HT (serotonin), ouabain, etc. The activity of the enzyme is inhibited by insulin and prostaglandins. It has been confirmed that insulin inhibits the activation of adenylcyclase in liver and fat cells and PG-E that of fat cells.

'Adenyl Cyclase' System— Stimulation and Inhibition

Interaction of the hormone with its receptor results in the activation or inactivation of adenyl cyclase.

Process is mediated by at least two GTP-dependent regulatory proteins.

- **Gs** (stimulatory)—also called as Ns.
- **Gi** (inhibitory)—Ni.

Each of the regulatory protein is composed of 3 subunits—α, β and γ.

Two parallel system, a stimulatory (S) one and an inhibitory (i) one, converge upon a single catalytic molecule C. Each consists of a receptor Rs or Ri and regulatory complex—Gs and Gi.

Gs and Gi are each trimers composed of α, β and γ-subunits. β and γ subunits in Gs appear to be identical to their respective counterparts Gi. α subunit in Gs differs from that of Gi, designated as α_s (MW = 45,000) and α_i (MW = 41,000).

The binding of a peptide hormone to Rs or Ri results in a receptor-mediated activation of G, which entails Mg^{++}-dependant binding of GTP by α and concomitant dissociation of β and γ from α.

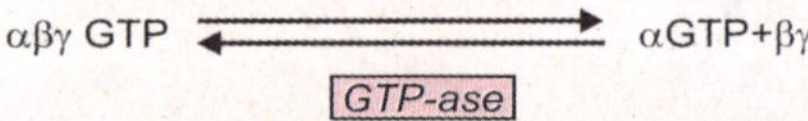

α_s has intrinsic *GTP-ase* activity and the active form of α_s-GTP is inactivated upon hydrolysis of GTP to → GDP and the trimeric Gs complex (α β γ) is reformed.

Recently, it has also been shown that *adenylate cyclase* activity is also modulated by a heatstable calcium-dependent regulatory protein ('CDR') which appears to be major calcium binding protein within the cell.

Phosphodiesterase: c-AMP is rapidly inactivated by an enzyme, a cyclic nucleotide ***phosphodiesterase*** which opens the 3′, 5′-phosphate bond at the 3′ position leaving ordinary 5′-AMP as the product and thus inactivating c-AMP.

- Certain activators and inhibitors of the enzyme are known.
  - ***Activators:*** Promotes degradation of c-AMP and, thus reduce its level.
  - ***Inhibitors:*** Prevent degradation and, thus increase c-AMP level.

Known activators and inhibitors of the enzymes are listed below.

Activators	*Inhibitors*
• Imidazoles • Mg^{++}ions • NH_4^+ ions	• Methylxanthines theophylline> caffeine> theobromine • Papaverine • Bromolysergic acid diethyl amide • Reserpine

FUNCTIONS OF C-AMP

- Mediator of hormone action—acts as "Second messenger" in the cell.
- Regulates glycogen metabolism: increased c-AMP produces breakdown of glycogen (glycogenolysis).
- Regulates TG metabolism: increased c-AMP produces lipolysis (breakdown of TG).
- Cholesterol biosynthesis is inhibited by c-AMP.
- c-AMP stimulates protein kinases so that inactive protein kinase is converted to active protein kinase.
- c-AMP modulates both transcription and translation in protein biosynthesis.
- c-AMP activates different steps of steroid biosynthesis.
- c-AMP also regulates permeability of cell membranes to water, sodium, potassium and calcium.
- Plays an important role in regulation of insulin secretion, catecholamine biosynthesis, and melatonin synthesis.
- Histamine increases c-AMP production in parietal cells which in turn increases gastric secretion.
- Decrease in c-AMP level is involved in the excitation of bitter taste receptors in tongue.
- c-AMP plays an important role in cell differentiation: ***Addition of c-AMP to malignant cell lines "in vitro" reduces growth rates and restores their morphology to normal.***

2. c-GMP

Formation: c-GMP is made from GTP by the enzyme ***guanylate cyclase*** which exists in soluble and membrane-bound form. The enzyme requires Mn^{++} as a cofactor. Guanylate cyclase is also reported to be stimulated by Ca^{++}

Fate: c-GMP is hydrolyzed by cyclic nucleotide ***phosphodiesterase***. The cyclic nucleotide phosphodiesterase is trimeric consisting of three subunits, α, β and γ. γ-subunit is inhibitory and binding of γ-subunit activates the ***phosphodiesterase*** (α, β).

The activated phophodiesterase (α, β) then catalyzes the hydrolysis of c-GMP to 5′-AMP.

Phosphodiesterase (α, β, γ)
("inactive")
↓
Phosphodiesterase (α, β)
("active")

Excretion: About 20% of plasma c-GMP appears to be excreted in urine by kidney, and the rest is taken up by other cells different from original cells in which it was formed and metabolized.

FUNCTION OF C-GMP

1. ***Role of c-GMP in phosphorylation of proteins:*** "Muscarinic action" of acetyl choline on smooth muscles is mediated through c-GMP dependent phosphorylation.
2. ***Role of c-GMP in vasodilation:*** Compounds like nitroglycerine, sodium nitrite, etc. cause smooth muscle relaxation and vasodilation by increasing c-GMP level.
3. ***Role of c-GMP in action of neurotransmitters:*** Gamma aminobutyric acid (GABA) has been claimed to change c-GMP level in cerebellar tissues.
4. ***Role of c-GMP in PG's:*** PG-$F_{2\alpha}$ has been shown to use c-GMP as second messenger for its action.
5. ***Role of c-GMP in insulin actions:*** Insulin action in certain tissues may be mediated through c-GMP which activate the *'protein kinases'*, which in turn phosphorylates some enzymes to modulate their activities.
6. ***Role of c-GMP in retinal light-dark adaptations:*** It has been claimed that c-GMP as second messenger regulates the opening and closing of Na^+ channels. ***In the dark, there are high level of c-GMP which binds to Na^+ channels causing them to open. Reverse occurs in the light.***

☞ SALIENT POINTS TO REMEMBER

- Purine bases are mainly two—adenine and guanine and are found in both DNA and RNA.
- Pyrimidine bases are mainly three—cytosine is found both in DNA and RNA, thymine is found in DNA only and uracil is found in RNA only.
- A nucleoside is composed of purine or pyrimidine base linked to either D-ribose (in RNA) or D-2-deoxy ribose (in DNA). The base and the sugar are joined by β-N-glycosidic linkage.
- A nucleotide is a nucleoside to which a phosphoric acid group is attached to the sugar molecule by esterification at a definite –OH group.
- ***General composition of a nucleotide is base-sugar-PO_4.*** Thus necleotides are nucleoside-P.
- Bond between the nucleotides is the phosphoric acid diester bond.
- Certain synthetic derivatives, viz. 6-mercaptopurine, cytarabine, azathioprine, vidarabin, etc have been found to be useful in cancer chemotherapy and certain viral infections.
  Allopurinol, a synthetic analogue, inhibits the enzyme ***xanthine oxidase*** by competitive inhibition and prevents uric acid formation. It is ***used in treatment of gout.***
- 5-iodo-deoxyuridine has been found useful in the treatment of herpetic keratitis (infection of cornea by herpes simplex virus).
- Adenosine triphosphate (ATP) is the "storage battery" of the tissues (store house of energy).
- ***Two of the three phosphate residues are high energy phosphates (~P) and on hydrolysis each high energy bond releases 7.6 Kcal.*** The energy is utilized for "endergonic processes."
- Two cyclic nucleotides of biological importance are: Cyclic AMP and cyclic GMP. Both

are synthesized in the tissues from ATP and GTP respectively.

- c-AMP is synthesized by an enzyme *"adenyl cyclase"*. Activity of the enzyme is regulated by at least two GTP—dependant regulatory proteins.
- c-AMP is degraded by the enzyme *"phosphodiesterase"*.
- c-GMP is formed from GTP and in presence of the enzyme *"Guanylate Cyclase"* and degraded by the enzyme *"phosphodiesterase"*.
- Both cyclic nucleotides act as "second messenger" and help to mediate various biochemical processes and hormone action.

MULTIPLE CHOICE QUESTIONS

Give one correct answer:

1. Nucleoproteins are conjugated proteins containing nucleic acid and:
(a) Albumins
(b) Globulins
(c) Histones or protamines
(d) Prolamines
(e) Gliadins

2. Which of the following is an amino pyrimidine?
(a) Thymine (b) Adenine
(c) Guanine (d) Cytosine
(e) Uracil

3. Which compound is present in RNA but not in DNA?
(a) Uracil (b) Adenine
(c) Guanine (d) Thymine
(e) Cytosine

4. RNA does not contain:
(a) Ribose
(b) Uracil
(c) Adenine
(d) Hydroxymethyl cytosine
(e) Phosphate

5. Pyrimidines occur besides nucleic acids in:
(a) Adenine (b) FMN
(c) Uric acid (d) Inosinic acid
(e) Thiamine

6. Complete acid hydrolysis of nucleic acids will not yield:
(a) Ribose (b) Adenosine
(c) Phosphate (d) Guanine
(e) Adenine

7. Cyclic AMP is a cyclic nucleotide formed from:
(a) ADP (b) ATP
(c) Adenylic acid (d) GTP
(e) AMP

8. The synthesis of adenyl cyclase is increased by
(a) Epinephrine (b) Parathormone
(c) ACTH (d) Thyroid hormones
(e) Glucagon

9. Cyclic GMP is a cyclic nucleotide formed from:
(a) UTP (b) GTP
(c) CTP (d) ATP
(e) Guanylic acid

10. In formation of cyclic AMP the stimulation of adenyl cyclase by the hormone receptor complex requires the presence of:
(a) UTP (b) CTP
(c) GTP (d) UMP
(e) CDP

11. The enzyme cyclic nucleotide "Phosphodiesterase" is inhibited by following as a result increasing c-AMP level in cells.
(a) Ammonium ions
(b) Mg^{++}
(c) Imidazoles
(d) Theophylline
(e) None of the above

ANSWERS

1. (c)	2. (d)	3. (a)
4. (d)	5. (e)	6. (b)
7. (b)	8. (d)	9. (b)
10. (c)	11. (d)	

Chemistry of Nucleic Acids

NUCLEIC ACIDS

INTRODUCTION

Among all the properties of living organisms, one is absolutely important for continuance of life: a living system must be able to replicate itself. To do so an organism must possess a complete description of itself. In living organisms this description is stored in the substances called *nucleic acids. These are nonprotein nitrogenous substances made up of a monomeric unit called a nucleotide. Two different types* of nucleic acids exist in living organisms, namely deoxyribonucleic acid or DNA and ribonucleic acid or RNA. *The monomeric unit of DNA is deoxyribonucleotide while that of RNA is ribonucleotide.*

DEOXYRIBONUCLEIC ACID (DNA)

DNA is a polymer of deoxyribonucleotides and is found in chromosomes, mitochondria and chloroplasts. The nuclear DNA is found bound to basic proteins called histones. ***DNA is present in every nucleated cell and carries the genetic information.*** It is conveniently isolated from viruses, thymus gland, leucocytes, etc.

Structure of DNA:

1. *Primary structure of DNA:* Chromosomal DNA consists of very long DNA molecules (mol. Wt. 1.6×10^6 to 2×10^9).

- Each DNA is a polymer of about 10^{10} deoxyribonucleotides.
- Normally, there are only four different types of deoxyribonucleotides that are found in DNA molecule, namely adenine deoxyribonucleotide (dA), thymine deoxyribonucleotide (dT), guanine deoxyribonucleotide (dG), and cytosine deoxyribonucleotide (dC).
- Nucleotides of each of the two helical strands are ***bound to each other by covalent 3′-5′ phosphodiester linkage***. Each such bond is formed by the ester linkages of a single phosphate residue with 3′-OH (i.e. C-3′-OH group of the ribose sugar) of one nucleotide with the C-5′-OH group of ribose of the next nucleotide.
- This kind of bonding gives rise to a linear polydeoxyribonucleotide strand with 2 free ends on both sides.
- That end of the strand which bears a free 5′ phosphate group without phosphodiester linkage is called the **5′ end.** The opposite end bears a free 3′-hydroxyl or 3′ phosphate group and is called the **3′ end.**
- The primary structure is the number and sequence of different deoxyribonucleotides in its strands joined together by phosphodiester linkages.
- The backbone of the primary structure is the linear strand of interconnected sugar phosphate residues while the purine or pyrimidine connected with the sugar residue projects laterally from the backbone.

2. *Secondary structure of DNA:* This consists of a **double stranded helix** formed by the two polydeoxyribonucleotide strands around a central axis. This type of model was first proposed by

Watson and Crick in their paper in Nature in 1953. Later on, they were awarded the Nobel prize in 1962 alongwith Maurice Wilkins.

- DNA is a ***double helix. (Fig. 6.1)*** Each of its two strands is coiled about a central axis, ***usually a right handed helix***. The two sugar phosphate backbones wind around the outside of the bases like the banisters of a spiral staircase and are exposed to the aqueous solution. The phosphodiester bonds in the two interwoven strands run in opposite directions. Therefore the strands are called **antiparallel**. Thus the polarity of the two strands will be 3′-5′ and 5′-3′. ***The 3′-5′ strands is called coding or "template strand" and 5′-3′ strand is called non-coding 'strand'***. The aromatic rings of bases are hydrophobic and they are stacked in the interior, nearly perpendicular to the long axis of the helix.
- ***Adenine base of one strand of DNA is hydrogen bonded to a thymine in the opposite strand; while the guanine is hydrogen bonded to a cytosine (Fig. 6.2).***
- The hydrogen atoms in the bases of DNA can shift from one ring nitrogen or oxygen atom to another. These proton shifts called tautomerization reactions-interconvert the positions that can serve as hydrogen-bond donors and acceptors in base pairs. There are ***two hydrogen bonds present between adenine and thymine, while three hydrogen bonds present between guanine and cytosine.*** The length of hydrogen bond is around 3.0Å.
- ***The ratio of purine to pyrimidine bases in the DNA molecule is always around 1 (i.e. G+A/T+C≈1)***. This is known as ***Chargaff's rule.***
- In DNA, the glycosidic bonds between sugar and bases are not directly opposite each other and two grooves of unequal width form around the double helix. The edge of the helix that measures more than 180° from glycosidic bond to glycosidic bond is called the ***major groove*** and if it is less the 180° it is called ***minor groove.***
- DNA can exist in several conformation depending upon the base composition and

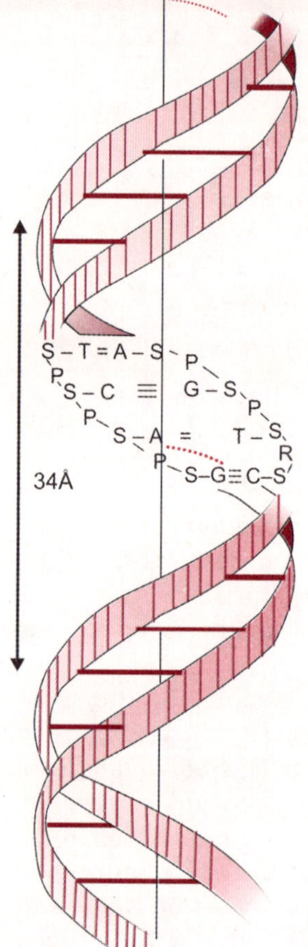

Fig. 6.1: Double-helix DNA

Fig. 6.2: Hydrogen bonds between (A) adenine and thymine and between (B) cystosine and guanine

under different physical conditions. In all these conformations, the same base pairing rules apply, changes do not alter the information content of the DNA. The conformations of DNA have been determined by X-ray crystallography. By far the most common conformation is B-DNA. Other conformations are A-DNA and Z-DNA.

Table 16.1: The major structural features of A, B and Z DNA

Property	*A-DNA*	*B-DNA*	*Z-DNA*
• **Helix Handedness**	right	right	left
• **Repeating Unit Base pairs**	1 base pair	1 base pair	2 base pair
• **Per turn**	10	11	12
• **Rotation/base pair**	32.7°	34.6°	30°
• **Inclination of basepair to helix axis**	19°	1.2°	9°
• **Rise per base pair along helix axis**	0.23 nm	0.33 nm	0.38 nm
• **Pitch**	2.46 nm	3.40 nm	4.56 nm
• **Diameter**	2.55 nm	2.37 nm	1.84 nm
• **Conformation of Glycosidic bond**	anti	anti	anti at C syn at G
• **Major groove**	present	present	non-existent or convex shaped
• **Minor groove**	present	present	deep cleft

Denaturation of DNA: Two strands of DNA's double helix can separate or unwind during processes such as DNA replication, RNA transcription and genetic recombination. Complete unwinding of DNA can take place *in vitro* and is called denaturation of DNA, or it is also known as ***"a helix to coil transition"***. Denaturation occurs when the hydrogen bonds between bases break and the base pairs separate when DNA is treated above a certain temperature or melted.

Temperature of DNA: The temperature at which DNA is half denatured is called the ***melting temperature-Tm of DNA.*** At this temperature the absorbance of DNA at 260 nm is increased by 18.5%, i.e. half the 37% increase in absorbance where DNA is completely denatured. This phenomenon is called ***hyperchromicity or hyperchromic effect.*** The melting temperature of DNA is determined by its base composition. Since there are two hydrogen bonds between A and T while three between G and C, **increasing G-C base pairs raises Tm**. ***Tm is strongly influenced by the base composition of the DNA. DNA rich in G-C pairs has a higher Tm than DNA with high proportion of A-T pairs.***

Mammalian DNA, which has about 40% G-C pairs, has a Tm of about 87 °C. The Tm of DNA extracted from different species and measured at pH 7 in ***an isotonic salt solution*** varies linearly with G-C content; with synthetic Poly-A-T having a Tm of about 65° and synthetic Poly G-C having a Tm of 105 °C.

Annealing: Once the strands are separated, they can be renatured. If a melted sample of DNA is slowly cooled, the absorbance of the solution decreases. This is indicative of complementary strands being paired again. This process is called as ***annealing. Annealing can occur only at a temp below Tm of DNA which is about 70°C.*** It is fastest at 20°C below Tm or 50 °C.

RIBONUCLEIC ACID (RNA)

Ribonucleic acid is a polymer of ribonucleotides of adenine, uracil, guanine and cytosine, joined together by 3′-5′ phosphodiester bonds. Thymine is absent in RNA. RNA is found in the nucleolus, Nissl granules, ribosomes, mitochondria and cytoplasm. The Pentose sugar of the nucleotide is D-ribose.

Structures of RNA

1. ***Primary structure of RNA:*** The primary structure of RNA is defined as the number and sequence of ribonucleotides in the chain. Each linear strand is held together by the ribonucleotides bound to each other by 3′, 5′ phosphodiester bonds joining 3′-OH of one nucleotide with the 5′-OH of the next.

2. ***Secondary structure of RNA:*** The secondary structure of RNA involves various coil formation of the polyribonucleotide chain.

- These coil structures are stabilized by hydrophobic interactions between the purine and pyrimidine bases.
- There are ***intrachain hydrogen bonds between G-C and A-U***. The hydrogen bonds are the same as in DNA for G-C while N^3 as well as C^4 oxo group of uracil (or dihydrouracil) which pairs with adenine.

3. ***Tertiary structure of RNA:*** The tertiary structure of RNA involves the folding of the molecules into three dimensional structure. The cross-linking also occurs at various sites stabilized by hydrophobic and hydrogen bonds producing a compactly coiled globular structure.

Types of RNA

There are mainly ***three types of RNAs*** found in human beings. They are:

- **Messenger RNA or m-RNA,**
- **Transfer or soluble RNA or t-RNA,** and
- **Ribosomal RNA or r-RNA.**

The main function of each of these RNA is protein synthesis. In human cells there are small nuclear RNA or Sn-RNA which are not involved in protein biosynthesis directly. They may have some role in processing of RNA and cellular architecture. They are found in nucleoplasm, nucleolus, perichromatic granules, and cytoplasm and vary in size from 90 nucleotides to 300 nucleotides. A large precursor of messenger RNA (m-RNA) called as heterogeneous nuclear RNA or hnRNA is also found in the nucleus.

1. ***Messenger RNA (m-RNA):*** This is the most heterogeneous class of RNA with respect to its size and stability.

- The molecular weight varies from 3×10^4-2×10^6. They consist of 10^3–10^4 ribonucleotides.
- It carries mainly adenine, guanine, cytosine and uracil as the major bases and methylpurines and methylpyrimidines as minor bases.
- The m-RNA molecules are formed with the help of DNA template strand (3′-5′) during the process called ***"transcription"***.
- The m-RNA carries a specific sequence of nucleotides in ***"triplets"*** called ***codons,*** responsible for the synthesis of a specific protein molecule.
- The 3′-OH end of most m-RNA molecules carries a polymer of adenylate ribonucleotides consisting of 20-250 residues in length. This is called as ***Poly A tail,*** the function of which is not yet fully understood, but it ***seems to maintain the intracellular stability of the specific m-RNA by preventing the attack of 3′-exonucleases.***
- On the other hand, the 5′-OH end of the m-RNA carries a cap structure consisting of 7 methylguanosine triphosphate. ***The cap is probably involved in recognition of protein biosynthetic machinery and it helps in stabilizing the m-RNA by preventing the attack of 5′-exonucleases.***
- The protein synthesis begins at 5′-end of the capped structure of m-RNA.

Heterogenous Nuclear RNA or hn-RNA: In mammalian cells, the m-RNA that comes to cytoplasm is the product of processing of a precursor called, heterogeneous nuclear or hnRNA. These molecules are very large and may have a molecular weight of more than 10^7.

Characteristics:

- It is synthesized in the nucleus.
- Has a half life of 23 minutes.
- Has 400 to 4000 nucleotides and it is 10 to 100 times bigger than m-RNA.
- Is bound to macromolecular proteins called ***"informofers"*** and exists as ***"heterogeneous*** ribonuclear proteins" ***(hn RNP)***.
- 75% of hn RNA is degraded in the nucleus. Only 25% of the hn RNA forms a precursor of m-RNA (Pre-mRNA).

PRE-mRNA

- Pre-mRNA is converted to m-RNA
- Pre-mRNA has regions called as ***"introns"*** transcripts-the sequences not required (inactive) and ***"exons"*** transcripts (active portion required for translation).
- Approximately 80% of length of pre-mRNA is removed as "introns transcripts" and only

20% of Pre-mRNA, the "exons transcripts" are spliced to form the m-RNA.

2. *Transfer RNA or t-RNA:* These are *also called as soluble or s-RNA.* They remain largely in cytoplasm. The t-RNAs are relatively small, single-stranded, globular molecules with molecular weight of 2-3 × 10^4. There are at least ***20 different t-RNA molecules.***

Primary structure of t-RNA: t-RNA molecules consist of approximately 75 nucleotides. Their bases include adenine, guanine, cytosine, uracil, pseudouridine (Ψ) or uracil 5-ribofuranoside and thymine are present in one loop

Secondary structure of t-RNA: Each single stranded t-RNA molecule remains folded to form a ***cloverleaf like*** secondary structure.

These folds of the secondary structure are stabilized by H-bonds between complementary bases in different portions of the same strand. These double stranded helical structures are called as ***stems.***

All t-RNA molecules contain *five* main arms or loops.

- ***Acceptor arm:*** This consists of unpaired sequences of cytosine-cytosine-adenine at the 3′ end also known as ***acceptor end.*** The 3′-OH terminal of adenine may bind with the α COOH of a specific amino acid and carry the latter as an aminoacyl-t-RNA complex to ribosomes for protein synthesis. The acceptor arm is borne by a base paired acceptor stem whose bases are hydrogen bonded with the last few bases at the 5′ end of t-RNA.
- ***Anticodon arm:*** This is another unpaired and nonbonded loop ***carrying specific sequences of three bases*** constituting the ***anticodon.*** The bases of anticodon are hydrogen bonded with three complementary bases of codon of m-RNA. The base pair stem leading to anticodon loop is called the ***"anticodon stem".***
- ***D-arm:*** The third is the D-arm because it contains the base dihydrouridine.
- ***TΨC arm:*** contains thymine, pseudouridine and cytosine.
- ***Variable arm or extra-arm:*** Extra-arm is most variable structure of t-RNA and it forms the basis of its classification ***(Fig. 6.3).***

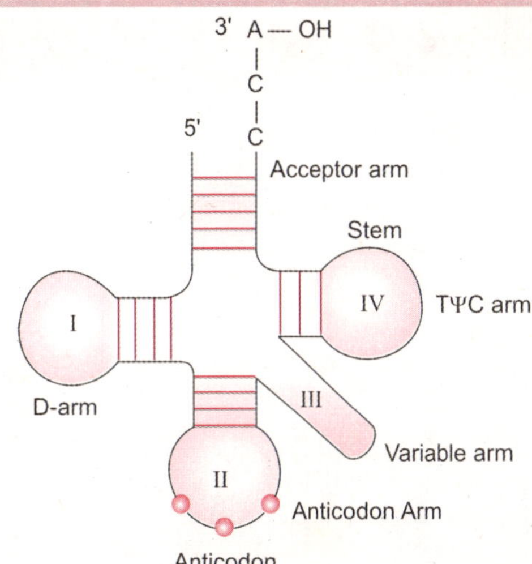

Fig. 6.3: Primary and secondary structure of t-RNA

3. ***Ribosomal or r-RNA:*** The ribosome is present in the cytoplasm and is a nucleoprotein. It is on the ribosome that the m-RNA and t-RNA interact during the process of protein biosynthesis. Ribosomes contain the third type of RNA known as r-RNA. The r-RNA forms 80% of the total cellular RNA.

- Ribosomes possess a sedimentation coefficient of 80s with a molecular weight of 4.2 × 10^6. Mammalian ribosomes are made up of **two subunits**:
  - ***Larger one*** with **60 s** and molecular weight 2.8 × 10^6.
  - ***Smaller subunit*** with **40s** and molecular weight of 1.4 × 10^6. The **60s** subunit carries 60% of r-RNA and is a combination of **5s** r-RNA, **5.8s** r-RNA and **28s** r-RNA. The **40s** subunits carries **18s** r-RNA and 33 different proteins. All the r-RNA molecules except **5s** r-RNA are processed from a precursor of **45s** r-RNA.

Function of r-RNA: The function of r-RNA in ribosome particle is still not clearly understood. However, they are necessary for ribosomal assembly and seem to play key roles in the binding of m-RNA to ribosomes and its translation.

Differentiating features of DNA and RNA are given in **Table 6.1** and differentiation of m-RNA and t-RNA is given in ***Table 6.2.***

Table 6.1: Differentiation of DNA and RNA

DNA	*RNA*
Similarities	
• Both have adenine, guanine, cytosine	
• The nucleotides are linked together by phosphodiester bonds.	
• The bonding is in 3′-5′ direction	
• Main function involves protein biosynthesis.	
Differences	
• In addition to A, G, C the fourth base T, ***Uracil is absent***	• In addition to A, G, C the fourth base is U, ***thymine absent***
• Pentose sugar is deoxyribose	• Pentose sugar is ribose
• Present in nucleus, mitochondria but never in cytoplasm	• In addition to nucleus RNA is found in cytoplasm
• They consist of 2 helical strands	• Single stranded
• There are A, B, C, D and Z forms of DNA	• There are t-RNA, m-RNA, r-RNA, hn RNA and Sn RNA
• Large molecules	• Only hn, m and r-RNA are large molecules
• One strand 3′-5′ carries genetic information	• m-RNA transcribed from DNA carries genetic information
• DNA can form RNA by the process of "transcription"	• RNA cannot give rise to DNA under normal conditions, but it can under special experimental conditions using ***reverse transcriptase***
• Purine and pyrimidine contents are almost equal	• Not equal
• Alkali hydrolysis does not give 2′-3′ cyclic diesters.	• Alkali hydrolysis gives 2′-3′cyclic mononucleotides.

Table 6.2: Differentiation of m-RNA and t-RNA

m-RNA	*t-RNA*
• Large molecular weight	• Low molecular weight
• Most heterogeneous	• Only about 20 different forms (less heterogeneous)
• Acts as a template for protein synthesis	• Acts as carrier of amino acid
• Carries codons	• Carries anticodon
• Shape and size is not constant	• Shape and size is constant for all t-RNA's "clover-leaf"
• The cap structure is found on 5′ OH end	• No such structure
• Poly A tail is found on 3′ OH end	• 3′ OH end carries C.C.A sequence where specific amino acid is bound.
• Precursor is hn-RNA	• No such precursor
• Unusual bases are not found	• Unusual bases such as pseudouridine, thymine, etc. are found.
• Stem and loop structure is not found	• Stem and loop structure is a consistent feature.

☞ SALIENT POINTS TO REMEMBER

- Nucleic acids are the polymers of nucleotides (Polynucleotides) held by 3' and 5' phosphodiester bridges.
- Nucleic acids are mainly two: DNA (Deoxyribonucleic acid) and RNAs (Ribonucleic acids).
- DNA is the chemical basis of heredity. DNA is organized into "genes", the fundamental units of genetic information. Genes control protein biosynthesis through the mediation of RNAs.
- RNAs (m-RNA, t-RNA and r-RNA) are produced by DNA which in turn carry out protein synthesis.
- Both DNA and RNAs contain the purines–Adenine (A) and Guanine (G) and the pyrimidine cytosine. The second pyrimidine

is Thymine (T) in DNA and it is uracil (U) in RNA.

- The pentose sugar deoxy-ribose is found in DNA, while the RNAs contain D-ribose.
- Structure of DNA is a double-helix as per Watson-Crick model, composed of two anti-parallel strands of polydeoxy-ribonucleotides twisted around each other.
- The strands, like a staircase, are held together by 2 or 3 hydrogen bonds formed between the bases.
- Adenine (A) is always joined to thymine (T) by two hydrogen bonds (A = T), while guanine (G) is joined to cytosine (C) by three hydrogen bonds (G ≡ C).
- The ratio of purine to pyrimidine bases in the DNA molecule is always around 1 (i.e., G + A/T + C = 1). This is called as **Changaff's rule.**
- DNA can exist in several conformations. **Most common conformation is B-DNA.** Other conformations are A-DNA and Z-DNA.
- Two strands of DNA's double helix can separate or unwind during processes such as DNA replication, RNA transcription and genetic recombination.
- The temperature at which DNA is half-denatured is called the "melting temperature" of DNA (or **Tm of DNA**).
- The joining of the two separated strands is called **"annealing".**
- ***RNA is usually single-stranded*** polyribonucleotide.
- m-RNA molecules are formed with the help of DNA template strand (3'-5') during the process called as transcription.
- m-RNA carries a specific sequence of nucleotides in 'triplets' called 'codons' responsible for synthesis of specific protein molecule.
- ***m-RNA is capped at 5′-terminal end by 7-methyl GTP while at the 3′ end contains a poly A-tail.***
- The cap is involved in recognition of protein biosynthetic machinery and helps in stabilizing the m-RNA by preventing the attack by ***"5′-exonuclease"***.
- The structure of t-RNA resembles that of a *"clover-leaf"* ***with four arms*** viz. acceptor arm, anticodon, D and T Ψ C, held by complementary base pairs.
- There are ***20 (twenty) t-RNAs for 20 L-amino acids*** required for protein synthesis, t-RNA picks up the specific amino acid and delivers for protein synthesis.
- r-RNAs are found in combination with proteins and are involved in binding of m-RNA to ribosomes for protein synthesis.

MULTIPLE CHOICE QUESTIONS

Give one correct answer:

1. **m-RNA is a complementary copy of:**
   (a) A single strand DNA
   (b) Double strand of DNA
   (c) Ribosomal RNA
   (d) Ribosomal DNA
   (e) None of the above
2. **A t-RNA molecule has the following:**
   (a) A loop containing minor base dihydrouracil
   (b) A clover-leaf structure
   (c) An anticoden arm
   (d) All of the above
   (e) None of the above
3. **The anticodon region is an important part of the structure of:**
   (a) m-RNA (b) t-RNA
   (c) r-RNA (d) hn RNA
   (e) Z-DNA
4. **Which pyrimidine nucleotide acts as the high energy intermediate?**
   (a) CTP (b) ATP
   (c) CMP (d) UTP
   (e) UDP-G
5. **In a DNA molecule guanosine nucleotide is held by the cylosine nucleotide by the number of hydrogen bonds:**
   (a) 1 (b) 2
   (c) 3 (d) 4
   (e) 5

6. **If the Percentage concentration of thymine in DNA is 40 percent, the concentration of cytosine will be:**
   (a) 10 percent (b) 20 percent
   (c) 30 percent (d) 40 percent
   (e) 60 percent
7. **In t-RNA molecules, there is a "loop" which contain a minor base:**
   (a) Cytosine (b) Dihydrocytosine
   (c) Uracil (d) Dihydrouracil
   (e) Thymine
8. **All the following are features of Watson Crick model of DNA *except:***
   (a) Double stranded helix
   (b) Each turn of the helix has about 10 base pairs
   (c) Adenine bonds with thymine
   (d) Strands are held by hydrogen bonds
   (e) Guanine bonds with uracil
9. **If the cytosine content of double stranded DNA is 20 percent of the total bases, the adenine content will be:**
   (a) 10 percent (b) 20 percent
   (c) 30 percent (d) 40 percent
   (e) 50 percent
10. **Which of the following nucleoside is found in DNA?**
    (a) Dihydrouridine
    (b) Deoxythymidine
    (c) Pseudouridine
    (d) Ribothymidine
    (e) None of the above
11. **The melting temperature of DNA (Tm) is:**
    (a) Directly proportiomal to the length of DNA
    (b) Directly proportional to A-T content
    (c) Directly proportional to G-C content
    (d) Not related to base composition at all
    (e) None of the above
12. **Unusual nucleotide bases are found in which of the RNAs:**
    (a) m-RNA (b) hn RNA
    (c) r-RNA (d) t-RNA
    (e) Pre-m-RNA

ANSWERS

1. (a)	2. (d)	3. (b)
4. (e)	5. (c)	6. (a)
7. (d)	8. (e)	9. (c)
10. (b)	11. (c)	12. (d)

Chemistry of Enzymes

INTRODUCTION

Enzymes are another important group of biomolecules synthesized by the living cells. ***They are catalysts of biological systems (hence are called as biocatalyst), colloidal, thermolabile and protein in nature.*** They are remarkable molecular devices that determine the pattern of chemical transformations. They also mediate the transformation of different forms of energy. The ***striking characteristics of enzymes are their catalytic power and specificity.*** Actions of most enzymes are under strict regulation in a variety of ways. Substances on which enzymes act to convert them into products are called ***substrates.***

Catalytic Activity of Enzymes: Enzymes have immense catalytic power and accelerate reactions at least a million times, ***by reducing the energy of activation.*** Before a chemical reaction can occur, the reacting molecules are required to gain a minimum amount of energy-this is called the ***energy of activation.*** It can be decreased by increasing the temperature of the reaction medium. But in human body which maintains a normal body temperature fairly constant, it is achieved by enzymes.

Protein Nature of Enzymes: In general with the exception of ***ribozymes*** which are few RNA molecules with enzymatic activity, ***all the enzymes are protein in nature*** with large molecular weight. Few enzymes are simple proteins while some are conjugated proteins. In such enzymes, the non-protein part is called ***prosthetic group or coenzyme*** and the protein part is called as ***apo-enzyme.*** The complete structure of *apoenzyme* and *prosthetic group* is called ***holoenzyme.***

Holoenzyme =	**Apoenzyme**	**+**	**Coenzyme**
	(Protein part)		**(Prosthetic group)**

Certain enzymes with only one polypeptide chain in their structure are called ***monomeric enzymes,*** e.g. *ribonuclease.* Several enzymes possess more than one polypeptide chain and are called ***oligomeric enzymes,*** e.g *lactate dehydrogenase, hexokinase, etc.* Each single polypeptide chain of oligomeric enzymes is called *subunit.* When many different enzyme catalyzing reaction sites are located at different sites of the same macromolecule, it is called ***multienzyme complex.*** The complex becomes inactive when it is fractionated into smaller units each bearing individual enzyme activity, *e.g. fatty acid synthase, carbamoyl phosphate synthetase II, pyruvate dehydrogenase complex, prostaglandin synthase, etc.*

Co-enzymes: Certain enzymes require ***a specific, thermostable, low molecular weight, non-protein organic substance called coenzyme.*** A co-enzyme may bind covalently or non-covalently to the *apo-enzyme.*

Since the involvement of coenzyme in a given reaction on a substrate is so intimate that coenzyme is often called as ***cosubstrate*** or second substrate.

Many coenzyme are derived as the physiologically active forms from the constituents of vitamin B-complex such as:

- **Pantothenic acid:** CoA
- **Vitamin B_{12}:** Cobamide

- **Folic acid:** Tetrahydrofolate
- **Niacin:** NAD^+, $NADP^+$
- **Riboflavin:** FMN, FAD
- **Pyridoxine:** Pyridoxal phosphate
- **Thiamine:** TPP

Biotin, lipoic acid act as such as coenzymes. In addition, heme acts as coenzymes in cytochromes, peroxidases. Many coenzymes contain adenine, ribose and phosphate and are derivatives of adenosine monophosphate (AMP) such as NAD^+, FAD (For details see Chapter on "Vitamins").

Role of Metal Ions in Enzymes: The activity of many enzymes depends on the presence of certain metal ions such as K^+, Mg^{++}, Ca^{++}, Zn^{++}, Cu^{++}.

- *Metal activated enzymes:* In certain enzymes the ***metals form a loose and easily dissociable complex.*** Such enzymes are called metal activated enzymes. The metal ion can be removed by dialysis or any other such method from the enzyme without causing any denaturation of apoenzyme.
- *Metallo-enzymes:* The second category of metal enzymes is called metallo-enzymes. In this case, metal ion is ***bound tightly to the enzyme*** and is not dissociated even after several extensive steps of purification. Metals play variety of roles such as:
  - They help in either maintaining or producing (or both) active structural conformation of the enzyme
  - Formation of enzyme-substrate complex
  - Making structural changes in substrate molecule
  - Accept or donate electrons
  - Activating or functioning as nucleophiles
  - Formation of tertiary complexes with enzyme or substrate.

NOMENCLATURE AND CLASSIFICATION OF ENZYMES

Enzymes are generally named after adding the suffix-*"ase"* to the name of the substrate, e.g. enzymes acting on nucleic acids are known as ***nucleases,*** enzymes hydrolyzing dipeptides are called ***dipeptidases***. Even though few exceptions such as trypsin, pepsin, and chymotrypsin are still in use.

Further, few enzymes exist in their inactive forms and are called as ***proenzymes or zymogens,*** e.g. ***pepsin*** has ***pepsinogen*** *as* its zymogen. The zymogens become active after undergoing some prior modification in its structure by certain agents. Many times the active form of enzyme acts on zymogen and catalyzes its conversion into active form and this process is called ***as autocatalysis.***

In order to have a uniformity and unambiguity in identification of enzymes, ***International Union of Biochemistry (IUB))*** adopted a nomenclature system based on chemical reaction type and reaction mechanism. According to this system, enzymes are grouped in ***six main classes.***

- Each enzyme is characterized by a code number (Enzyme code no or EC no.) comprising ***four figure (digits) separated by points:***
  - ***First*** being that of the main ***class (one of the six)***
  - ***Second figure*** indicates the type of group involved in the reaction
  - ***Third figure*** denotes the reaction more precisely indicating substrate on which the group acts
  - ***Fourth figure*** is the serial number of the enzyme briefly, the four digits characterize class, sub-class, sub-sub-class and serial number of a particular enzyme.

- ***Oxidoreductase:*** Enzymes involved in oxidations and reductions of their substrates, e.g. *alcohol dehydrogenase, lactate dehydrogenase, xanthine oxidase, glutathione reductase, glucose-6-phosphate dehydrogenase.*
- ***Transferases:*** Enzymes that catalyze transfer of a particular group from one substrate to another, e.g. *aspartate and alanine transaminase (AST/ALT), hexokinase, phosphoglucomutase, hexose-1-phosphate uridytransferase, ornithine carbamoyl transferase, etc.*
- ***Hydrolases:*** Enzymes that bring about hydrolysis, e.g. *glucose-6-phosphatase, pepsin, trypsin, esterases, glycoside hydrolases,* etc.

- ***Lyases:*** Enzymes that facilitate removal of small molecule from a large substrate, e.g. *fumarase, arginosuccinase, histidine decarboxylase.*
- ***Isomerases:*** Enzymes involved in isomerization of substrate, e.g. *UDP-glucose, epimerase, retinal isomerase, racemases, triosephosphate isomerase.*
- ***Ligases:*** Enzymes involved in joining together two substrates, e.g. *alanyl-t. RNA synthetase, glutamine synthetase, DNA ligases.*

Many times the word **OTHLIL** is used to recognise the six classes.

SPECIFICITY OF ENZYMES

Another important property of enzymes is their specificity. The specificity is of ***three different types*** namely:

- ***Stereochemical specificity***
- ***Reaction specificity***, and
- ***Substrate specificity***.

Since each enzyme has its own sets of specificity, it is understandable that there is a large number of different enzymes. In general, ***the stereospecificity is due to apoenzyme part of holoenzyme, while the reaction specificity is due to the coenzyme or prosthetic group.***

1. STEREOSPECIFICITY

- ***Optical specificity:*** There can be many optical isomers of a substrate. However, it is only one of the isomers which acts as a substrate for an enzyme action, e.g. for the oxidation of *D*- and *L*-amino acids, there are two types of enzymes which will act on *D*- and *L*-isomers of amino acids. Secondly, there can be a product of enzyme action which can have isomers. However, it is only one kind of isomer which will be produced as a product, e.g. *succinic dehydrogenase* while acting on succinic acid will give only fumaric acid and not malic acid which is its isomer.

2. REACTION SPECIFICITY

A substrate can undergo many reactions but in a reaction specificity, one enzyme can catalyze only one of the various reactions. **For example,** oxaloacetic acid can undergo several reactions, but each reaction is catalyzed by its own separate enzyme which catalyzes only that reaction and none of the others.

3. SUBSTRATE SPECIFICITY

The extent of substrate specificity varies from enzyme to enzyme. There are two types of substrate specificity : (i) ***Absolute*** and (ii) ***relative specificity***. Absolute specificity is comparatively rare such as *urease* which catalyzes hydrolysis of urea. Relative substrate specificity is further divided as

- Group dependent or
- Bond dependent.

- ***Group specificity***: Examples of group specificity are trypsin, chymotrypsin. *Trypsin* hydrolyzes the residues of only *lysine* and *arginine,* while chymotrypsin hydrolyzes residues of only aromatic amino acids.
- ***Bond specificity:*** Bond specificity is observed in case to *proteolytic enzymes, glycosidases* and *lipases* which act on peptide bonds, glycosidic bonds and ester bonds respectively.

MECHANISM OF ENZYME ACTION

Michaelis and **Menten** have proposed a hypothesis for enzyme action, which is the most acceptable. According to their hypothesis, ***the enzyme molecule (E) first combines with a substrate molecule (S) to form an enzyme-substrate (E S) complex which further dissociates to form product (P) and enzyme (E) back.***

$$E + S \underset{K_2}{\overset{K_1}{\rightleftharpoons}} \underset{\text{Complex}}{E-S} \underset{K_4}{\overset{K_3}{\rightleftharpoons}} E + P$$

Enzyme once dissociated from the complex is free to combine with another molecule of substrate and form product in a similar way. **The ES complex is an intermediate** or **transient complex** and the bonds involved are weak non-covalent bonds, such as H-bonds, van der Waal's forces, hydrophobic interactions.

Sometimes two substrates can bind to an enzyme molecule and such reactions are called as **bisubstrate reactions**. The site to which a substrate can bind to the enzyme molecule is extremely specific and is called ***active site or catalytic site.*** Normally the molecular size and shape of the substrate molecule is extremely small compared to that of an enzyme molecule. The **active site** is *made up of several amino acid residues that come together as a result of folding of secondary and tertiary structures of the enzyme.* So, the active site possesses a complex three-dimensional form and shape, provides a predominantly non-polar cleft or crevice to accept and bind the substrate. Few groups of active site amino acids are bound to substrate while few groups bring about change in the substrate molecule.

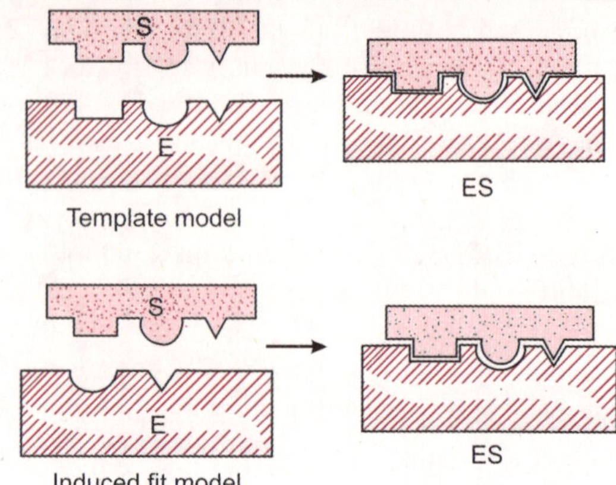

Fig. 7.1: Models for enzyme-substrate interaction

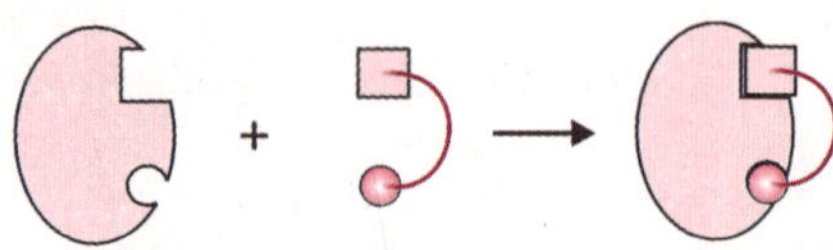

Fig. 7.2: Template or lock and key model

MODELS OF ENZYME-SUBSTRATE COMPLEX FORMATION

These interactions have been described basically of **two types** ***(Fig. 7.1).***

1. TEMPLATE OR LOCK-AND KEY MODEL

This model was originally proposed by **Fischer** which states that the active site already exists in proper conformation even in absence of substrate. **Thus the active site by itself provides a rigid pre-shaped template**, fitting with the size and shape of the substrate molecule. ***Substrate fits into active site of an enzyme as the key fits into the lock and hence it is called the lock and key model. (Fig. 7.2).*** This model proposes that substrate binds with rigid pre-existing template of the active site and provides additional groups for binding other ligands. But this cannot explain change in enzymatic activity in presence of allosteric modulators.

2. INDUCED-FIT OR KOSHLAND MODEL:

Because of the restrictive nature of lock-and-key model, another model was proposed by **Koshland** in 1963 which is known as induced-fit model. ***The important feature of this model is the flexibility of the region of active site (Fig. 7.3).*** According to this, active site does not possess a rigid, preformed structure on enzyme to fit the substrate. On the contrary, ***the substrate during its binding induces conformational changes in the active site to attain the final catalytic shape and form.*** This explains several matters related to enzyme action such as,

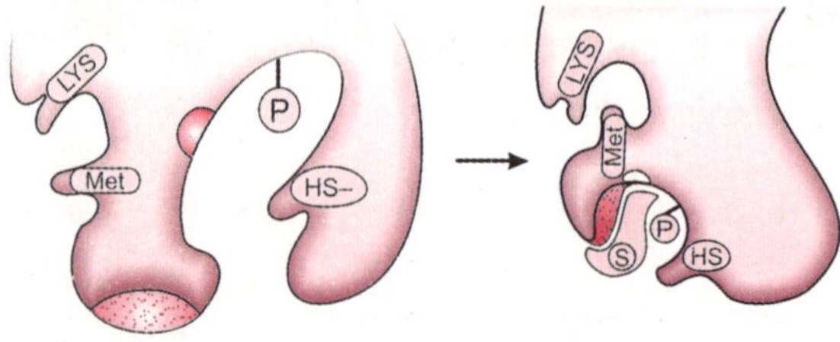

Fig. 7.3: Induced fit model

- Enzymes become inactive on denaturation
- Saturation kinetics,
- Competitive inhibition and
- Allosteric modulation.

KINETIC PROPERTIES OF ENZYMES

Kinetic analysis of enzymes was used for characterization of enzyme-catalyzed reactions even before enzymes had been isolated in pure form.

One of the first things that is measured in kinetic analysis is the variation in rate of reaction with substrate concentration. For this purpose, a fixed low concentration of enzyme is used in a series of parallel experiments in which only the substrate concentration is varied. Under these conditions, initial velocity increases until it reaches a substrate-independent maximum velocity at substrate concentration.

The saturation effect is believed to reflect the fact that all the enzyme binding sites are occupied with substrate. This interpretation of the substrate saturation curve led **Hensi, Michaelis and Menten** to develop a general treatment of kinetic analysis of enzyme catalyzed reactions.

Kinetics of enzyme-substrate reaction is expressed as:

$$V_0 = \frac{V_{max}\,[S]}{[S] + Km}$$

This is called the ***Michaelis-Menten equation,*** the rate equation for one substrate-enzyme catalyzed reaction. It is a statement of the quantitative relationship between the initial velocity V_0, the maximum velocity Vmax and the initial substrate concentration, all related through the Michaelis Menten constant Km.

- An important relationship is observed when the initial reaction rate is exactly one-half the V_{max}. Then,

$$\frac{V_{max}}{2} = \frac{V_{max}\,[S]}{Km + [S]}$$

Dividing by V_{max}

$$\frac{1}{2} = \frac{[S]}{Km + [S]}$$

Solving for Km, we get

$$Km + [S] = 2\,[S]$$

$$\mathbf{Km = [S]}$$

The Michaelis-Menten equation can be algebraically transformed into equivalent equations that are useful in the practical determination of Km and V_{max}.

Therefore, Km is equal to substrate concentration at which the velocity is half the maximum. The initial velocity V_0 is directly proportional to the molar concentration [S] of the substrate when substrate concentration is very low as compared to Km. In this stage, a single substrate enzyme reaction is a first order reaction and its rate depends on conc. of single reactant.

$$S << Km,$$

$$\therefore \quad Km + [S] \simeq Km,$$

$$\therefore \quad V_0 = \frac{V_{max}\,[S]}{Km + [S]} = \frac{V_{max}\,[S]}{Km} = K\,[S]$$

Where K is a new constant equalling $\frac{V_{max}}{Km}$ because both V_{max} and Km are constants for a particular enzyme.

When S>> Km, the initial velocity attains its *V*max and becomes independent of [S]. The reaction now turns into a zero-order reaction.

Hyperbolic curve of reaction velocity (V) against substrate concentration (S) is depicted in ***Figure 7.4.***

FACTORS AFFECTING ENZYME ACTION

Activity of enzymes is markedly affected by several factors such as temperature, pH, conc. of other substances, presence of activators or inhibitors, etc.

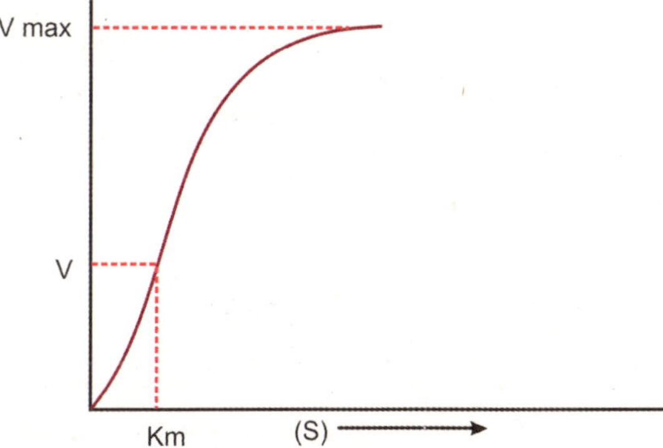

Fig. 7.4: The hyperbolic curve of reaction velocity (V) against substrate concentration (S). Km is the substrate concentration at ½ V_{max}

1. EFFECT OF TEMPERATURE

Each enzyme is most active at a specific temperature which is called its ***optimum temperature.*** Temperature increases the total energy of the chemical system with the result the activation energy is increased. The exact ratio by which the velocity changes of 10°C temperature. rise is the Q_{10} ***or temperature coefficient. Reactions velocity almost doubles with 10°C rise (Q_{10} = 2) in many enzymes.*** Activity of enzyme progressively decreases when the temperature of reaction is below or above the optimum temperature. However, increase in temperature also causes denaturation of enzyme. Note that the shape of the curve is ***bell-shape.*** Most of the enzymes of human system have an optimum pH within the range of 35-40°C. Thus, the ***optimum temperature*** is ***that temperature at which the activity of the enzyme is maximum (Fig. 7.5).***

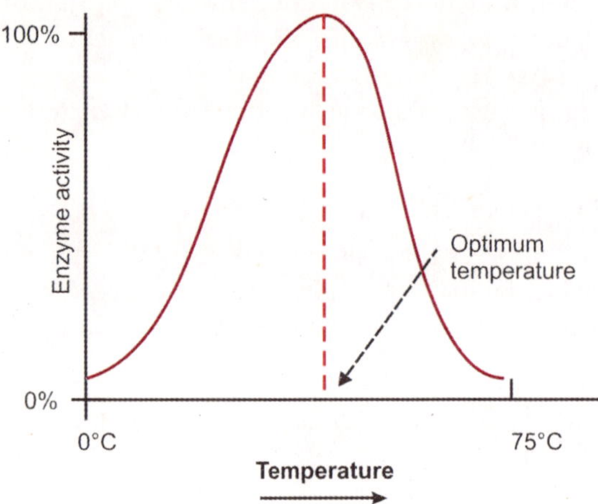

Fig. 7.5: Effect of temperature on enzymatic reaction

2. EFFECT OF PH

The rate of the enzymatic reaction also depends on pH of the medium. The enzymatic activity is maximum at a particular pH which is called its ***optimum pH. The optimum pH of most enzymes lies in the range of 4-9.***

- Hydrogen ions in the medium may alter the ionization of active site or substrates. Ionization is a requirement for ES complex formation,
- pH may influence the separation of coenzyme from holoenzyme complex ***(Fig. 7.6).***

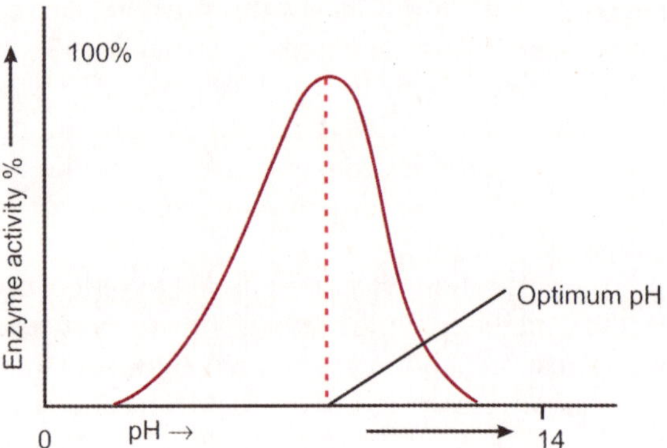

Fig. 7.6: Effect of pH on enzymatic 'reaction'

3. EFFECT OF ENZYME CONCENTRATION

In the beginning ***velocity of the enzymatic reaction is directly proportional to the enzyme concentration.*** When the substrate concentration is in large excess exceeding that of V_{max}, because enzyme is the limiting factor in the enzyme-substrate reaction and providing more enzyme molecules enables the conversion of progressively larger numbers of substrate molecules ***(Fig. 7.7).***

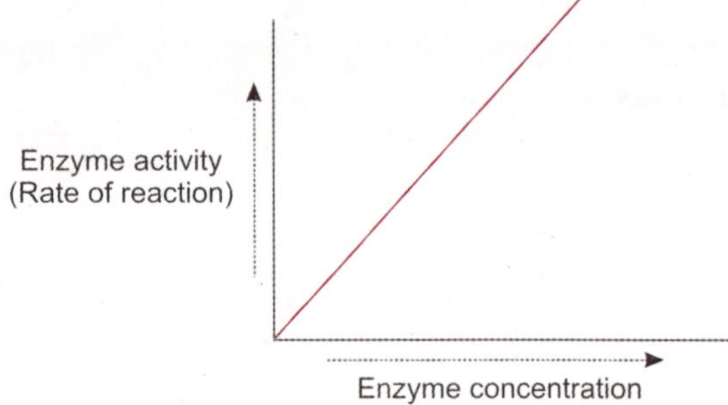

Fig. 7.7: Effect of enzyme concentration on enzymatic reaction

4. EFFECT OF PRODUCT CONCENTRATION

products formed as a result of enzymatic reaction may accumulate, and this excess of product may lower the enzymatic reaction by occupying the active site of the enzyme. It is also possible that under certain conditions of high concentration of products, a reverse reaction may be favoured forming back the substrate.

5. EFFECT OF SUBSTRATE CONCENTRATION

As already described a known quantity of enzyme, the reaction is directly proportional to the substrate concentration. However, ***this is true only up to a certain concentration after which the increasing concentration of substrate does not further increase the velocity of reaction*** (*Fig. 7.8*).

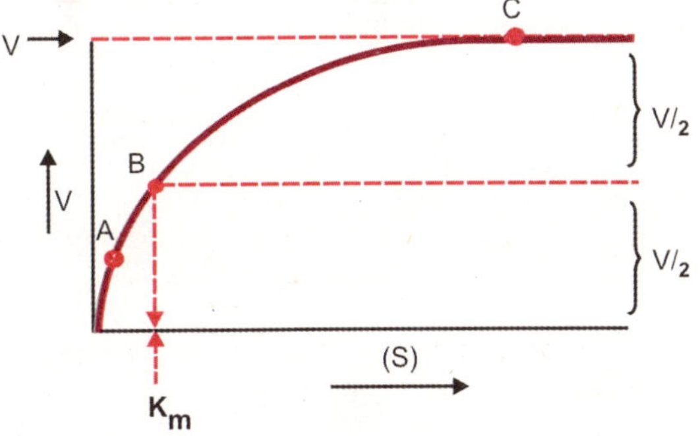

Fig. 7.8: Effect of substrate concentration on enzymatic reaction

6. EFFECT OF ACTIVATORS AND COENZYMES

The activity of certain enzymes is greatly dependent of metal ion activators and coenzyme. The role of metal ion and coenzymes is already discussed.

7. EFFECT OF MODULATORS AND INHIBITORS

Whenever the active site is not available for the binding of the substrate, the enzyme activity may be reduced. ***The substances which stop or modify the enzymatic reaction are called inhibitors or modulators.*** Presence of these substances in reaction medium can adversely affect the rate of enzymatic reaction.

8. EFFECT OF TIME

The time required for completion of an enzyme reaction increases with decreases in temperature from its optimum. However, under the optimum conditions of pH and temperature, time required for enzymatic reaction is less.

ENZYME INHIBITION

Enzymes are protein and they can be inactivated by the agents that denature them. The chemical substances which inactivate the enzymes called as ***inhibitors*** and ***the process is called as enzyme inhibition.*** Inhibitors are sometimes referred to as ***negative modifier***, they may be small inorganic ions, or organic substances. Enzyme inhibitions is classified under ***three*** major groups.

- ***Competitive inhibition (reversible).***
- ***Non-competitive inhibition (irreversible or reversible)***
- ***Allosteric inhibition.***

1. COMPETITIVE INHIBITION

When the active site or catalytic site of an enzyme is occupied by a substance other than the substrate of that enzyme, its activity is inhibited. The type of inhibition of this kind is known as competitive inhibition. This is a type of ***reversible inhibition.*** In such inhibition, both the ES and EI (enzyme inhibitor) complexes are formed during the reaction. However, the actual amounts of ES and El will depend on:

- Affinity between enzyme and substrate/ inhibitor
- Actual concentration (amounts) of substrate and inhibitor present, and
- Time of preincubation of enzyme with the substrate or inhibitor.

So, the affinity of the substrate for the enzyme is progressively decreased with the increase in concentration of inhibitor lowering the rate of enzymatic reaction. ***Thus the Km is high, but V_{max} is the same in competitive inhibition.*** However, when the concentration of substrate is increased, the effect of inhibitors can be reversed forcing it out from EI complex. Few examples of competitive inhibitors are given in ***Table 7.1.***

Example of Competitive Inhibition in Biological System—Used Clinically

- ***Allopurinol***
  - Uric acid is formed by oxidation of hypoxanthine by the enzyme ***"xanthine oxidase"***

Table 7.1: Some Competitive Enzyme Inhibitors

Enzyme	*Substrate*	*Competitive inhibitor*
• **Lactate dehydrogenase**	Lactate	Oxalate
• **Aconitase**	Cisaconitate	Trans-aconitate
• **Succinate dehydrogenase**	Succinate	Malonate
• **HMG-CoA reductase**	HMG-CoA	HMG
• **Dihydrofolate reductase**	7,8 Dihydrofolate	Amethopterin

- ***Allopurinol structurally resembles hypoxanthine***, and thus by competitive inhibition inhibits the enzyme xanthine oxidase thus ***reducing uric acid formation***
- Allopurinol is used for treatment of gout.

- ***MAO inhibitors***
  - The enzyme ***"monoamine oxidase" (MAO)*** oxidizes pressor amines, catecholamines, epinephrine and norepinephrine.
  - Ephedrine and amphetamine have similar structure to catecholamines, thus they can competitively inhibit the enzyme "MAO" and prolong the action of pressor amines.
- ***In bacteria***
  - Sulphonamides compete with para-amino benzoic acid (PABA).
  - PABA is essential for synthesis of folic acid by the enzyme action, where it is needed for growth of bacteria.
  - Sulphonamides compete with PABA and competitively inhibit enzyme action. Thus, ***folic acid is not synthesized and bacterial growth suffers.***
- *Methotrexate*
  - A drug used for cancer therapy. Chemically it is 4-amino-N^{10} methyl folic acid. The drug structurally resembles folic acid. Hence it competitively inhibits the enzyme ***"folate reductase" and prevents formation of F-H_4. Hence DNA synthesis suffers.***

Diagramatic presentation of competitive inhibition is given in *Figure 7.9.*

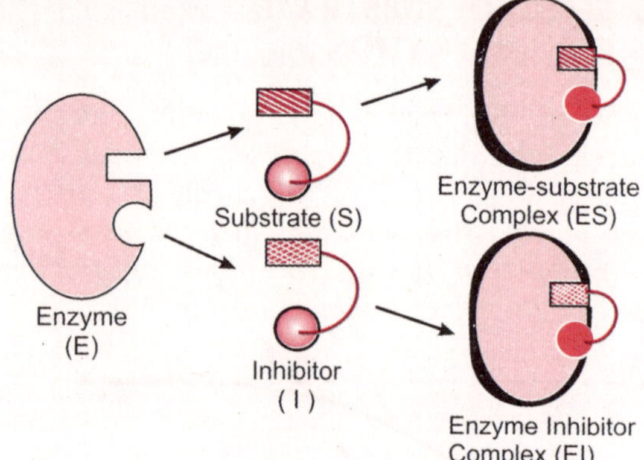

Fig. 7.9: Competitive inhibition

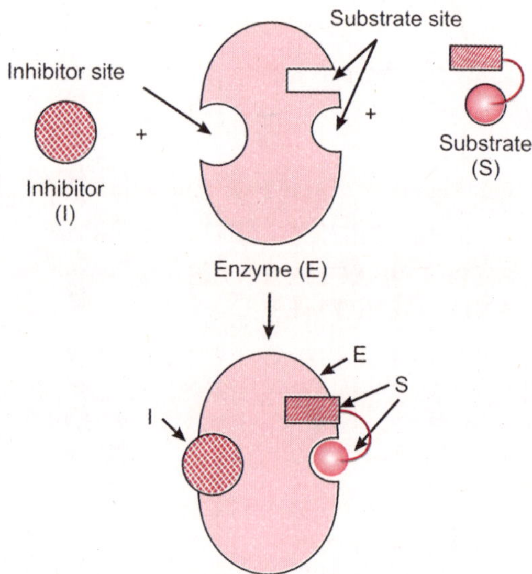

Fig. 7.10: Noncompetitive inhibition

2. NONCOMPETITIVE INHIBITION *(FIG. 7.10)*

This is of **two different types** namely:

- *Reversible* and
- *Irreversible.*

This occurs when the inhibitors not resembling the geometry of the substrate, do not exhibit mutual competition. Most probably, the ***sites of attachment of the substrate and inhibitor are different.*** The inhibitor binds reversibly with a site on enzyme other than the active site. So, the inhibitor may combine with both free enzyme and ES complex. This probably brings about the changes in three dimensional structure of the enzyme inactivating it catalytically. ***In non-competitive inhibition* Vmax *is lowered, but Km is kept constant.***

- If the inhibitor can be removed from its site of binding without affecting the activity of the enzyme, it is called as ***Reversible-Non-Competitive Inhibition.*** However, if the inhibitor can be removed only at the loss of enzymatic activity, it is known as ***irreversible non-competitive inhibition.*** However, the kinetic properties in case of both are the same.

Table 7.2 gives the differences that are observed between competitive and non-competitive inhibition.

3. ALLOSTERIC INHIBITION AND ALLOSTERIC ENZYMES:

There is a mixed kind of inhibition when the ***inhibitor binds to the enzyme at a site other than the active site but on a different region in the enzyme molecule*** called **allosteric site**. Allosteric inhibition does not follow the Michaelis-Menten hyperbolic kinetics. Instead it ***gives a sigmoid kinetics (Fig. 7.11).***

Allosteric inhibitors shift the substrate saturation curve to the right. However, as opposite to inhibitors, the presence of activators shifts the curve to the left. Allosteric enzymes are of *K* and *M* series according to their kinetics:

- ***In K-enzymes,*** e.g *aspartate carbamoylase* and *phosphofructokinase,* the ***allosteric inhibitor lowers the substrate affinity to raise the Km of the enzyme; but the Vmax is unchanged***

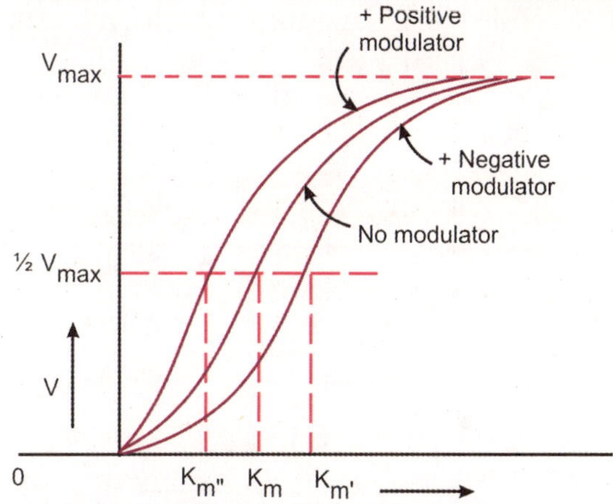

Fig. 7.11: Sigmoid kinetics, allosteric inhibition

- ***In M-enzymes,*** e.g. ***Acetyl-CoA carboxylase, the allosteric inhibitor reduces the maximum velocity but no change in Km or substrate affinity.*** Allosteric activators produce a fall in K enzymes and a rise in *V*max in *M enzymes*.

When the final product allosterically inhibits the enzyme, it is called as ***feedback allosteric inhibition***, e.g. pyrimidine nucleotide CTP inhibits *aspartate transcarbamoylase* allosterically in the synthesis of pyrimidine A metabolite may also cause feed-forward allosteric activation of an enzyme for a subsequent step of its metabolism, e.g. F 1, 6 biphosphate allosterically activates *pyruvate kinase* catalyzing subsequent step.

An allosteric effector oppositely influences two allosteric enzymes catalyzing reverse reactions. For example, AMP allosterically activates

Table 7.2: Differentiation of Competitive and Non-competitive Inhibitions

Competitive inhibition	*Non-competitive inhibition*
• Reversible	• Reversible or irreversible
• Inhibitor and substrate resemble each other in structure	• Does not resemble
• Inhibitor binds the active site	• Inhibitor does not bind the active site
• ***Vmax* is same**	• ***Vmax* lowered**
• **Km is increased**	• **Km unaltered**
• Inhibitor cannot bind with ES complex	• Inhibitor can bind with ES complex
• Lowers the substrate affinity to enzyme	• Does not change substrate affinity for the enzyme
• Complex is E-1.	• Complex is E-S-I or E-I.

phosphofructokinase and allosterically inhibits *fructose, 16-biphosphatase.*

Table 7.3 gives some examples of allosteric modulation.

Table 7.3: Examples of Allosteric Modulation

Name of enzyme	*Allosteric activator*	*Allosteric inhibitor*
• **Glutamate dehydrogenase**	ADP	ATP, NADH
• **Hexokinase, ICD**	ADP	G-6-P, ATP
• **Protein kinases**	c-AMP	—
• **Pyruvate carboxylase**	Acetyl CoA	ADP

In oligomeric enzymes, the allosteric site and active site are located on different subunits. Changes in the enzyme-substrate interaction due to the allosteric effects of regulatory molecules other than the substrate are called ***heterotrophic allosteric modulations.*** Allosteric activators and inhibitors exhibit respectively positive and negative cooperativities with the substrates. Binding of a substrate to one promoter enhances the binding of the same to another promoter or another substrate binding site on the same enzyme molecule. When the binding of a substrate enhances the interaction between the allosteric enzyme and more molecules of the same substrate it is ***homotropic allosteric effect.***

THERAPEUTIC USES OF ENZYMES:

Enzymes have been used therapeutically for treatment purposes. Some of the enzymes used therapeutically are:

I. Used Systematically:

- ***Streptokinase and urokinase:*** used in acute myocardial infarction, deep vein thrombosis, pulmonary embolism.
- ***Digestive enzymes like amylase, lipase and protease:*** used as replacement therapy in pancreatic insufficiency in chronic pancreatitis, cystic fibrosis, following pancreatectomy.
- ***L-asparaginase:*** used in acute leukaemia, malignant lymphomas. Tumor cells require L-asparagine for growth. The enzyme hydrolyzes L-asparagine and thus growth of tumor cells suffer.
- ***Serrato-peptidase:*** used as adjunct therapy in managements of inflammatory oedema due to injury, postsurgical infections. Also used in subconjunctival bleeding.
- ***α-chymotrypsin:*** has mucolytic and proteolytic activity used as adjunct therapy in inflammatory oedema after injury or postsurgical infections and dental procedures.

II. Used Locally:

- ***Hyaluronidase:*** promotes diffusion of fluids given subcutaneously.

ENZYMES AND ISOENZYMES OF CLINICAL IMPORTANCE

The investigation and interpretation of changes in serum enzymes in diseases is one of the most rapidly expanding fields in clinical biochemistry. **Wröblewski** and his coworkers in 1956 published their first papers on serum Glutamate-oxaloacetate transaminase (SGOT) and followed by serum lactate dehydrogenase (LDH) and brought the possibilities of these enzymes assays in general notice. Thus began the present efforescence of clinical enzymology and large number of enzymes have been used for diagnosis and prognosis of various diseases.

Unit of serum enzyme activity: Various workers have used various units. It is better to have uniformity, the serum enzyme activity is expressed in '**International Units' (IU).**

Definition: One IU is defined as the activity of the enzyme which transforms one μ mole of substrate per minute under optimal conditions and at defined temperature, and expressed as IU/ml. When milli-micromole of the substrate is transformed/mt, it is IU/L or m-IU/ml.

VALUE OF SERUM ENZYME ASSAY IN CLINICAL PRACTICE

Single or serial assay of the serum activity of a selected enzyme or enzymes may provide information on the nature and extent of a disease process.

- ***Value in diagnosis:*** An enzyme assay of serum creatine phosphokinase (CPK) on the day of a suspected case of myocardial infarction will be helpful for diagnosis if ECG changes are doubtful.
- ***In differential diagnosis:*** When the differential diagnosis lies between a disease that is known to cause a particular pattern of serum enzyme change and one that does not, e.g. as an aid in differentiating myocardial infarction and pulmonary embolism both presenting with chest pain.

	SGOT	LDH
• **Myocardial infarction**	↑	↑
• **Pulmonary embolism**	Normal	↑

- ***In ascertaining prognosis:*** Serial enzyme assay is required:
  - To ***ascertain progress*** in ***viral hepatitis:*** Serial enzyme assay of serum glutamate pyruvate transaminase SGPT are of great help.
  - ***Response to endocrine therapy of carcinoma of prostate*** is shown by degree of reduction of the elevated serum acid phosphatase.
- ***Early detection of a disease:*** When damage to tissue is suspected which is so slight that it cannot be detected otherwise.

For example:

- Minimal hepatotoxic effects of antidepressant drugs can be detected by a raised serum ICD/or OCT before the patient is clinically ill.
- Increased SGPT in early stage of viral hepatitis when jaundice has not appeared (subclinical stage).

CLINICAL SIGNIFICANCE OF ENZYME ASSAYS

Various enzyme assays used in different diseases are shown in ***Table 7.4.***

VALUE OF ENZYMES IN MALIGNANCIES

Chief enzyme assays useful in malignancies are listed in ***Table 7.5.***

Different serum enzymes, their normal values alongwith increase/decrease in different diseases is given in ***Table 7.6.***

ISOENZYMES

Definition: Isoenzymes (or isozymes) are the ***physically distinct forms of the same enzyme, but catalyze the same chemical reaction*** or reactions and differ from each other structurally, electrophoretically and immunologically.

Table 7.4: Various Enzyme Assays used in Different Diseases

Diseases	*Commonly used enzyme assay*	*Enzyme assays not commonly done*
1. **In myocardial infarction**	• Creatine phosphokinase (CK) • Aspartate transaminase (GOT/or AST) • Lactate dehydrogenase (LDH)	• γ-glutamyl transpeptidase (GGTP) • Histaminase • Pseudo-cholinesterase
2. **Liver diseases**	• Alanine transminase (GPT/or A-LT) • Aspartate transaminase (GOT/or A-ST) • Alkaline phosphatase (ALP) • γ-Glutamyl transpeptidase (γGT) (carboxylase GT)	• Aldolase • Cholinesterase • Isocitrate dehyhydrogenase (ICD) • Leucine amino peptidase (LAP) • 5′- nucleotidase • Ornithine carbamoyl transferase (OCT)
3. **GI diseases**	• Amylase	• Lipase
4. **Muscle diseases**	• Creatine phosphokinase (CK) • Aldolase • SGOT/SGPT	
5. **Bone diseases**	• Alkaline phosphatase (ALP)	
6. **In malignancies (See Table 7.5)**		

Table 7.5: Chief Enzyme Assays Useful in Malignancies

Enzymes assayed	*Diseases*
• **Serum acid phosphatase (ACP)**	• Cancer of prostate with/without metastasis
• **Serum alkaline phosphatase (ALP)**	• Metastasis in liver • Osteoblastic metastasis in bone • Jaundice due to carcinoma of head of pancreas
• **Serum LDH, aldolase, phosphohexose isomerase**	• Widespread malignancies • Advanced leukaemias
• **β-Glucuronidase in urine**	• Cancer of urinary bladder • Cancer head of pancreas
• **LDH in effusion fluids**	• Local malignancies
• **LAP**	• Liver cell carcinoma • Primary or secondary superimposed on cirrhosis liver.

Table 7.6: Increase/decrease of Different Enzymes in Diseases

Serum enzymes	*Normal value*	*Concentrations increased in*	*Concentrations decreased in*
• *Aspartate transaminase (AST) (SGOT)*	4-17 IU/L	***Myocardial infarction,*** elevation slight to moderate in muscle disease, acute liver disease, toxic liver cells necrosis, haemolytic anaemia	
• *Alanine transaminase (ALT) (SGPT)*	3-15 IU/L	***Marked increase-viral hepatitis.*** Slight to moderate-obstructive jaundice, cirrhosis liver, toxic liver cells necrosis, skeletal muscle disease.	
• *Lactate dehydrogenase (LDH)*	60 to 250 IU/L	Acute myocardial infarction, acute hepatitis, also raised in -muscle diseases, leukaemias, renal tubular necrosis, carcinomatosis, cerebral infarction, pernicious anaemia.	
• *Alkaline phosphatase (ALP)*	3 to 13 K.A. units % (23-92 IU/L). Infants and growing children 12-30 KA units per 100 ml	***Marked increase-Obstructive jaundice (>35 KAunits%)***, bone diseases: rickets, Paget's disease, hyperparathyroidism. Slight to moderate increase-acute liver diseases, metastatic carcinoma, "space-occupying" lesions of liver, kidney disease, osteoblastic sarcoma.	
• *Creatine kinase (CK or CPK)*	4-60 IU/L	***Marked increase-acute myocardial infarction*** muscular dystrophies; mild to moderate rise-muscle injury, severe physical exertion, hypothyroidism.	
• *Aldolase*	2 to 6 m-IU	Muscular dystrophies, acute liver disease, myocardial infarction, diabetes mellitus, leukaemias, etc.	

Contd...

Contd...

Serum enzymes	*Normal value*	*Concentrations increased in*	*Concentrations decreased in*
• ***Amylase***	80 to 180 Somogyi units %	***Acute pancreatitis***, acute parotitis (mumps), perforated peptic ulcer, intestinal obstruction, macroamyla-saemia, renal failure.	Acute liver diseases, diabetes mellitus
• ***Lipase***	1. Colorimetric assay 9.0 to 20 m-IU (Seligman and Nachlas) 2. Titrimetric method 0.06 to 1.02 ml of 0.05 (N) NaOH. 3. Cherry-Krandall units. 1.0 to 1.5 units%	***Acute pancreatitis*** perforated peptic ulcer, cirrhosis liver, pancreatic carcinoma	Acute liver diseases, diabetes mellitus, vitamin A deficiency
• ***Cholinesterase***	2.17 to 5.17 IU/ml (130-310 units, dela Huerga)	Nephrotic syndrome, acute myocardial infarction	Acute liver diseases, Malnutrition,- acute infectious diseases. organo-phosphorous poisoning (diazinon poisoning)
• ***Acid phosphatase (ACP)***	0.6 to 3.1 KA units/100 ml: Tartarate-labile ACP- 0 to 0.8 KA units%	***Metastasizing prostatic*** carcinoma, marked rise seen in Gaucher's disease, slight to moderate rise seen in Paget's disease, hyperparathyroidism, osteolytic lesions from breast carcinoma, thrombocytosis. Slight increases after rectal examination (PR), chronic granulocytic leukaemia, myeloproliferative lesions.	
• ***Caeruloplasmin (Ferroxidase)***	3 to 58 mg%	Cirrhosis, bacterial infections, pregnancy	Wilson's disease (Hepato-lenticular degeneration)
• ***Isocitrate dehydrogenase (ICD)***	0.9 to 4.0 IU/L	Marked increase seen in viral hepatitis, slight to moderate rise in cirrhosis liver	
• ***Ornithine carbamoyl transferase (OCT)***	8 to 20 m-IU	Marked elevation in viral hepatitis; slight elevation in cirrhosis liver, obstructive jaundice, metastatic carcinoma	
• ***Leucine amino-peptidase (LAP)***	15 to 56 m-IU	Moderate rise-viral hepatitis slight increase in cirrhosis liver, ***marked rise in superimposed hepatoma in cirrhosis liver***, in liver cell carcinoma	
• ***γ-Glutamyl transpeptidase (γ-GT)***	1 to 47 IU/L	Marked rise seen in acute hepatobiliary diseases, ***alcohol abuse***, alcoholic cirrhosis slight to moderate increase seen-epileptic patients with drug therapy with anticon-vulsants, pancreatic diseases	
• ***5′-Nucleotidase***	2 to 17 IU/L	Acute liver diseases, ***obstructive jaundice***, tumours.	

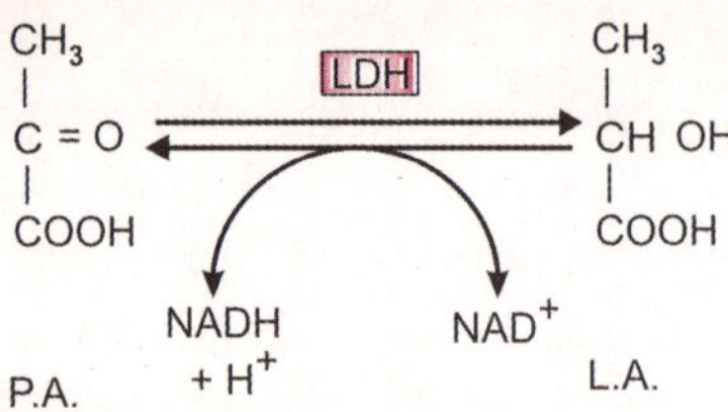

VALUE AND SIGNIFICANCE OF DIFFERENT ISOENZYMES

1. **LDH isoenzymes:** LDH catalyzes the reversible oxidation of lactate to pyruvate.

- In blood serum as many as *5 (five) physically distinct isoenzymes* of this enzyme exist and are known as **LDH-1**, **LDH-2**, **LDH-3**, **LDH-4** and **LDH-5.**
- All these isoenzymes though different physically they catalyze the same reaction of oxidation of LA to PA.
- The different forms can be separated by electrophoresis.
    - **LDH-1** has the highest negative charge and hence ***moves fastest*** during electrophoresis.
    - **LDH-5** is the *slowest moving* fraction.
- The isoenzymes may have different physical properties also, e.g. LDH-4 and LDH-5 are easily destroyed by heat, whereas LDH-1 and LDH-2 are not, if heated up to about 60°C *("Heat-resistant")*
- The isoenzymes have different pH optima and Km values.

STRUCTURE OF LDH ISOENZYMES:

- In man, there are five principal isoenzymes of LDH as mentioned above.
- A sixth atypical isoenzyme LDH has been found in male genital tissues called LDHx.
- Each isoenzyme protein is made up of four polypeptide subunits, thus, each is a *"tetramer"*.
- Each subunit may be one of two types termed H and M, and the different isoenzymes contain H and M in different proportions.
- Thus, **five possible combinations** occur as shown in *Table 7.7.*

Clinical Significance

- After damage to either of these tissues, viz. myocardium or liver, total serum LDH is increased, and it may be useful to know the origin of this increase in enzyme.
- In normal serum, LDH_2 (H_3M) is the most prominent isoenzyme and the slowest peak of LDH-2 is rarely seen.
- After myocardial infarction, the faster isoenzymes LDH-1 and LDH-2 predominate.
- In active viral hepatitis, the slowest isoenzymes LDH-5 and LDH-4 (M_2 and HM_3) predominate.

LDH isoenzymes in malignancy

Total serum LDH is frequently elevated in neoplastic diseases.

- ***In malignancies, isoenzyme pattern shifts towards slower migrating zone***-there is usually an increase in LDH-3, LDH-4 and LDH-5.
- An increase in LDH-5 is seen in breast carcinoma, malignancies of CNS, prostatic carcinoma.
- In leukaemias, rise is more in LDH-2, and LDH-3.
- Malignant tumours of testes and ovary show rise of LDH-2, LDH-3, and LDH-4.

Table 7.7: Structural Pattern of Principal Isoenzymes

Type	*Polypeptide chains*	*Electrophoretic mobility*	*Tissue rich in isoenzyme type*
LDH-1	(H_4) H H H H	Fast moving (fastest)	Found in myocardium
LDH-2	(H_3M) H H H M		
LDH-3	(H_2M_2) H H M M		
LDH-4	(HM_3) H M M M		
LDH-5	(M_4) M M M M	Slowest moving	Found in liver (hepatic)

2. Isoenzymes of CPK: In human tissues, CPK exists as **three different isoenzymes.**

- Each isoenzyme is a *"dimer"*, composed of **two protomers 'M' (for muscle) and 'B' (for brain).** Thus three possible isoenzymes are:

Type	*Polypeptide chains*	*Electrophoretic mobility*	*Tissues found*
CPK-1	BB	Fast moving (more -ve charge)	Brain
CPK-2	MB		Myocardium
CPK-3	MM	Slow moving	Skeletal muscle

CK isoenzymes can be separated by:

- Electrophoresis.
- Ion exchange chromatography techniques.

Clinical Significance

- Normally CK-2 (MB) isoenzymes is very small, (accounts for about 2% of total CK activity of plasma), and almost undetectable.
- ***In myocardial infarction-increase of CK-2 (MB) occurs within 4 hours, maximum in 24 hrs then falls rapidly.***
- MB accounts for 4.5 to 20% of the total CK activity in plasma of patients with a recent myocardial infarction and the total MB isoenzyme level is elevated up to 20-fold above normal.

ATYPICAL CPK ISOENZYMES

In addition to above three distinct forms CK-BB, CK-MB and CK-MM, as stated above, ***two atypical isoenzymes of CPK*** have been reported. They are:

- **Macro-CK (CK-macro)**
- **Mitochondrial CK (CK-Mi)**

(a) Macro-CK (CK-macro):

- *Formation:* It is formed by aggregation of CK-BB with immunoglobulin usually with IgG but sometimes IgA. It may also be formed by complexing CK-MM with lipoproteins.
- *Electrophoresis:* Electrophoretically migrates between CK-MB and CK-MM.
- *Incidence:* 0.8 to 1.6%
- *Age and sex:* Occurs frequently in women above 50 years of age.
- *Clinical significance:* No specific disease has been found to be associated with this isoenzyme.

(b) CK-Mi (Mitochondrial CK-isoenzyme):

- *Formation:* It is present bound to the exterior surface of inner mitochondrial membrane of muscle, liver and brain. It can exist in dimeric form or as an oligomeric aggregates having high molecular weight of approximately 35,000.
- *Electrophoresis:* Electrophoretically, it migrates towards cathode and is behind CK-MM band.
- *Incidence:* It is not present in normal serum. Incidence is from 0.8 to 1.7%.

Clinical Significance

It is only present in serum when there is extensive tissue damage causing breakdown of mitochondrial and cell wall. Thus its presence in serum indicate severe illness and cellular damage.

It is not related with any specific disease states, but it has been detected in case of malignant tumours.

3. Isoenzymes of Alkaline Phosphatase (ALP): ALP exists as a number of isoenzymes, the major isoenzymes found in serum are derived from liver, bone, intestine and placenta.

Assay: The techniques used most frequently for separating the isoenzymes are:

- **Electrophoresis.**
- **Chemical inhibition.**
- **Heat inactivation.**

Electrophoresis is considered the most useful single technique for ALP isoenzyme analysis. By starch gel electrophoresis at pH 8.6, at least ***six* isoenzyme bands** have been delineated.

- *Hepatic isoenzyme:* travels fastest towards the anode and occupies the same position as the fast α_2-globulin.
- *Bone isoenzyme:* the hepatic isoenzyme is closely followed by bone isoenzyme in β-globulin region.

- *Placental isoenzyme:* follows bone isoenzyme.
- *Intestinal isoenzyme:* Slow moving and follows the placental isoenzyme.

REMARKS:

- ***The major ALP isoenzyme in normal serum of adult healthy person is derived from liver, and it shows main liver band.*** In growing child, bone isoenzyme predominates.

The presence of intestinal isoenzyme in serum depends on blood group and secretor status. Individuals who have B or O blood group and are secretors are more likely to have intestinal isoenzyme.

- Nearly all tissues show a ***"subsidiary band"*** near the point of insertion, this approximates in position of serum β-lipoproteins.
- ***Liver isoenzyme*** can actually be divided into ***two* fractions:**
  - The ***major liver band.***
  - A subsidiary smaller fraction, called ***'fast' liver or α_1-liver,*** which migrates anodal to the major band and corresponds to α_1-globulin.

When total ALP levels are increased, it is the major liver fraction that is most frequently elevated.

Clinical Significance

- The major liver band increased in many hepatobiliary diseases.
- 'Fast' liver band is found in many hepatobiliary diseases and in metastatic carcinoma of liver. The two subsidiary bands form a ***"doublet"*** which ***is of diagnostic significance in extrahepatic obstructive jaundice.***
- ***Bone isoenzyme: increases due to osteoblastic activity*** and is normally elevated in children during periods of growth and in adults over the age of 50. In these cases, an elevated ALP level may cause difficulty in interpretation.
- ***In pregnancy:*** during last six weeks of pregnancy, placental isoenzyme of ALP increases. Placental isoenzyme is ***"heat stable"*** and resists heat denaturation at 65°C for ½ hour. ***It is inhibited by L-phenylalanine.***
- Increases of intestinal isoenzyme occurs after consumption of fatty meal. It may increase in several disorders of GI tract and cirrhosis of liver. Increased levels are also found in patients undergoing chronic haemodialysis.

Characteristics of intestinal isoenzyme are given below:

- Slow moving in electrophoresis.
- Inhibited by L-phenyl alanine.
- Resistant to neuraminidase.

Atypical ALP-isoenzymes-"oncogenic markers": In addition to four major ALP isoenzymes, two more abnormal fractions are seen associated with tumours. They are:

- **Regan isoenzyme.**
- **Nagao isoenzyme.**

They have been called as "**carcinoplacental ALP iso-enzymes**" as they resemble placental isoenzyme. Frequency of occurrence in cancer patients is 3 to 15%.

Properties:

- *Regan isoenzyme:* electrophoretically migrates to same position as bone fraction. It is extremely 'heat-stable' and resists heat denaturation of 65°C for ½ hour. It is inhibited by L-phenyl alanine.
- *Nagao isoenzyme:* may be considered as a variant of Regan isoenzyme. Other properties and electrophoretic mobility are similar to Regan isoenzyme. It can be inhibited by L-leucine.

Clinical Significance

- Regan isoenzyme is produced by malignant tissues. It has been detected in various carcinomas of breast, lungs, colon and ovary. Highest incidence of positivity found in cancers of ovary and uterus.
- Nagao isoenzyme has been detected in metastatic carcinoma of pleural surfaces and adenocarcinoma of pancreas and bile duct. Both have prognostic significance. They disappear on successful treatment.

☞ SALIENT POINTS TO REMEMBER

- Enzymes are proteins, synthesized by living cells and they act as biocatalysts.
- Few enzymes are simple proteins while some are conjugated proteins.
- In conjugated protein enzymes, the non-protein part is called prosthetic group or **coenzyme** and the protein part is called **apoenzyme**. The complete structure of apoenzyme and prosthetic group is called as **holoenzyme**.
- The enzymes are classified into **six major classes:** oxido-reductases, transferases, hydrolyses, lyases, isomerases and ligases.
- Certain enzymes require a specific, thermo-stable, low molecular weight, non-protein substance called as coenzyme.
- Most of the coenzymes are derivatives of B-complex vitamins, e.g. NAD^+, FAD, TPP, etc.
- The activity of many enzymes depends on the presence of certain metal ions, e.g. Mg^{++}, K^+, Zn^{++} etc.
- Factors like concentration of enzyme, substrate concentration, temperature, pH, etc. influence enzyme activity.
- The substrate concentration to produce half-maximal velocity is known as Michaelis constant (km).
- The exact ratio by which the velocity changes of 10°C temperature rise is the Q_{10} or temperature co-efficient.
- Reaction velocity almost doubles with 10°C rise ($Q_{10} = 2$) in many enzymes.
- An enzyme is specific in its action, possessing an active site, where the substrate binds to form enzyme-substrate complex (ES complex), before the product is formed.
- The mechanism of enzyme action is explained by Lock and Key model of Fischer, and by more recently induced fit model of Koshland.
- The important feature of Koshland induced fit model is the ***flexibility of the region of active site.***
- The chemical substances which inactivate the enzymes are called as "inhibitors" and the process is called as "inhibition".
- Enzyme inhibition is of three types: competitive inhibition (reversible), non-competitive inhibition (irreversible or reversible) and allosteric inhibition.
- Competitive inhibitors of certain enzymes are of great biological importance.
- Allopurinol, a drug used in treatment of gout competitively inhibits *"xanthine oxidase"* and decreases formation of uric acid.
- Methotrexate, a drug used in cancer therapy, competitively inhibits *"folate reductase"* enzyme.
- Other drugs which act by competitive inhibition are sulphomamides (antibacterial agent), dicoumarol as an anticongulant, MAO inhibitors like Ephedrine and amphetamine.
- In living organisms, the regulation of enzyme activities occurs through allosteric inhibition, activation of latent enzymes, control of enzyme synthesis and degradation.
- Feedback or end product inhibition is special type of allosteric inhibition that control several metabolic pathways, e.g. cholesterol inhibits *"HMG-CoA reductase"*, CTP inhibits *"aspartate transcarbamoylase"*.
- Certain enzymes are used as therapeutic agents, e.g. streptokinase and urokinase — used to dissolve clots as in Myocardial infarction. 1-Asparaginase is used in treatment of leukaemia and lymphomas.
- Locally the enzyme hyaluronidase is used to promote diffusion of fluids given subcutaneously (SC).
- Estimation of serum enzymes is of great help in the diagnosis of several diseases, e.g.
  - Aspartate transaminase (AST, SGOT) and creatine phosphokinase (CPK) in myocardial infarction.
  - Alanine transaminase (ALT/SGPT) in hepatitis for diagnosis and prognosis.
  - Alkaline phosphatase (ALP) in obstructive jaundice, and in bone diseases like Ricket's, Paget's disease.
  - Serum amylase and lipase in acute Pancreatitis.
  - Acid phosphatase (ACP) in prostatic cancer.

- γ-glutamyl transpeptidase (γ-GT) in alcoholism.
- Isoenzymes are the multiple forms of an enzyme catalyzing the same reaction which, however, differ in their physical and chemical properties.
- LDH has five isoenzymes: LDH-1 (H_4), LDH_2 (H_3M), LDH-3 (H_2M_2), LDH-4 (HM_3) and LDH-5 (M_4).
- CPK has three isoenzymes: CPK-1 (BB), CPK-2 (MB) and CPK-3 (MM)
- LDH-1 and CPK-2 are important for diagnosis of myocardial infarction.

MULTIPLE CHOICE QUESTIONS

Give one correct answer:

1. **An enzyme that catalyzes the conversion of an aldose sugar to a ketose sugar is classified as:**
   (a) Transferases (b) Ligases
   (c) Oxido reductases (d) isomerases
   (e) Hydrolases
2. **In non-competitive enzyme action:**
   (a) Concentration of active enzyme molecule is reduced
   (b) Apparent Km is increased
   (c) Apparent Km is decreased
   (d) Vmax is increased
   (e) None of the above
3. **In competitive inhibition of enzyme action:**
   (a) The apparent Km is decreased
   (b) The apparent Km is increased
   (c) Vmax is increased
   (d) Vmax is decreased
   (e) Apparent concentration of enzyme molecules decreased.
4. **An allosteric enzyme influences the enzyme activity by:**
   (a) Competing for the catalytic site with the substrate
   (b) Changing the specificity of the enzyme for the substrate
   (c) Changing the conformation of the enzyme by binding to a site other than catalytic site
   (d) Changing the nature of the products formed
   (e) All of the above
5. **Enzymes may be used for the following *except:***
   (a) For diagnostic pruposes,
   (b) For prognosis
   (c) As therapeutic agents
   (d) As nutrients
   (e) As tumor markers
6. **The following acts as competitive inhibitors *except:***
   (a) Methotrexate (b) Allopurinol
   (c) Cytabarine (d) Dicoumarol
   (e) Sulphonamides
7. **Serum enzymes helpful in the clinical diagnosis of myocardial infarction are the following *except:***
   (a) A-ST (Aspartate transaminase)
   (b) A-LT (Alanine transaminase)
   (c) CPK (Creatine phosphokinase)
   (d) LDH (Lactate dehydrogenase)
   (e) Pseudocholinesterase
8. **Digestive enzymes belong to the class of:**
   (a) Isomerases
   (b) Hydrolases
   (c) Oxido-reductases
   (d) Transferases
   (e) Ligases
9. **The most useful enzyme test for the diagnosis of acute haemorrhagic pancreatitis during the first few days is:**
   (a) Urinary lipase test
   (b) Serum calcium
   (c) Urinary amylase
   (d) Serum amylase
   (e) Serum inorganic phosphate
10. **The best enzyme test for the diagnosis of acute pancreatitis in the presence of mumps is:**
    (a) A serological test for mumps
    (b) Virus isolation
    (c) Serum amylase
    (d) Urinary amylase
    (e) Serum lipase

11. Which of the following enzyme typically elevated in alcoholism?
(a) Serum ALP (b) Serum γ-GT
(c) Serum ALT (d) Serum LDH
(e) Serum acid phosphatase

12. How many isoenzyme forms are there for lactate dehydrogenase (LDH) enzyme?
(a) Two
(b) Four
(c) Five
(d) Six
(e) Eight

13. Liver and skeletal muscle diseases are characterized by a disproportionate increase of which LDH isoenzyme fraction?
(a) LDH-1 (b) LDH-1 and LDH-2
(c) LDH-3 (d) LDH-4
(e) LDH-5

14. Cardiac muscle contains which of the following CK-isoenzyme?
(a) BB only
(b) MM and BB only
(c) MM, BB and MB all three
(d) MM and MB only
(e) MB only

ANSWERS

1. (d)	2. (a)	3. (b)
4. (c)	5. (d)	6. (c)
7. (b)	8. (b)	9. (d)
10. (e)	11. (b)	12. (c)
13. (e)	14. (d)	

8 Biological Oxidation

INTRODUCTION

Oxidation is a reaction with oxygen directly or indirectly or to lose hydrogen and/or electrons. Biologically it is carried out by the enzymes. In any case involvement of oxygen at one or the other state is observed. Oxygen is vital for all living organisms.

The biological oxidation and reductions are restricted to the following three simple classes:

- Loss of one or more electrons, e.g.

$$Fe^{++} \xrightarrow{-e^-} Fe^{+++}$$

- Loss of one or more hydrogen atoms, e.g.

$$CH_3CH_2OH \xrightarrow[\text{or } 2H^+,\ 2e^-]{-e^-} CH_3CHO.$$

- Addition of one or more oxygen atoms

$$CH_3CHO \xrightarrow{+O} CH_3COOH$$

Thus, biological oxidations and reductions can be represented as given below:

$$\text{A red} \xrightarrow{-ne^-} \text{A ox. (Oxidation)}$$

$$\text{A ox} \xrightarrow{+ne^-} \text{A red. (Reduction)}$$

Where ne^- is the number of electrons involved.

Since there is no involvement of free electrons or atoms, biological oxidations and reductions can be represented in the following way:

A red ⟷ B ox

A ox ⟷ B red

In biological oxidations, the terms exothermic and endothermic are replaced by *exergonic* and *endergonic*, e.g. suppose a substance A is oxidized to B with the release of energy and the oxidation is coupled to another reaction in which C is being converted to D. Now, some of the energy liberated in oxidative step A → B is transferred to the synthetic step C→D, in the form other than heat. This is free energy. Thus, ***in exergonic and endergonic reactions, free energy is released or absorbed respectively.***

The principles of biological oxidations of carbohydrates, proteins and fats may be summarized as given below:

- First of all complex organic molecules are degraded into 2-C compound.
- The 2-C fragments are then broken down by a series of steps. In each step, one CO_2 and 2H are removed.
- Decarboxylation of organic acids removes CO_2 without any considerable change in energy.
- The second end product, water arises from reduced coenzymes of respiratory chain and molecular O_2 of atmosphere with production of some energy.

A. Oxidation by Direct Action of Oxygen

A number of enzymes catalyzes direct interaction of substrates with molecular oxygen. Depending upon the fashion in which molecular O_2 is used, these enzymes can be further classified as, (i) ***Oxidases***, (ii) ***Oxygenases***, (iii) ***Hydroxylases*** and (iv) ***Hydroperoxidases***.

1. *Oxidases*: They are electron transferring oxidases and catalyze removal of hydrogen from substrate by directly using O_2 as hydrogen acceptor.

$$O_2 + 4e^- \longrightarrow 2O^- \xrightarrow{-4H+} 2H_2O$$

or

$$O_2 + 2e^- \longrightarrow O_2^- \xrightleftharpoons{2H+} H_2O_2$$

Thus, the product of oxidase action is either H_2O or ***H_2O_2***. Following are the examples of oxidases:

- **With H_2O as the product:** *Cytochrome oxidase, ascorbate oxidase, catechol oxidase.*
- **With H_2O_2 as the product:** *Urate oxidase, amino acid oxidase, xanthine oxidase, aldehyde oxidase, glucose oxidase.*

Some of them are copper-containing enzymes and oxidize the substrate by transferring reducing equivalents from it to molecular O_2. The Cu^{+2} of the enzyme receives the electron from the substrate and gets reduced to Cu^+. The latter subsequently donates the electron to molecular O_2 and gets re-oxidized to Cu^{+2}.

2. *Oxygenases:* These enzymes incorporate O_2 into their substrates, but are not concerned with energy production. They have **two subclasses:**

- ***Dioxygenases:*** These catalyze the incorporation of both the atom of O_2 into the substrate, *e.g. carotene 15-15′ dioxygenases, Tryptophan 2, 3 dioxygenases.*
- ***Monoxygenases or hydroxylases:*** These incorporate one oxygen atom into substrate to form hydroxyl group on it, *e.g. microsomal cyt-D5 mono-oxygenase, mitochondrial cyt P_{450} monooxygenase, etc.* These enzymes transfer reducing equivalents from NADPH or NADH.

3. *Hydroxylases*: There is another group of enzymes called *hydroxylase* which also fall under this. They are sometimes called as mixed function oxidases, *e.g. tyrosinase, phenylalanine hydroxylase, etc.*

4. *Hydroxyperoxidases:* They catalyze oxidation in which H_2O_2 acts as hydrogen acceptor and is reduced to water as:

$$AH_2 + H_2O_2 \rightarrow A + 2H_2O$$
$$A + H_2O_2 \rightarrow AO + H_2O$$

All peroxidases found in plants and milk, and *catalases* found in animals and plants are the examples.

$$H_2O_2 + H_2O_2 \xrightarrow{catalase} 2H_2O + O_2$$

- Both catalase and peroxidase, like glutathione peroxidase decompose $H_2O_2 \rightarrow H_2O + O_2$

Catalase vs Peroxidase

- Catalase can react directly with H_2O_2, but glutathione peroxidase requires reduced glutathione (G-SH).
- ***Km of catalase for H_2O_2 is much greater than glutathione peroxidase.***
- Glutathione peroxidase is the active enzyme to remove small amounts of H_2O_2 formed in cells, e.g. RBC's and lens of eye.

B. Oxidation as a Result of Loss of Hydrogen

Enzymes that remove hydrogen from the substrate fall under this class and are *called* ***dehydrogenases.*** When the hydrogen removed from the substrate is passed onto O_2 directly, it is called ***aerobic dehydrogenase***.

1. *Aerobic dehydrogenases*: These are flavoproteins bearing FMN or FAD as the prosthetic group. They accept 2 hydrogens ($2H^+$ and $2e^-$) from it on the FMN or FAD which is thereby reduced to $FMNH_2$ or $FADH_2$. These can be further reoxidized by donating the hydrogen to molecular oxygen forming H_2O_2.

$$AH_2 + FAD \rightleftharpoons FADH_2 + A$$

$$FADH_2 + O_2 \longrightarrow \mathbf{H_2O_2} + FAD$$

These enzymes can also donate hydrogens to artificial electron-acceptors like methylene blue, e.g. *L-amino acid oxidase, urate oxidase, xanthine oxidase.*

2. *Anaerobic Dehydrogenases:* In this group of enzymes there is direct transfer of electrons to molecular oxygen. They make use of intermediate electron acceptors. The latter reduced thereby transfers the electrons to some other electron acceptor.

- ***Pyridine-linked dehydrogenases:*** These oxidize the substrate by transferring a hydride ion (H^-) from the substrate to NAD^+ or NADP.

The second hydrogen removed from the substrate is released as free H^+. In the process the NAD and NADP get reduced to NADH and NADPH. The chain of reaction continues with another dehydrogenase enzyme.

- ***Flavin-linked dehydrogenases:*** FMN and FAD are the two flavin containing coenzymes that remain linked to specific dehydrogenase enzymes. Some also carry either heme or one or more iron-sulfur clusters. They oxidize the substrate by removing $2H^+$ and $2e^-$ from it and transferring them to the flavin coenzymes. In the process, the flavin coenzymes get reduced to either $FMNH_2$ and $FADH_2$ depending on the enzyme. The reduced flavin nucleotides then transfer the reducing equivalents to an electron acceptor other than molecular O_2. Most of these enzymes get reoxidized by transferring reducing equivalents to coenzyme Q, e.g.
- ***FAD linked enzymes:*** *D-amino acid oxidase, glycine oxidase, succinic dehydrogenase, diaphorase*
- **FMN-linked enzymes:** NADP-Cyt-c reductase, Cyt b_2.

Differences between Aerobic Dehydrogenases and Anaerobic Dehydrogenases

Aerobic dehydrogenase	*Anaerobic dehydrogenase*
• Can react directly with O_2	• Cannot transfer the hydrogen and electrons to O_2 directly. Transfers hydrogen and electrons from substrate to NAD or FP
• H_2O_2 is produced	• H_2O_2 not produced, NADH + H^+ or FpH_2 are produced
• ATP is not produced	• ATP is produced by oxidation of NADH/ Fp H_2 in electron transport chain

C. Iron-Sulfur Proteins and Ubiquinones or Coenzyme Q:

A group of quinones has been found to be present in the mitochondria. Following types of non heme iron-sulfur clusters are normally present.

- **FeS:** It has single Fe coordinated to the side chain-SH-groups of four cysteine residues
- **Fe_2S_2:** It contains two iron atoms, two inorganic sulfides and four-SH groups. Each iron is linked to 2-SH and 2 sulfur groups.
- **Fe_4S_4:** It consists of four iron atoms and four cysteine-SH groups and four inorganic sulfides, each iron remains linked to one-SH, 3 inorganic sulfides while each sulfide is coordinated to three iron atoms.
- **Fe_3S_4:** Comprises 3 Fe, 4-SH and 4 inorganic sulfides.

The enzymes may have one or more of the combinations of the clusters mentioned above. Fe^{+2} of a reduced iron-sulfur protein gets subsequently reoxidized by donating its electron to an electron acceptor such as CoQ or Cyt-c_1. Each iron-sulfur protein transfers only one electron at a time. It is also believed that vit E, vit D and plastoquinones in the plant tissues participate in the process of electron transfer.

D. Cytochromes

These are very important enzymes which contain heme and are involved in cellular oxidation. The oxidized form of cytochrome possesses a single Fe^{+3} ion and is called ***ferricytochrome***. It is reduced to ***ferrocytochrome*** having a Fe^{+2} ion, on accepting an electron. Cytochromes are identified by their characteristic absorption spectra.

1. ***Cytochrome-c:*** Since it is available in large quantities, it is the best studied of the cytochromes.

- It is water soluble and easily extractable.
- It shows characteristic absorption spectra in the reduced form at 550, 521 and 416 mμ. Oxidized form gives two diffuse bands at 530 mμ and 400 mμ.
- Cyt-c is incapable of combining with O_2 or CO. it is a basic protein with one polypeptide chain with 104 amino acids having mol. Wt of 12400 to 13000.

2. ***Cytochrome-c_1:*** Like Cyt-c, Cyt-c_1 also possesses an iron-protoporphyrin IX complex-haem-C. It has absorption maxima at 554, 524 and 418 mμ. This is also incapable of combining with O_2, CO, CN^-.

3. *Cytochrome b:* Cytochrome b also contains the same protoporphyrin IX complex (**haem b**). The apoprotein is however different.

- It is found to be tightly bound to flavoproteins and ubiquinones in the mitochondria.
- It is thermostable and not easily extractable.
- It also does not react with O_2, CO or CN^-.
- In normal course its oxidation requires the presence of Cyt c, a and a_3. Cyt-b is reduced by accepting an electron from reduced CoQ.

4. *Cytochromes a and a_3 (Cytochrome oxidases):* Cytochrome oxidases constitute the complex IV of the mitochondrial electron transport chain.

- Both possess an identical type of iron-porphyrin complex called ***haem-a.***
- In spite of identical haem groups, cytochromes a and a_3 differ in their electron affinity and biological activity because of their location of haem groups at different sites of the apoprotein.
- Cyt-a does not react with O_2, CO, or CN^- whereas ***Cyt-a_3 is autooxidizable and forms compounds with CO and CN^-.***

REDOX POTENTIAL AND FREE ENERGY

In the discussion so far, we have made it clear that an oxidizing or reducing agent may exist in two forms:

- The oxidized form or oxidant which can accept electrons
- The reductant which can donate its electrons to a substrate. Each oxidizing or reducing agent exist as a conjugated pair of electron acceptor oxidant and electron donor reductant forms.

$$\text{Oxidant} + ne^- \rightarrow \text{reductant}$$

Where 'n' is the number of electrons. ***The pair consisting of the oxidant and reductant forms of an oxidizing or reducing agent is known as a redox couple or conjugate redox pair, e.g.*** $NAD^+/NADH$, $FMN/FMNH_2$, Cyt c Fe^{++}/Cyt c Fe^{+++}. ***Oxidizing agents differ in their electron affinity. The standard redox potential Eo is a measure of the tendency of a redox couple to donate or accept electrons under standard conditions.*** Redox potential of a given system is intimately related to its free energy change. If redox-potential of a given system is known, the corresponding free energy change which might occur in the system on oxidation or reduction may be found. If the sign of free-energy calculated is negative, it indicates free energy release and if positive, it indicates free energy consumption. The redox potentials of many biologically important redox couples are known and are as shown in ***Table 8.1.***

Table 8.1: Redox Potentials of Biologically Important Redox Couples

	System	*E'o volts*
α-Hydroxybutyrate	⇔ acetoacetate	–0.346
Isocitrate	⇔ α-ketoglutarate	–0.36
NADH	⇔ NAD^+	–3.20
$FMNH_2$	⇔ FMN	–0.30
Ubiquinol	⇔ Ubiquinone	+0.10
Cyt-b (Fe^{+2})	⇔ Cyt-b Fe^{+3}	+0.08
Cyt c_1 Fe^{+2}	⇔ Cyt-c_1 Fe^{+3}	+.022
Cyt c Fe^{+2}	⇔ Cyt-c Fe^{+3}	+ 0.254
Cyt a Fe^{+2}	⇔ Cyt-a Fe^{+3}	+ 0.29
Cyt a_3 Fe^{+2}	⇔ Cyt-a_3 Fe^{+3}	+ 0.386
O_2	⇔ H_2O	+0.816

MITOCHONDRIAL ELECTRON TRANSPORT CHAIN

Definition: ***This is the final common pathway in aerobic cells by which electrons derived from various substrates are transferred to oxygen.*** Electron transport chain (ETC) is a series of highly organized oxidation-reduction enzymes whose reactions can be represented as:

Reduced A + Oxidized B ⇔ Oxidized A + Reduced B.

Localization: The ETC is localized in the mitochondria. The outer membrane of mitochondria is permeable to most of the small molecules. There is an intermediate space which presents no barrier to passage of intermediates. The inner membrane shows a highly selective permeability. It has transport systems only for specific substances such as ATP, ADP, pyruvate, succinate, α-ketoglutarate, malate and citrate, etc. ***The enzymes of the electron transport chain are embedded in the inner membrane in association with the enzymes of oxidative phosphorylation.***

Table 8.2: Various Reactions and Enzymes Taking Place in the Mitochondrial Matrix

Reaction	*Enzyme*	*Oxidant*
• α Glycerophosphate → Dihydroxyacetone	α Glycerophosphate dehydrogenase	FAD
• Acyl CoA → Unsaturated acyl CoA	Acyl CoA dehydrogenase	FAD
• Glutamate → Ketoglutarate	Glutamate dehydrogenase	NAD^+
• Pyruvate → Acetyl CoA	Pyruvate dehydrogenase	NAD^+
• Succinate → Fumarate	Succinate dehydrogenase	FAD
• Malate → Oxaloacetate	Malate dehydrogenase	NAD^+
• α-Ketoglutarate → Succinyl CoA	α-Ketoglutarate dehydrogenase	NAD^+

The most accepted sequences of electron carriers in the mitochondria is as follows:

$$\text{Substrate} \rightarrow NAD^+ \rightarrow FAD \rightarrow CoQ \rightarrow 2\text{Cyt-b}$$
$$\downarrow$$
$$O_2 \leftarrow 2\text{Cyt}\ (a_3 + a) \leftarrow 2\text{Cyt-c} \leftarrow 2\text{Cyt-C}_1$$

As already mentioned the ***redox potentials in the ETC are in increasing order except in the case of ubiquinone.*** The chain actually consists of a series of redox couples, at ***each step electrons flow from the reductant of a redox couple with more negative redox potential to the oxidant of the next redox couple having a more positive redox potential.***

Dehydrogenation of substrate is the first step in the process of respiratory chain oxidation. Most of the dehydrogenases require NAD^+ which can accept a hydride ion (H^-) which is formed by one hydrogen atom and an electron. The electron is received from the second hydrogen atom releasing the second hydrogen atom in the form of a proton (H^+).

The second type of hydrogenase reaction makes use of FAD as the coenzymes. ***Table 8.2*** gives the various reactions and the enzymes that take place in the mitochondrial matrix. In these reactions the oxidants are reduced to NADH + H^+ or $FADH_2$. ***Figure 8.1*** shows the path of electron transport.

The electron transport chain (ETC) in the mitochondrial membrane has been **separated in 4 (four) complexes or components** as follows *(Fig. 8.2)*:

- **Complex I:** NADH-CoQ reductase
- **Complex II:** Succinate-CoQ reductase
- **Complex III:** CoQ - Cytochrome C reductase
- **Complex IV:** Cytochrome C oxidase

COMPLEX I: NADH-COQ REDUCTASE

This system has ***two functions:***

- ***Electron transfer***
- ***Acts as a proton pump.***

The system catalyzes transfer of two electrons from NADH to small lipid soluble CoQ via FMN and FeS clusters.

$$NADH + H^+ + FMN \rightarrow FMN.H_2 + NAD^+$$

From $FMN.H_2$ electrons are transferred to a group of FeS proteins. Fe atoms of FeS protein oscillate between Fe^{++} and Fe^{+++}. The electrons are then transferred to CoQ.

$$CoQ \xrightarrow{e^-} CoQ.H\ \text{(Semi-quinone)}$$

$$CoQ.H \xrightarrow{e^-} CoQ.H_2\ \text{(Quinol)}$$

The process is accompanied by pumping of protons from mitochondrial matrix into intermembrane space.

- ***Permits one ATP Formation (Site I).***

Note: Upto CoQ, H is transferred. But from CoQ onward only e^- is transferred, $2H^+$ goes into the medium.

COMPLEX II: SUCCINATE-COQ REDUCTASE:

Flow of electrons from succinate to CoQ occurs via $FAD.H_2$.

$$\textbf{Succinate + CoQ} \rightarrow \textbf{Fumarate + CoQ.H}_2$$

Standard reduction potential for transfer of electrons from $FAD.H_2$ to CoQ is + ***0.113V (much lower than +0.420 V energy change for the reaction of complex I).*** The small energy change does not allow *"succinate-CoQ reductase"* system to pump protons across the mitochondrial membrane, hence this protein complex does not contribute to proton gradient. ***Hence no ATP is formed.***

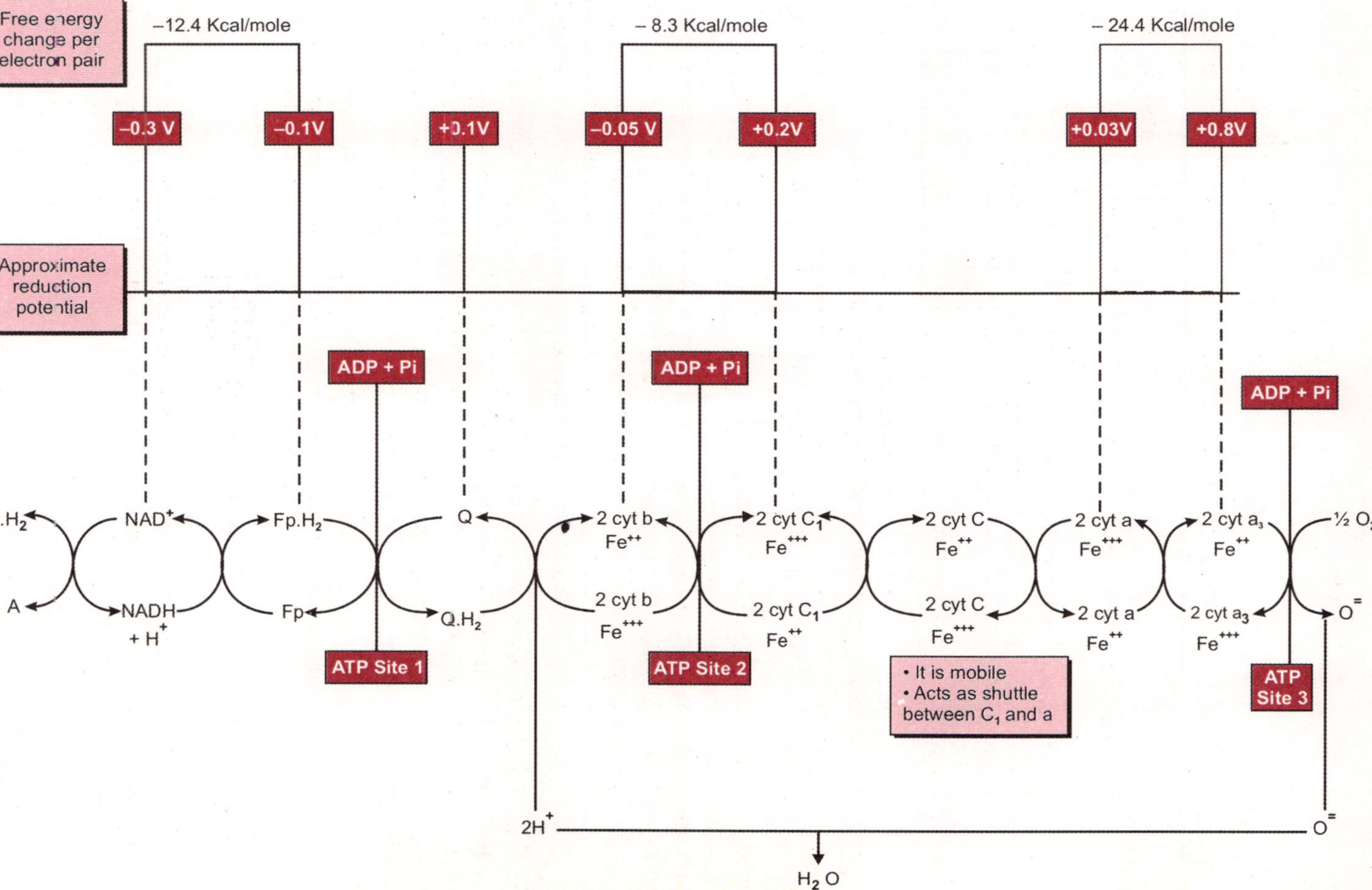

Fig 8.1: The electron transport system of the respiratory chain showing the sites of formation of 3ATP molecules

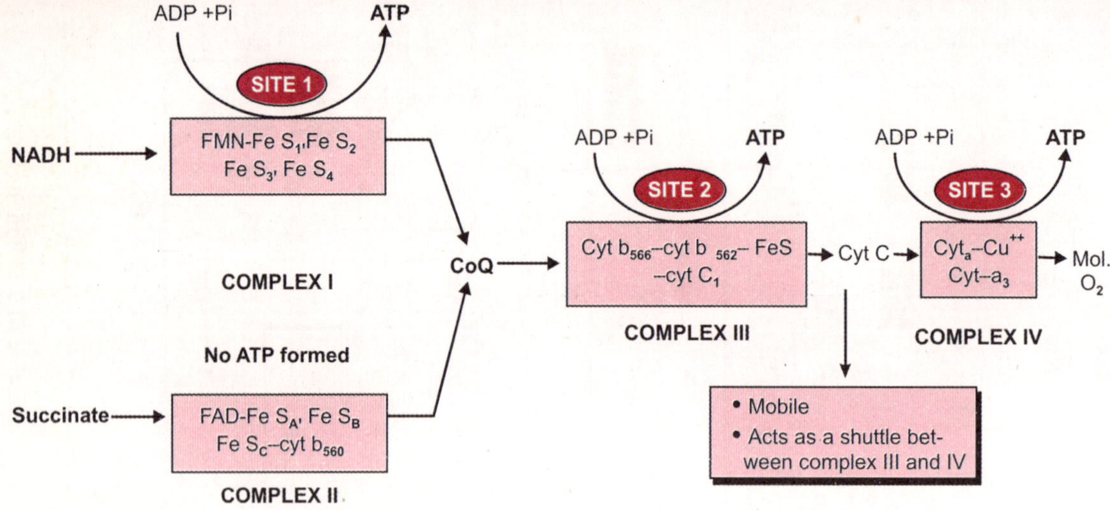

Fig. 8.2: Showing four complexes of electron transport chain

Note: CoQ is the electron acceptor in the reaction catalyzed by *"NADH-CoQ reductase"* (Complex I) and *"succinate-CoQ reductase"* (Complex II). The electrons received are subsequently transferred from $CoQ.H_2$, a lipid soluble mobile electron carrier to *"CoQ-cyt. C reductase"* (Complex III).

COMPLEX III: COQ-CYT.C REDUCTASE:

Functions as

- *Proton pump,* and
- *Catalyzes transfer of electrons*

This system catalyzes transfer of electrons from $CoQ.H_2$ to Cyt. c via Cyt. b and Cyt.c_1.

The electrons from $CoQ.H_2$ is first accepted by Cyt.b_{566} and then transferred to Cyt.b_{562}, which reduces

$$Co.Q.H_2 \rightarrow CoQ$$

Fe^{+++} accepts electron and is oxidized to Fe^{++}.

The **system also acts as a proton pump**. It is believed that 4 (four) protons are pumped across the mitochondrial membrane during the oxidation.

$$CoQ.H_2 + 2\,Cyt\text{-}c\,(Fe^{+++}) \rightarrow Co.Q + 2\,Cyt.c\,(Fe^{++}) + 2\,H^+$$

The energy change permits ATP formation (Site II).

COMPLEX IV: CYT-C OXIDASE:

The system **functions:**

- **As proton pump**
- **Catalyzes transfer of electrons to molecular O_2 to form H_2O.**

This is the terminal component of ETC. It catalyzes the transfer of electrons from Cyt.c to molecular O_2 via cyt.a, cu^{++} ions and cyt a_3.

$$4\,Cyt\,c\,(Fe^{++}) + 4H^+ + O_2 \rightarrow 4\,cyt\,c\,(Fe^{+++}) + 2H_2O$$

The flow of electrons is as follows:
$Cyt\,c \rightarrow Cyt\,a \rightarrow Cu^{++} \rightarrow Cyt\text{-}a_3 \rightarrow O_2$

Role of Cu Ions: Cu atom adjacent to cyt. heme a is Cu-A (Sub unit II) and Cyt-heme a_3 is close to CuB (Sub unit I). From Cyt-c, the electrons are transferred to heme-a-CuA cluster and then heme a_3-CuB cluster.

The ***system also acts as a proton pump,*** it pumps two protons into intermembrane space. ***The energy change permits ATP formation (Site III)*** between cyt a_3 and molecular O_2.

Note: Cyt c does not form a part of any complexes. It is ***mobile*** and ***acts as a shuttle*** between complex-III and complex-IV to transfer e^- (electron).

FREE ENERGY CHANGES AND SITE OF ATP FORMATION

Free energy changes calculated from the oxidation, reduction potential differences of various reactions of respiratory chain are as given in *Table 8.3. Thus the span of the respiratory chain is 1.14 V which corresponds to 52.6 K Cal/mole.* There is decline in free energy as electrons flow down the electron transport chain. At *three sites* free energy released per electron pair transferred is sufficient *to support the phosporylation of ADP to ATP which requires about 7K Cal/mole.*

The **three sites where ATP is produced** in respiratory chain are as follows by a process called oxidative phosphorylation.

- **NADH → CoQ**
- **Cyt-b → Cyt-c_1**
- **Cyt-a → O_2**

The details of this process called as oxidative phosphorylation will be described later.

- Thus, the electrons that enter the transport chain through the NADH-Q reductase complex support the synthesis of 3 mols of ATP per pair of electrons.
- By contrast electrons entered at the level of CoQ as they would be donated by $FADH_2$ only support the synthesis of 2 mol of ATP per pair of electrons.

Table 8.3: Free Energy Changes Calculated from Redox Potential Differences

Step			*Differences in Redox Potential*	*Free energy changes K cal.*
• NAD	$\xrightarrow{2H}$	FP	+0.26 V	–12.004
• FP	$\xrightarrow{2e^-}$	2Cyt b	+0.10 V	–4.617
• Cyt b	$\xrightarrow{2e^-}$	2Cyt C_1	+0.23 V	–10.619
• Cyt C_1	$\xrightarrow{2e^-}$	Cyt a_1	+0.02 V	–0.923
• Cyt a_1	$\xrightarrow{2e^-}$	Cyt a_3	+0.21 V	–9.695
• 2Cyt a_3	$\xrightarrow{2e^-}$	0	+0.32 V	–14.774
Total			1.14V	52.63 K cal

ADP : O or P : O Ratio: The NAD-dependant dehydrogenases such as malate, pyruvate, α-keto-glutarate, isocitrate, etc. produce three high energy phosphate bonds for each pair of electrons transferred to O_2 because they have P: O ratio of 3 *Thus, P : O ratio is the measure of how many moles of ATP are formed from ADP by phosphorylation per gram atom of oxygen used.* This is usually measured as the number of moles of ADP (or Pi) that disappear per gram atom of oxygen used.

$$\text{P : O ratio} = \frac{\text{Phosphate group esterified}}{\text{Electron pairs transferred}}$$

$$\text{Efficiency} = \frac{\text{P/O ratio} \times 7.3}{\text{51 Kcal}} \times 100$$

However, P : O ratio in case of $FADH_2$ is 2, and therefore efficiency is lower in that case.

INHIBITORS OF ELECTRON TRANSPORT CHAIN

Transfer of electrons is selectively inhibited at various components of the electron transport chain by a variety of substances. Some of these are used as poisons, (e.g. insecticides) and some of which are used as drugs.

INHIBITORS OF ETC

Site-I (Complex I)

- ***Rotenone:*** A fish poison and also insecticide inhibits transfer of electron through complex NADH-Q reductase
- ***Amobarbital (Amytal) and secobarbital:*** Inhibits electron transfer through NADH-Q reductase
- ***Piericidin A:*** An antibiotic blocks electron transfer by competing with CoQ.
- ***Drugs:*** Like chlorpromazine and hypotensive drug like guanethidine.

Site-II (Complex III)

- ***Antimycin A:*** (Antibiotic)
- ***BAL*** (Dimercaprol)
- ***Hypoglycaemic drug:*** like phenformin

} blocks electron transfer from Cyt b to C_1

Site-III (Complex IV)

- Cyanide
- *H_2S:* } Inhibits terminal transfer of electron to molecular O_2
- *Azide*
- ***CO (Carbon monoxide):*** Inhibits Cyt oxidase by combining with O_2 binding site. It can be reversed by illumination with light.

Complex II (Succinate dehydrogenase-FAD)

- *Carboxin:* } Specifically inhibit transfer of reducing equivalent from succinate dehydrogenase
- *TTFA*
- ***Malonate:*** A competitive inhibitor of succinate dehydrogenase

Mitochondrial Shuttle Systems

Glycolysis produces NADH in the cytoplasm which cannot enter mitochondria. Shuttles between cytoplasm and mitochondria operate. ***Two such shuttles*** are of considerable importance.

- ***Glycerophosphate shuttle***
- ***Malate shuttle***

(For details-Refer Chapter on Carbohydrate Metabolism).

OXIDATIVE PHOSPHORYLATION

The process of oxidative phosphorylation is closely associated with the functioning of the electron transport chain. This was studied by fragmentation of mitochondria. In the first fragmentation step, the outer membrane is removed by treatment with various detergents such as saponin, digitonin. The two particulate fractions that result are:

1. The outer membrane, either in the form of vesicles or completely solubilized.
2. The inner membrane and the mitochondrial matrix enzymes. This fraction is found to contain the enzymes of:
   - **The electron transport chain**
   - **Oxidative phosphorylation**
   - **The TCA cycle.**

In oxidative phosphorylation ATP is produced by combining ADP and Pi with the energy generated by the flow of electrons from NADH to molecular oxygen in the electron transport chain. There are **three sites** in the respiratory chain where ATP is formed by oxidative phosphorylation. These sites have been proved by the free energy changes of the various redox couples. Since hydrolysis of ATP to ADP + Pi releases around 7.3 K. Cal/mole, ***the formation ATP from ADP + Pi requires a minimum of around 8 K Cal/mole.*** The formation of ATP is therefore not possible at the sites where free energy released is less than 8 K. Cal/mole.

Whenever two systems or redox couple of the respiratory chain differ from each other by 0.22 volts in standard redox potential (E'o), the free energy is sufficient to form ATP.

$$G^o = -n\,F\,Eo$$

$$G^o = -2 \times 23.06 \times 0.22 = -10.15 \text{ K.Cal}$$

Sites of ATP Formation: There are **three sites** in the respiratory chain where ATP can be formed.

- *Site I:* This involves the transfer of electrons from NADH –CoQ. Obviously this step is omitted by *succinic dehydrogenase* whose $FADH_2$ prosthetic group transfers its electrons directly to CoQ bypassing NADH. ***This step is blocked by piericidin, rotenone, amobarbital, certain drugs like chlorpromazine, guanethidine.***
- *Site II:* This involves the transfer of electrons from cyt b–cyt c_1. This step as well as the previous one is bypassed in oxidation of L-ascorbate whose electrons are directly transferred to cyt c. ***This step is blocked by BAL, Antimycin A, Hypoglycaemic drug like phenformin.***
- *Site III:* Transfer of electrons from cyt a_3 to molecular oxygen ***which is blocked by CO, CN, H_2S, and azide.***

MECHANISM OF OXIDATIVE PHOSPHORYLATION

Three major proposals for the mechanism of oxidative phosphorylation have been considered. The synthesis of ATP is carried out by a molecular assembly in the inner mitochondrial membrane. ***This enzyme complex is called Mitochondrial ATPase or H^+-ATPase. It is also called ATP-synthase.***

Theories:

The three hypothesis do make use of the information available on *ATP synthase*.

A. The Chemical Coupling Hypothesis: This is developed from the concept of a high energy intermediate common to both electron transport and phosphorylation of ADP. However, such intermediate has not been identified so far.

B. The Conformational Coupling Hypothesis: According to this hypothesis the mitochondrial cristae undergo conformational changes and these changes in architecture of the mitochondrial cristae reflect the changes in the different components of the electron chain to one another. It is believed that these conformational change represents the formation of high energy state.

C. Chemiosmotic Theory: This is the most accepted view of oxidative phosphorylation postulated by **Peter Mitchell in 1961**. Mitchell's chemiosmotic theory postulates that the energy from oxidation of components in the respiration chain is coupled to the translocation of hydrogen ions (Protons, H^+) from the inside to the outside of the inner mitochondrial membrane. **Each of the respiratory chain complexes I, III and IV acts as a proton pump.** The inner membrane is impermeable to ions in general but particularly to protons, which ***accumulate outside the membrane, creating an electrochemical potential*** difference across the membrane ($\Delta\mu H^+$). This consists of a chemical potential **(difference in pH)** and an electrical potential.

The electrochemical potential resulting from the asymmetric distribution of the hydrogen ion is used to ***drive the mechanism responsible for the formation of ATP.***

Experimental Evidences to Support the Chemiosmotic Hypothesis

- Addition of protons H^+ (acid) to the external medium of intact mitochondria leads to the generation of ATP.
- Oxidative phosphorylation does not take place in soluble system where there is no possibility of a vectorial ATP synthase.
- A closed membrane is a must to achieve oxidative phosphorylation.

ATP SYNTHASE

Much information is now available regarding ATP synthase and its role in ATP formation.

Structure: (Fig. 8.3)

It is an ***enzyme complex present in the inner mitochondrial*** membrane. It is now referred as **COMPLEX V** the enzyme complex has **two subunits – F_0 and F_1.**

- **F_0 unit or subcomplex:**
  It spans inner mitochondrial membrane and **serves as a proton channel** through which protons enter into mitochondria.
  It is a **disk of "C-subunits"**. Attached to it is a **γ-subunit** in the form of a ***"bent axle". The γ-subunit fits inside the F_1 subcomplex.***
- **F_1 unit or subcomplex:**
  This projects into the mitochondrial matrix. It catalyzes the ATP synthesis. F_1 subcomplex consists of **3β chains (β_3)** and **3α chains (α_3).**

γ subunit fits inside the F_1 subcomplex of 3α and 3β subunits which are fixed to the membrane.

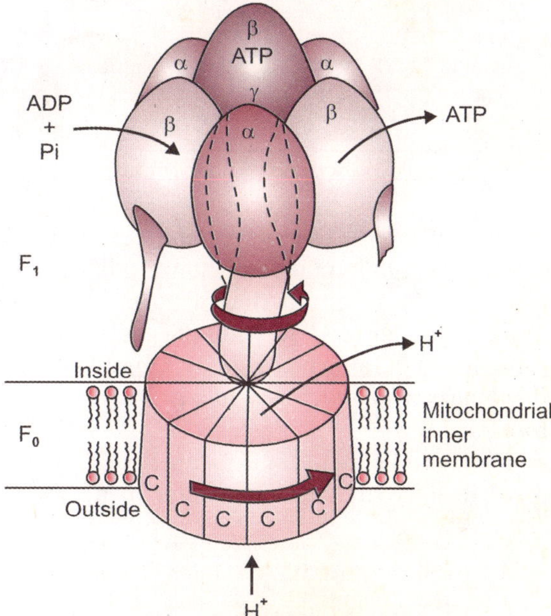

Fig. 8.3: Schematic representation of ATP synthase

In addition, the complex has **sigma** and **epsilon subunits**, the function of which are not known.

Mechanism of ATP Synthesis (Boyer's hypothesis):

Paul Boyer originally proposed a **"binding change" mechanism.**

According to this hypothesis 3β subunits (catalytic sites) though structurally similar, but functionally not same at a particular time.

It is envisaged that **b subunits** occur in **3 forms:**

- **'O' form (Openform):** It has low affinity for substrates ADP + Pi.
- **'L' form (Looseform):** Can bind substrates ADP and Pi with more affinity but ***catalytically it is inactive.***
- **'T' form (Tight form):** Binds substrates ADP and Pi tightly and ***catalyzes ATP synthesis***.

Protons entering the system cause conformational changes in the β subunits.

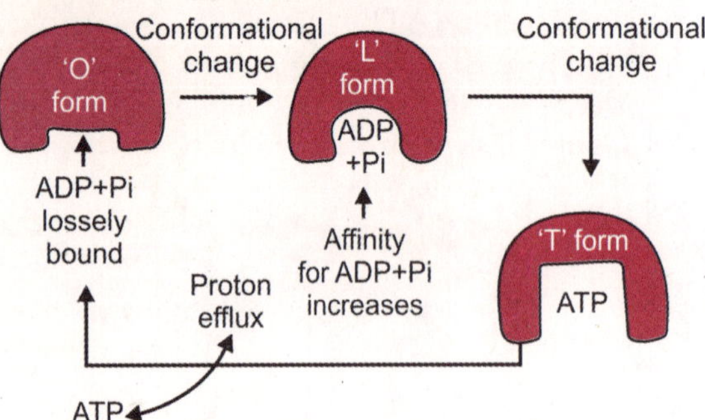

Rotary or Engine Driving Model:

Original Boyer's hypothesis is now modified. It is now widely accepted that protons passing through the disk of 'C' subunits of F_0 subcomplex cause it and the attached γ-subunit **to rotate**. The ***β-subunits which are fixed to membrane do not rotate.***

ADP and Pi are taken up sequentially by the β-subunits which undergo conformational changes

'O' form → 'L' form → 'T' form
↑________________↑

and forms ATP, which is expelled as the rotating γ-subunit squeezes each β-subunit inturn.

Thus 3 ATP molecules are generated per revolution.

Inhibitors of Oxidative Phosphorylation

- *Oligomycin:* It ***binds with the enzyme ATP synthase and blocks the proton channels.*** It thus prevents the translocation of H^+ into the mitochondrial matrix, this leads to accumulation of H^+ at higher concentration in intermembrane space. Since protons cannot be pumped out against steep proton gradients, electron transport stops (respiration stops).
- *Atractyloside:* It is a **glycoside, it blocks the translocase that is responsible for movement of ATP and ADP,** across the inner mitochondrial membrane. Adequate supply ot ADP is blocked thus preventing phosphoglation and ATP formation.
- *Bongregate:* Toxin produced by Pseudomonads. It acts similarly to atractyloside.

UNCOUPLERS OF OXIDATIVE PHOSPHORYLATION

These are the compounds that allow mitochondria to use oxygen regardless of whether or not there is any phosphate (ADP) available. When an uncoupler is added, there is marked increase in O_2 uptake.

Uncouplers of Oxidative Phosphorylation

- *2, 4 Dinitrophenol:* a classic uncoupler of oxidative phosphorylation (mechanism see below).
- *Dicoumarol (Vitamin K analogue):* Used as anticoagulant
- *Calcium:* Transport of Ca^{++} ion into mitochondria can cause uncoupling.
  - Mitochondrial transport of Ca^{++} is energetically coupled to oxidative phosphorylation.
  - It is coupled with uptake of Pi.
  - When Ca^{++} is transported into mitochondria, electron transport can proceed but energy is required to pump the Ca^{++} into the mitochondria. Hence, no energy is stored as ATP.

- ***CCCP: Chloro carbonyl cyanide phenyl hydrazone***—most active uncoupler.
- ***FCCP:*** Trifluorocarbonyl cyanide pheyl hydrazone. As compared to DNP it is hundred times more active as uncoupler.
- ***Valinomycin:*** Produced by a type of Streptomyces. Transports K^+ from the cytosol into matrix and H^+ from matrix to cytosol, thereby decreasing the proton gradient.
- ***Physiological Uncouplers:***
  - Excessive thyroxine hormone
  - EFA deficiency
  - Long chain FA in Brown adipose tissue
  - Unconjugated hyperbilirubinaemia

Figure 8.4 shows the inhibitors of ETC and oxidative phosphorylation.

☞ SALIENT POINTS TO REMEMBER

- The most important function of food is to supply energy to the living cells. This is finally achieved through biological oxidation.
- $NAD.H_2$ and $FAD.H_2$ produced during oxidation of foodstuffs get oxidized to NAD^+ and FAD, by the respiratory chain or Electron transport chain (ETC).
- Respiratory chain or electron transport chain (ETC) located in the inner mitochondrial membrane represents the final stage of oxidizing reducing equivalents $NADH + H^+$ and $FADH_2$ derived from the metabolic intermediates to water.
- The enzymes of ETC are arranged in increasing redox potential except ubiquinone (CoQ) as follows:

$$\text{Substrate} \rightarrow NAD^+ \rightarrow FAD \rightarrow CoQ$$
$$\downarrow$$
$$O_2 \leftarrow 2\text{ cyt }(a_3 + a) \leftarrow 2\text{ cyt c} \leftarrow 2\text{ cyt }c_1 \leftarrow 2\text{ cyt.b}$$

- ETC is arranged in ***four complexes:***
  Complex I: NADH → CoQ reductase
  Complex II: Succinate → CoQ reductase
  Complex III: CoQ → cyt.c reductase
  Complex IV: Cyt c oxidase

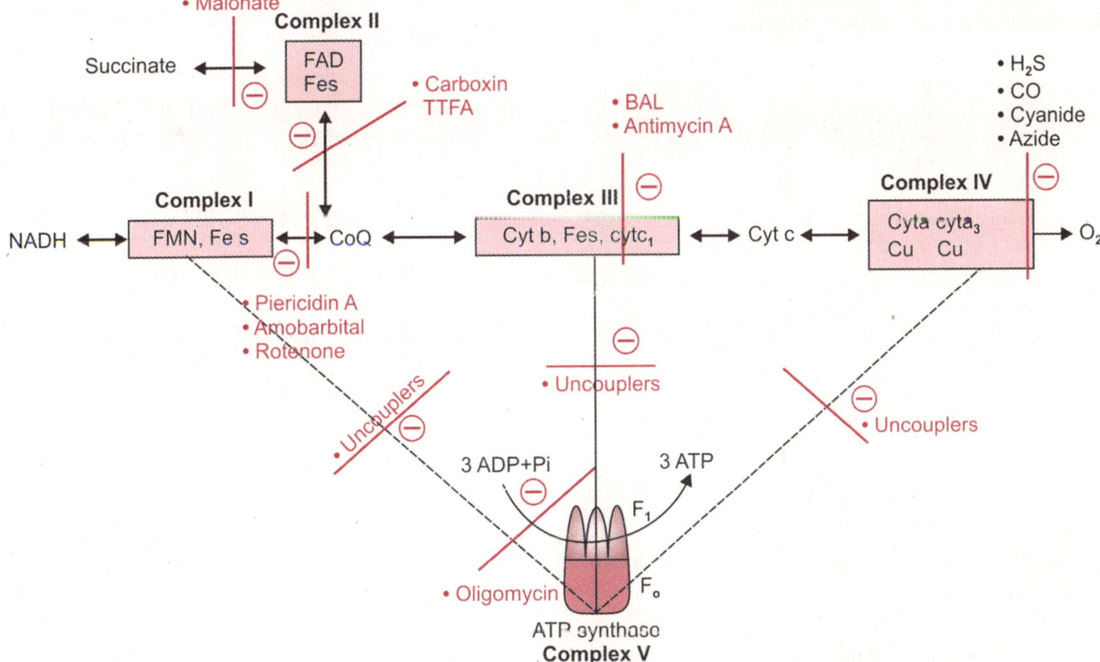

Fig 8.4: Inhibitors of respiratory chain and oxidative phosphorylation

- CoQ and cytochrome c are not included in any of the complexes.
- ***Cytochrome c is mobile and acts as a shuttle between complex III and IV.***
- The **three sites** where ATP is produced in respiratory chain by a process called oxidative phosphorylation are:
  - Site I: NADH → CoQ
  - Site II: cyt b → cyt c_1
  - Site III: cyt a_3 → O_2
- The free energy release per electron pair transferred at these three sites is sufficient to support phosphorylation of ADP to ATP ***which requires about 8 kcal/mole.***
- The process of synthesizing ATP from ADP + Pi, coupled with ETC is known as oxidative phosphorylation.
- NADH oxidation (P : O ratio 3) indicates that 3 ATPs are synthesized while $FAD.H_2$ oxidation (P : O ratio 2) result in formation of 2 ATP.
- NADH produced in the cytosol cannot directly enter mitochondrion. Two shuttle systems are available—glycerophosphate shuttle and malate shuttle for transferring the reducing equivalents to mitochondria.
- Among the hypothesis put forth to explain the mechanism of oxidative phosphorylation, the chemiosmotic hypothesis of Mitchell is accepted.
- The flow of electrons through ETC causes proton (H^+) gradient across the inner mitochondrial membrane which leads to the synthesis of ATP from ADP and Pi catalyzed by *ATP synthase (Complex V).*
- There are many inhibitors of ETC—
  Site I: Rotenone, Piericidin, Amobarbital, Certain drugs like chlorpromazine, guanethidine
  Site II: BAL, antinyacin, Hypoglycaemic drugs like phenformin.
  Site III: CO, CN^-, H_2S and azide
- Inhibitors of oxidative phosphorylation are: oligomycin, atractyloside, bongregate.
- Uncouplers like dinitrophenol, valinomycin etc delink ETC from oxidative phosphorylation.
- Physiological uncouplers are: excessive thyroxine hormone, EFA deficiency, long chain FA in brown adipose tissue, unconjugated hyperbilirubinaemia.

MULTIPLE CHOICE QUESTIONS

Give one correct answer:

1. **All of the following electron carriers are components of the mitochondrial electron transport chain *except:***
   (a) NAD^+ (b) $NADP^+$
   (c) FAD (d) FMN
   (e) CoQ
2. **Which of the following vitamins is not a component of ETC?**
   (a) Nicotinamide (b) Riboflavin
   (c) Ubiquinone (d) Biotin
   (e) All of the above
3. **Aerobic dehydrogenases have the prosthetic group:**
   (a) NAD^+
   (b) $NADP^+$
   (c) FAD
   (d) ATP
   (e) AMP
4. **Electrons from pyruvic acid enter the mitochondrial electron transport chain at**
   (a) Coenzyme Q
   (b) NADH → Q reductase
   (c) QH_2 → Cyt.c reductase
   (d) Between CoQ and cytochrome b
   (e) Cyt.c oxidase
5. **Which of the following respiratory chain enzymes contain copper?**
   (a) Coenzyme Q
   (b) Cytochrome c
   (c) Cytochrome oxidase
   (d) Cytochrome P_{450}
   (e) Cytochrome b
6. **Which of the following compounds inhibits electron flow at site 2?**
   (a) Cyanide (b) Antimycin
   (c) Rotenone (d) Azide
   (e) H_2S

7. Which of the following inhibitor acts at site 1 of respiratory chain?
(a) BAL (b) Cyanide
(c) Azide (d) Carboxin
(e) Piericidin A

8. Oxidative phosphorylation is inhibited by the following *except:*
(a) Oligomycin, (b) Hydrogen cyanide
(c) Atractyloside (d) Pyrophosphate
(e) Bongregate

9. Which of the following statements describing cytochrome oxidase is true?
(a) It is inhibited by copper
(b) It transfers electrons from CoQ to cyt. b
(c) It is a single cytochrome
(d) It is also known as cytochrome c
(e) It transfers four electrons and four protons to form H_2O molecule.

10. Dinitrophenol (DNP) causes which of the following in biologic oxidation?
(a) Increased hydrolysis of ATP
(b) Increased synthesis of ATP
(c) Prevents electron transfer
(d) Lowers the body heat production
(e) All of the above

11. In oxidative phosphorylation, one molecule of reduced flavoprotein produces how many ATPs:
(a) zero (b) 1
(c) 2 (d) 3
(e) 4

12. All the following can act as physiological uncouplers *except:*
(a) Excessive Thyroxine hormone
(b) Catecholamines
(c) EFA deficiency
(d) Unconjugated hyperbilirubinaemia
(e) Long chain fatty acids in brown adipose tissue.

13. Which of the following acts as inhibitor at site 3 of ETC?
(a) Carboxin (b) Sodium azide
(c) BAL (d) Rotenone
(e) Antimycin

14. In oxidative phosphorylation the oxidation of one molecule of NADPH produces how many ATPs?
(a) zero (b) 2
(c) 3 (d) 4
(e) 5

ANSWERS

1. (b)	2. (d)	3. (c)	4. (b)
5. (c)	6. (b)	7. (e)	8. (d)
9. (e)	10. (a)	11. (c)	12. (b)
13. (b)	14. (a)		

Vitamins

DEFINITION

Vitamins have been defined as organic compounds occurring in natural foods either as such *as utilizable "precursors"*, which are *required in minute amounts for normal growth, maintenance and reproduction,* i.e. for normal nutrition and health.

- They **differ from other organic foodstuffs** in following aspects:
  - They do not enter into tissue structures, unlike proteins.
  - Vitamins do not undergo degradation for providing energy unlike carbohydrates and lipids.
  - Several B-complex vitamins play an ***important role as "coenzymes"*** in several energy transformation reactions in the body.
- Vitamins differ from hormones as they are not produced within the organism, and most of them have to be provided in the diet.

CLASSIFICATION

All vitamins are broadly divided into **two groups** according to solubility.

1. **Fat-soluble vitamins are:**
   - *Vitamin A*
   - *Vitamin D*
   - *Vitamin E and*
   - *Vitamin K*
2. **Water-soluble vitamins are:**
   a. **Vitamin C** (Ascorbic acid),
   b. **Vitamin B-complex group that includes:**
      - *Vitamin B_1 (Thiamine)*
      - *Vitamin B_2 (Riboflavin)*
      - *Niacin (Nicotinic acid)*
      - *Vitamin B_6 (Pyridoxine)*
      - *Pantothenic acid*
      - *α-Lipoic acid*
      - *Biotin*
      - *Folic acid group*
      - *Vitamin B_{12} (Cyanocobalamine)*

Other water-soluble vitamins included in this group are:

- Inositol
- Para-amino benzoic acid(PABA)
- Choline

FAT-SOLUBLE VITAMINS

VITAMIN A

Chemistry

In general, the term vitamin A is now used when reference is made to the biological activity of more than one vitamin A active substance. **Three important forms** of vitamin are shown below:

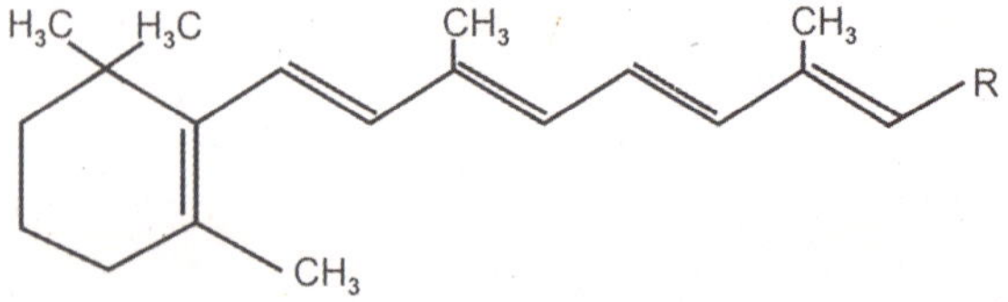

When

R = —CH_2OH ***Retinol*** or vitamin A alcohol

R = —CHO ***Retinal*** or vitamin A aldehyde

R = — COOH ***Retinoic*** acid or vitamin A acid.

All three compounds contain as ***common structural unit a trimethyl cyclohexenyl ring (β-ionone)*** and an all *trans* configurated polyene chain, (isoprenoid chain) **with four double bonds**. They are crystalline substances with limited stability. As already shown above these three forms are

- ***Vitamin A alcohol or retinol***
- ***Vitamin A aldehyde or retinal or retinene*** and
- ***Vitamin A acid or retinoic acid.***

These forms are sometimes referred to as ***retinoids.***

Vitamin A is a derivative of certain carotenoids which are hydrocarbon (polyene) pigments (yellow, red). These are widely distributed in the nature. These are called ***"Provitamins A"*** and are ***α, β and γ carotenes.*** Carotenes are $C_{40}H_{56}$ hydrocarbons.

Note: ***Two mols of vitamin A*** are formed by symmetrical oxidative scission of ***β-carotene*** while only ***one mole of vitamin A*** is obtained from ***α and γ carotenes*** or ***cryptoxanthine.***

Forms of vitamin A: Vitamin A occurs in nature in different forms. The usual form vitamin A_1 predominates except in fresh water fish, in them another form namely vitamin A_2 is present. Differences between vitamin A_1 and A_2 are shown below in ***Table 9.1.***

Neovitamin A: Is a stereoisomer of A_1 and it has about 70 to 80% of the biological activity of vitamin A_1.

Properties of vitamin A: It is yellow coloured oil in appearance, which is insoluble in water. Crystal forms prism. It shows an absorption maximum at 325-328 mμ. Molecular wt is 286.4 and melting point is about 62°-64°C. It is heat labile. Alcoholic hydroxyl group forms esters.

Dietary Sources

Animal sources: Liver oil, butter, milk, cheese, egg yolk.

Plant sources: In the form of provitamin carotene tomatoes, carrots, green-yellow vegetables, spinach, and fruits such as mangoes, papayas, corn, sweet potatoes. Recently, ***spirulina species,*** an algae, have been found to be a good source of vitamin A.

Unit of activity: Activity is expressed as International Unit (IU)

IU = 0.3 μg of retinol or
= 0.344 μg of retinylacetate or
= 0.6 μg of β-carotene.

It is also expressed now as ***"retinal equivalent",*** one Retinal equivalent=1 μg of retinol.

Daily requirement: Adult male and female require about 3000 IU per day. However, a recommended allowance is around 5000 IU per day. It is higher in growing children, pregnant women and lactating mothers. The requirement is also higher in hepatic disease.

Table 9.1: Differences between Vitamins A_1 and A_2

Vitamin A_1	*Vitamin A_2*
• Found predominantly in major species of animal	• Found in fresh water fish liver and other tissues
• Shows absorption maximum at 693 mμ when treated with $SbCl_3$	• Shows absorption maximum at 620 mμ on treatment with $SbCl_3$
• Only one double bond present in β-ionone ring	• Two double bonds in β-ionone ring (additional double bond between (C_3-C_4)
• More potent in its activity than vitamin A_2	• Less potent, biological activity is approximately 40% that of A_1
• Can be obtained from carotenes.	• Carotenes cannot give rise to vitamin A_2.

Absorption, Storage and Transport

- Vitamin A and its carotene precursors are absorbed in the small intestine.
- It is believed that the presence of tocopherols (vitamin E) and other anti-oxidants protect them against oxidation and destruction in intestinal lumen.
- Dietary vitamin A is chiefly in ester form which is hydrolyzed by cholesterol esterase into fatty acid and free vitamin A. Free retinol is absorbed and undergoes re-esterification in the intestinal epithelial cells. It is stored in the liver as retinyl ester normally as retinol palmitate.
- Conversion of carotenes to retinol occurs in intestinal epithelial cells in few animals, although liver may also participate in conversion. However, *in man liver is the only organ where carotenes are converted to vitamin A.*
- Retinol is transported in the blood in association with a ***specific retinol binding protein (RBP). There is another Retinoic acid binding protein (RABP)*** specific for retinoic acid.
- About 95% of vitamin A is stored as its ester mainly as palmitate in the liver. It is released in the plasma as and when required. About 10-20 mg of vitamin A is present per 100 g of liver.
- ***Normal blood level of vitamin A*** is found to be 18-60 μg/dl and that of carotenoids 100-300 μg/dl.

FUNCTIONS OF VITAMIN A

1. *Role in vision:* Perhaps the only function of vitamin A which is clearly understood to its molecular details is its role in vision. The overall mechanism through which vitamin A functions in visual system is known as ***Wald's visual cycle or Rhodopsin cycle (Fig. 9.1)*** discovered by George Wald for which he was awarded Nobel prize.

Retina contains 2 types of receptor cells:

- **Cones:** which are specialized for colour and detail vision in bright light contains **iodopsin**.
- **Rods:** which are specialized for visual activity in dim light (night vision), contains **rhodopsin**.

Light waves striking these receptors produce chemical changes which in turn give rise to nerve impulses. ***Vitamin A plays significant role in the photo-chemical phase of this process.*** Visual activity of rod cells is dependent on their content of photosensitive pigment called ***"rhodopsin"*** or ***"visual purple"*** which is a conjugated protein with a molecular weight of 40,000. It contains ***Opsin*** as its apoprotein and ***retinene*** as its prosthetic group. Retinene or retinal or retinaldehyde present in rhodopsin is ***11-cis-retinal.*** The aldehyde group of 11-cis-retinal is bound to $\varepsilon - NH_2$ group of lysine of opsin. Rhodopsin has a light absorbing property due to polyene group of 11-*cis* retinal. Even dim light can break rhodopsin.

When the light falls on rhodopsin it is split into ***opsin*** and ***all-trans-retinal*** in a series of events. ***It first forms photorhodopsin, bathorhodopsin, then lumirhodopsin, then metarhodopsin I, II and III. Finally metarhodopsin gets split into opsin and all-trans-retinal.***

At this stage the eye becomes less sensitive to light. ***All-trans-retinal is inactive in synthesis of rhodopsin, it has to be converted to 11-cis-retinal.*** It can take place in the following ways:

- All-*trans*-retinal may be isomerized to its 11-*cis*-isomer ***in presence of blue light—but in the eye this isomerization is not significant.***
- The all-*trans*-retinal can be converted to all-*trans*-retinol by ***retinene reductase*** by making use of NADH and all-*trans*-retinol then can be isomerized to its *cis* isomer.
- All-*trans*-retinol from blood can be first isomerized to 11-*cis*-retinol. All 11-*cis*-retinol then can be converted to 11-'cis'-retinal by ***retinol dehydrogenase,*** in presence of NAD^+.
- ***Now 11-cis-retinene (retinal) which is active, can combine with opsin to form back rhodopsin in dark.*** Thus the visual process involves continual removal of the active cis-retinol from blood into retina.
- ***Role of Cyclic GMP in Retinal Light-Dark Adaptation*** (Refer to chapter on Chemistry of Nucleotide).

The closing of Na^+ channels occur by a light-regulated enzymatic reactions in which the original signal-absorption of a single photon by *'rhodopsin'* is amplified manifold. The regulatory protein ***transducin*** is involved in this process. Transducin is a guanine-nucleotide binding protein (G protein), the structure and function of which is similar to those of G-proteins that take part in hormonal signals across biological membranes.

Transducin binds to GDP when it is "inactive", and in "active state" it binds to GTP. Transducin is "trimeric" and composed of three subunits, α, β and γ. GDP/GTP binding site is associated with α-subunit.

Mechanism of Action of Transducin

- Photoactivated rhodopsin, metarhodopsin II, initiates a guanine nucleotide amplification. It interacts with the α-subunit of *"transducin"* catalyzing the exchange of bound GDP for GTP.
- When transducin binds to GTP, the α-subunit gets dissociated from β and γ-subunits, activating the transducin (Tα-GTP complex).

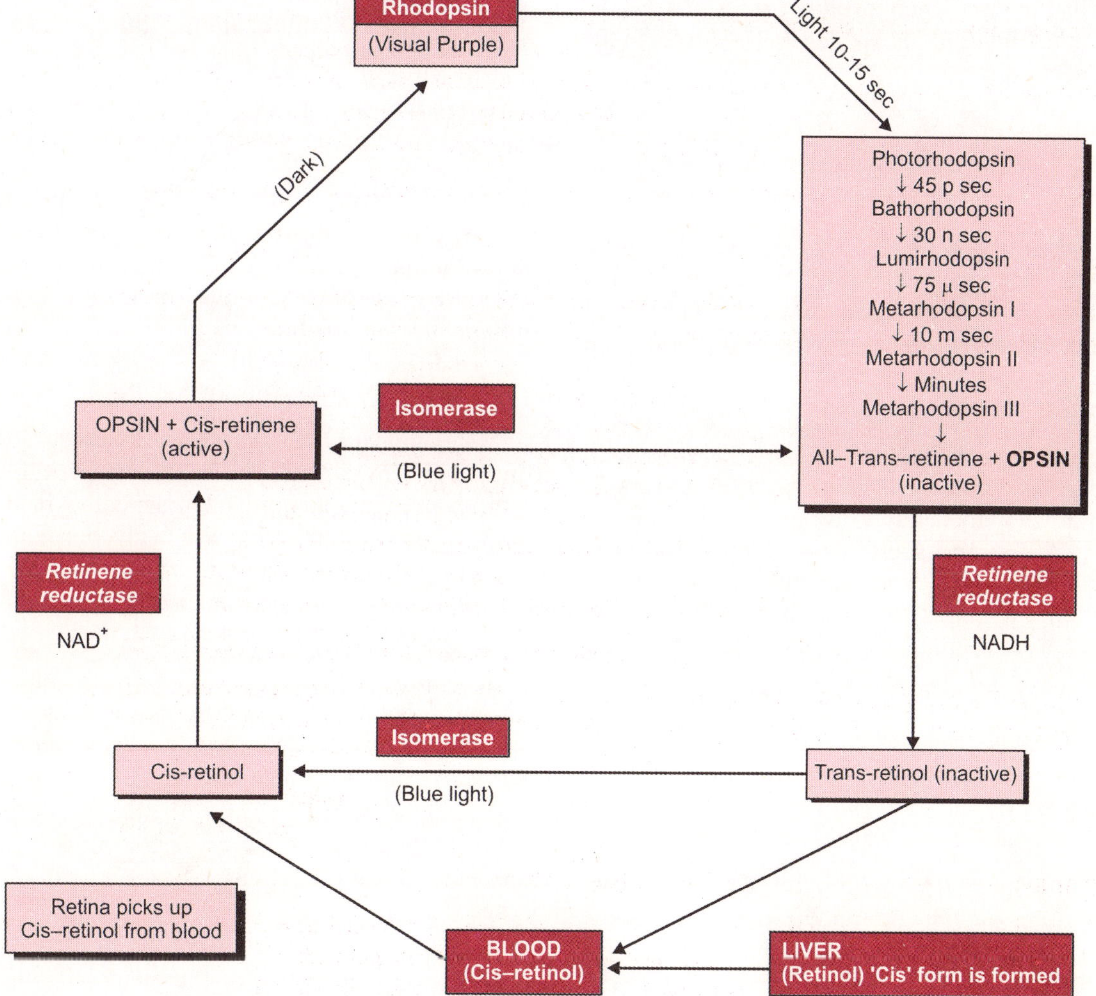

Fig. 9.2: Wald's visual cycle (Rhodopsin cycle)

- The activated transducin now activate ***phosphodiesterase** (PDE)* by binding to inhibitory γ-subunit and removing this; thus activating the α, β subunit of PDE (PDE α β).
- The activated PDE α β then catalyzes the hydrolysis of second messenger c-GMP to 5′–AMP, *lowering the c-GMP level to the plasma membrane of the outersegment, causing the Na^+ channels to close.*

The c-GMP is the second messenger that regulates the opening and closing of Na^+ channels.

Conclusion

- **In the dark**, there are ***high level of c-GMP**, which binds to the Na^+ channels*, causing **them to open**.
- **In the light**, photo-activated rhodopsin, through transducin and phosphodiesterase, ***lowers the levels of c-GMP***, thus ***closing the*** *most of Na^+ channels.*

2. ***Night blindness (Nyctalopia):*** This is one of the earliest signals of vitamin A deficiency which is ***impairment of dark adaptation***. Retinol deficiency depresses the resynthesis of rhodopsin and interferes with the function of rods resulting in night blindness.

3. ***Role in reproduction:*** Experimental work with rats shows that vitamin A deficient male rats do not develop their testes properly in that they are oedematous and sperm cells do not develop to state of maturity. When such male rats are allowed to mate with normal fertile females, no conception takes place. In contrast, vitaminA deficient female rats maintain normal oestrous cycle and do conceive, but are unable to carry the pregnancy to full term. Pregnancy is terminated by gestation resorption beginning on the 14th day of pregnancy. Steroid hormone synthesis is found to be adversely affected in avitaminosis A.

4. ***Role in epithelialization:*** The epithelial structures of skin and mucous membrane show gross structural changes in ***deficiency. Skin becomes dry, scaly and rough***. These ***changes*** are called as ***keratinization.***

- ***Lacrimal glands:*** Similar changes occur in these glands leading to dryness of conjunctivae and cornea, a condition described ***xerophthalmia.***
- ***Cornea:*** White opaque spots called ***Bitot's spots*** appear in the conjunctiva on either side in each eye. Corneal epithelium becomes keratinized, opaque and may become softened and ulcerated, condition described as ***keratomalacia.***
- ***Respiratory tract:*** Keratinization occurring in the mucous membrane of respiratory tract ***leads to increased susceptibility to infection*** and lowered resistance to disease.
- ***Urinary tract:*** Keratinization of urinary tract leads of ***"calculi formation"***

5. ***Role in bone and teeth formation:*** It plays a role in the construction of normal bone. Deficiency results in slowing of endochondral bone formation and decreased osteoblastic activity, the bone becomes cancellous losing their fine structural details. ***Mechanical damage to the brain and cord due to arrested limits of bony framework and cranium and vertebral column in which it has to grow.*** Teeth become unhealthy due to thinning of enamel and chalky deposits on surface.

6. ***Role in glycoprotein synthesis:*** Retinoic acid found to be more involved in glycoprotein synthesis probably forming its phosphate which acts as carrier of oligosaccharides in glycoprotein synthesis. Thus, ***vitamin A is involved in the development and maintenance of the ground substance in collagenous tissues.***

7. ***Mucopolysaccharide synthesis:*** The ground substance contains mucopolysaccharides as an important constituent. ***Vitamin A is involved in synthesis of chondroitin sulphate.***

8. ***Growth:*** Vitamin A along with other vitamin is principally involved in growth. Its role in cell differentiation and cell division has been proved beyond doubt.

9. ***Metabolism:*** It may be involved in protein synthesis and may play a role in metabolism of DNA.

10. ***Antioxidant and anticancer activity:*** β-carotene and vitamin A have ***antioxidant and anticancer activity.***

FUNCTIONS OF RETINOIC ACID

- Prevents keratinization of epithelium: respiratory tract, urogenital tract, lacrimal duct, etc.
- Plays important role in synthesis of glycoproteins as carriers of oligosaccharide chains.
- Role in synthesis of mucopolysaccharides.
- Inhibits the enzyme collagenase.

EFFECT OF EXCESS OF VITAMIN A (HYPERVITAMINOSIS A)

- Excess of vitamin A induces series of toxic effects known under the name of ***hypervitaminosis A syndrome.*** In man, the main symptoms are alterations of the skin and mucous membrane, hepatic dysfunction and headache, drowsiness, ***peeling of skin about the mouth*** and elsewhere. These syndromes were recognized by Eskimos as occurring after eating the livers of polar bears and arctic foxes which are extremely rich in vitamin A.
- Chronic effects of continued intake of excessive amounts of vitamin A produces roughening of skin, irritability, coarsening and falling of hair, anorexia, loss of weight.

VITAMIN D

Chemistry: Vitamin D_3 or cholecalciferol occurs in fish liver, and is also produced in human skin by ultraviolet light. The inactive natural precursors of the vitamin D, the corresponding ***provitamins*** are cyclopentanoperhydrophenanthrene derivatives classified as steroids. At least 10 such substances are known differing only in the side chain. Only two of these have been found in nature.

- *Ergosterol:* **Provitamin D_2** is found in plants.
- *7-dehydrocholesterol:* **Provitamin D_3** is found in animals.

Transformation from inactive provitamin to the active vitamin is accomplished by the ultraviolet rays. The photochemical activation, photolysis results only in intramolecular rearrangement.

Properties: It is a white powder, mol wt 384. Its melting point is 84°C. Absorption spectra can be seen with 265 mμ. αD^{20} =+ 102.5°. Important group of activity is C_{10}-C_{18} methylene. Resistant to heat and oxidation.

Dietary sources: Fish liver oil is the richest source of vitamin D. Egg yolk, margarine, lard, also contain considerable quantity of vitamin D. Some quantity is also present in butter, cheese, etc.

- **Ergosterol** is widely distributed in plants. It is not absorbed well hence is not of nutritional importance. Calciferol is readily absorbed.
- **7-dehydrocholesterol** is formed from cholesterol in the intestinal mucosa, passed on to the skin where it undergoes activation to vitamin D_3 by the action of solar U V rays.

Daily requirement: 1 USP unit = IU = 0.025 μg of vitamin D_3. About 100 IU or 2.5 μg of vitamin D_3 is the daily requirement in adult man. Pregnant and lactating mother as well as infants and children require about 220 IU per day. ***Vitamin is easily supplied by cutaneous synthesis in sunlight in tropical countries.***

Absorption and transport: Like most other fat-soluble vitamins, bile salts help in absorption of vitamin D from duodenum and jejunum. After absorption, it is carried in chylomicron droplets of the lymph in combination with serum globulin in blood plasma.

BIOLOGICALLY "ACTIVE" FORM OF VITAMIN D (CALCITRIOL)

Formation of calcitriol: The biologically active form of vitamin D is called **calcitriol** which is synthesized in **liver** and **kidneys** ***(Fig.9.2).*** Vitamin D_2 or vitamin D_3 binds to a specific D binding protein and is transported to the ***liver. It undergoes hydroxylation at 25 position.*** It normally takes place in the endoplasmic reticulum of the mitochondria. The requirement of Mg^{++} and NADPH and molecular O_2 is obligatory. A cytoplasmic factor is also found to be required

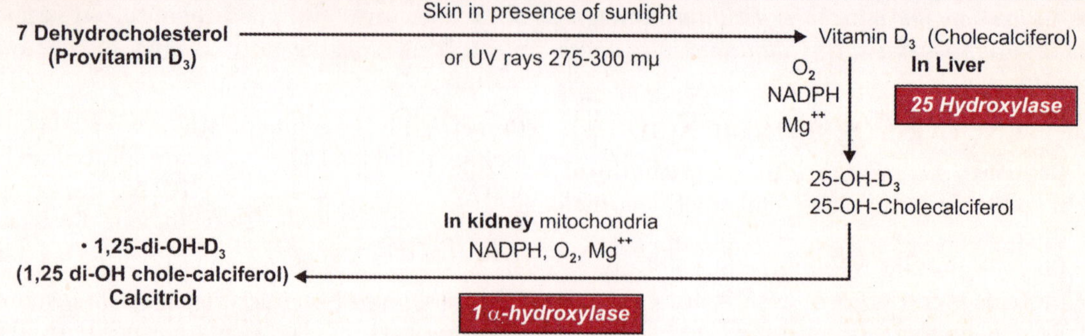

Fig. 9.2: Synthesis of calcitriol

which is not known. **Two enzymes**, an NADPH-dependent cytochrome P-450 reductase and a cytochrome-450 are involved. The 25-OH-D_3 is the major storage site of vitamin D in the liver and found in appreciable amounts in circulation. A specific vitamin D binding protein carries 25-OH-D_3 to the ***Kidneys*** where it undergoes further hydroxylation at position 1. This again is carried out by the mitochondria of the renal proximal convoluted tubule. The **reaction is a complex mono-oxygenase reaction** requiring NADPH, Mg^{++}, molecular O_2 and at least **three enzymes:**

- ***Ferredoxin reductase***
- ***Ferrodoxin and***
- ***Cytochrome P-450.***

This system produces 1,25 dihydroxy vitamin D_3 which is the most potent metabolite of vitamin D. Renal hydroxylation at position C_1 is the most significant, although similar hydroxylation is found to take place in placenta and bone.

Regulation:

- Its own concentration
- Parathyroid hormone
- Serum phosphate level
- Serum calcium level.

It is tight feedback regulation. Hypocalcaemia leads to marked increase of *1-α-hydroxylase* activity, and requires PTH. Calcitriol regulates its own concentration since high levels of calcitriol inhibit 1α-hydroxylation and stimulate the formation of 24,25 $(OH)_2$-D_3 which is not potent as calcitriol and is now supposed to be a storage form.

Mode of Action of Calcitriol:

- ***Calcitriol acts in a similar way as the steroid*** hormone receptors. This binding is specific and reversible. The receptors has a specific binding site on DNA that appears to contain zinc-finger motif characteristic of other steroid receptors.
- The receptors carries calcitriol in target cell such as intestinal mucosa, kidneys, etc.
- Calcitriol receptor binds to chromatin in the nucleus stimulating the gene transcription and formation of m-RNAs that codes for the calcium binding protein. There are several cytosolic proteins with high binding affinity for calcium.
- The increased synthesis of calcium binding protein helps in absorption and reabsorption of calcium in intestines and kidneys.

Since calcitriol is synthesized in the body and acts like steroid hormone and has a basic sterol nucleus in its structure, ***it is now regarded as a hormone.***

FUNCTIONS OF VITAMIN D

Vitamin D is found to act *on target organs* like bones, kidneys, intestinal mucosa to regulate calcium and phosphate metabolisms.

- ***Intestinal absorption of calcium and phosphate:*** It binds to the chromatin of target tissue and expresses the genes for calcium binding protein as well as Ca^{++}ATPase in intestinal cells. This increases the Ca^{++} absorption by actively transporting Ca^{++}

across the plasma membrane against electrochemical gradients. Phosphate absorption is facilitated probably through gene expression of intestinal alkaline phosphatase.

- *Mineralization of bones:* Mineralization of bones is promoted by 1,25, $(OH)_2D_3$ as well as 24,25 $(OH)_2D_3$. It is believed that the synthesis of Ca^{++}-binding proteins like osteocalcin and alkaline phosphatase is promoted which increase calcium and phosphate ion in the bone. These ions enhance the mineral deposition in the bone. 24,25 $(OH)_2D_3$ helps the deposition of hydroxyapatite in bone.

Other functions:

- Vitamin D is also believed to promote bone resorption and calcium mobilization to raise the levels of Ca and P in blood in association with PTH.
- Renal reasorption of calcium and phosphorous is also done by 1,25 $(OH)_2D_3$ in similar way.
- It lowers the pH in certain parts of the gut such as colon and produces increase in urinary pH.
- It counteracts the inhibitory effect of calcium ions on the hydrolysis of phytate. In adequate amounts and in case of high calcium intake, it suppresses the anticalcifying and rachitogenic effect of phytate.
- In physiologically compatible intake, it is found to increase the citrate content of bone, blood tissues and urinary level.

DEFICIENCY OF VITAMIN D

1. *Rickets: Deficiency produces rickets in growing children and osteomalacia in adults.* Vitamin D is required for the normal growth and mineralization of bones. In its absence, instead of growth occurring normally, the osteoblasts proliferation does not take place in an orderly fashion and is not accompained by vascularization and mineralization at the normal rate. This results in irregularity in the zone of provisional calcification. The cartilage cells do not degenerate as they should, and *ends of the long bones become bulky and soft.*

The bone mineral may be reasorbed away from shaft of long bones making it soft. Bending of long bones gives rise to deformities such as ***bow legs*** and ***knock knees.*** The ankles, knees, wrists and elbow are swollen due to swelling of epiphyseal cartilages.

The fontanelles do not close properly giving ***hot-cross-bun*** appearance of head.

Ribs give beaded appearance and chest gives a ***pigeon breast*** appearance. Tooth erupts late and are deformed.

2. *Osteomalacia:* The deficiency of vitamin D in adults is Osteomalacia which is rare.

- Pregnancy and lactation: Where there is additional requirement of this vitamin and drainage of it in milk.
- In women who observe *purdah* or in climate where sunshine is scanty, calcium and phosphorous absorption is decreased. Consequently mineralization of osteoid to form bone is impaired. Such bones become soft. This particularly affects pelvic bones.

3. *Renal Osteodystrophy*: When renal parenchyma is lost or diseased quite significantly, it is unable to form calcitriol and calcium absorption is impaired. Hypocalcaemia leads to increase in PTH which acts on bone to increase Ca^{++}. Consequently, there is excessive bone turnover and structural changes. This condition is known as renal osteodystrophy.

Hypervitaminosis D

Normally, vitamin D is well tolerated if taken in large doses, but serious deleterious effects may be produced if taken in extremely large doses, i.e. 500 to 1000 times of normal requirements for prolonged periods.

Effects are mainly due to induced hypercalcaemia:

- **Immediate effects** and
- **Delayed effects.**

1. *Immediate effects:* Include anorexia, thirst, lassitude, constipation and polyuria. Later on, it is followed by nausea, vomiting and diarrhoea.

2. *Delayed effects:* Persistent hypercalcaemia and hyperphosphataemia may produce:

- *Urinary lithiasis*
- ***Metastatic calcification*** which may affect kidneys, bronchi, pulmonary alveoli, muscles, arteries and gastric mucosa. Renal failure may develop and can lead to death.
- In growing children, there may be excessive mineralization of the zone of provisional calcification at the expense of the diaphysis which may undergo deminerlization.

Note: Certain clinical disorders have been attributed to states of hypervitaminosis D due to increased sensitivity to the vitamin, e.g.

- *"Idiopathic hypercalcaemia" of children*
- *Boeck's sarcoidosis.*

VITAMIN E (TOCOPHEROLS)

Chemistry: The tocopherols differ from each other in the number or position of methyl groups.

- Structure of tocol (see ahead)
  - α- tocopherol : 5,7,8 trimethyl tocol
  - β- tocopherol : 5,8 dimethyl tocol
  - γ- tocopherol : 7,8 dimethyl tocol
  - δ- tocopherol : 8 methyl tocol
- ***The α-tocopherol is the most active in vitamin E activity.***
- ***The presence of the phenolic-OH group on the 6th carbon of the chromane ring is the most important group for its anti-oxidant activity.***

Properties: Heat labile, acid-stable, alkali-labile, oxidation labile yellow oil. Mol wt: 430.7, melting point: 2.5°-3.5°C, photolabile. It forms salts, esters with-OH group of chromane ring at 6 position. Absorption maxima at 292 mμ. It is an optically active aromatic quinoid with $\alpha^{25}{}_{D}$ = + 0.32°

Dietary Sources and Recommended Allowance:

Cotton seed oil, corn oil, sunflower oil, wheat germ oil and margarine are the richest sources of vitamin E. It is also found in fair quantities in dry soyabeans, cabbage, yeast, lettuce, apple seeds, peanuts.

Units: 1 mg of d-a-tocopherol = 1.49 IU

1 mg of dl-α-tocopherol acetate = 1.0 IU

Normal blood level = 1.2 mg/dl.

Recommended Allowance: Children 10-15 IU/day; Adults 20-25 IU/day

Special attention has to be given to the dietary intake of unsaturated fatty acids in which case the daily requirement is increased. It is also more in pregnancy and lactation.

Absorption, Distribution and Excretion: Free tocopherols and their esters are readily absorbed in small intestine with the help of bile acids. ***Vitamin E is stored in adipose tissue.*** Absorbed vitamin E is transported to liver where it gets incorporated into lipoproteins and carried by blood to muscle tissues and to adipose tissue for storage. ***The normal value of blood level is around 1 mg/dl*** and it is transported chiefly in the α-lipoprotein fraction. Under normal dietary conditions, there is no significant excretion of tocopherols in urine or faeces as it rapidly and extensively undergoes destruction in the GI tract and in tissues. Placental transfer of vitamin E is limited; mammary transfer is much more extensive. Thus, the serum α-tocopherol level of breast fed infants increases more rapidly than that of bottle-fed infants.

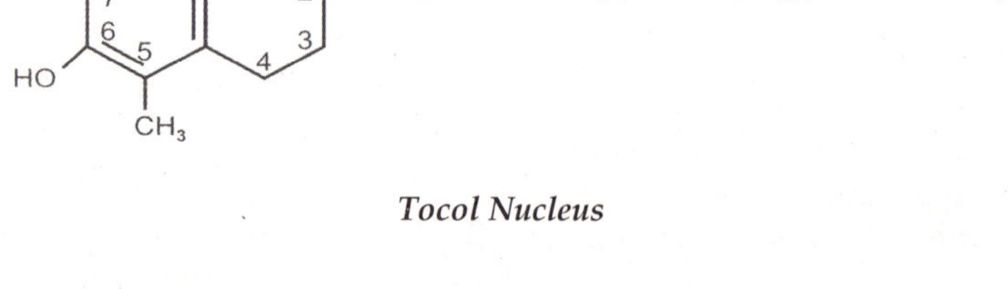

Tocol Nucleus

FUNCTIONS OF VITAMIN E

1. ***Antioxidant property:*** This is the most important functional aspect of vitamin E.

- ***Removal of free radicals:*** Vitamin E is involved in removal of free radicals and prevents their peroxidative effects on unsaturated lipids of membranes and thus helps in maintaining the integrity of cell membrane. Free radicals like OH^-, superoxide anion O_2^- are formed during the action of some oxidoreductases such as the microsomal NADPH oxidase. The free radicals peroxidate the unsaturated fatty acids of the cell membranes, mitochondrial membranes, etc and cause their rupture. ***Vitamin E prevents this peroxidation.***
- Antioxidant action of vitamin E along with other factors prevents the peroxidative effects of O_3, H_2O_2 and NO_2 on respiratory membrane, and thus prevents their damage.
- Factors 3 has been identified as a selenium compound (selenoprotein) which gives a complete protection against necrosis. Vitamin E helps to protect selenide at the active sites of membrane selenoproteins against the effects of free radicals.
- Vitamin E prevents the peroxidative changes in membrane of mitochondria and helps in maintaining the smooth translocation of phosphate ions into mitochondria. Thus the oxidative phosphorylation is enhanced. In addition, the oxidation of sulfhydryl enzymes is also prevented by tocopherols.
- Tocopherols prevents oxidation of vitamin A and carotenes and reduces their wastage.

2. ***Role in reproduction in rats:*** Vitamin E helps in maintaining seminiferous epithelium intact. However, its deficiency leads to irreversible degenerative changes leading to permanent sterility. Motility of sperms is lost and spermatogenesis is impaired.

In female rats, the ovary is unaffected by vitamin E deficiency; but the foetus does not develop normally, dying *in utero* undergoing resorption.

3. *Other Functions:*

- Tocopherol derivative tocopheranolactone may be involved in synthesis of coenzymes Q or ubiquinone.
- Vitamin E may have some role in nucleic acid synthesis.

DEFICIENCY OF VITAMIN E

1. ***Muscular dystrophy:*** Vitamin E deficiency leads to the increased oxidation of polyunsaturated fatty acids in the muscle with a consequent rise in O_2 consumption and peroxide production. Peroxides may then cause an increase in intracellular hydrolase activity by affecting the lysosomal membranes. Those hydrolases may then catalyze such breakdowns in muscle and produce muscular dystrophy. The muscle creatine is low and creatinuria occurs.

2. *Haemolytic anaemia:* Low tocopherol diet may produce low plasma tocopherol, ***increased susceptibility to haemolysis due to peroxides and dialuric acid.*** This could be the reason of haemolytic or microcytic anemia. Extensive oedema, reticulocytosis, thrombocytosis and thrombus formation in blood vessels, increased susceptilbility of the RBC to haemolysing effects of peroxides and dialuric acid is observed. These symptoms are often aggravated by diets rich in essential fatty acids.

Clinical cases of vitamin E deficiency may be found in lipoproteinaemia and in disease like sprue, obstructive jaundice, pancreatitis, and steatorrhoea.

3. ***Dietary hepatic necrosis: Diets low in cystine and rich in polyunsaturated fatty acids can cause hepatic necrosis.*** Fall in acetate utilization and in respiration of necrotic liver is more effectively cured or prevented by tocopherols. Vitamin E and factor 3 a selenite compound are complementary to each other in preventing hepatic necrosis or muscular dystrophies (Refer to "Selenium metabolism").

Clinical and Therapeutic Uses: vitamin E has been used in following diseases.

- *Nocturnal muscle cramps (NMC)*
- *Intermittent claudication (IC)*
- *Fibrocystic breast disease (FBD)*
- *Atherosclerosis*

VITAMIN K

Chemistry: All vitamin K forms are the napthoquinone derivatives. It is closely related to a compound ***pthiocol,*** a constituent of tubercle bacteria with slight vitamin K activity.

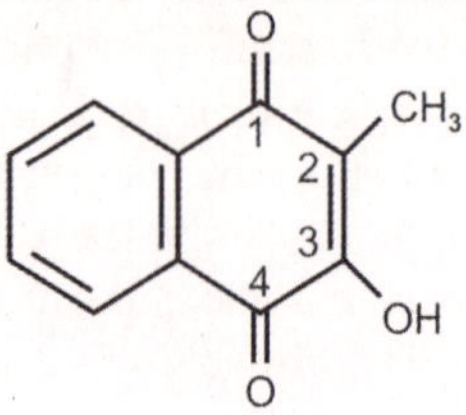

Pthiocol
(2-methyl, 3-hydroxy, 1,4-Naphthoquinone)

- Vitamins *K_1 and K_2* are the two naturally occurring forms of vitamin K that have been identified. ***The third form vitamin K_3 is the synthetic analogue.***

1. Vitamin K_1: It is ***phylloquinone*** or phytonadione ***isolated from alfalfa leaves.*** It is also called **mephyton.** Thus, vitamin K_1 is 2 methyl, 3 phytyl-1, 4 naphthoquinone. It is a light yellow oil, mol wt = 450.7, melting point 20°C. it is heat-stable, acid-alkali labile, photolabile. It absorbs UV light with 243-260 mμ as absorption maxima. Optically active $\alpha^{20}_{D} = +0.4°$.

2. Vitamin K_2: Vitamin K_2 is known as ***farnoquinone,*** it was isolated from **putrid fish meal-*synthesized by bacteria,*** and has a longer difarnesyl chain attached at position 3.

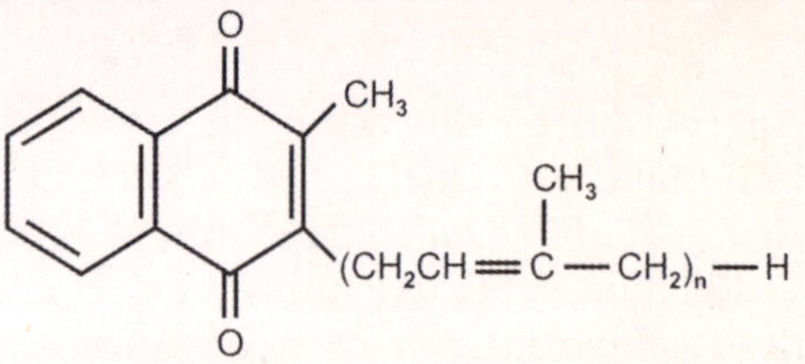

Vitamin K_2 (farnoquinone): 2 methyl-3-difarnesyl-1, 4 naphthoquinine. It is a yellow oil, melting point 54°C. thermostable, photolabile, alkalilabile. It absorbs UV light at 269 mμ.

3. Vitamin K_3: It is also known as **menadione,** is 2 methyl, 1,4 naphthoquinone ***without any side chain or OH group,*** is the synthetic analogue of vitamin K. It is ***three times more potent than*** natural varieties. It is water-soluble and ***can be given parenterally. Its activity is related to the presence of methyl group at position 2.***

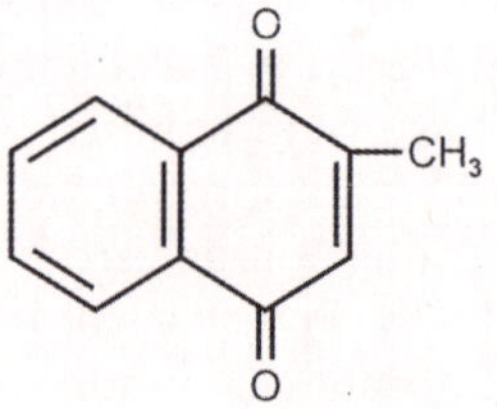

Vitamin K_3 (Menadione)

Dietary Sources and Daily Requirement:

- Both vitamin K_1 and K_2 are mainly found in plants and synthesized by bacteria respectively.
- Vitamin K_1 is present ***chiefly in green leafy vegetables,*** such as ***alfalfa, spinach, cauliflower, cabbage, soyabeans, tomatoes.***
- Vitamin K_2 is a product of metabolism of most bacteria ***including the normal intestinal bacteria*** of most higher animal species.
- Dietary requirement of vitamin K is of not much importance under normal circum-

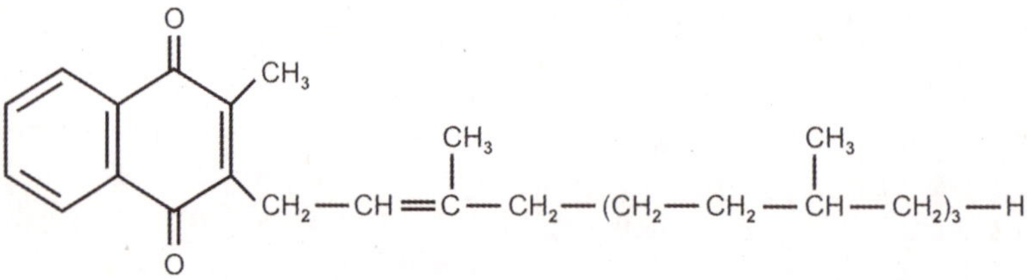

Vitamin K_1 (Phylloquinone) $C_{31}H_{46}O_2$

stances, as it is provided by intestinal bacteria in adequate quantities.

Absorption: It is ***readily absorbed from the small intestine in presence of bile salts.*** It is not stored to any appreciable extent. It can cross the placental barrier and is available to the foetus. Vitamin K is not excreted in the urine or bile. Faeces contain large quantities. This may be of the bacterial origin. It may also represent actual excretion by the intestinal mucosa.

FUNCTIONS OF VITAMIN K

- ***Blood coagulation:*** The main function of vitamin K is the ***promotion of blood coagulation*** by helping in the post-transcriptional modifications of blood factors such as pro-thrombin, and factors II, VII, IX, X.
- ***Calcium binding proteins:*** Vitamin K is found to carboxylate specific glutamate residues of calcium binding proteins of bones, spleen, placenta and kidneys. This enhances the capacity of those proteins to deposits calcium in the tissues concerned.
- ***Role in oxidative phosphorylation:*** Vitamin K is a ***necessary cofactor in oxidative phosphorylation being*** associated with mitochondrial lipids. UV irradiation of isolated mitochondria destroys their vitamin K content and ultimately their ability for oxidative phosphorylation. The normal process of oxidative phosphorylation is restored when vitamin K is added to them. ***Further dicumarol an antagonist of vitamin K is known to act as uncoupler of oxidative phosphorylation.***

DEFICIENCY OF VITAMIN K

Deficiency of vitamin K is very rare, since most common foods contain this vitamin. In addition intestinal flora of microorganisms synthesize adequate quantity of vitamin K. However, a deficiency may occur as a result of:

- ***Prolonged use of antibiotics and sulfa drugs.*** This suppresses the growth of vitamin K producing bacteria thus making vitamin K not available. ***This leads to fall in prothrombin level in plasma,*** an abnormally long blood coagulation time and a tendency to spontaneous hemorrhage which may even be fatal.
- ***Malabsorption*** and biliary tract obstruction, sprue, steatorrhoea and coeliac disease can lead sometimes to vitamin K defieciency. Vitamin K being a fat soluble vitamin, is absorbed with the help of bile salts. The biliary obstruction impairs the delivery of bile hence vitamin K is not able to get absorbed. Malabsorption syndromes such as steatorrhoea and sprue have similar effect.
- ***Spoilt sweet-clover hay*** when consumed by cattle, causes a bleeding disease. In such cases fall in O_2 consumption, poor oxidative phosphorylation, low prothrombin, proconvertin and stuart factor activities are observed, Spoilt sweet-clover hay contain dicoumarol- a vitamin K antagonist.
- ***Short circuiting of the bowel*** as a result of surgery may also foster deficiency which may not respond even to large oral doses of vitamin K. Water- soluble form of vitamin K, i.e. vitamin K_3 alone is useful in such cases.
- ***Hypoprothrombinaemia:*** In immediate postnatal infants, hypoprothrombinaemia and bleeding in many tissues occurs in vitamin K deficiency. Relatively small amounts of vitamin K are obtained from the mother through placental transfer and also because the intestinal microflora has not yet been established, this leads to vitamin K deficiency, and its consequent effects. If prothrombin is significantly low this may result in ***haemorrhagic disease of the newborn.*** Hypoprothrombinaemia can be prevented by administering vitamin K to the mother before parturition or by giving the infant a small dose of vitamin K.

☞ SALIENT POINTS TO REMEMBER

- Vitamins are accessory food factors required in small quantities in the diet as most of them cannot be synthesized in the body ***(exception- bacterial synthesis of vitamin K and some B-complex vitamins in the gut, formation of vit***

A from carotenes, vit D_3 from 7-dehydro-cholesterol in skin, niacin synthesis from aminoacid tryptophan).

- Vitamins are classified into two major groups:
  (a) Fat soluble vitamins: A, D, E and K
  (b) Water soluble vitamins: B-complex group and vitamin C.
- Vitamin A is involved in vision (Wald's rhodopsin cycle), proper growth, differentiation and maintenance of epithelial cells.
- Deficiency of vitamin A produces nyctalopia (Night-blindness) and keratinization of epithelia.
- Biological active form of vitamin D is calcitriol (1, 25 - di-OH cholecalciferol) which functions like a steroid hormone and regulates plasma levels of Ca and P.
- Vitamin D deficiency produces a disease called rickets in children and osteomalacia in adults.
- ***Vitamin E is a natural anti-oxidant and mops up "free radicals"*** and prevents damage of cell membranes.
- Vitamin E is necessary for normal reproduction in many animals.
- Vitamin K has a specific coenzyme function. It catalyzes the carboxylation of glutamic acid residues of blood clothing factors, viz. prothromlin, factors VII, IX and X.
- Fat-soluble vitamins are not excreted in urine, hence excess of consumption can lead to hypervitaminosis A and D with toxic effects.

WATER-SOLUBLE VITAMINS

Vitamin C (Ascorbic Acid)

Synonyms: Antiscorbutic vitamin.

Chemistry: Ascorbic acid is an "enediol-lactone" of an acid with a configuration similar to that of the sugar L-glucose.

- It is a comparatively **Strong acid,** stronger than acetic acid, owing to dissociation of enolic H at C_2 and C_3.

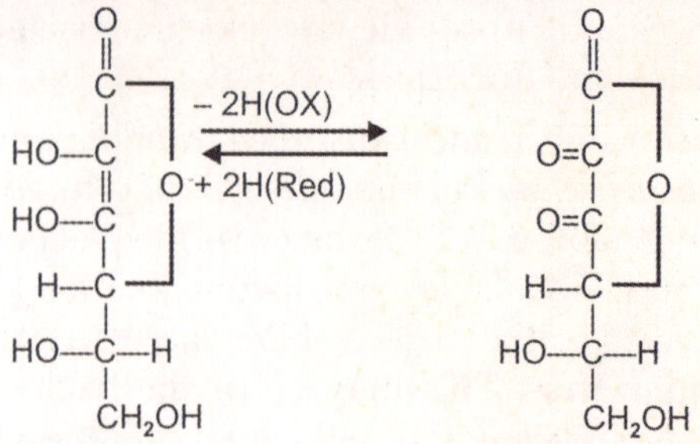

– 2H(OX) / + 2H(Red)

L-Ascorbic acid (reduced form) ⇌ ***L-dehydroascorbic acid (oxidized form)***

- ***Strong reducing property:*** Depends on the liberation of H-atoms from the enediol-OH groups, on C_2 and C_3; the ascorbic acid being oxidized to dehydroascorbic acid, e.g. by air H_2O_2, $FeCl_3$, methylene blue, ferricyanide, 2,6 dichlorophenol indophenol, etc.
- The above reaction is readily reversible by reducing agents *'in vitro'* by H_2S and *'in vivo'* by -SH compounds, such as "glutathione".
- It is stable in solid form and in acidic solutions but is rapidly destroyed in alkaline solutions.
- Oxidative destruction of ascorbic acid is accelerated by increasing pH. Silver (Ag^{++}) and cupric (Cu^{++}) ions accelerate process.

BIOSYNTHESIS

- Some lower mammals like rats can synthesize the vitamin from glucose by the uronic acid pathway.
- ***Man, monkey and guinea pigs lack the enzymes necessary for the synthesis.*** They cannot convert keto-gulonolactone to ascorbic acid. ***Hence the entire human requirement must consequently be supplied by the diet.***

Metabolism-Absorption, Distribution and Excretion: It is absorbed readily from the small intestine, peritoneum and subcutaneous tissues.

- It is widely distributed throughout the body. Some tissues contain high concentrations as compared to others. ***Local concentration roughly parallels the metabolic activity,*** found in descending order as given below:

Pituitary gland, adrenal cortex, corpus luteum, liver, brain, gonads, kidney, heart, skeletal muscle, etc.

- From maternal blood, it can cross the placental barrier and supplies the foetus.
- Normal human blood plasma contains approximately 0.6 to 1.5 mg of ascorbic acid per 100 ml.
- The vitamin exists in the body largely in the "reduced " form, with reversible equilibrium with a relatively small amount of "dehydro-ascorbic acid" (oxidized form). **Both forms are physiologically and metabolically active** (See below).
- Under normal dietary intake (of 75 to 100 mg)

50 to 75% are converted to inactive compounds	25 to 50% is excreted in urine as such.

It is also secreted in milk.

- *Metabolites:* (i) Chief terminal metabolites in the rat and guinea pig are CO_2 and oxalic acid. (ii) **In human beings,** decarboxylation of ascorbic acid does not occur, the chief ***terminal metabolites being-oxalic acid and diketogulonic acid,*** which are excreted in urine. ***Conversion of ascorbic acid to oxalate in man may account for the major part of the endogenous urinary oxalate.***

Occurrence and Food Sources: Vitamin C is widely distributed in plants and animal tissues. In animal tissues, there is no storage site that is why, it contains small amount but highest concentration found in metabolically highly "active" organs, e.g. adrenal cortex, corpus luteum, liver etc.

Dietary Sources: These are chiefly vegetables sources. **Good sources** are citrous fruits: orange/ lemon/lime, etc; other fruits like papaya, pine-apple, banana, strawberry. Amongst vegetable, leafy vegetables like cabbage and cauliflower, germinating seeds, green peas and beans, potatoes, and tomatoes are good source. ***Amla is the richest source.*** Considerable amount of vitamin C activity is lost during cooking, processing and storage-because of its irreversible oxidative degradation to inactive compounds.

Metabolic Role and Functions

- ***Role in cellular oxidation-reduction:*** The fact that vitamin C is very sensitive to reversible oxidation, Ascorbic acid ⇄ dehydroascorbic acid, suggest that it may be involved in cellular oxidation-reduction reactions, perhaps serving as hydrogen transport agent.
- ***Role in collagen synthesis:*** hydroxyproline and hydroxylysine are important constituents of mature collagen fibres. Pre-collagen molecules contain the amino acids proline and lysine. They are hydroxylated by corresponding *hydroxylases* in presence of vitamin C, Fe^{++} and molecular O_2. Thus:

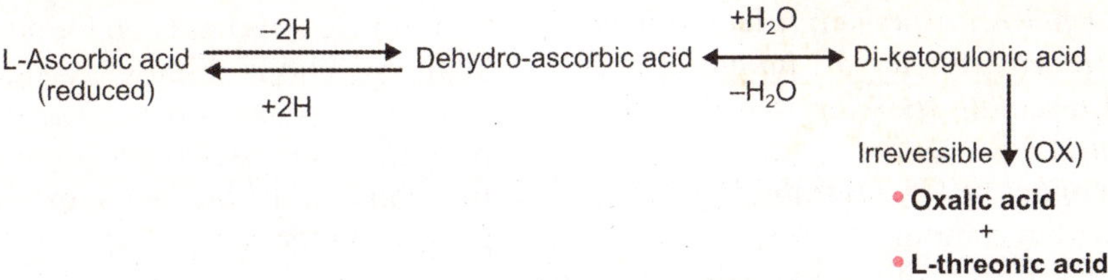

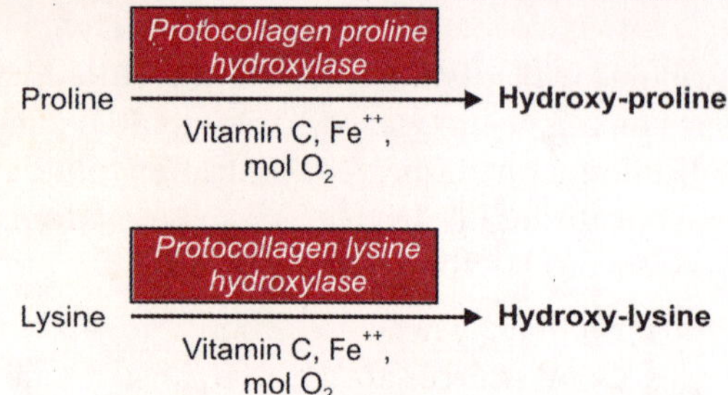

Note: In scurvy, failure of conversion of procollagen to collagen due to the failure of hydroxylation may lead to a rapid destruction of the collagen intermediates.

- ***Functional activity of fibroblasts/osteoblasts:*** Ascorbic acid is required for functional activities of fibroblasts, and osteoblasts, and consequently for formation of MPS of connective tissues, osteoid tissues, dentine and intercellular cement substance of capillaries.
- ***Role in tryptophan metabolism:*** Vitamin C is required as a cofactor for hydroxylation of tryptophan to form 5-OH derivative, in the pathway of biosynthesis of serotonin (5-HT).
- ***Role in tyrosine metabolism:*** It is required as a cofactor with enzyme ***p-OH phenyl pyruvate hydroxylase*** which is necessary for hydroxylation and conversion of p-OH phenyl pyruvate to homogentisic acid.

Note:

Scorbutic guinea pigs and premature infants given a high protein and ascorbic acid deficient diet excrete increased amounts of – OH-phenyl pyruvate and p-OH phenyl lactic acid. Administration of vitamin C corrects this condition.

Vitamin C deficiency in premature infants may increase urinary excretion of "homogentisic acid" and resemble the inherited disorder "alkaptonuria".

- ***Formation of active FH_4 (Tetrahydrofolate):*** Ascorbic acid in combination with folic acid helps the maturation of the RB cells. It has been suggested that vitamin C by maintaining the *folic acid reductase* **in its "active" form keeps the folic acid in the reduced tetrahydrofolate FH_4 form.**
- ***Absorption of Fe:*** Ascorbic acid in food helps ***in the absorption of Fe by converting the inorganic ferric iron to the ferrous form.*** It is also formed by forming water-soluble Fe-ascorbate chelate. It also helps in mobilization of Fe from its storage form "Ferritin". Disturbances of these functions may contribute to the development of hypochromic microcytic anaemia in scurvy. Absorption of Fe both in normal or Fe-deficient patients is increased by over 10% after administration of vitamin C.
- ***Role in electron transport system:*** Ascorbic acid seems to take part in electron transport system of mammalian 'microsomes'. The detailed mechanism of role of vitamin C is not definitely known but is has been suggested that the reaction is coupled with hydroxylation.
- ***Role in formation of catecholamines:*** Vitamin C is required as a coenzymes with the enzyme ***dopamine hydroxylase*** which catalyzes the conversion of dopamine to norepinephrine.
- ***Role in formation of carnitine:*** Formation of "carnitine" in liver by ***hydroxylation of γ-butyrobetaine is helped by vitamin C,*** α-keto glutarate, Fe^{++} and a dioxygenase.
- ***Effect on cholesterol level:*** Relation of ascorbic acid with hypocholesterolaemia in man and guinea pigs has been reported.
- ***Role in stress:*** The adrenal cortex contains a large quantity of vitamin C and this is rapidly depleted when the gland is stimulated by ACTH. Increased losses of the vitamin accompany infection and fever. Circulating vitamin C levels has been found to be low in acute infectious diseases, congestive heart failure, in renal and hepatic diseases and malignancies. ***All these suggest that the vitamin C may play an important role in the reaction of the body to "stress".***

Deficiency Manifestations: Scurvy

In the humans, its deficiency produces a disease called *scurvy.The main defect is a failure to deposit intercellular cement substance.*

- Capillaries are fragile and there is tendency to haemorrhages-petechial, subcutaneous, subperiosteal and even internal haemorrhages can occur.
- ***Wound healing is delayed*** due to deficient formation of collagen.
- Poor dentine formation in children, leads to poor teeth formation.
- ***Gums are swollen and becomes spongy*** and bleeds on slightest pressure-Hyperaemia, swelling, sponginess and bleeding of gums are seen. In severe scurvy, it may lead to secondary infection and loosening and falling of teeth.
- Osteoid of bone is poorly laid and mineralization of bone is poor. The bones are weak and readily fractures. Haemorrhages occurring below the periosteum and into the joints may cause extremely painful swellings of bones and joints.
- Anaemia may be associated which is ***hypochromic microcytic type.***

"Bachelor" scurvy: Elderly bachelors and widowers who may prepare their own foods are particularly prone to development of vitamin C deficiency.

Requirement: ***A daily intake of about 100 mg is quite adequate*** in normal adults.Official recommended minimal daily intakes are:

- Adults - 75 mg per day
- Infants - 30 mg per day
- Adolescence - 80 mg per day
- Pregnant women - 100 mg per day
- Lactating women - 150 mg per day

Requirement is increased in presence of infections and stress.

Hypervitaminosis (Effects of excess ascorbic acid). Administration of large amounts of ascorbic acid is not known to produce any effects in humans. But in rats, dehydroascorbic acid in enormous doses (1.5 gm/kg body wt) produces permanent diabetes, similar to that produced by the glycoside alloxan; it ***produces probably destruction of β-cells of islets of Langerhans.*** This action is prevented by immediate antecedant IV injection of-SH compounds like cysteine, glutathione as in the case of alloxan, which resembles dehydroascorbic acid in chemical structure.

B-COMPLEX VITAMINS
THIAMINE (VITAMIN B_1)

Synonyms: Anti beri-beri factor, anti-neuritic vitamin, aneurin.

Chemistry: Free thiamine is a basic substance and contains *(i)* **A pyrimidine,** and *(ii)* **A thiazole ring.**

- ***It contains sulphur*** (sulphur containing vitamin). Refer Figure below)
- ***Solubility:*** Soluble in water (1 gm/ml) and 95% alcohol (1 gm/100 ml). Not soluble in fat solvents.
- ***Stability:*** Resistant to heat (boiling/autoclaving) in solution <pH 3.5, but loses activity at pH>5.5.

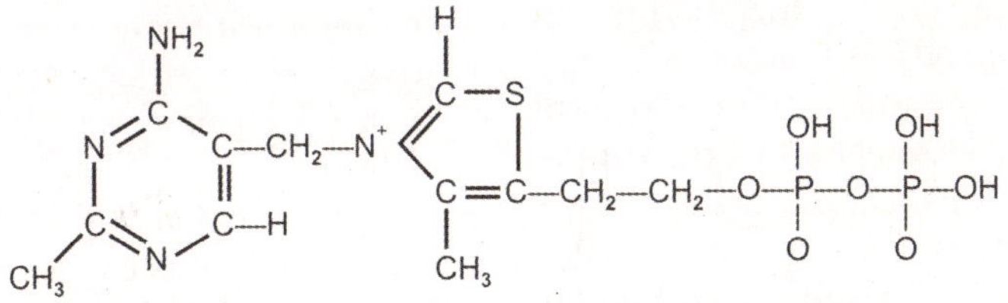

2,5-dimethyl, 4, methyl-6, amino pyrimidine 5-OH ethyl thiazole
Thiamin pyrophosphate (Thiamin diphosphate).

Thiamine content of vegetables well preserved by freezing and by storage below 0°C. Rapidly destroyed in alkaline medium.

Biosynthesis: Thiamine is synthesized by plants yeast and bacteria, but not synthesized by human beings, hence ***it should be supplied in diet.*** Intestinal bacterial flora can synthesize the vitamin.

Metabolism

Absorption: Free thiamine is absorbed readily from the small intestine, but the pyrophosphate (esterform) is not. Bulk of the dietary vegetable thiamine is in the "free" form. ***In tissues, it is***

actively phosphorylated to form Thiamine pyrophosphate (TPP) in liver, and to a lesser extent in other tissues like muscle, brain and nucleated RB Cells.

Plasma/Blood Level and Storage and Excretion
It is present in plasma and CS fluid in the "free" form, approx. 1 µg/100 ml. Blood cells contain 6 to 12 µg/100 ml where it occurs as TPP.

Storage: The capacity to store is limited. It is present in both free and combined forms in heart (highest concentration), liver and kidneys and in lower concentration in skeletal muscle and brain. The total amount of vitamin *Thiamine* in body is approx. 25 mg.

Excretions: If normal amount of thiamine is taken in the diet:

- About 10% is excreted in the urine.
- The remainder is (i) partly phosphorylated and is used as coenzyme, and (ii) partly degraded to neutral sulphur compounds and inorganic SO_4 which are excreted in urine.
- It is secreted in milk as thiamine-protein complex and in certain species, e.g. goats as mono and di-phosphothiamine.

OCCURRENCE AND FOOD SOURCES

- ***Plant source:*** It is widely distributed in plant kingdom. In ***cereal grains, it is concentrated in outer germ/bran layers, e.g. rice polishings (Richest source).*** Other good sources are peas, beans, whole cereal grains, bran, nuts, prunes, etc. ***Whole white bread is a good source.***
- ***Animal source:*** Thiamine is present in most animal tissues. Liver, meat and eggs supply considerable amounts. Ham/pork meats are particularly rich. ***Milk has low concentration,*** but a good source as large quantities are consumed.

Metabolic Role and Functions

Biological "active" forms: ***Thiamine pyrophosphate (TPP) acts as a coenzyme*** in several metabolic reactions.

- ***It acts as coenzyme to the enzyme pyruvate dehydrogenase complex (PDH)*** which converts pyruvic acid to acetyl CoA (oxidative decarboxylation).

$$\text{Pyruvate} \xrightarrow[\text{TPP}]{\text{PDH}} \text{Acetyl COA}$$

- Similarly, it ***acts as a coenyme to α-oxoglutarate dehydrogenase complex*** and converts α-oxoglutarate to succinyl CoA (oxidative decarboxylation).

$$\alpha\text{-Oxoglutarate} \xrightarrow[\text{TPP}]{\alpha\text{-oxo-glutarate dehydrogenase}} \bullet\ \textit{Succinyl CoA}$$

- TPP also acts as a coenzyme with the enzyme ***transketolase*** in transketolation reaction in HMP pathway of glucose metabolism.

$$\text{Ribose -5-P + xylulose-5-p} \xrightarrow[\text{TPP}]{\textit{Transketolase}} \text{Sedoheptulose -7-P + Glyceraldehyde -3-p}$$

- B_1 is also required in amino acid tryptophan metabolism for the activity of the enzyme ***Tryptophan pyrrolase.***

Deficiency Manifestations: Beri-beri

The deficiency of thiamine produces a condition called ***beri-beri.*** It is characterized by the following manifestations.

- ***CV manifestations:*** These include palpitation, dyspnoea, cardiac hypertrophy and dilatation, which may progress to congestive cardiac failure.
- ***Neurological manifestations:*** These are predominantly those of ascending, symmetrical, peripheral polyneuritis. These neurological features may be accompanied occasionally by an acute haemorrhagic polioencephalitis which is then called as ***Wernicke's encephalopathy.***
- ***GI symptoms:*** Amongst these, anorexia is an early symptom. There may be gastric atony,

with diminished gastric motility and nausea; fever and vomiting occur in advanced stages.

Dry beri-beri: When it is not associated with oedema.

Wet beri-beri: Oedema is associated. It is probabaly in part to congestive cardiac failure and in part to protein malnutrition (low plasma albumin).

Deficiency in Animals: Deficiency in animals produces symptoms resembling beri-beri as described above, with certain important additional features in certain species:

- ***In rats,*** It is associated with marked bradycardia.
- ***Pigeons*** develop a characteristic rigid retraction of head-opisthotonos.

The above two are utilized for bio-assays.

Chastek paralysis: It is observed in foxes eating raw fish. It is characterized by extreme, board-like rigidity with retraction of head.

Reason: Raw fish contains heat-labile thiamine splitting enzyme ***thiaminase*** which destroys thiamine.

Bracken disease: A similar condition which has been reported in grazing animals feeding on ferns and related species of plants which contain the enzyme *thiaminase.*

BIOCHEMICAL FEATURE IN THIAMINE DEFICIENCY

- Decreased level of thiamine and cocarboxylase TPP is found in blood and urine. Determination of amount of thiamine excreted in 4 hours urine is used.
- ***Accumulation of pentose sugars in RB cells*** due to retardation of transketolation reaction.
- ***Increased level of pyruvic acid and lactic acid*** is found in blood due to retardation of oxidative decarboxylation of pyruvic acid.

LA/PA ratio: Abnormal blood LA/PA ratio is said to be more specific indicator of B_1 deficiency.

Daily Requirements

Adult: 0.5 mg for each 1000 calories; 1.0 to 1.5 mg for diets providing 2000 to 3000 C. Minimum requirement is 1.0 mg. ***Actual requirement is related more directly to carbohydrates content of diet than to calorie value of diet.***

Children: It ranges from 0.4 mg for infants to 1.5 mg for preadolescents (10 to 12 years of age).

Requirement increases:

- In anoxia-shock and haemorrhage,
- Serious illness and injury,
- ***During prolonged administration of broad-spectrum oral antibiotics,***
- In increased calorie expenditure like fever, hyperthyroidism,
- ***Increased carbohydrate intake,***
- ***Increased alcohol intake, and***
- ***In pregnancy and lactation.***

RIBOFLAVIN (VITAMIN B_2)

Synonyms: Lactoflavin

Chemistry:

- It is an orange-yellow compound containing,
  - A ribose alcohol-**D-ribitol**
  - A heterocyclic parent ring structure **"Isoalloxazine" (Flavin nucleus).**
- ***1-Carbon of ribityl group is attached at the 9th position of iso-alloxazine nucleus.***
- Ribityl is an alcohol derived from pentose sugar D-ribose.
- ***Stability:*** It is stable to heat in neutral acid solution but not in alkaline solutions. Aqueous solutions are unstable to visible and UV light.

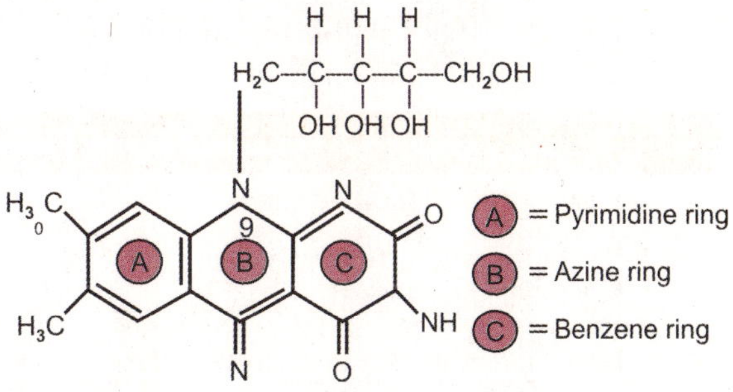

A = Pyrimidine ring
B = Azine ring
C = Benzene ring

6,7-dimethyl-9-D-ribityl iso-alloxazine

Biological Active Forms

The biological "active" forms, in which riboflavin serves as the prosthetic group (as co-enzyme) of a number of enzymes are the phosphorylated derivatives.

Two main derivatives are:

- **FMN-Flavin Mononucleotide:** In this, phosphoric acid is attached to ribityl alcoholic group in position 5.

Flavin-Ribityl-PO_4

- **FAD-Flavin Adenine Dinucleotide:** It may be linked to an adenine nucleotide through a pyrophosphate linkage to form FAD.

Flavin-ribityl-P-P-ribose-adenine.

Thus, FMN and FAD are two coenzymes of this vitamin.

F_P(holoenzyme) = FMN/FAD + Protein
(coenzyme) (Apoenzyme)

FP may also unite with metals like Fe and Mo thus forming Metallo-flavoproteins.

BIOSYNTHESIS

- ***All higher plants and micro-organisms can synthesize riboflavin.***
- ***Riboflavin content of seeds increases with germination,*** e.g. germinating grams/dals are rich in riboflavin.
- Human beings and animals cannot synthesize and hence ***solely dependent on dietary supply.***

In man, considerable amounts can be synthesized by intestinal bacteria, but the quantity absorbed is not adequate to maintain normal nutrition.

METABOLISM

Absorption: Flavin nucleotides are readily absorbed in small intestine. ***Free riboflavin undergoes phosphorylation, a prerequisite for absorption (cf. Thiamine).***

Blood/plasma level: Human blood/plasma contains 2.5 to 4.0 µgm%, two-third as FAD and bulk of remainder as FMN. Riboflavin present in all tissues as nucleotides bound to proteins (FP), highest concentration in liver and kidney.

Excretion: It is mainly excreted in free form, up to 50% as nucletides in urine. Daily urinary excretion is 0.1 to 0.4 mg (10 to 20% of intake).

Occurrences and food sources: It is widely distributed in nature. It is found in all plant and animal cells.

- ***Plant souces:*** It occurs in high concentration in yeasts.
  Appreciable amount present in whole grain, dry beans and peas, nuts, green vegetable. Germinating seeds, e.g. grams/dals are very good source.
- ***Animal source:*** Liver (2-3 mg/100 gm), kidney, milk, eggs, crab meat has high content.

Metabolic Role

FMN and FAD act as coenzyme in various H-transfer reactions in metabolism. The hydrogen is transported by reversible reduction of the coenzyme by two hydrogen atoms added to the 'N' at position 1 and 10, thus, forming dihydro or leucoriboflavin. The principal enzyme reactions catalyzed are as shown in ***Table 9.2.***

Deficiency manifestations: There is ***no definite disease entity.*** Deficiency is usually associated

Table 9.2: Principal Enzyme Reactions Catalyzed by FMN and FAD

FMN	*FAD*
• Warburg's yellow enzyme	• Xanthine oxidase (Xanthine → uric acid)
• Cytochrome-C reductase	• D-amino acid oxidase
• L-amino acid oxidase	• Aldehyde oxidase
(FP is autooxidizable at substrate level by molecular O_2 forming H_2O_2)	• Fumarate dehydrogenase (Succinate→fumarate)
	• Glycine oxidase
	• Acyl CoA dehydrogenase
	• Diaphorase

with deficiencies in other B-vitamins. **In human beings,** lesions of the mouth, tongue, nose, skin and eyes with weakness, and lassitude are reported. They include:

- *Lips:* Redness and shiny appearance of lips.
- *Cheilosis:* Lesions at the mucocutaneous junction at the angles of the mouth leading to painful fissures are characteristic.
- *Tongue:* Painful glossitis, the tongue assumes a red-purple (magenta) colour.
- *Seborrhoeic dermatitis:* Scaly, greasy, desquamation chiefly about the ears, nose and nasolabial folds.
- *Eyes:* May lead to corneal vascularization and inflammation with cloudiness of cornea, watering, burning of eyes, photophobia, scleral congestion and cataract has also been reported.
- *Protein synthesis:* This is impaired in severe riboflavin deficiency; since protein malnutrition interferes with utilization and retention of riboflavin.

Daily requirement: Exact human requirement is not known ***Related to degree of protein utilization (cf. Thiamine).***

Recommended daily intake:

- Adults: 1.5 to 1.8 mg
- Women: in later half of pregnancy: 2.0 mg during lactation: 2.5 mg
- Infants: 0.6 mg
- Children: 1.0 to 1.8 mg
- Adolescence: 2.0 to 2.5 mg.

Requirement increases:

- After severe injury, burns, etc.
- During acute illness and during convalescence
- During increased protein utilization
- In ***pregnancy and lactation***
- ***During oral broad spectrum antibiotic therapy.***

NIACIN

Synonyms: Nicotinic acid, P-P factor, pellagra preventing factors of Goldberger

Chemistry: Nicotinic acid (Niacin is chemically Pyridine-3-carboxylic acid.

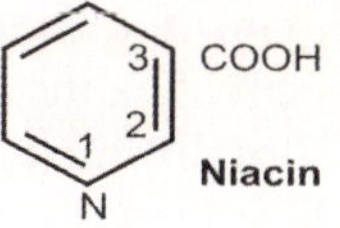

In ***tissues, it occurs principally as the "amide" (nicotinamide, niacinamide).*** In this form, it enters into physiological active combination.

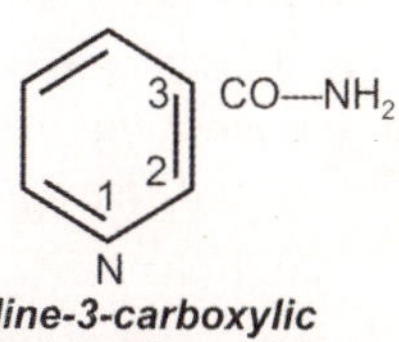

Pyridine-3-carboxylic amide (nicotinamide)

Biological Active Forms

In tissues, nicotinamide is present largely as a "dinucleotide", the pyridine 'N' being linked to a D-ribose residue. **Two such neucleotide active forms are known.**

1. *Nicotinamide adenine dinucleotide* (NAD^+). Other names are: DPN^+, *coenzyme I, cozymase,* or *codehydrogenase*

   The compound contains:

   - One molecule of nicotinamide,
   - Two molecules of D-ribose,
   - Two molecules of phosphoric acid, and
   - One molecule of adenine.

   Structure may be shown schematically as given below:

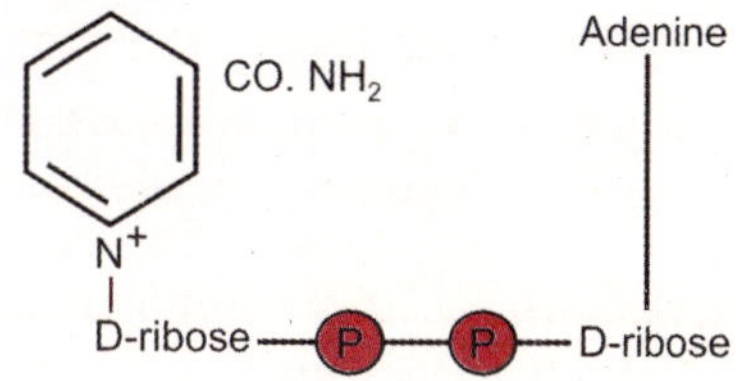

2. ***Nicotinamide adenine dinucleotide phosphate (NADP^+^).*** Others names are: TPN^+, *Co-enzyme II.*

This compound differs from NAD^+ in that it contains an additional molecule of phosphoric acid attached to 2-position of D-ribose attached to N-9 of Adenine

The reduced form of either coenzymes is designated by the prefix "dihydro", e.g. reduced NAD^+ is called dihydro-nicotinamide adenine dinucleotide (NADH).

BIOSYNTHESIS

- *Amino acid tryptophan is a precursor of nicotinic acid* in many plants, and animal species including human beings. ***60 mg tryptophan can give rise to 1 mg of niacin.*** Pyridoxal-P is required as a coenzyme in this synthesis.
- It *can be synthesized also by intestinal bacteria.*

Applied aspect: In *high corn diet, requirement of dietary niacin increases, as synthesis from tryptophan cannot take place*. The reason is that the maize protein **"Zein"** lacks the amino acid tryptophan. ***Hence pellagra is more common in persons whose staple diet is maize.***

Formation of nicotinamide: Nicotinamide is not formed directly from nicotinic acid. It is formed by degradation of NAD^+ and $NADP^+$.

METABOLISM

Absorption: Nicotinic acid and its amide are absorbed from the small intestine.

Blood/plasma level:

- ***Whole blood:*** 0.2 to 0.9 mg/100 ml (average 0.6 mg%).
- ***RB Cells:*** 1.3 mg%.
- ***Plasma:*** Total activity 0.025 to 0.15 mg% (average 0.075 mg%).

Note:

- Most of the nicotinic acid and its amide in the blood is in RB cells presumably as coenzyme.
- Values in the blood are not altered significantly even in severe niacin deficiency. ***Hence its determination is of no value in the detection of clinical deficiency states.***

Excretion: **In urine,** it is excreted as follows:

- As nicotinic acid and nicotinamide
  Normal adults on normal diet excretes both nicotinic acid and its amide in urine.
  Nicotinic acid: 0.25 to 1.25 mg daily.
  Nicotinamide: 0.5 to 4 mg daily.
- **As N′-methyl nicotinamide:** *Major urinary metabolite derivative-N′-methyl nicotinamide.* The methylation occurs in liver, by the enzyme ***niacinamide methyl transferase.*** CH_3 group is given by "Active methionine".

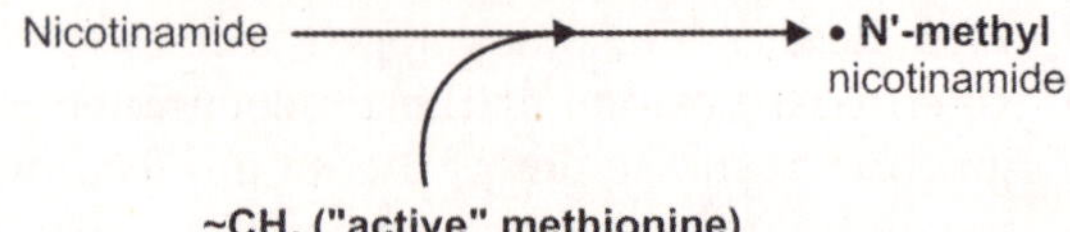

Occurrence and Food Sources

- Both nicotinamide and coenzyme forms are distributed widely in plants and animals.
- Important food sources are:
  - *Animal source:* Liver, kidney, meat, fish
  - *Vegetable source:* Legumes (peas, beans, lentils), nuts, certain green vegetables, coffee and tea.

Nicotinamide is present in highest concentration in germ and pericarp (bran) in cereal grains. Yeasts are also particularly rich. ***Poor sources are fruits, milk and eggs.***

Metabolic Role and Functions

- ***The coenzymes NAD^+ and $NADP^+$ operate as hydrogen and electron transfer agents by virtue of reversible oxidation and reduction.***
- The mechanism of the transfer of Hydrogen from a metabolite to oxidized NAD^+, thus completing the oxidation of the metabolite and the formation of reduced NAD ($NADH + H^+$) is shown as follows:
  Reduction of NAD^+ occurs in para position: one H loses an electron and enters the medium as H^+.
- Functions of $NADP^+$ is similar to that of NAD^+ in hydrogen and electron transport.
- The two coenzymes are interconvertible.

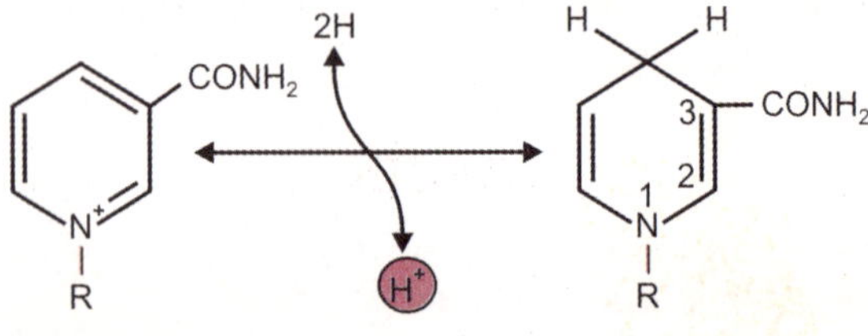

Reduction of NAD^+

Table 9.3: Action of NAD^+ and $NADP^+$ as Coenzyme on Some Important Enzymes

NAD^+	*$NADP^+$*
• *Alcohol dehydrogenase (Ethanol→Acetaldehyde)* • *Lactate dehydrogenase* (LDH) (P.A.↔L.A.) • *Malate dehydrogenase (Malate↔O.A.A.)* • Glyceraldehyde-3-P dehydrogenase (Gly-3-P→1,3-di-phosphoglycerate) • α-Glycero-P-dehydrogenase • *Pyruvate dehydrogenase complex* (PDH) (PA→Acetyl CoA) • α-Ketoglutarate dehydrogenase complex (α-ketoglutarate→succinyl CoA	• *Glucose-6-P-dehydrogenase* (G-6-P-D) *(G-6-P→6-Phosphogluconate)* • Glutathione reductase ***Either NAD^+ or $NADP^+$*** • *Glutanate dehydrogenase* (Glutamate→ α-ketoglutarate + NH_3) • *(Isocitrate-dehydrogenase* (ICD) (Isocitrate→ Oxalosuccinate)

- The important enzymes to which NAD^+ and $NADP^+$ act as coenzymes are listed as given in ***Table 9.3.***

Deficiency Manifestations: Pellagra

Nicotinic acid deficiency produces a disease called **"pellagra"** (Pelle=skin; agra = rough)

Cardinal features described as **"3 D's"** are:
- **Dermatitis,**
- **Diarrhoea, and**
- **Dementia.**

Precipitating factors are:
- High-corn diet and
- Alcoholism

Clinical Features

- ***Skin lesions:*** Typically involves areas of skin exposed to sunlight and subjected to pressure, heat or other types of trauma or/irritation. These include face, neck, dorsal surfaces of the wrist, forearms, elbows, breasts and perineum. The skin becomes reddened, later brown, thickened and scaly.
- ***GI manifestations:*** Include ***anorexia, nausea, vomiting,*** abdominal pain, with alternating constipation diarrhoea. Diarrhoea becomes intractable later.
  - **Gingivitis** and **stomatitis** with reddening of the tip and margin of the tongue, which become swollen and cracked.
  - **Achlorhydria** present in about 40% cases.
  - Thickening and inflammation of the colon, with cystic lesions of the mucosa, which later becomes atrophic and ulcerated.
- ***Cerebral manifestations:*** These include headache, insomnia, depression and other mental symptoms ranging from mild psycho-neuroses to severe psychosis.
- ***General effects:*** These include:
  - Inadequate growth
  - Loss of weight and strength
  - Anaemia which may be due to associated deficiency of other vitamins
  - Dehydration and its consequences resulting from diarrhoea.

Daily Requirement

- ***In adult:*** 17 to 21 mg daily
- ***Infants:*** 6 mg
- ***Pre-adolescence:*** 17 mg.

Requirement increases in:
- Increased calorie intake or expenditure
- Acute illness or early convalescence
- After severe injury, infection and burns

- *High corn or maize diet*
- *Pregnancy and lactation*

OTHER CLINICAL ASPECTS AND EXPERIMENTAL STUDIES

- *Development of fatty liver:* In rats, administration of large amounts of nicotinic acid or amide produced fatty liver, which is prevented by simultaneous administration of methionine, choline or betaine.

  Explanation: There occurs diversion of —CH_3 group for the ***formation of excessive amount of N′-methyl nicotinamide producing relative deficiency of choline.***
- *Effect on plasma lipids:* Nicotinic acid and ***not amide*** have been found ***to reduce the plasma lipid concentration in certain cases of hyperlipidaemia.*** Large doses of nicotinic acid from 3 to 6 grams per day have been found to reduce the levels of cholesterol, β-lipoproteins and TG in blood.

PYRIDOXINE (VITAMIN B_6)

Synonyms: Rat antidermatitis factor

CHEMISTRY: Pyridoxol (pyridoxine), also called as "adermin" is chemically 2-methyl-3-OH-4,5-di (hydroxymethyl) pyridine.

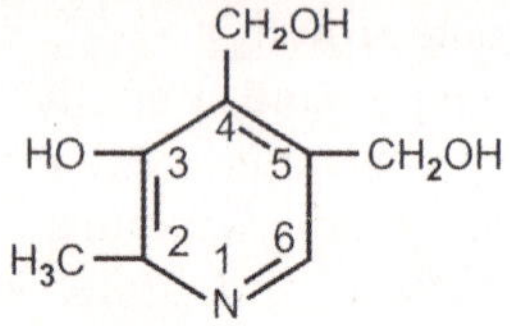

Pyridoxine (pyridoxol)

- It occurs in association, perhaps in equilibrium, with an aldehyde-"**Pyridoxal**" and an amine "**Pyridoxamine**" form.

All these forms exhibited vitamin B_6 activity.

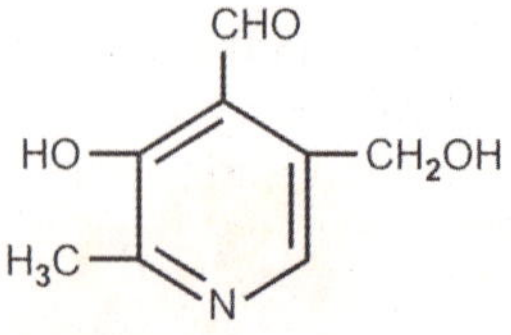

Pyridoxal

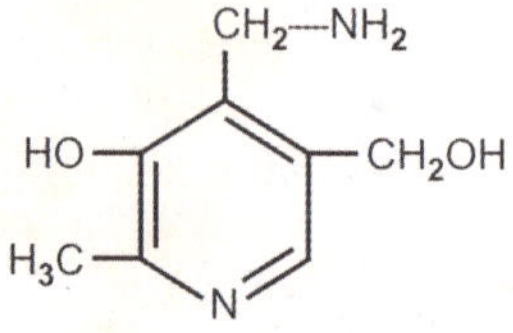

Pyridoxamine

Biological Active Forms

- Biological active forms of the vitamin are:
  - *Pyridoxal-PO_4, and*
  - *Pyridoxamine-PO_4*
- The active forms are the phosphorylated derivatives: phosphorylation involves the hydroxy-methyl group -CH_2OH at position 5 in the pyridine ring.
- These forms occur in nature largely in combination with protein (apoenzyme).

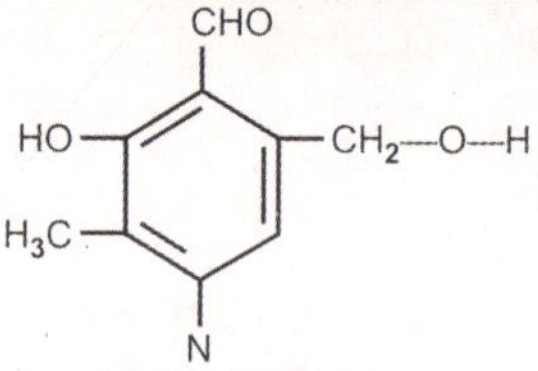

Pyridoxal-P

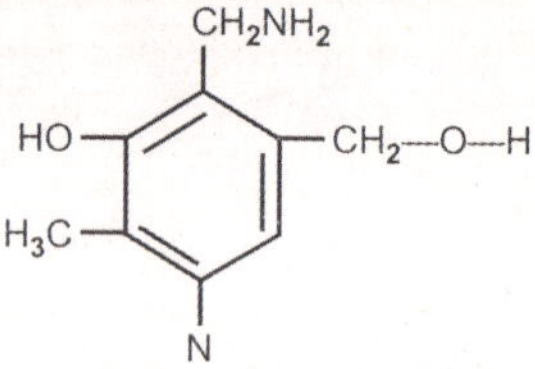

Pyridoxamine-P

BIOSYNTHESIS

- Vitamin B_6 can be formed by many micro-organisms and probably also by plants.
- ***Human beings cannot synthesize the vitamin hence has to be provided in the diet.***
- Intestinal bacteria can synthesize the vitamin.

METABOLISM

Absorption: Dietary vitamin B_6 is readily absorbed by the intestine.

Excretion

- Pyridoxal and pyridoxamine are excreted in urine in small amounts 0.5 to 0.7 mg daily.
- Majority urinary metabolite, about 3 mg daily is the biologically inactive form 4-pyridoxic acid.

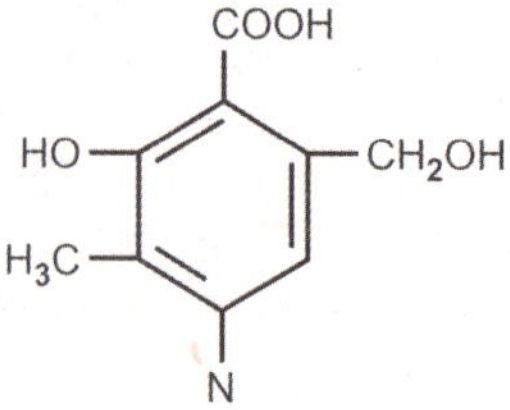

Pyridoxic acid

Occurrence and Food Sources

- The vitamin is distributed widely in animal and plant tissues. Rich sources of the vitamin are yeast, rice polishings, germinal portion of various seeds and cereal grains and egg-yolk.

- Moderate amounts are present in liver, kidney, muscle, fish.
- *Milk is a poor source.* Highest concentration occurs in royal jelly (bee).

Metabolic Role and Functions

Pyridoxal P acts as a coenzyme. It is principally involved with metabolism of amino acids.

- *Co-transaminase:* Acts as a coenzyme for the enzyme *transaminases* (aminotransferases) in transamination reaction.
- *Co-decarboxylase:* Acts as coenzyme for the enzyme *decarboxylases* in decarboxylation reaction. Amino acids are decarboxylated to form corresponding amines. (Biogenic amines).
- *Coenzyme for kynureninase:* In tryptophan metabolism, pyridoxal-P acts as a coenzyme for the enzyme *kynureninase* which converts 3-OH-kynurenine to 3-OH-anthranilic acid which ultimately forms nicotinic acid. *Thus in B_6-deficiency niacin synthesis from tryptophan does not take place.* **In B_6 deficiency** kynurenine and 3-OH kynurenine levels increase and they are converted to *"Xanthurenic" acid* in extrahepatic tissues, which is excreted in urine *(Fig. 9.3). "xanthurenic acid" index is a reliable criterion for B_6 deficiency.*
- *Transulfuration:* It takes part in transulfuration reaction involving transfer of -SH group, e.g.

Homocysteine + Serine→Homoserine + cysteine.

- As coenzyme for *desulfhydrases:* Catalyzes non-oxidative deamination of cysteine in which H_2S is liberated.
- In *interconversion of glycine and serine by serine hydroxy methyl transferase:* In this both $F.H_4$ and B_6 are required as coenzymes.
- Pyridoxal-P is required as a conenzyme in the *biosynthesis of arachidonic acid* from "linoleic acid".
- *Synthesis of Sphingomyelin:* Pyridoxal-P is required as a coenzymes for activation of serine which is required for synthesis of sphingomyelin.

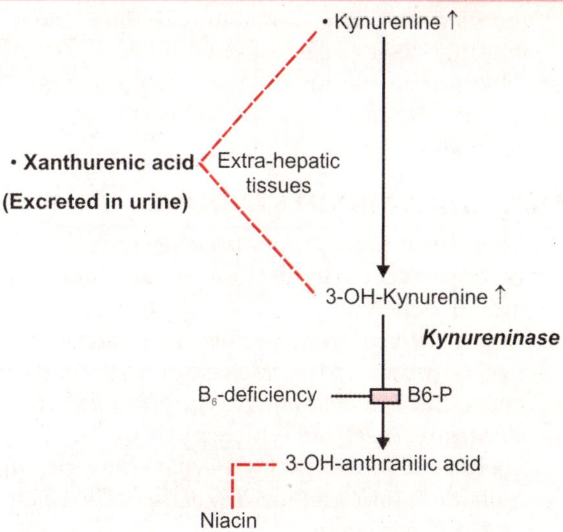

Fig. 9.3: Conversion of kynurenine and 3-OH-kynurenine to xanthurenic acid

- *Intramitochondrial FA synthesis:* It is required as a coenzyme with *condensing enzyme* for chain elongation of FA in intramitochondrial FA synthesis.
- It is also required *for "active transport" of amino acids* through cell membrane and intestinal absorption of amino acids.
- *Muscle phosphorylase:* As a constituent of *muscle phosphorylase,* 4 molecules of pyridoxal-(P)per molecule of enzyme (tetramer).
- *Transport of K^+:* Vitamin B_6 has been reported to promote transport of K^+ across the membrane from exterior to interior.
- *Synthesis of CoA-SH (Coenzyme A):* Vitamin B_6 is involved in synthesis of coenzyme A from pantothenic acid. **In B_6 deficiency,** coenzyme A level in liver is reduced.
- *In porphyrin synthesis:* Pyridoxal-P is required for conversion of *α-amino-β-keto adipic acid to δ-ALA,* an important step in hemesynthesis. *In B_6-deficiency heme synthesis suffers and leads to anaemia.*
- *Hypercholesterolaemia:* Relationship of B_6-deficiency and hypercholesterolaemia and atherosclerosis in monkey has received considerable attention, although the exact role of vitamin B_6 is not clear.

- *Immune response:* In vitamin B_6 deficiency, immune response is impaired.
- *Oxaluria:* Vitamin B_6 deficiency has been observed to produce oxaluria in experimental animals.

DEFICIENCY MANIFESTATIONS

No deficiency disease has been described. But following clinical manifestation are attributed to vitamin B_6 deficiency.

- ***"Epileptiform" convulsions in infants*** have been attributed to pyridoxine deficiency. It is related to lowered activity of ***glutamic acid decarboxylase,*** for which pyridoxal-P is a coenzyme. As a result ***there occurs lowering of γ-amino butyric acid (GABA) in the brain which causes convulsions.***
- ***Pyridoxine responsive anaemia:*** A **hypochromic microcytic anaemia with high serum Fe level** and haemosiderosis of liver, spleen and bone marrow may occur with B_6-deficiency. Pyridoxal-P is required as a coenzyme in the reaction by which α-amino-β-keto adipic acid is decarboxylated to form δ-ALA in heme synthesis. In ***B_6-deficiency, hence synthesis suffers and Fe cannot be utilized.***
  - ***Isonicotinic acid hydrazide treatment in tuberculosis:*** A syndrome due to vitamin B_6 deficiency has been observed in humans during the treatment of tuberculosis with high doses of tuberculostatic drug "isonicotinic acid hydrazide" or "isoniazid" (INH). Signs and symptoms were alleviated by administration of pyridoxine to these patients. ***50 mg of pyridoxine per day completely prevented the development of neuritis and neuropathies.***

  Mechanism of Action: It is believed isoniazid forms a "hydrazone complex" with pyridoxine resulting in incomplete activation of the vitamin.
- ***Vitamin B_6 has been found empirically to be of value in treatment of:***
  - Nausea and vomiting of pregnancy ("morning sickness"),
  - Radiation sickness,
  - Muscular dystrophies,
  - Treatment of hyperoxaluria, and recurring oxalate stones of kidney.
- Mild forms of pyridoxine deficiency have been reported to occur sometimes in women taking oral contraceptives containing oestradiol.

Daily Requirement: It has been difficult to establish definitely the human requirement of vitamin B_6 due to the fact that

- Quantity needed is not large, and
- Bacterial synthesis in intestine provides a portion of the requirement.

There is evidence that requirement of vitamin B_6 is related to dietary protein intake, as it is involved as coenzyme in many metabolic reactions of amino acid metabolism.

- An adult 2 mg per day has been recommended.
- Infants: 0.3 to 0.4 mg/day.
- During second half of pregnancy: 2.5 mg/day.
- In patients receiving antitubercular treatment with INH, requirement of vitamin B_6 increases much.

LIPOIC ACID (THIOCTIC ACID)

Synonyms: Protogen, acetate replacement factor.

Chemistry: It is a ***sulphur containing*** fatty acid called 6,8-dithiooctanoic acid (α-lipoic acid or thioctic acid). ***It contains eight carbon and two sulphur atoms.***

- Oxidized and reduced forms of the compound is shown as follows:

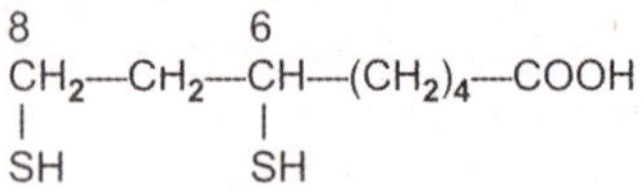

8 6
$CH_2—CH_2—CH—(CH_2)_4—COOH$ (SH on C8 and C6)

α–Lipoic acid (reduced form)

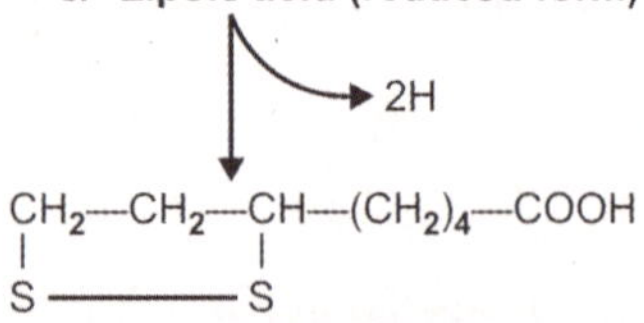

↓ → 2H

$CH_2—CH_2—CH—(CH_2)_4—COOH$ (C8 and C6 joined through S—S)

α–Lipoic acid (oxidized form)

Metabolic Role

It is recognized as an essential component in metabolism although it is active in extremely minute amounts.

- As a coenzyme of *pyruvate dehydrogenase* complex (PDH), it is required along with other coenzymes in oxidative decarboxylation of pyruvic acid to acetyl CoA.
- As a coenzyme of α-*oxoglutarate dehydrogenase* complex, it is required along with other coenzymes in oxidative decarboxylation of α-oxo-glutarate to succinyl CoA.
- Lipoic acid is also required for the action of the enzyme *sulfite oxidase* required for conversion of SO_2 to SO_4^{-2}. Hypoxanthine is also required for the action.

SO_2^-

Lipoic acid ↓ ***Sulfite oxidase***
Hypoxanthine

$SO_4^=$

Deficiency Manifestations: Not known. Lipoic acid occurs in a wide variety of natural materials. Its requirement in the diet of higher animals has not yet been demonstrated. Attempts to induce lipoic acid deficiency in animals have so far been unsucessful.

PANTOTHENIC ACID

Synonyms: Filtrate factor, chick antidermatitis factor.

Chemistry: Pantothenic acid consists of **β-alanine in peptide linkage** with a **di-hydroxy di-methyl butyric acid (pantoic acid).**

β-alanine + Pantoic acid→ Pantothenic acid

- The free acid is soluble in water and is hydrolyzed by acids/or alkalies. It is thermolabile and destroyed by heat. Its sodium and calcium salts are fairly soluble in water and are somewhat more stable to heat than the free acid.

Biological Active Form

Active form is coenzyme A. In tissues, this vitamin is present almost entirely in the form of the coenzyme, (coenzyme A is also known as *Coacetylase)* and largely bound to proteins (apoenzyme).

Structure of coenzyme A has been delineated and can be represented schematically below in the box

- Pantothenic acid is joined in one hand to adenosine-3′-P by a pyrophosphate bridge, and on the other hand,
- Joined by peptide linkage to β-mercapto-ethanol amine which is obtained from amino acid cysteine.

  ***The terminal-SH group (thiol group) of β-mercapto ethanol amine is the reactive site of the coenzyme molecule ("Active site" or group). Hence, for convenience coenzyme A is represented* CoA.SH.**

BIOSYNTHESIS AND METABOLISM:

Human tissues cannot synthesize pantothenic acid, hence, it has to be obtained from diet.

- In addition to dietary source, synthesis by intestinal bacteria supply fair amount of pantothenic acid.

Structure of Coenzyme A

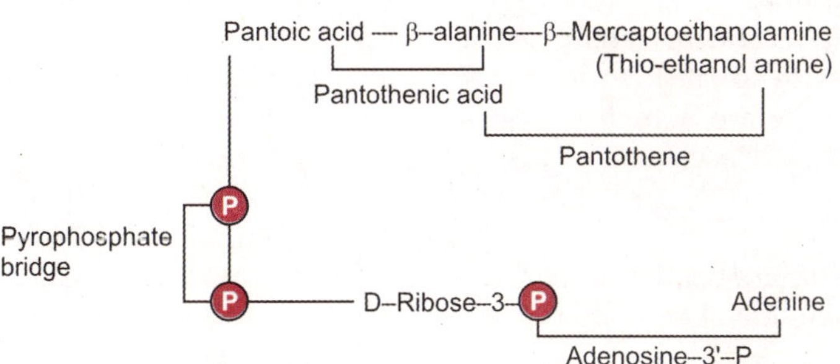

Source in humans (Pantothenic acid)
- Dietary
- Synthesis by intestinal bacteria

- *Synthesis of Coenzyme-A:* Complete synthesis of coenzyme A was described by **Khorana** in 1959. Human tissues as well as plants and bacteria can synthesize COA-SH.

Whole blood level: The concentration of pantothenic acid in whole blood is 15-45 μg/100 ml (average 30 μg%). It is present in all tissues in small amounts, the highest concentration occurring in liver (40 μg per gram wt) and kidney (30 μg/gm).

Excretion: Catabolic products of pantothenic acid are not known. Under ordinary dietary condition about 2.5 to 5 mg are excreted daily in the urine.

Occurrence and Food Sources: It is widely distributed in plants, animal tissue and food materials.

- **Excellent food sources** (100 to 200 μg/gm of dry materials): include kidney, liver egg yolk, yeast, cereals and legumes.
- **Fair sources** (35 to 100 μg/gm) include skimmed milk, chicken, certain fishes, sweet potatoes, molasses.
- Most vegetables and fruits are rather poor source.
- Richest known source of pantothenic acid is Royal Jelly(also rich in biotin and pyridoxine)

Metabolic Role and Functions

Only demonstrated metabolic function of pantothenic acid is as a constituent of CoA-SH, pantothenic acid is essential to several fundamental metabolic reactions.

- *Formation of active acetate (Acetyl CoA):* It readily combines with acetate to form Acetyl CoA or "Active" acetate, which is metabolically active. Acetyl-CoA chemically is:

$$CH_3—\overset{\overset{O}{||}}{C}\sim S.CoA$$

, the sulphur bond of acetyl CoA is a high energy bond equivalent to that of the high energy PO_4 bond of ATP.

In the form of active acetate, it participates in a number of important metabolic reactions, e.g.

- ***Utilized directly by combination with oxaloacetate (OAA) to form citric acid, which initiates TCA cycle.*** Thus acetyl-CoA derived from carbohydrates, Lipids and many amino acids undergo further metabolic breakdown via this "final common metabolic pathway".
- *Acetyl choline formation:* Acetyl-CoA combines with choline to form Acetyl-choline.
- *For acetylation reaction:* Used in acetylation reactions with drugs/chemicals, like sulphonamides before their excretion.
- *Synthesis of cholesterol:* Acetyl CoA is the starting material for cholesterol biosynthesis via HMG-CoA.
- *Formation of ketone bodies:* Acetyl CoA is the starting material for formation of ketone bodies.
- Acetyl CoA and malonyl CoA are used in the ***synthesis and elongation of fatty acids.***

- *Formation of active succinate (succinyl CoA):* Product of oxidative decarboxylation of α-oxo-glutarate in TCA cycle is a coenzyme derivative called **"Active" succinate (succinyl-CoA).** Succinyl-CoA is involved in certain important metabolic reactions.
  - *Heme synthesis:* In heme synthesis, "active" succinate and glycine combines to form δ-ALA, the first step in the pathway of heme formation.

    Applied aspects: Anaemia may occur in pantothenic acid deficiency probably due to deficiency in formation of succinyl CoA. Due to non-availability of the substrate the heme synthesis sufferes.
  - *Degradation of ketone bodies by extra-hepatic tissues:* Succinyl CoA combines with acetoacetate to form acetoacetyl CoA and succinic acid catalyzed by the enzyme *CoA-transferase (thiophorase).*
- *Role in lipid metabolism:*
  - *Oxidation of FA (β-oxidation):* First step in oxidation of FA catalyzed by ***thiokinase (acyl synthases)*** involves the activation of

the FA by formatoin of CoA derivatives. Removal of a 2-C fragment in β-oxidation is acomplished by a "thiolytic" cleavage, which utilizes another molecule of CoA-SH.

- *Biosynthesis of FA:* Pantothenic acid is a constituent of a compound called as "acyl-carrier protein" (ACP) and also a constituent of "multienzymes complex" in mammals, which is used in the extramitochondrial *"de Novo"* fatty acid synthesis.
- *Role in Adrenocortical function:* Pantothenic acid appears to be involved in adrenocortical activity, being essential to the f*ormation of adrenocortical hormones from "active" acetate and cholesterol.*

Deficiency Manifestations: ***No deficiency disease has been recognised in man.*** This may be due to:

- Its widespread distribution in foodstuffs and
- Supply from synthesis by bacterial flora of intestines.

Deficiency manifestations observed in experimental animal are:

- **Dermatitis**
- ***Loss of hair (alopecia):*** Circumocular "spectacle" alopecia and greying of hairs.
- ***GI manifestations:*** Include gastritis and enteritis with ulceration and haemorrhagic diarrhoea.
- **Fatty liver** develops in dogs and rats
- **Anaemia** develops in certain species and in severe cases, hypoplasia of bone marrow.
- ***Nervous system manifestations:*** Include myelin degeneration of peripheral nerves and degenerative changes in posterior root ganglia.

Daily Requirement: The human requirement of pantothenic acid is not known due to its widespread distribution.

- For adults it is recommended a daily intake of 5 to 12 mg per 2500 cal.
- In infants: 1 to 2 mg
- In children: 4 to 5 mg.

Requirement Increases:

- In presence of severe stress, e.g. acute illness, burns, severe injury, etc.
- **In oral administration of broad spectrum antibiotics.**
- **In pregnancy and lactation.**
- In growing children.
- In convalascence.

BIOTIN

Synonyms: Bios, vitamin H, Coenzyme R, anti egg white injury factor.

Chemistry: Biotin is a heterocyclic monocarboxylic acid.

- It is a ***sulphur-containing*** water soluble B vitamin.
- Structure of the compound was worked out by **du Vigneud**, which is as follows:

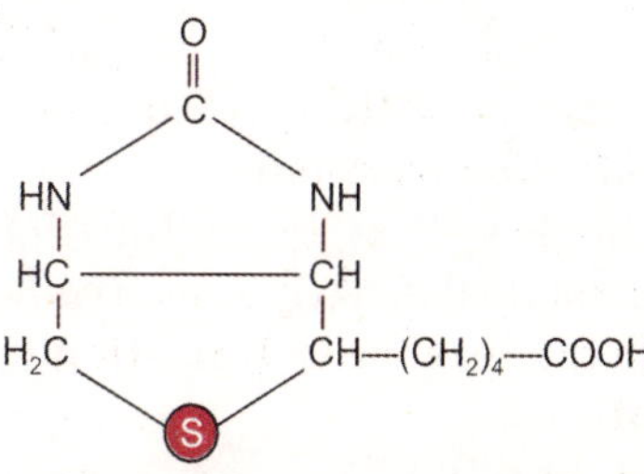

Biotin

It consists of two fused rings—one ***imidazole*** and the other ***thiophene*** derivative. Biotin ($C_{10}H_{16}O_3N_2S$) is chemically ***hexahydro-2-oxo-1-thieno-3,4-imidazole-4 valeric acid.***

- Biotin crystallizes in long needles. It is soluble in water and ethyl alcohol, but insoluble in ether and chloroform. It is heat-stable. Biotin is destroyed by acids and alkalies and by oxidizing agents such as peroxide and permanganates.

Occurrence and Food Sources: Biotin is widely distributed in plants and animal tissues. It occurs chiefly as:

- ***"Water-soluble"*** form in most plant materials, except cereals and nuts, and
- Mainly in a ***"water-insoluble"*** form in animal tissues.

Foods rich in biotin include animal and plant sources

- *Animal sources:* are liver, kidney, milk and milk products and egg-yolk.
- *Vegetable sources:* Include vegetables, legumes, and grains which are good sources. Molasses contain good amount of biotin. Exceptionally large amounts are present in royal jelly (bee).
- Human beings cannot synthesize the vitamin and hence it has to be supplied in diet. But bacterial flora in intestine can synthesize the vitamin and is a good source.

Source in humans
- Dietary source
- Synthesis by bacterial flora of intestine.

Metabolic Role and Functions

- Biotin is the prosthetic group of certain enzymes that catalyze CO_2-transfer reaction (***CO_2-fixation reaction).***
- In biologic system, biotin functions as the coenzyme for the enzyme called *carboxylases,* **which catalyze the CO_2-fixation (Carboxylation).**

Examples of carboxylation or "CO_2-fixation" reaction in biologic system are given below:

- ***Conversion of acetyl CoA to malonyl CoA:*** In the first step of extra-mitochondrial *'de Novo'* FA synthesis, the acetyl CoA is converted to malonyl CoA, the reaction is catalyzed by the enzyme ***acetyl-CoA carboxylase.***
- ***Conversion of propionyl CoA to methylmalonyl CoA:*** The enzyme catalyzing the reaction is ***Propionyl-CoA carboxylase.***
- ***Conversion of pyruvic acid to oxaloacetate:*** The enzyme that catalyzes the reaction is ***pyruvate carboxylase.***

Deficiency Manifestations: Biotin deficiency may be induced in experimental animals:

- ***By inclusion of large amounts of raw egg-white in the diet.***
- By using sulphonamide drugs or broad spectrum oral antibiotics for prolonged periods.

The ***features include:***

- Dermatitis
- "Spectacle-eyed" appearance due to circum-ocular alopecia
- Thinning or loss of fur/and hairs
- Greying of hairs/fur of black or brown colours,
- Paralysis of hind legs.

Human volunteers: Deficiency has been produced by excluding dietary biotin and **feeding large amounts of raw egg-white** (30% of total calories). ***Egg-white produces injury as it contains an antivitamin called "avidin".***

Such individuals developed following symptoms beginning after 5 to 7 weeks.

- Dermatitis of the extremities
- Pallor of skin and mucous membranes
- Anorexia and nausea
- Muscle pains and hyperaesthesia
- Depression, lassitude and somnolence
- Anaemia, and
- Hypercholesterolaemia.

Prompt relief of symptoms occurred when biotin concentrates was given.

Daily Requirement: It is difficult to arrive at a quantitative requirement of this vitamin as it is ubiquitous, and secondly intestinal bacteria synthesize and supply the vitamin.

- Human adults: 25 to 50 μg daily
- Infants: 10 to 15 μg daily
- Children: 20 to 40 μg daily

Requirement Increases:

- In pregnancy and lactation
- In oral antibiotic therapy for prolonged periods.

FOLIC ACID GROUPS

Synonyms: Liver lactobacillus caseifactor, vitamin M, *Streptococcus lactis* R (SLR) factor, vitamin Bc, fermentation residue factor, pteroyl glutamic acid (PGA).

Chemistry: The designation "folic acid" is applied to a number of compounds which contain the following groups:

- *A "pteridine" nucleus (pyrimidine and pyrazine rings)*
- *Para-aminobenzoic acid (PABA) and*
- *Glutamic acid.*

- Structure of folic acid is shown below. Chemically called **"pteroyl glutamic acid" (PGA).**

Pteroyl (pteroic acid) folic acid (folacin)

- There are at least three chemically related compounds of nutritional importance which occur in natural products-all may be termed "**pteroyl glutamates**". These ***three compounds differ only in the number of glutamic acid residues*** attached to pteridine PABA complex (pteroic acid).
  - ***Monoglutamate:*** Having one glutamic acid. it is synonymous with vitamin Bc.
  - ***Triglutamate:*** Having three glutamic acid residues. This substance once designated as ***"fermentation factor".***
  - ***Heptaglutamate:*** Having seven glutamate rsidues-synonymous with vitamin Bc conjugate of yeast.

    Pteroyl glutamic acid is liberated from these conjugates by enzymes called ***conjugases.***
- Folic acid is soluble in water.
- It is fairly resistant to heating. It is destroyed if heated to above 100°C in the acid medium.

Biological Active Forms

- Active "coenzyme" form of the vitamin is the reduced tetra-hydroderivative. ***"Tetrahydrofolate"*-F.H$_4$**, obtained by addition of four hydrogens to the pteridine moiety at 5,6,7 and 8 position.
- Structure of tetrahydrofolate is shown below:

5,6,7,8,—Tetrahydrofolate (F.H$_4$)

- Because of their lability, these occur naturally only in small quantities, being present mainly in the form of N^5-formyl or N^5-methyl derivatives.

Formation of F.H$_4$ Folic acid, before functioning as a coenzyme, must be reduced first to 7, 8-dihydrofolic acid ***(F.H$_2$)*** and then to 5,6,7,8 tetrahydrofolate ***(F.H$_4$).***

- Both the reactions are catalyzed by ***folic acid reductases enzyme,*** which use NADPH as hydrogen donor. It also requires vitamin C (ascorbic acid) as cofactor.

The steps of the reactions are as follows:

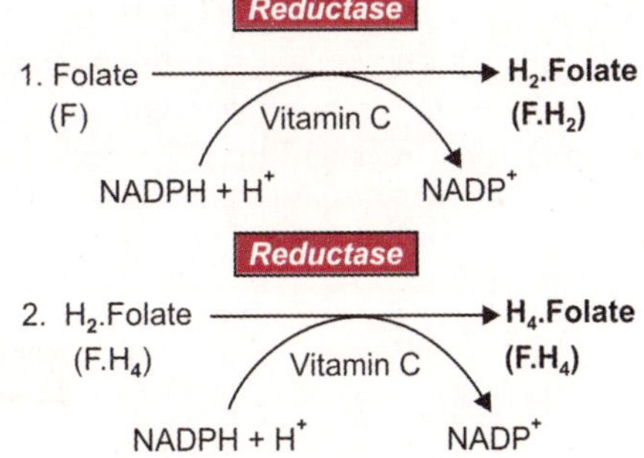

Clinical Importance

Some of clinically described cases of folic acid deficiency anaemias may actually be due to inherited deficiency of *Folic acid reductase.*

Folinic Acid

- This is one of the active forms of folic acid-a **"formyl" derivative.** It is reduced tetrahydrofolate ($F.H_4$) with a "formyl" group on position 5 ($f^5.F.H_4$). Folic acid when added to liver slices is converted to the "formyl" derivative in presence of NADPH. Ascorbic acid enhances the activity of the liver in this reaction.
- This form of folic acid was first discovered in liver extracts when it was found to supply an essential growth factor for a *Lactobacillus* called *Leuconostoc citrovorum* and it was termed as ***"citrovorum factor"*** and when its chemical structure was determined the name ***"folinic acid"*** was applied.
- Structure of folinic acid is similar to folic acid, ***except***
  - It is the reduced tetrahydroform ($F.H_4$) and
  - With a "formyl group" at position-5. It is also called as ***leucovorin*** earlier and a similar synthetic form "Folinic acid-SF" (synthetic factor) has same structure and function.

Conversion of f^5 to f^{10}:

- The f^5 can be converted to f^{10} by the action of an enzyme system ***formyltetrahydrofolate isomerase*** in presence of ATP, first $f^{5\text{-}10}$ FH_4 is formed, which by the action of ***cyclohydrase*** is converted to $f^{10}\cdot FH_4$ (see box below).
- This is also present in a variety of natural materials, e.g. pigeon liver, many bacteria, an enzyme *formyl tetrahydrofolate synthetase,* catalyzes the direct addition of "formate" (H-COOH) to $F.H_4$. The enzyme is specific for formate.

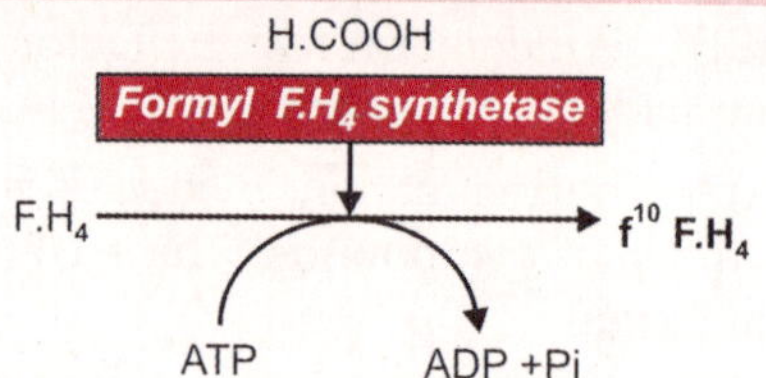

Formation of N^5-methyl $F.H_4$ form $f^{5\text{-}10}$ $F.H_4$: $f^{5\text{-}10}$ FH_4 can be converted to N^5-methyl $F.H_4$ by an NAD^+***-dependant reductase*** and this—CH_3 group is then transferable to "De-oxyadenosyl B_{12}" (Cobamide coenzyme) to form methyl-B_{12}, an important donor of $-CH_3$ group as occurs in methylation of homocysteine to form methionine.

Biosynthesis and Metabolism

- Many microorganisms including those inhabiting the intestinal tract can synthesize folic acid.

Effect of drugs: Sulphonamide drugs and antibiotics inhibit their growth by blocking the incorporation of PABA in the synthetic pathway (by competitive inhibition).

- Higher animals including human beings cannot synthesize folic acid and it has to be supplied in diet.
- In human beings, intestinal bacteria can synthesize and is a good source.

Absorption: Folic acid absorption occurs along the whole length of mucosa of small intestine. Polyglutamates ingested in diet are converted to monoglutamates and dihydrofolates are reduced to tetrahydrofolates by *folate reductase.* Tetrahydrofolates are then converted to methyl tetrahydrofolates which enter the portal blood and then carried to liver.

Transport: Transported in blood as methyl tetrahydrofolate bound to a specific protein.

Conversion of f^5 to f^{10}

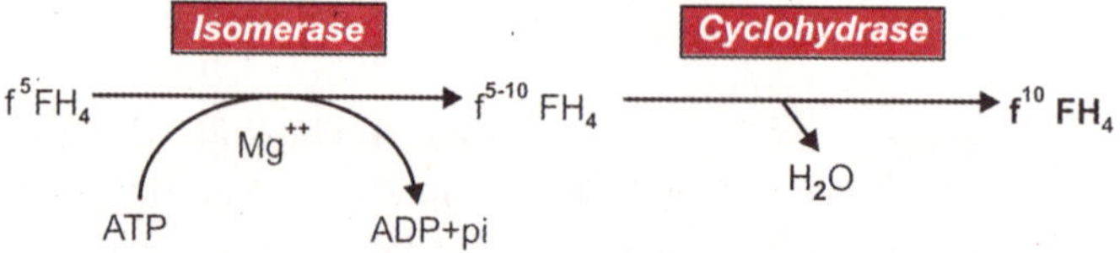

Plasma level: In normal individuals, it varies from 3 to 21 ng/ml.

Excretion:

- *Urine:* 2 to 5 μg/day. This is much increased after an oral dose of folate if the tissues are saturated.
- *Faeces:* 20% of the ingested folates that remains unabsorbed + 60 to 90 μg in the bile that is not reabsorbed + some unabsorbed synthesis of folate by bacterial flora of intestine.

Tissue folate: About 70 mg in the whole body, of which about 1/3 (5 to 15 μg) is in the liver.

RB cells folate: Folate is incorporated into the RB cells during erythropoiesis, and is retained there during their entire life span except for only a slight fall in concentration. ***Red cell folate is a reliable indicator of the folate status of the body.*** Average level is 300 ng/ml of whole blood on a PCV of 45% (range 160-640 ng/ml)

Occurrence and Food Sources: Folates are widely distributed in nature being present in many animal and plant tissues and in microorganisms. These are particularly abundant in liver, yeast, kidney and green leafy vegetables. ***Spinach and cauliflower are also good sources.*** Other good sources are meat, fish, wheat. Fair sources are milk and fruits.

Metabolism Role ("One-carbon" Metabolism)

- The folic acid coenzymes are specifically concerned with metabolic reactions involving the transfer and utilization of the one carbon moiety (C_1).
- ***"One carbon moiety"*** (C_1) may be either methyl (—CH_3), formyl (—CHO), formate (H.COOH), "formimino" group (—CH = NH) or hydroxymethyl (—CH_2OH).
- Most of them are metabolically "interconvertible" and catalyzed by an NADP-dependant ***hydroxymethyl dehydrogenases*** (see ahead in the box).
- As discussed above, folinic acid is 5-formyl F.H_4 (f^{5-10} FH_4). However except for the formylation of glutamic acid in the course of the metabolic degradation of histidine, the f^5 compound is metabolically inert.
- On the other hand, the f^{10} tetrahydrofolate (f^{10} FH_4) or f^{5-10}. FH_4 are the active forms of the folic acid coenzymes in metabolism.

Table 9.4 provides a comparative study of C_1-moiety (donors) and C_1-moiety (acceptors).

Clinical significance—Folic acid (antagonists): Several antagonists to this vitamin have been found out. They are of much clinical interest,

Table 9.4: Comparison of C_1-moiety (Donors) and C_1-moiety (Acceptors)

C_1-moiety (Donors)	*C_1-moiety (Acceptors)*
• Formimino group (—CH =NH) of formimino glutamic acid (formed from Histidine)	• Positions 2 and 8 of purine ring
• Methyl group (—CH_3) of methionine, choline, betaine and thymine. All of which are oxidized to hydroxymethyl	• N-formly methionine of t-RNA (given by f^{10} FH_4)
• (—CH_2OH) group are carried as such on f^{5-10} FH_4. The hydroxymethyl group is then oxidized in an NADP-dependant reaction to a 'formyl' group. h^{5-10} FH_4 → f^{5-10} FH_4 (NADP⁺ → NADPH + H⁺)	• Glycine→to serine conversion; formation of β-carbon of serine
• β-carbon of serine as a hydroxymethyl group may contribute single carbon moiety.	• Homocysteine→ to form methionine
	• Uracil → to form thymine
	• Ethanolamine → to form choline
	• Histidine synthesis

Interconversion of One-carbon Moiety

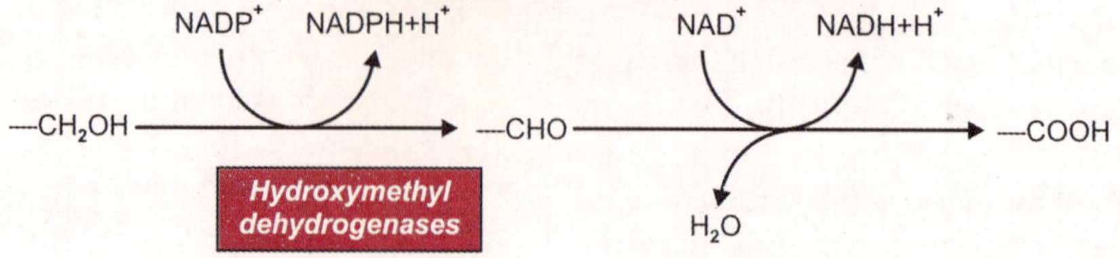

NADP$^+$ → NADPH+H$^+$; NAD$^+$ → NADH+H$^+$

—CH_2OH → (Hydroxymethyl dehydrogenases) → —CHO → —COOH (+ H_2O)

- On account of their ability to inhibit cell division and multiplication.
- Thus, they have been used in the treatment of conditions where there is unrestricted cell growth, e.g.
  - *In leukaemias,*
  - *In erythraemias, and*
  - *In malignant growths.*

Two folic acid antagonists are important:

- *Aminopterin:* NH_2 group is substituted for the -OH group in position 4 of the pteridine nucleus. Chemically, it is 4-aminofolate. It has maximal inhibitory action.
- *Amethopterin or methotrexate:* It is 4-amino 10 methyl folate. In animals, the inhibitory effect of aminopterin and amethopterin cannot be reversed by folic acid, but only by folinic acid. This suggests that the amino pterin interferes with the formation of folinic acid from folic acid or with the utilization of formyl group.

Recent work suggests that the interference of the antimetabolites occur in the reduction of folic acid to the tetrahydroderivatives. In tissue cultures, it has been found that both aminopterin and amethopterin block the synthesis of nucleic acids, presumably by preventing the reduction of folic acid to the tetrahydroderivative and thus prevents the transport of the "formyl" carbon into the purine rings, such inhibited cells fail to complete their mitoses.

Deficiency Manifestations: Deficiencies have been produced and studied in experimental animals as well as in human volunteers.

- *In experimental animals, deficiency produced most readily in two ways:*
  - By feeding sulphonamides and broad spectrum antibiotics for prolonged periods-to inhibit growth of intestinal bacteria.
  - By administration of folic acid antagonists
- Outstanding features is abnormalities of blood formation. Other manifestations include growth retardation, weakness, lethargy, reproduction difficulties (infertility in females) and inadequate lactation.
- Produces a *Macrocytic type of anaemia.*
- *Bone marrow shows:* arrested development of all elements erythroid, myeloid and thrombocytes. Megaloblasts and myeloblasts accumulate at the expense of more mature cells, viz. erythroblasts, normoblasts and myeloblastes. The number of megakaryocytes decreases.
- *The peripheral blood picture:* Reflects these production defects, being characterized by one or more of the following, depending mainly on the degree of deficiency.
  - A *macrocytic type of anaemia* at times with normoblasts, erythroblasts, and megloblasts.
  - Granulocytopenia, occasionally with myelocytes, and
  - Thrombocytopenia

On the basis, chiefly of prompt response to specific replacement therapy, the following clinical conditions have been attributed to folic acid deficiency:

- *Nutritional macrocytic anaemia* (cause dietary deficiency of folic acid).

- *Megaloblastic anaemia of infancy* (also mainly due to dietary deficiency).
- ***A congenital (irherited) type*** may be due to *reductase* deficiency: 'familial" type.
- ***Megaloblastic anaemia of pregnancy:*** mechanism not clear, may be due to relative deficiency.
- ***Macrocytic anarmia in liver diseases*** (may be due to inadequate storage/conversion).
- ***Megaloblastic anaemia*** in caeliac disease and sprue (inadequate absorption). In this there may be B_{12} deficiency also ***associated with neurological manifestations.***
- ***Macrocytic anaemia after extensive intestinal resection*** (inadequate absorption)

Figlu test-to detect folate deficiency:

- In the metabolism of the amino acid histidine there is folic acid dependent step at the point where formimino-glutamic acid ("Figlu")is converted to glutamic acid (GA).

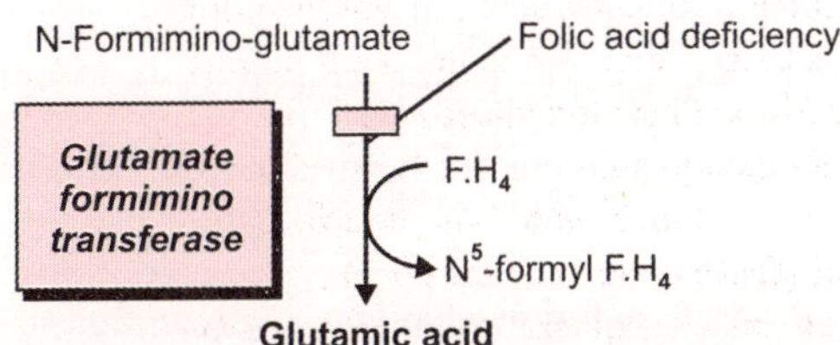

- In folic acid deficient patients, this reaction cannot be carried out, as a result, 'figlu' accumulates in the blood and excreted in urine. ***Figlu excretion in urine is an index of folic acid deficiency.***
- When a "loading dose" of histidine is given, the excretion of 'Figlu' in urine is increased further (***Histidine loading test***).

Daily Requirement: The exact requirement is difficult to ascertain due to two reasons.

- Available in nature-ubiquitous.
- Most of human need is supplied by bacterial synthesis in intestine.

Recommended dietary daily allowance:

- Adult 400 to 500 μg daily
- Infants—50 μg
- Children—100 to 300 μg

Requirement increases in pregnancy and lactation

- Pregnant women—800 μg
- Lactating women—600 μg

VITAMIN B_{12} (CYANOCOBALAMINE)

Synonyms: Anti-pernicious anemia factor, extrinsic factor of castle, animal protein factor

Chemistry: The central portion of the molecule consists of four reduced and extensively substituted ***"pyrrole rings"***, surrounding a single cobalt atom (Co). This central structure is called as ***"Corrin ring" system"***. The system is similar to porphyrins, but differs in that ***two of pyrrole rings, rings I and IV are joined directly.***

- Below the corrin ring system, is **DBI ring**—5, 6-dimethyl benzimidazole riboside which is connected
  - At one end to central cobalt atom, and
  - At the other from the riboside moiety to the ring IV of corrin ring system.
- One PO_4 group connects ribose moiety to **"aminopropanol"** (esterified), which in turn is attached to propionic acid side chain of ring IV.
- A **cyanide group** is coordinately bound to the cobalt atom and then it is known as cyanocobalamine.

Varieties of Vitamin B_{12}

- ***When cyanide is bound to cobalt atom it is called "cyanocobalamine"***, but if cyanide group is removed, then it is called "cobalamine". Cyanocobalamine is identical with originally isolated vitamin B_{12}.
  B_{12} which occurs in natural materials does not contain cyanide group. In the original isolation, cyanide group was added only to promote crystallization.
- —OH group, NO_2, Cl^- and SO_4^{2} may replace cyanide group in which case, it is called respectively as:
  - ***hydroxycobalamine ($B_{12}a$) (hydroxocobalamine)***
  - ***nitrito-cobalamine ($B_{12}c$)***
  - ***chlorocobalamine***
  - ***sulphato-cobalamine, in that order.***

- Biologic actions of these derivatives are similar to cobalamine, but ***Hydroxocobalamine ($B_{12}a$) is superior as,***
  - It is more active in enzyme systems
  - It is retained longer in the body when given orally.

Hence, $B_{12}a$ is more useful for therapeutic administration of B_{12} by mouth.

Metabolism—Absorption and Excretion

- Vitamin B_{12} is **"extrinsic factor"** of Castle
- Vitamin B_{12} is absorbed from ileum, for its proper absorption it requires:
  - Presence of HCl, and
  - **"Intrinsic factor" (IF) of Castle:** a constituent of normal gastric juice.

Intrinsic Factor (IF)

- It is secreted by parietal cells found in *"Cardiac"* end and *fundus of stomach,* but not in the pylorus.
- It is a *"glycoprotein"*, a constituent of gastric mucoproteins. In addition to amino acids, it contains hexoses, hexosamines and sialic acid.
- It is *non-dialyzable* and *thermolabile,* destroyed by heating at 70° to 80°C for ½ hour.

Note:

- ***Atrophy of fundus of stomach and a lack of free HCl (achlorhydria) is usually associated with pernicious anaemia, caused by B_{12} deficiency.***

Mechanism of Absorption *(see Fig.9.4)*

Recently, it has been shown that *two binding proteins* are required for absorption of Vit B_{12}. They are:

- **Cobalophilin:** a binding protein secreted in the saliva.
- **Intrinsic factor (IF),** a glycoprotein secreted by parietal cells of gastric mucosa.
- Gastric acid (HCl) and pepsin release the Vit B_{12} from protein binding in food and make it available to bind to salivary protein, cobalophilin.

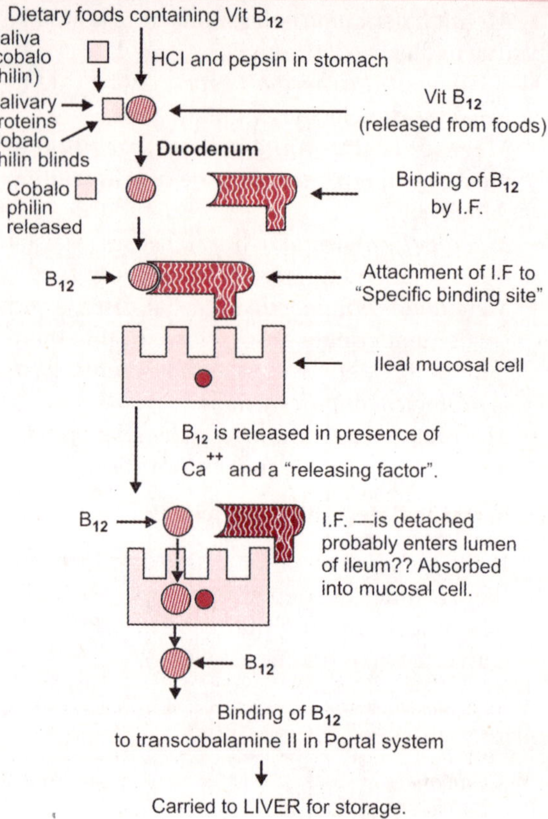

Fig. 9.4: Showing mechanism of absorption of vitamin B_{12}

- In the duodenum, cobalophilin is hydrolyzed, releasing the vitamin for binding to "Intrinsic factor" (IF).

Clinical Aspect

In pancreatic insufficiency, the ***"cobalophilin-bound vitamin B_{12}"*** may not be split and the complex is excreted in faeces resulting to development of vitamin B_{12} deficiency.

- Vitamin B_{12} is absorbed from the distal third of the ileum via **"specific binding site" (receptors)** that binds the "B_{12}-IF complex". The removal of B_{12} from 'intrinsic factor' (IF) in presence of Ca^{++} ions and a ***"releasing factor"*** (RF) secreted by duodenum take place and B_{12} enters the ileal mucosal cells for absorption into the circulation. If ileal absorptive mechanism is functioning, it can adequately transport 0.5 to 10.0 μg of B_{12}. It is also shown that a small amount, about 1 to 3% may be absorbed by "simple diffusion".

Transport in the Blood: Vitamin B_{12} is transported in blood in association with specific proteins named (***transcobalamine*** I and ***transcobalamine II and III***). Physiologically transcobalamine II is more important. Transcobalamines have α_2 to β mobility.

Normal Serum Level of B_{12}: Normal serum level varies from 0.008 to 0.42 μg/dl. Average = 0.02 μg/dl.

Excretion: Normally there is practically no urinary excretion. But following parenteral administration there is urinary excretion up to 0.3 μg/day.

Transcobalamine I	*Transcobalamine II*
• Source-probably leucocytes. Increased in myeloproliferative states.	• Source is liver
• Plasma level = 60 μg/L	• Plasma level = 20 μg/L

Storage: Main storage site is liver. A man on normal non-vegetarian diet may store several mg. (=4 mg). ***As storage is high, development of deficiency state takes long time.***

Biological "Active" Forms of B_{12}

- Biologically active forms are ***cobamide coenzymes***—acts as coenzyme with various enzymes.
- Cobamide coenzyme do not contain the "cyano" group attached to cobalt but instead there is an ***"adenine nucleoside" (5′-deoxyadenosine) which is linked to cobalt by a C–CO bond (Fig. 9.5).*** 5′-adenosyl moiety is derived from ATP, which after donating the "adenosyl" group, releases all three PO_4 groups as inorganic "tripolyphosphates".
- ***In formation of "adenosyl coenzyme" cobalt undergoes successive reduction in a series of steps catalyzed*** by the enzyme *B_{12a} reductase* which requires NADH and FAD. B_{12} (CO^+) reacts with ATP to form "adenosyl coenzyme".

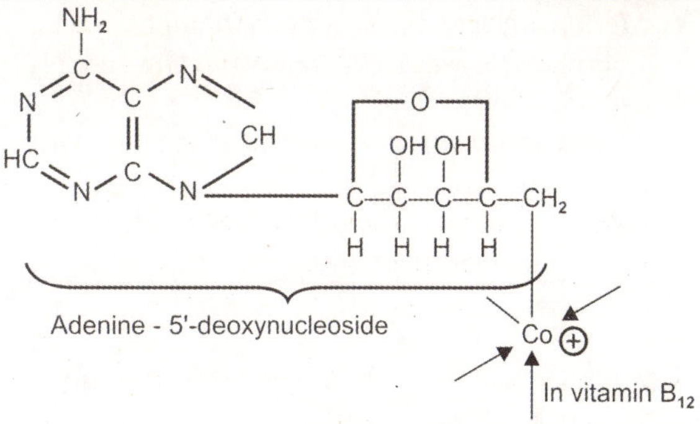

Fig. 9.5: Attachment of adenosyl moiety to vitamin B_{12} through 5′C to cobalt in the cobamide coenzymes

B_{12a} — Red coloured (Co^{+++})
B_{12r} — Orange (Co^{++})
B_{12s} — Grey-green (Co^{+})

Varieties of cobamide coenzymes: At least **four varieties** have been isolated:

- **DBC:** Contains 5,6-dimethyl benzimidazole (called dimethyl-benzimidazole cobamide)
- **BC:** Benzimidazole cobamide; this contains an unsubstituted methyl free benzimidazole
- **AC:** Adenyl cobamide, which contains an adenyl group.
- **MC:** Methyl cobamide. CH_3 group is attached to cobalt atom rather than adenosyl moiety. These coenzymes do not contain the cyanide group and hence called as ***"Corrinoid coenzymes".***

Metabolic Role of Cobamide Coenzymes

- ***Methyl malonyl CoA to succinyl CoA conversion:*** Vitamin B_{12} is required as a coenzyme for the conversion of L-methyl malonyl CoA to succinyl CoA. The reaction is catalyzed by the enzyme ***isomerase***.

$$\text{L-Methyl malonyl CoA} \xrightarrow{B_{12}} \text{Succinyl-CoA}$$

Isomerase

Normal healthy individual excretes less then 2 mg/day which is not detectable. In **B_{12} deficiency,** methyl malonic acid accumulates and excretion of methyl malonic acid in urine is increased. ***Methyl malonic aciduria is a sensitive index for B_{12} deficiency***

- ***Methylation of homocysteine to methionine:*** This requires tetrahydrofolate ($F.H_4$) as a-CH_3 carrier.
- ***Methylation of pyrimidine ring:*** to form thymine.
- ***Conversion of ribonucleotides to deoxyribonucleotides:*** It is of importance in DNA synthesis.

$$\text{Ribonucleotides} \xrightarrow{B_{12}} \text{Deoxy-ribonucleotides}$$

Reductase

- Cobamide coenzymes play an essential role as a "H-transferring agent".
- ***Required for metabolism of 'Diols':***

$$\begin{matrix} CH_2OH \\ | \\ CH_2OH \end{matrix} \xrightarrow{B_{12}} \underset{\text{Acetaldehyde}}{CH_3.CHO} + H_2O$$

Ethylene glycol

- ***In bacteria:*** Interconversion of glutamate and β-methyl aspartate.

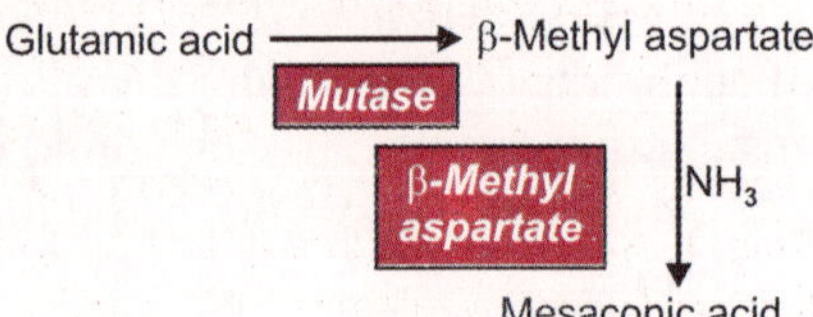

Folate Trap ***(Methyl Trap Hypothesis):***

- B_{12} is necessary as coenzyme for conversion of N^5–methyl $F.H_4$ to form methyl–B_{12} which is required for conversion of homocysteine to methionine.

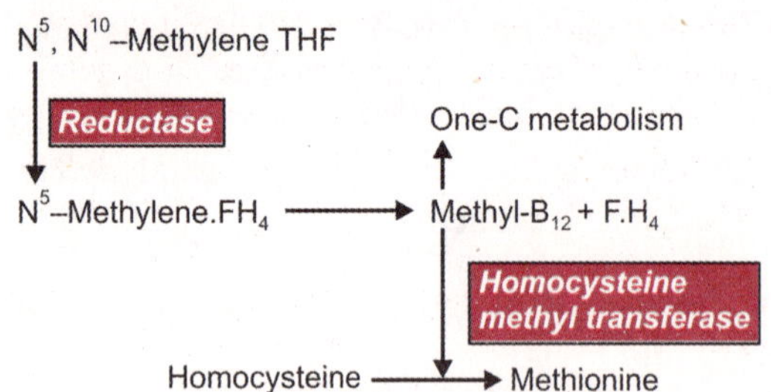

- **In B_{12} deficiency,** the above reactions cannot take place and folate is permanently trapped as N^5–methyl. FH_4 and is therefore not available for C_1-transfer. It is called as ***"folate trap"***. This results in diminished synthesis of thymidylate and DNA. Increased folate levels are observed in plasma and the activity of the enzyme ***"homocysteine methyl transferase"*** is low.

DEFICIENCY MANIFESTATIONS

1. ***Adult pernicious anaemia:*** Produces **macrocytic megaloblastic anaemia.** ***In addition to haematological manifestation, it is combined with neurological features (subacute combined degeneration of the cord).*** It is an **autoimmune disease:** ***Antibodies to IF and parietal cells found.***

In addition to haematological changes, the following changes are seen.

- Mucosal atrophy of stomach and inflammation of tongue ***glossitis,*** inflammation of mouth (***stomatitis***)***,*** and pharynx ***pharyngitis***
- Absence of HCl ***achlorhydria***
- Degenerative changes of posterior and lateral columns of the spinal cord, resulting in peripheral sensory disturbances, hyperactive reflexes, ataxia, paralysis.
  Cause: Increased concentration of methyl malonic acid, which competes with malonyl CoA leading to impairment of FA synthesis.

Haematological changes: Peripheral blood picture is:

- ***Macrocytic type of anaemia with megaloblasts,*** erythroblasts, and normoblasts
- Granulocytopenia with occasional myelocytes
- Thrombocytopenia
- Reduction in RB cells count and Hb content.

Other Biochemical Changes are:

- Serum B_{12} level is decreased
- Urinary B_{12} level is decreased
- Rise in faecal B_{12} excretion
- ***"Schilling test"*** shows decrease in labelled B_{12} absorption
- Urinary excretion of methyl malonic acid is increased
- Autoantibodies to IF (intrinsic factor) and parietal cells (canalicular lipoproteins).

Bone Marrow

- Shows evidences of arrested development of all elements: Erythroid, myeloid and thrombocytes.
- Megaloblasts and myeloblasts accumulate at the expense of more mature cells, viz. erythroblasts, normoblasts and myelocytes.
- Number of megakaryocytes decrease.

DNA synthesis: In pernicious anaemia, DNA synthesis in maturing red blood cells is depressed, due to

- Failure in conversion of ribonucleotides to deoxyribonucleotides, and
- Partly owing to the failure in forming the thymidylic acid by the methylation of deoxyuridylic acid.

The fall in DNA synthesis results in prolongation of resting phases between successive mitoses of maturing RB cells as also a rise in the RNA levels in those cells so that ***the resulting macrocytic RB cells have a much higher RNA:DNA ratio than the normal RB cells.*** The lengthening of resting phase may be the ultimate reason for the formation of megaloblasts in pernicious anaemia.

2. *Congenital pernicious anaemia:*
   - Occurs in postnatal period, before 2 ½ years of age.
   - Due to lack of intrinsic factor (IF).
   - It is not accompanied by gastric acid secretion/or abnormalities of gastric mucosa.
3. *Juvenile pernicious anaemia:*
   - Failure to secrete intrinsic factor (IF).
   - Associated achlorhydria and atrophic gastritis.
   - Antibodies to IF/and/or parietal cells have been demonstrated ("autoimmune" in nature).
4. *Following surgical operations:* Pernicious anaemia may occur in following:
   - Total gastrectomy
   - Extensive resections of small intestine.
5. *Tapeworm infection of GI tract:* A megaloblastic anaemia, responsive to vitamin B_{12} therapy occurs with infestation with **"Fish tape worm"**- ***Diphyllobothrium latum,*** which eats up unusually large amounts of vitamin B_{12} from the gut, creating B_{12} deficiency to the host.

Methyl malonic aciduria: This is of **two types:**

1. ***Due to vitamin B_{12} deficiency:*** Vitamin B_{12} is required as a coenzymes for *"isomerase"* which converts methyl malonyl CoA to succinyl CoA. In ***vitamin B_{12} deficiency,*** this conversion cannot take place, as a result methyl malonic acid ↑ accumulates in blood and tissues and excreted in urine. Excretion of methyl malonic acid in urine is a sensitive index for vitamin B_{12} deficiency.
2. ***Inherited deificiency of the enzyme isomerase:*** In this vitamin B_{12} deficiency is not there. It is observed as inherited disorders in infants and young children, with severe metabolic acidosis.

Occurrence and Sources of Vitamin B_{12}: ***It is present in foods of animal origin only*** and is ***not present in foods of vegetables sources.*** In nature, it is obtained via synthesis by bacteria in soil, water, and animal intestine.

- ***Good and rich animal sources are:*** liver, eggs, fish, meat, kidney. ***Fair sources*** are: milk, and dairy products

  Note: Those people who are purely vegetarians should take enough milk/and milk products and one egg twice a week so that they do not develop B_{12} deficiency in long run.

Daily Requirements

- In normal adults: 3 µg/day
- Infants: 0.3 µg/day
- Children: 1 to 2 µg/day
- In pregnancy and lactation: requirement is increased approx 4 µg/day.
- In pernicious anaemia, 0.5 to 1.0 µgm/day given parenterally will maintain in complete haematologic and neurologic remissions.

☞ SALIENT POINTS TO REMEMBER

- Water soluble vitamins are: (i) Vitamin B-complex group and (ii) Vitamin C.
- Thiamine or vitamin B_1 contains sulphur in its molecule. Biological active form is TPP which acts as a coenzyme.

- Two important reactions in which TPP acts as coenzyme are: (i) Oxidative decarboxylation of pyruvic acid (P-A) and α-Oxoglutarate and (ii) Transketolation reaction in HMP shunt.
- Deficiency of vit B_1 produces a disease called beri-beri, which can be wet type or dry type.
- Coenzymes of riboflavin, vit B_2 (FAD and FMN) and niacin (NAD^+ and $NADP^+$) take part in dehydrogenase reactions.
- Riboflavin deficiency does not produce a disease entity but manifests as cheilosis, redness of lips, glossitis, seborrhoeic dermatitis, etc.
- Niacin deficiency produces a disease called as Pellagra manifested as 3 D's—Dermatitis, Diarrhoea and Dementia.
- Niacin is one of the vitamins which can be synthesized in the body from the amino acid L-tryptophan.
- ***60 mg of tryptophan can give rise to 1 mg of niacin in the body.***
- Maize protein "Zein" lacks the amino acid tryptophan. Hence ***pellagra is more common in persons whose staple diet is maize.***
- Pyridoxal-P and pyridoxamine-P are the biological active forms of vitamin B_6 (Pyridoxine). They act as coenzyme in various amino acid metabolism viz., in transamination, transulfuration, decarboxylation, deamination and condensation reactions.
- Prolonged therapy of Isonicotinic acid hydrazide (INH) in treatment of Tuberculosis can cause B_6 deficiency.
- Biotin participates as coenzyme in "CO_2 - fixation reactions", e.g. conversion of acetyl CoA to malonyl-CoA, conversion of propionyl CoA to methyl malonyl CoA, conversion of pyruvic acid to oxaloacetate, etc.
- High consumption of raw eggs which contain anti-vitamin **'avidin'** may lead to biotin deficiency.
- Biological active form of pantothenic acid is coenzyme A which is involved in formation of "active acetate" (acetyl CoA) and "active succinate" (Succinyl CoA).
- Biological active form of folic acid is tetrahydrofolate ($F.H_4$). **It participates in the transfer of "one carbon moiety" (methyl, formyl, formimino group, formic acid, etc.) in amino acid and nucleotide metabolism.**
- Deficiency of folic acid produces megaloblastic anaemia, in which there is no neurological involvement.
- ***"FIGLU" excretion in urine is an index of folic acid deficiency.***
- Folic acid antagonists are aminopterin, amethopterin (methotrexate)—used in treatment of leukaemias and other malignancies.
- Vitamin B_{12} is called as cyanocobalamine. It is called as "extrinsic factor of Castle".
- B_{12} is absorbed from ileum. For its proper absorption it requires: (i) presence of HCl and (ii) "Intrinsic factor" of Castle (IF), a glycoprotein secreted by parietal cells of stomach.
- Biological active forms of B_{12} are "cobamide coenzymes". B_{12} is required for conversion of L-methyl malonyl CoA to succinyl CoA.
- Absence of B_{12} coenzyme produces the condition called methyl malonic aciduria.
- ***Increased excretion of methyl malonic acid (methyl malonic aciduria) is a sensitive index for B_{12} deficiency.***
- B_{12} deficiency produces the disease called pernicious anaemia (Megaloblastic anaemia + subacute combined degeneration of the cord).
- Diphyllobothrium latum (fish tapeworm) infection of the gut produces B_{12} deficiency as the worm eats up B_{12} in the gut.
- A combined therapy of B_{12} and folic acid is commonly employed to treat megaloblastic anaemias.
- Ascorbic acid (vit C) is another water soluble vitamin. It ***must be supplied in the diet as it cannot be synthesized in the body.***
- Various citrous fruits are good source of vitamin C. ***Amla is very rich source of vit C.***
- Vit C takes part in cellular oxidation - reduction, hydroxylation of proline and lysine in collagen synthesis, in absorption of Fe, as

coenzyme required in tyrosine and tryptophan metabolism, formation of active $F.H_4$, etc.

- Vitamin C deficiency produces a disease called "*Scurvy*" in which ***collagen is grossly affected.***
- Prolonged administration of oral antibiotics destroys the bacterial flora of the gut hence vitamin synthesis stops. Supplementation of vitamins is necessary during prolonged oral antibiotic therapy.

MULTIPLE CHOICE QUESTIONS

Give one correct answer:

1. **Which of the following vitamin is associated with synthesis of coagulation factor prothrombin?**
(a) Vitamin A (b) Vitamin C
(c) Vitamin D (d) Vitamin E
(e) Vitamin K

2. **Retinal is reduced to retinol by the enzyme retinene reductase in presence of which coenzyme?**
(a) NAD^+ (b) $NADH^+ H^+$
(c) $NADP^+$ (d) $NADPH + H^+$
(e) FAD

3. **Increased carbohydrate consumption increases the dietary requirement for**
(a) Thiamine (b) Riboflavine
(c) Niacin (d) Pyridoxine
(e) Biotin

4. **Deficiency of vitamin K can occur in the following conditions *except:***
(a) Obstructive jaundice
(b) After gastrectomy
(c) Malabsorption syndrome
(d) Prolonged antibiotic therapy
(e) Administration of dicoumarol

5. **Vitamin K_2 was originally isolated from:**
(a) Soyabean (b) Alfalfa
(c) Putrid fish meal (d) Wheat germs
(e) Oysters

6. **Which coenzyme is not involved in oxidative decarboxylation of pyruvic acid?**
(a) CoA - SH (b) Pyridoxal-P
(c) Mg^{++} (d) Lipoic acid
(e) TPP

7. **The disease pellagra is due to the deficiency of**
(a) Niacin (b) Pantothenic acid
(c) Thiamine (d) Pyridoxine
(e) Riboflavine

8. **The antiegg-white injury factor is:**
(a) Avidin (b) Biotin
(c) Choline (d) Lipoic acid
(e) Folic acid

9. **'Chastek paralysis' described in foxes is due to eating of:**
(a) Leguminous plants
(b) Ferns
(c) Raw Polar Bear's liver
(d) Raw fish (e) Soybeans

10. **Xanthurenic acid is excreted in urine in the deficiency of:**
(a) Pyridoxal-P (b) Niacin
(c) Thiamine (d) Pantothenic acid
(e) Vitamin B_{12}

11. **Which of the following vitamin would most likely become deficient whose staple diet is maize?**
(a) Thiamine (b) Riboflavine
(c) Niacin (d) Lipoic acid
(e) Ascorbic acid

12. **Biotin is involved in which of the following types of reactions?**
(a) Carboxylation (b) Decarboxylation
(c) Deamination (d) Oxidation
(e) Hydroxylation

13. **A biochemical indication of vitamin B_{12} deficiency can be obtained by measuring the urinary excretion of:**
(a) Pyruvic acid (b) Lactic acid
(c) Malic acid (d) Methyl malonic acid
(e) Urocanic acid

14. **Increased protein intake is accompanied by an increased dietary requirement for**
(a) Thiamine (b) Niacin
(c) Riboflavine (d) Pyridoxine
(e) Cyanocobalamine

15. Which of the following coenzyme is involved in the formation of hydroxy proline during collagen synthesis?
(a) TPP (b) FAD
(c) Biotin (d) Vitamin C
(e) Cyanocobalamine

16. Pyridoxal-P is a coenzyme for which of the following enzymatic reaction?
(a) Deamination (b) Decarboxylation
(c) CO_2-fixation (d) Dehydrogenation
(e) Transmethylation

ANSWERS

1. (e)	2. (b)	3. (a)
4. (b)	5. (c)	6. (b)
7. (a)	8. (b)	9. (d)
10. (a)	11. (c)	12. (a)
13. (d)	14. (c)	15. (d)
16. (b)		

10 Chemistry of Haemoglobin

HAEMOGLOBIN

INTRODUCTION

- The red colouring matter of the blood is a conjugated protein, haemoglobin, a chromoprotein, containing *heme* as prosthetic group and *globin* as the protein part-apoprotein. ***Heme-containing proteins are characteristic of the aerobic organisms,*** and are altogether absent in anaerobic forms of life.
- The normal concentration of Hb in an adult male varies from 14.0 to 16.0 gm percent, and there are about 750 gm of Hb in the total circulating blood of 70 kg man. ***Approximately 6.25 gm (90 mg/kg) of Hb are produced and destroyed in the body each day.***
- The structure of *heme* remains the same in Hb from animal source, the ***basic protein globin varies from species to species*** in its amino acid composition and sequence and thus responsible for the ***species-specificity.***

BIOMEDICAL IMPORTANCE

- Hb is important in O_2-binding and its transport and delivery to tissues which is required for metabolism.
- Part of CO_2, a waste-product of metabolism, is also carried by the globin part of Hb.
- *2,3 biphosphoglycerate (BPG)* produced in RB cells by Rappoport-Leubering shunt is necessary for stabilization of Hb-conformation at quarternary level by holding salt bridges and is important for understanding of high-altitude sickness and changes that take place in adaptation at high altitudes.
- Cyanide poisoning and carbon-monoxide poisoning are fatal because they combine and inhibit heme-protein ***cytochrome oxidase*** in electron transport chain, and stops cellular respiration.
- ***Conversion of Hb to methaemoglobin by $NaNO_2$/or sodium thiosulfate forms the basis of treatment of cyanide poisoning,*** as cyanide combines readily with methaemoglobin to form cyanmethaemoglobin which is not toxic, and thus spares the cytochrome oxidase.
- Study of Hb chemistry provides an insight into the molecular basis of genetic diseases such as haemoglobinopathies and abnormal haemoglobins.

STRUCTURE OF Hb

The structure of Hb molecule has been extensively studied. It can be discussed ***under two headings:***

- ***Structure of heme the prosthetic group, and***
- ***Structure of globin, the protein part-apoprotein.***

1. Heme: It is a **Fe-porphyrin compound.** The porphyrins are complex compounds with a ***tetrapyrrole structure***, each pyrrole ring having the following structure.

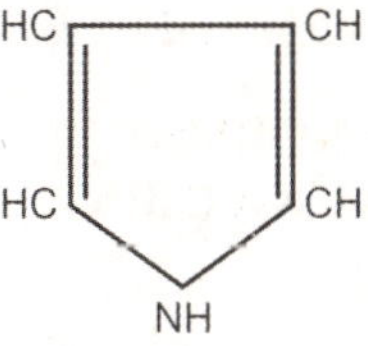

Pyrrole ring

- Four such pyrroles called I to IV, are combined through –CH= bridges, called as ***methyne or methylidene*** bridges to form a porphyrin nucleus.
- ***Fe is in the centre of four pyrrole and is in Fe⁺⁺ (ous) state.*** The Fe, besides its linkages to four nitrogens of the pyrrole rings, is also linked internally (5th linkage) to the nitrogen of the imidazole ring of histidine (His) of the polypeptide chains ***(hemelinked group).*** The sixth valence is directed outwards from the molecule and is linked to a molecule of H_2O in de-oxygenated Hb.
- When Hb is oxygenated, the H_2O is displaced by O_2.

$$Hb.\ H_2O + O_2 \rightleftharpoons Hb.O_2 + H_2O$$

- If the central Fe is oxidized and converted to Fe(ic) state (Fe^{+++}), ***it will carry a surplus +ve charge*** which is balanced by taking an-OH group from the medium.

2. Globin (Protein Part): It is ***composed of four polypeptide chains, two identical α-chains and two identical β-chains,*** in normal adult Hb, arranged in the configuration of a ***"tetrahedron"***. Thus there are six edges of contact.

Polypeptide Chains: Each polypeptide chain contains a "heme" in the so-called "heme-pocket". ***Thus, one Hb molecule contains four heme units.*** In other normal haemoglobins, in place of two β chains are replaced by either two δ-chains, or two γ-chains, or two ε-chains, forming different types.

FORMATION OF "HEME-POCKETS"

- Each subunit contains one "heme" moiety hidden within the subunit.
- The heme pockets of α-subunits are of size just adequate for entry of O_2 molecule, ***but the entery of O_2 into the heme-pockets of the β-subunits is blocked by a valine residue.***

VARIETIES OF NORMAL HUMAN HAEMOGLOBIN

Normal human Hb is of several types, containing four subunits made up of various combination of possibly five different yet related polypeptide chains, designated as α, β, γ, δ and ε chains. Most normal human Hb contains two α-chains plus two other chains, which may be β, γ, δ, or ε depending on the type.

1. **Hb-A_1:** Noraml adult Hb, commonly called Hb-A, consists of two α- and two β-chains and designated as **$\alpha_2^A \beta_2^A$ (or simply $\alpha_2 \beta_2$).** 90 to 95% of Hb of normal adult is of this type.
2. **Hb-F:** Human foetal Hb is designated as Hb-F and it is $\alpha_2 \gamma_2$. Hb-F differs in many respects from adult Hb-A_1 (Refer Box below).
3. **Hb-A_2:** A minor component of normal adult Hb, present usually to the extent of 2.5 percent. Electrophoretically, it is a slowly migrating fraction. It contains two α-chains and two δ-chains and thus it is **$\alpha_2 \delta_2$.**
4. **Embryonic Hb:** Another form which is found in first three months of intrauterine life of the baby. It contains two α-chains and two ε-chains and thus, it is **$\alpha_2 \varepsilon_2$.**
5. **Hb-A_3:** An electrophoretically fast fraction also appears, amounting to between 3 and 10 percent of the total. This is designated as A_3 and it appears to be ***an altered form of Hb-A,*** found chiefly in old red cells.
6. **Hb-A_{1C} (Glycosylated Hb):** In addition to Hb-A_1 the major form of normal adult Hb, a minor glycosylated form is also found in adult red blood cells. In normal individuals, it is present in concentration of 3 to 5 percent of total Hb. ***However, in patients with diabetes mellitus it may be increased to as much as 6 to 15 percent of total Hb.*** This minor glycosylated Hb is designated as HbA_{1C}.

Differences of HbF and HbA

Hb-F differs in many respects from adult Hb-A_1 viz.

- Structurally $\alpha_2 \beta_2$
- Resistance to alkali denaturation
- Electrophoretically moves behind Hb-A
- BPG content ↓
  - Affinity O_2↑
  - Delivery power of O_2↓
  - Present in foetal life and disappears after one year.

Chemistry: Amino acid sequence of Hb-A_{1C} is exactly the same as that of Hb-A_1. The chemical difference consists of attachment of 1-amino-1-deoxy fructose to the $-NH_2$ terminal of valine of the β-chain of Hb-A_1. Addition of sugar moiety to valine occurs nonenzymatically, either by addition of glucose directly to the protein, or by formation by G-6-P of an adult with Hb-A_1 (Hb-A_{1b}) which is subsequently dephosphorylated to form Hb-A_{1c}.

Clinical Importance

- The ***level of glycosylated Hb appears to be an index of the levels of blood sugar*** for a period of several weeks prior to the time of sampling. ***Once the RB cells get glycosylated, it remains for the lifespan of the RB cells.***
- ***Its measurement would be a more reliable indicator*** of the adequacy of control of the diabetic state as compared to occasional measurement of blood and urine glucose.

Properties of Hb

- ***Crystallizable protein:*** Each species has its own crystalline form, which is related to variations in the amino acids of the globin part.
- ***Molecular wt:*** Approximately 65,000 as determined by osmotic pressure and ultracentrifugation measurements.
- ***Shape:*** The overall shape resembles a spheroid, having a length of 64 Å, a width of 55 Å and a height of 50Å.

DERIVATIVES OF HAEMOGLOBIN

1. Action of Acids and Alkalies: Acids and alkalies act upon Hb to form the acid haematin and alkali haematin. The essential differences and similarities between the two are given in Table 10.1

2. Haemin: It is chemically haematin hydrochloride. It is prepared by boiling oxy-Hb with NaCl and glacial acetic acid. It is a ferric compound. Haemin crystallizes in characteristic brown crystals, which can be seen under the microscope.

3. Haemochromogen: Heme and the ferrous prophyrin complexes react readily with basic substances such as hydrazines, primary amines, pyridines, or an imidazole such as the amino acid histidine, resulting compound is called a *"haemochromogen" (haemochrome)*. On spectroscopy, this compound shows

- A *"**soret band**"*- a sharp absorption band near 400 mμ.

Note: It is a distinguishing feature of porphyrin ring and is characteristic of all porphyrins.

- In addition it ***shows two additional absorption bands: α-band–a*** narrow band at 559 mμ and ***β-band***–a broader band at 527 mμ. Both bands are in green part of the spectrum nearer to "D" line.

4. Methaemoglobin: It is a derivative in which Fe is in the ***ferric state and it is a true oxidation product of Hb.*** Increased amount of methaemoglobin in blood above normal is called as ***methaemoglobinaemia***

Table 10.1: Essential Differences and Similarities between Acid Haematin and Alkali Haematin

Acid haematin	*Alkali haematin*
• Dilute HCl/other acids split Hb into heme and globin, hence is "ferro-heme"	• Alkalies also split Hb into globin and "ferro-heme"
• In presence of O_2 heme is quickly oxidized to *"ferri-heme"*	• In presence of O_2 "ferro-heme" is converted to *"**ferri-heme**"*
• Additional + ve charge is balanced by Cl^- ion in case of HCl and forms "acid haematin" which is chemically, **"Ferri heme chloride"** Hb+HCl → globin +ferro-heme 2 ferro heme + ½ O_2 +2 HCl → 2 ferri-heme chloride **(acid haematin)**	• Additional +ve charge is balanced by-OH ion in case of NaOH or KOH and forms **'alkaline haematin**, which is chemically **"ferri-heme hydroxide"** Hb+NaOH→globin +ferro-heme 2 ferro-heme+ ½ O_2 + – OH ions → ferri-heme hydroxide **(alkali haematin)**
• **Absorption bands:** By spectroscopy-shows a thinner band at 650 mμ between C and D line, but nearer to C line	• By spectroscopy-shows a broader band at 600 mμ between C and D line, but near to D line

Formation of Methaemoglobin and its Conversion to Haemoglobin

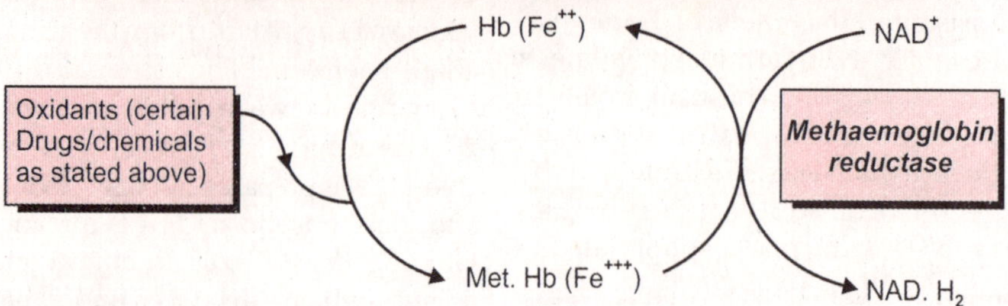

Causes: Methaemoglobin can be produced as follows:

- ***In vitro*** is produced by treating blood with potasium ferricyanide.
- ***In vivo*** is produced by certain drugs or exposure to certain poisons, e.g. chlorates, acetanilid, nitrites, nitrobenzene, antipyrin, phenacetin, sulfonal, and perhaps most important, the sulphonamide drugs.
- ***Familial methaemoglobinaemia:*** An inherited disorder due to to lack or absence of the enzyme ***methaemoglobin reductase***, which is responsible for conversion of methaemoglobin to normal Hb (Fe^{++}).
- ***Hb-M:*** Methamoglobinaemia may also be found in individuals with abnormal haemoglobin as Hb-M.

Mechanism of Methaemoglobin Formation:

- In methaemoglobin formation, ***iron is oxidized to ferric state***
  - As such it cannot bind O_2.
  - The additional +ve charge per heme molecule is balanced with negative group, presumably-OH group.

Mechanism of reconversion of methaemoglobin to Hb in normal health: In normal healthy adult, small amount of methaemoglobin may be present approx 0.3 gm/100 ml (about 1.7% of total Hb). This is converted to normal Hb by an enzyme called ***methaemoglobin reductase*** which requires NADH as coenzyme.

- Recently, an additional enzyme *diaphorase I*, has been found out, which is NADPH-dependant, which can also perform the same function.
- ***Glutathione*** and ***ascorbic acid***, reducing substances present in significant amounts in erythrocytes, may also be involved in reduction of Met-Hb **(Refer box above).**

Absorption spectra: By spectroscopy, methaemoglobin gives characteristic absorption spectra. Dilute neutral Met-Hb gives ***four absorption bands***

- One broad band at 490 mμ in green part nearer to "F" line
- A narrow band at 540 mμ in green part
- Another narrow band at 575 mμ in yellow part of the spectrum
- A band at 634 mμ at red part of the spectrum. ***This band is the characteristic one and is used for detection of Met-Hb.***

Alkaline Met-Hb gives only three bands: band at 490 mμ is missing.

COMBINATION OF HAEMOGLOBIN WITH GASES

1. Oxy-haemoglobin: Combination with Oxygen (Oxy-Hb)

The physiological importance lies in the fact that ***Hb can readily combine with O_2***. The combination is ***loose*** and ***reversible.*** The gas is taken up readily at high partial pressures (e.g. in the lungs) and is released as readily at low O_2 pressures (e.g. in tissues), thus providing an effective system for transport of O_2 from the atmosphere to the cells of the body. ***At O_2 tensions of 100 mm Hg or more,*** Hb is virtually 100 percent saturated ***approximately 1.34 ml of O_2 is combined with each gram of Hb.*** De-oxygenated Hb can loosely combine with forming Oxy-Hb, the attachment with O_2 occur with Fe in the heme portion.

Fe remains in the "ferrous" state both in deoxygenated Hb and oxy-Hb. O_2 remains attached with the unpaired electrons of Fe. ***Each heme can bind only one molecule of*** O_2. Since each molecule of Hb contains 4 mols. of heme; hence ***one mol of Hb can maximally combine with four mols of*** O_2.

Factors: The combination is ***loose*** and ***reversible*** and ***governed by the following factors:***

- Partial pressure of O_2 (pO_2) favours oxygenation
- Partial pressure of CO_2 (pCO_2) favours dissociation
- pH of the medium-acidosis favours liberation of O_2.

Absorption Spectrum of Oxy-Hb: On spectroscopy, it shows ***two characteristic bands***

- ***α-band:*** Narrow-band in yellow portion of the spectrum at 597 mµ nearer to D-line.
- ***β-band:*** Wider broad-band, nearer to E-line in green part of spectrum at 542 mµ.

2. Carboxy-Hb: Combination with CO

- CO combines with heme portion of Hb to form ***carbon monoxide Hb*** (also called as ***carboxy-Hb*** or ***carbonyl Hb).***

Characteristics

- It is a much ***firmer*** combination, as compared to oxy-Hb.
- ***Not reversible.***
- ***Affinity*** of Hb to CO is ***210 times more*** than O_2.
- ***Lethal action is due to inhibition of cytochrome oxidase*** of electron transport chain and thus stops cellular respiration.

Poisoning by CO is a common danger of modern life. The victim frequently becomes unconscious in a few minutes and death often follows quickly—

Causes:

- Incomplete combustion of carbonaceous materials.
- Automobile exhaust gas (4 to 7 percent).
- Chimney gases and smoke.
- Found as a constituent of illuminating gas (derived from coal or oil) in which its presence varies from 4 to 40 percent.

An individual inhaling CO from above mentioned sources can become a victim.

BIOCHEMICAL TESTS:

- ***Physical exmination of blood:*** It shows a ***cherry-red colour.***
- ***Chemical test: Dilution test:*** To dilute the suspected blood, after treating it with a little NaOH and compare the colour with normal blood similarly treated. Normal blood shows a greenish hue after such treatment whereas ***blood containing carboxy-Hb remains pink.***
- ***Absorption spectra:*** These resemble like oxy Hb, but the two bands are slightly nearer to violet end of the spectrum. On treatment of blood sample with sodium hydrosulphite, there is no change of absorption bands (two bands persists) in case of carboxy-Hb while the two bands of oxy-Hb are changed to one broad **β-band** ***(α-band disappears) as oxy-Hb is reduced to deoxy Hb.***

Figure 10.1 gives absorption spectra of different derivatives.

3. Combination with CO_2: A different type of combination is that of Hb with CO_2 to form ***carbaminohaemoglobin.*** In this case, ***the combination is with the globin*** rather than with the heme. CO_2 combines with NH_2 group.

$$Hb.NH_2 + CO_2 \rightleftharpoons Hb.NHCOOH \rightleftharpoons Hb.NH.COO^- + H^+$$

It is a ***reversible*** process. This is a normal and constant physiologic reaction and accounts for 2 to 10 percent of CO_2 transported by the blood.

4. Action of HCN and Cyanides: HCN and cyanides ***do not react directly with haemoglobin but they react with methaemoglobin to form cyanmethaemoglobin, which is not toxic.*** The lethal and toxic action of cyanides resides in the fact, that it **inhibits** ***cytochrome oxidase*** a_3 of electron transport chain and stops cellular respiration.

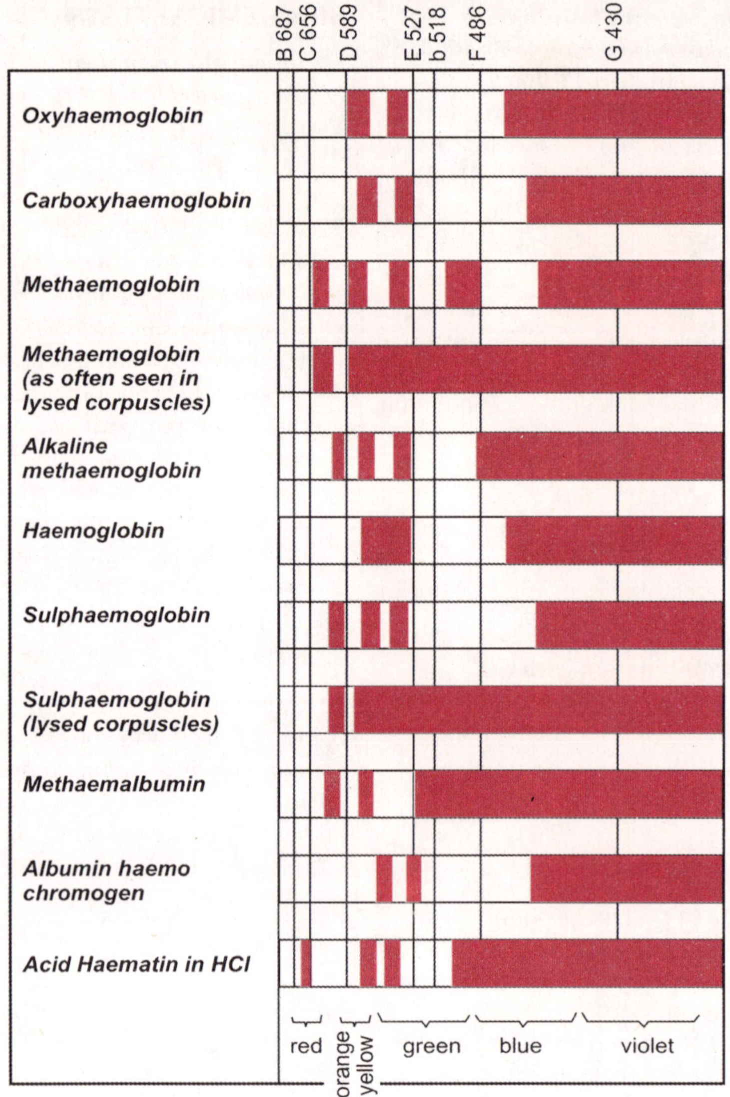

Fig. 10.1: Showing absorption spectra of different Hb-derivatives

Biochemical Basis of Treatment of Cyanide Poisoning:

a. To enhance formation of met-Hb in the body so that the cyanides combine with met-Hb and spares cytochrome oxidase a_3. This is achieved by ***administering sodium nitrite*** intravenously to the patient. *It induces the production of methaemoglobin which quickly combines with cyanide to produce cyanmethaemoglobin which is non-toxic* and slowly converted subsequently to Hb and cyanate, which is non-toxic and is excreted.

b. To administer a drug which will combine with cyanides and thus spares cytochrome oxidase a_3. This is achieved by giving ***sodium thiosulfate IV. Sodium thiosulfate reacts with cyanides, yielding thiocyanate, an inocuous substance, which is readily excreted out.***

ABNORMAL HAEMOGLOBINS AND HAEMOGLOBINOPATHIES

In addition to normal adult Hb and other varieties discussed earlier, more than 30 abnormal types have been described.

ABNORMAL HAEMOGLOBINS

The occurrence of these abnormal haemoglobins which are best differentiated by their characteristic electrophoretic mobilities, has given rise to the concept of *"molecular disease"*. These abnormalities are ***genetically transmitted and are each due to a single mutant gene.***

They are of ***two types:***

1. If the mutation affects ***structural gene,*** it results in replacement of a single amino acid residue of Hb-A_1 by some other amino acid resulting into abnormal Hb.

   Example: ***Hb-S, Hb-M, Hb-C, Hb-D (Panjab) and others.***
2. If the mutation affects the ***regulator gene,*** which ***affect the rate of synthesis of the peptide chains,*** the amino acid sequence remains unaffected. This produces ***Thalassaemias.*** Depending on the chains affected, it can be (a) **α-chain thalassaemias** and (b) **β-chain thalassaemias.**

Effects of Abnormal Haemoglobins: The presence of abnormal Hb in the blood is often associated with the following:

- Abnormalities in red cell morphology
- Definite clinical manifestation like haemolytic anaemia and/or jaundice, and other features pertaining to the property of that abnormal Hb.

If the genetic defect is "heterozygous" the patient will have so-called "**trait**" (**e.g.** sickle-cell trait) and may be free from clinical manifestations although the presence of abnormality can be detected electrophoretically/biochemically by certain tests. On the other hand, if the defect is ***"homozygous"*** the patient will have full-blown disease.

HAEMOGLOBINOPATHIES

Hb-S: In Hb-S, both the α-chains have the same amino acid sequence as those of normal Hb-A, but in both β-***chains glutamic acid in sixth position is replaced by valine.*** Thus, its formula will be—$\alpha_2^A\ \beta_2^{6val}$

Note: ***One single amino acid substitution valine for glutamic acid at sixth position*** is the only chemical difference between Hb-A and Hb-S among the total of 574 amino acids and ***that is responsible for such a dreadful disease.***

Solubility: The solubility of Hb-S in oxygenated state is not very different from that of Hb-A; but in the deoxygenated state, ***deoxygenated Hb-S is only 2 percent as soluble as de-oxygenated Hb-A, and about 1 percent as soluble as its own-form.*** It is likely that the loss of the glutamate residue with its two carboxyl groups alters the distribution of +ve and –ve charges on the protein surface and thus changes its solubility. As a result of this insolubility of Hb-S, a significant increase in viscosity occurs, which results in precipitation of Hb-S resulting into ***crescent-shaped RB cells (Sickle cells).*** The process is called ***sickling*** which can be demonstrated *in vitro* from the patient's blood. This hypothesis is not tenable now. ***Biochemically, it is explained now by the formation of "sticky patch" on the outside of the β-chains.***

Biochemical basis of sickling of RB cells in sickle cell disease: Replacement of a "non polar" residue valine in β-chain to "polar residue" glutamic acid generates the formation of ***sticky patch*** on the outside of the β-chains. The sticky patch develops on the oxygenated ("R" form) of Hb-S and deoxygenated ('T' form) of HbS, ***but never present on oxy-HbA ("R" form).***

On the surface of deoxygenated Hb-S ('T' form), there exists a ***"complementary site"*** to the sticky patch, but in the oxygenated Hb-S ('R' form) the complementary site is masked and not present (Refer Fig. 10.2).

When Hb-S is deoxygenated, the sticky patch can bind to the complementary patch or site on

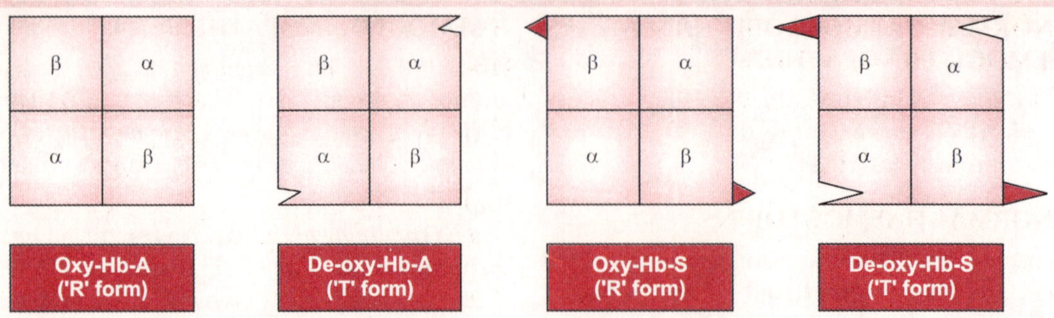

Fig. 10.2: Diagrammatic representation of 'sticky patch'

another deoxygenated Hb-S molecule. This binding causes ***polymerization of deoxy-Hb-S, forming long fibrous precipitates*** these extend throughout the RB cells and mechanically distort it, causing lysis and multiple secondary clinical effects.

Thus, if Hb-S can be maintained in an oxygenated state, or if the concentration of deoxygenated Hb-S can be minimized, then formation of these polymers will not occur and "sickling" can be prevented. ***Because it is the 'T' form of Hb-S that polymerizes, low oxygen tension exacerbates sickling of RB cells.***

Although the deoxy Hb-A contain the receptor sites for the sticky patch present on oxygenated or deoxygenated Hb-S, the binding of sticky Hb-S to deoxy-Hb-A cannot extend the polymer, since the latter (deoxy Hb-A) does not have a sticky patch to promote binding to another Hb molecule. Hence, ***the binding of deoxy Hb-A to either the 'R' or 'T' form of Hb-S will terminate the polymerization.***

Nature of polymer: The polymer forms a twisted helical fibre whose cross-section contains 14 Hb-S molecules. These tubular fibres distort the RB cells so that they take the shape of a **"sickle"** and are vulnerable to lysis as they penetrate the interstices of the splenic sinusoids.

Sickle-Cell Anaemia/and Trait

A hereditary haemolytic anaemia characterized by presence of Hb-S.

In ***Homozygous:*** Full blown picture of sickle cell anaemia is seen. They have 80-100 percent Hb-S and 0 to 20 percent Hb-A.

In ***heterozygous:*** Manifests ***trait*** without clinical manifestation. The patients usually have 20-40% Hb-S and 60 to 80 percent Hb-A. Some patients may inherit more than one haemoglobinopathy and produce not only Hb-S but Hb-C, Hb-D, or some other abnormal Hb as well. The genetic defect is virtually limited to Negroes. In USA 8 to 11% of Negroes carry the hereditary abnormality, only 1 in 40 of these is homozygous. In native populations in Africa, incidence of genetic abnormality may be 45%.

Effects of sickle Erythrocytes:

- *"Sickle" cells are more fragile due to their shape* ***and predisposes to haemolysis*** leading to haemolytic anaemia and jaundice.
- ***Packing of these abnormal red cells into vessels,*** specially capillaries of organs, causes ***vascular stasis*** and ***anoxic damage*** to the tissues, giving rise to clinical manifestations of the particular organs affected.

RELATION WITH OTHER DISEASES

- ***Protection from malaria:*** Persons suffering from sickle cell anaemia/trait ***show an increased resistance to malaria.*** It has been shown that world distribution of sickle cell anaemia closely parallels the distribution of malarial mosquitoes.

- ***Increased incidence to Salmonella infections:*** On the other hand, incidence of *Salmonella* infections has been found to be more in sickle cell anaemia.

Other Abnormal Haemoglobins: Some of the other abnormal haemoglobins are Hb-C, Hb-D (Panjab), Hb-E, etc. Substitution of amino acid and molecular formulas are given below. Hb-C is confined amongst Negroes in West Africa. All of them bring about change in red cell morphology, affect solubility and may produce mild haemolytic anaemia. Hb-C and Hb-D can occur with Hb-S.

THALASSAEMIAS

Impairment of synthesis of a single kind of Hb chain results in ***"thalassaemias"***, so called because the conditions are more common in Mediterranean countries (***thalasa***=derived from Greek word meaning "sea"). The α-chain thalassaemia is also prevalent in SE Asia with an occurrence of 1 in 100 in Thailand. ***They occur due to mutation of "regulator gene"***.

1. α-chain Thalassaemias: Synthesis of α-chains are repressed and there occurs a compensatory increase in synthesis of other chains of which the cell is capable either β-chains or γ-chains.

Type	*Chain affected*	*Change in amino acid sequence*	*Formula*
• ***Hb-C***	β-chain	Glutamic acid at 6 replaced by lysine	$\alpha_2^A\ \beta_2^{6Lys}$
• ***Hb-D (Panjab)***	β-chain	Glutamic acid at position 121 is replaced by glutamine	$\alpha_2^A\ \beta_2^{121\ Gln}$
• ***Hb-E***	β-chain	Glutamic acid at 26 is replaced by lysine	$\alpha_2^A\ \beta_2^{26Lys}$

- **Hb-H (β_4):** In Hb-H (β_4), there is ***inhibition of α-chain synthesis*** and rate of β-chain production increases. The excess of β-chains form a large intracellular pool and presumably aggregate to form β_4 molecules (tetramer) and called Hb-H.

Hb-H disease is characterized by:

- Moderate degree of haemolytic anaemia.
- Red cell morphological appearance of thalassaemia (see β-chain thalassaemia).
- Variable amount of Hb-H (usually 10 to 20%).

Inclusion bodies: After incubation of blood sample with brilliant cresyl blue and then drawing a smear on the slide, when seen under microscope, ***numerous "inclusion bodies" can be seen which represent denatured Hb-H.***

- **Hb-Barts (γ_4):** In Hb-Barts (γ_4), gross defect in repression of α-chain synthesis result in great excess of γ-chains, which aggregate to γ_4 molecules (tetramer).

Clinical Significance

Pregnant ladies suffering from this haemoglobinopathy delivers stillborn infants with clinical picture of ***Hydrops foetalis***. This disorder is found in SE Asia. Eighty percent of stillborn infants are due to Hb-Barts.

2. β-chain Thalassaemia (Thalassaemia Major)

- When the thalassamia gene represses β-chain synthesis, an excess of α-chains occur which can combine with δ-chains ***producing an increase in Hb-A_2***, or γ-chains producing an ***increase in Hb-F***.

  This is the group of thalassaemias associated with severe anaemias of infancy or early childhood which was first described by **Cooley**, called ***Cooley's anaemia***. Infants suffering from this disease have ***"Mongoloid"*** features and have stunted growth. They suffer from ***severe haemolytic anaemia***.
- ***On examination,*** marked pallor is seen; icterus is variable; enlargement of spleen (splenomegaly) is found.

- ***Blood:*** Hb very low may be 3 to 5 gm percent; ***hypochromic microcytic anaemia; osmotic fragility increased.***
- ***Blood smear:*** Shows hypochromasia, polychromasia, basophilic stippling, **target cells** ++, nucleated cells+.
- ***Radiological examination:*** Lateral view of skull-shows ***"hair-on-end"*** appearance. This is a characteristic feature.
- ***Biochemically:*** Serum Fe level is normal. Rise in Hb-F 5 to 80 percent. Hb-A_2 is significantly increased.

☞ SALIENT POINTS TO REMEMBER

- Haemoglobin is a conjugated protein containing protein called "Globin" and the non-protein prosthetic group called "heme".
- Globin is a tetramer, consisting of four polypeptide chains. In normal adult Hb A_1 have 2 α chains and 2 β chains ($\alpha_2\ \beta_2$).
- Heme is a tetrapyrrole. It is hexavalent. Four pyrroles are joined to Fe^{++} (Ferrous) in centre by four bounds, fifth is joined to globin and sixth to water molecule.
- Each peptide chain (sub unit) contains one "heme" in so-called "heme-pockets". Thus ***one Hb molecule contains 4 heme units.***
- Human foetal Hb is called Hb-F and it is $\alpha_2 r_2$. It disappears from blood after birth (after one year). ***Persistence of HbF is pathological.***
- Glycosylated Hb designated as Hb A_{1C} found to the extent of 3 to 5 percent of total Hb in normal individuals but it is increased to as much as 6 to 15 percent of total Hb in patients of diabates mellitus.
- Hb can readily combines with O_2; the combination is loose and reversible.
- O_2 is readily taken up in the lungs due to high pO_2 and released readily in tissue due to low pO_2. This provides an effective system for transport of O_2 from lungs to tissues.
- Hb actively participates in the transport of CO_2 from tissues to lungs.
- Increased partial pressure of CO_2 (pCO_2) accompanied by elevated H^+ decreases the binding of O_2 to Hb, a phenomenon known as Böhr effect.
- Methaemoglobin is a derivative in ***which Fe is in the "Ferric" state*** and it is a true oxidation product of Hb. It can be produced *"in vivo"* by certain oxidant group of drugs.
- Increased concentration of Met-Hb produces methaemoglobinaemia. As Fe is in ferric state, it cannot bind O_2.
- Carbon monoxide (CO) combines with 'heme' portion of Hb to form carboxy-Hb or carbonyl Hb.
- It is much firmer combination, not reversible and lethal due to inhibition of cytochrome oxidase of ETC.
- Sickle cell anaemia due to Hb-S is a classical example of abnormal Hb. ***Glutamic acid at 6 position in β chain is replaced by valine.***
- Hb-S is characterized by haemolytic anaemia, tissue damage and increased susceptibility to infection.
- ***Hb-S offers protection to Plasmodium falciparum infection.***
- Thalassaemias are a group of hereditary haemolytic disorders characterized by impairment in the synthesis of globin, α or β chains.
- α-thalassaemia can be of 2 types: Hb-H (β_4) or (ii) Hb-Barts (γ_4).
- Pregnant ladies suffering from Hb-Barts (α-chain thalassaemia) suffer from hydrops foetalis.
- β-chain thalassaemia (also called Cooley's anaemia) presents as a severe form of haemolytic anaemia. **Biochemically, it is characterized by increased Hb-F and Hb-A_2.**

MULTIPLE CHOICE QUESTIONS

Give one correct answer:

1. **The iron in heme is linked to the globin through**
   (a) Valine (b) Histidine
   (c) Arginine (d) Lysine
   (e) Serine
2. **One gram of Hb can carry how much oxygen?**
   (a) 1.84 ml (b) 3.4 ml
   (c) 11.34 ml (d) 1.34 ml
   (e) 13.4 ml

3. **In methaemoglobin formation, the iron in heme is:**
   (a) In ferrous form (b) is attached to H_2O
   (c) Ferric form (d) None of the above
   (e) Both ferrous and ferric form

4. **The type of polypeptide chains present in globin of Hb A_2 are:**
   (a) $\alpha_2\ \beta_2$ (b) $\alpha_2\ \gamma_2$
   (c) $\beta_2\ \gamma_2$ (d) $\alpha_2\ \delta_2$
   (e) $\gamma_2\ \delta_2$

5. **All of the following are associated with formation of methaemoglobinaemia, *except:***
   (a) Nitrites (b) Primaquin
   (c) Acetanilid (d) Hb-M
   (e) Methylene blue

6. **In sickle-cell Hb the position 6 of glutamic acid residue of β-chain of normal adult Hb is replaced by:**
   (a) Tyrosine (b) Valine
   (c) Lysine (d) Glutamine
   (e) Threonine

7. **The protective effect against malaria by *Plasmodium falciparum* is related to which of the following?**
   (a) Hb-H (b) Hb-S
   (c) Bart's Hb (d) Hb-F
   (e) Hb-A_3

8. **All the following manifestations are seen in sickle cell anaemia, *except:***
   (a) Severe haemolytic anaemia
   (b) Pain and swellings in joints
   (c) Sickled cells in peripheral circulation
   (d) Impairment of growth
   (e) Inclusion bodies in RB cells

9. **Carbon monoxide inhibits mitochondrial electron transport by:**
   (a) Inhibiting the electron transfer of NADH-Q reductase
   (b) Binding to Hb in RB cells and so blocking the transport of O_2 to tissues
   (c) Binding to the O_2 binding site of cytochrome oxidase
   (d) Blocking electron transport at the level of cyt b $\rightarrow$ cyt c_1
   (e) Combining with CoQ

10. **Which of the following globin chains are not synthesized during intrauterine life?**
   (a) α-chains (b) β-chains
   (c) γ-chains (d) δ-chains
   (e) Eta-chains

11. **Sickle cell anaemia is characterized by all of the following *except:***
   (a) Presence of Hb-S
   (b) Increased osmotic fragility
   (c) Normocytic red blood cells
   (d) Sickling of erythrocytes *in vitro*
   (e) Hyperbilirubinaemia

12. **The incidence of *Salmonella* infections is most often increased in patients with:**
   (a) Sickle cell anaemia
   (b) Hb-C disease
   (c) α-chain thalassaemia
   (d) G-6-PD deficiencies of RB-cells
   (e) β-chain thalassaemia

ANSWERS

1. (b)	2. (d)	3. (c)
4. (d)	5. (e)	6. (b)
7. (b)	8. (e)	9. (c)
10. (d)	11. (b)	12. (a)

Digestion and Absorption of Carbohydrates, Lipids and Proteins

DIGESTION OF CARBOHYDRATES

Dietary carbohydrates principally consists of the

- ***Polysaccharides:*** starch and glycogen. It also contains • ***disaccharides:*** sucrose (cane sugar), • lactose (milk sugar) and • maltose and in small amounts ***monosaccharides*** like • fructose and • pentoses. Liquid food materials like milk, soup, fruit juice escape digestion in mouth as they are swallowed, but solid foodstuffs are masticated thoroughly before they are swallowed.

1. Digestion in Mouth: Digestion of carbohydrates start at the mouth, where they come in contact with saliva during mastication.

- Saliva contains a carbohydrate splitting enzyme called salivary ***amylase (ptyalin)***.
- ***Action of Ptyalin (salivary amylase):*** It is ***α-amylase***, requires Cl^- ion for activation and optimum pH 6.7 (range 6.6 to 6.8). The enzyme hydrolyzes α-1-4 glycosidic linkages at random deep inside polysaccharide molecule like starch, glycogen and dextrins, producing smaller molecules *maltose, glucose* and trisaccharide *maltotriose.* Ptyalin action stops in stomach when pH falls to 3.0.

$$\text{Starch, Glycogen and Dextrins} \xrightarrow{\alpha\text{-Amylase}} \text{Glucose, Maltose and Maltotriose}$$

2. Digestion in Stomach: Practically no action. No carbohydrate splitting enzymes available in gastric juice. Some dietary sucrose may be hydrolyzed to equimolar amounts of glucose and fructose by HCl.

3. Digestion in Duodenum: Food bolus reaches the duodenum from stomach where it meets the pancreatic juice. Pancreatic juice contains a carbohydrate-splitting enzyme ***pancreatic amylase*** (also called ***amylopsin***) similar to salivary amylase.

Action of Pancreatic Amylase: It is also an ***α-amylase***, optimum pH 7.1. Like *ptyalin* it also requires Cl^- for activity. The enzyme hydrolyzes α-1→4 glycosidic linkage situated well inside polysaccharide molecule. Other criteria and end products of action are similar to ptyalin.

4. Digestion in small Intestine: ***Action of Intestinal Juice:***

- ***Intestinal amylase:*** This hydrolyzes terminal α-1→4, glycosidic linkages in polysaccharides and oligosaccharide molecules liberating free glucose molecule.
- ***Lactase:*** It is a β-galactosidase, its pH range is 5.4 to 6.0. Lactose is hydrolyzed to equimolar amounts of glucose and galactose.

$$\text{Lactose} \xrightarrow{\text{Lactase}} \text{Glucose + Galactose}$$

- ***Isomaltase:*** It catalyzes hydrolysis of α-1→6 glycosidic linkage, thus splitting α-limit dextrin at the branching points and producing maltose and glucose.
- ***Maltase:*** The enzyme hydrolyzes the α-1→4 glycosidic linkage between glucose units in maltose molecule liberating equimolar quanti-

ties of two glucose molecules. Its pH range is 5 8 to 6.2.

Maltose —**Maltase**→ Glucose + Glucose

Five maltases have been identified in intestinal epithelial cells.

Maltase V can act as *isomaltase* over and above its action on maltose.

- ***Sucrase:*** pH range 5.0 to 7.0. It hydrolyzes sucrose molecule to form equimolar quantities of glucose and fructose.

  Maltase III and ***maltase IV*** also **have *sucrase* activity**

Sucrose —**Sucrase**→ Glucose + Fructose

ABSORPTION OF CARBOHYDRATES

It is observed from above that carbohydrate digestion is complete when the food materials reach small intestine and all complex dietary carbohydrates like starch and glycogen and the disaccharides are ***ultimately converted to simpler monosaccharides.***

- All monosaccharides, products of digestion of dietary carbohydrates, are practically completely absorbed almost entirely from the small intestine.
- Rate of absorption diminishes from above downwards; proximal jejunum three times greater than that of distal ileum.
- It is also proved that some disaccharides, which escape digestion, may enter the cells lining the intestinal lumen may be by "***pinocytosis***"; and are hydrolyzed within these cells.

Note: No carbohydrates higher than the monosaccharides can be absorbed directly into the blood stream in normal health and if administered parenterally, they are eliminated as foreign bodies.

Experimental Studies: Absorption of glucose has been studied in dogs; average rate of absorption of glucose in dog is 1 gm/kg body weight/hour. A portion enters in thoracic lymph, but the major portion passes into the portal blood, and carried directly to liver.

- **Cori** studied the rate of absorption of different sugars from small intestine in rat. Taking glucose absorption as 100, comparative rate of absorption of other sugars were found as follows:

Galactose >	Glucose >	Fructose >	Mannose
110	100	43	19
> Xylose >	Arabinose		
15	9		

- The above study proves that ***glucose and galactose are absorbed very fast;*** fructose and mannose intermediate rate and the pentoses are absorbed slowly. ***Galactose is absorbed more rapidly than glucose.***

MECHANISMS OF ABSORPTION

Two mechanisms are involved.

1. **Simple Diffusion:** This is dependent on sugar concentration gradients between the intestinal lumen, mucosal cells, and blood plasma. All the monosaccharides are probably absorbed to some extent ***by simple "passive" diffusion.***

2. **Active Transport Mechanisms:**

- ***Glucose*** and ***galactose*** are absorbed very rapidly and hence it has been suggested that they are ***absorbed actively*** and ***it requires energy.***
- Fructose absorption is also rapid but not so much as compared to glucose and galactose, but it is definitely faster than pentoses. Hence, fructose is not absorbed by simple diffusion alone and it is suggested that some mechanism facilitates its transport, called as ***facilitated transport.***

WILSON AND CRAINE'S HYPOTHESIS OF ACTIVE TRANSPORT

Wilson and **Craine** have shown that sugars which are ***"actively" transported*** have several chemical features in common. They suggested that to be actively transported, sugar must have the following:

- They must have a ***six-membered ring***
- Secondly, they **must have one or more carbon atoms attached to C5,** and
- Thirdly, they must have ***α-OH group at C-2*** with the same stereoconfiguration as occurs in D-glucose.

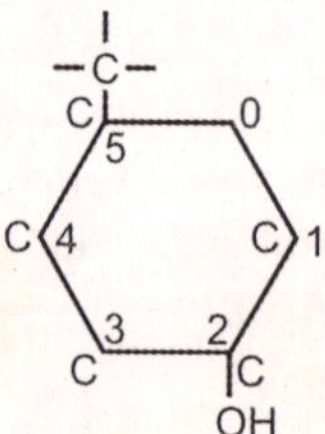

Note: -OH group on carbon 2 and 5 hydroxymethyl or methyl group on the pyranose ring appear to be essential structural requirements for the active transport mechanism.

Craine and his collaborators explain active transport by envisaging the presence of a ***Carrier protein (transport protein)*** in the brush border of intestinal epithelial cell. The "carrier protein" has the following characteristics:

- It has ***two binding sites one for sodium and another for the glucose***
- The carrier protein is ***specific for sugar.***
- It is ***mobile***
- It is ***sodium-dependent***
- It is ***energy-dependent***

Energy: Energy is provided by ATP.

- It is believed that ***sodium binding by the carrier protein is a prerequisite for glucose binding.*** Sodium binding changes the conformation of the protein molecule, enabling the binding of glucose to take place and thus the absorption to occur. It is presumed that analogous "carrier protein" exists for D-galactose also ***(Fig. 11.1).***

Absorption of Other Sugars

- Sugars like D-fructose and D-mannose are probably absorbed by ***facilitated transport*** which requires the presence of carrier protein but ***does not require energy.***
- Other sugars like pentoses and *L*-isomers of glucose and galactose are absorbed passively by simple diffusion.

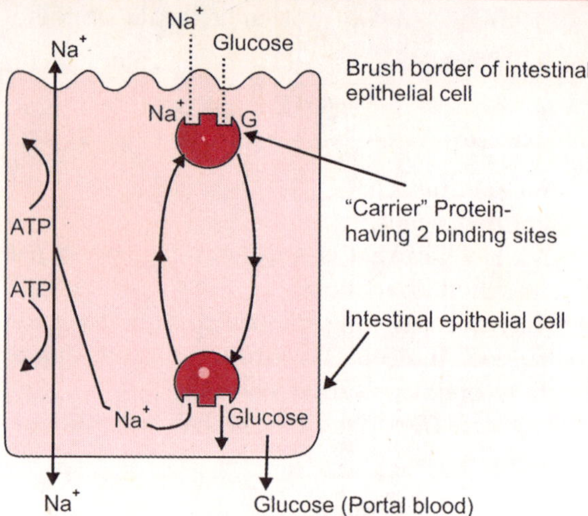

Fig. 11.1: Showing 'carrier protein' and transport of glucose

Factors Influencing Rate of Absorption

1. ***State of mucous membrane and length of time of contact:*** If mucous membrane is not healthy absorption will suffer. Similarly in hurried bowel, length of contact is less as such absorption will be less.
2. ***Hormones:***

- ***Thyroid hormones:*** These increase absorption of hexoses and act directly on intestinal mucosa.
- ***Adrenal cortex:*** Absorption decreases in adrenocortical deficiency, mainly due to decreased concentration of sodium in body fluids
- ***Anterior pituitary:*** This affects absorption mainly through its influence on thyroids. Hyperpituitarism induces thyroid overactivity and *vice versa.*
- ***Insulin: This has no effect on absorption of glucose.***

3. ***Vitamins:*** Absorption is diminished in states of deficiency of B-vitamins, viz. thiamine, pyridoxine and pantothenic acid.
4. ***Inherited enzyme deficiencies:*** Inherited enzyme deficiency like sucrase and lactase can interfere with hydrolysis of corresponding disaccharides and their absorption.

DIGESTION OF LIPIDS

The digestion of fats and other lipids poses a special problem because of:

- The ***insolubility of fats in water,*** and
- Because ***lipolytic enzymes,*** like other enzymes, are ***soluble in an aqueous medium.***

The above problem is solved in the ***gut by emulsification of fats, particularly by bile salts, present in bile and PL.*** The breaking of large fat particles or oil globules, into smaller fine particles by emulsification increases the surface exposed to interaction with lipases and, thus, the rate of digestion is proportionally increased.

PHASES OF DIGESTION AND ABSORPTION

The whole process of digestion of dietary lipids and its subsequent absorption may be arbitrarily divided into ***three phases:***

- ***Preparatory phase:*** Which includes the digestion of lipids in the intestine. The large lipid particles are broken down into smaller particles with the help of lipolytic enzymes.
- ***Transport phase:*** Which includes the transport of digested fats across the membrane of intestinal villous layer into intestinal epithelial cells.
- ***Transportation phase:*** Which includes the events of action that take place inside intestinal epithelial cells and its passage through lacteals to Lymph/or in portal blood.

Dietary Sources of Lipids: The chief dietary sources of lipids in human beings:

- ***Animal source:*** Dairy products like milk, butter, ghee, etc. meat and fish, especially pork, eggs.
- ***Vegetable source:*** Various cooking oils from various seeds, viz. sunflower oil, groundnut oil, cotton seed oil, mustard oil, etc. and fats from other vegetable sources.

A. PREPARATORY PHASE

1. Digestion in Mouth and Stomach: It was believed earlier that little or no fat digestion takes place in the mouth. Recently, a *lipase* has been detected called ***lingual lipase*** which is secreted by the dorsal surface of the tongue ***(Ebner's gland).***

Lingual Lipase:

- The pH range of activity is 2.0 to 7.5 (optimal pH value is 4.0 to 4.5). *Lingual lipase* activity is continued in the stomach also where the pH value is low. Due to retention of food bolus for 2 to 3 hours, about 30 percent of dietary triacyl glycerol (TG) may be digested.
- ***Lingual lipase*** is more active on TG having shorter FA chains and is found to be more specific for ester linkage at 3-position rather than position-1.
- Milk fats contain short and medium chain FA which tend to be esterified in the 3-position. Hence, ***milk fat appears to be the best substrate for this enzyme.*** The released short chain fatty acids are relatively more soluble and hydrophilic and can be absorbed directly from the stomach wall and enter the portal vein.

Gastric Lipase: There is evidence of presence of small amounts of *gastric lipase* in gastric secretion. The overall digestion of fats, brought about by gastric lipase is negligible because:

- No emulsification of fats takes place in stomach,
- The enzyme secreted in small quantity,
- pH of gastric juice is not conducive which is highly acidic, whereas gastric lipase activity is more effective at relatively alkaline pH (average pH 7.8).
- *Gastric lipase* activity requires presence of Ca^{++}. Activity of gastric lipase is seen when intestinal contents are regurgitated into the gastric lumen.
- Recent studies have shown that gastric lipase is not capable of hydrolyzing fats containing long-chain FA. Whatever minimal action of gastric lipase is there, it is confined to highly emulsified fats, viz. those of milk fats or fats present in egg-yolk or fats with short chain fatty acids present in egg-yolk or fats with short chain fatty acids, as these are somewhat relatively more soluble and hydrophilic.

Role of Fat in Stomach: Fats play one important role in the stomach in that they delay the rate of emptying of the stomach, presumably by way of the hormone ***enterogastrone,*** which inhibits gastric motility and retards the discharge of bolus of food from the stomach. ***Thus, fats have a high satiety value.***

2. Digestion in Small Intestine: The major site of fat digestion is the small intestine. This is due to presence of a powerful lipase, ***steapsin*** in the pancreatic juice and presence of bile salts which acts as an effective emulsifying agent for fats.

Pancreatic juice and bile enter the upper small intestine, the duodenum, by way of the pancreatic and bile ducts respectively. Secretion of pancreatic juice is stimulated by the

- Passage of an acid gastric contents (acid chyme) into the duodenum, and
- By secretion of the GI hormones, *secretin* and CCK-PZ.

Secretin increases the secretion of electrolytes and fluid components of pancreatic juice, whereas ***pancreozymin of CCK-PZ,*** stimulates the secretion of the pancreatic enzymes. ***Cholecystokinin*** of ***CCK-PZ,*** in turn, cause contraction of the gall bladder and discharge the bile into the duodenum. Discharge of bile is also stimulated by *secretin* and bile salts themselves.

Hepatocrinin released by the intestinal mucosa stimulates more bile formation which is relatively poor in the bile salt content.

The above sequence of events prepares the small intestine for the digestion of fats.

LIPOLYTIC ENZYMES IN PANCREATIC JUICE

Pancreatic juice has been shown to contain a number of lipolytic enzymes:

- ***Pancreatic lipase (steapsin),***
- ***Phospholipase A_2 (lecithinase),*** and
- ***Cholesterol esterase.***

The pancreatic lipase is the most important which hydrolyzes TG containing short-chain FA as well as long-chain FA. Other two enzymes are required for phospholipids/and cholesterol respectively.

Pancreatic Lipase (Steapsin): It is an *esterase* with optimum pH value of 6.

1. Role of Bile Salts in Pancreatic Lipase Activity: Bile salts are required for proper functioning of the enzyme.

- Bile salts help in combination of *"lipase"* with two molecules of a small protein called as ***colipase*** (mol wt = 10,000) in the intestinal lumen. ***This combination of lipase with colipase has two effects:***
  - enhances the lipase activity of the intestinal pH,
  - also protects the enzyme against inhibitory effects of bile salts and against surface denaturation
- Bile salts also help in emulsification of fats.

2. Role of Ca^{++}: In the presence of Ca^{++} in the intestine, the FFA are immediately precipitated as "soaps" (insoluble Ca-soaps) and are thereby prevented from inhibiting further lipase action. Thus, ***Ca^{++} facilitates lipase action.***

Mode of Action of Pancreatic Lipase: The complete hydrolysis of fats (TG) produces glycerol and FA. ***Pancreatic lipase is virtually specific for the hydrolysis of "primary ester linkage". It cannot readily hydrolyze the ester linkage of position-2(β), if it does so it occurs at a very slow rate.***

- Digestion of TG molecule by pancreatic lipase proceeds:
  - First by removal of a terminal FA to produce an ***"α, β-diglyceride"***, and
  - The other terminal FA is then removed to produce a ***"β-monoglyceride"***.
- Since the last FA at position (Sn-2) is linked by a secondary ester group and as it cannot be hydrolyzed easily by pancreatic lipase, the ***β-monoglyceride is first converted to α-monoglyceride*** by isomerization ***by an isomerase enzyme.*** Then the α-monoglyceride is hydrolyzed by pancreatic *lipase.*
- Sequence of events that occurs in the intestinal lumen is shown schematically in ***Fig. 11.2.***
- As it is seen from above, by the action of ***pancreatic lipase*** and **isomerase** α and β-monoglycerides are the major end-products of fat digestion, and less than one-fourth of the ingested fat (25% or less) is completely broken down to glycerol and FA.

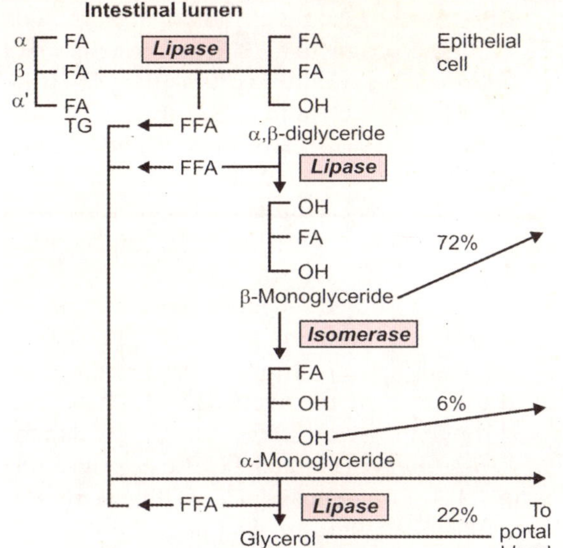

Fig. 11.2: Sequence of events in intestinal lumen

"Micelle" Formation:

- Bile salts and soaps formed in the intestinal lumen and bicarbonates of pancreatic and intestinal juices, collect the molecules of higher FA, mono- and diglycerides, lecithins, cholesterol, etc. in the form of ***water-soluble molecular aggregates*** called ***mixed micelles,*** which are much smaller than the droplets of emulsified fats (size 0.1 to 0.5 μ in diameter) and are absorbed mainly from duodenum and jejunum.
- Bile salts of the "micelles" are not absorbed at this point but are redissolved in other emulsoid particles. ***They are reabsorbed later in the lower part of the small intestine and return to the liver*** via the portal vein for resecretion into the bile. This is known as ***entero-hepatic circulation of bile salts.***

B. TRANSPORT PHASE

- Current evidences, based on electron microscopic studies, indicate that the products of fat digestion, FFA, α and β-monoglycerides mainly enter the microvilli and the apical pole of absorptive epithelial cells by *simple diffusion* through the cell membrane.
- Short and medium chain FA (6 to 10 C) and unsaturated FA are more readily absorbed than the long chain FA (12 to 18 C). Also, the short chain FA appears to enhance the absorption of fats in general, whereas long-chain FA tend to impair the process.
- *Pinocytosis* does not appear to play a significant role in fat absorption as was formerly believed; probably less than 5 per cent absorbed in emulsified forms may be absorbed by pinocytosis.
- The products of digestion next appear to be taken up by the smooth endoplasmic reticulum and ***re-synthesized into TG*** again by enzymes present in the membrane and/or cavities of the reticulum.

Activation of FFA

$$\text{R–COOH} + \text{CoA–SH} \xrightarrow[\text{Mg}^{++},\ \text{ATP} \rightarrow \text{ATP+Ppi}]{\text{Thiokinase}} \text{R–}\overset{\text{O}}{\overset{\|}{\text{C}}}\sim\text{S.CoA}$$

Acyl - CoA

- There is a merging of the smooth endoplasmic reticulum into rough endoplasmic reticulum, in which probabaly enzymes for TG resynthesis are formed as well as the protein component (apo-B_{48}) of lipoprotein complex ***chylomicron.***

C. TRANSPORTATION PHASE

Sequence of events inside the intestinal mucosa cell is as follows:

- Within the intestinal epithelial cell, α-monoglycerides (6%) are further hydrolyzed by *intestinal lipase* to produce freeFA and glycerol. ***Intestinal Lipase:*** A lipase distinct from that of the pancreatic lipase is present in the intestinal mucosal cell. Principal action of this enzyme is confined within epithelial cell.
- FA absorbed from intestinal lumen and FA formed from hydrolysis of α-monoglycerides, are activated to "Acyl-CoA". An ATP-dependant *thiokinase* has been shown to be present in the mucosal cells of the intestine (shown above).

- ***Note that glycerol released within the intestinal wall cells are reutilized for TG resynthesis.*** Glycerol is converted to α-glycerol-(P) by *glycerokinase* in presence of ATP. Some amount of α-glycero-(P) can be contributed from glycolysis operating in intestinal epithelial cell. α-glycero (P) thus formed combines with "acyl-CoA" to form TG molecule.
- β-monoglyceride (72%) which is absorbed from intestinal lumen can combine directly with "acyl CoA" to reform TG. Sequence of events that takes place in resynthesis of TG is shown in *Fig. 11.3.*

ABSORPTION OF LIPIDS

ABSORPTION OF RESYNTHESIZED TG AND OTHER PRODUCTS

1. Glycerol: Free glycerol (22%) released in the intestinal lumen is ***not*** utilized for synthesis of TG in intestinal epithelial cell *(Fig.11.3). It directly passes to the portal vein and taken to liver.*

2. Fatty Acids (FA): Behaviour of absorption of FA differs according to the carbon contents.

- Short-chain FA and medium-chain FA (less than 8 to 10 C) and unsaturated FA ***are absorbed to portal blood directly and taken to liver.***
- Normally, all FFA present in the intestinal wall are ultimately reincorporated in TG after activtion.
- Some of absorbed FA, more than 10C atoms in lengths, irrespective of the form, in which they are absorbed, are found as "esterified FA" in the lymph of the lacteals, which passes through thoracic duct to systemic circulation.

3. Fate of Resynthesized TG: Re-esterification to form TG molecule takes place in the cisternae of endoplasmic reticulum of the mucosal cells. Resynthesized TG cannot pass to lymphatics (lacteals) nor to portal blood as it is insoluble in water (hydrophobic). ***Hence, it is converted to water soluble lipoprotein complex called chylomicrons.*** Each droplet of hydrophobic and water insoluble TG gets covered with a layer of hydro-

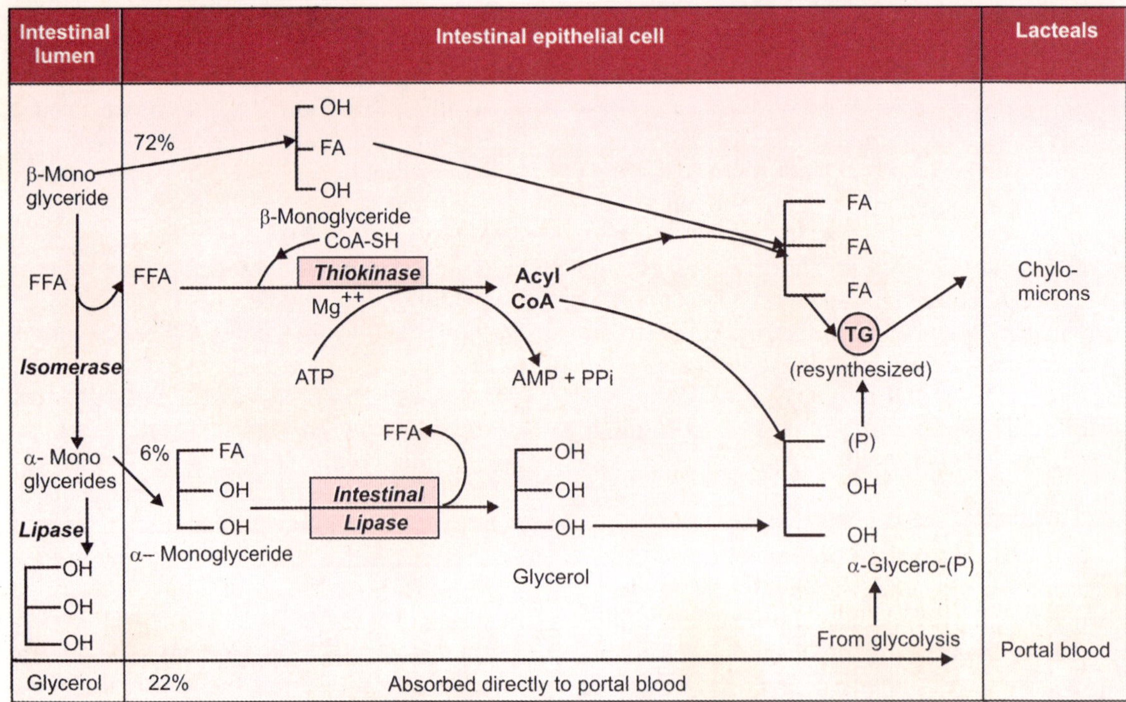

Fig. 11.3: Resynthesis of TG in intestinal epithelial cells

philic PL, cholesterol/cholesterol esters and an apoprotein called *apo-B_{48}. Addition of the "polar" ions make it relatively soluble and hydrophilic.*

Chylomicrons: They are synthesized in the intestinal wall. Size of chylomicrons range from 0.075 to 1 mμ (average 0.5 mμ in diameter)

- It is composed largely of TG, cholesterol (both "free" and esterified), PL and a smaller percent less than 2 percent, of specific protein, called "**apo-B_{48}**".
- Average composition of chylomicron molecule is 87 to 88 percent TG, about 8 percent PL, about 3 percent free/and esterified cho-lesterol, and 0.5 percent to 2 percent specific "apo-B_{48}" protein.
- Chylomicrons pass out through the cell membrane of bases and lateral walls of intestinal epithelial cells, and moves through extracellular spaces between those cells to enter lymphatic vessels of abdominal region, and later goes to systemic circulation through the thoracic duct.

DIGESTION AND ABSORPTION OF CHOLESTEROL:

- Pancreatic juice contains an enzyme ***cholesterol esterase***, which may either catalyze the esterification of free cholesterol with FA or it may also catalyze the opposite reaction, i.e. hydrolysis of cholesterol esters. In the intestinal lumen, depending on the equilibrium, the "cholesterol-esters" are hydrolyzed by this enzyme. ***Thus, cholesterol appears to be absorbed from the intestine almost entirely in "free" (unesterified) form.*** Nevertheless, 85 to 90 percent of the cholesterol in the lymph is found to be in esterified form, indicating that esterification of cholesterol, like that of FFA, must take place within the intestinal mucosal cell.
- Certain plant sterols like sitosterol and stigmasterol are not absorbed, rather their presence can inhibit cholesterol absorption. (Thus acts as cholesterol lowering agents).

DIGESTION AND ABSORPTION OF PHOSPHOLIPIDS:

- Dietary phospholipids may be absorbed from intestine without any digestion. Due to its polar structure and hydrophilic properties, they are ***absorbed directly to portal blood and taken to liver.***
- Pancreatic juice contains an enzyme called ***phospholipase A_2* (or *lecithinase*)**. It is an *esterase,* and secreted as an inactive zymogen "proenzyme", which is changed to active form by hydrolysis of a peptide molecule with the help of *trypsin.*
- In the presence of bile salts and Ca^{++}, the active *phospholipase* B_2 hydrolyzes the ester linkage between a FA and secondary alcohol group of position 2 of glycerol in a phospholipid molecule so that free FA and lysophospholipid are formed and are absorbed. Some lysophospholipid may be resynthesized to PL again in mucosal cell.
- Some PL is incorporated in "chylomicrons" synthesis and also for VLDL synthesis in intestinal mucosal cell and carried in lymphatic vessels.

DIGESTION OF PROTEINS

Dietary Proteins: Proteins which we take in our diet are either from animal source or vegetable source.

- ***Animal sources:*** Milk and dairy products, meat,fish, liver, eggs.
- ***Vegetable sources:*** Cereals, pulses, peas and beans, nuts.

DIGESTION IN MOUTH

There are ***no proteolytic enzymes in mouth***. After mastication and chewing, the bolus of food reaches stomach where it meets the gastric juice.

DIGESTION IN STOMACH

Gastric juice contains a number of proteolytic enzymes. They are:

- *Pepsin,*
- *Rennin,*
- *Gastriscin,*
- *Gelatinase.*

1. **Pepsin:** It is a potent proteolytic enzyme and is present in gastric juice of different species including the mammals.

- It is secreted as inactive ***zymogen*** form, ***pepsinogen,*** having a mol wt of 42,500 approx. it is synthesized in **"chief cells"** of stomach, and 99 percent is poured in gastric juice as *pepsinogen*. Remaining 1 percent is secreted in the blood stream from where it is ultimately excreted in the urine. ***Urinary pepsin is known as uropepsin.***
- Pepsinogen is hydrolyzed in the stomach with the help of HCl or pepsin itself ***(autocatalytically)*** to form the "**active**" ***pepsin*** (mol wt = 34,500).
- In the process of activation,
  - An inactive peptide called as ***"pepsin inhibitor".*** (mol wt 3242), and
  - 5 smaller peptides are liberated.

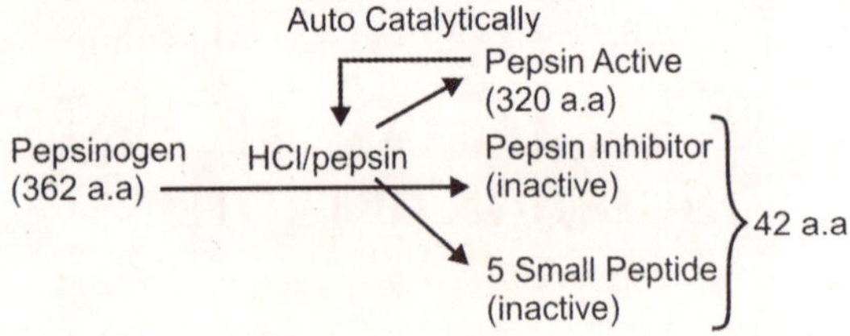

- HCl maintains the gastric pH at about 1 to 2 and ensures maximum pepsin activity. Optimum pH for pepsin is 1.6 to 2.5 and pepsin gets denatured if the pH is greater than 5.
- ***Pepsin is a proteinase,*** a nonspecific endopeptidase, and it hydrolyzes peptide bonds well inside the protein molecule and produces *proteoses* and *peptones*.

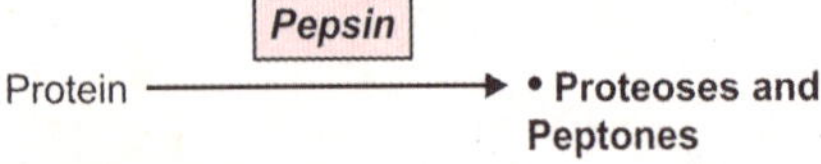

- Pepsin cannot act on proteins like keratins, silkfibroins, mucoproteins, mucoids, and protamines.

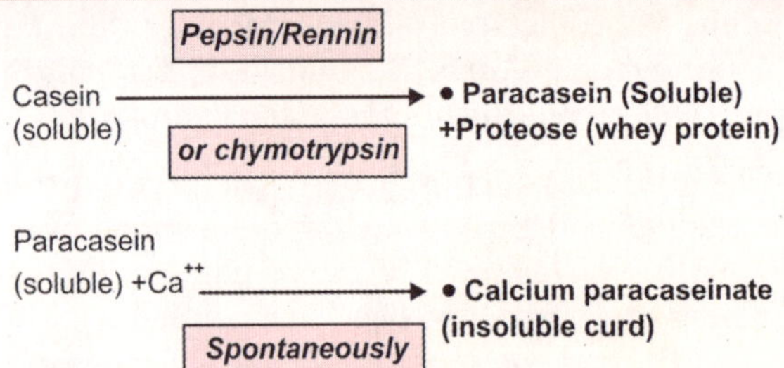

Action of Pepsin on Milk: Pepsin can act on milk. It hydrolyzes the soluble phosphoprotein "casein" of milk to produce ***"paracasein"*** and a proteose, the latter is the whey protein. Paracasein is then precipitated as ***"ca-paracaseinate"*** which is further digested by pepsin to peptones.

2. **Action of Rennin:** ***Rennin is absent in adult humans,*** and many non-ruminants. Certain amount of rennin activity is seen in babies in infancy. In the calf, it is secreted in zymogen form ***prorennin,*** which is activated in the stomach to form ***active rennin*** (mol wt 40,000) and in the process of activation an inactive peptide is split off. Optimum pH for activity is 4.0 and specificity of action is very similar to pepsin, in that it ***hydrolyzes peptide bonds connected with L-aromatic amino acids.*** Like pepsin, it also acts on casein of milk to form paracasein which is immediately precipitated by Ca^{++}. Thus it also coagulates milk like *pepsin* (see above).

3. **Gastricin:** The enzyme is secreted in the gastric juice of humans as inactive zymogen form, which is activated in presence of HCI. Optimum pH is 3 to 4. It acts as *Proteinase* and requires an acidic medium for its activity.

4. **Gelatinase:** Gelatin is hydrolyzed by the enzyme *gelatinase* present in gastric juice to form polypeptides. It acts in an acidic medium.

DIGESTION IN DUODENUM

The bolus of blood after leaving stomach reaches duodenum, where it meets with pancreatic juice. A number of proteolytic enzymes are present in pancreatic juice to act on proteins and partly digested products. Chief enzymes are:

- *Trypsin,*
- *Chymotrypsin,*
- *Carboxy peptidases,*
- *Elastases, and Collagenases.*

1. Trypsin: Trypsin, a ***proteinase***, is secreted as an inactive zymogen form ***trypsinogen***, which is activated to form ***active Trypsin***, which has strong proteolytic activity and an inactive hexapeptide which is produced and liberated during the process of activation ***(Fig. 11.4).***

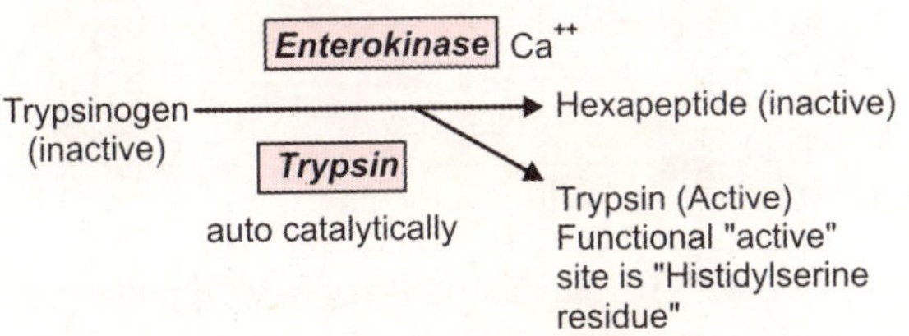

Fig. 11.4: Process of activation of trypsin

- Activation is brought about by:
  - A glycoprotein enzyme known as ***entero kinase*** of the intestinal juice at a pH of 5.5 and
  - Also by ***trypsin itself*** once it is formed, ***autocatalytically***, at a pH of 7.9.
  - Ca^{++} also is required for the activation.
- Trypsin acts in an alkaline medium pH 8 to 9 (optimum pH 7.9).

Note:

- Though trypsin is a strong proteolytic enzyme, it cannot hydrolyze any peptide bond with proline residue.
- ***Trypsin-inhibitors:***
  Our food may contain trypsin-inhibitors, for example;
  - Egg-white contains water soluble muco-protein, a very potent trypsin inhibitor,
  - Human and bovine colostrum and raw soyabeans have also been shown to contain trypsin inhibitors.
  - Trypsin inhibitors have also been reported recently from lung tissues and blood.
  - Experimentally, trypsin can be inhibited by di-iso propylfluorophosphate (DEP).

2. Chymotrypsin: Chymotrypsin, a ***proteinase*** is secreted as inactive zymogen ***chymotrypsinogen***, which is activated by trypsin and completed by chymotrypsin which ***acts autocatalytically. Three chymotrypsinogens A, B and C are found in pancreatic juice*** of vertebrates. During its activation two inactive peptides are liberated in two stages:

- Seryl-arginine dipeptide (a.a 14 to 15) and
- Threonyl-asparagine (a.a 147 and 148)

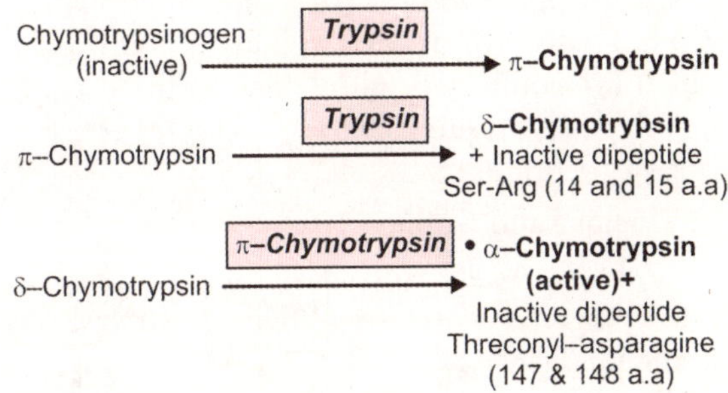

α-Chymotrypsin: Also included under ***serine proteases*** like trypsin.

- Optimum pH = 7 to 8
- α-Chymotrypsin converts the proteoses, peptones and peptides to smaller peptides and amino acids.

Action of Chymotrypsin on Milk: α-Chymotrypsin can hydrolyze milk protein casein to paracasein and a proteose (whey protein). Paracasein is then precipitated by a spontaneous reaction with Ca^{++} and forms Ca-paracaseinate.

3. Carboxypeptides: There are **two types** of carboxy peptidases.

- *Carboxypeptidase A*
- *Carboxypeptidase B*

a. ***Carboxy Peptidase A***: It is a metallo-enzyme, contains zinc (*Zn-protein).*

- Secreted as inactive zymogen ***Pro-carboxy peptidase A,*** which has three subunits, III, II, and I.
  - Trypsin converts subunit II to a proteinase and subunit III is degraded.
  - Then both trypsin and proteinase formed from subunit II, changes subunit I of

procarboxy peptidase A to *active carboxy peptidase A* (see ahead).

- It is an *exopeptidase* and cannot act on peptide bonds well inside the protein molecule. ***The enzyme hydrolyzes the terminal peptide bond*** connected to an end a.a bearing free α-COOH group, particularly if the end a.a is ***Tyr, Phe or Trypt. It liberates the end a.a as "free" form, so that the peptide becomes shorter by one a.a.***

b. ***Carboxypeptidase B***: It is also an ***"exopeptidase"***. Also hydrolyzes terminal peptide bonds, which are connected with "basic" amino acids e.g. *Arg, lysine* bearing free COOH gr. (cf. Carboxypeptidase A)

4. Elastase and Collagenase

*a. **Elastase***: A serine protease. Secreted as inactive zymogen ***proelastase***. Activated by trypsin to ***active elastase***.

- The enzyme has maximum activity on peptide bonds connected to carbonyl groups of neutral aliphatic a.a.

*b. **Collagenase***: An enzyme which can act on proteins present in collagen.

Both the enzymes can digest yellow and white connective tissue fibres respectively to yield peptides.

Formation of active carboxy peptidase

Procarboxypeptidase A
↓
3 subunits III, II and I
↓ *Trypsin*
Subunit III is degraded | Subunit II is changed to active proteinase
↓ + *Trypsin*
Subunit I | Active Carboxypeptidase A (Exopeptidase)

DIGESTION IN SMALL INTESTINE

Proteolytic enzymes present in intestinal juice are

- *Enterokinase*
- *Amino peptidases*
- *Prolidase*
- *and tri and Di-peptidases.*

1. Enterokinase: Also Known as *enteropeptidase*. A glycoprotein enzyme, also present in the epithelial cells of brushborder of duodenal mucosa and secreted in duodenum.

- **Action:** It converts trysinogen to active trypsin.

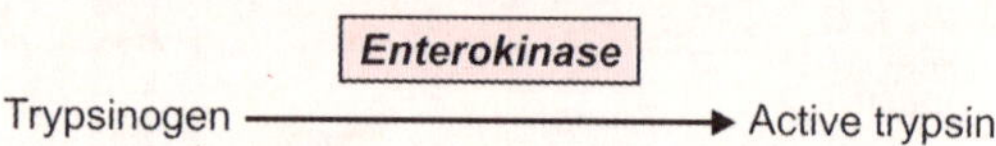

- Ca^{++} is required for this activation.
- ***Bile salts*** help in liberation of ***enterokinase*** from the brush border membrane of intestinal epithelial cells to intestinal lumen.

2. Aminopeptidases: Best example of aminopeptidase is LAP (leucine aminopeptidase)

- Can hydrolyze peptides to tripeptides.
- Cannot hydrolyze a dipeptide
- Requires presence of Zn^{++}, Mn^{++} and Mg^{++} which help in formation of a metal-enz-substrate coordination complex for the catalysis.

3. Prolidase: An *exopeptidase*, can hydrolyze a proline peptide of collagen molecule, acts on terminal peptide bond connected to proline as end a.a, liberating a proline molecule.

4. Tri and Di-peptidases: These enzymes hydrolyze the peptides at either of two places:

- In microvillus membrane of intestinal epithelial cells, or
- Inside the epithelial cells after the peptides have been absorbed inside the cell.

- ***Tri-peptidase*** acts on a tripeptide and produces a dipeptide and free a.a.
- A ***dipeptidase*** hydrolyzes a dipeptide to produce two molecules of amino acids.
- They require the presence of Mn^{++}, Co^{++}, or Zn^{++} as cofactors for their activity.

ABSORPTION OF AMINO ACIDS

Under normal circumstances, the dietary proteins are almost completely digested to their constituent amino acids. But some amounts of oligopeptides like tri and dipeptides may remain as such. The above products of digestion are rapidly absorbed.

Site of Absorption: ***Amino acids are absorbed from ileum and distal jejunum.*** Oligopeptides like di and tri peptides are absorbed from duodenum and proximal jejunum.

How they Reach Liver?: Amino acids and other products of digestion like di- and tripeptides, if any, after absorption are carried by portal blood to Liver. There is a marked rise in amino acid level in portal blood after a protein meal.

Rate of Absorption: There is difference in rate of absorption from the intestine of the two isomers.

- ***L-amino acids and L-peptides are absorbed more rapidly than D-isomers*** and they have been shown to be absorbed by ***active transport*** process. *L*-aminoacids are actively transported across the intestine from mucosa to serosal surface. Pyridoxal-(P) (B_6-PO_4) is probably involved in this process.
- *D*-amino acids are absorbed slowly and they are absorbed by ***simple passive diffusion.***

Mechanism of Absorption of L-amino acids-Ion gradient hypothesis:

L-amino acids are absorbed from small intestine by ***sodium (Na^+) dependent, carrier-mediated process.*** This transport is ***energy dependent*** and ***energy is provided by ATP*** (similar to absorption of glucose and galactose).

Note: Different classes of *L*-amino acids viz. diamino acids, small neutral a.a., iminoacids, and large neutral a.a are believed to be absorbed by different "carrier" protein molecules present in the microvillus membrane of intestinal cells.

- High concentration of one *L*- aminoacid sometimes reduces the rate of absorption of some other *L*- amino acids, indicating several *L*-amino acids may share a common "carrier" molecule and may compete with each other.
- Basic and dicarboxylic aminoacids are generally more slowly absorbed than neutral amino acids.

Absorption of *L*-Oligopeptides: *L*- oligopeptides are ***also actively transported.*** Intracellular peptidases hydrolyze them into a.a. This hydrolysis within the intestinal epithelial cells is rapid enough to keep peptide concentration low in these cells. Transport mechanisms for *L*-peptides appear to be independent of *L-amino acids.*

Role of Glutathione in Amino Acid Absorption: **Meister** has proposed that ***glutathione participates in an "active group translocation" of L-amino acids (except L-proline)*** into the cells of small intestine, kidneys, seminal vesicles, epididymis and brain. He proposed a **"cyclic"** pathway, in which the glutathione is regenerated again, and it is called as ***γ-glutamyl cycle (Fig. 11.5).***

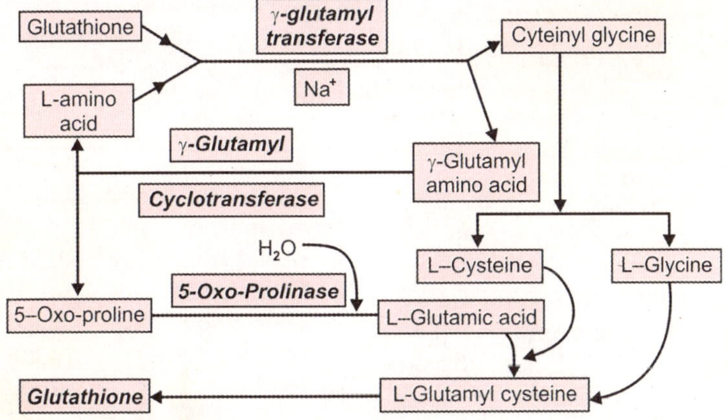

Fig. 11.5: Shows diagrammatically-γ-Glutamyl cycle

☞ SALIENT POINTS TO REMEMBER

- Digestion is a process that converts complex large molecules foodstuffs to simpler ones by the enzymes present in the G.I. tract so that they can be readily absorbed.
- Stomach, duodenum and upper part of small intestine are the major sites of digestion. The small intestine is the principal site for the absorption of digested foods.
- The digestion of carbohydrates is initiated in the mouth by *α-amylase* present in the saliva, but duration of stay of food is very short.
- It is completed in the duodenum and the small intestine by the *α-amylase* present in Pancreatic juice and the disaccharidases (*Sucrase, maltase* and *lactase*) respectively.
- Monosaccharides - Glucose, galactose and fructose are the final absorbable products of carbohydrate digestion.
- Glucose and Galactose are absorbed rapidly from the small intestine by a 'carrier mediated, Na^+ - dependant, energy requiring process. ***("active" transport).***
- Fructose is absorbed by ***"facilitated"*** transport which requires a "carrier" protein but ***does not require any energy.***
- Digestion of lipids occurs in the duodenum and small intestine. Digestion in mouth and stomach is limited.
- ***Lingual lipase*** is secreted by the dorsal surface of the tongue (Ebner's glands). Its activity is continued in the stomach and is more active on TG having shorter F.A. chains.
- ***Emulsification of lipids brought about by bile salts, is a prerequisite of the digestion of fats.***
- ***Pancreatic Lipase,*** aided by a colipase degrades T.G. to diglyceride and then to monoglycerides.
- β-monoglyceride is converted to α-monoglyceride by an isomerase.
- One-fourth of the ingested fats (25 percent or less) is completely broken down to glycerol and F.A.
- Thus end-products of fat digestion are two monoglycerides β and α, glycerol and 3 FFA.
- Cholesterol esterase and Phospholipases respectively hydrolyze cholesteryl esters and phospholipids.
- Lipid absorption occurs through "mixed micelles", formed by bilesalts in association with producets of lipid digestion (mentioned above).
- In the intestinal mucosal cells, lipids are resynthesized to T.G. from the absorbed components.
- ***T.G. is hydrophobic, it is converted to hydrophillic "chylomicrons"***, a lipoprotein, being packed with P.L., cholesterol and cholesterol esters and a ***specific protein apo-B_{48} (Polar substances).***
- Chylomicrons enter the lymphatic vessels and then through thoracic duct to systemic circulation.
- Free glycerol (22 percent) released in intestinal lumen is not utilized for T.G. in intestinal mucosal cell. It directly passes to the portal vein and taken to liver.
- Protein digestion begins in the stomach by the enzyme "pepsin".
- Pepsin is secreted as inactive zymogen form "Pepsinogen" and converted to active pepsin by dil HCl and autocatalytically.
- Principal pancreatic proteases are trypsin, chymotrypsin and elastase. They are all secreted as inactive zymogen forms.
- Trypsinogen, the inactive form, is activated to 'active trypsin' by the enzyme *"enterokinase"* and then autocatalytically.
- Intestinal proteolytic enzymes are amino peptidases and dipeptidases. They complete the degradation of proteins to amino acids and some dipeptides (may escape).
- The intestinal absorption of amino acids occurs by different transport system and require Na^+ - dependant carrier protein and energy (process similar to active transport of glucose and galactose).
- γ-Glutamyl cycle is a cyclic pathway proposed by Meister which states the role of Glutathione in amino acid absorption. Glutathione participates in an "active group translocation" of L - amino acids, in intestinal epithelial cells. ***Glutathione is regenerated again at the end of the cycle.***

MULTIPLE CHOICE QUESTIONS

Give one correct answer:

1. **Amylase present in saliva is:**
   (a) α amylase (b) β - amylase
   (c) δ - amylase (d) γ - amylase
   (e) None of the above
2. **Which of the following sugars is absorbed by facilitated transport?**
   (a) Glucose (b) Fructose
   (c) Galactose (d) Xylose
   (e) Arabinose
3. **For activity of salivary amylase, which of the following is required as activator?**
   (a) Na^+ ions (b) HCO_3^- ions
   (c) K^+ ions (d) Cl^- ions
   (e) Mg^{++} ions
4. **Which of the following hormone increases the absorption of glucose from G.I. tract?**
   (a) Glucagon
   (b) Insulin
   (c) Gluco-corticoides
   (d) Thyroid hormones
   (e) Progesterone
5. **Delay in the rate of gastric emptying is due to the action of:**
   (a) Enterogastrone (b) Enterokinase
   (c) Gastric Lipase (d) Pancreozymin
   (e) CCK
6. **The absorption of glucose is decreased by the deficiency of:**
   (a) Vitamin A (b) Vitamin D
   (c) Thiamine (d) Riboflavine
   (e) Niacin
7. **Dietary T-Gs are absorbed from the intestinal lumen after hydrolysis mainly as:**
   (a) FFA and glycerol
   (b) FFA and two monoacyl glycerol
   (c) FFA and α, β-diglyceride
   (d) Acyl CoA and glycerol
   (e) Glycerol-P and fatty acids.
8. **Bite salts help in the absorption of dietary lipids by:**
   (a) incorporating cholesterol into chylomicrons
   (b) Converting triglycerides into monoglycerides
   (c) Providing optimum pH for lipase activity
   (d) Producing the "micelles"
   (e) None of the above
9. **Ca^{++} facilitates action of Lipase**
   (a) by emulsification
   (b) by inhibiting emulsion
   (c) by soap formation
   (d) by formation of tiny droplets
   (e) None of the above
10. **The milk protein in the stomach in an adult is digested by:**
    (a) Pepsin (b) Rennin
    (c) Trypsin (d) HCl
    (e) Gastriscin
11. **The zymogen form trypsinogen of pancreatic juice is converted to 'active' trypsin by:**
    (a) Pepsin (b) Enterokinase
    (c) enterokrinin (d) dil HCl
    (e) Rennin
12. **Pancreatic juice contains all of the following *except:***
    (a) Lipase (b) Trypsinogen
    (c) Amylase (d) Elastase
    (e) Amino peptidases
13. **Active chymotrypsin is:**
    (a) π-chymotrypsin
    (b) γ - chymotrypsin
    (c) α - chymotrypsin
    (d) δ - chymotrypsin
    (e) all of the above
14. **Rennin acts on casein of milk in infants in presence of:**
    (a) Mg^{++} (b) Ca^{++}
    (c) Zn^{++} (d) Mn^{++}
    (e) Co^{++}

ANSWERS

1. (a)	2. (b)	3. (d)
4. (d)	5. (b)	6. (c)
7. (b)	8. (d)	9. (c)
10. (a)	11. (b)	12. (e)
13. (c)	14. (b)	

Metabolism of Carbohydrates

INTRODUCTION

Utilization of Glucose in the Body-General Outline

After absorption of monosaccharides into the portal blood, it **passes through the liver (the first "filter") before entering the systemic circulation,** a fact of considerable physiological and biochemical importance.

In liver, two mechanisms operate:

- ***"Withdrawal"*** of carbohydrates from blood.
- ***"Release"*** of glucose by liver to the blood.

These two mechanisms are shown in ***Table 12.1.*** All the above processes are finely regulated in the liver cells, control exerted at substrate level, by the end products and by hormones. ***The amount of glucose reaching the systemic circulation at any instant, will be the resultant of operation of these two groups of opposing forces.*** Once glucose is in systemic circulation, it becomes available for its utilization by ***"extrahepatic tissues".*** Thus, extrahepatic tissues are presented with carbohydrates which have already been "picked over" by the liver in a selective manner. ***Hence functional state of the liver will be prime importance*** and will have a profound influence on the carbohydrate metabolism on the entire organism. Glucose is taken up by intestinal mucosal cells and kidney tubule cells by "active" transport. ***Hepatic cells are freely permeable to glucose.*** Insulin increases uptake of glucose by many extrahepatic tissues as skeletal muscle, heart muscle, diaphragm, adipose tissue, lactating mammary gland, etc.

Utilization of Glucose

1. Oxidation

- ***For provision of energy:*** In response to physiological needs, human body requires energy. Oxidation of glucose or glycogen to pyruvate and lactate by EM pathway is called ***"glycolysis".*** Glucose is degraded in this

Table 12.1: Mechanisms operating in liver

Withdrawal of carbohydrates from blood	*Release of glucose by liver to the blood*
• Uptake of hexoses by liver cells such as galactose and fructose and their conversion to glucose by liver cells.	• Formation of blood glucose from hexoses other than glucose by liver and its release from liver cells.
• Conversion of glucose to glycogen for storage in liver (*"glycogenesis"*).	• Conversion of liver glycogen to blood glucose (*"Glycogenolysis"*).
• Utilization of glucose, by oxidation (*glycolysis*) for energy production.	• Formation of blood glucose by the liver from non-carbohydrate sources, viz. amino acids (glucogenic), pyruvates and lactates, glycerol and propionyl CoA (*"Gluconeogenesis"*).
• Utilization of glucose for synthesis of other compounds, viz. FA and certain amino acids.	

pathway to pyruvate, which in presence of O_2 is completely oxidized to CO_2 and H_2O. ***Glycolysis occurs in all tissues.***

- *HMP shunt:* An alternative pathway for oxidation of glucose. ***It is not meant for energy.*** The pathway **provides NADPH** which is used for reductive synthesis and **pentoses** which is used for nucleic acids synthesis. This pathway ***operates only in certain special tissues and not all tissues.***
- *Uronic acid pathway:* This is another alternative pathway for oxidation of glucose. It **provides D-glucuronic acid** which is used for synthesis of mucopolysaccharides and conjugation reaction.

2. *Storage:* Excess of glucose taken is converted to glycogen in various tissues *(glycogenesis)* specially liver and skeletal muscle and stored there for future needs. **Amount of glycogen storage in liver and muscles is limited.** Liver can store approximately 108 gm (5 to 6% of the weight of liver) and muscles can store approximately 245 gm (0.7% of total weight).

3. *Conversion to Fats:* As mentioned above, since the amount of glycogen that can be stored is limited, excess of glucose is converted to FA and stored as "triacyl glycerol" (TG) in fat depots **(lipogenesis).**

4. *Conversion to Other Carbohydrates:* Small amounts of glucose are used directly or indirectly, in the synthesis of certain other carbohydrates or derivatives, which play important role in the body.

- ***Formation of ribose and deoxy ribose***: This is required for synthesis of nucleic acids. It is formed by HMP shunt.
- ***Formation of fructose from glucose***: Seminal fluid is rich in fructose and it is required for the metabolism of spermatozoa. Fructose is formed from glucose in seminiferous tubular epithelial cells by "sorbitol" (polyol) pathway.
- ***Mannose, fucose, glucosamine and neuraminic acid***: Form parts of mucopolysaccharides (MPS) and glycoproteins.
- ***Galactose***: A component part of glycolipids. Galactose required for synthesis of lactose (milk sugar) in lactating mammary gland is synthesized from glucose.
- ***D-Glucuronic acid:*** Required in the formation of mucopolysaccharides (MPS) and in conjugation reaction for detoxication. It is produced in the body from glucose by uronic acid pathway.

5. *Conversion to Amino Acids:* Certain amino acids are not required in the diet, although they occur in tissue proteins. These amino acids are synthesized in the body. This group is called as "dispensable" or "non-essential amino acids".

Fat of Glucose and its Utilization

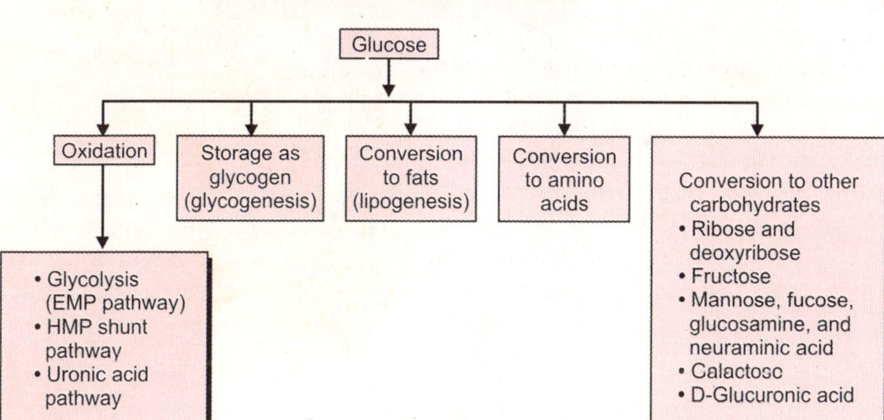

The C-skeletons of such amino acids are derived form glucose or its metabolites.

GLYCOLYSIS

Definition: Oxidation of glucose or glycogen to pyruvate and lactate is called glycolysis.

Note:

- This was described by **Embden, Meyerhof and Parnas.** Hence it is also called as *Embden-Meyerhof-Parnas pathway.*
- It *occurs virtually in all tissues.* Erythrocytes and nervous tissues derive their energy mainly from glycolysis.
- This pathway is unique in the sense that it can utilise O_2, if available, (*aerobic*) and it can function in absence of O_2 also (*anaerobic*). Anaerobic phase limits the amount of energy per mol of glucose oxidized. ***Hence, to provide a given amount of energy, more glucose must undergo glycolysis under anaerobic as compared to aerobic.***
- *Enzymes:* Enzymes involved in glycolysis are *extramitochondrial*.

BIOMEDICAL IMPORTANCE

- This pathway is *meant for provision of energy.*
- *Heart muscle* as compared to skeletal muscle, is adapted for aerobic performance. It has relatively poor glycolytic activity and poor survival under conditions of ischaemia.
- *Role in cancer therapy:* In fast-growing cancer cells, rate of glycolysis is very high. It produces more pyruvic acid (PA) than TCA cycle can handle. Accumulation of pyruvic acid leads to excessive formation of lactic acid producing ***local lactic acidosis. Local acid environment may be congenial for certain cancer therapy.***
- *Haemolytic anaemias:* Inherited enzyme deficiencies like hexokinase deficiency and pyruvate kinase deficiency in glycolytic pathway enzymes can produce haemolytic anaemia.

REACTIONS OF GLYCOLYTIC PATHWAY

Series of reactions of glycolytic pathway ***(Fig. 12.1)*** which degrades glucose/glycogen to pyruvate/lactate are discussed below. For discussion and proper understanding, the various reactions can be arbitrarily divided ***into four stages.***

Stage I: This is ***a preparatory stage.*** Before the glucose molecule can be split, the rather ***asymmetric glucose molecule is converted to almost symmetrical form*** fructose-1,6-biphosphate by donation of $2PO_4$ groups from ATP.

1. ***Uptake of Glucose by Cells and its Phosphorylation***

- **Glucose is freely permeable to liver cells.** In intestinal mucosa and kidney tubules, Glucose is taken up by "active" transport.
- In other tissues, like skeletal muscle, cardiac muscle, diaphragm, adipose tissue, etc. Insulin facilitates the uptake of glucose.
- Glucose is then phosphorylated to form glucose-6-P. The reaction is catalyzed by the specific enzyme ***glucokinase*** in liver cells and by non-specific ***hexokinase*** in liver and extra hepatic tissues.

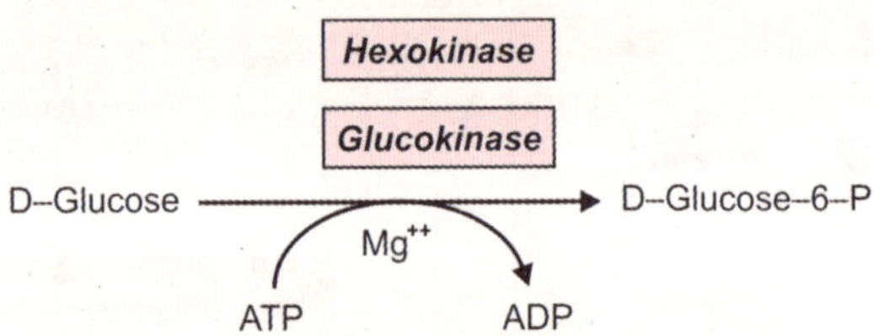

Note:

- Reaction is ***"irreversible"***.
- ATP acts as PO_4 donor. One high energy PO_4 bond is utilized and ADP is produced.
- Glucose-6-P formed is an important compound at the junction of several metabolic pathways like glycolysis, glycogenesis, glycogenolysis, gluconeogenesis, HMP shunt, uronic acid pathway. Thus, it is a ***committed step*** in metabolic pathways.

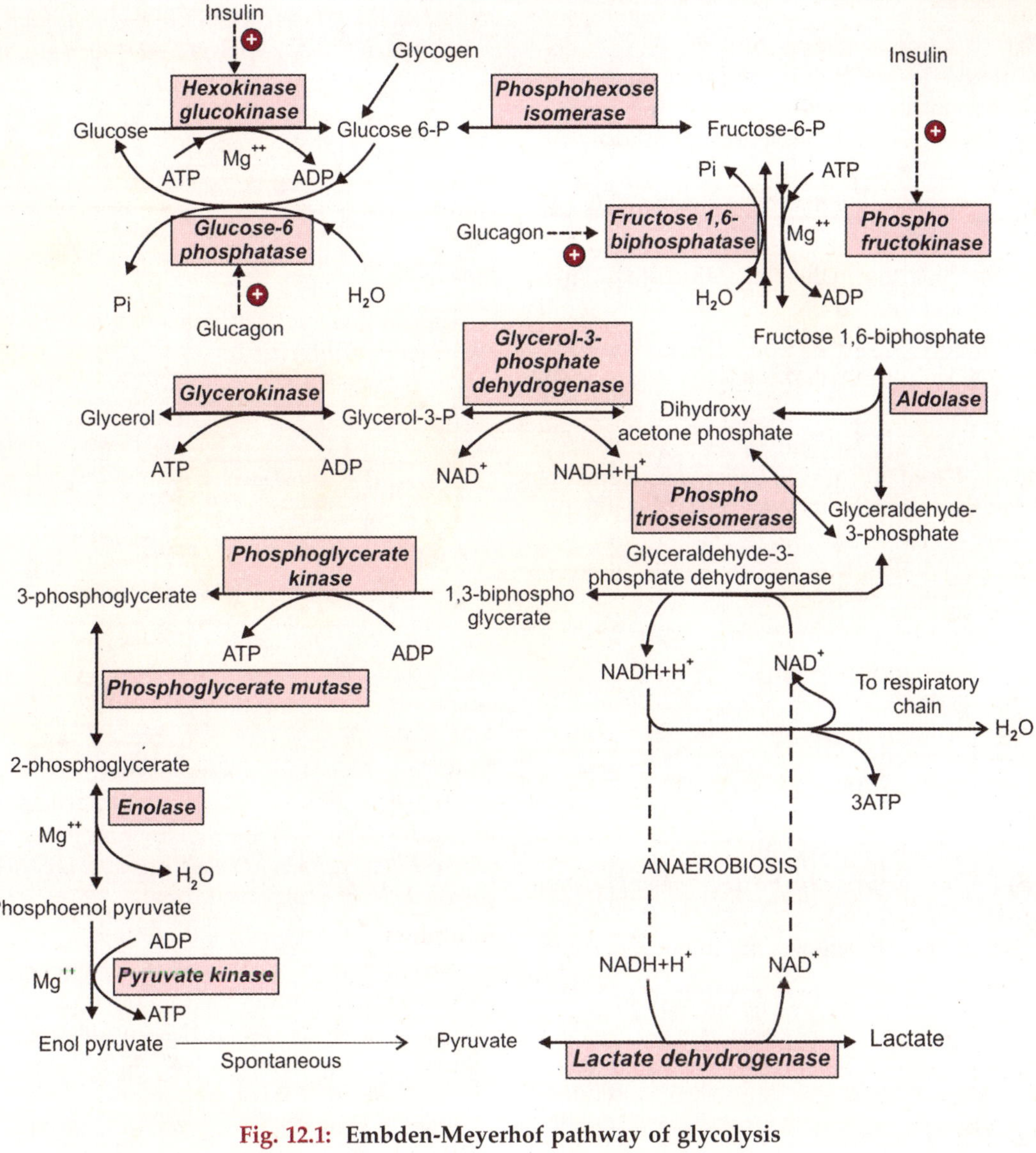

Fig. 12.1: Embden-Meyerhof pathway of glycolysis

2. ***Conversion of G-6-P to Fructose 6-P:*** G-6-P after formation is converted to fructose 6-P by ***phosphohexose isomerase.***

3. ***Conversion of Fructose-6-P to Fructose-1-6-bi-P:*** The above reaction is followed by another phosphorylation. Fructose-6-P is phosphorylated with ATP at 1 –position catalyzed by the enzyme ***phosphofructokinase-I*** to produce the symmetrical molecule fructose-1,6-biphosphate.

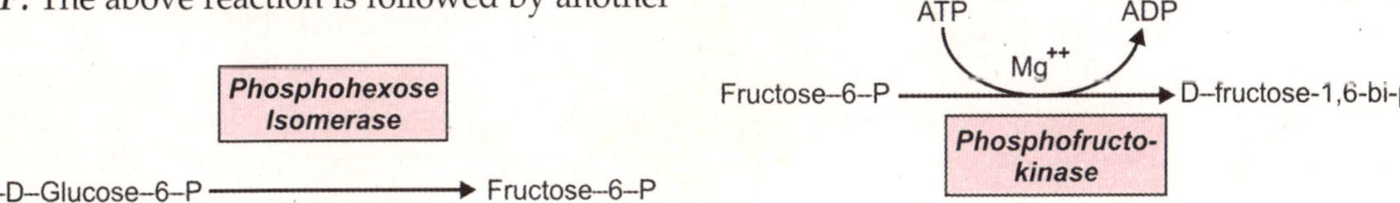

Note:

- The reaction is *irreversible*
- One ATP is utilized for phosphorylation
- Phosphofructokinase-1 is the ***key enzyme*** in glycolysis which regulates breakdown of glucose.
- The enzyme is ***inducible*** as well as allosterically modified.

Energetic: Note that in this stage, glucose oxidation does not yield any useful energy rather there is **expenditure of two ATP molecules for two phosphorylations (-2 ATP).**

–2ATP

Stage II: ***Actual Splitting of Symmetrical Fructose 1-6-bi-P***: It is split by the *enzyme aldolase* into two molecules of triose-phosphates-an aldotriose glyceraldehyde-3-P, and one ketotriose dihydroxy acetone-P.

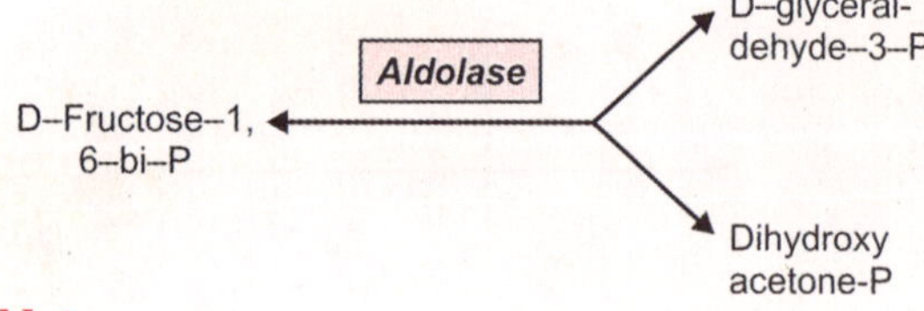

Note:

- The reaction is **reversible**
- There is ***neither expenditure of energy nor formation of ATP.***
- Both triose phosphates are interconvertible.

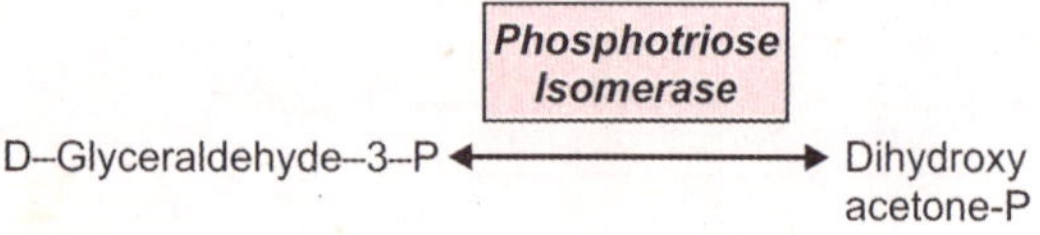

Stage III: ***It is the Energy-Yielding Reaction.*** Reaction of this type in which ***an aldehyde group is oxidized to an acid is accompanied by liberation of large amounts of potentially useful energy.***

This stage consists of the following **two reactions:**

1. ***Oxidation of Glyceraldehyde-3-P to 1,3-Biphosphoglycerate:*** Glycolysis proceeds by the oxidation of glyceraldehyde-3-P to form 1,3-biphosphoglycerate. Dihydroxyacetone-P also forms 1,3-bi-phosphoglycerate via glyceraldehyde-3-P. Enzymes responsible is ***glyceraldehyde-3-P dehydrogenase which is NAD⁺ dependant.***

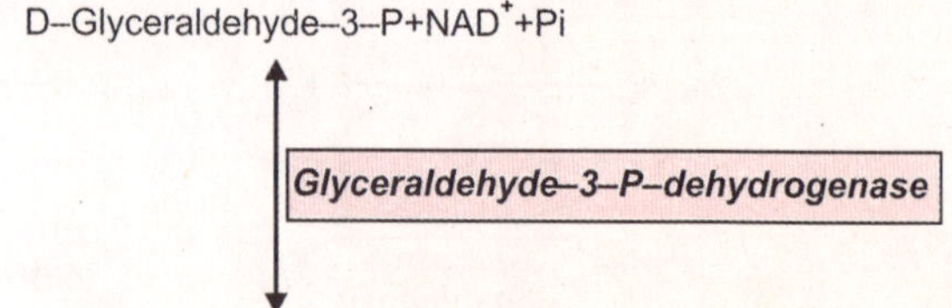

2. ***Conversion of 1,3-Biphosphoglycerate to 3-Phosphoglycerate:***

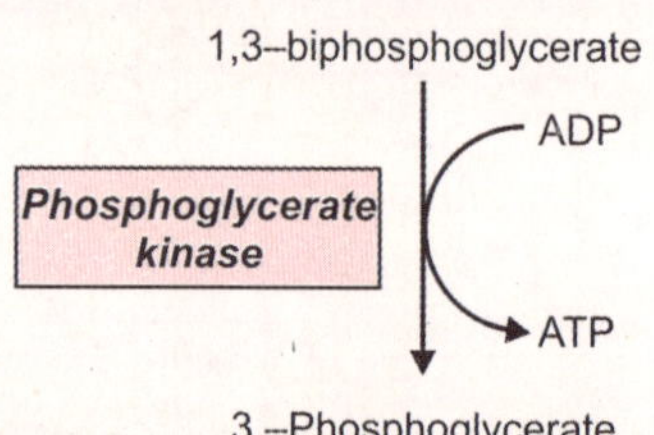

The reaction is catalyzed by the enzyme ***phosphoglycerate Kinase.*** The high energy PO_4 bond at position 1 can donate the PO_4 to ADP and forms ATP molecule.

Note: This is a unique example where ATP can be produced at *substrate level* without participating in electron transport chain. ***This type of reaction where ATP is formed at substrate level is called as substrate level phosphorylation.***

Inhibitors

- ***Arsenite:*** If present, arsenite competes with inorganic Pi in the reaction of conversion of glyceraldehyde-3-P to 1,3-biphosphoglycerate and produces 1-arseno-3-phosphoglycerate which hydrolyzes spontaneously to yield 3-phosphoglycerate and heat. Thus, in the next step no ATP is produced.
- ***Iodoacetate and Iodoacetamide:*** They bind with-SH group and alkylate the-SH group of the enzyme glyceraldehyde-3-P dehydrogenase. They bind irreversibly with the enzyme and inhibits glycolysis. This leads to accumulation of glyceraldehyde-3-P.

Energetics: In first reaction of this stage, NADH produced, in presence of O_2, will be oxidized in electron transport chain to produce 3 ATP. Since two molecules of triose-P are formed per molecule of glucose oxidized, 2 NADH will produce 6 ATP.

+6 ATP

- The second reaction will produce one ATP. Two molecules of substrate will produce 2 ATP.

+ 2 ATP

Net gain at this stage per molecule of glucose oxidized = **+8 ATP.**

Stage IV: It is the ***recovery of the PO_4 group*** from 3-phosphoglycerate. The two molecules of 3-phosphoglycerate, the end-product of the previous stage, still retain the PO_4 group originally derived from ATP in Stage I. ***Body wants back the two ATP spent in first stage for two phosphorylations.***

The above is achieved by the following ***three reactions:***

1. ***Conversion of 3-Phosphoglycerate to 2-Phosphoglycerate:*** 3-Phosphoglycerate formed by the above reaction is converted to 2-phosphoglycerate, catalyzed by the enzyme ***phosphoglycerate mutase.***

2. ***Conversion of 2-Phosphoglycerate to Phosphoenol Pyruvate:*** The reaction is catalyzed by the enzyme ***enolase,*** the enzyme requires the presence of either Mg^{++} or Mn^{++} for activity. The reaction involves ***dehydration*** and ***redistribution of energy*** within the molecule raising the PO_4 in position 2 to a ***"high-energy state".***

3. ***Conversion of Phosphoenol Pyruvate to Pyruvate:*** Phosphoenol pyruvate is converted to "enol" pyruvate, the reaction is *catalyzed* by the enzyme ***pyruvate kinase.*** The high energy PO_4 of phosphoenol pyruvate is directly transferred to ADP producing ATP.

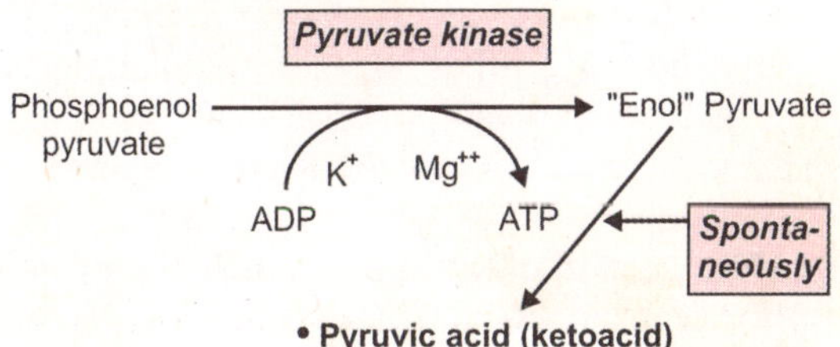

Note:

- Reaction is ***irreversible***
- ATP is formed at the substrate level without electron transport chain. This is another example of ***substrate level phosphorylation*** in glycolytic pathway. "Enol" pyruvate is converted to "Keto" Pyruvate spontaneously.

Inhibitors: Fluoride inhibits the enzyme "enolase".

Clinical Importance

Sodium fluoride is used along with K-oxalate for collection of blood for glucose estimation. If K-oxalate is used alone, then *in vitro* glycolysis will reduce the glucose value in the sample

Functions of fluoride:

- Inhibits in *vitro* glycolysis by inhibiting enzyme *enolase;*
- Also acts as anticoagulant; and
- Antiseptic.

Energetics: In this stage two molecules of ATP are produced per molecule of glucose oxidized.

+2 ATP

ENERGY YIELD PER GLUCOSE MOLECULE OXIDATION

A. In Glycolysis: in Presence of O_2 (Aerobic Phase)

Reaction catalyzed by	*ATP Production*
Stage I	
• Hexokinase/glucokinase reaction (for phosphorylation)	–1 ATP
• Phosphofructokinase-I (for phosphorylation)	–1 ATP
Stage III	
• Glyceraldehyde-3-P dehydrogenase (oxidation of 2 NADH in electron transport chain)	+ 6 ATP
• Phosphoglycerate kinase *(substrate level phosphorylation)*	+ 2 ATP
Stage IV	
• Pyruvate kinase *(substrate level phosphorylation)*	+ 2 ATP
Net gain	= 10 – 2
	= 8 ATP.

B. In Glycolysis: in Absence of O_2 (Anaerobic Phase)

- In absence of O_2, ***re-oxidation of NADH at glyceraldehyde-3-P dehydrogenase stage can not take place in electron transport chain.***
- But the cells have limited coenzymes. Hence to continue the glycolytic cycle, NADH must be oxidized to NAD^+. This is achieved by re-oxidation of NADH by conversion of pyruvate to lactate ***(without producing ATP)***

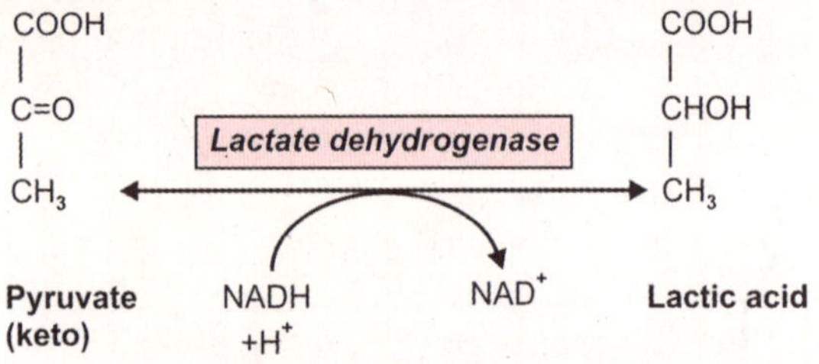

- It is to be noted that in this reaction catalyzed by glyceraldehyde-3-P dehydrogenase, therefore, no ATP is produced.
  In anaerobic phase per molecule of glucose oxidation 4 – 2 = 2 ATP will be produced

+2 ATP

Note:

- ***Tissues that function under hypoxic circumstances will produce lactic acid from glucose oxidation, producing local acidosis. If lactate production is more it can produce metabolic acidosis.***
- Vigorously contracting skeletal muscle will produce realtive anaerobiosis, and glycolysis will produce lactic acid.
- ***Whether O_2 is present or not, glycolysis in erythrocytes always terminate in pyruvate and lactate.***

REGULATIONS OF GLYCOLYSIS

Regulation of glycolysis is achieved by **three types of mechanisms:**

- Changes in the rate of enzyme synthesis-induction/repression.
- Covalent modification by reversible phosphorylation
- Allosteric modification

1. ***Induction and Repression of key Enzymes:*** This is not rapid and takes several hours to come into operation.

- ***Glucose:*** When there is increased substrate, i.e. glucose, the enzymes involved in utilization of glucose are activated, on the other hand enzymes responsible for producing glucose (gluconeogenesis) are inhibited. Glucose also increases the activity of the key enzymes *glucokinase, phosphofructokinase-I and pyruvate kinase.*
- ***Insulin:*** The secretion of insulin which is responsive to blood glucose concentration enhances the synthesis of the key enzymes responsible for glycolysis.

2. ***Covalent Modification by Reversible Phosphorylation:*** Hormones like epinephrine and glucagon which increase c-AMP level activate c-AMP-dependent *protein kinase* which can phosphorylate and inactivate the key enzyme *pyruvate kinase* and, thus, inhibit glycolysis. This is a ***rapid process*** and occurs quickly.

3. ***Allosteric Modification:*** *Phosphofructokinase-I* is the key regulatory enzyme and is subject to "feedback" control.

- ***Inhibition of the enzyme:*** The enzyme is inhibited by citrate and by ATP
- ***Activator of the enzyme:*** The enzyme is activated by AMP.

PECULIARITIES OF GLUCOSE OXIDATION BY RB CELLS

Red blood cells are structurally and metabolically unique as compared to other cells.

A. Structural Peculiarities: Structurally mature erythrocytes do not possess " nucleus" nor "cytoplasmic subcellular structures".

B. Metabolic Peculiarities: Metabolically mature erythrocytes

- ***Entirely depends on glucose for its energy, i.e glycolysis.*** More than 90 percent of total energy is met by glycolysis.
- Glucose is ***freely permeable to erythrocytes*** like liver cells.
- Glucose oxidation always ends in the formation of pyruvic acid (PA) and lactic acid (L,A), wheather O_2 is available or not.

- *The enzyme pyruvate dehydrogenase complex is absent hence pyruvic acid is not converted to "acetyl CoA"*
- Maintains a high steady state concentration of "2,3-biphosphoglycerate-(2,3-BPG)-produced by a diversion in glycolytic pathway.

The diversion is called as *Rapaport-Leubering cycle or shunt*-**(RLC or RLS)**. A supplementary to glycolysis.

FUNCTIONAL SIGNIFICANCE OF THIS SHUNT PATHWAY

1. *Factor which "waste" energy are not present in RB cells:*
   - Energy demanding "endergonic" reactions utilizing ATP is not present in mature human red blood cells.
   - *ATPase* activity which controls ATP/ADP ratio is not active in mature RB cells.

RB cells utilize more glucose than it requires to maintain cellular integrity, resulting in accumulation of ATP and 1,3-BPG, causing cessation of glycolysis. ***RLC or RLS provides a mechanism to dissipate the excess energy.*** RL shunt/cycle is shown in ***Fig.12.2***

2. *Role in Hb:* In adult Hb-A_1, 2,3-BPG concentration is high, affinity to O_2 less and unloading/dissociation is more.

In Hb-F, 2,3-BPG concentration is low, affinity to O_2 is more, and unloading/dissociation is less.

3. *Role in hypoxia:* Tissue hypoxia has an important effect on the level of red cells BPG. Pulmonary hypoxic hypoxia, stagnant hypoxia either as a result of CV failure or shock, and anaemic hypoxia, as in a deficit of red cells mass, ***all favour an increase in red cells BPG level, thus enhancing unloading of O_2 in tissues.***

Behavior of red cells in these inherited deficiencies is shown below:

4. *Inherited enzyme deficiency:* Several hereditary defects in enzyme of red-cell glycolysis that affect red cell BPG concentration, such as rare *"hexokinase deficiency"* and much more commonly occurring *"Pyruvate kinase (PK) deficiency"*, also exhibit alterations of red cells BPG concentration.

	Hexokinase deficient red cells	*Pyruvate kinase deficient red cells*
• *2,3 BPG*	↓	↑
• **Affinity to O_2**	↑	↓
• **Unloading of O_2**	↓	↑

FORMATION AND FATE OF PYRUVIC ACID

1. **Formation of Pyruvic Acid:** Pyruvic acid is a key substance in phase-II metabolism.
   - Principally, it is formed from oxidation of glucose (glycolysis) by EM pathway (discussed above). In addition to that, pyruvic acid can be formed in the body from various other sources. They are:
     - Conversion of lactic acid to pyruvic acid (see below).
     - Also formed from deamination of amino acid alanine.
     - Certain other amino acids during their catabolism produces puruvic acid, e.g. glycine, serine, cysteine/and cystine and threonine.

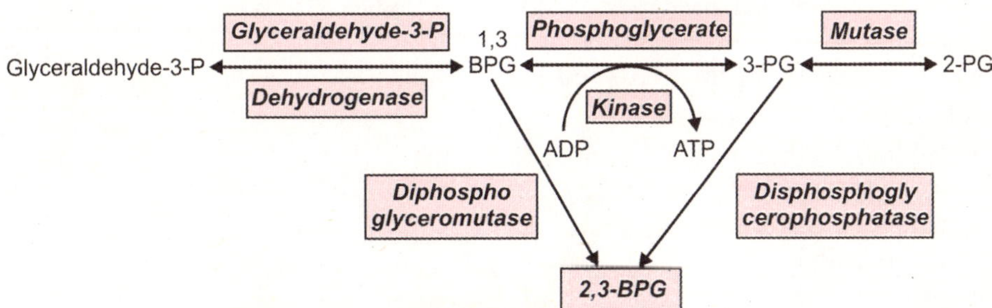

Fig. 12.2: RL shunt/cycle

- Pyruvic acid can also be formed from decarboxylation of dicarboxylic ketoacid "oxaloacetic acid", which can be spontaneous decarboxylation or can be catalyzed by the enzyme *oxaloacetate decarboxylase*.
- Lastly, pyruvic acid can be formed in the body from "malic acid" by **"malic enzyme"**.

2. Fate of Pyruvic Acid: Fate of pyruvic acid *depends on the redox state of the tissues.*

- **In presence of O_2,** pyruvic acid is oxidatively decarboxylated ***to two-carbon unit "acetyl-CoA".***
- **In absence of O_2,** pyruvic acid is converted to lactic acid (LA)

Other fates of pyruvic acid can be summed up as follows:

- Pyruvic acid can be aminated to form the amino acid ***alanine*** (see transamination reaction).
- Pyruvic acid can be converted to form ***glucose*** in the body (see ***gluconeogenesis***).
- Pyruvic acid can be converted to ***malic acid,*** which in turn can form ***oxaloacetic acid (OAA).***
- Pyruvic acid can be converted directly to oxaloacetic acid in the body by "CO_2-fixation" ("CO_2- assimilation") reaction.
  Last two reactions are important in the body as OAA can be formed and supplied to TCA cycle in case of relative deficiency (***"Anaplerotic" reactions***).

Conversion of Pyruvic Acid to Lactic Acid:

- **In anaerobic glycolysis,** pyruvate acts as a temporary H-store. It dehydrogenates (oxidizes), the reduced NADH+H^+ back to oxidized NAD^+, so that glycolysis can continue even in absence of O_2. **Pyruvate is thus reduced to lactic acid.**
- **In presence of O_2,** lactic acid can be oxidized to pyruvic acid again.

  Characteristics of this reaction:
  - *Reversible* reaction
  - Oxidation-reduction
  - Same enzyme and coenzyme required

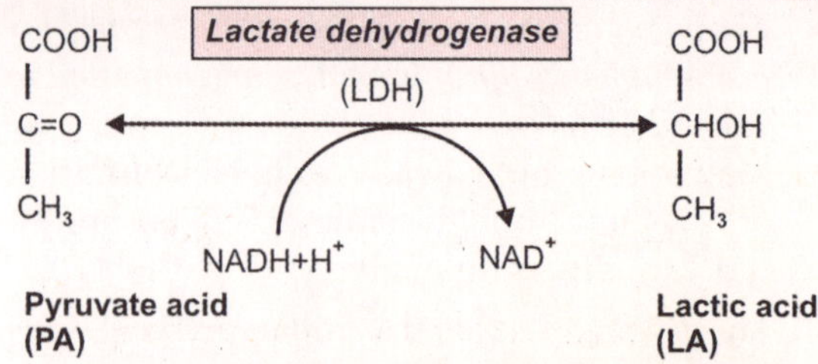

CONVERSION OF PA TO ACETYL-COA:

- **In presence of O_2,** pyruvate undergoes oxidative decarboxylation to form 2-C compound *"acetyl CoA".*
- ***Pyruvate formed in cytosol is transported to mitochondrion by a "transport" protein.***
- Since the overall reaction involves both oxidation and loss of CO_2 (decarboxylation), it is **termed oxidative decarboxylation.** The mechanism of the reaction is one of the most complex involved in metabolism of carbohydrates.
- The reaction is catalyzed by a **multienzyme complex** called ***pyruvate dehydrogenase complex*** which can exist both as ***"inactive form"*** and the ***"active" form*** (see regulation below).
  The enzyme complex consists of:

  29 Molecules of *pyruvate dehydrogenase* (PD)
  +8 Molecules of flavoprotein containing *dihydrolipoyl dehydrogenase*, and
  + 1 Molecule of *dihydrolipoyl transacetylase*

- The enzyme complex for its activity requires at least ***six coenzymes/cofactors:***
  - Thiamine pyrophosphate (TPP)
  - Lipoic acid
  - CoA-SH
  - FAD
  - NAD^+ and
  - Mg^{++}
- The overall reaction can be represented as follows:

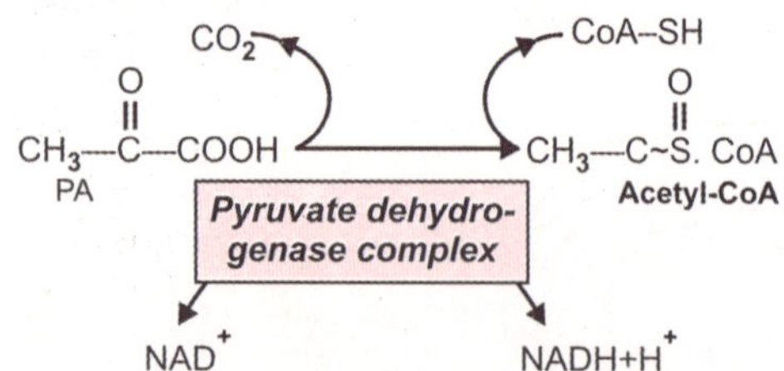

- "Acetyl" moiety of PA is transferred to CoA-SH.
- Carbon of COOH group is liberated as CO_2 (decarboxylation).
- Remaining two H atoms, one from-COOH group of PA and another from CoA-SH.
- SH group are transferred to NAD^+, by way of a mechanism involving lipoic acid and FAD.

Energetics:
- One molecule of glucose produces two molecules of PA which, in turn, by oxidative decarboxylation produces 2 molecules of acetyl CoA and 2 NADH.
- Two molecules of NADH will be oxidized to 2 molecules of NAD^+ producing 6 ATP molecules in respiratory chain.

+ 6 ATP

Regulation: Activation and inactivation of pyruvate dehydrogenase complex (PDH).
- *Conversion of inactive to active PDH:* Insulin, stimulates phosphatase and converts "inactive" to "active" form by dephosphorylation.
- *Conversion of "active" to "inactive" PDH: "PDH kinase"* enzyme is activated by
  - Rise in ATP/ADP ratio ↑
  - $NADH/NAD^+$ ratio ↑
  - Acetyl CoA/CoA-SH ratio ↑
  - Increased cyclic AMP ↑ in cells.

PDH-kinase is inhibited by increased pyruvic acid (PA) by carbohydrate diet, i.e. "active" PDH is formed.

Formation of pyruvate and its fate shown diagrammatically in *Fig. 12.3.*

CITRIC ACID CYCLE

Synonyms: TCA cycle (tricarboxylic acid cycle), Krebs' cycle, Krebs' citric acid cycle

Characteristic Features:

- It is a *cyclic process.* The cycle involves a sequence of compounds interrelated by oxidation-reduction, and other reactions which finally produces CO_2 and H_2O.
- It is the *final common pathway of breakdown/ catabolism of carbohydrates, fats and protein (phase III of metabolism).*
- **Acetyl-CoA** derived mainly from oxidation of either glucose or β-oxidation of FA and partly from certain amino acids, **combines with oxaloacetic acid (OAA) to form *"citrate"*** the first reaction of citric and cycle. In this reaction, acetyl-CoA transfers its acetyl-group (2-C) to OAA.
- By stepwise dehydrogenations and loss of two molecules of CO_2, accompanied by internal rearrangements, the citric acid is reconverted to OAA, which again starts the cycle by taking up another acetyl group from acetyl-CoA. *A very small "catalytic" amount of OAA can*

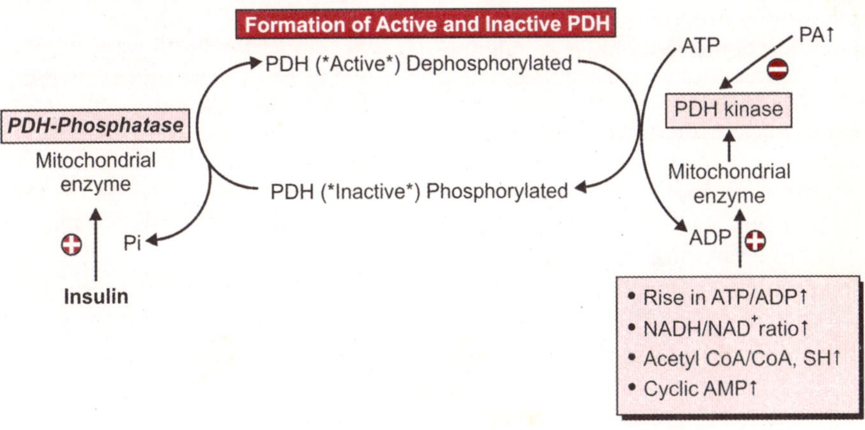

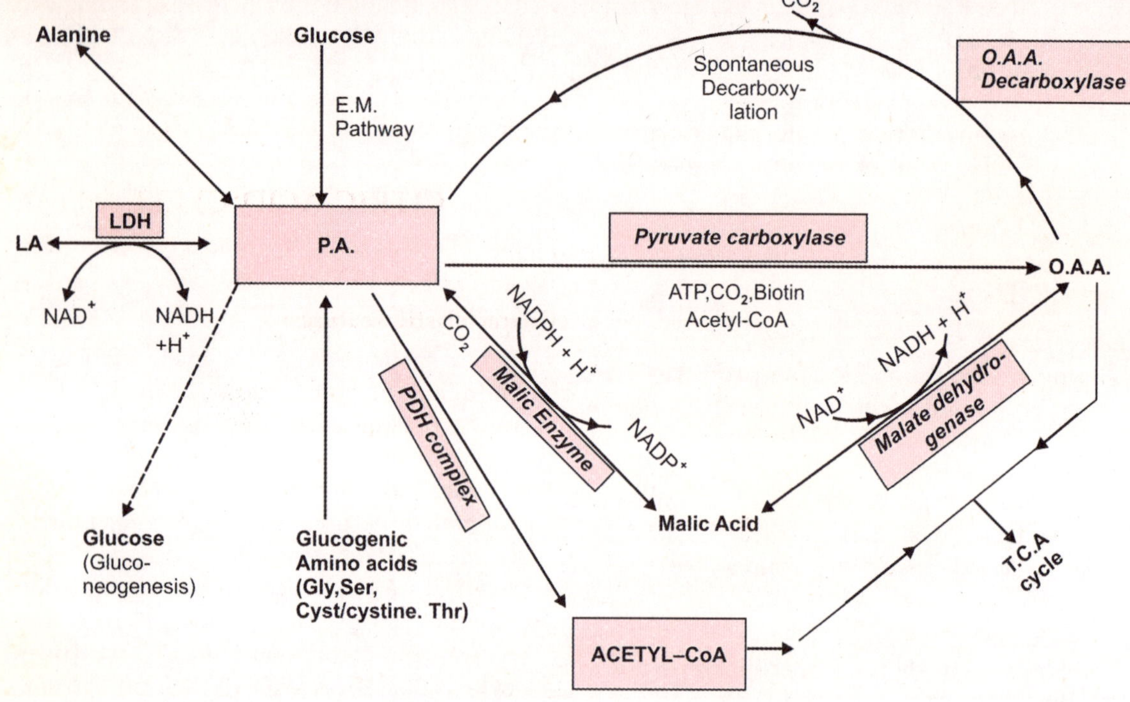

Fig. 12.3: Formation and fate of pyruvic acid

bring about the complete oxidation of active acetate.

- Enzymes are located in ***mitochondrial matrix,*** either free or attached to the inner surface of the inner mitochondrial membrane, which facilitates the transfer of reducing equivalents to the adjacent enzymes of the respiratory chain.
- The whole process is ***aerobic,*** requiring O_2 as the final oxidant of the reducing equivalents.

Absence of O_2(anoxia)or partial deficiency of O_2 (hypoxia) causes total or partial inhibition of the cycle.

- The H atoms removed in the successive dehydrogenations are accepted by corresponding coenzymes. Reduced coenzymes transfer the reducing equivalents to electron-transport system, where oxidative phosphorylation produces ATP molecules.

BIOMEDICAL IMPORTANCE OF CITRIC ACID CYCLE

- Final common pathway for carbohydrates, proteins and fats, through formation of 2-carbon unit acetyl-CoA.
- Acetyl- CoA is oxidized to CO_2 and H_2O giving out energy (III phase of catabolism).
- ***Intermediates of TCA cycle play a major role in synthesis also, like heme formation, formation of non-essential amino acids, FA synthesis. Cholesterol, and steroid synthesis.***

REACTIONS OF CITRIC ACID CYCLE

Reactions of citric acid cycle ***(Fig. 12.4)*** are arbitrarily divided into ***four stages*** for discussion:

Stage 1

1. ***Formation of Citric Acid from Acetyl-CoA and OAA***

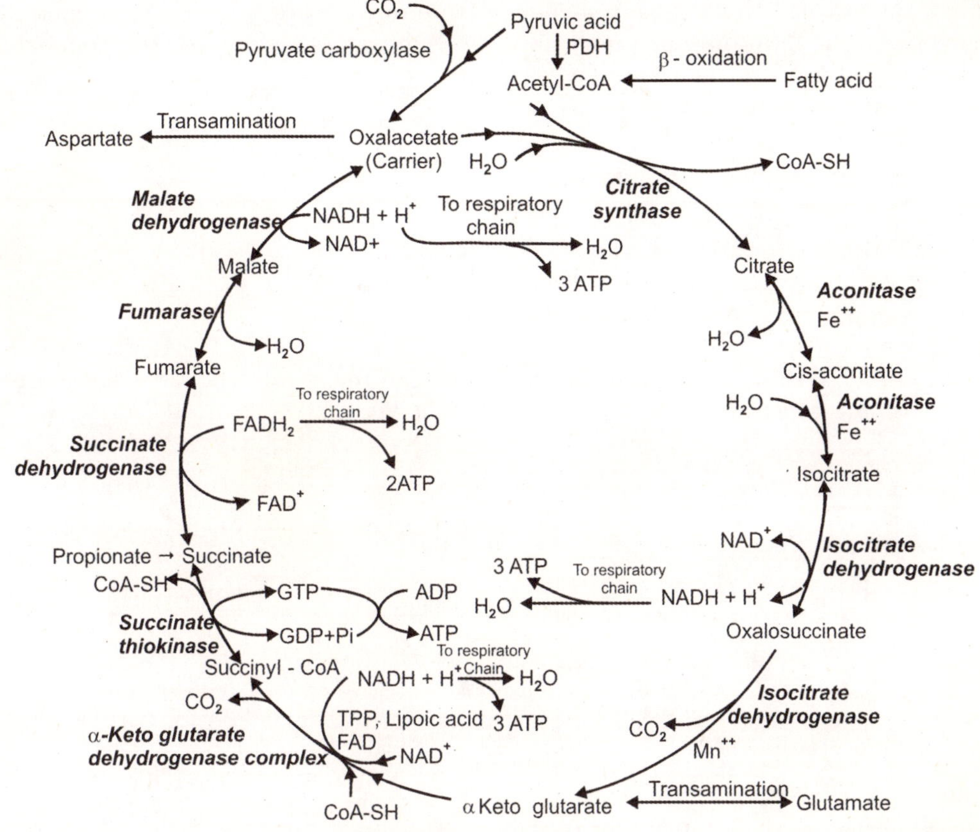

Fig. 12.4: Citric acid cycle

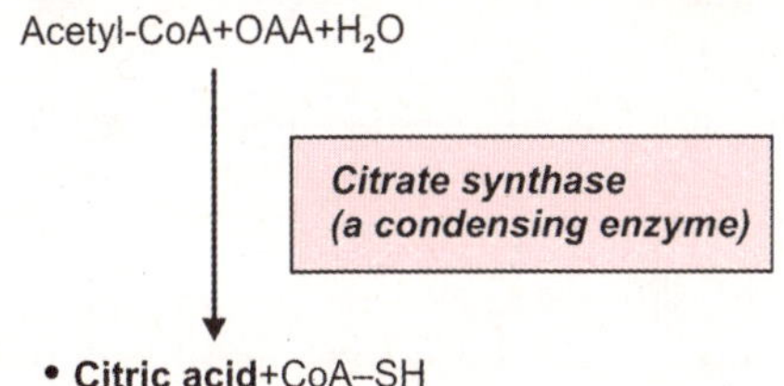

- An *irreversible* reaction
- Exergonic reaction—gives out 7.8 K cal.
- Acetyl group of acetyl-CoA is transferred to OAA.
- No oxidation or decarboxylation involved.

CoA-SH released is re-utilized for oxidative decarboxylation of P.A.

2. *Formation of cis-Aconitic Acid and Isocitric Acid from Citric Acid:* Citric acid is converted to isocitric acid by the enzyme ***aconitase***. This conversion takes place in **two steps:**

- Formation of cis-aconitic acid from citric acid as a result of ***"Asymmetric dehydration"***.
- Formation of isocitric acid from cis-aconitic acid as a result of ***stereospecific rehydration***.

Both processes are catalyzed by the same enzyme *aconitase* which requires Fe^{++}.

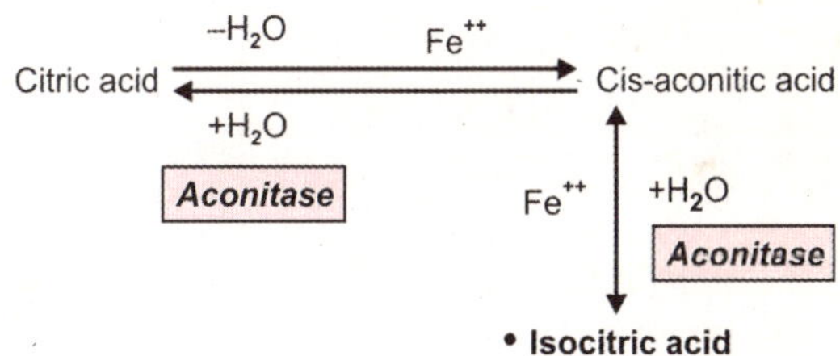

Inhibitor: "Fluoroacetate" is inhibitor of aconitase: Fluoroacetate, in the form of fluoroacetyl CoA condenses with OAA to form fluorocitrate which, in turn, inhibits the enzyme *aconitase* and allows citrate to accumulate.

Energetics: No ATP formation at this stage.

Stage II: The six-carbon *isocitric* acid is converted to a derivative of the four carbon succinyl-CoA. The isocitric acid undergoes oxidation followed by decarboxylation to give **α-oxoglutarate (5 C)** (α-ketoglutarate).

1. ***Formation of Oxalo-Succinic Acid and α-Oxoglutarate from Isocitric Acid***

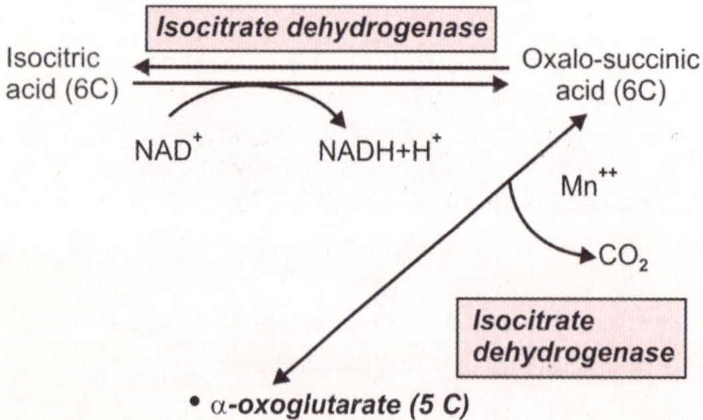

Respiratory chain-linked oxidation of isocitrate proceeds almost completely through the NAD$^+$ dependant ICD in mitochondrion.

2. ***Oxidative Decarboxylation of α-Oxoglutarate to Succinyl-CoA:*** This reaction is analogous to oxidative decarboxylation of pyruvic acid to acetyl-CoA.

- Enzyme is ***α-ketoglutarate dehydrogenase complex.***
- It requires identical coenzymes and cofactors: TPP, Lipoic acid, CoA-SH, FAD, NAD$^+$ and Mg^{++}. Reaction steps are similar to PDH reaction.
  - The reaction is *irreversible.*

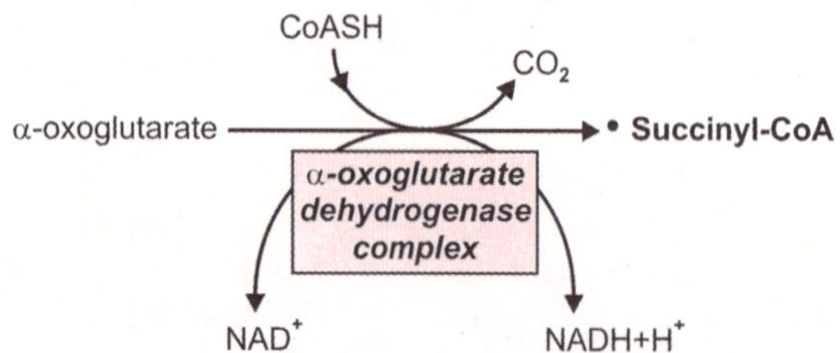

Inhibitor: Arsenite inhibits the reaction causing the substrate α-oxoglutarate to accumulate.

Energetics: NADH produced is oxidized in respiratory chain yielding 3 ATP, from 2 NADH → 6 ATP will be produced.

+ 6 ATP

Stage III: The product of preceding stage succinyl CoA is converted to succinic acid to continue the cycle.

- Enzyme catalyzing this reaction is **succinate thiokinase** (also called as ***succinyl CoA synthase***).

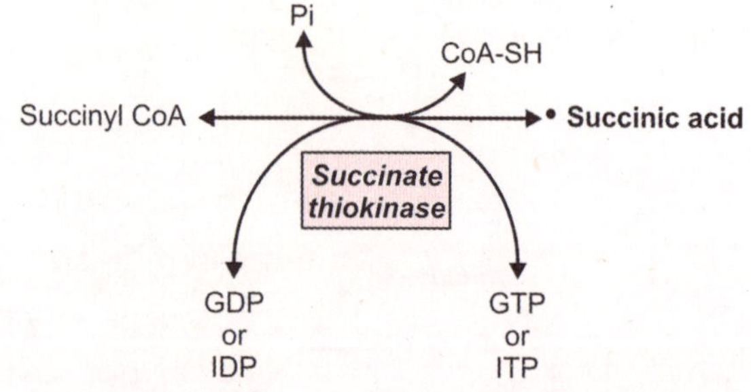

- Reaction requires GDP or IDP, which is converted in presence of Pi to either GTP or ITP.
- In presence of enzyme ***nucleoside diphosphate kinase,*** ATP is produced either from GTP or ITP.

GTP + ADP or ITP ⟶ ATP + GDP or IDP (Nucleoside diphosphokinase)

Thus, ***ATP is produced at substrate level*** without participation of elctron transport chain. This is the only example of "***substrate level phosphorylation***" in TCA cycle.

Energetic: One ATP is produced in this reaction at substrate level. So, from two succinyl CoA → 2 ATP will be produced.

+2 ATP

Stage IV: This ***involves three successive reactions in which succinic acid is oxidized to oxaloacetate (OAA).***

1. *Oxidation of Succinic Acid to Fumaric Acid:* It is a dehydrogenation reaction catalyzed by the enzyme ***succinate dehydrogenase,*** hydrogen, acceptor is FAD.

- The enzyme is 'ferri-flavo protein", mol. wt=200,000 containing FAD and Iron-sulphur (Fe:S), contains 4 atoms of non-hemin Fe and one FAD per mol of enzyme. In contrast to other enzymes of TCA cycle, this enzyme is bound to the inner surface of the inner mitochondrial membrane.

Note:

- This is the only dehydrogenation in citric acid cycle which involves direct transfer of H from substrate to a flavoprotein without the participation of NAD^+.

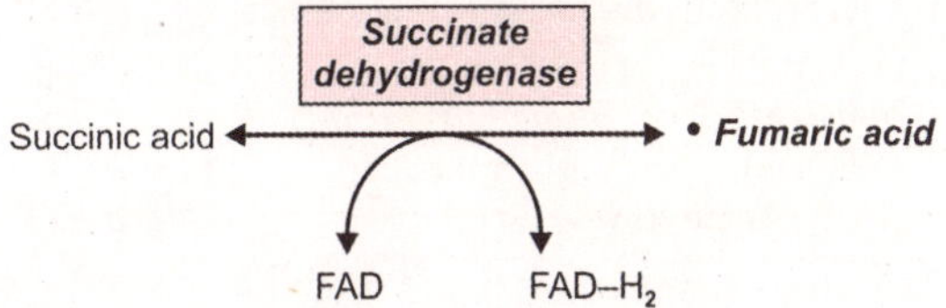

Inhibitor: Addition of malonate/or OAA inhibits succinate dehydrogenase competitively resulting in accumulation of succinate.

Energetic: Oxidation of FAD. H_2 through ETC yields 2 ATP. Hence, 2 molecules of succinic acid will give 4 ATP.

+4 ATP

2. *Formation of Malic Acid from Fumaric Acid*

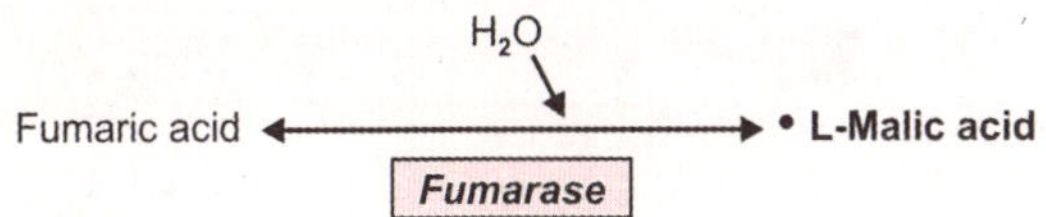

3. *Oxidation of Malic Acid to Oxaloacetate (OAA):* The reaction is catalyzed by the enzyme *malate dehydrogenase* which requires NAD^+ as H-acceptor.

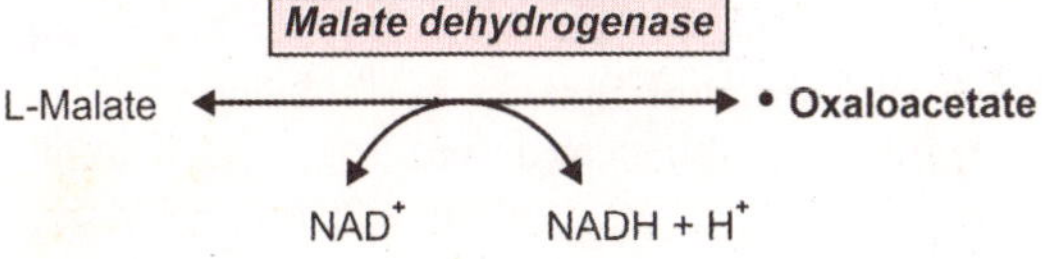

OAA produced, acts 'catalytically', combines with a fresh molecule of acetyl-CoA and the whole process is repeated.

Energetic: Oxidation of NAD. H_2 through ETC produces 3 ATP. Hence, two molecules of NADH. H_2 will give 6 ATP

+6 ATP

TCA CYCLE IS CALLED AMPHIBOLIC IN NATURE–WHY?

TCA cycle has dual role:

- *Catabolic, and*
- *Anabolic.*

1. *Catabolic role:* The two carbon compound acetyl-CoA produced from metabolism of carbohydrates, lipids and proteins are oxidized in this cycle to produce CO_2, H_2O and energy as ATP.

2. *Anabolic or synthetic role:* Intermediates of TCA cycle are utilized for synthesis of various compounds.

Examples:

- *Trasamination: Synthesis of non-essential Amino Acids:* TCA cycle serves as a source of C-skeletons for the synthesis of non-essential amino acids.

Asparate + PA ⟷ OAA + Alanine
Glutamate + PA ⟷ α-Ketoglutarate + Alanine

- *Formation of Glucose: (Gluconeogenesis):* Other amino acids contribute to gluconeogenesis because all or part of their C-skeletons enter TCA cycle after deamination or transamination.
- *Pyruvate forming amino acids:* Glycine, alanine, serine, cysteine/cystine, threonine, hydroxyproline and tryptophan.
- *α-Ketoglutarate forming amino acids:* Arginine, histidine, glutamine, proline, lysine, glutamate.
- *Oxatoacetate forming amino acid:* Aspartic acid.
- *Fumarate forming amino acids:* Phenylalanine and tyrosine
- *Succinyl CoA forming amino acids:* Valine, methionine and isoleucine.

- ***Fatty Acid Synthesis:*** Acetyl CoA formed from PA by the action of PDH complex is the starting material for ***long chain FA synthesis (palmitic acid).*** But this synthesis is extra-mitochondrial, whereas acetyl CoA is formed in mitochondria. Acetyl CoA is transported out in the form of citrate to cytosol, where by the action of the enzyme ***"citrate cleavage enzyme"*** it reforms acetyl-CoA.
- ***Synthesis of Cholesterol and Steroids:*** Acetyl-CoA is used for synthesis of cholesterol, which, in turn, is required for ***synthesis of steroids.***
- ***Heme Synthesis:*** Succinyl CoA produced in TCA cycle takes part in ***heme synthesis*** (see heme synthesis)
- Succinyl CoA is utilized for ***formation of "aceto-acetyl CoA"*** from acetoacetate in extra hepatic tissues (see ketolysis).

Regulation of TCA Cycle: As the primary function of TCA cycle is to provide energy, respiratory control via the ETC and oxidative phosphorylation exerts the main control. Activity is immediately dependent on the supply of NAD^+, which in turn, will depend on supply of ADP for ATP formation. Hence provided there is adequate O_2, the rate of doing work via utilization of ATP determines both the rate of respiration and the activity of TCA cycle.

- In addition to this overall and coarse control, several enzymes of TCA cycle are also important in the regulation.

Three key enzymes are:

- ***Citrate synthase***
- ***Isocitrate dehydrogenase (ICD)***
- ***α-Oxoglutarate dehydrogenase***

These enzymes are responsive to the energy status as expressed by the [ATP]/[ADP] ratio and [NADH]/[NAD^+] ratio.

- ***Citrate synthas***e enzyme is allosterically inhibited by ATP and long-chain acyl CoA.
- NAD^+- dependent mitochondrial ***isocitrate dehydrogenase*** **(ICD)** is activated allosterically by ADP and is inhibited by ATP and NADH.
- α-Ketoglutarate dehydrogenase regulations is analogous to PDH complex (see regulation of PDH-complex).
- In addition to above, *succinate dehydrogenase* enzyme is inhibited by OAA and the availability of OAA is controlled by *malate dehydrogenase,* which depends on [NADH]/[NAD^+] ratio.

Bioenergetics

Overall energy production in glycolysis cum TCA cycle in presence of O_2 is summarised below:

A. Glycogenolysis ATP yield per hexose unit

- Glycogen→ Fructose-1, 6bi-P **–1 ATP**

Glycolysis

- Glucose→ Fructose-1, 6 bi-P **–2 ATP**
- Glycereldehyde- 3P-dehydrogenase (2 NADH → 2 NAD^+) **+ 6 ATP**
- ***Substrate level phosphorylation***
  (a) 2-phosphoglycerate kinase **+ 2 ATP**
  (b) Pyruvate kinase **+ 2 ATP**

Net gain
For Glucose = +8 ATP
For glycogen = + 9 ATP

B. Oxidative decarboxylation of PA

- Pyruvate dehydrogenase complex (2 NADH → 2 NAD^+) **+ 6 ATP**

C. TCA cycle

- Isocitrate dehydrogenase 2 (NADH→NAD^+) **+ 6 ATP**
- α-Ketoglutarate dehydrogenase complex 2 (NADH→NAD^+) **+ 6 ATP**
- ***Substrate level phosphorylation*** succinate thiokinase 2 GTP or 2 ITP→2 ATP **+ 2 ATP**
- Succinate dehydrogenase 2 ($FAD.H_2$→FAD) **+ 4 ATP**
- Malate dehydrogenase 2 (NADH→NAD^+) **+ 6 ATP**

1. Total per mol. of glucose (under aerobic condition) **30+ 8 = 38 ATP**
2. Total per mol of glycogen (glycogenolysis provides G-1-P (G-1-P→G-6-P) **30+ 9 = 39 ATP**
3. Total per mol of glucose (under anaerobic condition) **= 2ATP** (only in anaerobic glycolysis)

Efficiency: Complete oxidation of glucose to CO_2 and H_2O in a "Bomb calorimeter" yields 6,86,000 calories which is liberated as heat. When oxidation occurs in tissues, some of this energy is not lost immediately as 'heat but captured as "high energy PO_4 bonds". At least 38 high energy PO_4 bonds are generated per molecule of glucose oxidized to CO_2 and H_2O.

- Assuming each high energy bond to be equivalent to 7,600 calories. Total energy captured in ATP per mol of glucose oxidized
  = 7,600 × 38
  = 2,88,800 calories

$$\text{Hence, } \textbf{efficiency} = \frac{2,88,800}{686,000} \times 100$$

= **42 percent** of energy of combustion.

Pasteur Effect: Anaerobic oxidative reactions (glycolysis) ***may be decreased by aeration.*** This was first observed by **Pasteur** in studies of the fermentation of glucose by yeast cells. Pasteur also noted that in the presence of O_2, less glucose was broken down by the yeast cells and less alcohol was formed, whereas under anaerobic conditions more alcohol was formed and more glucose was fermented.

Definition: ***The phenomenon of inhibition of glycolysis by O_2 is termed as the Pasteur effect.***

"Carb-tree" Effect: This is opposite of Pasteur effect, which represents decreased respiration of cellular systems caused by high concentration of glucose.

SHUTTLE SYSTEMS

- ***NADH produced in the glycolysis is extra-mitochondrial, whereas the electron transport chain, where NADH has to be oxidized to NAD^+ is in the mitochondrion.***
- ***NADH is not permeable to mitochondrial membrane.*** It is envisaged that NADH produced in cytosol transfer the reducing equivalents through the mitochondrial membrane via substrate pairs, linked by suitable dehydrogenases by shuttle systems. It is important that the specific dehydrogenases which act as "shuttle " be present on both sides of mitochondrial membrane.
- ***Two such shuttle systems are:***
  - ***Glycerophosphate shuttle***
  - ***Malate shuttle***

1. Glycerophosphate Shuttle: The α-glycerophosphate shuttle is shown in ***Fig. 12.5.*** α-glycero-P in mitochondrion is FP-dependent. Hence ***produces 2 ATP per mole of NADH oxidized.***

2. Malate Shuttle: Malate shuttle is shown in *Fig. 12.6.* This shuttle system is more common and universal. Reduced NADH+ H^+ is reformed in mitochondrion, which being oxidized in respiratory chain produces 3 ATP.

Energetics:

- When body utilizes α-glycero-P-shuttle, net ATP produced by glycolysis-TCA cycle per molecule glucose oxidized will be **36 ATP** (2 ATP less) and **(NOT 38 ATP)**
- Use of malate shuttle will form **38 ATP.**

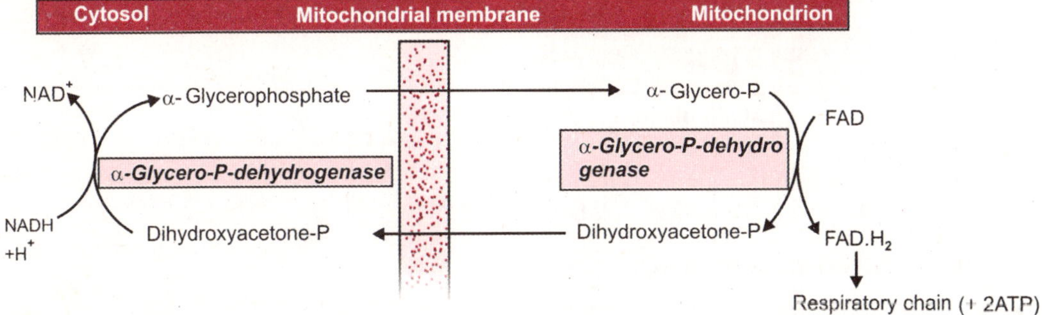

Fig. 12.5: Glycerophosphate shuttle

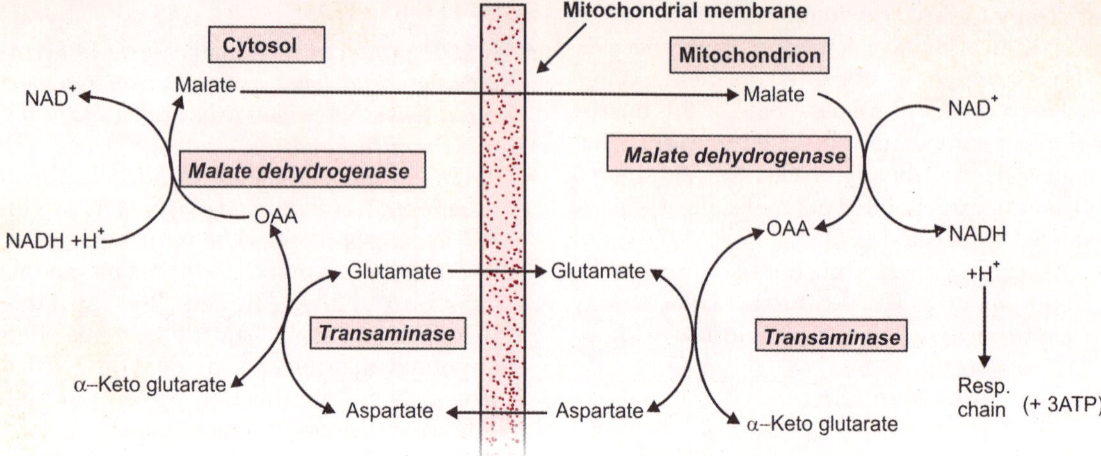

Fig. 12.6: Malate shuttle

METABOLISM OF GLYCOGEN

Glycogen is the storage form of glucose which is stored in animal body specially in liver and muscles. it is mobilized as glucose whenever body tissues require.

Role of Liver Glycogen:

- ***It is the only immediately available reserve store of blood glucose.***
- ***A high liver glycogen level protects the liver cells against the harmful effects of many poisons and chemicals,*** e.g. CCl_4, ethyl alcohol, arsenic, various bacterial toxins.
- Certain forms of detoxication, e.g. conjugation with glucuronic acid; and acetylation reactions, are directly influenced by the liver glycogen level.
- The rate of deamination of amino acids in the liver is depressed as the glycogen level rises, so that amino acids are preserved longer in that form and so remain available for protein synthesis in the tissues.
- Similarly, a high level of liver glycogen depresses the rate of ketone bodies formation.

BIOMEDICAL IMPORTANCE

- Liver glycogen is largely concerned with storage and supply of glucose-1-P, which is converted to glucose, for maintenance of blood glucose, ***particularly in between meals.***
- Muscle glycogen on the other hand, is to act as readily available source of intermediates of glycolysis for provision of energy within the muscle itself. ***Muscle glycogen cannot directly contribute to blood glucose level.***
- Inherited deficiency of enzymes in the pathway of glycogen metabolism produces certain inherited disorders called as ***glycogen storage diseases (GSDs).***

Metabolism of glycogen can be discussed under **two headings.**

1. *Synthetic phase: formation of glycogen*
2. *Catabolic phase: breakdown of glycogen*

Note: The ***above two pathways are different from each other Breakdown pathway is not a "reversal" of synthetic pathway.***

- ***Glycogen in any tissue is not static.*** It is being constantly used up and resynthesized. ***So at any time, the glycogen of the tissue should be considered as a balance between constant production and loss.*** Both the processes are finely controlled at substrate level, by end-products and hormones.
- **When glycogenesis occurs, glycogenolysis does not take place and *vice versa.***

GLYCOGENESIS

Definition: It is the formation of glycogen from glucose.

Sites: Principally, it *occurs in liver* and *skeletal muscles*, but it can occur in every tissue to some extent.

Limitations of Storage: In humans, the liver may contain as much as 4 to 6 percent of glycogen as per weight of the organ *(Table 12.2)*, when analyzed shortly after a meal, high in carbohydrate. After 12 to 18 hours of fasting, the liver becomes almost totally depleted of glycogen.

Table 12.2: Storage capacity of glycogen in a normal adult man (70 kg)

Organ	*Amount*		*Normal weight of the organ*
• Liver glycogen	4 to 6%	= 72-108gm	1800 gm (liver)
• Skeletal muscles	0.7%	= 245 gm	35 kg (muscle)
• Extra cellular glucose	0.1%	= 10 gm	Total volume= 10 litres
	Total	= 327-363 gms	

Reactions of Synthetic Pathway

- Glucose is first phosphorylated to glucose-6-P by *glucokinase (or hexokinase).*
- Glucose-6-P converted to glucose-1-P by the enzyme *phosphoglucomutase.*
- Glucose-1-P then reacts with one molecule of uridine-triphosphate (UTP) to form the "active" nucleotide *uridine-diphosphateglucose" (UDP-Glc),* under the influence of the enzyme ***UDP-Glc pyrophosphorylase*** with elimination of a molecule of "pyrophosphate" (PPi).
- By the action of the enzyme *glycogen synthase,* C-1 of the activated glucose of UDP-Glc forms a glycosidic bond with C-4 of a terminal glucose residue of glycogen "**primer**", liberating UDP. ***A pre-existing glycogen molecule, or "primer" must be present to initiate this reaction.***
  From where this 'primer' comes?: The glycogen "Primer" is supposed to be synthesized on a protein backbone, which is a process similar to synthesis of other glycoproteins.
- UDP liberated, as above, is converted to UTP as given below so that it can be re-utilized

$$\text{UDP + ATP} \xrightarrow[\textit{Nucleoside diphosphokinase}]{} \text{UTP + ADP}$$

In this way, ***an existing glycogen chain can be repeatedly extended by one glucose unit at a time. In each extension, 2 ATP molecules are expended:***

- One in phosphorylation of glucose to form G-6-P.
- Another in the regeneration of UTP.

Glycogen synthase requires glucose-6-P as an activator.

Glycogen synthase is the principal key enzyme which reglulates the glycogen formation (see regulation).

- When the chain has been lengthened to minimum of 11 glucose residues, a second enzyme, ***branching enzyme (amylo-1,4→1,6-transglucosidase)*** comes into play and ***transfer a part of α 1→ 4 chain, minimum length 6 glucose residues, to a neighbouring chain to form α 1 → 6 linkage thus establishing a branch point in the molecule.*** The branches grow by further additions of α 1→4 glycosyl units and further branching.

  Regulation of Glycogenesis: *Glycogen synthase* is the key enzyme which regulates the process of glycogenesis. It is present as **"active"** and **'inactive'** forms, which are interconvertible.
  - **Active form is GS "a"** (previously called as GS-I).
  - **Inactive form is GS "b"** (previously called as GS-D).
- ***Active GS "a" is converted to inactive GS "b" by phosphorylation,*** which is modulated by cyclic-AMP dependant *protein kinase.* When glycogen synthase is converted to inactive form, the glycogenesis is inhibited.
- ***Inactive GS "b" is converted to active GS "a" by dephosporylation*** catalyzed by the enzyme ***protein phosphatase-1;*** when glycogen synthase is converted to active form glycogenesis occurs.
- The interconversion of active to inactive and *vice versa* is controlled by substrate level, end products and hormones.

The interconversion of "glycogen synthase" "a" and "b" and its regulation is shown schematically in *Fig.12.7.*

Role of Cyclic AMP Dependant Protein Kinases: Protein kinases exist in cells, the enzyme is of wide specificity and c-AMP dependant. It can be in "active" and "inactive" forms. ***Increase in cyclic AMP converts inactive protein kinase to active form.***

"Active" protein kinase formed due to increased cyclic AMP in the cell has ***two effects*** on glycogenesis:

- It brings about phosphorylation of *glycogen synthase* with the help of ATP and thus converts "active" GS "a" (desphosphorylated) to "inactive" GS "a" (phosphorylated). Thus, glycogen synthesis is inhibited.
- At the same time, "active" protein kinase (C_2), stimulates a protein factor called "inhibitor – 1" ('inactive') and phosphorylates it to form "active" inhibitor-1–P, which, in turn, inhibits *protein phosphatase-1* thus conversion of inactive GS 'b' to active GS "a" does not take place. Thus, glycogenesis in the cells is inhibited.

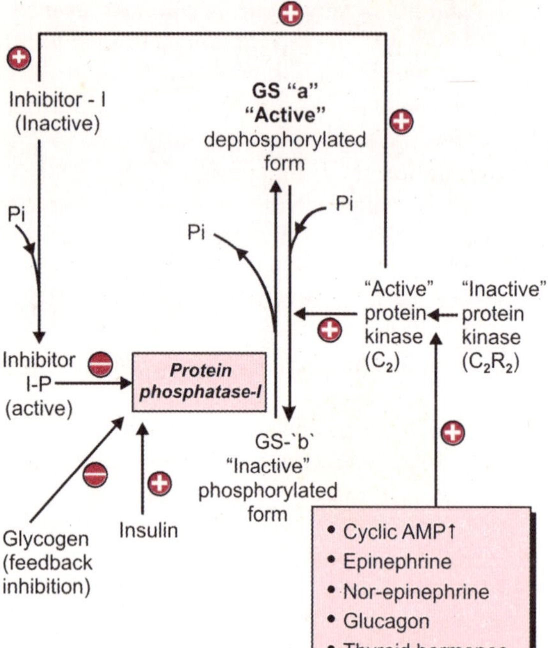

Fig. 12.7: Showing activation and Inactivation of glycogen synthase

Clinical Aspect

Relation of glycogenesis with K^+ influx into the cell:

- Clinical importance in ***treatment of hyperkalaemia***, when insulin and glucose are adminstered.
- Importance in treatment of diabetic ketoacidosis, with insulin and glucose, danger of ***"hypokalaemia"*** to precipitate. The ***patient should be monitored for potassium level in blood while treating diabetic ketoacidosis with insulin and glucose infusion.***

GLYCOGENOLYSIS

Definition: Breakdown of glycogen to glucose.

"Phosphorylase" Enzyme: It is initiated by the action of a specific enzyme *phosphorylase*, which brings about "phosphorolytic" cleavage of $\alpha 1 \rightarrow 4$ linkage to yield glucose-1-P. Liver and muscle both contain the enzyme *phosphorylase.* In both, the enzyme can be in "active" and "inactive" forms and both are interconvertible.

Differences of Muscle Phosphorylase from Liver Phosphorylase

- There is no cleavage of structure with liver phosphorylase as compared to muscle phosphorylase.
- *Muscle phosphorylase* is not affected by glucagon ***(no receptor on muscle).***
- ***4 molecules of pyridoxal-P (B_6-P)*** is required for activity of muscle phosphorylase.
- Ca^{++}. can bring about glycogenolysis in muscle/and liver, independent of cyclic-AMP (similarities).
- "Active" liver phosphorylase is phosphorylated form and "inactive" form is dephosphorylated.

For activation of phosphorylases. (See regulation of glycogenolysis.)

STEPS OF GLYCOGENOLYSIS

- Phosphorylase step is the first step which is the ***rate-limiting*** and ***key enzyme*** in glycogenolysis. With proper activation and in presence of inorganic phosphate (Pi), the enzyme breaks the glucosyl α-1→4 linkages and removes by phosphorolytic cleavage the 1→4 glycosyl residues from outermost chains of the glycogen molecule until approximately four (4) glucose residues remain on either side of a α-1 → 6 branch (Limit dextrin).

  Note: Students should note that by phosphorylase activity ***glucose is liberated as glucose-1-P and not as free glucose.***
- When ***four glucose residues are left from the branch point,*** then another enzyme, ***"α-1,4→ α-1,4 glucan transferase"*** transfer a ***"trisaccharide" unit*** from one side to the other ***thus exposing α-1→6 branch point.***
- The hydrolytic splitting of α-1→6 glucosidic linkage requires the action of a *specific* ***debranching enzyme (amylo-1→6- glucosidase).*** As the α-1→6 linkage is hydrolytically split, ***one molecule of free glucose is produced,*** rather than one molecule of glucose-1-P as is the case with phosphorolytic cleavage with the enzyme phosphorylase.

Clinical Significance

In this way, it is possible for some rise in blood glucose to take place even in absence of glucose-6-phosphatase, in Von Gierke's disease, after epinephrine or glucagon is administered.

Fate of Glucose-1-P

- The combined action of phosphorylase and other enzymes convert glycogen to glucose-1-P mostly.
- By the action of *phosphoglucomutase* enxyme, glucose-1-P is easily converted to glucose-6-P, as the reaction is reversible.
- In ***liver and kidney*** a **specific enzyme** ***glucose-6-phosphatase*** is present, that removes PO_4 from glucose-6-P, enabling "free glucose" to form and diffuse from the cells to extracellular spaces including blood. This is the final step in hepatic glycogenolysis, which is reflected by a rise in blood glucose.
- In ***muscles, enzyme glucose-6-phosphatase is absent.*** Hence, glucose-6-P enters into glycolytic cycle and ***forms pyruvte and LA. Muscle glycogenolysis does not contribute to blood glucose directly.*** But indirectly, lactic acid can go to glucose formation in liver (Cori cycle).

REGULATION OF GLYCOGENOLYSIS

Cyclic AMP dependant protein kinase has dual effects, on glycogenolysis regulation.

Activation of Phosphorylase Enzyme:

- Catecholamines, glucagon and thyroid hormones bring about glycogenolysis, by increasing the cyclic AMP level in cells, which in turn, activates "protein kinase".
- "Active" protein kinase (C_2), in turn phosphorylates *"inactive" phosphorylase-kinase "b"* and converts it to *active phosphorylase kinase "a"*.
- "Active" *phosphorylase-kinase "a"* now with the help of ATP, phosphorylates *"inactive" dephosphophosphorylase "b"* to *"active" phosphophosphorylase "a"*, which brings about phosphorolytic cleavage of α-1→4 glucosidic linkage as stated above.
- At the same time, *active protein kinase,* phosphorylates the protein factor called "inhibitor-1" (inactive) and converts it to "active" inhibitor-1-P, which inhibits *protein phosphatase-I* which, in turn, inhibitis conversion of ***phosphorylase kinase "a"*** to ***"b"***. Phosphorylase kinase "a" in turn phosphorylates "dephosphosphorylase" "b" to "active" phosphophosphorylase "a".

Note:

- Catecholamines cause breakdown of liver and muscle glycogen, acting through β-adrenergic cell receptors on cell membrane.
- ***Glucagon breaks down liver glycogen only, and not muscle glycogen*** as β-adrenergic cell receptors for glucagon are not present on muscle cell membrane.

Regulation of Glycogen Metabolism

- Regulation of glycogen metabolism is achieved ***by a balance in activities between glycogen synthase and phosphorylase, which are as follows:***
  - Substrate control (through " allostery") as well as
  - Hormonal control; and by
  - end products.
- Not only *"phosphorylase"* enzyme is activated by a rise in concentration of c-AMP ↑ via phosphorylase kinase, but " glycogen synthase" enzyme is at the same time converted to "inactive" form, ***both the effects are mediated via "c-AMP-dependant proteinkinase"***.
- ***Thus inhibition of glycogenolysis increases net glycogenesis and inhibition of glycogenesis increases net glycogenolysis. Both processes cannot occur simultaneously together.***
- Dephosphorylation of phosphorylase "a", phosphorylase kinase "a" and glycogen synthase "b" is accomplished by a single enzyme of wide specificity ***"protein phosphatase-1"***, which, in turn, is inhibited by c-AMP dependant protein kinase via the protein "inhibitor-1". ***Thus, glycogenolysis can be terminated and glycogenesis can be stimulated synchronously, or vice versa, because both processes are geared to the activity of c-AMP dependant proteinkinase.***

INHERITED DISORDERS

Glycogen Storage Diseases (GSDs): These are a group of inherited disorders associated with glycogen metabolism, familial in incidence and characterized ***by deposition of normal or abnormal type and quantity of glycogen in the tissues.*** **Six classical types** of GSDs will be considered, though there are quite a number of additions in the list. ***Table 12.3*** shows the six types of GSDs.

☞ SALIENT POINTS TO REMEMBER

- Carbohydrates are the major source of energy for the living cells. Glucose, normal fasting level 60 to 100 mg/dl ("true glucose") is the central molecule in carbohydrate metabolism.
- Glucose actively participates in a number of metabolic pathways, viz. Glycolysis, Glycogenesis/Glycogenolysis, Gluconeogenesis, hexosemonophosphate shunt, uronic acid pathway etc.
- Oxidation of Glucose or glycogen to form pyruvate and lactate is called glycolysis. It occurs in all tissues and is meant for energy.
- Glycolysis can occur in presence of O_2 (aerobic glycolysis) producing 8 ATP and in absence of O_2 (anaerobic glycolysis) producing 2 ATP.
- One glucose molecule on oxidation produces 2 moles of pyruvic acid.
- A diversion in glycolytic pathway, called Rapaport - Leubering cycle or shunt (RLC/RLS) produces 2:3 biphosphoglycerate (2, 3 - BPG). In presence of 2, 3-BPG, oxy-Hb unloads more O_2 to the tissues.
- The occurrence of glycolysis is increased very much in rapidly growing cancer cells producing local lactic acidosis.
- In Alcoholics with thiamine deficiency, more pyruvic acid is diverted to Lactate formation resulting to Lactic acidosis.
- Fate of pyruvate depends on the redox state of the tissues.
- In absence of O_2 (anaerobiosis), the pyruvic acid is converted to lactic acid, the reaction is reversible.
- In presence of O_2, the pyruvic acid is oxidatively decarboxylated to two carbon unit "acetyl CoA". This occurs in presence of a multienzyme complex, *"Pyruvate dehydrogenase complex"* requiring six coenzymes/cofactors viz. TPP, Lipoic acid, CoASH, FAD, NAD^+ and Mg^{++}.
- Acetyl CoA thus produced from pyruvate is completely oxidized in citric acid cycle (also called Krebs's cycle or TCA cycle), the final common oxidative pathway for all food stuffs. The complete oxidation of glucose in Glycolysis - TCA cycle generates 38 ATP.
- TCA cycle has dual role (amphibolic):

Table 12.3: Glycogen Storage Diseases (GSDs)

Types Name	Deficient enzyme (Enzyme)	Inheritance	Structure of glycogen	Organs affected	Clinical features
1. *von Gierke's disease*	*G-6-Pase*	Autosomal recessive	Normal (metabolically NOT available)	Liver, Kidney, intestine	Hypoglycaemia, ketosis and acidosis LA↑, uric acid↑, failure to thrive, hepatomegaly
II. *Pompe's disease*	*Acid maltase* (Present in lysosomes. Catalyzes breakdown of oligosaccharides)	Autosomal recessive	Normal	Liver, heart, smooth and striated muscles	Cardiomegaly, muscle hypotonia, no hypoglycaemia
Note: Infants die of cardiac failure and bronchopneumonia. Death usually before 9 months. A few survive 2 ½ years.					
III. *Limit dextrinosis (Forbe's disease)*	*Debranching enzyme*	Autosomal recessive	*Abnormal, "Limit dextrin type"* short missing outer branches	Liver (18%) heart, and muscle (6%)	Moderate hypoglycaemia, acidosis, Progressive myopathy, hepatomegaly
Note: Patients survive well to adult life.					
IV. *Amylopectinosis (Andersen's disease)*	*Branching enzyme*	Not known	*Abnormal ("amylopectin" type)* very long inner and outer unbranched chains, very few branch point	Liver heart, muscle, RE system	Moderate hypoglycaemia, hepatosplenomegaly, Ascites, Nodular Cirrhosis of liver, hepatic failure
Note: Prognosis Fatal, Longest survival reported as 4 years.					
V. *Mac Ardle's disease*	*Muscle phosphorylase*	Autosomal recessive	Normal	Skeletal muscle (excess normal glycogen muscles)	Muscle cramps on exercise, pain in muscle, weakness and stiffness of muscle
Note: Affects children and adults, muscle recovers with rest—Due to utilization of FA for energy., after inj. Epinephrine/glucagon → Blood sugar ↑ (Shows liver phosphorylase not affected)					
VI. *Her's disease*	*Liver Phosphorylase*	Autosomal dominant	Normal	Liver, leucocytes	Hypoglycaemia, mild to moderate acidosis, hepatomegaly
Note: Present like a mild case of Type-1, the condition has also been reported to occur in association with Fanconi syndrome.					

1. ***Catabolic role:*** oxidation of acetyl CoA to CO_2 and H_2O.
2. ***Anabolic role:*** intermediates of TCA cycle play a major role in various synthesis like heme formation, FA synthesis, formation of nonessential amino acids, cholesterol and steroid synthesis.

- Enolase enzyme of glycolytic pathway is inhibited by fluoride. Fluoride is used as anticoagulant for blood sugar estimation.
- Glycogen is the storage form of glucose. Mainly stored in liver and muscles. The capacity of storage is limited.
- Liver can store 4 to 6 percent (72 to 108 gm) and Muscle can store 0.7 percent (245 gm).
- ***Formation of glycogen from glucose is called glycogenesis. The breakdown of glycogen to glucose is called glycogenolysis.***

- ***In glycogenolysis, glucose is liberated as Glucose-1-P and not as glucose.***
- Liver glycogenolysis produces Glucose-1-P. Which is converted to Glucose-6-P and forms glucose by the enzyme *"Glucose-6-Phosphatase"* present in Liver. Liver glycogenolysis thus provides glucose immediately, and it is meant for maintenance of blood glucose particularly in between meals.
- ***Muscle glycogenolysis produces Glucose-1-P which is converted to Glucose-6-P.***, but it cannot form glucose immediately as the muscle lacks the enzyme *"Glucose-6-phosphatase"*. Thus muscle glycogen cannot directly contribute to blood glucose level.
- Muscle glycogenolysis act as readily available source of intermediates of glycolysis for provision of energy within the muscle itself.
- Inherited enzyme defects in synthesis or degradation of glycogen lead to "Glycogen storage Diseases" (GSDs). von Gierke's disease (Type 1) is due to the defect in the enzyme *"Glucose-6-phosphatase."*
- Glycogen storage diseases are characterized by deposition of normal or abnormal type of glycogen in one or more tissues resulting to abnormal function of the particular organ or tissues.

HEXOSE MONOPHOSPHATE (HMP) SHUNT

An alternate pathway for oxidation of glucose.
Synonyms: Variously called as:

- ***Hexose monophosphate pathway or shunt***
- ***Pentose phosphate pathway (PP pathway)***
- ***Pentose cycle***
- ***Phosphogluconate pathway***
- ***Warburg-Dickens-Lipman pathway.***

BIOMEDICAL IMPORTANCE

- Though it is oxidation of glucose, but it is ***not meant for energy.***
- ***Provides NADPH*** which is required for various reductive synthesis in metabolic pathways.
- ***Provides pentoses*** required for nucleic acid synthesis.
- Deficiency of a particular enzyme leads to haemolytic anaemia, which is of great clinical importance.

MAJOR DIFFERENCES WITH EM PATHWAY *(Table 12.4)*

- This pathway ***occurs in certain specialized tissues only to serve specific functions,*** e.g. liver, adipose tissue, RB cells, testes and ovary, adrenal cortex and lactating mammary gland. Also lens and cornea of eye. It is unimportant for skeletal muscle and does not operate in non-lactating mammary gland.
- It is a ***multicyclic process,*** 3 molecules of glucose-6-P enter the cycle, producing 3 mols of CO_2 and 3 mols of 5-C residues, which rearrange to give 2 mols of Glucose-6-P and one mol of glyceraldehyde-3-P.
- Oxidation is achieved by dehydrogenation but ***$NADP^+$ is used as hydrogen acceptor*** and **NOT NAD^+.**
- CO_2 is produced in this pathway which is never produced in EM pathway.

Table. 12.4: Difference of EM pathway and HMP shunt

EM Pathway	*HM Pathway*
• Occurs in all tissues	• Occurs in certain special tissues for special function
• Not a multicyclic process	• Multicyclic process
• Oxidation by dehydrogenation but, NAD^+ is H-acceptor	• Oxidation achieved by dehydrogenation but $NADP^+$ is used as H-acceptor
• ATP is required and ATP is produced	• Not meant for energy: ATP is not produced. ATP is required for glucose to glucose-6—P (for phosphorylation) and for interconversion of pentoses.
• CO_2 is never formed	• CO_2 is produced.

Similarity: The only similarity is that enzymes are extramitochondrial (cytosol) and it operates in cytosol.

Summary of the reactions:

$$3\text{-Glucose-6-P+NADP}^+ \rightarrow 3\ CO_2\uparrow + \text{Glucose-6-P} + \text{1-Glyceraldehyde 3p} + 6\ \text{NADPH} + 6H^+$$

METABOLIC PATHWAYS

Reactions of this pathway can be considered arbitrarily in **2 stages** (See *Fig. 12.8)*.

Stage I (Oxidative Phase): Oxidation of glucose and formation of pentose phosphates.

Stage II (Non-oxidative phase): Pentose-phosphate reactions (interconversion of pentoses) and conversion of pentose phosphates to hexose phosphates.

Stage I: Oxidation of Glucose and Formation of Pentose Phosphates (Oxidative Phase)

1. ***First Oxidation:*** Dehydrogenation of glucose-6-P to form 6-phosphogluconate via the formation of intermediate unstable compound 6-phosphogluconolactone, catalyzed by the first enzyme in this pathway ***glucose-6-P dehydrogenase (G-6-PD) an NADP-dependent enzyme.*** Hydrolysis of 6-phosphogluconolactone is accomplished by the enzyne *gluconolactone hydrolase.*

- G-6-PD enzyme is the first enzyme in the pathway which is ***"rare-limiting"***.

2. ***Second Oxidative Step:*** The second oxidative reaction takes place in 2 steps:

First 6-phosphogluconate is converted to 3-keto 6-phosphogluconate, catalyzed by the enzyme *"6-phosphogluconate dehydrogenase"*, in which $NADP^+$ acts as H-acceptor.

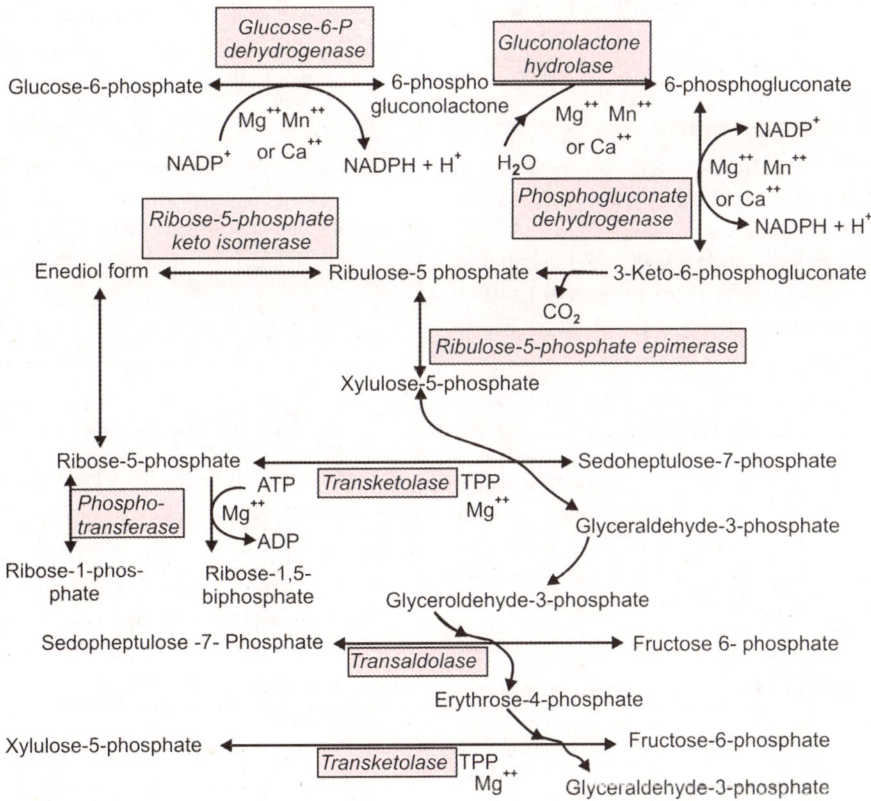

Fig. 12.8: The hexose monophosphate shunt or pentose phosphate pathway

- Secondly, 3-keto-6-phosphogluconate undergoes decarboxylation, first carbon is removed as CO_2 and form ketopentose, "D-ribulose-5-P".

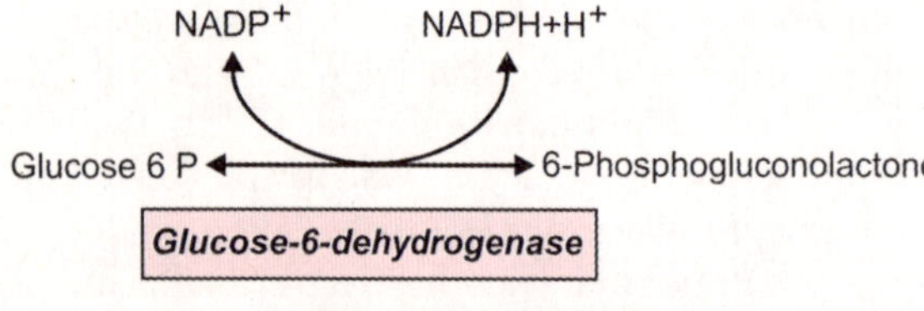

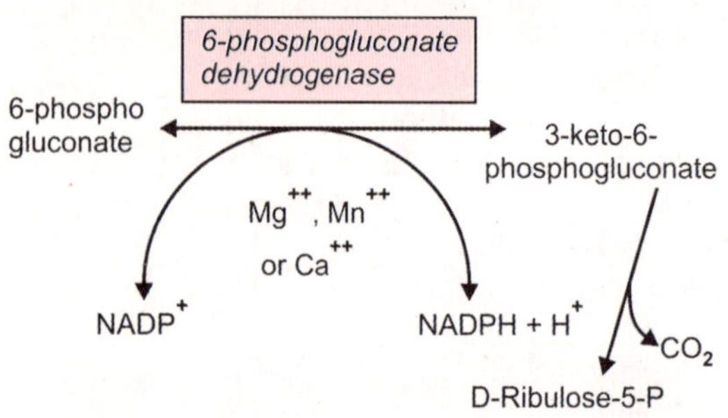

Stage II: Non-Oxidative Phase

1. *Pentose P Reactions (Interconversions of Pentoses):* D-ribulose-5-P is readily converted into a variety of pentoses.

- D-ribulose-5-P is acted upon by a *keto-isomerase* and forms *D-ribose-5-P* (aldopentose) which can be converted to D-ribose-1, 5-di P and D-ribose-1-P.

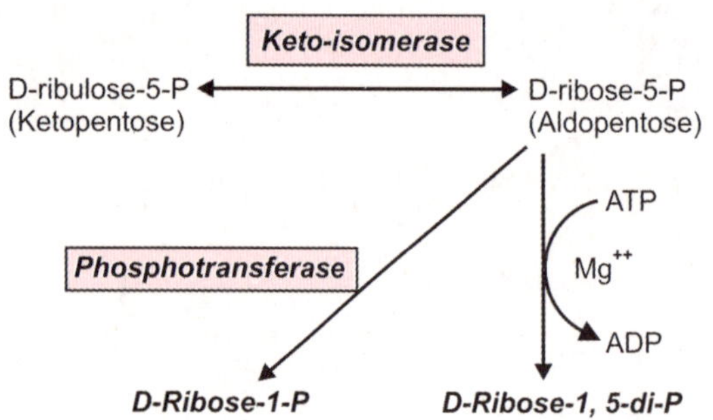

- D-ribulose-5-P can be converted to D-xylulose-5-P, another keto pentose, the reaction being catalyzed by an "*epimerase*".

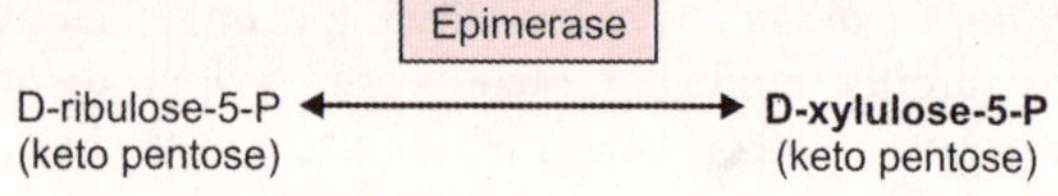

- Some ribose-5-P may be epimerized by ***phosphopentose-2-epimerase*** to form "**arabinose 5-P**".

2. *Conversion of Pentose Phosphates to Hexose Phosphates:* Reactions in this stage involves the conversion of pentose phosphates to fructose-6-P which is isomerized to glucose-6-P to begin the cycle over again. This is achieved by two peculiliar reactions dependant on two enzymes- *transketolase* and *transaldolase* and reactions are called transketolation and transaldolation, respectively. In the HMP shunt, two transketolase reactions and one transaldolase reaction are involved.

Fate of Fructose-6-P and Glyceraldehyde-3-P: Two molecules of Glyceraldehyde-3-P can form one molecule of fructose-1,6,bi-P, which is converted to fructose-6-P by the enzyme Fructose-1,6-bi Phosphatase Fructose-6-P is converted to glucose-6-P. by isomerase.

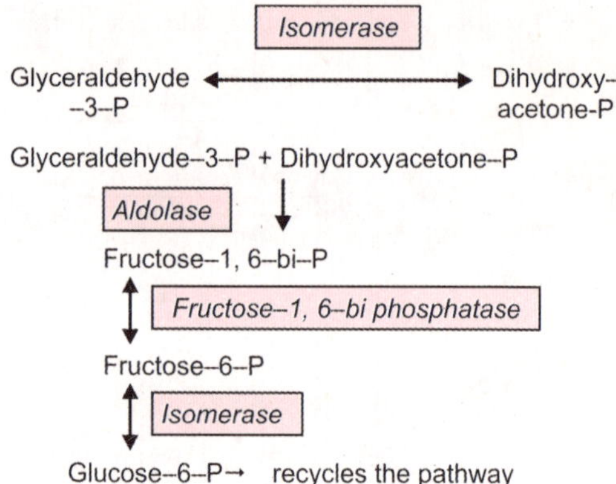

REGULATION OF HMP SHUNT

- ***Reaction catalyzed by G-6-PD, the first reaction of the pathway constitutes the rate-limiting step.*** It is primarily regulated by cytoplasmic levels of $NADP^+$ and NADPH, thus the ratio of the two, i.e. $[NADP^+]/[NADPH]$.
- If the cytoplasmic ratio is high, i.e. a rise in $NADP^+$ enhances the "rate-limiting" reaction as well as the shunt pathway.

- A decrease in the ratio, i.e. a rise in NADPH level inhibits both ***G-6-PD*** and ***6-phosphogluconate dehydrogenase*** by making less $NADP^+$ available for their catalytic reactions and also by competing with $NADP^+$ to occupy the enzyme binding site of G-6-PD.
- Activities of both dehydrogenases and the rate of the pathway are enhanced on feeding high carbohydrate diets and are reduced in starvation and dibetes mellitus.
- Increase in FA synthesis and steroid synthesis re-oxidizes NADPH to $NADP^+$ and cytoplasmic ratio of $NADP^+$/NADPH is increased which enhances the shunt pathway.
- *Hormones:*
  - ***Insulin*** induces the synthesis of both the dehydrogenases and thus enhances the activity of the pathway.
  - ***Thyroid hormones*** enhance the activity of G-6-PD and thus the shunt pathway.

METABOLIC SIGNIFICANCE OF HMP SHUNT

1. Formation of NADPH: ***NADPH is produced in this pathway which is used as electron donor in many reductive syntheses in the body.*** Some examples of such reactions where NADPH is used are:

- ***Extramitochondrial de novo fatty acid synthesis.***
- ***Synthesis of cholesterol***
- ***Synthesis of steroidal hormones***
- ***Conversion of oxidized glutathione G-S-S-G to reduced glutathione G-SH.***

2. Provision of Pentoses: Provision of pentoses for nucleotide and nucleic acid synthesis; the source of the D-ribose is the D-ribose-5-P, an intermediate in this pathway.

3. Role in RB Cells Fragility: HMP shunt in erythrocytes provides NADPH for:

- ***Reduction of oxidized glutathione (G-S-S-G) to reduced glutathione (2 G-SH)*** catalyzed by the enzyme *glutathione reductase.*
- Reduced glutathione (G-SH) thus formed in turn, removes H_2O_2 from the erythrocytes in a reaction catalysed by *glutathione peroxidase* (Se-containing enzyme).

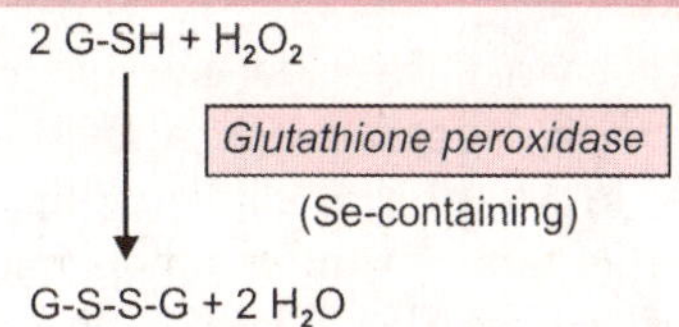

This reaction is important, since accumulation of H_2O_2 may decrease the lifespan of RB cells by increasing the rate of oxidation of Hb to methaemoglobin. ***An inverse correlation exists between the activity of "G-6-PD" enzyme and the fragility of red cells (susceptibility to haemolysis).***

4. Role in Lens Metabolism: In studying lens metabolism, it has been observed, at least 10 percent of glucose is metabolized by shunt pathway and provides NADPH, which is necessary to convert oxidized glutathione to reduced glutathione, which is necessary for maintenance of lens proteins.

5. Oxidation: Oxidation in this pathway is different from EM pathway. Oxidation occurs in the first reaction and third reaction, by specific *dehydrogenase* and NADPH is produced. Carbon-1 of glucose is removed as CO_2 by decarboxylation, which is never formed in EM pathway.

6. Role in Tissue Anoxia: Tissues subjected to extended periods of anoxia develop fatty infiltration. This is due to increased formation of NADPH due to enhanced HMP shunt, which increases FA-synthesis.

7. Role in CO_2-Fixation Reaction: Carbon dioxide produced in HMP shunt may be used in "CO_2-fixation" reactions. In plants, CO_2 produced in HMP shunt which is utilized for glucose formation by photosynthesis.

Clinical Aspects

A. Haemolytic Anaemia Due to G-6-PD Deficiency: A mutation present in some populations causes a deficiency of the enzyme G-6-PD with impairment of generation of NADPH that is manifested as red cells haemolysis when the susceptible individuals are subjected to oxidant group of drugs such as antimalarials, like primaquine and aspirin etc.

Inheritence: Generally transmitted by a sexlinked gene of intermediate dominance.

Race: Defect has a high incidence in Negroes. Also found in non-Negro races and seen most frequently in Mediterranean peoples, namely Italians particularly Sardinians and some Greeks. Other races known to be affected include: Indians, Chinese, Malayan and Thais. In India, the genetic disorder is relatively frequent in Parsis, Punjabis, Sindhis and Kutchi-Lohans. In general, the deficiency of the enzyme is more marked in non-Negroes.

Clinically: Develops acute haemolytic episode after administration of oxidant group of drugs. First described with primaquine administration, hence, called also as ***"primaquine-sensitive haemolytic anaemia"***

Severity of haemolysis related to dose of the drug. Haemolysis is shown by:

- *Anaemia*
- *Fall in blood Hb* ↓
- *May be jaundice, and*
- *Blackenning of urine.*

This type of haemolysis is "self-limiting"; older cells are destroyed whereas the younger cells are resistant.

Mechanism of haemolysis: Discussed above.

Oxidant drug: which may cause haemolysis in G-6-PD deficient subject are:

- **Antimalarials:** Primaquine, pamaquin
- **Analgesics:** Acetyl salicyclic acid, phenacetin
- **Sulphonamides** group of drugs
- **Sulphones:** Dapsone, sulphoxone, etc.
- **Nitrofurans:** Furadantin; furoxone
- **Miscellaneous:** Vit K, Probenecid, PAS, phenylhydrazine, methylene blue, etc.

Relationship with Other Diseases

- ***Relation of P. falciparum infection:*** There is evidence to suggest that the defect confers some protection against *P. falciparum* infection, where this genetic disorder is prevalent. It may lessen the severity of malarial infections in young children and infants.
- ***Relation with colour blindness:*** It has been shown that the disorder shows a close linkage with colour blindness.

B. Favism: A disorder characterized by an acute haemolytic anaemia of sudden onset, often with haemoglobinuria, occurs in G-6-PD deficient subjects ***sensitive to the fava beans (Vicia fava)*** either

- On ingestion with uncooked or lightly cooked beans; or
- On inhalation of pollens from the blossom of the plant.

Although favism occurs typically with Mediterranean people, it may also occur in certain non Mediterranean subjects with G-6-PD deficiency including Chinese and Jews.

URONIC ACID PATHWAY

It is an alternate pathway for oxidation of glucose.

BIOMEDICAL IMPORTANCE

- In this pathway ***energy is not produced.***
- ***Major function is to produce D-glucuronic acid*** which is mainly utilized for detoxication of foreign chemicals (xenobiotics).
- Inherited deficiency of an enzyme in this pathway produces ***essential pentosuria.***
- Total absence of one particular enzyme in primates, accounts for the fact that ***ascorbic acid (vitamin C) cannot be synthesized by humans***, and requires to be provided in the diet.

METABOLIC PATHWAY

For an outline pathway see ***Fig:12.9.***

1 (a) Formation of UDP-G from Glucose: The steps are similar to glycogenesis.

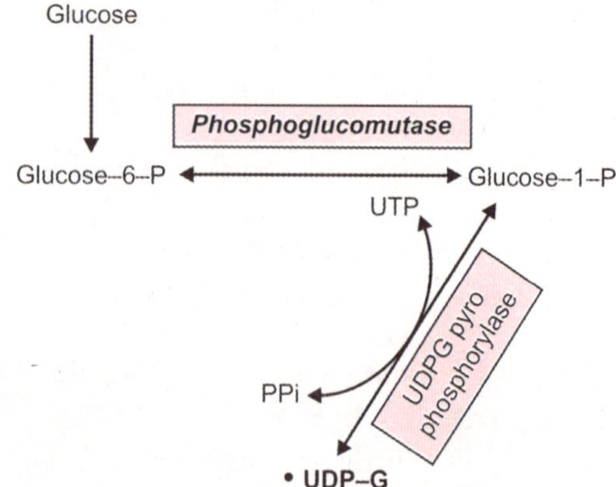

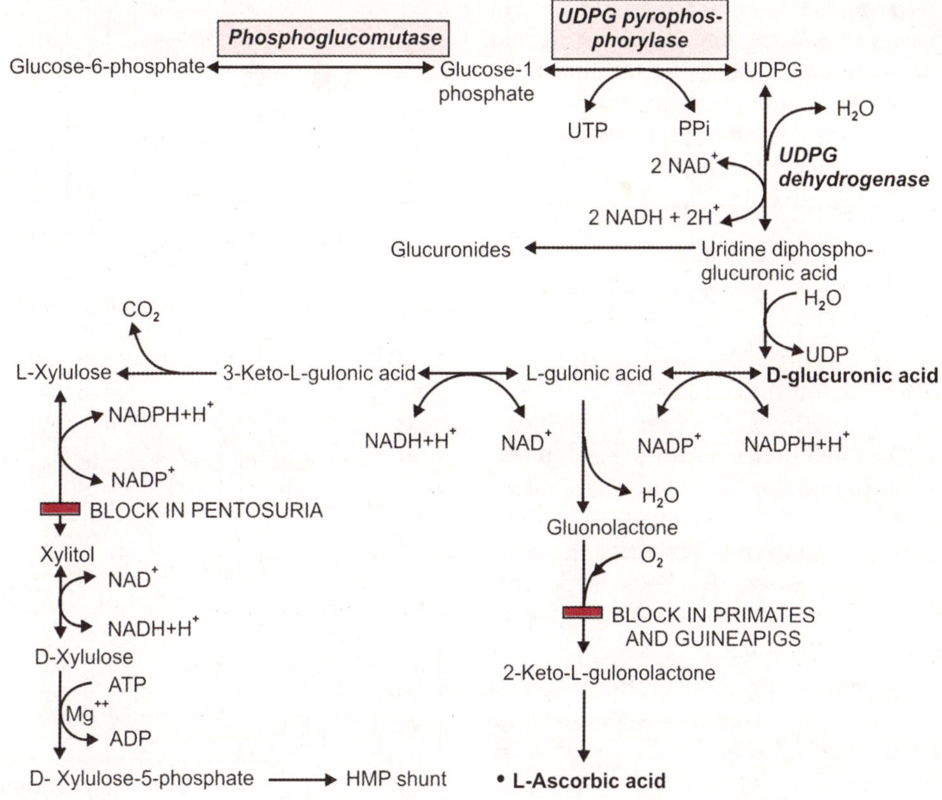

Fig.12.9: Uronic acid pathway

(b) Formation of D-Glucuronic Acid: UDP-G is now oxidized at carbon-6-by a two-step process to form "D-glucuronic acid"

- UDP-G is oxidized by an enzyme *UDP-G dehydrogenase* and forms **"UDP-glucuronic acid"**. The enzyme requires NAD^+ as hydrogen aceptor.
- UDP-glucuronic acid is hydrolyzed to form D-glucuronic acid.

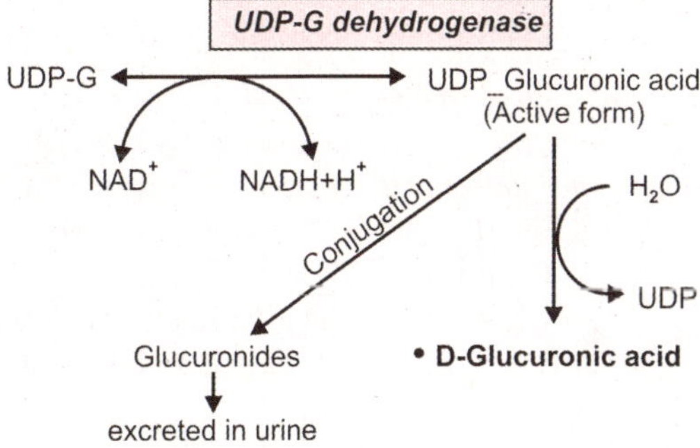

UDP-glucuronic acid is the "active" form which takes part in conjugation to form "glucuronides" or in formation of proteoglycans. Further metabolism of D-glucuronic acid varies according to animals.

II. Formation of L-Gulonic Acid: In an NADPH-dependant reaction D-glucuronic acid is first reduced to "L-gulonic acid"

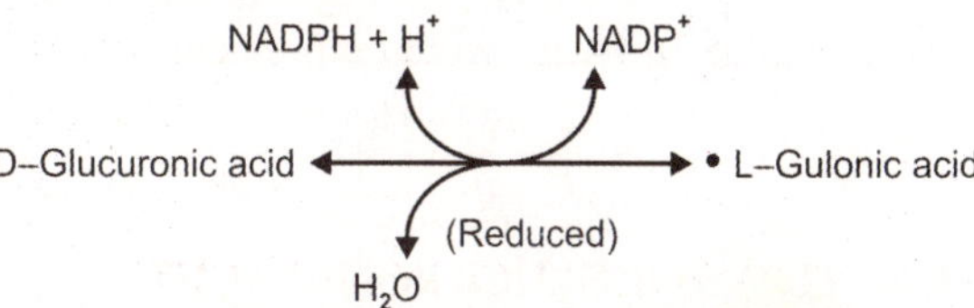

III. Fate of L-Gulonic Acid: Fate of L-gulonic acid is different according to the animals.

Synthesis of Ascorbic Acid: L-gulonic acid is the direct precursor of ascorbic acid, in those animals which are capable of synthesizing this vitamin.

***Fate of L-Gulonic Acid in Humans: In man and other primates as well as guineapigs* ascorbic acid cannot be synthesized** and L-gulonic acid is oxidized to 3-keto L-gulonic acid, which is then decarboxylated to the pentose "**L-xylulose**". Fate of L-xylulose is shown in *Fig 12.10.*

Clinical Importance of Uronic Acid Pathway

Disruption of uronic acid pathway can be caused by enzyme defects and administration of certain drugs.

1. **Essential Pentosuria:** An inherited disorder
- ***Inheritance*** is autosomal recessive.
- ***Enzyme deficiency:*** *L-xylitol dehydrogenase.*
- Due to inherited deficiency of the enzyme *L-xylitol dehydrogenase,* L-xylulose cannot be converted to xylitol. As a result L-xylulose accumulates and excreted in urine. In some cases, L-arabitol is also excreted in urine. This pentose sugar may be derivved from L-xylulose by reduction.

2. **Oxalosis:** Parenteral administration of xylitol may lead to *oxalosis* involving calcium oxalate deposition in brain and kidneys. This results from the conversion of D-xylulose to oxalate as shown below:

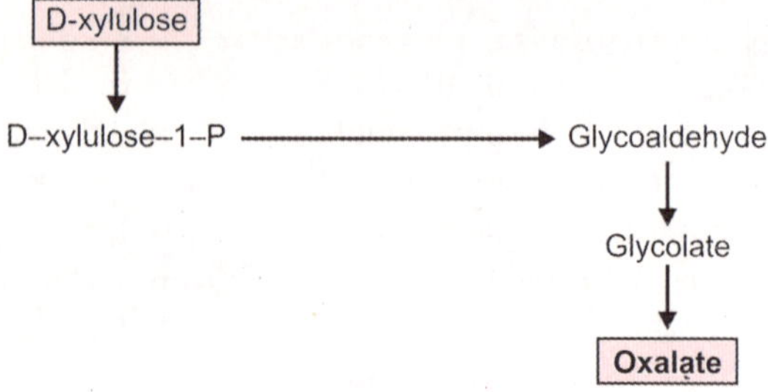

Other sources of oxalates in body are:
- Ascorbic acid (vitamin C)
- Glycine

FUNCTIONS OF GLUCURONIC ACID

1. **Conjugation:** Glucuronic acid takes part in conjugation reaction with various xenobiotics like drugs, chemicals, pollutants, food additives, carcinogens and endogenous hormones. (Refer chapter to Detoxication).

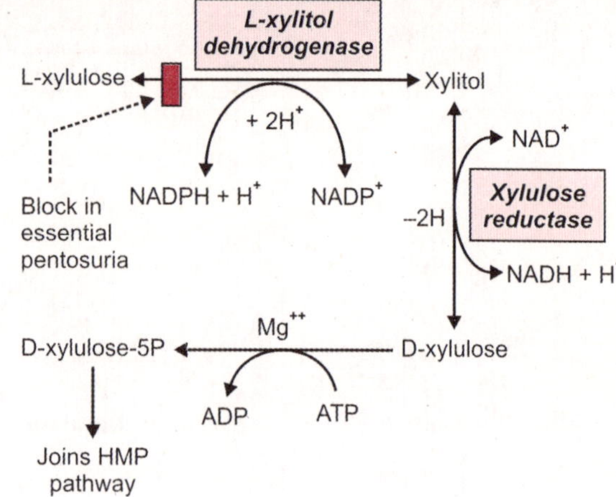

Fig. 12.10: Fate of L-xylulose

Important substances that undergo conjugation are as follows.

- ***Aromatic acid, e.g. benzoic acid:***
  Benzoic acid + D-Glucuronic acid→Benzoyl glucuronide
- ***Phenols and secondary/tertiary aliphatic alcohols:*** In which coupling occurs with OH group ("ether" linkage).
  Phenol + D-Glucuronic acid→Phenyl glucuronide
- ***Bile pigments:*** Bilirubin is conjugated with D-glucuronic acid to form mono and di-glucuronides (see hemecatabolism for details).
- ***Drugs and other xenobiotics:*** They are first hydroxylated by mono-oxygenase cyt-p-450 system and then conjugated with D-glucuronic acid.
- ***Antibiotics:*** Certain antibiotics like chloramphenicol is also conjugated with D-glucuronic acid.
- ***Hormones:*** Derivatives of certain steroid hormones and certain hormones like thyroid hormones are detoxicated by D-glucuronic acid.

2. **Synthesis of MPS**
- ***Incorporation of D-glucuronic acid in mucopolysaccharides (MPS):*** Incorporation of D-glucuronic acid in mucopolysaccharides like hyaluronic acid, chondroitin, chondroitin SO_4 and heparin. UDP-glucuronic acid acts as a donor in liver and matrices of cartilages and bones.

- UDP- glucuronic acid may be changed to UDP-L-iduronic acid with the help ***UDP-glucuronic acid-5-epimerase***. L-iduronic acid is incorporated in forming Dermatan SO_4 (chondroitin SO_4 B) in skin.
- UDP-xylose may be formed by the decarboxylation of UDP-glucuronic acid in cornea, cartilage, etc. with the help of NAD^+ and a specific enzyme and is used in mucoprotein synthesis.

GLUCONEOGENESIS

Definition: The formation of glucose or glycogen ***from non-carbohydrate sources*** is called gluconeogenesis.

BIOMEDICAL IMPORTANCE

Why gluconeogenesis is necessary in the body?

1. ***Gluconeogenesis meets the requirements of glucose in the body when carbohydrates are not available in sufficient amounts from the diet.*** Even in condition, where fat is utilized for energy still certain *basal level of glucose* is required to meet the need for glucose for special uses, e.g.
   - Source of energy for nervous tissue and erythrocytes.
   - Required for maintaining level of intermediates of TCA cycle
   - Source of glyceride-glycerol-P required for adipose tissue,
   - It is a precursor of milk sugar (lactose) for lactating mammary gland; and
   - It serves as only fuel for skeletal muscles in anaerobic conditions.
2. Gluconeogenic mechanisms are required to clear the products of metabolism of other tissues from the blood, e.g.
   - *lactic acid:* Produced by muscles and erythrocytes; and
   - *Glycerol:* Continuously produced by adipose tissue by lipolysis of TG (triacyl glycerol).

Site of Gluconeogenesis: In mammals, the principal organs involved in gluconeogenesis are *liver* and *kidneys*, as they possess the full complement of enzymes necessary for gluconeogenesis.

SUBSTRATES FOR GLUCONEOGENESIS

Principal substrates as per priorities are listed below

- *Glucogenic amino acids:* Amino acids which form glucose are pyruvate forming amino acids and those that produce intermediates of TCA cycle, e.g. oxaloacetic acid and α-ketoglutarate.
- *Lactates* and pyruvates
- *Glycerol* obtained from lipolysis of fats.
- *Propionic acid* (important in ruminants): In human beings, Propionyl-CoA is formed in metabolic pathways, which can form glucose.

METABOLIC PATHWAYS INVOLVED IN GLUCONEOGENESIS

Gluconeogenesis involves glycolysis, the citric acid cycle and some special reactions.

A. Main Pathway of Gluconeogenesis

For the outline pathway see ***Fig. 12.11. Main pathway is a reversal of glycolytic pathway*** but thermodynamic ***"barriers"*** prevent a simple reversal of glycolysis, certain modifications and adaptations are necessary in the EM Pathway. Kerbs showed that energy barriers obstructs a simple reversal of glycolysis. There are ***four such energy barriers which are irreversible.***

- ***Between pyruvate and phosphoenol pyruvate.***
- ***Between fructose-1 6-bi-phosphate and fructose-6-P.***
- ***Between glucose-6-P and glucose.***
- ***Between glucose-1-P and glycogen***

The above energy barriers and irreversible reactions are circumvented by special adaptations which are discussed below:

1. *Between Pyruvate and Phosphoenol Pyruvate:* The conversion of pyruvic acid (thus also lactic acid which can be converted to PA) to phosphoenolpyruvate is achieved by **two important enzymes:**
   - ***Pyruvate carboxylase,*** a mitochondrial enzyme,

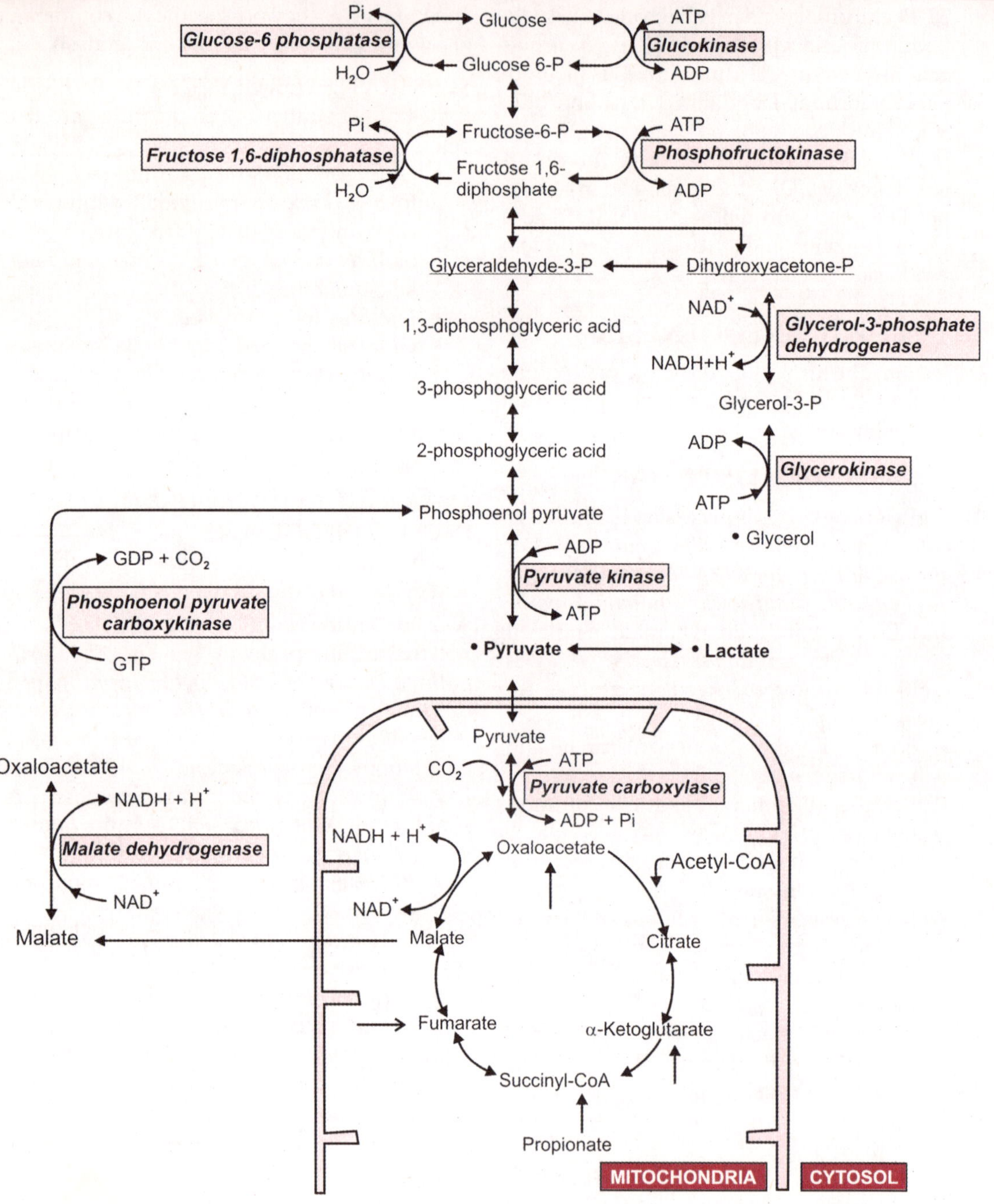

Fig. 12.11: Major pathway of gluconeogenesis in the liver. Entry points of glucogenic amino acids are shown by arrows

- *Phosphoenol pyruvate carboxykinase* an enzyme present principally in cytosol, but also in small amount present in mitochondrion.

Functions of these enzymes are:

- *Pyruvate carboxylase* in mitochondrion, in presence of ATP, Biotin and CO_2 converts pyruvate to OAA (CO_2 fixation reaction).

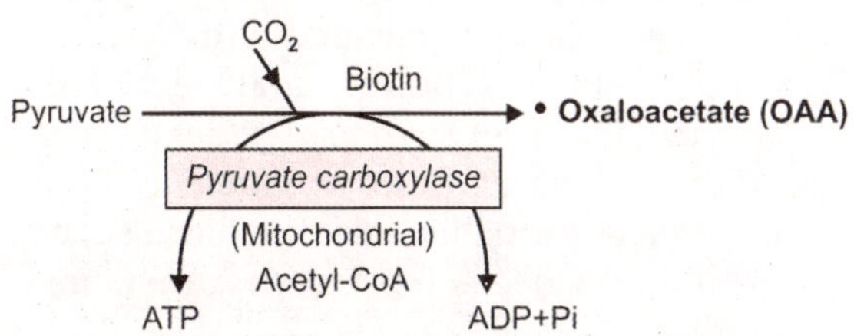

- ***Phosphoenol pyruvate carboxykinase*** enzyme present chiefly in cytosol, catalyzes the conversion of OAA to phosphoenol pyruvate. High energy phosphate in the form of GTP or ITP is required in this reaction and CO_2 is liberated. ***Once phosphoenol pyruvate is formed from pyruvic acid by the action of above two enzymes, it can go into reverse glycolytic pathways.***

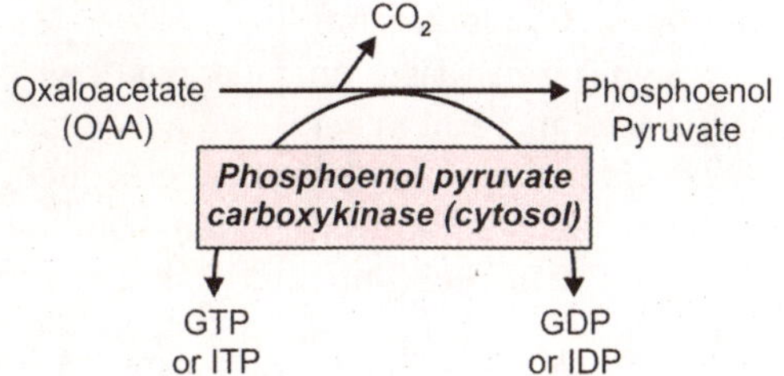

Note:

- It is to be noted that OAA is formed inside the mitochondrion, but the other reaction occurs in the cytosol. ***OAA is not permeable to mitochondrial membrane.*** OAA is transferred to cytosol by **two mechanisms:**
  - **Mainly as malate** which then in cytosol is converted to OAA again *(Fig. 12.12).*
  - Secondly, ***OAA can combine with acetyl CoA to form citrate, which is permeable to mitochondrial membrane. Citric acid is cleaved by citrate-cleavage enzyme and reforms OAA.***

- In addition to pyruvate carboxylase, PA can be converted to OAA via the formation of malate.

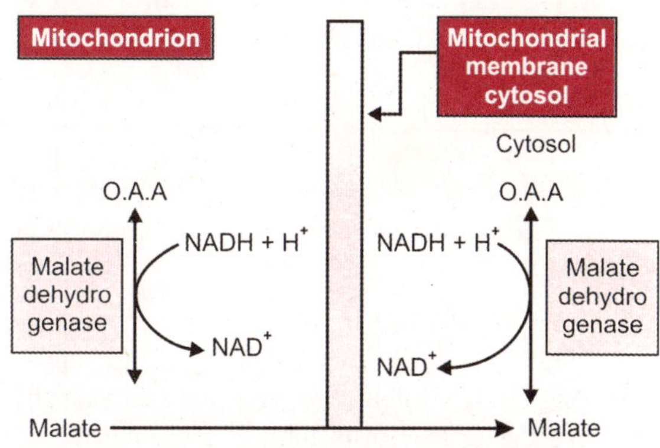

Fig. 12.12: Conversion of malate to OAA

2. ***Between Fructose-1, 6-Biphosphate to Fructose-6-P***

The conversion of fructose-1, 6-biophosphate to fructose 6-phosphate, the next energy barrier; is circumvented as follows to achieve a reversal of glycolysis. The above reaction is ctalyzed by a specific *enzyme* ***fructose-1, 6-biophosphatase.*** This is a *key enzyme* in gluconeogenic pathway, and its presence determines whether or not a tissue is capable of forming glucose/and glycogen not only from pyruvate/lactate but also from triosephosphates.

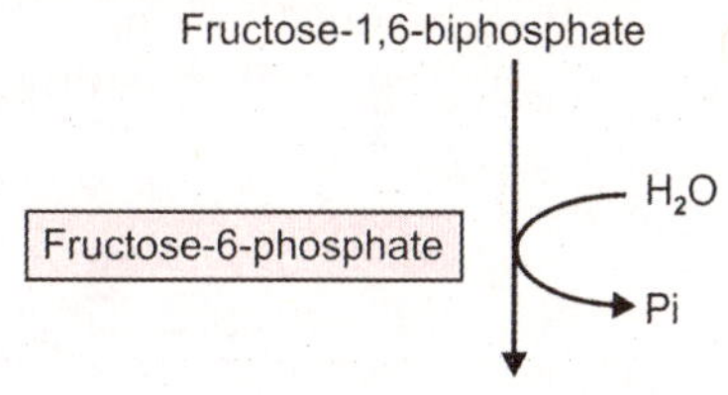

Site: The enzyme is present in liver, kidneys and intestine.

Recently it has been shown to be present also in striated muscles. The enzyme is absent in adipose tissue, cardiac muscle and smooth muscles.

3. ***Between Glucose-6-P and Glucose***

The conversion of glucose-6-P to glucose, the third energy barrier in the glycolytic pathway is circumvented as follows:

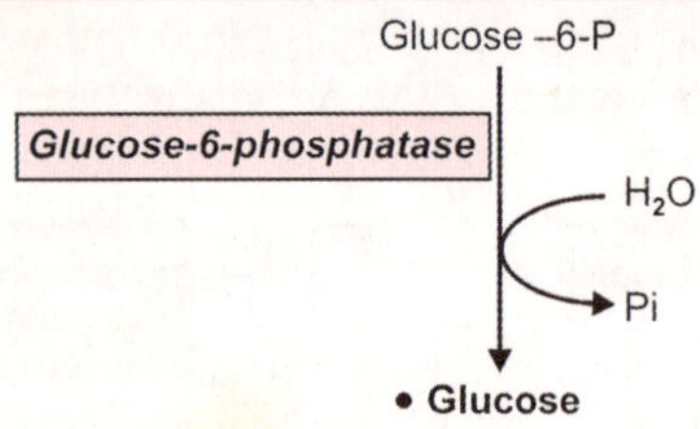

The above reaction is catalyzed by a specific enzyme ***glucose-6-phosphatase.*** The enzyme is microsomal and also possesses "pyrophosphatase" activity.

Site: The enzyme is present in liver, kidneys, intestine and platelets. The enzyme is absent in adipose tissue and muscles. **As the enzyme is absent in muscles, it cannot contribute to blood glucose directly by glycogenolysis.**

B. Other Special Pathways for Gluconeogenesis

1. ***Conversion of Glycerol to Glucose:*** Glycerol is a product of metabolism of adipose tissue and is produced by lipolysis. Tissues which possess the activating enzyme ***glycerokinase*** can utilize glycerol.

Sites: The enzyme is present in liver, Kidneys, heart muscle, lactating mammary gland, and intestinal mucosa. ***The enzyme is absent in adipose tissue.***

*Reaction of this pathway are shown in **Fig.12.13.***

This pathway, thus connects with the triose-phosphate stages of the glycolytic pathway and triose-P can enter "reverse" glycolysis after conversion to fructose-1,6-biphosphate and then it can form glucose.

2. ***Conversion of Propionic Acid to Glucose:*** Propionic acid is a major source of glucose in ruminants, and enters the main gluconeogenic pathway via TCA cycle after conversion to succinyl-CoA.

- Propionate is first activated with ATP and CoA-SH, the reaction is catalyzed by the enzyme ***Acyl-CoA synthase*** (earlier called as ***thiokinase)*** and converted to "***propionyl-CoA***".
- In humans, propionic acid is not formed, but propionyl-CoA is formed as a metabolic product.

Chief sources of propionyl-CoA in humans are:

- Catabolism of L-methionine via α-keto butyrate (see methionine catabolism).
- Catabolism of amino acid isoleucine.
- β-oxidation of odd-chain fatty acids
- Biosynthesis of bile acids.

Fate of propionyl CoA in humans is shown in ***Fig.12.14.***

Hormones in Gluconeogenesis

- ***Glucagon:*** It increases gluconeogenesis from lactic acid and amino acids.
- ***Glucocorticoids:*** They stimulate gluconeogenesis by increasing protein catabolism in the peripheral tissues and increasing hepatic

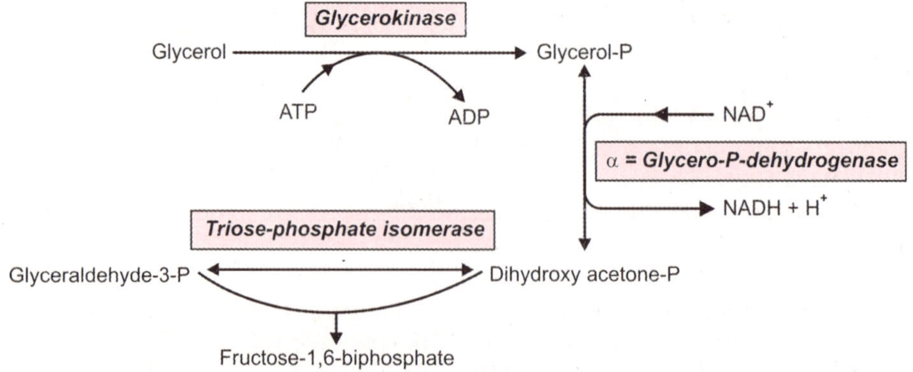

Fig. 12.13: Reactions of the pathway for gluconeogenesis

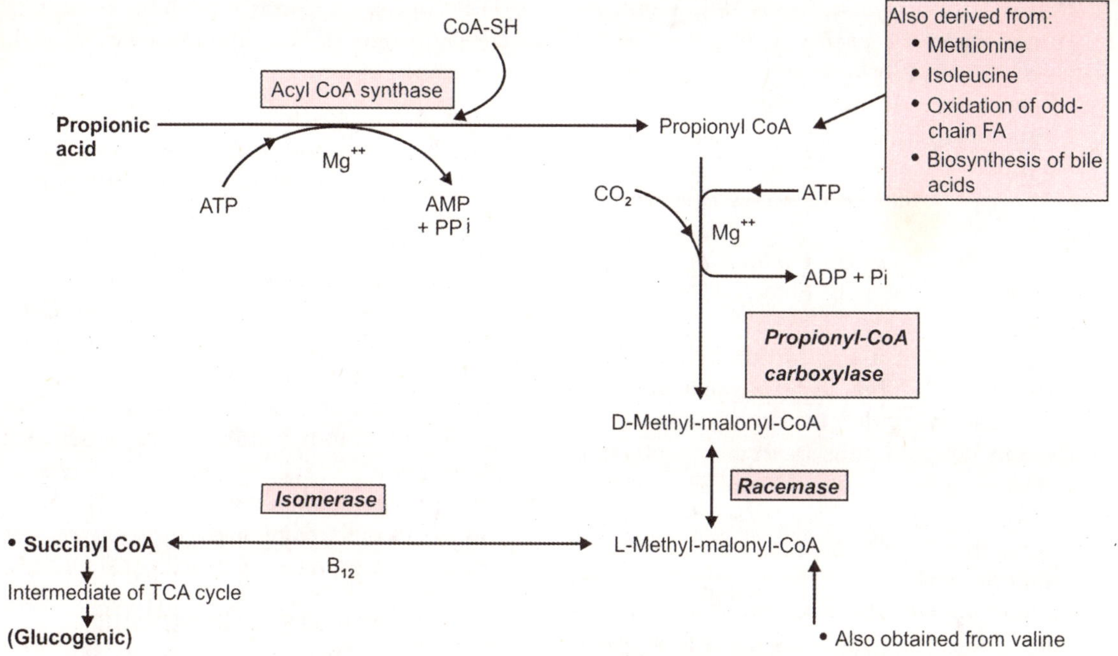

Fig. 12.14: Metabolism of propionic acid

uptake of amino acids and increases activity of transaminases and other enzymes concerned in gluconeogenesis.

Regulation of Gluconeogenesis

1. *Key enzymes* which regulate gluconeogenesis are:
   - *Pyruvate carboxylase*
   - *Phospho-enol pyruvate carboxykinase (PEPCK)*
   - *Fructose-1,6-biphosphatase and*
   - *Glucose-6-phosphatase.*

2. *High Carbohydrate Diets:* These reduce gluconeogenesis by increasing the insulin/glucagon ratio and thereby reducing the activities of all four key gluconeogenic enzymes.

3. *Glucose-6-Pase:* This enzyme is induced by the hormones glucagon and glucocorticoids, which are secreted during starvation thus enhancing gluconeogenesis. Insulin represses the enzyme

4. *Fructose-1,6-Biphosphatase:* This enzyme is stongly and allosterically inhibited by AMP, but is activated by citrates. Hence, ***gluconeogenesis is increased when there is increased ATP and citrate levels.*** Gluconeogenesis is decreased by inhibition of this enyzyme when liver cells are rich in AMP and low in citrate concentration.

5. *Role of Fructose-2,6-Biphosphate:* Fructose-2,6-bi-P is formed by phosphorylation of fructose-6-P by the enzyme *phosphofructokinase-2*. The same enzyme protein is also responsible for its breakdown since it also contains *fructose-2,6-biphosphatase activity*. ***This bifunctional enzyme is under the allosteric control of fructose-6-P.*** Under conditions of glucose shortage, gluconeogenesis is stimulated by glucagon by decreasing the concentration of fructose-2,6, bi-P, which, in turn, inhibits *phosphofructokinase-1* and activates the enzyme *fructose-1,6-biphosphatase*

6. *Phosphoenol Pyruvate Carboxykinase:* The enzyme is induced by glucagon, during starvation, thus increaisng gluconeogenesis. Insulin reduces gluconeogenesis as it represses the enzyme.

7. *Pyruvate Carboxylase:* This is the **key enzyme in gluconeogenetic pathway.** The enzyme is activated allosterically by acetyl CoA. It binds with the allosteric site of the enzyme, brings about conformational change at teritary level, so that the affinity of the enzyme for CO_2 increases.

8. *Fatty Acid Oxidation Promotes Gluconeogenesis:*

- It *provides acetyl CoA which acts as +ve allosteric modifier* of the enzyme **Pyruvate carboxylase**.
- Increased acetyl CoA and NADH from β-oxidation inhibits *pyruvate dehydrogenase complex* so that oxidative decarboxylation of PA does not occur thus sparing its conversion to OAA.
- It provides energy, thus, it spares PA from degradation

9. *Other factors*

- *Increased ADP allosterically inhibts pyruvate carboxylase* and this decreases gluconeogenesis
- *Insulin represses the enzyme pyruvate carboxylase and reduces gluconeogenesis*
- On the other hand, hormones like glucagon, adrenaline and glucocorticoids induce the synthesis of the enzyme *pyruvate carboxylase* and enhances gluconeogenesis.

FATES OF LACTIC ACID IN THE BODY

1. **Chief fate is conversion to pyruvate** and its utilizsation as puryvate which either undergoes oxidative decarboxylation to form acetyl CoA, or it can be glucogenic (For other fates see pyruvate metabolism).

2. **What is "Cori Cycle"?**

- Once formed *lactic acid can be further metabolized only by its reconversion to pyruvate* as stated above.
- In contrast to the phosphorylated intermediates of glycolysis which are locked in the cells, *lactates and pyruvates can readily diffuse out from the cells* in which they are produced and pass into the circulation.
- From circulation, they are removed by the liver and in liver cells they are reconverted to form glucose and glycogen by gluconeogenesis
- Muscles cannot convert glucose-6-P to glucose due to lack of the enzyme *glucose-6-phosphatase.*

This cycle is referred to as **Cori cycle *(Fig. 12.15)*.**

☞ SALIENT POINTS TO REMEMBER

- Hexose monophosphate shunt or pathway is an alternate pathway for direct oxidatioan of glucose.
- The *pathway is not meant for energy.* It is of importance since this pathway ***provides NADPH and Pentoses.***
- NADPH is required for various reductive synthesis in metabolic pathways and pentoses are required for nucleic acid synthesis.
- HMP shunt does not occur in all the tissues of the body. It only operates in certain

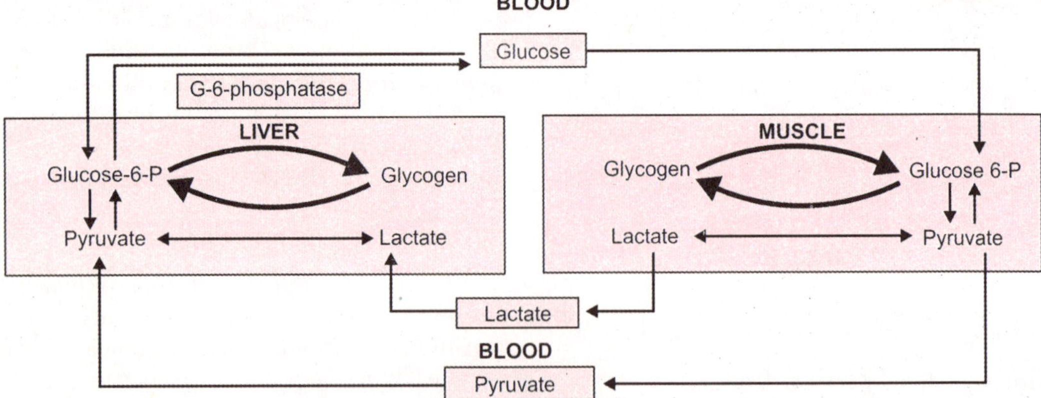

Fig. 12.15: Cori cycle

specialized tissues viz. Liver, adipose tissue, R.B. cells, adrenal cortex, testes/ovary, lactating mammary glands and lens of the eye, to serve specific functions.

- The absence of the first enzyme in the metabolic pathway, glucose-6-phosphate dehydrogenase (G-6-PD), results in haemolysis of R.B. cells by oxidants resulting to haemolytic anaemia.
- ***G-6-PD deficient people are resistant to Plasmodium falciparum infection.***
- Uronic acid pathway is another alternative pathway for oxidation of glucose. This pathway is also not meant for energy. The pathway provides formation of D-Glucuronic acid.
- Glucuronate is involved in the conjugation of bilirubin, steroid hormones and detoxification of drugs. Also required for synthesis of Muco-Polysaccharides (MPs).
- Absence of an enzyme *gluconolactone oxidase* in this pathway in humans, primates and guineapigs make them incapable to synthesize ascorbic acid (vitamin C), whereas other animals can synthesize due to the presence of the enzyme.
- Inherited deficiency of the enzyme *"L-xylitol dehydrogenase"* produces the disease **essential pentosuria**.
- Gluconeogenesis is the synthesis of glucose from non carbohydrate sources.
- The substrates are Glucogenic amino acids, Pyruvates/and Lactates, Glycerol and Propionate.
- The reversal of glycolysis from Pyruvate with alternate arrangements to circumvent the three irreversible reactions in glycolytic pathway is the hallmark of gluconeogenesis.
- In ruminants, propionic acid formed during the course of carbohydrate digestion is a good precursor for gluconeogenesis.
- In humans, propionate is not a good source and constitutes minor pathway. The main sources of propionic acid in humans are: catabolism of methionine and isoleucine, oxidation of odd-chain fatty acids. and biosynthesis of bile acids.

METABOLISM OF GALACTOSE

- Galactose is derived from the hydrolysis of the disaccharide "lactose" (sugar of milk) in the intestine by the enzyme *"lactase"*.
- Galactose is "actively" transported, to portal blood. ***Galactose absorption is faster than glucose.*** Galactose reaches liver by portal blood where it is readily converted to glucose. This property is used as test of liver function called "galactose tolerance test".
- Most of the dietary galactose is converted to glucose and goes to systemic circulation as glucose. Very little galactose as such goes to systemic circulation.
- ***Tissues requiring galactose synthesizes it from glucose, taken up by tissues from systemic circulation.***

BIOMEDICAL IMPORTANCE

- Galactose is required in lactating mammary gland ***for synthesis of lactose for breast milk.***
- Galactose is utilized in brain and nervous tissues for synthesis of glycolipids-cerebrosides and gangliosides.
- Galactose is required for synthesis of chondromucoids and mucoproteins.
- Inherited deficiency of certain enzymes in pathway of galactose metabolism produces inherited disorder ***galactosaemia.***

METABOLIC PATHWAY

The pathway by which galactose is converted to glucose and lactose is synthesized is shown in *Fig. 12.16.*

- ***In reaction 1:*** Galactose is phosphorylated with the enzyme ***galactokinase***, an ***adaptive enzyme***, using ATP as phosphate donor, and produces galactose-1-P. The reaction is **irreversible**.
- ***In reaction 2:*** Galactose-1-P reacts with UDP glucose to form UDP-galactose and glucose-1-P, in presence of the enzyme ***"galactose-1-P-uridyl transferase"***.
- ***In reaction 3:*** UDP-galactose and UDP-glucose are interconvertible and catalyzed by the enzyme ***epimerase***, which requires NAD^+. The reaction is freely ***"reversible".***

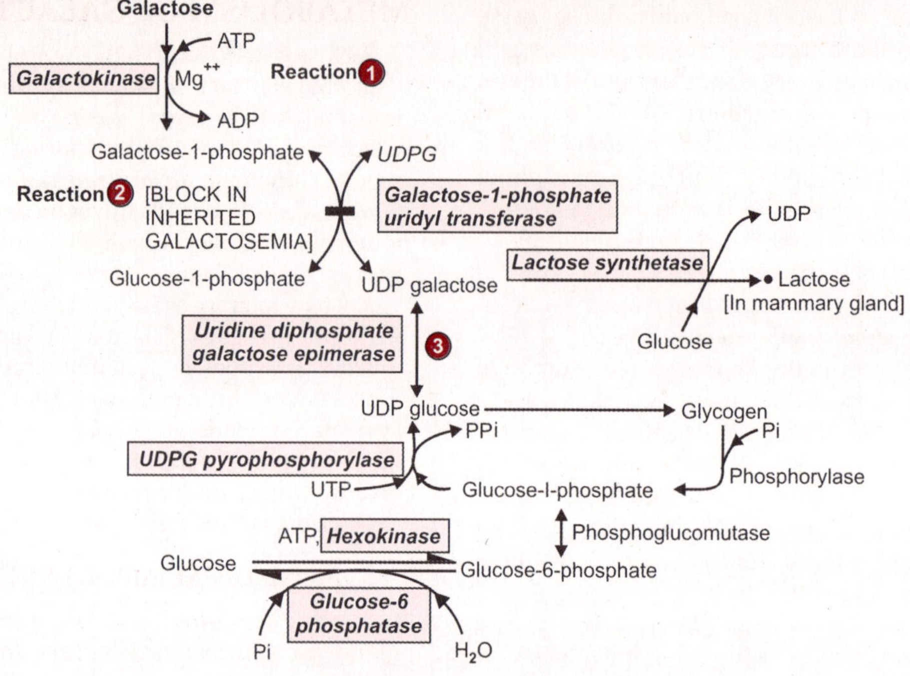

Fig. 12.16: Metabolism of galactose

- In this manner, glucose can be converted to galactose, so that preformed galactose is not essential in the diet.

Note: Formation of UDP-glucose from glucose is similar to steps in glycogenesis (see the reactions in glycogenesis).

BIOSYNTHESIS OF LACTOSE

- In synthesis of lactose in lactating mammary gland, UDP glucose is converted to UDP-galactose by the enzyme *epimerase.*
- UDP-galactose condenses with one molecule of glucose, to form "lactose", the reaction is catalyzed by the enzyme *lactose synthetase.* Lactose synthetase also called as *galactosyl transferase.*

INHERITED DISORDER OF GALACTOSE METABOLISM

Galactosaemia: An inherited disorder, in which there is inability to convert galactose to glucose in normal manner.

- *Incidence:* 1 in 18,000 live births.
- *Enzyme defects:*
  - *Galactose-1-P-uridyl transferase* enzyme is deficient **(classical type):** In this both galactose and galactose-1-P accumulate in blood and tissues.
  - *Galactokinase deficiency* **(minor type):** In this galactose accumulates in blood and tissues.
  - It is claimed that there may be *epimerase* deficiency, which is rare.
- *Inheritance:* autosomal recessive
- *Clinically:*

a. *Infants appear normal at birth but later,*
  - Fail to thrive; become lethargic; and may vomit
  - *Hypoglycaemia:* causes may be:
    - Due to enzyme deficiency galactose cannot be converted to glucose; and
    - Increased galactose level increases insulin secretion; and
    - Galactose-1-P inhibits *phosphogluco-mutase* enzyme.

- May manifest jaundice, which may be prolonged in neonatal period.

b. *After 2 to 3 months:*
- ***Liver*** may show ***fatty infiltration*** and ***lead to cirrhosis liver.***
- ***Mental retardation*** due to accumulation of galactose and galactose-1-P in cerebral cortex;
- Development of ***cataracts*** because:
  - excess of galactose in lens is reduced to **"galactitol" (Dulcitol)** by the enzyme *"aldose reductase"*
  - galactitol cannot escape from lens cells. **Osmotic effect** of the sugar alcohol contributes to injury to lens proteins and development of cataracts.
  - excess of galactose inhibits *glucose-6-P-dehydrogenase* (G-6-PD) leading to less NADPH which results to ***less of reduced glutathione (G-SH).***

- ***Biochemical and Urinary Findings:***
  - Increase blood galactose level ↑
  - Blood sugar level decreases ↓ (hypoglycaemia)
  - Inorganic P decreases ↓ due to utilization of PO_4 for galactose-1-P.
- ***Urine:*** Increased excretion of galactose in urine ↑ ***(galactosuria), albuminuria, amino aciduria:*** amino acids excreted usually are serine, alanine and glycine.
- ***Prognosis:*** Not fatal. Can survive to puberty and adulthood.

REGULATION OF BLOOD (HOMEOSTASIS)

Blood glucose level is maintained within physiological limits 60 to 100 mg percent ***(true glucose)*** in fasting state and 100 to 140 mg per cent following ingestion of a carbohydrate containing meal, by a balance between ***two sets of factors:***
- Rate of glucose entrance into the blood stream
- Rate of its removal from the blood stream *(Table 12.5).*

RATE OF SUPPLY OF GLUCOSE TO BLOOD

Except for a possible minor contribution by the kidney, which probabaly does not occur under physiological conditions, the blood glucose may be derived directly from the following sources:
- By absorption from the intestine.
- Breakdown of glycogen of liver, (hepatic glycogenolysis).
- By gluconeogenesis in liver source being glucogenic amino acids, lactate and pyruvate, glycerol and propionyl CoA.
- Glucose obtained from other carbohydrates e.g. fructose, galactose, etc.

RATE OF REMOVAL OF GLUCOSE FROM BLOOD

- Oxidation of glucose by the tissues to supply energy.
- Glycogen formation from glucose in liver *(hepatic glycogenesis).*

Table 12.5: Regulation of blood glucose level

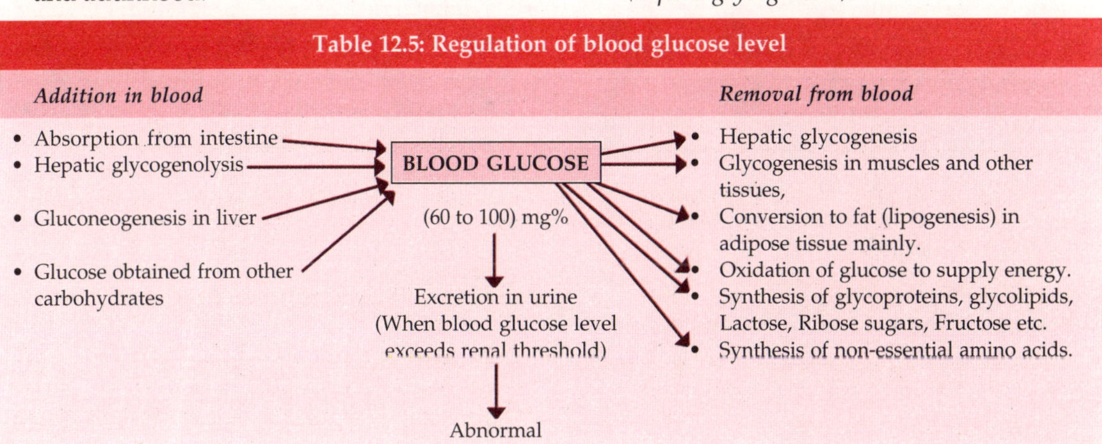

- Glycogen formation from glucose in muscles *(muscle glycogenesis)*.
- Conversion of glucose to fats *(lipogenesis)* specially in adipose tissue.
- Synthesis of compounds containing carbohydrates-blood glucose is utilized, e.g.
  - Formation of fructose in seminal fluid,
  - Formation of lactose (sugar of milk) in lactating mammary gland;
  - Synthesis of glycorproteins and glycolipids and
  - Formation of ribose sugars from glucose required for nucleic acid synthesis.
- Excretion of glucose in urine (glycosuria), when blood glucose level exceeds the renal threshold.

  All the above processes are under substrate, endproduct, nervous and hormonal control.

1. CONDITION OF BLOOD GLUCOSE IN POST-ABSORPTIVE STATE

What is Post-absorptive State?

- This is ***fasting state, approximately 12 to 14 hours after last meal.*** There is practically no intestinal absorption. It is not prolonged starvation, as there are no metabolic abnormalities.
- It is the condition of a subject between 8 to 10 AM, if he had his dinner previous evening about 8 PM and had taken nothing thereafter. Under such a situation only source of glucose is Liver glycogen.
- At rest, tissues utilize approximately 200 mg of glucose per miniute from blood.

2. CONDITION OF BLOOD GLUCOSE IN POSTPRANDIAL STATE

- ***Condition following ingestion of food is called postprandial state.*** Absorbed monosaccharides are utilized for oxidation to provide energy. Remaining in excess is stored as glycogen in liver and muscles.

I. AUTOREGULATION

(Fundamental Regulatory Mechanisms)

- Process of hepatic glycogenesis, glycogenolysis, and tissue utilization of glucose are sensitive to relatively slight deviation from the normal blood sugar concentration.
- ***As blood sugar tends to increase:***
  - Glycogenesis is accelerated; and
  - Utilization of glucose by tissues is increased, resulting to fall in blood glucose level.
- The reverse occurs as the blood glucose level tends to fall.
- Normal balance between production and utilization of blood glucose, at a mean level of circulating glucose of approximately 80 mg percent is, therefore, dependant upon the sensitivity of these processes to variations above and below this concentration.
- This level of sensitivity is determined to a considerable extent by the balance between-
  - **Insulin in one hand,** and
  - **Hormones of adrenal cortex** and **anterior pituitary on the other hand.** Overall effect of insulin is to lower the blood glucose level and adrenocortical/and growth hormone to raise it.
- In as much as these two sets of factors are mutually antagonistic to each other. ***It is the ratio between them rather than their absolute amounts that is of prime importance in this connection.***
- The processes of hepatic glycogenesis, glycogenolysis, and glucose utilization and also the blood glucose concentration are continually exposed to disturbing influences under physiological conditions. These include absorption of glucose from intestine, physical and mental activity, emotional states, etc.
- ***Primary effect of majority of these is to cause a rise in blood glucose. This results in:***
  - ***decrease in delivery of glucose by liver,*** and
  - ***acceleration of utilization by tissues.***
- Simultaneous increase in insulin secretion, stimulated by elevated blood glucose concentration results in increase in ratio of insulin/adrenocortical hormones and growth hormone.
- ***This change in ratio and hormonal balance results in:***
  - ***Increased hepatic glycogenesis;***
  - ***Decreased gluconeogenesis;***
  - ***Decreased output of glucose from liver and***
  - ***Increased utilization of glucose.***

As a result of above, the blood glucose concentration ***tends to fall.***

- A drop in blood glucose concentration below the normal resting level causes:
  - Decrease in secretion of insulin;
  - Resulting to decrease in ratio of insulin/ glucocorticoids and GH;
  - Increased production of blood glucose mainly by gluconeogenesis; and
  - Decreased glucose utilization.

Due to the above actions, blood glucose tends to rise.

- If the blood glucose falls below to hypoglycaemic levels, additional ***emergency mechanisms*** come into play:
  - ***Stimulation of secretion of catecholamines*** by hypoglycaemia resulting in hepatic glycogenolysis and rise in blood glucose.
  - The ***increase in catecholamines*** may also stimulate production of ACTH, hence of adrenocortical hormones, causing increased gluconeogenesis.

Conclusion: The ***blood glucose concentration in normal health regulates itself (autoregulation).*** Efficient operation of this autoregulation at physiological levels, however, requires a normal balance between *(i)* Insulin and *(ii)* the carbohydrate active adrenocorticoids and anterior pituitary hormones, and also to normal responsiveness of the pancreatic islet cells to variation in blood glucose concentration. This constitutes the ***autoregulation*** or central regulatory mechanism.

II. HORMONAL INFLUENCES (ENDOCRINE INFLUENCES) ON CARBOHYDRATE METABOLISM

Endocrine organs play an important key role in this homeostatic mechanism. There are ***two categories of endocrine influences:***

- Those which exert a fundamental regulatory influence, their normal function being essential for normal carbohydrate metabolism, for example, hormones of pancreatic islet cells specially insulin, and hormones of adrenal cortex and anterior pituitary.
- Those which influence carbohydrate metabolism, but are not essential for its autoregulation under normal physiological conditions, e.g. hormones of adrenal medulla and hormones of thyroid gland.

1. ***Insulin:*** Administration of insulin is followed by **a fall ↓** in ***blood glucose concentration*** to hypoglycaemic levels, if adequate amounts are given. This results from:
   - Net decrease of delivery of glucose to systemic blood by liver, and
   - Increase in the rate of utilization of glucose by tissue cells.

a. ***Diminished supply of glucose to blood is due to:***

- Decreased hepatic glycogenolysis
- Increased hepatic glycogenesis.
- Decreased gluconeogenesis
- The liver glycogen tends to increase although this may be obscured by the hypoglycaemia, which itself tends to accelerate hepatic glycogenolysis.

b. ***Increase in the rate of utilization of glucose by tissue cells:***

Glucose is removed from the blood more readily and is utilized more actively for:

- Oxidation for energy production
- Increases lipogenesis
- For glycogenesis

The overall effect of insulin is antagonistic to that of adrenal glucocorticoids and growth hormone.

2. ***Adrenocortical Hormones:*** Adrenal cortex produces a number of steroid hormones, of which the ***glucocorticoids*** are important in carbohydrate metabolism. The predominant glucocorticoids in man is ***"cortisol"***. Glucocorticoids:

a. ***Increases blood glucose level:***

- By gluconeogenesis, as a result of
  - Increased protein catabolism in the peripheral tissues, so that **more amino acids are available**;
  - Increased hepatic uptake of amino acids and increasing the activity of *transaminases* and all the enzymes concerned with gluconeogenesis, e.g. *pyruvate carboxylase,*

PEP-carboxykinase, fructose-1, 6-biphosphatase and *glucose-6-phosphatase;* and
- by diminishing peripheral uptake and utilization of glucose.

b. ***Increases liver glycogen:*** Attributable in part to increased activity of glycogen synthase, "b" to "a" conversion. ***Glucocorticoids are catabolic to peripheral tissues but anabolic to liver.***

3. ***Anterior Pituitary Gland:*** Secretes hormones that ***tend to elevate the blood glucose level*** and therefore, antagonize the effect of insulin.These are ***growth hormone*** and **ACTH** (corticotrophin) and possibly other "diabetogenic" principles. ***Growth hormone secretion is stimulated by hypoglycaemia.***
- Growth hormone decreases glucose uptake in certain tissues, e.g. muscles.
- ***Liver: there is increase in liver glycogen due to increased gluconeogenesis.***

Chronic administration of GH leads to diabetes. By producing hyperglycaemia, leads to stimulation of secretion of insulin, which eventually produces exhaustion of β-cells.

4. ***Catecholamines:*** These are hormones produced by adrenal medulla:
- Produces an increase in blood glucose level and also blood lactic acid level. It stimulates glycogen breakdown (glycogenolysis) in liver as well as in muscle.
- In muscle due to absence of ***glucose-6-pase,*** glycogenolysis does not directly contribute to blood glucose. It increases the pyruvate and lactate. Pyruvate and lactates diffuse into the blood and in liver are converted to glucose and glycogen. (See *Cori cycle*).
- Catecholamines also stimulate ACTH formation, which increase glucocorticoids, enhancing gluconeogenesis.
- Epinephrine has direct inhibitory action on insulin release.

5. ***Glucagon:*** Glucagon is a protein hormone, a polypeptide containing 29 amino acids. It is produced by α-cells of islets of Langerhans. It is ***also known as HGF (hyperglycaemic glycogenolytic factor)***
- In response to hypoglycaemia, α-cells produce glucagon which produces ***rapid glycogenolysis in liver.***

  Note: ***Glucagon cannot produce glycogenolysis in muscle as it lacks the receptor.***
- Glucagon also enhances "gluconeogenesis" from amino acids and pyruvates and lactates.

6. ***Thyroid Hormones: Thyroxine accelerates hepatic glycogenolysis, with consequent rise in blood glucose.***

This may ***be due in part to:***
- ***Increased sensitivity of the tissues to catecholamines;*** and
- ***In part to accelerated destruction of insulin.***
- ***Thyroid hormones may also increase the rate of absorption of hexoses from the intestine.***
- Increased hepatic *glucose-6-phosphatase* activity.
- Rate of protein catabolism is increased by excessive thyroid hormones and thus increases gluconeogenesis from amino acids.

BLOOD SUGAR LEVEL AND ITS CLINICAL SIGNIFICANCE

A. Normal Values: The range for normal fasting or postabsorptive blood glucose taken at least three hours after the last meal:
- As per *glucose-oxidase method* ("true" glucose) 60 to 100 mg per cent. Some authorities give as 60 to 95 mg per cent.
- As per "Folin and Wu's method" 80 to 120 mg percent.

B. Abnormalities in Blood Glucose Level
- Increase in blood glucose level above normal is called ***hyperglycaemia.***
- Decrease in blood glucose level below normal is called ***hypoglycaemia***

1. Hyperglycaemia: Causes of hyperglycaemia:
- Most common cause is ***diabetes mellitus*** (DM) in which the highest values for fasting blood glucose is obtained, in which it may vary from normal to 500 mg percent and over, depending on the severity of the disease.

- ***Hyperactivity of the thyroids, pituitary, and adrenal glands,*** Except in DM, fasting blood glucose rarely exceeds 200 mg percent. There may be increased incidence of DM in hyperthyroidism and hyperpituitarism.
- ***Emotional "stress"*** can increase the blood glucose level.
- ***In diffuse diseases of pancreas,*** e.g. in pancreatitis and carcinoma of pancreas, some increase in fasting blood glucose may occur.
- Increase of blood glucose in appreciable amount may be seen ***in sepsis*** and in a number of infectious diseases.
- A moderate hyperglycaemia may also be found in some ***intracranial diseases*** such as meningitis, encephalitis, intracranial tumours and haemorrhage.
- ***Anaesthesia*** can also increase blood glucose, depending on the degree and duration of anaesthesia.
- ***Asphyxia*** may also increase blood sugar level.
- Increase in blood sugar, rarely exceeding 150 to 180 mg percent may be seen ***in convulsions*** and ***in the terminal stages of many diseases.***

2. Hypoglycaemia: Causes of hypoglycaemia: Hypoglycaemia may be considered to be present when the blood glucose is below 40 mg percent ("true" glucose value by glucose oxidase method)

- Most common cause and clinically important to be considered first is ***overdosage of insulin*** in treatment of diabetes mellitus.
- ***Insulin-secreting tumour (insulinoma) of pancreas*** produces a severe hypoglycaemia in which blood glucose is very low or may be almost completely absent. It is extremely rare.
- Fasting blood glucose may be reduced in ***hypoactivity of thyroids*** (myxoedema, and cretinism), ***hypopituitary*** (Simmond's disease) and ***hypoadrenalism*** (Addison's disease).
- ***In severe liver diseases,*** low blood glucose levels are often found.
- In childhood, an ***idiopathic hypoglycaemia,*** due to sensitivity to the amino acid leucine has been recognized ***(leucine-sensitive hypoglycaemia).***
- An ***acquired leucine sensitivity*** has also been stated to exist.
- ***Spontaneous hypoglycaemia*** in childhood may be due to deficiency of glucagon production.
- ***Severe exercise*** may produce hypoglycaemia due to depletion of liver glycogen.
- Hypoglycaemia is also found in some of the ***"glycogen storage diseases (GSDs),*** e.g. in von Gierke's disease, liver phosphorylase deficiency. Due to impaired ability to produce glucose from glycogen.
- Impaired absorption of glucose in some types of ***steatorrhoea.*** The blood glucose may be in the lower part of the normal range, it is rare to be subnormal.
- ***Transient postprandial hypoglycaemia ("reactive" hypoglycaemia),*** may occur in an occasional case, some one and a half to three hours after taking food, and more commonly in patients with partial gastrectomy.
- Hypoglycaemia has also been found to be associated with ***alcohol ingestion.***
- Recently, it has been seen that a ***variety of tumours of non-endocrine origin,*** particularly, ***retroperitoneal fibrosarcoma*** may produce hypoglycaemia by secreting insulin-like hormones.

GLYCOSURIA

Under ordinary dietary conditions, glucose is the only sugar present in the free state in blood plasma in demonstrable amounts. Although normal urine contains virtually no sugar; under certain circumstances, glucose or other sugars may be excreted in the urine. This condition is called ***melituria (excretion of sugar in urine).*** The terms glycosuria, fructosuria, galactosuria, lactosuria, and pentosuria are applied specially to the urinary excretion of glucose, fructose, galactose, lactose, and pentose respectively.

Definition: Glycosuria is *defined* as the *excretion of glucose in urine* which is *detectable by Benedict's qualitative test.*

Note: In normal subjects, a small amount less than 0.5 gm of glucose may escape reabsorption by the tubules and be excreted by urine. But **this amount is not detected by Benedict's qualitative test.**

MECHANISM OF GLYCOSURIA

Excretion of abnormal amounts of glucose in the urine may be **due to two types of abnormalities:**

- *Increases in the amount of glucose entering in the tubule/mt.*
- *Decrease in the glucose reabsorption capacity of the renal tubular epithelium.*

1. The quantity of glucose entering the tubules is the product of:

  - The minute volume of glomerular filtrate and
  - The concentration of glucose in the filtrate, i.e. in the arterial blood plasma.

In as much as glomerular filtration is rarely increased markedly, *glycosuria of this type is due almost invariably to an increase in the blood glucose concentration above the "renal threshold level"* and called as *hyperglycaemic glycosuria.*

2. Reabsorption of glucose by renal tubular epithelium is accomplished mainly by an *"active transport" mechanism, by transport carrier protein.* The capacity for reabsorption may be diminished by:

  - *Hereditary cause:* absence of carrier protein or defective carrier protein
  - *Acquired:* due to certain types of kidney diseases specially involving the tubules or damage of tubules by chemicals/poisons.
  - *Lowering of renal threshold.*
  - *Induced:* experimental glycosuria, e.g. by *administration of glycoside "phloridzin".*

The above type of glycosuria is called as **renal glycosuria.** *Blood glucose level in this type is normal or even may be subnormal.*

TYPES OF GLYCOSURIAS

From above the glycosuria can be divided into **two main groups:**

- *Hyperglycaemic glycosuria*
- *Renal glycosuria*

1. Hyperglycaemic Glycosuria

- *Alimentary Glycosuria:* When a large carbohydrate diet is taken, blood sugar rises and may cross renal threshold in occasional case and may produce glycosuria. This condition does not seem to be a normal process, as homeostatic control is so efficient in normal healthy person that such glycosuria should not occur. Alimentary glycosuria, therefore, is only possible in those subjects in whom the power of glucose utilization is impaired and such people should be kept under observation and should be screened regularly for diabetes.
- *Nervous or "Emotional" Glycosuria:* Stimulation of the sympathetic nerves to the liver or of the splanchnic nerves, break down of liver glycogen occurs and produces hyperglycaemia and glycosuria.

  Nervous stimulation mentioned above causes
  - Glycogenolysis directly, and
  - Also by increased secretion of catecholamines, producing glycogenolysis.
- *Glycosuria Due to Endocrine Disorders*: Deranged function of a number of endocrine glands produces hyperglycaemia which may result in glycosuria.

Examples:

- *Diabetes mellitus-clinical:* In this case β-cells of islets of Langerhans fail to secrete adequate amount of insulin, ***producing absolute or relative deficiency of insulin.*** Lack of insulin produces hyperglycaemia and glycosuria (see diabetes mellitus).
- *Hyperthyroidism:* Hyperactivity of thyroid is always attended with low sugar tolerance, hyperglycaemia and may be glycosuria. ***In 25 to 35 percent of cases, hyperthyroidism and diabetes mellitus can coexist.***
- *Epinephrine:* Increased secretion of epinephrine or prolonged administration through subcutaneous route can increase the breakdown of liver glycogen leading to hyperglycaemia and glycosuria.

- *Hyperactivity of anterior pituitary:* Hyperactivity of anterior pituitary as in acromegaly is attended with hyperglycaemia and glycosuria (20 to 30% cases), due to increased secretion of GH and adrenocortical hormones.
- *Adrenal cortex:* Hyperactivity of adrenal cortex as in Cushing's syndrome/disease, may cause hyperglycaemia and glycosuria. Glucocorticoids stimulate gluconeogenesis and increased resistance to insulin (glucose uptake by peripheral tissues inhibited).
- *Glucagon:* Increased secretion of glucagon by α-cells of islets of Langerhans can cause glycogenolysis producing hyperglycaemia and glycosuria.

EXPERIMENTAL HYPERGLYCAEMIC GLYCOSURIAS:

- *"Piqure" glycosuria:* Certain injuries to the nervous system can cause hyperglycaemia and glycosuria. ***Claude Bernard*** found that puncture of a particular spot in the floor of the IV ventricle of rabbits produces hyperglycaemia and glycosuria ***("puncture" diabetes).*** This glycosuria persists for 24 hours or more and is accompanied by marked hyperglycaemia.

  Mechanism: It is suggested that experimental procedure stimulates a group of nerve cells at the floor of IV ventricle which sends impulses through the splanchnic nerves to adrenal medulla and liver, increasing glycogenolysis by increased secretion of catecholamines.
- *'Alloxan' diabetes and glycosuria:* Injection of "alloxan" to an experimental animal like dog, a substance related chemically to "Pyrimidine" bases, produces permanent diabetes. ***Diabetes is due to degeneration, necrosis and resorption of β-cells of islets of Langerhans***. The α-cells and acinar cells are unaffected. ***The alloxan acts directly, promptly and specifically on β-cells.*** Its effect can be prevented by administration of cysteine, glutathione, BAL, or thioglycolic acid immediatley before or within a few minutes after injection of the alloxan. This protective action is due to apparently to the –SH content of these compounds, the alloxan being probably reduced to an inactive substance.

A similar diabetogenic effect is produced experimentally by dehydroascorbic acid and dehydroisoascorbic acid when ***administered in large doses*** (see vitamin C).

2. Renal Glycosurias

- ***Hereditary:*** A milder glycosuria occurs spontaneously, as hereditary familial traits, persisting throughout life, ***due to absence of "carrier protein: or altered kinetics of the carrier system due to failure of development.***
- *Acquired:*
  - ***Diseases of renal tubules:*** In some cases of kidney diseases, the renal tubules may be grossly damaged, thus the tubules fail to reabsorb glucose producing glycosuria.
  - ***Due to heavy metal poisoning:*** The heavy metals like lead (Pb), cadmium (Cd), mercury (Hg), etc. can damage the renal tubules thus interfering with the reasorption of glucose resulting in glycosuria.
- *Lowering of Renal Threshold:* About 15 to 20 percent cases of pregnancy may be associated with the physiological glycosuria with advancement of pregnancy ***due to lowering of renal threshold.*** But pregnancy may be associated with diabetes mellitus in which there will be hyperglycaemic glycosuria. ***These two can be differentiated by performing a fasting blood sugar level.***
- *Renal Glycosuria:* It may also occur in association with evidences of other renal tubular transport defects, e.g. aminoacidurias, renal tubular acidosis, hyperphosphaturia as in Fanconi syndrome.
- *'Experimental' Renal Glycosuria: "Phloridzin" glycosuria:* Phloridzin is a glycoside found in roots of apple tree; when hydrolyzed it gives glucose and aglycone **"phloretin".** When Phloridzin is administered subcutaneously, it gives rise to intense glycosuria. The dose given to dogs is 1 gm/day, in oil, SC. Certain other glycosides, such as "Arbutin" have similar effects.

Mechanism: Phloridzin displaces sodium from the sodium binding site from "carrier protein" and hence glucose cannot be bound to the glucose binding site, thus inhibiting glucose reabsorption.

DIABETES MELLITUS

Diabetes mellitus is a common disease in man. A predisposition to the diseases is probably inherited as an autosomal recessive trait. About 25 percent of the relatives of diabetics show abnormal glucose tolerance curves as compared to 1 percent in the general population.

Definition: A chronic disease due to primarily to a disorder of carbohydrate metabolism, cause of which is deficiency or diminished effectiveness of insulin, resulting in hyperglycaemia and glycosuria. Secondary changes may occur in the metabolism of proteins, fats, water and electrolytes and in tissues/organs sometimes with grave consequences.

CLINICAL TYPES AND CAUSES

These are **two main groups:**

- *Primary (Idiopathic):* Constitute major group: exact cause is not known; metabolic defect is insufficient insulin which may be absolute or relative.
- *Secondary:* Constitute minor group where it can be secondary to some disease process.

1. **Primary (Idiopathic): Two clinical types:**
   - *"Juvenile" onset diabetes:* now called as Type-I (insulin dependent) **(IDDM).**
   - *" Maturity" onset diabetes:* Type-II Non-insulin Dependent **(NIDDM)**

Differences between the two clinical types are listed in ***Table 12.6.***

Other Factors

- *Heredity:* In both types, familial tendency noted. Genetic factors more important in those who develop after 40 years. In younger, "juvenile" type, susceptibility ***is associated with particular HLA phenotype.*** Risk is two to three times more in those who are **HLA phenotype B_8 or BW_{15}.**
- *Auto-immunity: **Insulin-dependent juvenile type may be an autoimmune disorder*** and has been found to coexist with other autoimmune disorders.

  Evidences in favour of autoimmunity:
  - Lymphocytic and plasma cells infiltrations in pancreas,
  - Detection of autoantibodies by immuno-fluorescence.
- *Infections: **Certain viral infections may precipitate juvenile type.*** Experimentally it

Table 12.6: Clinical types of primary (idiopathic) diabetes mellitus

"Juvenile onset" diabetes-Types –I	*"Maturity onset" diabetes –Types II*
• *Frequency: less*	• *Frequency:* more common
• Commences usually before 15 years of age. Males suffer more then females	• Occurs in middle aged individuals. Women are more prone
• *Onset:* rapid and abrupt	• *Onset*—is insidious
• Speedy progression to ketoacidosis and coma	• Usually mild. Ketoacidosis is rare
• Usually patients are thin and underweight	• Associated with obesity in 2/3 of cases. Usually detected during routine check-up of urine.
• Deficient insulin—at first juvenile diabetics produce more insulin than normal, but the β-cells soon become exhausted and patient becomes "overt" diabetic with atrophied β-cells and practically no insulin	• β-cells respond normally. Relative deficiency of insulin, which may be due to ***"insulin" antagonism"***
• ***Plasma insulin:*** There is practically if any, circulating insulin. It is almost absent. No insulin response is shown to glucose load.	• ***Plasma insulin*** levels may be normal or even raised
• Insulin therapy is necessary for control of these cases	• Oral hypoglycaemic agents and ***dietary control*** are useful in treatment

has been shown that certain viruses can induce diabetes. Incidence is high after mumps. ***Antibodies to Coxsackie B_4 virus have been found in young juvenile type.***

- ***Obesity:*** Majority of middle aged maturity onset diabetics are obese, ***"stress" like pregnancy may precipitate.***
- ***Diet:*** Overeating and under activity are also predisposing factors in elderly middle aged maturity onset diabetes.
- ***Insulin antagonism:*** In "maturity onset" diabetes, the deficiency of insulin is relative and glucose-induced insulin secretion may be greater and more prolonged than normal. This relative deficiency may be due to ***"insulin antagonism"***, exact cause for the same is not known, but various factors have been incriminated from time to time.

  Possible causes proposed:
  - ***Insulin "antibodies".***
  - ***Secretions of "abnormal" and "less active" insulin or "altered" insulin.***
  - ***A "tissue barrier" to the transport of insulin to the cells, probably receptor deficiency.***
  - ***Lack of cellular response to insulin.***

2. Secondary

This forms a minor group. Diabetes is secondary to some other diseases.

- ***Pancreatic diabetes:***
  - Pancreatitis
  - Haemochromatosis
  - Malignancy of pancreas.
- ***Abnormal concentrations of antagonistic hormones, for example:***
  - Hyperthyroidism.
  - Hypercorticism, like Cushing's disease and syndrome
  - Hyperpituitarism, like acromegaly.
  - Increased glucagon activity.
- ***Iatrogenic:*** In genetically susceptibles, it may be precipitated by therapy like corticosteroids, thiazide diuretics.

Presentation of Diabetes Mellitus

The disease has a varied presentation:

- ***Glycosuria*** may be detected during routine examination of urine like annual check-up, or when doing routine examination due to some other diseases. There may not be any symptoms/signs.
- Some may present with all classical symptoms like thirst, polydipsia, polyuria, polyphagia, loss of weight, etc. ***("overt" diabetics).***
- Some women present during pregnancy (stress)
- A few specially Type-1 cases may present as fulminant ketoacidosis and a few with complications.

CLINICAL FEATURES AND BIOCHEMICAL CORRELATIONS

- Large amount of glucose my be excreted in urine (may be 90 to 100 gm/day in some cases) loss of solute produces osmotic diuresis thus large volume of urine ***(polyuria).***
- Loss of fluid leads to thirst and ***polydipsia.***
- ***Polyphagia,*** a patient eats more frequently and is more fond of sweets. The above symptoms may persist for many months in maturity onset diabetes. In juvenile onset type-1, further symptoms develop if treatment is not started.
- Tissues including muscles received liberal supply of glucose but cannot use glucose due to absolute or relative deficiency of insulin/or transport defect to cells. This causes ***weakness*** and ***tiredness.***
- As glucose cannot be used for fuel, fat is mobilized leading to ***increased FFA*** ↑ in blood and liver.
- Increased acetyl CoA is diverted for cholesterol synthesis-***hypercholesterolaemia*** and ***atherosclerosis***. ***Xanthomas*** may develop.
- Increased ketone bodies leads to ***acidosis***, which leads to hyperventilation (air-hunger).
- If ketosis is severe, acetone will be breathed out, giving characteristic ***"fruity" smell in breath*** (due to acetone).
- Alongwith above, there may be excessive breakdown of tissue proteins. Deaminated amino acids are catabolized to provide energy, which accounts for ***loss of weight.***
- Due to ketosis, develops anorexia, nausea, and vomiting. Continued loss of water and electrolytes increases ***dehydration.***
- Ketoacidosis produces increasing drowsiness, leading to ***diabetic coma*** in untreated cases.

GLUCOSE TOLERANCE TEST (GTT)

What is Carbohydrate Tolerance?: The ability of the body to utilize carbohydrates may be ascertained by measuring its carbohydrate tolerance. It is indicated by the nature of blood glucose curve following the administration of glucose. Thus, ***glucose tolerance is a valuable diagnostic aid.*** A 70 kg man can ingest approximately 1500 gm/day.

Decreased glucose tolerance is seen in:
- Diabetes mellitus.
- Hyperactivity of anterior pituitary and adrenal cortex
- Hyperthyroidism.

Increased tolerance is seen in:
- Hypopituitarism.
- Hyperinsulinism.
- Hypothyroidism.
- Adrenal cortical hypofunction (such as Addison's disease).
- Also if there is decreased absorption, like sprue, caeliac disease.

TYPES OF GLUCOSE TOLERANCE TEST

GTT is of **two types:**
- **Standard oral glucose tolerance test.**
- **IV glucose tolerance test.**

A. Standard Oral GTT

Indications:
- In patients with transient or sustained glycosuria, who have no clinical symptoms of diabetes with normal fasting and PP blood glucose.
- In patients with symptoms of diabetes but with no glycosuria and normal fasting blood glucose level.
- In persons with strong family history but no overt symptoms.
- In patients with glycosuria associated with thyrotoxicosis, infections/sepsis, liver diseases, pregnancy, etc.
- In women with characteristically large babies 9 lbs or individuals who were large babies at birth.
- In patients with neuropathies or retinopathies of undetermined origin.
- In patients with or without symptoms of DM, showing one abnormal value.

Pre-requisites: *Precautions to be taken on the day prior to the test:*
- The individual takes usual supper at about 2000 hours and does not eat or drink anything after that. Early morning if so desires, a cup of tea/or coffee may be given without sugar or milk. No other food or drink is permitted till the test is over.
- ***Should be on normal carbohydrate diets at least for three days prior to test*** (approximately 300 gm daily), ***otherwise "false" high curve may be obtained.***
- Complete mental/and physical rest.
- No smoking is permitted.
- All samples of blood should be venous preferably. If capillary blood from 'finger prick' is used, all samples should be capillary blood.

Procedure
- A fasting sample of venous blood is collected in fluoride bottle ***(fasting sample).***
- The bladder is emptied completely and urine is collected for qualitative test for glucose and ketone bodies ***(fasting urine).***
- The individual is given 75 gm of glucose dissolved in water, about 250 ml, to drink. Lemon can be added to make it palatable and to prevent nausea/vomiting. Time of oral glucose administration is noted.
- A total of ***five specimens*** of venous blood and urine are collected every ½ hour after the oral glucose viz. ½ hr, 1 hr, 1 ½ hr, 2 hr, and 2 ½ hr.
- Glucose content of **all the six** (including fasting sample) samples of blood are estimated and corresponding urine samples are tested qualitatively for presence of glucose and ketone bodies.

A curve is plotted which is called as ***glucose tolerance curve.***

Explanation and Significance of a Normal Curve

1. A sharp rise to a peak, averaging about 50 percent above the fasting level within 30 to 60 minutes. Extent of the rise varies considerably from person to person, but maximum should not exceed 160 to 180 mg per cent in normal subjects.

Reason: rise is due directly to the glucose absorbed from the intestine, which temporarily exceeds the capacity of the liver and tissues to remove it.

- As the blood glucose concentration increases, ***regulatory mechanisms*** come into play:
  - Increased insulin secretion due to hyperglycaemia.
  - Hepatic glycogenesis is increased.
  - Hepatic glycogenolysis is decreased.
  - Glucose uptake and utilization in tissues increased.

2. A sharp fall to approximately the fasting level at the end of 1 ½ to 2 hours.

Reason: Glucose now leaves the circulation faster than it is entering. This is due to:

- Continuing stimulation of the mechanisms stated above, i.e. increased utilization and hepatic glycogenesis.
- To slowing or completion of glucose absorption from the intestines.

3. Hypoglycaemic dip: Continued fall to a slightly subfasting (10 to 15 mg lower than fasting value) at 2 hours and subsequent rise to fasting level at 2 ½ to 3 hours.

Reason: The hypoglycaemic "dip" is due to "inertia" of the regulatory mechanisms. The decreased output of glucose by liver and increased utilization induced by the rising blood glucose are not reversed as rapidly as the blood sugar falls.

Characteristics of Different Types of GTC Fig. 12.17 depicts

1. A Normal GTC:

- Fasting blood glucose within normal limits of 60 to 100 mg percent ("True" glucose).
- The highest peak value is reached within one hour.
- The highest value does not exceed the renal threshold, i.e 160 to 180 mg percent.
- The fasting level is again reached by 2 ½ hour.
- No glucose or ketone bodies are detected in any specimens of urine.

2. Diabetic Type of GTC:

- Fasting blood glucose is definitely raised 110 mg percent or more ("true" glucose).
- The highest value is usually reached after 1 to 1 ½ hour.
- The highest value exceeds the normal renal threshold.

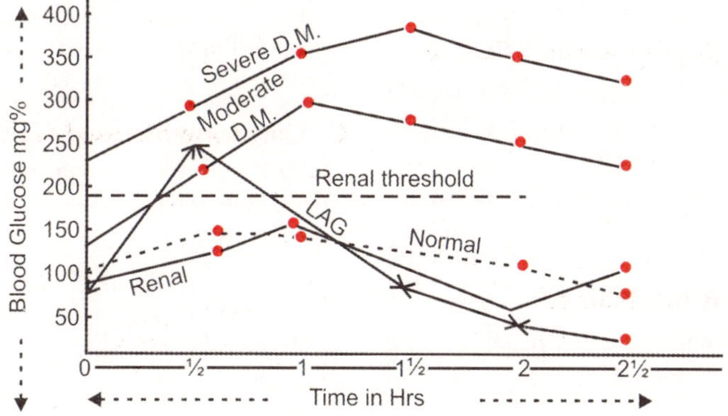

Fig. 12.17: Showing different glucose tolerance curves

- Urine samples always contain glucose except in some chronic diabetics or nephritis who may have raised renal threshold ("dangerous type"), hyperglycaemia but no glycosuria. Urine may or may not contain ketone bodies depending on the type of diabetes and severity.
- ***The blood glucose does not return to the fasting level within 2 ½ hours. This is the most characteristic feature of true DM.***

According to severity, it may be:

- ***Mild diabetic curve.***
- ***Moderately severe diabetic curve*** and
- ***Severe diabetic curve.***

3. *Renal Glycosuria Curve:* Glucose appears in the urine at levels of blood glucose much below 170 mg percent. Patients who show no glycosuria when fasting may have glycosuria when the blood glucose is raised.

The condition may be:

- Idiopathic without any pathological significance.
- Occasionally occurs in certain renal diseases and in pregnancy (when there may be lowering of renal threshold)
- May be found in case of "early" diabetes with low renal threshold
- It has been reported in children of diabetic parents.

These cases should be reviewed from time to time (every six months).

4. *Lag Curve (or Oxyhyperglycaemic Curve):*

- Fasting blood glucose is normal, but it rises rapidly in the ½ to 1 hour and ***exceeds the renal threshold*** so that the corresponding urine specimens show glucose.
- The return to normal value is rapid and complete.

This type of GTC may be obtained:

- ***In hyperthyroidism,***
- ***After gastroenterostomy,***
- ***During pregnancy***
- ***Also in "early" diabetes.***

A patient showing "lag curve" should be reviewed from time to time after every six months.

Value of GTT

- Most valuable in investigating a case of "symptomless" glycosuria, such as renal glycosuria, and lag type glycosurias.
- Helpful in recognizing milder cases of DM and "early DM".
- Rarely necessary for diagnosis of DM of moderately severe or severe intensity, where if characteristic symptoms alongwith high fasting blood glucose and glycosuria are present.
- But helpful in following course and treatment in established DM. In such cases, modified GTT, can be done in two specimens, one fasting and the other, post-prandial (PP), 2 hours sample.
- May be of use in certain endocrine dysfunction and patients with steatorrhoeas.

B. Intravenous GTT: ***Preferred where there are abnormalities in absorption of glucose. Thus, IV GTT is indicated:***

- ***In hypothyroidism***
- ***In sprue and caeliac disease.***

Dose: 1/3 gm of glucose/kg body wt. given as 50 percent solution IV within 3 to 5 minutes.

Procedure: Similar to oral GTT. Blood glucose estimations are done on "fasting" and ½ hourly intervals for 2 hours after IV injection of glucose.

Observations:

- All normal cases required less than 60 minutes for the blood glucose to return to normal.
- In diabetes mellitus, even mild cases take more than 120 minutes to return to initial level.

C. Cortisone-Stressed GTT: ***Used for detecting "latent" diabetes or prediabetes.***

Basis: It is based on the fact that while a large dose of ACTH or a suitable corticosteroid will produce a raised "glucose tolerance curve" and glycosuria in normal persons. Smaller doses will do so only in "pre-diabetic" persons.

Dose:

- ***Two doses*** of 50 mg ***cortisone*** orally.
  First dose is given 8 ½ hours before GTT, and ***second dose*** 2 hours before GTT or alternatively.

- *Two doses of prednisolone* 0.4 mg/kg body wt, ½ the dose at midnight and ½ at 6 AM before carrying out GTT at 8 AM.

D. Extended GTT: Instead of ending at 2 ½ hours after taking glucose, ½ hourly blood sugars are done for periods upto 4 to 5 hours.

Partial gastrectomy cases and patients with islet cell tumours may have attacks suggesting hypoglycaemia some 2 to 3 hours after food.

Extended GTT are sometimes used:

- ***To differentiate transient attacks of hypoglycaemia*** from those due to insulin secreting tumours of islet of Langerhans in the pancreas, and other abnormal endocrine conditions such as Simmond's disease which cause hypoglycaemia.
- ***In the endocrine disorders,*** fall in blood glucose at the end of tolerance test tends to be progressive. However, the fasting blood glucose particularly early morning sample before breakfast may be low enough for diagnosis.

☞ SALIENT POINTS TO REMEMBER

- Galactose is required in lactating mammary gland for synthesis of Lactose, the milk sugar in breast milk.
- Galactose is utilized in brain and nervous tissues for synthesis of Glycolipids - Cerebrosides and gangliosides. Also required for synthesis of chondromucoids and mucoproteins.
- The inherited deficiency of the enzyme ***"Galactose-1-Phosphate uridyl transferase"*** produces the classical type of the disease Galactosaemia.
- Severe cases of galactosaemia are associated with the development of cataract, which is due to accumulation of 'galactitol.'
- In health, the normal blood sugar is maintained at level of 60 to 100 mg/dl ("true" glucose). Auto regulation of blood sugar is done by the balance of insulin in one hand and hormones of adrenal cortex and growth hormone on the other hand.
- It is the ratio between them rather than their absolute amounts is important.
- Glycosuria is defined as the exeretion of glucose in urine which is detectable by Benedict's qualitative test.
- Glycosuria are of 2 main types:
  (1) Hyperglycaemic glycosuria where the blood glucose increases and crosses the renal threshold.
  (2) Renal glycosuria where the blood glucose is normal but glucose is excreted in urine due to renal diseases.

MULTIPLE CHOICE QUESTIONS

Give one correct answer:

1. **In the normal resting state of humans, most of the blood glucose burnt as 'fuel' is consumed by:**
   (a) Liver (b) Kidneys
   (c) Muscles (d) Brain
   (e) Adipose tissue
2. **All of the following compounds are intermediates of TCA cycle *except:***
   (a) Pyruvate (b) Oxaloacetate
   (c) Malate (d) Succinate
   (e) Fumarate
3. **UDP-glucose is converted to UDP-glucuronic acid by:**
   (a) ATP (b) GTP
   (c) NAD^+ (d) $NADP^+$
   (e) FAD
4. **Which of the following compound is positive allosteric modifier of the enzyme pyruvate carboxylase?**
   (a) Glucose-6-P (b) Oxaloacetate
   (c) Biotin (d) Acetyl-CoA
   (e) ATP
5. **A specific inhibitor of the enzyme succinate dehydrogenase is:**
   (a) Citrate (b) Malonate
   (c) Fluoride (d) Arsenite
   (e) Cyanide

6. **The hydrolysis of Glucose-6-P is catalyzed by an enzyme phosphatase that is not found in which of the following?**
(a) Kidney (b) Liver
(c) Muscle (d) Spleen
(e) Brain

7. **Which of the following hormones is not involved in carbohydrate metabolism:**
(a) Insulin (b) Cortisol
(c) Glucagon (d) Growth hormone
(e) Vasopressin

8. **An essential for converting glucose to glycogen in liver is:**
(a) Lactic acid (b) Pyruvic acid
(c) UTP (d) GTP
(e) CTP

9. **Which of the following enzymes in glycolytic pathway is inhibited by fluoride?**
(a) Aldolase
(b) Enolase
(c) Pyruvate kinase
(d) Hexokinase
(e) Phsophoglycerate kinase

10. **Dehydrogenases involved in HMP shunt are specific for:**
(a) FAD (b) FMN
(c) NAD^+ (d) $NADP^+$
(e) TPP

11. **The ratio that approximates the number of net molecule of ATP formed per mole of glucose oxidized in presence of O_2 to the net number formed in absence of O_2 is:**
(a) 4:1 (b) 10:2
(c) 12:1 (d) 18:1
(e) 24:1

12. **How many ATP molecules will be required for conversion of 2 molecules of Lactic acid to glucose?**
(a) Two (b) Four
(c) Six (d) Eight
(e) Ten

13. **An allosteric enzyme responsible for controlling the rate of TCA cycle is:**
(a) Aconitase
(b) Isocitrate dehydrogenase
(c) Fumarase
(d) Succinate Thiokinase
(e) Malate Dehydrogenase

14. **A regulator of the enzyme glycogen synthetase is:**
(a) Pyruvate (b) Citric acid
(c) 2:3 BPG (d) GTP
(e) Glucose-6-P

15. **Out of 24 molecules of ATP formed in citric acid cycle, two molecules of ATP can be formed at "Substrate level," by which of the following reaction?**
(a) Succinyl CoA → Succinic acid
(b) Succinic acid → fumarate
(c) Malate → Oxaloacetate (O.A.A)
(d) Citric acid → Isocitric acid
(e) Isocitrate → oxalosuccinate

ANSWERS

1. (d)	2. (a)	3. (c)
4. (d)	5. (b)	6. (c)
7. (e)	8. (c)	9. (b)
10. (d)	11. (d)	12. (c)
13. (b)	14. (e)	15. (a)

13 Metabolism of Lipids

PLASMA LIPIDS

In mammals, **principal lipids** that have **metabolic significance** are as follows.

- ***Triacyl glycerol (TG)***, also called neutral fats (NF)
- ***Phospholipids***
- ***Steroids***, chief of which is ***cholesterol.***

Plasma lipids also constitute the products of the metabolism.

- Fatty acids long-chain and short-chain (free FA)
- Glycerol.

Extraction of plasma lipids with a suitable lipid solvent and subsequent separation of the extract into various classes of lipids shows the presence of:

- Triacyl glycerol (TG)
- Phospholipids (PL)
- Cholesterol

} approximately in equal quantities.

- Much smaller fraction of non-esterified long chain fatty acid (NEFA) or free fatty acid (FFA), which constitutes less than 5% of total FA present in plasma.

NEFA is now known to be metabolically most active of the plasma lipids and ½ life being approximately 2 to 3 minutes. ***Plasma lipids at any time may be considered to represent the net balance between production, utilization and storage.*** Lipids of the blood plasma in humans are listed in ***Table 13.1.***

Table 13.1: Showing lipid fractions in plasma

Lipid fraction	*Plasma level in mg/100ml* *Range*	*Mean*
• Total lipids	360-820	560
• Triacyl glycerol (TG)	80-180	150
• Total phospholipids (PL)	125-390	210
(i) Phosphatidyl choline (lecithin)	50-200	
(ii) Phosphatidyl ethanolamine (cephalin)	50-130	
(iii) Sphingomyelins	15-35	
• Total cholesterol	150-250	200
• Free cholesterol (non-esterified)	25-105	55
• Free fatty acids or Non-esterified FA (NEFA)	6-16	10

TRANSPORTATION OF PLASMA LIPIDS

Principal lipid, triacyl glycerol (TG), is ***hydrophobic material.*** To transport them in blood in an aqueous medium poses a problem, which is solved by associating the more insoluble lipids with more "polar" ones, such as phospholipids, cholesterol and combining with a specific, protein molecule (called as apoprotein). Thus, the hydrophobic and insoluble triacyl glycerol (TG) ***is converted by above combination into a hydrophilic and soluble lipoprotein complex.***

Thus:

- TG derived from intestinal absorption of fats are transported in the blood as a lipoprotein complex called ***chylomicrons.*** Chylomicrons are small microscopic particles of fats, about 1μ in diameter and ***are responsible for transport of exogenous TG in the blood***
- Similarly, TG that are synthesized in liver cells are converted to lipoprotein particles, called ***very low density lipoproteins (VLDL)*** and thrown into the circulation. VLDL is mainly concerned ***with transport of endogenous TG.***

- Fatty acids released from adipose tissue by hydrolysis of TG are thrown in the circulation as free fatty acid (FFA). They are carried in non-esterified state in plasma hence also called NEFA. In circulation, FFA/NEFA combines with albumin and are carried as ***albumin-FFA complex.*** Some 25 to 30 mols of FFA are present in combination with one mol of albumin.

SEPARATION OF PLASMA LIPIDS

1. Ultracentrifugation: Pure fat is less dense than water. As the proportion of lipid to protein in lipoprotein complex increases the density of the molecule decreases. This property has been utilized in separation of plasma lipids, the various lipoprotein fractions, by ultracentrifugation.

2. Electrophoresis: Lipoproteins may also be separated according to their electrophoretic properties and identified more accurately using immunoelectrophoresis. **Fredrickson and others (1967)** identified lipoproteins into **4 groups** by electrophoresis as follows:

- **HDL:** Moves fastest and occupies position of α-globulin, called ***α-lipoproteins***
- **LDL:** ***(β-lipoproteins)***
- **VLDL:** ***(Pre-β or α_2-lipoproteins)***
- **Chylomicrons:** Slowest moving and remains near the origin.

Table 13.2 shows the normal value of lipoprotein fractions in health.

Table 13.2: Normal values of lipoproteins (normal lipid profile)

Lipid fraction	*Normal values*
• Total cholesterol	150 to 240 mg/dl
• Serum HDL cholesterol	Males: 35 to 60 mg/dl Females: 40 to 70 mg/dl
• Serum TG	Males: 60 to 165 mg/dl
• (Triacyl glycerol)	Females: 40 to 140 mg/dl
• Serum chylomicrons	upto 28 mg/dl (14 hours Post-absorptive state)
• Serum pre-β lipoproteins (VLDL)	Males: upto 240 mg/dl Females: upto 210 mg/dl
• Serum β-lipoproteins (LDL)	Upto 550 mg/dl
• Serum LDL-cholesterol	Upto 190 mg/dl

Serum LDL cholesterol can be calculated by the *Friedewald formula:*

(i) LDL cholesterol in mg/dl =

$$\text{Total cholesterol} - \text{HDL cholesterol} - \frac{\text{TG}}{5}$$

(ii) LDL cholesterol in mmol/l =

$$\text{Total cholesterol} - \text{HDL cholesterol} - \frac{\text{TG}}{2.2}$$

Note: The formula is not much reliable at TG concentration > 4.5 mmol/l (> 400 mg/dl)

METABOLISM OF ADIPOSE TISSUE

The lipids in the body physiologically exist in *two forms:*

- **"Element constant"** or *structural lipids.*
- **" Element variable"** *stored lipids (depot fats).*

Although a sharpline of demarcation cannot be made between the two, it has been generally observed that the value of the former remains constant even under extremes of starvation, whereas the latter varies.

A. *Composition of Element Constant:* Cytoplasm and cell membranes of all organs are composed of "element constant", so that ***their fat content does not diminish in starvation.*** Element constant is composed chiefly of phospholipids (PL), along with smaller amounts of other lipids, including cholesterol. It is independent of previous feeding. It remains an integral part of the cell protoplasm and is essential for its life.

B. *Composition of Element Variable:* The lipids which are stored in the body in excess of above. The ***amount fluctuates*** and it is ***composed mainly of triacylglycerol (TG),*** also ***called as neutral fats (NF).***

Dynamic State of Adipose Tissue: Adipose tissue is not just a static lump of fats; it is in ***dynamic state; breakdown of fats and synthesis take place all the time.***

METABOLISM

TG stores in the body is continually undergoing:

- *Esterification (synthesis)*
- *Lipolysis (breakdown).*

These two processes are not the forward and reverse processes of the same reaction. They are entirely different pathways involving different reactants and enzymes. Many of the nutritional, metabolic and hormonal factors regulate either of these two mechanisms, i.e. esterification and lipolysis. Resultant of these two processes determine the magnitude of free fatty acid pool in adipose tissue and this, in turn, ***will determine the level of free fatty acid (FFA) circulating in the blood.***

Esterification (Synthesis of TG)

In adipose tissue, for TG synthesis ***two substrates are required:***

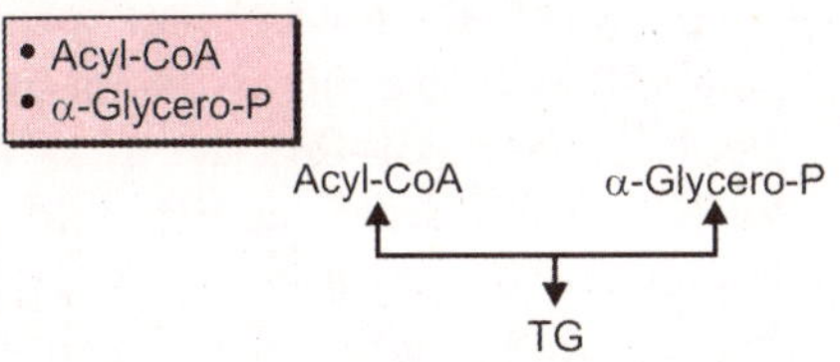

1. ***Sources of Acyl-CoA:*** Source of FFA in blood are:
   - Dietary
   - Synthesis of FA (palmitic acid) from Acetyl CoA-*de novo* synthesis (extramitochondrial). Further elongation to form other fatty acids in microsomes
   - Acyl-CoA obtained from lipolysis taking place in adipose tissue
   - FFA obtained from lipolysis of TG of circulating chylomicrons and VLDL by *lipoprotein lipase* enzyme present in capillary wall, which are taken up by adipose tissue.
2. ***Source of α-Glycerol-P:*** Mainly **two sources:**
   - Conversion of glycerol to α-glycerol-P by the enzyme *glycerokinase* in presence of ATP
   - The other source is from glucose oxidation. Dihydroxy acetone-P is converted to α-glycero-P.

The ***enzyme glycerokinase is practically absent in adipose tissue.*** If any glycerokinase is present, it has very low activity. Hence, ***glycerol produced by lipolysis in adipose tissue cannot be utilized for provision of α-glycero-P*** and thus glycerol passes into the blood, from where it is taken up by liver, kidney and other tissues which possess glycerokinase and is utilized for gluconeogenesis. ***Thus, for provision of α-glycero-P in adipose tissue for TG synthesis, the tissue is dependent on a supply of glucose and glycolysis.***

B. Lipolysis (Breakdown of TG):

TG in adipose tissue undergoes hydrolysis by a *hormone-sensitive lipase* enzyme to form free fatty acids and glycerol. ***Adipolytic lipases* are three:**

- "Hormone sensitive" ***triacyl glycerol lipase:*** key regulating enzyme
- Two others are not hormone-sensitive:
  - ***Diacyl glycerol lipase***
  - ***Monoacyl glycerol lipase.***

These lipases are distinct from *lipoprotein lipase* that hydrolyzes lipoprotein TG present in chylomicrons and VLDL. The free fatty acids formed by lipolysis can be reconverted in the tissue to acyl-CoA by *Acyl-CoA synthase* and re-esterified with α-glycero-P to form TG. Thus, there is a continuous cycle of lipolysis and reesterification within the tissue.

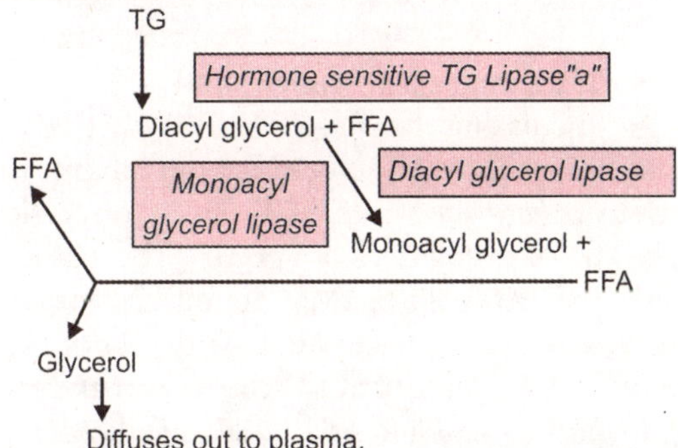

Note: When the rate of re-esterification is less than rate of lipolysis. FFA accumulates and diffuses into the plasma where it raises the level of FFA ↑ in plasma.

Effect of Glucose: Under conditions of adequate nutritional intake or when utilization of glucose by adipose tissue is increased, then more α-glycero-P will be available. ***Reesterification will be greater than lipolysis;*** as a result FFA outflow decreases and ***plasma FFA ↓ level falls.***

Adipose tissue metabolism in diabetes mellitus and in starvation: In diabetes mellitus and in starvation, availability of glucose in adipose tissue is grossly reduced, ***resulting to lack of α-glycero-P.*** Thus, rate of reesterification is decreased ↓. Lipolysis is greater than reesterification, resulting to accumulation of FFA and ***increase in plasma FFA level*** ↑.

INFLUENCE OF HORMONES ON ADIPOSE TISSUE

Rate of release of FFA from adipose tissue, is affected by many hormones which influence either the:

- *Rate of esterification or*
- *The rate of lipolysis*

A. *List of hormones that increase the rate of esterification:*

- **Insulin** is the principal hormone.
- **Prolactin:** effective in large doses.

1. **Insulin:** ***Net result of insulin on adipose tissue is to inhibit the release of free FA from adipose tissue,*** which results in ***fall of circulating plasma FFA*** ↓. This is brought about by decreasing the level of cyclic AMP ↓ in the cells. This is achieved by:

- Inhibiting *adenyl cyclase;* and
- Increasing the *phosphodiesterase* activity.

Lowered cyclic AMP level in the cell inhibits the activity of *hormone-sensitive-TG lipase* (conversion from "b" → to "a" does not occur). The action is mediated through c-AMP-dependant *protein kinase,* which is not activated. Thus, it not only decreases the release of free FA but also of glycerol.

Insulin also enhances the uptake of glucose into adipose cells. Glucose oxidation provides α-glycero-P through dihydroxyacetone-P, ***enhancing esterification.***

2. **Prolactin:** Effect of prolactin is similar to insulin provided it is given in larger doses.

B. *List of hormones that increases the rate of lipolysis:*

- *Catecholamines*-epinephrine and norepinephrine are the principal hormones
- *Other lipolytic hormones* are:
  - *Glucagon,*
  - *Growth hormone,*
  - *Glucocorticoids,*
  - *ACTH, α and β MSH, TSH and vasopressin.*

These hormones accelerate the release of FFA from adipose tissue and ***raise the plasma FFA*** ↑ level by increasing the rate of lipolysis of TG stores. Most of them act by activating *adenyl cyclase,* thus increasing the cyclic AMP level in cells.

Note:

- For an optimal effect most of these lipolytic process requires the presence of **glucocorticoids (GC) and "thyroid hormones"** ***in minimal amounts.*** On their own, these hormones, i.e. GC and thyroid hormones do not increase the lipolysis markedly but act in a ***"facilitatory"*** or ***"permissive"*** capacity with other lipolytic endocrine hormones.
- ***Hormones that act rapidly in promoting lipolysis are the catecholamines.*** They stimulate the activity of *adenyl cyclase* and increase cyclic-AMP level. Thyroid hormone in minimal amount is necessary for its full lipolytic activity.

Mechanism of action of the hormones is shown diagrammatically in ***Fig. 13.1.***

ASSIMILATION OF TG FA BY ADIPOSE TISSUE

- Major chemical forms in which plasma lipids interact with adipose tissues is TG as:
  - "Chylomicrons" derived from intestinal absorption of fats (see chylomicron formation)
  - "Very low-density lipoprotein" complex (VLDL) by liver.
- TG of circulating chylomicrons and VLDL is acted upon by an enzyme called ***lipoprotein lipase*** to hydrolyse TG to form FFA and glycerol
- The enzyme lipoprotein lipase is located in the walls of blood capillaries in various organs
- Activity of *lipoprotein lipase* in adipose tissue is high in the fed state and "low" in starvation and diabetes mellitus

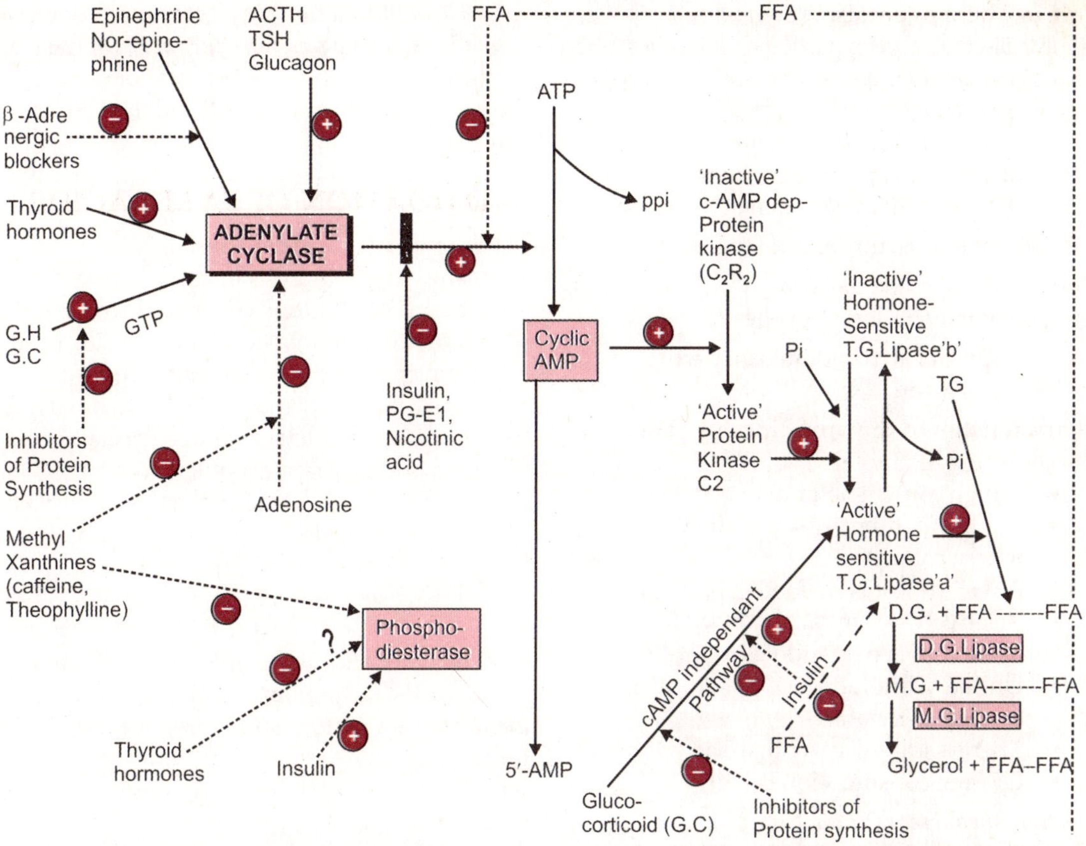

Epinephrine
Nor-epine-
phrine
ACTH
TSH
Glucagon
FFA
FFA
ATP
β-Adre
nergic
blockers
ppi
'Inactive'
c-AMP dep-
Protein
kinase
(C_2R_2)
Thyroid
hormones
ADENYLATE
CYCLASE
'Inactive'
Hormone-
Sensitive
T.G.Lipase'b'
G.H
G.C
GTP
Cyclic
AMP
Pi
TG
Insulin,
PG-E1,
Nicotinic
acid
'Active'
Protein
Kinase
C2
Pi
Inhibitors
of Protein
Synthesis
Adenosine
'Active'
Hormone
sensitive
T.G.Lipase'a'
Methyl
Xanthines
(caffeine,
Theophylline)
cAMP independant
Pathway
D.G. + FFA ------FFA
D.G.Lipase
Phospho-
diesterase
?
Insulin
M.G + FFA--------FFA
M.G.Lipase
FFA
Thyroid
hormones
Insulin
5'-AMP
Glycerol + FFA--FFA
Gluco-
corticoid (G.C)
Inhibitors of
Protein synthesis

Fig 13.1: Showing influence of hormones on adipose tissue metabolism

- However, following injection of heparin, *lipoprotein* is released into the circulation and is accompanied by clearing of lipemia (hence called as ***"clearing factor")***.
- Both phospholipids (PL) and apolipoprotein-CII are required as cofactors for *lipoprotein lipase* activity
- TG of chylomicrons and VLDL are progressively hydrolyzed to give DG and then MG and finally glycerol and FFA (three molecules)

TG of
chylomicron
and VLDL
Heparin+
Lipoprotein lipase
PL
APO-C-II
FFA + glycerol

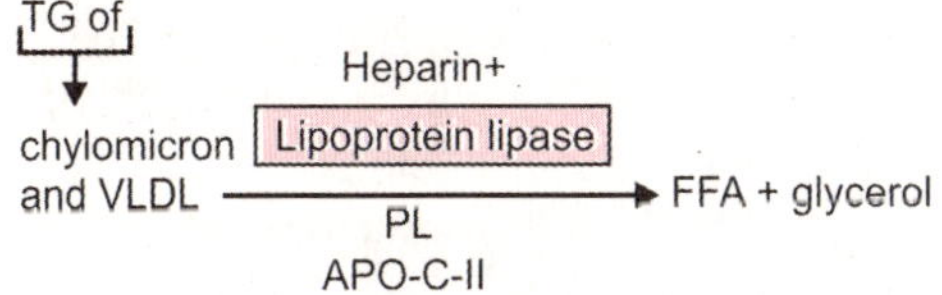

- Some of hydrolyzed FA returns to circulation being carried by albumin and bulk of FFA is taken up by tissues including adipose tissue.

Role of Hormones: In adipose tissue, insulin enhances the synthesis of lipoprotein lipase in adipose tissue cells and its translocation to luminal surface of capillary endothelium.

BROWN ADIPOSE TISSUE

Types of Storage Fats: There are **two types of storage fats:**

- Storage "white" fat present in depot fats-predominant
- In addition to usual white storage fat, another type of ***"pigmented" brown fat*** is stored in some species including humans.

Role in Thermogenesis: Brown adipose tissue is involved in metabolism particularly at times when *a heat generation is necessary.* Thus, *the tissue is extremely active:*

- *In arousal from hibernation;*
- *In animals exposed to cold;* and
- *In heat production in newborn animals.*

It is present in rats, throughout the life.

Note: It is to be noted that brown adipose tissue is reduced or may be absent in obese persons.

Location: It is located and present particularly in the thoracic region.

Characteristics of Brown Adipose Tissue:
It is characterized by:

- A high content of mitochondria;
- A high content of cytochromes (gives brown colour)
- A well-developed blood supply;
- Relatively rich in carnitine, which is significant for FA oxidation;
- Unlike white adipose tissue, it has the enzyme *glycerokinase;*
- There is low ATP-synthase activity; and
- Oxygen consumption is high.

Mechanism of Heat Production

- *Oxidation and phosphorylation are not coupled in mitochondria of this tissue.* Dinitrophenol has no effect and there is no respiratory control by ADP.
- Oxidation produces much heat and very little free energy is trapped as ATP due to decreased coupling of oxidation and phosphorylation.
- In terms of chemi-osmotic theory (see Biologic oxidation), it appears that the proton gradient, normally present across the inner mitochondrial membrane of coupled mitochondria, is *continually dissipated in brown adipose tissue by a thermogenic protein, called thermogenin,* which acts as a proton conductance pathway through the membrane. This explains the apparent lack of effects of uncouplers.

Function: Brown storage fat has a somewhat higher temperature than other tissues. *It plays a role in heat production for vital organs, serving as a sort of "heating pad" or "furnace"* for the local application of its heat to the vital organs of the thorax, the upper spinal cord, and the autonomic sympathetic chain.

OXIDATION OF FATTY ACIDS

Plasma free fatty acids are derived:

- Mainly from lipolysis in adipose tissue
- Portion of FFA is derived from degradation of circulating chylomicrons and VLDL by the action of the enzyme *lipoprotein lipase*
- A small portion of plasma FFA is derived from absorption of dietary source specially small chain and medium chain fatty acids.
- Also FFA is obtained from synthesis of acetyl CoA in liver cells, which are incorporated in TG.

In postabsorptive state, plasma contains 10 to 30 mg FFA percent, most of which is transported in plasma as a loose complex with albumin as ***"albumin-FFA complex"***, but in the ***cell they are attached to a fatty acid binding protein or "Z-protein".*** A small amount of FA is also associated with HDL. Shorter chain FAs are more water soluble and exist as the unionized acid or as a FA anion. Fatty acids exhibit a very rapid turnover rate with half life of only 1 to 3 minutes, they are rapidly taken up by tissues and metabolized.

Methods by which fatty acids are oxidized in the body are as follows:

A. *β-oxidation: Principal method of oxidation of FA.*

Other ancillary and **specialized methods are:**

B. *α-oxidation*
C. *ω-Oxidation*
D. *Peroxismal FA oxidation.*

A. β-OXIDATION:

Principal method by which FA are oxidized is called β-oxidation. Several theories have been proposed to explain the mechanism of the oxidation of FA chains. The classical theory of β-oxidation was the outcome of the work of **Knoop**.

Conclusion: **Knoop** proposed the β-oxidation theory. According to this mechanism, *FA chains*

are oxidized by the removal of 2 carbon atoms at a time. The carbon atom in the β-position to COOH group is assumed to be attacked with the formation of the corresponding β-keto acid; then the two terminal C atoms are split off as ***"acetyl-CoA".*** A new COOH group is formed at the site of the keto (=CO) grouping, so that a fatty acid remains ***with 2 carbon atoms less*** than the original. Again the new β-carbon atom is attacked and two more carbon atoms are split off as acetyl-CoA. In this way, the ***FA is degraded by the removal of 2 carbon atoms at a time, until finally the stage of acetoacetic acid is reached.***

Tissues in which β-Oxidation is Carried Out: The circulating FA are taken up by various tissues and oxidized. Tissues like liver, heart, kidney, muscle, brain, lungs, testes and adipose tissue have the ability to oxidize long-chain FA. In cardiac muscle, fatty acids are an important fuel of respiration (80% of energy derived from FA oxidation).

Enzymes Involved in β-Oxidation: ***β-oxidation takes place in mitochondrion.*** Several enzymes known collectively as ***FA-oxidase system*** are found in the mitochondrial matrix, adjacent to the respiratory chain, which is found in the inner membrane. These enzymes catalyze the oxidation of FA to acetyl-CoA.

Activation of FA: Fatty acids are in cytosol of the cell (extramitochondrial). As in the metabolism of glucose, fatty acids also must be first activated so that they participate in metabolic pathway. The activation requires energy which is provided by ATP. In presence of ATP, and coenzyme A, the enzyme ***acyl-CoA synthetase*** (previously called as ***thiokinases)*** catalyzes the conversion of a free fatty acid to an "**active" FA (acyl-CoA)**. Thus, in effect 2~P bonds are expended during activation of each FA molecule. Not only saturated FA but unsaturated FA and –OH fatty acids are also activated by these acyl CoA synthetases.

CARNITINE AND ITS ROLE IN FA METABOLISM

- "Active" FA (acyl-CoA) are formed in cytosol, whereas β-oxidation of FA occurs in mitochondrial matrix
- ***Acyl-CoA are impermeable to mitochondrial membrane.*** Long chain activated FA penetrate the inner mitochondrial membrane only in combination with carnitine

$$(CH_3)_3N^+-\underset{\gamma}{CH_2}-\underset{\beta}{\overset{OH}{\overset{|}{CH}}}-CH_2-COOH$$

- Carnitine is chemically ***"β-OH-γ-trimethyl ammonium butyrate".***
    - Carnitine is widely distributed in yeast, milk, liver and particularly large quantities in muscles and in meat extracts.
    - Carnitine level of tissues is also considerably influenced by dietary methionine and choline levels.
    - Carnitine is synthesized from lysine and methionine in liver principally, also in kidneys.

Function: Carnitine is considered as a ***"carrier molecule"***, it ***acts like a ferry-boat.*** It transports long-chain acyl-CoA across mitochondrial membrane which is impermeable to acyl-CoA.

- Facilitates transport of long-chain acyl-CoA for oxidation in mitochondria.
- Facilitates exit of acetyl-CoA and acetoacetyl CoA from within mitochondria to cytosol, where FA synthesis takes place.

Mechanism of Transport of Long-Chain Acyl-CoA

Activation of lower FA and their oxidation may occur within the mitochondria, independently, of cartinine; but long-chain acyl-CoA (or FFA) will not penetrate mitochondria and become oxidized unless they form ***"acyl carnitines"***.

- An enzyme ***carnitine palmitoyl transferase*** 1, present on the inner side of the outer mitochondrial membrane, converts long-chain acyl-CoA to *acyl carnitines;* which is able to penetrate mitochondria and gain access to the β-oxidation systems of the enzymes

$$\text{Acyl – CoA + carnitine} \xrightarrow{\text{Carnitine palmitoyl Transferase I}} \text{Acyl – carnitine + CoA}$$

- Another enzyme ***carnitine-acyl carnitine translocase*** acts as membrane-carnitine exchange transporter. Acyl carnitine is transported in, coupled with the transport out of one molecule of carnitine
- The acyl carnitine then reacts with CoA-SH, catalyzed by ***carnitine palmitoyl transferase II,*** attached to the inside of the inner membrane. Acyl-CoA is reformed in the mitochondrial matrix and carnitine is liberated.

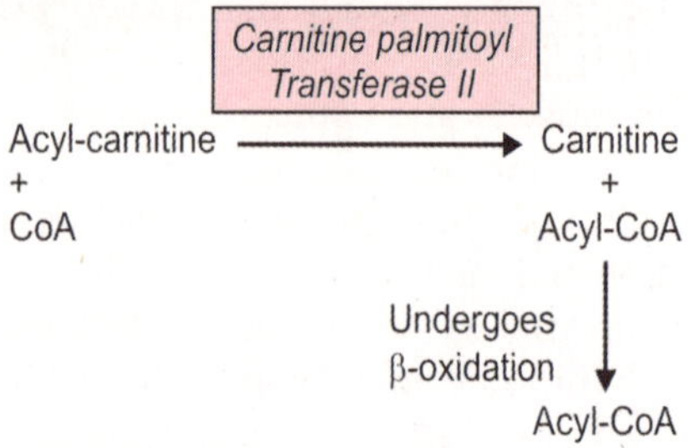

Steps of β-Oxidation *(Fig. 13.2)*

Once acyl-CoA is transported by carnitine in the mitochondrial matrix, it undergoes β-oxidation by ***fatty acid oxidase complex.*** The successive steps are as follows:

1. ***Dehydrogenation: Removal of 2 H Atoms***

- Removal of two hydrogen atoms from the 2 (α) and 3 (β) carbon atoms is catalyzed by the enzyme ***acyl-CoA dehydrogenase,*** resulting in formation of Δ^2-trans enoyl CoA (also called α, β-unsaturated acyl-CoA)
- Hydrogen acceptor, i.e. the coenzyme for this dehydrogenase is a *flavoprotein,* containing FAD as prosthetic group, whose reoxidation in the respiratory chain produces 2 ATP.

+ 2ATP

2. ***Hydration: Addition of One Molecule of H_2O***

- One molecule of water is added to saturate the double bond to form 3-OH acyl-CoA (also called as β-OH acyl-CoA), the reaction is catalyzed by the enzyme ***"Δ^2-enoyl-CoA hydratase"*** **(also called as *enoyl hydrolase;* earlier called as *crotonase*).**

3. ***Dehydrogenation: Removal of two Hydrogen Atoms***

- The 3-OH-Acyl-CoA undergoes further dehydrogenation on the 3 carbon, catalyzed by the enzyme ***3-OH-acyl CoA dehydrogenase,*** to form the corresponding 3-keto acyl-CoA (β-keto acyl-CoA).
- Hydrogen acceptor, i.e. coenzyme of this dehydrogenase is NAD^+. Reduced NAD when oxidized in respiratory chain produces 3 ATP.

+3 ATP

4. ***Thiolytic Cleavage:***

- Finally, 3-keto-acyl CoA is split at the 2, 3 position by ***thiolase*** (3-keto acyl thiolase or acetyl-CoA acyl transferase), which catalyzes a thiolytic cleavage involving another molecule of CoA.

End-products of this reaction: The thiolytic cleavage results in formation of:

- One molecule of acetyl-CoA; and
- ***An acyl-CoA molecule containing 2-carbons less than the original acyl-CoA molecule,*** which entered for oxidation by the enzyme *acyl-CoA dehydrogenase.*

- ***In this way, a long-chain FA may be degraded completely to "acetyl-CoA" (C-2 units).*** Acetyl-CoA can be oxidized to CO_2 and H_2O and thus complete oxidation of FA is achieved. Thus, end-product of β-oxidation of a long-chain FA will produce acetyl-CoA molecules (C-2 units).

How many acetyl-CoA are produced from β-oxidation of palmitic acid?

- Palmitic acid is $C_{15}H_{31}COOH$.
- Hence, in β-oxidation-for complete oxidation **it will undergo seven cycles,** producing 7 acetyl-CoA (in 7 cycles) + 1 acetyl CoA (last cycle—one extra).
- Therefore, ***total acetyl-CoA produced by β-oxidation of one molecule of palmitic acid is 8 acetyl-CoA.***

β-Oxidation of FA with an Odd Number of Carbon Atoms: Fatty acids with an odd number of carbon atoms are oxidized by β-oxidation pathway to produce acetyl-CoA until a 3-carbon residue ***propionyl CoA is left.*** Propionyl CoA is metabolized to succinyl CoA through methyl malonyl CoA. Succinyl CoA is an intermediate of TCA cycle.

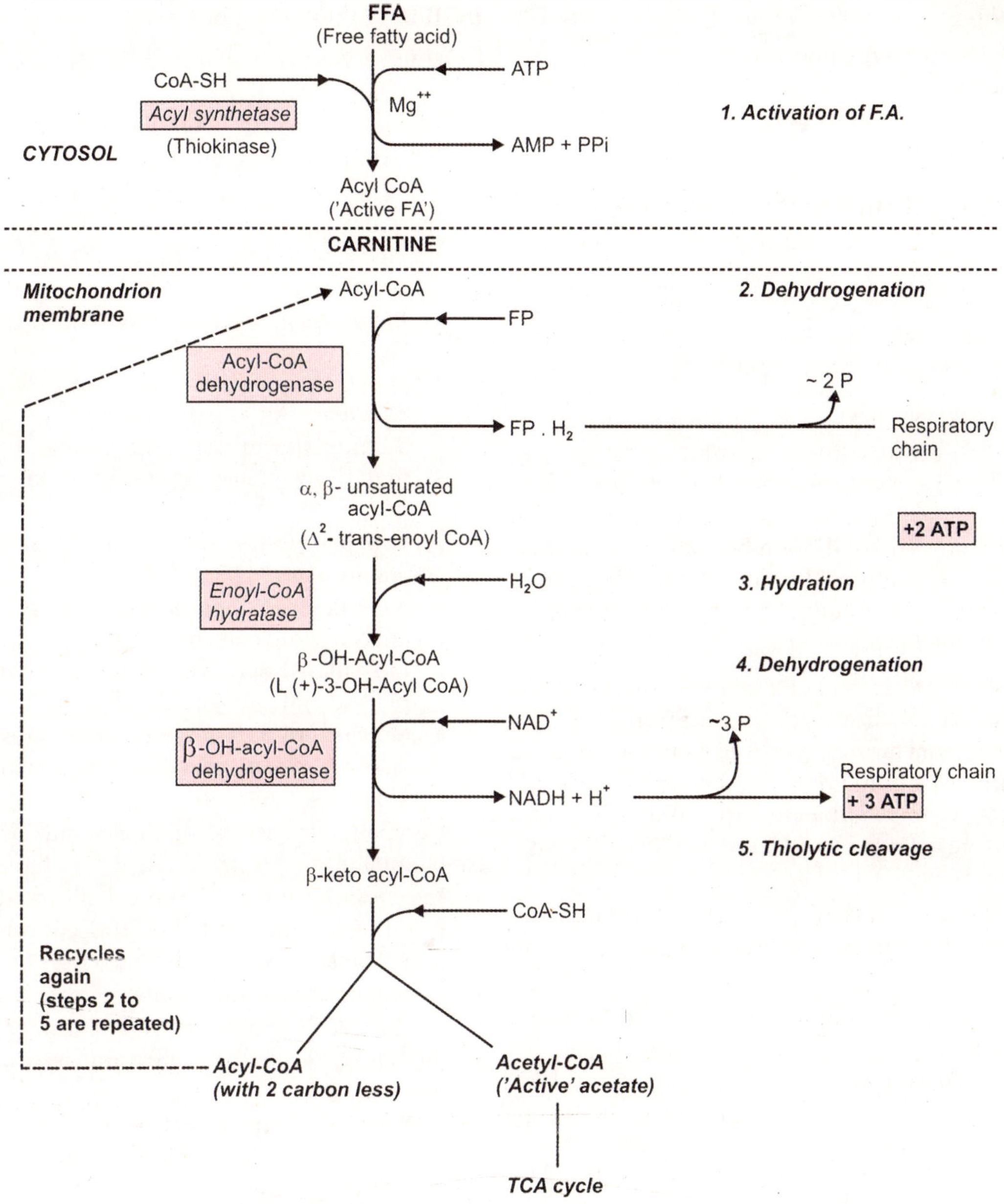

Fig.13.2: β-Oxidation of fatty acids

Note: Propionyl CoA formed from an odd-chain FA is the only part of the FA which is glucogenic; as it is converted to succinyl CoA.

Bio-Energetics of β-Oxidation and its Efficiency

Palmitic acid, $C_{15}H_{31}COOH$, on complete oxidation (β-oxidation) produces 8 acetyl-CoA (refer discussion above). Transport of electrons in respiratory chain from reduced Fp and NAD in each cycle produces five high energy phosphate bonds.

Hence, 7 cycles (7 acetyl-CoA = 7 × 5) =35~P.

Total 8 molecules of acetyl-CoA,

When oxidized in TCA cycle will

Produce = 12 × 8 = 96~P

Total high energy phosphate bonds
Produced = 131~P

In initial activation of FA
~ P bonds utilized −2 ~ P

Total = 129~ P

∴ Energy Production = 129 × 7.6 = 980 Kc
(or 129 × 30.5 = 3935 kj)

Caloric value of palmitic acid
(Bomb calorimeter) = 2340 Kc/mol
Hence, **efficiency** = 980/2340×100 = 41 percent of the total energy of combustion of FA.

B. α-OXIDATION: α-oxidation is another alternative pathway for oxidation of FA which involves decarboxylation of the COOH group after hydroxylation and the formation of a FA containing an "odd" number of carbon atoms, which subsequently undergoes repeated β-oxidation. ***No initial activation of FA is necessary in this process.***

C. ω-OXIDATION (VERKADE): In ω-oxidation, fatty acids undergo oxidation at the carbon atom farthest removed from the carboxyl group (ω-carbon) ***producing a dicarboxylic acid,*** which is then subjected to β-oxidation and cleavage to form successively smaller dicarboxylic acids.

Both processes occur principally in brain microsomes but are negligible in extent as compared to β-oxidation.

Purpose of α-Oxidation: In the body α-oxidation serves:

- ***To synthesize α-OH fatty acids like cerebronic acid*** to brain cerebrosides and sulfatides
- To form odd C long-chain FA required in brain sphingolipids
- Also helps to oxidize ***phytanic acid*** produced from dietary phytols, a constituent of chlorophyll of plant food stuffs. Phytanic acid is oxidized by α-oxidation with ***Phytate α-oxidase*** (an α-hydroxylase enzyme) to yield CO_2 and odd C chain FA ***"pristanic acid"*** which is then completely oxidized by β-oxidation.

INHERITED DISORDERS

Refsum's disease:

A rare genetic disorder.

- ***Enzyme deficiency: "phytanate α-oxidase",***
- ***Inheritance:*** autosomal recessive.
- ***Age:*** The disease may become manifest at any age from childhood to adult life. In some affected families there was consanguinity of the parents.
  - ***Biochemical defect:*** Phytanic acid cannot be converted to pristanic acid due to absence of the enzyme ***Phytanate α-oxidase.*** As a result phytanic acid accumulates in tissues and blood. Blood may show increase up to 20% of the total FA.
- ***Clinical manifestations:*** Principally manifestations are ***neurological.***
  - ***Neurological symptoms and signs:*** Early chronic polyneuropathy with distal muscular atrophy and progressive paresis of the distal parts of extremities.
  - ***Sensory disturbances:*** include paresthesiae, occasionally severe pain specially in knees.

Cerebellar involvement causes ataxia and nystagmus.

- ***Eye manifestations:*** Typical pigmentary retinitis, night blindness, and concentric narrowing of visual fields.
- ***Mental development:*** usually normal.
- ***CS fluid:*** CSF protein is always considerably increased, whilst the cell count is usually normal.
- ***Diagnosis:*** Demonstration of increased phytanic acid in plasma or in tissue lipids is pathognomonic.
- ***Treatment:*** Omit intake of dietary phytols which is the precursor of phytanic acid.

FATTY ACID SYNTHESIS

Earlier it was believed that fatty acid synthesis was reversal of fatty acid oxidation. But now it is clear that there are ***three systems*** for fatty acid synthesis.

A. Extra Mitochondrial System: This is radically different and ***highly active system*** responsible for ***"de novo" synthesis of palmitic acid from 2-carbon unit acetyl-CoA.***

B. Chain Elongation System:

1. *Microsomal System:* A system present in microsomes which can lengthen existing fatty acid chains. The palmitic acid formed in cytosol is lengthened to stearic acid and arachidonic acids.

2. *Mitochondrial System:* This system is mostly restricted to lengthening of an existing fatty acid of moderate chain length. It operates under *"anaerobiosis"* and is *favoured by a high NADH/ NAD^+ ratio*.

A. Extramitochondrial (Cytoplasmic) Synthesis of Fatty Acids: ("De Novo" sysnthesis)

The ***synthesis takes place in cytosol. Starting material is acetyl-CoA and synthesis always ends in formation of palmitic acid.***

Materials required for the synthesis

- *Enzymes:*
  - *Fatty acid Synthase* a multienzyme complex
  - *Acetyl-CoA carboxylase* also a multi-enzyme complex
- *Coenzymes and cofactors:* Biotin, NADPH, Mn^{++}
- **CO_2:** Sources of CO_2 is bicarbonate and
- **ATP:** for energy

Details of Enzymes

1. *Fatty Acid Synthase:* In yeast, mammals and birds, the enzyme system is called the **"fatty acid synthase" complex**—it is a **multienzyme complex.** It is made up of an ellipsoid dimer of two identical polypeptide monomeric units (monomer I and II), arranged in a "head to tail" fashion, ***Each monomeric unit contains six enzymes*** and ***an ACP molecule (Acyl carrier protein).***

Active site:

- The ACP has an-SH group in the 4-phospho-pantothene moiety, referred as **"Pantothenyl—SH " (Pan-SH)**
- Another active-SH group present in the cysteine moiety of the enzyme "Ketoacyl synthase" (condensing enzyme), referred as **"cysteinyl—SH" (Cys–SH).**

The "Pan –SH" of one monomeric unit is in close proximity to the "Cys-SH" group of other monomeric unit and vice-versa.

Following is the order of enzymes from end to end in each monomeric unit:

3-keto acyl synthase, transacylase, enoyl reductase, 3-OH acyl dehydratase, 3-keto acyl reductase, ACP and thioesterase (deacylase) (Fig.13.3).

It is found that complex is functional only when the two monomeric units are in association with each other. **The functional activity is lost when they are dissociated.** In a dimer form, the complex jointly synthesizes 2 molecules of pamitic acid simultaneously.

Note: In bacteria, plants and lower forms of life, the individual enzymes are separate and it is the **"Acyl carrier protein"** (ACP) which binds the acyl radicals. ACP is a single polypeptide chain of 77 amino acids, a serine moiety of this peptide chain is in combination with phosphopantothene. The –SH group of Pantothene moiety takes active part in synthesis of fatty acid.

- *Acetyl-CoA carboxylase:* Also a multienzyme complex containing:
  - *Biotin*
  - *Biotin carboxylase*
  - *Biotin carboxyl carrier protein*
  - *Trans carboxylase, and*
  - *A regulatory allosteric site.*

STEPS OF FA SYNTHESIS

The starting material for the synthesis is Acetyl CoA. Acetyl-CoA is formed in mitochondrion but synthesis occurs in cytosol. ***Acetyl-CoA is impermeable to mitochondrial membrane.*** The various means by which it is made available is discussed later.

1. *Formation of Malonyl CoA from Acetyl CoA:* ***In presence of the enzyme "acetyl-CoA Carboxylase"*** the acetyl-CoA is converted to malonyl CoA ***"CO_2-fixation reaction".*** Mn^{++} is required as a cofactor and ATP provides the energy.

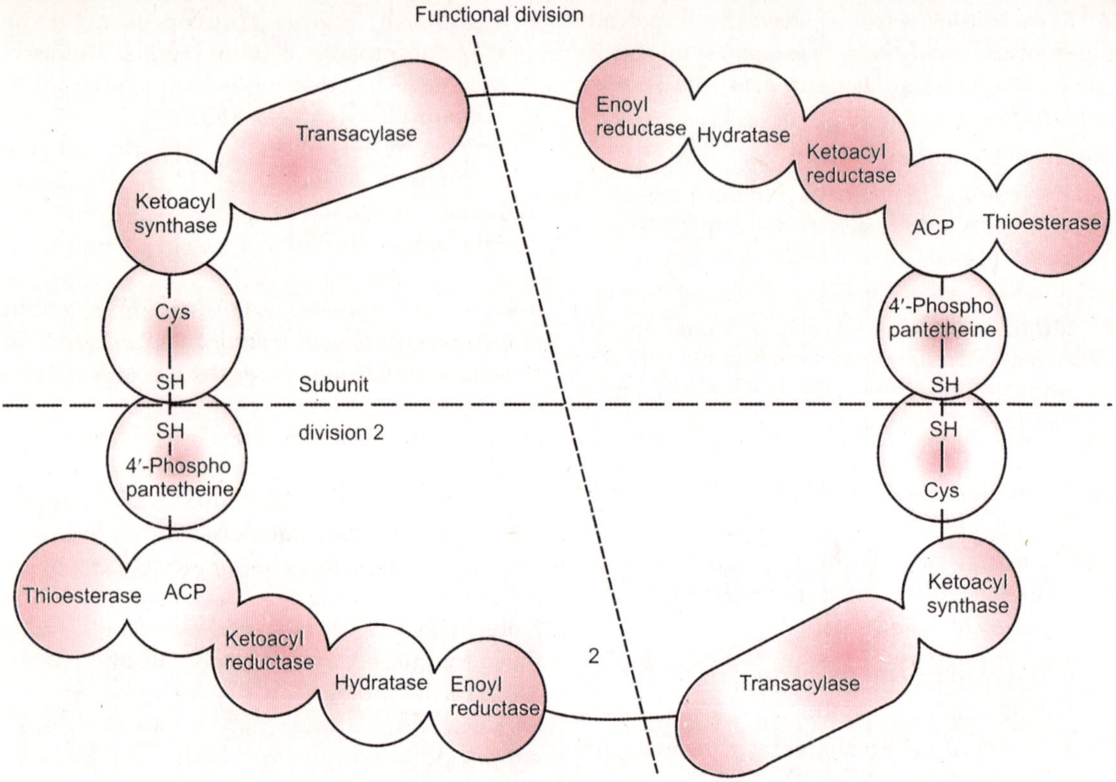

Fig.13.3: Fatty acid synthase multienzyme complex

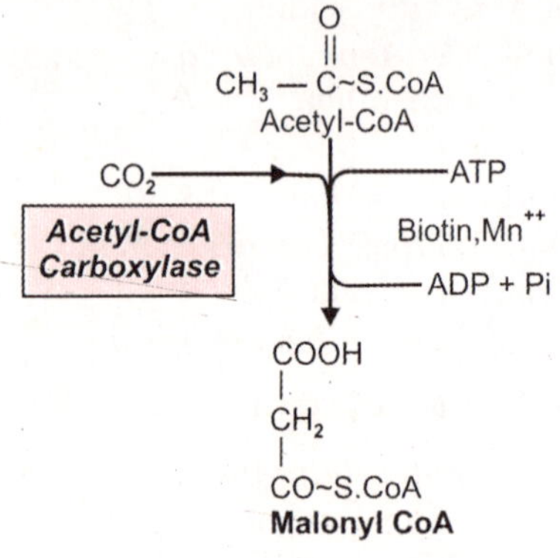

Reaction Occurs in Two Steps:

1. Biotin-enzyme + ATP + HCO_3^-
   ↓
   Carboxy-biotin-enz + ADP + Pi
2. Carboxy-biotin-enz + Acetyl-CoA
   ↓
   Malonyl CoA + biotin-enz

Characteristics:

- The reaction is ***irreversible***
- CO_2 is provided by HCO_3^-
- One high energy bond of ATP is utilized
- ***Acetyl-CoA carboxylase is a rate-limiting enzyme.*** Citrate is an activator of the enzyme and palmitidyl CoA is inhibitor.

2. *Subsequent Steps:*

Once malonyl CoA is synthesized, rest of fatty acid synthesis reactions take place with FA synthase complex.

"Cys—SH" and "Pan—SH" may be considered as two arms of the enzyme complex. 'Cys—SH' is the acceptor of Acetyl-CoA whereas "Pan–SH" takes up malonyl CoA.

- Initially, a molecule of acetyl-CoA combines with the **"Cys–SH"** of *"Keto acyl-synthase"* of one monomeric unit (monomer I). The coenzyme A is removed, the reaction is catalyzed by the enzyme *"transacylase"*.

- In a similar manner, a molecule of Malonyl CoA (formed as above) combines with the adjacent "Pan-SH" of ACP of opposite monomeric unit (Monomer II), to form "Malonyl-ACP enzyme". The coenzyme A of Malonyl CoA is also removed in this step and the reaction is catalyzed by the same *"transacylase"* enzyme.

3. *Condensation reaction:* Now, the acetate attacks malonate to form a "aceto-acetyl-ACP". The reaction is catalyzed by the enzyme ***"Ketoacyl Synthase" (condensing enzyme)*** and there is loss of one molecule of CO_2 (decarboxylation). ***The decarboxylation provides the extra thermodynamic push to make the reaction highly favourable.*** It also makes the central carbon a better nucleo-philic agent for attacking the carboxyl carbon of the acetyl group.

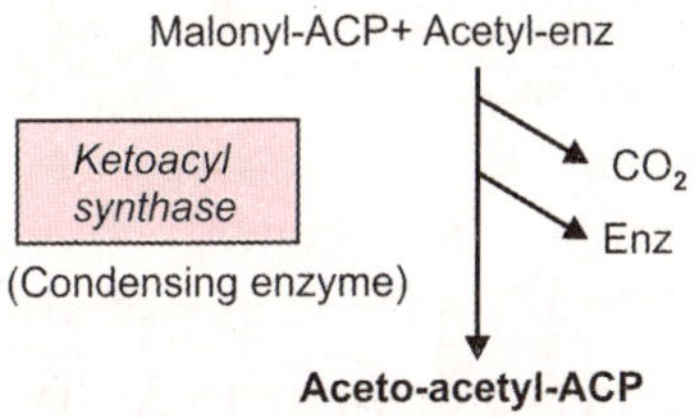

The aceto-acetate remains attached to Pan-SH of monomer II, ***the cys-SH of monomer I becomes free.***

4. *Other reactions:* While aceto acetate remains attached to ***"Pan–SH", three reactions*** take place, viz. ***reduction, dehydration,*** followed by another ***reaction***

a. ***First reaction (reduction):*** The keto-acyl group is reduced to hydroxy group(-OH) to form "β-OH bytyryl-ACP", catalyzed by the enzyme *"keto-acyl reductase"*.

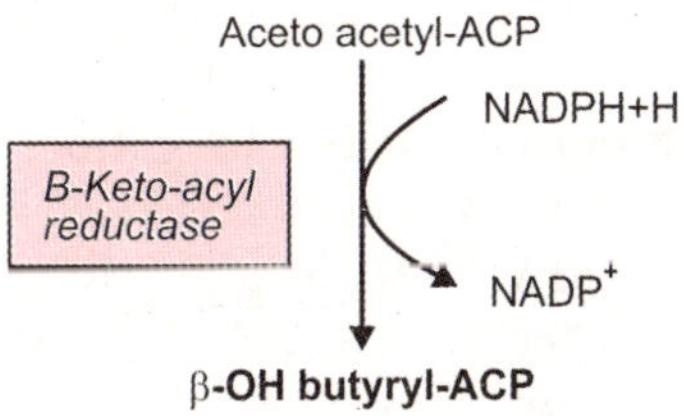

b. ***Second reaction (Dehydration):*** A molecule of H_2O is removed from β-OH-butyryl-ACP' to form "α, β-unsaturated butyryl-ACP" (also called crotonyl-ACP), catalyzed by the enzyme "β-*OH acyl dehydratase"*

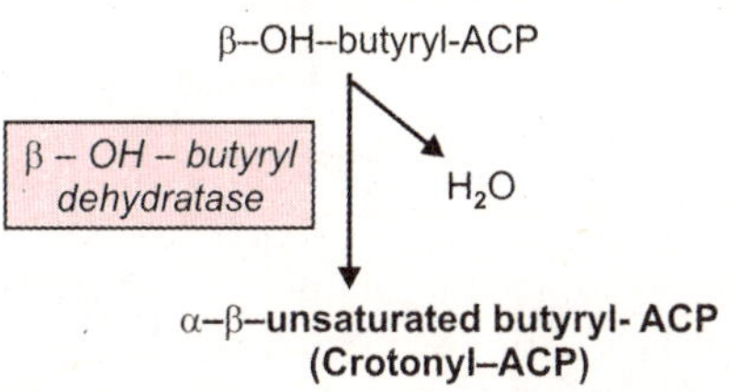

c. ***Third reaction (reduction):*** The third and final reduction is catalyzed by *"enoyl-reductase"*, using $NADPH+H^+$, as a result the double bond is ***saturated*** to form "butyryl-ACP" (**4 carbon). *All the above three reactions occur on "Pan–SH" of monomer II. Once saturated butyric acid is formed, it is now transferred to the "cys—SH" of monomer I which is free to accommodate.***

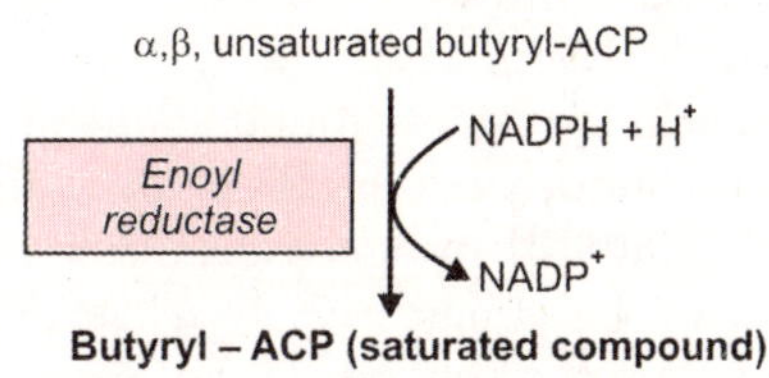

- ***Continuation reaction:*** Now a fresh molecule of ***Malonyl-CoA*** is taken up on to the ***free "Pan—SH"*** group of monomer II and the sequence of events is repeated to form a saturated **six carbon** fatty acid. Once formed this is again transferred to "Cys-SH" of monomer I.

  The set of reactions on each of the monomer is repeated till a ***16 carbon palmityl-ACP*** is formed on **"Pan–SH"** of monomer II.

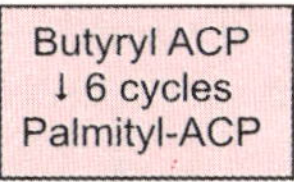

Note: The lengthening of the acyl group by each two carbon units at a time is brought about by one ATP-molecule which is used for formation of malonyl-CoA from acetyl-CoA.

6. *Termination reaction:* Palmityl-ACP is released as palmitic acid from the enzyme by the enzyme *"thioesterase" (deacylase).*

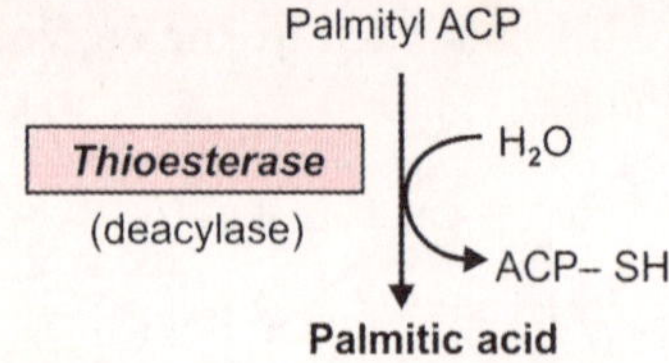

Note:

- The two carbons farthest away from the—COOH group are derived directly from "acetate" (acetyl-CoA)
- The remaining carbons are derived from Malonyl-CoA which adds two carbons at a time and the third is lost as CO_2 (decarboxylation).

SOURCES OF ACETYL-COA AND NADPH

As is clear from above, acetyl CoA and NADPH are substrates for fatty acid synthesis.

Sources are as follows:

1. *Sources of Acetyl-CoA:*

- Acetyl-CoA is mainly found in mitochondria which cannot pass out. It forms citrate by condensing with oxaloacetate. Citrate is transported out by a transporter protein in exchange of malate. Once in cytoplasm an enzyme *citrate lyase* cleaves citrate with the help of ATP to form acetyl-CoA and oxaloacetate
- ***Carnitine acetyl transferase*** may probably transfer acetyl group of acetyl-CoA to carnitine to form acylcarnitine in mitochondria. After translocation to cytoplasm acetyl group may be transferred to CoA to make it acetyl-CoA.

2. *Sources of NADPH:*

- ***Hexose monophosphate shunt or HMP pathway is the main source of NADPH.***
- Oxaloacetate produced by *citrate lyase* in the cytoplasm can be reduced to malate by NADH + H^+ and *malate dehydrogenase.* There is another cytoplasmic enzyme called *malic enzyme* (NADP-malate dehydrogenase). Malate is oxidatively decarboxylated to pyruvate and NADPH is produced.
- An enzyme called *isocitrate dehydrogenase* is present in the cytoplasm. It generates NADPH mainly in ruminants. It uses NADP as the coenzyme.

Regulation of Fatty Acid Synthesis

- In the biosynthesis of fatty acids, ***"acetyl-CoA carboxylase"* is the *rate-limiting*** step
- Citrate activates the enzyme
- Long chain acyl-CoA molecules inhibit the enzyme and this is an example of feedback inhibition
- The fatty acid synthesis is increased with high carbohydrate diets
- The enzyme decreases in the fasting state, in diabetes mellitus (DM) and in conditions of excessive dietary fat
- **Hormones:**
  - ***Glucagon:*** Inhibits the enzyme and thus induces inhibition of FA synthesis.
  - ***Insulin:*** Increases FA synthesis in several ways:
    - decreasing lipolysis
    - bringing about activation of *Protein phosphatase*
    - Stimulating synthesis of *citrate lyase*
    - Enhancing formation of acetyl-CoA from pyruvate by increasing glycolysis.

B. ELONGATION OF FATTY ACIDS

There are ***two types*** of elongation:

I. Microsomal Chain Elongation: The palmitic acid is synthesized in the cytoplasm. Higher fatty acids such as stearic acid (C_{18}) and others are formed from palmitate by enzymes of the microsomal elongase of chain elongation system in the smooth endoplasmic reticulum. It makes use of malonyl-CoA and NADPH to add 2-C at a time. Acyl-CoA group that acts as primer molecule may be saturated FA series C_{10} to C_{16} and some unsaturated C_{18} FA and are converted to next higher homologue. ***Molecular O_2 is necessary.***

II. Mitochondrial Chain Elongation: There is another elongation system found in mitochondria which is called as mitochondrial elongase. This makes use of acetyl-CoA, NADH, NADPH and ATP. Usually palmityl-CoA is the starting material and converted to stearyl-CoA. But other long-chain FA can also act as substrate. This system ***requires anaerobiosis*** and a high ratio of NADH/NAD^+ is favourable. ***Table 13.3*** shows similarities

Table 13.3: Showing similarities and differences between FA synthesis by mitochondrial system and microsomal system

Mitochondrial System	*Microsomal System*
• Not a common pathway	• Usual common pathway for chain elongation
• Operates in mitochondria	• Operates in "microsomal" system. Chain elongation of FA takes place in endoplasmic reticulum (ER)
• ***Palmityl-CoA is usually the starting material*** and converted to stearyl-CoA. Other long-chain FA may be elongated	• Acyl group that may act as "Primer" molecule; may be saturated FA series from C_{10} to C_{16} and some unsaturated - C_{18} FA. ***End-product is next higher homologue of the "Primer" acyl-CoA molecule"***
• Operates under ***"anaerobic"*** conditions. It is favoured by a high $NADH/NAD^+$ ratio in cells. Also in presence of excessive ethanol oxidation in liver	• ***Requires presence of*** O_2
• Acetyl-CoA (two carbon unit) is directly incorporated into the palmityl-CoA molecule.	• Acetyl moiety (two carbon) is added through malonyl-CoA and not directly by incorporating C-2 units
• NADPH is required which is provided by HMP shunt	• NADPH is required as a reductant provided by HMP shunt
• Pyridoxal-P is required as a coenzyme for the "condensing enzyme" in the first reaction to incorporate C-2 unit.	• Pyridoxal-P is not required.

and differences between FA synthesis by mitochondrial system and microsomal system.

CATABOLISM OF LECITHIN (PHOSPHATIDYL CHOLINE)

Steps

- Lecithin is degraded in the body by the enzyme *phospholipase* A_2, which catalyzes the hydrolysis of the ester bond in ***position-2 (β-position)*** to form a free fatty acid and ***lysolecithin*** (lysophosphatidyl choline).
- Lysolecithin is attacked by thc cnzyme *lysophospholipase (phospholipase B)* which hydrolyzes the ester bond at ***α-position (1-position),*** liberating another molecule of free fatty acid and forms ***'glycerol phosphoryl choline' (glyceryl phosphocholine).***
- Finally, glyceryl phospho-choline is hydrolyzed further by the enzyme *glyceryl phosphocholine hydrolase* to form the nitrogenous base **"choline"** and **α-glycero-P**. (Sn-glycerol-3-P). Degradation of lecithin is shown in ***Fig. 13.5.***

KETOSIS

Under certain metabolic conditions associated with a high rate of fatty acid oxidation, liver produces considerable quantities of compounds like **acetoacetate** and **β-OH butyric acid**, which pass by diffusion into the blood. Acetoacetate continually undergoes spontaneous decarboxylation to produce **acetone**. ***These three substances are collectively known as ketone bodies (or acetone bodies). Sometimes also called as "ketones",*** which is rather a misnomer. ***Interrelationship of these three substances are shown below:***

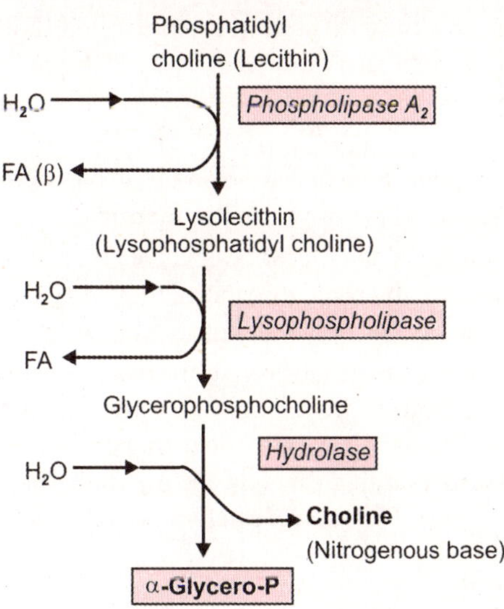

Fig.13.5: Showing degradation of lecithin

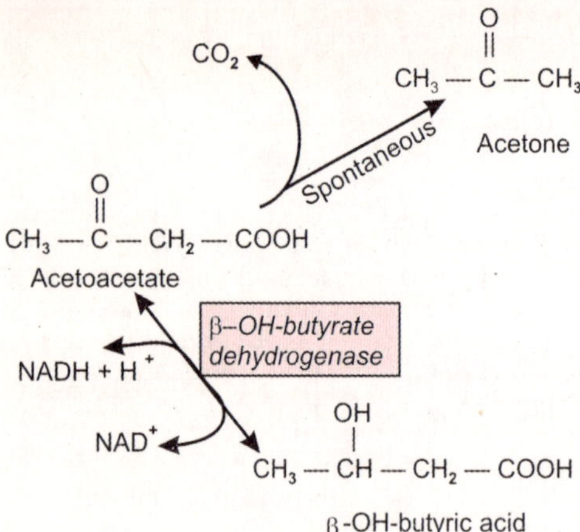

Concentration of Ketone Bodies: Concentration of total ketone bodies in the blood of well-fed individuals does not normally exceed 1 mg/100 ml (as acetone equivalents).

Urine: Loss via urine is usually less than 1 mg/ 24 hours in human.

KETOACIDOSIS

Acetoacetic acid and β-OH-butyric acid are moderately strong acids. They are buffered when present in blood and tissues, entailing some loss of buffer cations, which progressively depletes the "alkali reserve" ↓ causing ketoacidosis.

Note: This may be fatal in uncontrolled diabetes mellitus.

Certain Terminologies

Ketonaemia: Rise of ketone bodies in blood above normal level is known as ketonemia.

Ketonuria: When the blood level of ketone bodies rises above the renal threshold, they are excreted in urine and is called as ketonuria.

Ketosis: Accumulation of abnormal amount of ketone bodies in tissues and body fluids is termed as ketosis, where the urinary excretion of β-OH butyric acid exceeds 200 mg daily (normal 5 to 10 mg). ***The overall pattern is called ketosis.***

Causes:

- ***Starvation:*** Simplest form of ketosis occurs in starvation. Mechanism involves depletion of available carbohydrate reserve, coupled with mobilization of FFA and oxidation to produce energy.
- ***In pathologic states:***
  - ***In diabetes mellitus:*** Clinical and experimental
  - In some types of alkalosis, ketosis may develop
  - Pregnancy toxaemia in sheep and in lactating cattle
- In prolonged ether anaesthesia
- Other non-pathologic forms of ketosis are found under conditions of:
  - high fat feeding; and
  - after severe exercise in the post absorptive state.
- Injection of anterior pituitary extracts.

Site of Formation and Fate:

- ***Liver appears to be the only organ which produces ketone bodies and add to the blood***
- Extrahepatic tissues can pick up ketone bodies from the circulating blood and utilize them as respiratory substrates
- Net flow of ketone bodies from the liver to extrahepatic tissues results from an active enzymatic mechanism in the liver which exists, for the production of ketone bodies, coupled with very low activity of the enzymes rather their absence, responsible for their degradation or utilization
- The reverse situation exists in extrahepatic tissues ***(Fig. 13.6).***

A. KETONE BODY FORMATION IN LIVER (KETOGENESIS)

- ***Enzymes are mitochondrial***

Steps

1. ***Acetoacetyl-CoA: Acetoacetyl-CoA is the starting material for ketogenesis.*** This can arise in **two ways:**

- Directly during the course of β-oxidation of fatty acids, or
- As a result of condensation of two C-2 units, i.e. "active acetate" (acetyl-CoA) by reversal of *thiolase* reaction.

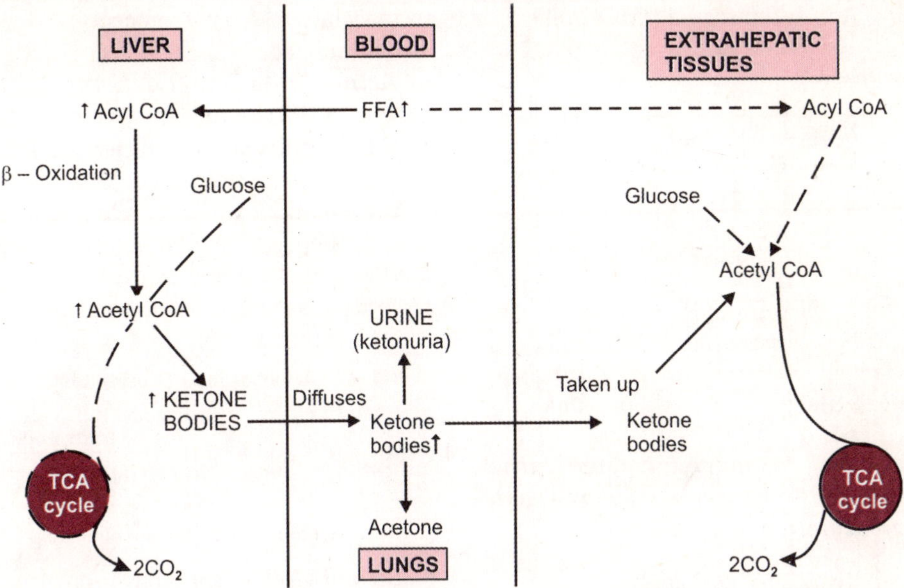

Fig.13.6: Formation, utilization and excretion of ketone bodies

2. ***Formation of Acetoacetate: Acetoacetate is the first ketone body to be formed.***

This can occur in **two ways:**

- ***By deacylation:*** Acetoacetate can be formed from acetoacetyl CoA by simple deacylation catalyzed by the enzyme *acetoacetyl CoA deacylase.*

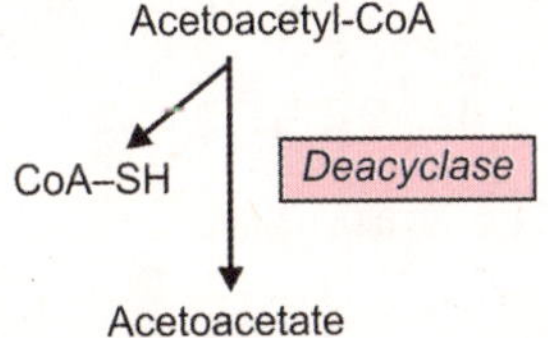

The above does not seem to be the major pathway when excessive amount of ketone bodies are formed, the deacylation reaction is not enough to cope up.

- ***Second pathway:*** Formation of acetoacetate via intermediate production of ***"β-OH-β-methylglutaryl-CoA" (HMG-CoA).***
  Present opinion favours the HMG-CoA pathway as the major route of ketone body formation.

Steps: It involves **two steps:**

- Condensation of acetoacetyl-CoA with another molecule of acetyl-CoA to form β-OH-β methyl glutaryl-CoA (HMG-CoA) catalyzed by the enzyme *HMG-CoA synthase* (mitochondrial enzyme)
- HMG-CoA is then acted upon by an another enzyme, *HMG-CoA lyase,* which is also mitochondrial enzyme, to produce one molecule of **"acetoacetate"** and one molecule of acetyl-CoA.

Note:

- Both the enzymes *HMG-CoA synthase* and *HMG-CoA lyase* are mitochondrial and must be available in mitochondrion for ketogenesis to occur. Both the enzymes are present in liver cells mitochondria only
- A marked increase in activity of *HMG-CoA lyase* has been noted in fasting
- **HMG-CoA is a "committed step"** cholesterol can also be formed by "HMG CoA reductase".

Formation of Acetoacetate (via HMG-CoA)

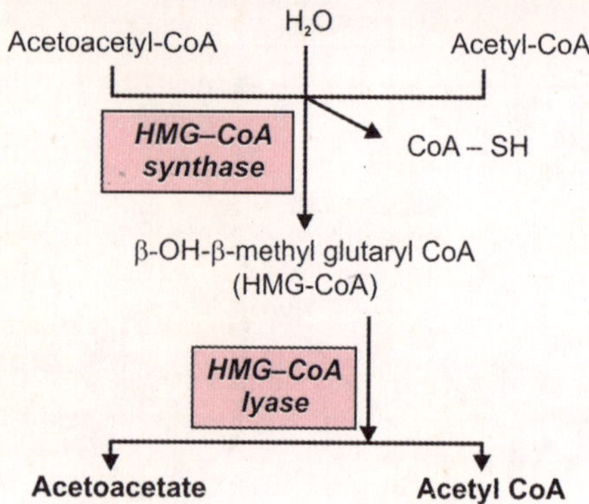

3. ***Formation of Acetone:*** As stated earlier, acetone is formed from acetoacetate by ***spontaneous decarboxylation*** (non-enzymatic).

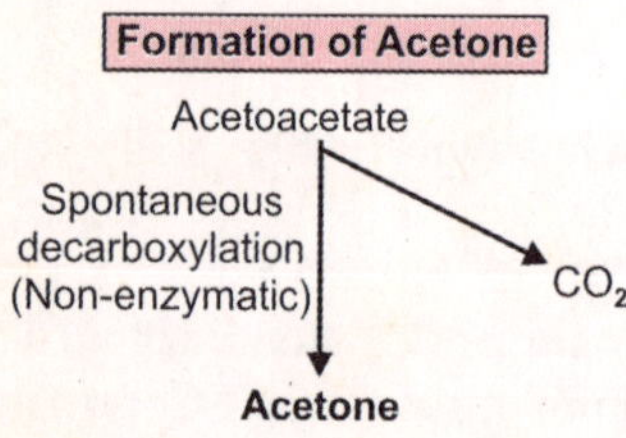

4. ***Formation of β-OH Butyrate:*** Acetoacetate once formed is converted to β-OH-butyric acid. The reaction is catalyzed by the enzyme *β-OH-butyrate dehydrogenase, present* in liver and also found in many other tissues. ***β-OH-butyrate is quantitatively the predominant ketone body present in blood and urine in ketosis***

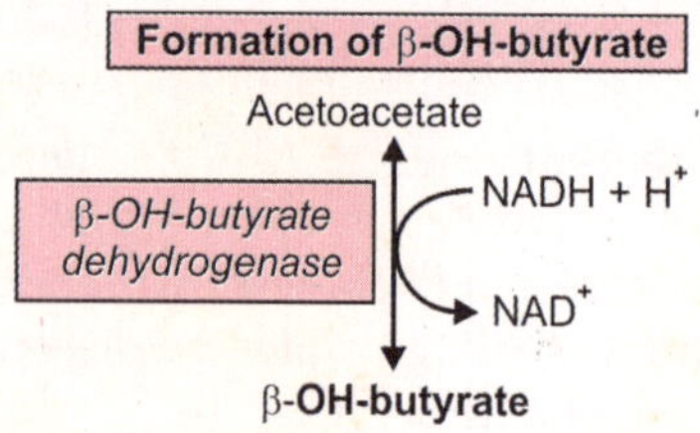

B. UTILIZATION OF KETONE BODIES (KETOLYSIS)

Ketone bodies are utilized by extrahepatic tissues as "fuel".

1. **Activation of Acetoacetate:** ***Two reactions*** take place in extrahepatic tissues which activate acetoacetate to form acetoacetyl-CoA, which is further utilized.

- ***Action of Acetoacetate with Succinyl-CoA: Major Pathway*** by which acetoacate is activated in extrahepatic tissues. Acetoacetate reacts with one molecule of succinyl-CoA (intermediate of TCA cycle), catalyzed by the enzyme *CoA transferase* (also called *thiophorase),* which transfers CoA from succinyl-CoA to acetoacetate, thus forming acetoacetyl-CoA and succinate.

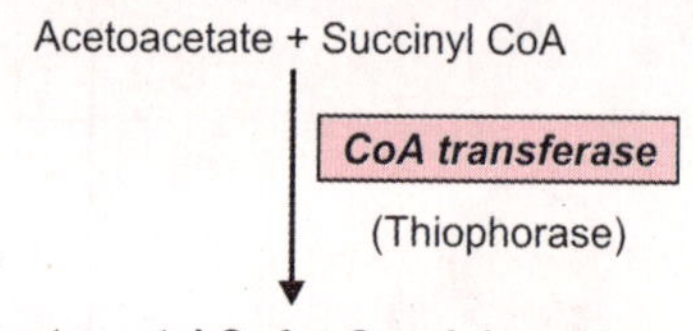

- ***Second Mechanism:*** Activation of acetoacetate with ATP and CoA-SH, catalyzed by the enzyme *acetoacetyl-CoA synthetase.* This is probably not a major pathway, can occur to some extent.

2. **Fate of β-OH-Butyrate:** β-OH-butyrate may be activated directly in extrahepatic tissues by a *synthetase,* similar to a reaction stated above, to form β-OH-butyryl-CoA, which can reform "acetoacetyl-CoA". ***This does not appear to be the major route.***

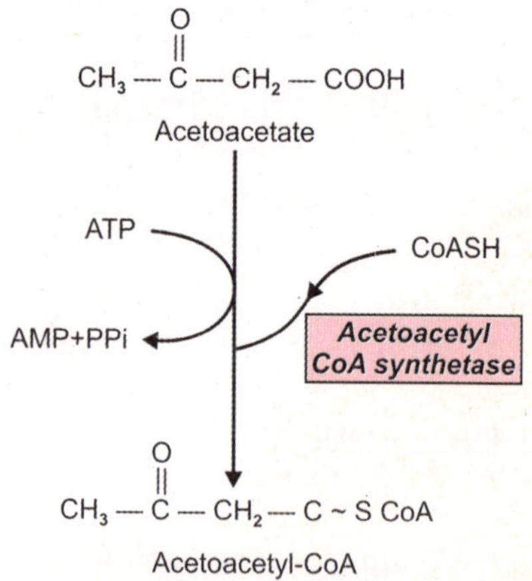

On the other hand, β-OH-butyrate can be converted back to "acetoacetate" by the enzyme *β-OH-butyrate dehydrogenase* and NAD^+, as the reaction is "reversible". Then acetoacetate can be activated to acetoacetyl-CoA, as stated above. This appears to be the major route.

Acetoacetyl-CoA thus formed by the above mechanisms is split to "acetyl CoA" by *thiolase* and oxidized in the TCA cycle.

3. Fate of Acetone: Acetone is difficult to be oxidized ***in vivo***. Experimental evidences show very slow rate of utilization.

- Some authorities propose a reversal of the reaction, in which acetone is converted back to acetoacetate
- Excess of acetone can be breathed out and also excreted in urine. This gives a ***fruity smell,*** in the breath and in urine
- Another possible pathway proposed is the ***"propanediol pathway", which is glucogenic.*** This may provide a route for the net conversion of FA to carbohydrates.

Note:

- The utilization of ketone bodies by the extrahepatic tissues is considerable. They are oxidized proportionately to their concentration in the blood. They are also oxidized in preference to glucose and FFA. If the blood level is raised, oxidation of ketone bodies increases until ***at a concentration of approximately 70 mg/100 ml, they saturate oxidative machinery*** and any further increase in the rate of ketogenesis raises the blood concentration producing ***ketonemia*** and ketosis and excess

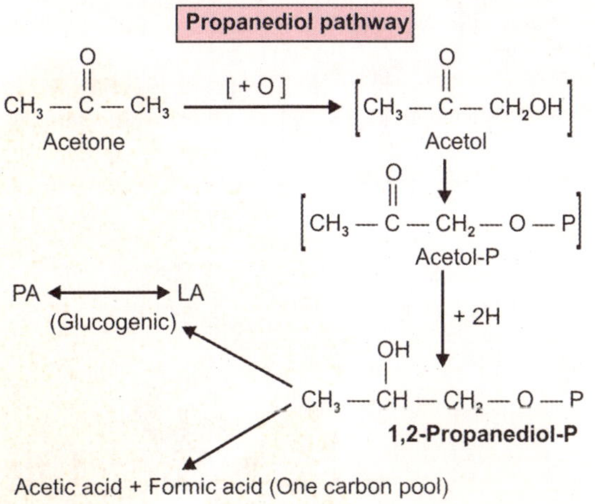

Propanediol pathway

$CH_3-CO-CH_3$ (Acetone) $\xrightarrow{[+O]}$ $[CH_3-CO-CH_2OH]$ (Acetol)

↓

$[CH_3-CO-CH_2-O-P]$ (Acetol-P)

↓ + 2H

$CH_3-CH(OH)-CH_2-O-P$ (**1,2-Propanediol-P**)

→ PA ⟷ LA (Glucogenic)

→ Acetic acid + Formic acid (One carbon pool)

amount excreted in urine called ***ketonuria.*** At this point, 90 percent of O_2 consumption in the animal may be accounted for by the oxidation of ketone bodies

- When carbohydrates are not being utilized, fats alone cannot supply the "fuel" needs of the tissues, and such needs are met in part by ketone body utilization in muscles, brain, kidney, heart, and adrenal gland
- It has been shown that human brain can utilize ketone bodies to the extent of 20 percent of the total energy requirement after an overnight fast, 60 percent after an eight-day fast and 80 percent after a forty-day fast.

SUSCEPTIBILITY TO KETOSIS

- Susceptibility to ketosis varies widely with animal species with age as well as sex. ***The decreasing order of susceptibility with species may be given as follows: humans and monkeys > goats > rabbits and rats > dogs. Dogs have been found to be exceedingly resistant to starvation ketosis.***
- ***Sex:*** The females are much less able to withstand starvation ketosis as compared to males.
- *Age:* Infants and young children are more susceptible than adults.

Factors Determining Magnitude of Ketogenesis

- Though ketone bodies are being formed constantly and being utilized, ***in vivo*** ketosis does not occur unless there is a concomitant rise in the level of circulating FFA. ***Severe ketosis is accompanied invariably by very high concentration of plasma FFA.*** Numerous experiments ***in vivo*** have demonstrated that fatty acids are the precursors of ketone bodies and liver is the main site of ketone body formation
- ***Liver in both fed and fasting conditions, is capable of extracting 30 percent or more of FFA passing through it.*** So, when FFA concentration in plasma is very high, substantial amount of FFA passes through the liver

- *Two fates* await the FFA, taken up by the liver cells after activation to acyl-CoA. Either
  - They are esterified to form TG, phospholipids and cholesterol esters, or
  - They undergo β-oxidation to form acetyl-CoA. The two fates are shown in *Fig. 13.7.*
- Acetyl-CoA, in turn, is oxidized in TCA cycle to form CO_2 and water. But if in excess, they are used for ketone bodies formation.

Note:

- Control is exercised initially in adipose tissue. As stated above, ketosis does not occur *in vivo* unless there is a concomitant rise in free fatty acid (FFA) level arising from lipolysis in adipose tissue
- Hence, factors regulating mobilization of FFA from adipose tissue are important in controlling ketogenesis.

ANTIKETOGENIC MECHANISMS

1. Esterification to Form TG: Once FFA, derived from lipolysis of TG in adipose tissue are esterified in the liver, they become negligible source of ketone bodies. ***Hence, esterification of FFA can be regarded as a significant antiketogenic mechanism in the liver.*** From ***Fig. 13.7*** it will be seen that if pathway (i) predominates, there will be less acyl-CoA to be diverted to pathway (ii) and (iii) Precursor substance for esterification is "α-glycero-P". ***Hence capacity for esterification by liver depends on the availability of the precursor substance "α-glycero-P".***

2. Role of Oxaloacetate: Theoretically, a fall in concentration of "oxaloacetate" particularly within the mitochondria could cause impairment of TCA cycle to metabolize acetyl-CoA. ***Since oxaloacetate is main pathway of gluconeogenesis, enhanced gluconeogenesis leading to a fall in concentration of OAA may account for severe forms of ketosis.*** Role of OAA is shown schematically in ***Fig.13.8.***

Glucose-FA Cycle of Randle: The suppression of glucose oxidation during periods of carbohydrates deprivation leading to release of NEFA (non-esterified fatty acid)/or FFA, from the fat depots into the blood and their subsequent oxidation has been termed by **Randle** as the ***"Glucose-FA cycle".***

Summary:

- Ketosis arises as a result of deficiency in available carbohydrates.
- Two principal actions in fostering ketogenesis are:
  - An imbalance between esterification and lipolysis in adipose tissue with consequent release of FFA in circulation.

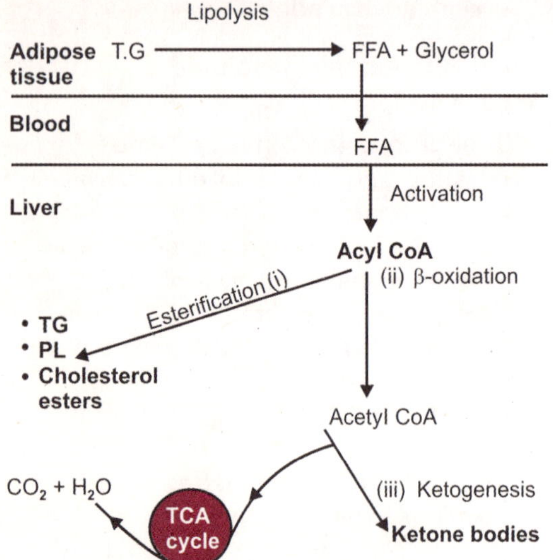

Fig. 13.7: Showing fate of FFA in liver

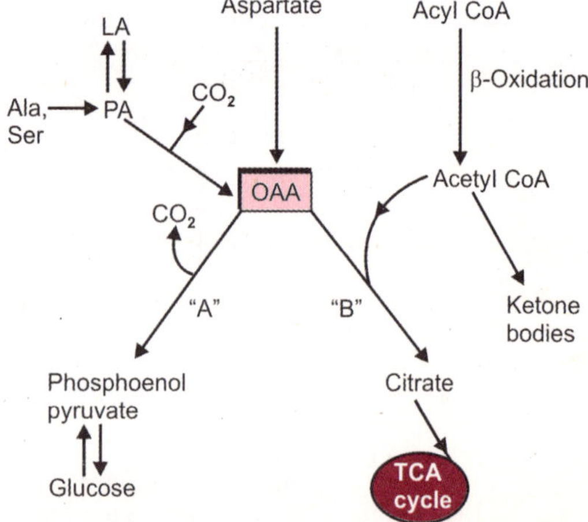

Fig. 13.8: Role of OAA in ketone bodies formation

- FFA are principal substrates for ketone bodies formation in liver.

Hence, all factors, metabolic or endocrine affecting the release of FFA from adipose tissue influence ketogenesis.

- Availability of carbohydrates in liver provides α-glycero-P, which determines the extent to which the large influx of FFA into the liver is esterified. FFA which remains unesterified is oxidized to CO_2 and to form ketone bodies.
- As quantity of FFA undergoing oxidation increases in starvation and DM, more form ketone bodies and less is oxidized in TCA cycle to form CO_2 and H_2O. This is regulated in such a manner that the total energy production remains constant.
- ***Ketone bodies produced in liver are not oxidized by liver, and they diffuse into the circulation from where they are extracted by extrahepatic tissues preferentially to other tissues.***

KETOGENIC/ANTIKETOGENIC RATIO IN DIET

While prescribing diets the proportion of the ketogenic and antiketogenic substances should be so regulated that ketosis may be avoided.

It is found that if the ratio between the molecules of the ketogenic substances and the molecules of the antiketogenic substances exceeds 2, ketone bodies appear in urine. ***The clinical rule is that the total fat (F) content of the diet must not exceed the sum of twice the carbohydrates (C) and half of the protein (P), i.e***

$$F = \text{or} < (2C + 1/2P)$$

Ketosis is abolished by increasing the metabolism of carbohydrates in the liver. In diabetes mellitus, this is achieved by giving insulin, and in ketosis due to carbohydrate deprivation by giving glucose or substances readily convertible to glucose or glycogen.

1. **Ketogenic Substances:** The ketogenic substances are:
   - All FFA (i.e. 90% of food fats)

     Note: *Glycerol part, the product of hydrolysis of TG, is glucogenic and hence, it is antiketogenic.*
   - ***Proteins:*** ketogenic amino acids (40%).

     The above are the sources from which ketone bodies are formed.
2. **Antiketogenic Substances:** These are substances which prevent the formation of ketone bodies. They provide glucose, which, in turn, can provide α-glycero-P, required for esterification.
   - All carbohydrates.
   - Insulin.
   - 60 percent of proteins, glucogenic amino acids.
   - 10 percent of dietary fats, glycerol part which is glucogenic.

☞ SALIENT POINTS TO REMEMBER

- Principal plasma lipids that have metabolic significance are T.G (triacyl glycerol), P-L (Phospholipids), and cholesterol/Cholesterol esters.
- Plasma lipids also include metabolic products like Glycerol and fatty acids. Fatty acids are carried in Plasma in combination with albumin.
- Less than 5 percent of total F.A. of Plasma is a smaller fraction of free fatty acid (FFA), also called non-esterified FA (NEFA) or unesterified FA (UFA).
- ***NEFA is now known to be metabolically most active of the plasma lipids.***
- Plasma lipids can be separated into different fractions by ultracentrifugation or more commonly by electrophoresis.
- Triacyl glycerol (TG) are highly concentrated form of energy stored in adipose tissue.
- ***TG of adipose tissue is not static lump of fat, it is in dynamic state,*** breakdown of fat (Lipolysis) and esterification (synthesis) take place.
- Hormone-sensitive lipase hydrolyses TG of adipose tissue to free fatty acids, which are activated to acyl-CoA and transported by carnitine to mitochondria where they are oxidized, mostly by β-oxidation to liberate energy.
- ***Complete oxidation of one molecule of Palmitic acid produces 129 ATP.***

- Insulin enhances esterification (synthesis), whereas catecholamines, Glucagon, GH, Glucocorticoids bring about lipolysis.
- Brown adipose tissue is a special type of adipose tissue. It is characterized by a high content of mitochondria.
- Brown adipose tissue is involved in metabolism particularly at a time when heat generation is necessary. In this, oxidation and phosphorylation are not coupled resulting to liberation of heat.
- Some individuals with active brown adipose tissue do not become obese despite over eating since whatever they eat is liberated as heat due to uncoupling of oxidation and phosphorylation in the mitochondria.
- Fatty acid biosynthesis occurs from acetyl CoA in the cytosol through the involvement of a multienzyme complex, ***Fatty acid synthase,*** associated with acyl carrier Protein (ACP), called as "denovo synthesis", the ***end result of synthesis is formation of palmitic acid.***
- The reducing equivalents NADPH required in the synthesis is provided by HMP shunt principally.
- Elongation of fatty acid chain is done by 2 ways:
  (1) Mitochondrial chain elongation system: occurs in mitochondria, palmityl CoA is the starting material, the system operates ***under anaerobic conditions*** and is favoured by a high $NADH/NAD^+$ ratio in cells. Acetyl-CoA is added directly and NADPH is required.
  (2) Microsomal chain elongation system; common pathway, operates in "microsomal" system. ***Requires presence of*** O_2 (aerobic). Acetyl-CoA is added through malonyl CoA and reducing equivalent is provided by NADPH.
- Degradation of Lecithin (Phosphatidyl choline) is initiated by the enzyme "***Phospholipase*** A_2". End products of catabolism are α-glycero-P and nitrogenous base choline.
- Excessive utilization of fatty acids occur in uncontrolled Diabetes mellitus and starvation.
- The above results in the over production of ketone bodies in liver (ketogenesis).
- ***Ketonebodies are mainly three: acetoacetic acid, β-OH butyric acid and acetone.***
- Acetoacetate is the first ketone body to be formed. β-OH butyric acid is the predominant ketone body found in plasma and urine of a case of uncontrolled DM and starvation ketosis.
- Acetone can be glucogenic through formation of 1, 2-propanediol-P (Propanediol pathway).
- ***Ketone bodies once formed in the liver can not be degraded in that organ and passes to blood.***
- Ketone bodies are utilized by extrahepatic tissues as "fuel" (Ketolysis).
- Esterification of FFA can be regarded as a significant anti ketogenic mechanism in liver.
- Ketogenic substances are all FFA (i.e. 90 percent) of food fats, and ketogenic amino acids.
- Antiketogenic substances are insulin, all carbohydrates, 60 percent of proteins (glucogenic amino acids) and Glycerol part of fats.

METABOLISM OF CHOLESTEROL

For chemistry of cholesterol, its properties and occurrence/distribution-refer to Chapter on Chemistry of Lipids. For absorption of cholesterol refer to Chapter on Digestion/Absorption of lipids.

BIOSYNTHESIS OF CHOLESTEROL

A number of established facts regarding cholesterol biosynthesis are as follows:

1. Site of Synthesis: Essentially, all tissues form cholesterol. ***Liver is the major site of cholesterol biosynthesis,*** other tissues are also active in this regard, e.g. adrenal cortex, gonads, skin, and intestine are most active. Low order of synthesis: adipose tissue, muscle, aorta and neural tissues. ***Brain of new born can synthesize cholesterol while the adult brain cannot synthesize cholesterol.***

- Efficiency of formation of cholesterol from labelled ^{14}C acetate:

Tissues	*Efficiency of cholesterol formation (liver = 100)*
Liver	100
Adult skin	90
Small intestine	60
Gonads	31
Kidney	4
Adult brain	0
Newborn brain	185

2. **Enzymes:** Enzyme system involved in cholesterol biosynthesis are associated with:
   - Cytoplasmic particles "microsomes"
   - Soluble fraction cytosol
3. **Acetate:** ***"Active acetate (acetyl CoA) is the starting material and principal precursor".*** The entire carbon-skeleton, all 27C of cholesterol in humans can be synthesized from active acetate.

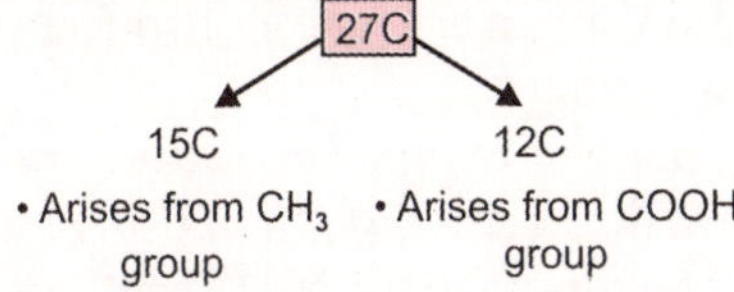

Steps of Biosynthesis

Cholesterol biosynthesis can be thought of as occurring in **five groups of reactions.** They are:

- ***Synthesis of mevalonate,*** a 6-C compound from acetyl CoA.
- ***Formation of "iso-prenoid units" (5-C)*** from mevalonate by successive phosphorylations and followed by loss of CO_2.
  Note: The isoprenoid units are regarded as the building blocks of the steroid nucleus.
- **Formation of squalene** a 3-carbon aliphatic chain-formed by condensation of six isoprenoid units.
- **Cyclization of squalene to form lanosterol.**
- **Conversion of lanosterol to form cholesterol.**

I. Synthesis of Mavalonate from Acetyl-CoA

(a) Formation of HMG-CoA (β-OH-β-methyl glutaryl CoA): HMG-CoA can be formed in the cytosol from acetyl-CoA in **two steps** catalyzed by the enzyme *"thiolase"* and *"HMG-CoA synthase"*. (See also ketone body formation).

Note:

- HMG-CoA may also be produced as an intermediate in the metabolic degradation of amino acid L-leucine
- There are **two pools of HMG-CoA:**
  - **Mitochondrial:** concerned with ketogenesis
  - **Extramitochondrial (cytosolic):** concerned with synthesis of mevalonate and isoprenoid units.

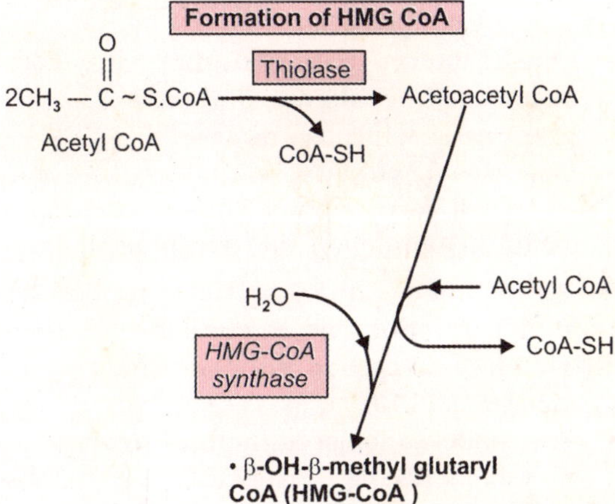

(b) In the next step, which is the ***rate-limiting step.*** HMG-CoA is converted to mevalonic acid (mevalonate) catalyzed by the enzyme *HMG-CoA reductase.*

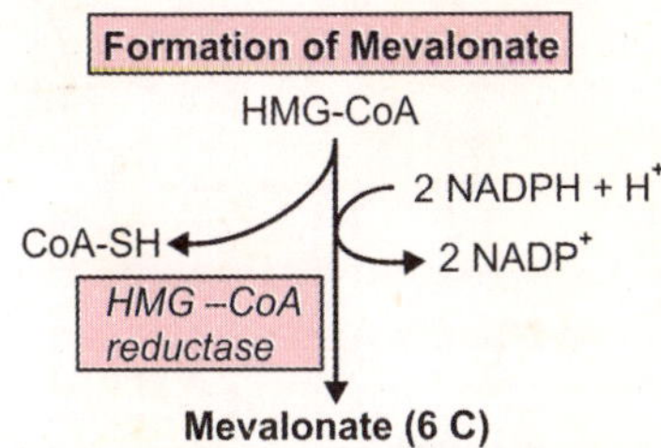

Characteristics of this reaction:

- Most important and ***"rate limiting"*** step.
- **Irreversible reaction.**
- NADPH required as cofactor-supplied by HMP-pathway.
- Dietary cholesterol and endogenously synthesized cholesterol inhibits this "rate-limiting" step ***("feedback" inhibitions)***

- ***Hormones: Insulin and thyroid hormones increase*** reductase activity, ***glucagon*** and ***glucocorticoids reduce the activity.***
- Also inhibited by cyclic AMP (see regulation).

II. Formation of Isoprenoid Units: (Fig. 13.9)

- Mevalonate is phosphorylated by ATP to form several "active" phosphorylated intermediates.
- Three such phosphorylated compounds are formed and it is followed by decarboxylation to form first "active" isoprenoid unit, *isopentenyl pyrophosphate" (5 C).*
- One of intermediate phosphorylated compound is "mevalonate-3-phospho-5-pyrophosphate" which is **unstable**.
- Isopentenyl pyrophosphate undergoes isomerization to form another 5 C isoprenoid unit, called 3,-3′-dimethyl allyl pyrophosphate.

III. Formation of Squalene: The pyrophosphorylated isoprenoid units condense to form ultimately a 30-carbon aliphatic chain called ***squalene (Fig. 13.10).***

- The condensation occur in ***three steps:***
  - One molecule of isopentenyl pyrophosphate first condenses with one molecule of 3,-3-dimethyl allyl pyrophosphate to form a 10-C compound called *geranyl pyrophophate,* the reaction is catalyzed by the enzyme *geranyl pyrophosphate synthetase.*
  - Another molecule of isopentenyl pyrophosphate reacts with geranyl pyrophosphate to form the 15 C compound *farnesyl pyrophosphate,* the reaction is catalyzed by the enzyme *farnesyl pyrophosphate synthetase.*
  - Finally, two molecules of farnesyl pyrophosphate condenses at pyrophosphate end to form 30 C aliphatic compound called squalene. Reaction is catalyzed by the enzyme *squalene synthetase*

Characteristics of this Reaction:

- The enzymes *squalene synthetase* is microsomal liver enzyme is firmly bound to microsomes.
- ***NADPH is required as a coenzyme*** as electron donor, provided by HMP pathway.
- ***Cofactors required:*** Mg^{++}, Mn^{++} and CO^{++}

IV. Cyclization of Squalene to Form Lanosterol: The formation of lanosterol from squalene ***(Fig. 13.11)*** takes place in **two steps:**

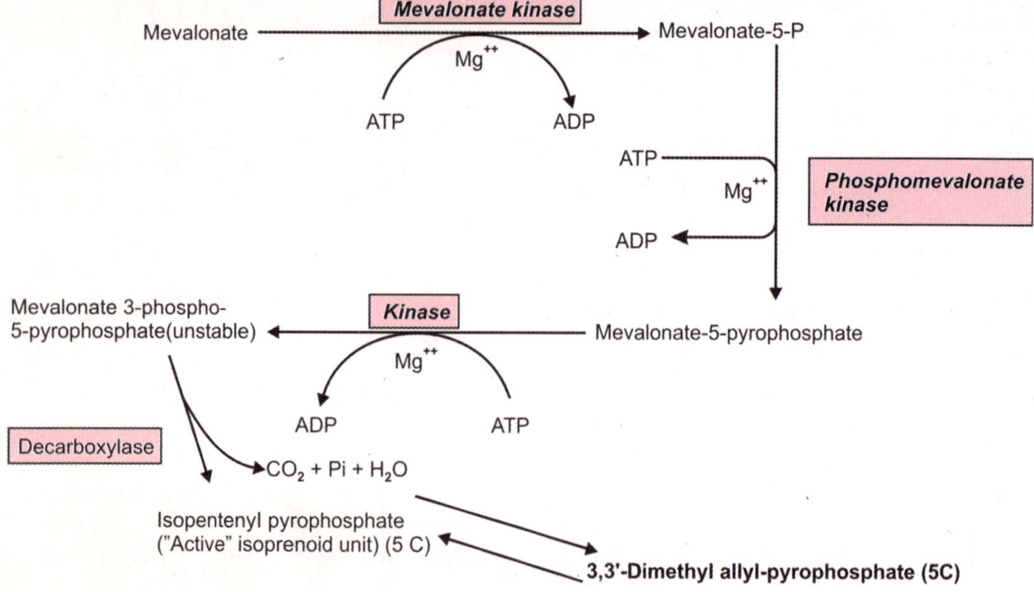

Fig. 13.9: Formation of isoprenoid units

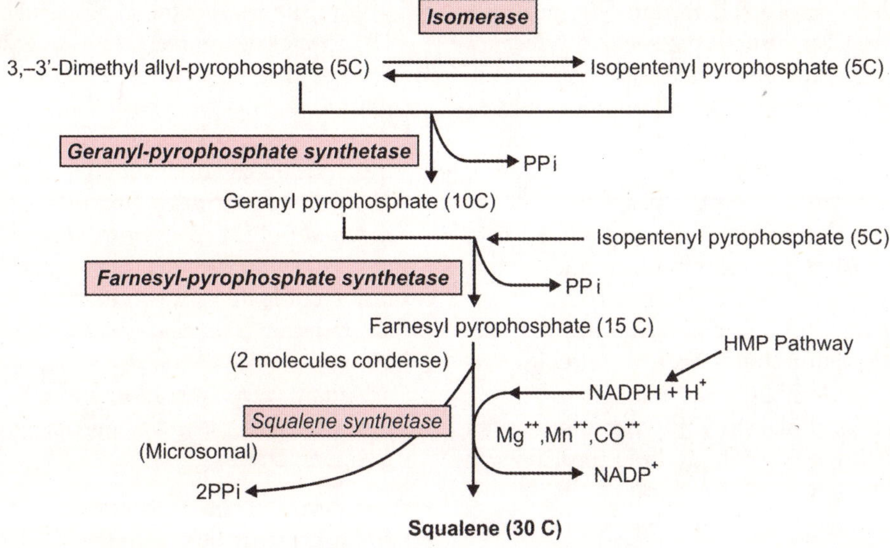

Fig. 13.10: Formation of squalene

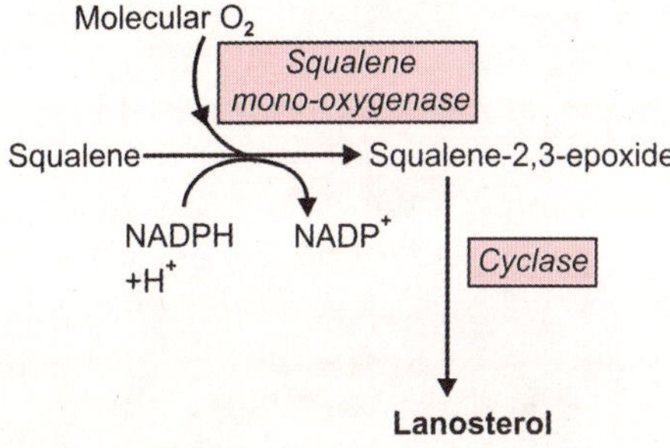

Fig.13.11: Formation of lanosterol from squalene

- **In the first step** squalene-2,3-epoxide is formed catalyzed by the enzyme *squalene mono-oxygenase;* which requires NADPH and molecular O_2.
- In the next step, an enzyme *cyclase* brings about the cyclization of squalene to form lanosterol.

V. Conversion of Lanosterol to Cholesterol: Main changes that are brought about are:

- ***Removal of three angular-CH_3 groups.*** This involves a series of reactions. Mechanism of demethylation is not properly known.
- ***CH_3 group at 14 C is first eliminated.***
- ***Shift of double bond*** between 8C and 9C to 5C and 6C, and
- ***Saturation of double bond*** in side chain. **Two possible pathways** have been suggested as follows:

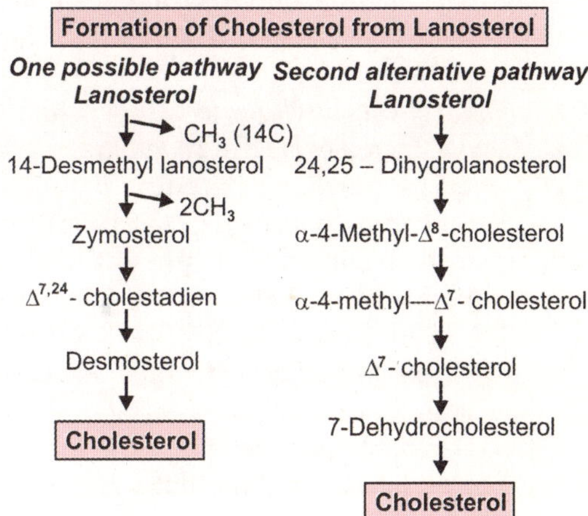

Control of Biosynthesis

- The steps in the biosynthesis of cholesterol to HMG-CoA are reversible. The formation of mevalonate, however, in the next step is ***"irreversible"*** and is the ***committed step.***
- The ***rate-limiting step*** in the biosynthesis of cholesterol is the ***conversion of HMG-CoA to mevalonate*** by the enzyme *HMG-CoA reduc-*

tase. Cholesterol itself inhibits the enzyme, providing an effective product *"feedback inhibition"* controlling the synthesis.
- Fasting/starvation also inhibits the enzyme and activate *HMG-CoA lyase* to form ketone bodies.
- A second control point appears to be at the cyclization of squalene and conversion to lanosterol, but details of the regulation at this step is not clear.
- The feeding of cholesterol reduces the hepatic biosynthesis of cholesterol by reducing the activity of *HMG-CoA reductase.*

Note: Intestinal cholesterol biosynthesis does not respond to the feeding of high cholesterol diets. In contrast, feeding of diets high in fat or carbohydrates tend to increase hepatic cholesterol biosynthesis.

- ***Role of Cyclic AMP:*** *HMG-CoA reductase* may exist in "active" and "inactive" forms, which is reversibly modified by phosphorylation/dephosphorylation mechanisms, which may be mediated by cAMP dependant *protein kinases.* ***Cyclic AMP inhibits cholesterol biosynthesis by converting HMG-CoA reductase to inactive form.***
- ***Hormonal effects on cholesterol biosynthesis:***
  - ***Insulin:*** Increases *HMG-CoA reductase*↑ activity. The hormone is required for the diurnal rhythm (diurnal variation) that occurs in cholesterol biosynthesis, a phenomenon probably related to feeding cycles and the need for bile acid synthesis.
  - ***Glucagon** and **glucocorticoids:*** decreases the activity of *HMG-CoA reductase* ↓ and reduces the biosynthesis ↓
  - ***Thyroid hormones:*** Stimulates *HMG-CoA reductase* activity ↑.

TRANSPORT OF CHOLESTEROL

- Cholesterol in the diet is absorbed from the intestine, and in company with other lipids, are incorporated into *chylomicrons* and also to some extent *VLDL.* Of the cholesterol absorbed, 80 to 90 percent in the lymph is esterified with long-chain FA. Esterification may occur in the intestinal mucosa.
- In man, the total plasma cholesterol varies from 150 to 250 mg percent (average 200 mg%), rising with age, although there are wide variations between individuals. The greater part is found in the "esterified" form and is transported as "lipoproteins" in plasma.
- ***Highest proportion of circulating cholesterol is found in LDL (β-lipoproteins) which carry cholesterol to tissues*** and also in HDL, which takes cholesterol to liver from tissues for degradation ***(scavenging action).***
- However, under conditions, where the VLDL are quantitatively predominant, an increased proportion of plasma cholesterol will reside in this fraction.

CONSIDERATION OF OTHER FACTORS THAT INFLUENCE CHOLESTEROL LEVEL IN BLOOD

1. *Dietary Fats:*

- Increased of fats in the diet increases level of cholesterol by increased synthesis.
- Greater amount of saturated fatty acids increases cholesterol level.
- Substitution in the diet of saturated FA by polyunsaturated FA has beneficial effect and lowers cholesterol level ***(Table 13.4).***

Table 13.4: Fats and Oils Rich in Saturated and Unsaturated Fatty Acids

Fats rich in saturated FA	*Oils that are rich in Polyunsaturated FA*
Butter fat, ghee, dalda vanaspati, beef fat, coconut oil are rich in saturated FA	Sunflower oil, cottonseed oil, mustard oil, soyabean oil, groundnut oil

Mechanism by which polyunsaturated FA lowers cholesterol level is not known exactly but possibilities are:

- It stimulates oxidation of cholesterol to bile acids
- Stimulation of cholesterol excretion in intestine
- May be a shift of cholesterol from plasma to tissues.
- Cholesterol esters of polyunsaturated FA are more rapidly metabolized by liver and other tissues.

2. *Dietary Cholesterol:* (See control of biosynthesis above)

- Increased feeding of cholesterol in diet decreases endogenous synthesis and reduces cholesterol level.
- It is difficult to lower the normal blood cholesterol level by taking food of low cholesterol. ***Restricted dietary intake of cholesterol is usually balanced by increased biosynthesis.***
- *Table 13.5* shows the percentage of cholesterol in some common food substances.

Table 13.5: Percentage of Cholesterol in Some Common Food Substances

Food items	*Cholesterol content in mg%*
Butter	280
Fresh whole egg	468
Fresh yolk of egg	2000
Hen meat	70
Lamb	70
Pork	60

- *Experimental evidence:* **Morries** and **Chaikoff** (1951) carried out experiments on rats. When only 0.05 percent of cholesterol included in diet, 70 to 80 percent of cholesterol in liver and adrenal cortex were synthesized in the body; when 2 percent cholesterol included in diet, endogenous production fell to 10 to 30 percent.
- *Table 13.6.* Shows the diets that are rich or poor in cholesterol content.

3. *Dietary Carbohydrates:* Increased consumption of carbohydrates increases cholesterol level. ***Consumption of excessive amount of sucrose and fructose cause increase in plasma lipids particularly TG and also cholesterol.*** A diet providing 50 percent carbohydrates, if ratio of starch: sucrose is 4:1, plasma cholesterol level is not much affected. ***When ratio between starch: sucrose is 1:4, an increase of plasma cholesterol is observed.***

4. *Heredity:* Hereditary factors play the greatest role in determining individual blood cholesterol concentrations. Persons who are prone to become obese, have a high level of plasma cholesterol.

5. *Blood Groups:* Cholesterol level found to be slightly, higher in persons belonging to blood groups "A" and "AB", than those belonging to "O" and "B" groups.

6. *Calorie Intake:* Intake of excess calories increases cholesterol level.

7. *Vitamin B-Complex:*

- ***Nicotinic acid in large doses has cholesterol lowering effect.***
- Pyridoxine deficiency produces increase in blood cholesterol level and atherosclerosis in monkeys.

8. *Minerals:*

- ***In vitro*** acetate to cholesterol conversion in tissue cell cultures ***depressed ↓ by addition of vanadium and increased by chromium and manganese salts.***
- Conversion of mevalonate to cholesterol was inhibited by "vanadyl SO_4".

9. *Dietary Fibres:* Increased fibres in the diet, caused an increased excretion of cholesterol and bile acids in faeces in experimental animals and produced significant reduction in serum cholesterol.

Table 13.6: Showing Cholesterol Rich and Poor Diets

Cholesterol rich food items	*Cholesterol poor food items*

• Milk, cream, cream soups
• Egg yolk,
• Liver, brain, heart and kidney
• Animal fats:
pork, bacon, lard, etc
	• Skimmed milk
	• Butter milk without fat
	• White of egg
	• Lean meats, lean fish
	• Cooked and raw vegetables and dry cereals
	  • Fruits, lemon juice
	  • Vinegar, tea, coffee
	  • Tomato juice/soup
	  • Vegetables fats/oils, margarine contain practically no cholesterol

10. ***Physical Exercise:*** Studies on human volunteers showed hard physical exercise brought about lowering in serum cholesterol ↓ level and increased level of HDL.↑

11. ***Lifestyle of the Individual:*** Lifestyle of the individual also affects serum cholesterol level. Additional factors which play a part in coronary heart disease include:

- ***Obesity;***
- ***Lack of exercise and sedentary habits;***
- ***Smoking;***
- ***High blood pressure;***
- ***Associated diabetes mellitus; and***
- ***Drinking of soft as opposed to hard water.***

12. ***Elevation of Plasma FFA:*** Elevation of plasma FFA due to any cause will enhance increased VLDL secretion by the liver by enhancing endogenous TG synthesis involving extra TG and cholesterol output to the circulation.

Table 13.7 depicts the important factors which increase or decrease the cholesterol level and synthesis. Factors leading to higher or fluctuating levels of FFA include:

- ***Emotional stress;***
- ***Nicotine from cigarette smoking;***
- ***Coffee drinking; and***
- Partaking a few large meals rather than more continuous feeding.

Note: Premenopausal women appear to be protected against these deleterious factors probably due to the hormone oestrogens and high HDL, as compared to men and postmenopausal women.

Hypolipidaemic Drugs: Several drugs are known to block the formation of cholesterol at various stages in the biosynthetic pathway. Some may increase the catabolism/excretion of cholesterol also; many of the drugs have also harmful side effect ***(see Table 13.8).***

Table 13.7: Factors Increasing/Decreasing Cholesterol Level and Synthesis

Increase	*Decrease*
• ***Dietary cholesterol:*** A reduction in dietary cholesterol enhances synthesis and increases in cholesterol	• ***Cholesterol feeding*** "feedback" inhibition: inhibits *HMG-CoA reductase*
• ***Dietary fats:*** Feeding of more saturated fatty acids increases cholesterol	• ***Fasting/starvation*** inhibits *HMG-coA reductase* activity. Increases *HMG-CoA lyase* activity and formation of ketone bodies ↑
• ***High carbohydrate diet*** and Increase in dietary sucrose and fructose	• ***Administration of analogues of mevalonate or squalene***
• ***Loss of Bile:*** Drainage of bile by fistula increases synthesis major factor is bile acid concentration in liver.	• ***Administration of cholate*** Increases bile acid concentration in liver will decrease synthesis
• ***Administration of plant sterols-sitosterol:*** Competes with esterification, decreases absorption lowering cholesterol level which enhances endogenous synthesis	• ***Presence of fats and bile acids in intestinal lumen*** increases intestinal absorption which in turn decrease synthesis
• ***Lack of dietary fibres.***	• ***Feeding of polyunsaturated fatty acids decreases synthesis.***
• ***Pyridoxal deficiency***	• ***Cyclic AMP:*** Increased cyclic AMP inhibits synthesis by converting "HMG-CoA reductase" to inactive form
• ***Hormones:*** • Insulin • Thyroid hormones. Both increase *HMG-CoA reductase* activity.	• ***Hormones:*** Glucagon and glucocorticoids decreases ↓ synthesis
	• ***Hypolipidaemic drugs:*** Lower the cholesterol level by inhibiting synthetic pathways/or catabolism.

Table 13.8: Hypolipidaemic Drugs and Possible Mechanism of Action

Drugs	*Mechanism of action*
• *Nicotinic acid* In large doses has hypocholesterolaemic effect.	• Reduces the flux of FFA by inhibiting adipose tissue lipolysis, thereby inhibiting VLDL production in liver. In large doses may produce fatty liver.
• *Oestrogen*	• Lowers cholesterol level and increases HDL.
• *Clofibrate* (Atromid S) Gemfibrozil CPIB (ethyl-p-chlorophenoxy isobutyrate) (commonly used drug)	• Acts by various ways: • Inhibiting secretion of VLDL by liver, • Inhibiting hepatic cholesterol synthesis, • Probably also increases faecal excretion, • They facilitate hydrolysis of VLDL triacyl glycerol by *lipoprotein lipase*
• *Certain resins, e.g.* • Colestipol • Cholestyramine (Questran)	• Prevent the reabsorption of bile salts by combining with them, increasing their faecal loss.
• *Probucol*	• Increases catabolism of LDL by receptor independent pathway.
• *Mevastatin* • *Lovostatin* (Recent drugs-obtained from fungi)	• Reduces LDL cholesterol level Few adverse effect (most commonly used)

FATE OF CHOLESTEROL

Fate of cholesterol in body is shown in ***Fig. 13.12.*** About 1.0 gm of cholesterol is eliminated from the body per day. Fate of cholesterol has been studied in rats by giving labelled ^{14}C cholesterol and ^{3}H cholesterol. Ring-labelled cholesterol has been shown to be transformed to:

- ***Degradation to CO_2:*** Some radioactive CO_2 is formed in a relatively short time, particularly if the terminal carbons are labelled. However, some CO_2 is also derived from others parts of molecule. ***In human tissues-conversion to CO_2 does not occur.***
- ***Conversion to Bile Acids:*** Major pathways, more than 50% is converted to bile acids and excreted in faeces. A large proportion of biliary excretion of bile salts is reabsorbed into the portal circulation, taken up by the liver and

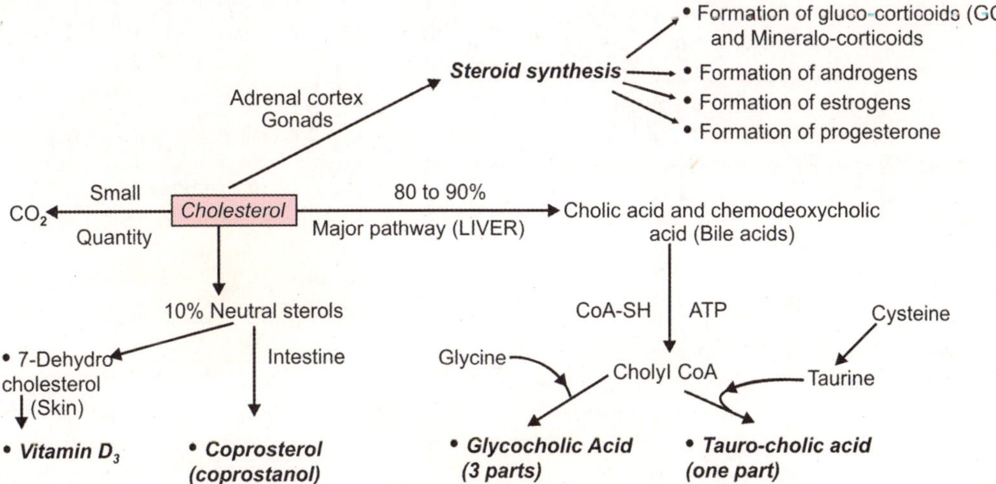

Fig. 13.12: Showing fate of cholesterol in the body

re-excreted in the bile. This is known as the ***enterohepatic circulation of bile salts.*** Bile salts undergo changes brought about by intestinal bacterial flora to form secondary bile acids.

- ***Conversion to Neutral Sterols:*** Ten percent of cholesterol is converted to neutral sterols called ***coprosterol (coprostanol),*** which is formed in lower part of intestine by the bacterial flora and excreted in faeces.
- ***Conversion to 7-Dehydrocholesterol:*** In skin, by UV light of sun's rays, 7-dehydrocholesterol is converted to vitamin D_3 [(cholecalciferol)].
- ***Formation of Adrenocortical Hormones:*** Glucocorticoids and mineralocorticoids are formed from cholesterol in adrenal cortex.
- ***Formation of Androgens***
- ***Formation of Estrogens***
- ***Formation of Progesterone***

BILE ACIDS

Bile acids are formed from cholesterol.

Types

- ***Primary bile acids:*** They are synthesized in the liver from cholesterol. They are ***mainly two:***
    - ***Cholic acid,*** quantitatively the largest amount in bile.
    - ***Chenodeoxycholic acid.***
- ***Secondary bile acids:*** They are produced in intestine from the primary bile acids by the action of intestinal bacteria, they are produced by deconjugation and 7-α-dehydroxylation. **They are mainly two:**
    - ***De-oxycholic acid,*** formed from cholic acid.
    - ***Lithocholic acid:*** formed from chenodeoxycholic acid.

BILE

- Bile is a viscous fluid produced by the liver cells. Strictly speaking it is not a digestive secretion as it does not contain any digestive enzymes but it helps in digestion and absorption of lipids. It is secreted continuously by the liver and through bile canaliculi and bile duct it accumulates in the gallbladder, where it is stored.
- In gallbladder, certain changes take place by reabsorption of large amount of water leading to concentration of bile. Water is absorbed along with inorganic components as isotonic solution. Mucin is added and bicarbonate and chloride are reabsorbed. Hence, organic constituents like cholesterol, bile pigments—bilirubin get concentrated in gallbladder bile. ***Table 13.9*** depicts the differences in composition of hepatic and gallbladder bile.
- During digestion, gallbladder contracts by the stimulation of the GI hormone "**cholecystokinin**" which is produced by small intestine and release bile rapidly to the intestine by the way of common bile duct.
- Approximately 500 to 1000 ml of bile is secreted by liver in a day.

Table 13.9: Differences in Composition of Hepatic Bile and Gallbladder Bile

	Hepatic bile	*Gallbladder bile*
pH	7.0 to 8.2	6.0 to 7.0
Specific gravity	1.010	1.040
Water	97.2%	88.0%
Solids	2.7%	12.0%
Bile acids	1.2%	6.2%
Mucin & bile pigments	0.58%	3.2%
Total lipids	0.3%	2.5%
TG	0.1%	0.4%
Phospholipids	< 0.1%	0.2%
Cholesterol	0.08%	0.5%
Inorganic salts	0.84%	0.75%

FUNCTIONS OF BILE SALTS

- ***Lowering of surface tension:*** Because of their power of lowering surface tension, ***they aid in the emulsification of fats*** and tend to stabilize such emulsions. ***The emulsification is a prerequisite for action of pancreatic lipase on fats.***
- ***Bile salts accelerate the action of pancreatic lipase:*** In the presence of bile salts, a ***colipase*** (molecular wt=10,000) binds to lipase and shifts the optimal pH of the enzyme from 9.0 to 6.0.

- ***Bile salts form 'micelles'*** with fatty acids, mono and diacyl glycerols and also TG which are made water soluble and helps absorption.
- Bile salts aid in the ***absorption of fat soluble vitamin*** (A, D, E and K) and also carotene by forming complexes more soluble in water ***("hydrotropic" action).***
- ***Stimulate intestinal motility.***
- Have great ***choleretic action.*** Thus, the liver is stimulated to secrete bile as long as bile salts are absorbed. **("Enterohepatic circulation" of bile salts).**
- Bile salts ***keep cholesterol in solution.*** Cholesterol remains soluble in gallbladder bile by bile salts.

Clinical Aspect

1. **Estimation of Bile Acids and Bile Salts in Blood:**
   - This has been used for liver function test.
   - ***Bile salts in blood are increased greatly in obstructive jaundice.***
   - After prolonged obstruction, the concentration of bile salts in blood may decrease due to diminished synthesis as a result of progressive parenchymal damage.
2. **Cholelithiasis (Gallstones):**
   - Bile salts keep cholesterol in solution in gallbladder bile. In the absence of bile salts, cholesterol may get precipitated producing *"gallstones"*
   - In the gallbladder, the cholesterol is solubilized and help in "micelles" with the help of conjugated bile salts and phospholipids. ***Solubility depends on ratio of cholesterol with the conjugated bile salts.***
   - Secretion of PL into the bile depends on availability of the conjugated bile salts.
   - If bile salts content is decreased due to any cause, the phospholipids also decreases leading to an imbalance of the ratio. The solubility of cholesterol is hampered and as a result it crystallizes out. The crystals grow to form the stones.

Conditions which Favour Stone Formation

1. ***Infection:*** favours stone formation

Infection causes:

- deconjugation of bile acids leading to decrease in solubility; and
- production of phospholipase which converts lecithin to lysolecithin.

  Thus, the ratio is disturbed leading to precipitation of cholesterol.

2. ***Decreased availability of bile salts:*** (Reduction in bile salt pool)
   - Defect in enterohepatic circulation.
   - Diseases of terminal ileum.
   - In patients with cirrhosis liver.

Types of Gallstones: Gallstones can be of mainly **three types:**

- ***Cholesterol stones:*** They are single or multiple, mainly formed of cholesterol, mulberry-shaped and are ***not radiopaque.***
- ***Pigment stones:*** Consists of bile pigments and calcium with other organic substances. Small multiple stones, dark green or black, ***not radiopaque.***
- ***Mixed stones:*** Consist of mixture of cholesterol plus pigments, calcium and organic material. Most common form, may be ***radiopaque.*** Stones are faceted and dark brown.

PATHOLOGICAL VARIATIONS OF SERUM CHOLESTEROL

1. **Normal Value:** Normal serum total cholesterol varies widely, though different values by different methods have been given by different workers. Normal range in young adults is 150 to 250 mg/100 ml (average 200 mg/100 ml).

2. **Increase:** Increase of serum cholesterol level above normal is called ***"hypercholesterolaemia"*** which is found most characteristically in:

- ***Nephrotic syndrome*** (Type II nephritis): in earlier stages when associated with oedema, values up to 600 to 700 mg percent are common. Sometimes it may reach up to 1000 mg percent or more.

- *Diabetes mellitus:* values up to 400 to 550 mg percent are commonly found when treatment is inadequate .
- *Obstructive jaundice:* Increase is found most commonly. Increases parallels with increase in serum bilirubin.
- *Myxoedema:* High values are obtained usually ranging from 500 to 700 mg percent. Helps in diagnosis.
- *Xanthomatous biliary cirrhosis:* Very high values are seen.
- *Hypopituitarism:* Small increases ranging from 250 to 350 mg percent may be seen.
- *Xanthomatosis:* Frequently found to be associated with high cholesterol values.
- *Coronary thrombosis* and *angina pectoris* value between 300 to 400 mg percent are rather of frequent finding.
- **Idiopathic hypercholesterolaemia** has also been described.

3. **Decrease:** Decrease in blood cholesterol below normal is called *hypocholesterolaemia*. Hypocholesterolaemia is characteristically seen in:

- *Thyrotoxicosis: Values as low as 80 to 100 mg percent may be seen.* But quite a number of hyperthyroidism cases may have a serum cholesterol within normal range.
- *Low values are also seen in:*
  - *Pernicious anaemia* and in other anaemias
  - *Haemolytic jaundice*
  - *Malabsorption syndrome*
  - *Wasting diseases*
  - *Acute infections* and in a number of terminal states.

RELATION OF CHOLESTEROL AND OTHER LIPIDS AS RISK FACTOR IN CORONARY HEART DISEASE (CHD)

Of the serum lipids, *cholesterol has been the one most often incriminated as the risk factor.* However, other parameters such as serum TG, VLDL and LDL have been incriminated. Patients with CHD can have *any one of following abnormalities:*

- *Elevated concentrations of VLDL with normal concentrations of LDL.*
- *Elevated LDL with normal VLDL.*
- *Elevation of both VLDL and LDL.*

1. **Role of cholesterol:** An elevation of the total cholesterol in plasma is considered to be a ***prime risk factor*** for CHD. The ***Framingham study*** has demonstrated a linear increase in coronary "risk" with increment of total plasma cholesterol level from 180 mg percent upwards. The Lipid Research Clinics Coronary Primary Prevention Trial had presented firm proof that in humans, a lowering of plasma cholesterol level reduces the coronary thrombosis and myocardial infarction and mortality. One conclusion deduced from this pioneering work is: ***a 1 percent fall in cholesterol predicts a 2 percent reduction in CHD risk.***

2. **Role of LDL and HDL:** Recent studies have shown that atherogenic significance of the total cholesterol concentration must be viewed with restrictions. From numerous studies, it is now concluded that ***LDL is the carrier of 70 percent of total cholesterol*** and it transports cholesterol to tissues and thus most potential atherogenic agent **(Bad cholesterol)**.

On the other hand, an increase of second cholesterol rich class HDL is not associated with *"risk" at all (Good cholesterol).*

An inverse relation between CHD and HDL concentration has been found. A raised HDL concentration is beneficial and protective against CHD. This protective mechanism is explained by the following **two mechanisms operating in parallel.**

- ***"Reverse transport" of cholesterol from peripheral tissues into the liver by way of HDL*** which thus reduces the intracellular cholesterol content (*Scavenging action of HDL*).
- Control of catabolism of TG rich lipoproteins. High HDL concentrations are associated with a faster elimination from the plasma of TG rich lipoproteins and their atherogenic intermediate.

3. **Control of TG and VLDL:**

- Elevated VLDL and hypertriglyceridaemia may also be considered a primary "risk" factor because it is associated in specific cases with an increased atherogenic risk.

- A low blood TG level is suggestive of efficient intravascular lipolysis and thus of enhanced formation of HDL by this route.
- Hypertriglyceridaemia, on the other hand, indicates less effective intravascular lipolysis and hence a reduced formation of HDL which is, in turn, associated with a higher atherogenic risk.

FORMATION AND FATE OF ACTIVE ACETATE (ACETYL-COA) (TWO C METABOLISM)

"Active" acetate or acetyl-CoA is the C-2 compound, ***a key substance in third phase of metabolism.*** It is produced from various sources, viz. metabolism of carbohydrates, lipids and proteins and is metabolized to CO_2 and water. It also produces large number of "biologically" important compounds (refer ***Fig. 13.13***). Formation and fate of active acetate is shown in ***Table 13.9.***

☞ SALIENT POINTS TO REMEMBER

- Cholesterol is synthesized in the body (endogenous synthesis) from 2C unit "active acetate" (acetyl-CoA).
- The entire carbon skeleton is formed from active acetate, 15 C arises from CH_3 group and 12 C from COOH group.
- Formation of HMG-CoA from acetyl-CoA involves reversible reactions. But formation mevalonate from HMG-CoA is irreversible, which requires HMG-CoA reductase enzyme.
- ***HMG-CoA to mevalonate is a committed step.*** Reductase forms mevalonate whereas lyase forms ketone bodies.
- ***HMG-CoA reductase is the rate-limiting enzyme.*** The end-product cholesterol inhibits the enzyme ("feedback" inhibition).
- Squalene is an intermediate 30-Carbon aliphatic chain formed by condensation of six isoprenoid units.
- Cyclization of squalene forms cyclic compound Lanosterol which is further converted to cholesterol.
- Cholesterol is degraded in liver to form Bile acids-Glycocholic acid (3 parts) and Taurocholic acid (one part).
- Cholic acids form the bile salts-Sodium Glycocholic acid and sodium taurocholic acid.
- Bile salts in the gut emulsifies the dietary fats, emulsification of fats is a pre-requisite for absorption of fats from intestine.
- Cholesterol is converted to 7-dehydro-cholesterol principally in liver, which is present in skin. UV lights of sun's rays converts 7-dehydrocholesterol to vit-D_3 (cholecalciferol).

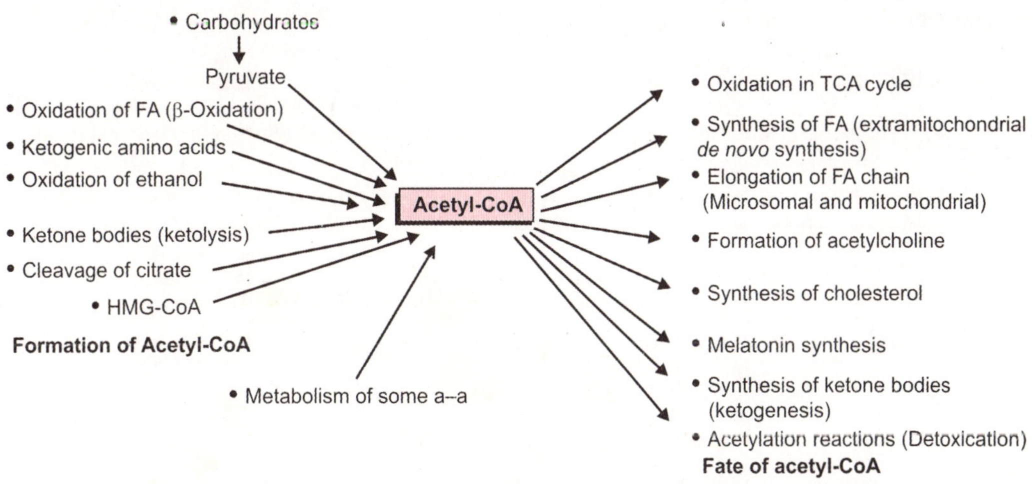

Fig. 13.13: Shows different sources and fate of acetyl-CoA schematically

Table 13.9: Sources of Acetyl CoA and its Fate

Formation	*Fate*
• **From metabolism of glucose:** Glucose forms pyruvate by glycolysis. Pyruvate is oxidatively decarboxylated in mitochondria by *pyruvate dehydrogenase complex to* Form acetyl-CoA.	• **Principal fate is oxidation in TCA cycle:** Most of acetyl-CoA combines with OAA to form citrate and further oxidized to CO_2 and H_2O in TCA cycle.
• ***β-oxidation of FA:*** Acetyl-CoA is produced in mitochondria from β-Oxidation of FA.	• ***In cholesterol biosynthesis:*** Acetyl-CoA is the starting material for cholesterol biosynthesis. All the 27 carbon atoms are derived from acetyl-CoA (see Cholesterol Biosynthesis).
• ***Cleavage of citrate:*** In the cytosol, acetyl-CoA is produced from citrate. Which is cleaved by *ATP citrate lyase* in presence of ATP and CoA to form OAA and acetyl-CoA.	• ***Ketogenesis:*** 'Acetyl-CoA' is the starting material required for the formation of first ketone body 'aceto-acetate' in liver (see Ketogenesis)
• ***Oxidation of ethanol:*** Alcohol is oxidized by the enzyme *alcohol dehydrogenase* to form acetyl-CoA. • ***Thio-esterification of Acetate:*** Acetate can be activated to acetyl-CoA by the enzyme *acetyl-CoA-synthase* in presence of ATP and CoA-SH. Acetate can be formed in ruminants from cellulose. In humans, small amount of acetate may be obtained from oxidation of ethanol, hydrolysis of aspirin, and catabolism of amino acid threonine.	• ***Fatty acid synthesis:*** • Cytoplasmic *de novo* fatty acid synthesis (extramitochondrial): Acetyl-CoA is the starting material for synthesis of palmitic acid (see Extramitochondrial de novo FA synthesis). • Microsomal elongation system: uses malonyl CoA synthesized from acetyl-CoA by carboxylation reaction for elongation of pre-existing acyl-CoA molecules by addition of C-2 units • Mitochondrial elongase system: Uses acetyl-CoA itself in incorporating C-2 units into acyl-CoA.
• ***From metabolism of certain amino acids.*** Catabolism of certain amino acids produces "acetyl-CoA" (ketogenic amino acids) e.g. phenylalanine, tyrosine, leucine, isoleucine, lysine and tryptophan.	• ***Acetylation reactions: (Detoxication)*** Acetyl-CoA is used in detoxication of many substances by "acetylation" reaction. *Acetyl transferases (acetylases)* transfer the acetyl group from acetyl-CoA to many substrates, e.g.
• ***By ketolysis:*** Aceto acetyl-CoA is formed from acetoacetate in extrahepatic tissues which is further split to form acetyl-CoA by thiolase	• Sulfanilamide is detoxicated to N-acetyl sulfanilamide in the liver by the enzyme *sulfanilamide acetylase* with acetyl-CoA, and excreted in urine • Bromobenzene is detoxicated by cysteine and acetyl-CoA to form para-bromophenyl mercapturic acid and excreted in urine.
• ***HMG-CoA:*** Forms acetyl-CoA by the action of the enzyme HMG-CoA lyase.	• ***Formation of acetyl choline from choline*** in cholinergic neurons. The enzyme *choline acetylase* transfers acetyl group of acetyl-CoA to choline.
	• **In melatonin synthesis:** Formation of N-acetyl serotonin from serotonin (see Melatonin Synthesis).

- In adrenal cortex, adrenocortical hormones are synthesized from cholesterol.
- Similarly in Gonads, the Gonadal hormones- – androgens, oestrogens and progesterones are synthesized from cholesterol.
- Bacterial flora of intestine converts cholesterol to a neutral sterol, called coprosterol (coprostanol) which is excreted in the faeces.
- Hypercholesterolaemia is associated with atherosclerosis and coronary heart disease (CHD).
- Consumption of Polyunsaturated fatty acids and fibres in the diet decreases cholesterol in circulation.
- Drugs such as Lovostatine, cholestyramines, clofibrate, large dosage of Nicotinic acid reduces plasma cholesterol level.
- Cholelithiasis, a cholesterol gallstone disease is caused by a defect in the absorption of bile salts from the intestine or biliary tract obstruction.

PLASMA LIPOPROTEINS AND METABOLISM

- *Hypercholesterolaemia*
- *Hypertension*
- *Cigarette smoking*
- ***Obesity have been identified as major independent risk factors for the development of premature cardiovascular disease.*** The clear delineation of hypercholesterolaemia, in the beginning, as a risk factor has stimulated active investigation into the metabolism of cholesterol and TG in normal healthy man and in patients with disorders of lipid metabolism and atherosclerosis.

What are Lipoproteins? In plasma, cholesterol and TG form integral components of macromolecular complexes called *as* ***lipoproteins*** which are conjugated proteins; lipids part is the prosthetic group and lipid-free proteins are designated as ***apolipoproteins or apoproteins.***

Structure of a Lipoprotein Complex: Extraction of plasma lipids with a suitable lipid solvent and subsequent separation of the extract into various classes of lipids, shows the presence of:

- *TG (triacyl glycerol)*
- *Phospholipids (PL)*
- *Cholesterol and cholesterol esters*
- *A specific protein called apoprotein,* and
- *The existence of a much smaller fraction of "unesterified long-chain" FA (Free FA)* that accounts for less than 5 percent of total FA present in the plasma. Free fatty acid is also called as unesterified FA (UFA) or non-esterified FA (NEFA). ***FFA is now considered to be metabolically most active of plasma lipids*** (see ***Fig. 13.14:*** Structure of Lipoprotein complex).

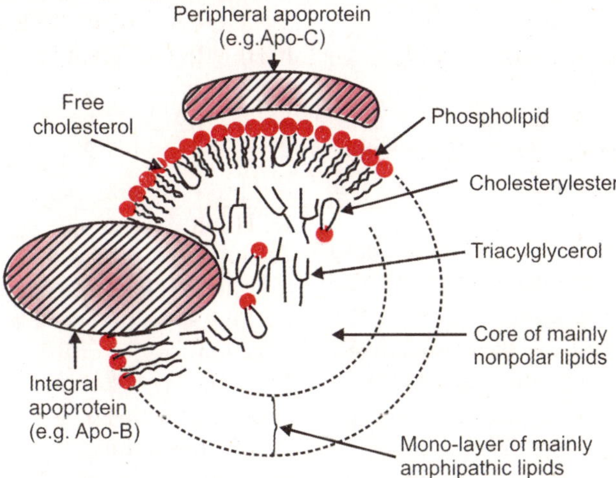

Fig. 13.14: Structure of lipoprotein molecules

Lipoproteins serve as 'carrier' of lipids in plasma: This is *achieved* by ***associating the more insoluble lipids with more "polar" ones,*** such as PL and then combining with cholesterol/and cholesterol esters and a specific protein called "apoprotein" to form the so called ***"hydrophilic lipoprotein complexes".***

It is in this way that TG formed in intestinal epithelial cells (exogenous TG) and TG formed in liver by synthesis ("endogenous" TG) are carried as lipoprotein complexes "chylomicrons" and VLDL (very low density lipoprotein) respectively.

Thus, ***chylomicrons are the chief carriers of exogenous TG, and hepatic VLDL for endogenous hepatic TG.***

CLASSIFICATION OF LIPOPROTEINS

Lipoproteins can be classified according to their hydrated density and electrophoretic mobility.

1. Classification as Per Hydrated Density

- Pure fat is less dense than water, as the proportion of lipid to protein in lipoprotein complexes increases ↑, the density of the macromolecule decreases ↓.
- Use of the above property has been made in separating various lipoproteins in plasma by ultracentrifugation.

Gofman and colleagues *(1954)* separated lipoproteins by ultracentrifugation into ***four*** major density classes:

- ***Chylomicrons:*** density lowest, floats.
- ***Very low density lipoproteins (VLDL or VLDLP).***
- ***Low density lipoproteins (LDL).***
- ***High density lipoproteins (HDL):*** settles below.

LDL has been further divided into LDL 1 or IDL (intermediate density lipoprotein) and LDL-2. *HDL* has been further separated into HDL-1 (this fraction is quantitatively insignificant), HDL-2 and HDL-3. Recently HDL c has been described.

2. Classification Based on Electrophoretic Mobility (Fredrickson and colleagues, 1967).

The most widely used and simplest classification for lipoproteins is based on the separation of major ***four classes*** by electrophoresis. The most frequently employed electrophoretic media are "paper" and "agarose". Plasma lipoproteins separated by this technique are classfied in relation to comparable migration of serum proteins. On electrophoresis, the different fractions according to mobility appear at:

- The origin is chylomicrons;
- Migrating into β-globulin region is called β-lipoprotein (LDL);
- Migrating into pre-β-globulin region, called as "pre-β-lipoproteins" (VLDL); and
- Migrating to α_1-globulin region called "α-lipoproteins" (HDL).

Migration is shown diagrammatically in ***Fig. 13.15.***

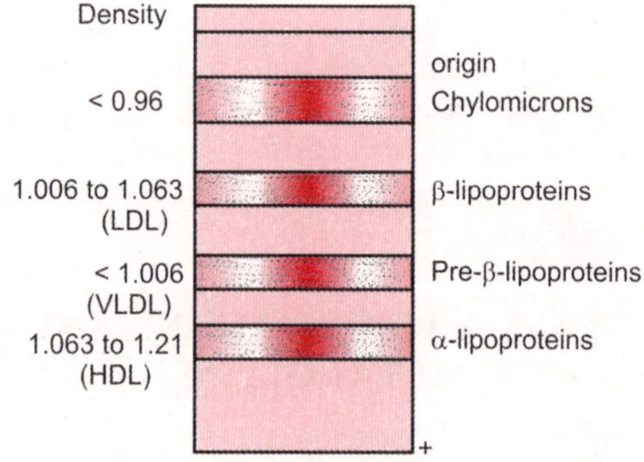

Fig. 13.15: Showing electrophoretic separation of plasma lipoproteins

TYPES OF APOPROTEINS PRESENT IN VARIOUS LIPOPROTEIN FRACTIONS (CHEMISTRY OF APOPROTEINS)

As stated above, lipoproteins are characterized by the presence of one or more proteins or polypeptides known as apoproteins.

According to ABC nomenclature:

1. **HDL:** Two major apoproteins of HDL are designated as **apo-A-I** and **apo-A-II**. In addition to above, **HDL also contains apo-C-I, C-II** and **C-III**. HDL-3 is characterized by having **apo-D** and HDL may also acquire arginine-rich **apo-E**.
2. **LDL:** The main apoprotein of LDL is **apo-B 100,** which is also present in VLDL.
3. **Chylomicrons:** Principal apoprotein of chylomicrons is **Apo-B-48** (mol wt=200 kdal). In addition, chylomicrons also contain **Apo-A (AI**

and AII) and **apo-C (C-II and C-III)**, Also arginine rich **Apo-E** (34 KD).

Apo-C seems to be freely transferable between chylomicrons and VLDL on one hand and HDL on the other.

4. VLDL and LDL: Principal apoproteins of VLDL, IDL and LDL is **apo-B-100** (350 Kd). They **also contain apo-C (C-I, C-II and C-III),** and **apo-E.** IDL carries some apo-E apoprotein.

Apo-E: Arginine rich apo-E, isolated from VLDL. It contains arginine to the extent of 10 percent of the total amino acids and accounts for 5 to 10 percent of total VLDL apo-proteins, in normal subjects but is present in excess in the **"broad" β-VLDL** of patients of type III hyperlipoproteinaemia.

Carbohydrate content: Carbohydrates account for approximately 5 percent apo-B and include mannose, galactose, fucose, glucose, glucosamine, and sialic acid. So, some of lipoproteins are glycoproteins.

Apo-J (Apolipoprotein J): It is a ***glycoprotein a dimer found in association with HDL-2.*** Its molecular weight is approximately 50,000.

- Two monomeric units are α and β. **α-subunit** consists of 205 a.a. and **β-subunit** has 222 a.a. It is found in atheromatous plaques.
- Apo-J has been found to **inhibit macrophage mediated cell damage** and it is **anti-atherogenic** and offers protection to endothelial and smooth muscle cells from injury **(Protective function).**

Difference of "Nascent" Chylomicrons and VLDL from "Circulating" Chylomicrons and VLDL.

"Nascent" chylomicrons and VLDL contains the principal apoprotein B-48 and B-100, respectively. During circulation they acquire apo-C principally by interaction with HDL and the other apoproteins like apo-E. "Nascent" chylomicrons may have also apo-A.

FUNCTIONS OF APOPROTEINS

1. By entering into the "polar" surface layer, they make the lipoprotein molecules "water-miscible" (hydrophilic).
2. Some apoproteins may act as "activator" /or "inhibitor" of some specific enzymes, e.g.
   - Apo-A-I and A-II acts as LCAT activator
   - Apo-C-I and C-II act as activator of *lipoprotein lipase.*
   - Apo-C-III act as inhibitor of *lipoprotein lipase.*
3. Some apoproteins like apo-B 100 and apo-E may bind with specific membrane "receptors" on hepatic cells leading to hepatic uptake of corresponding lipoproteins.
4. Apoprotein-D functions as "cholesteryl ester transfer protein" for transferring cholesteryl esters between different lipoproteins.

Characteristics of Human Plasma Lipoproteins

Fig. 13.16 shows the characteristics of human plasma lipoproteins.

1. **Chylomicrons:** TG is resynthesized in intestinal mucosal cells. Hydrophobic TG molecules get a coating composed of apoprotein, PL and cholesterol esters to form the lipoprotein particle chylomicron.

- Chylomicrons are transported in membrane bound vesicles to the lateral cell membranes of the mucosal cells, where they are released by *"exocytosis"* into the extracellular space. ***Chylomicrons then enter the lacteals and are transported by the lymphatic system to the thoracic duct,*** which empties into the left *subclavian vein* and then to systemic circulation. Chylomicrons are the carrier of exogenous T.G and while circulating are acted upon by *"lipoprotein lipase"*. The enzyme hydrolyzes the TG. Continued delipidation produces smaller particles called ***"chylomicron remnants"***
- ***Chylomicron remnants which remain after delipidation are rich in cholesterol and cholesterol ester.*** They are cleared by liver, where most of the cholesterol is used for bile acid formation, and fatty acids are used for PL biosynthesis.

2. **VLDL:** ***Main bulk of VLDL is synthesized in liver.*** A small amount is synthesized in intestinal mucosal cells.

- TG synthesized in liver cells (endogenous TG) being hydrophobic gets a coating of apo-

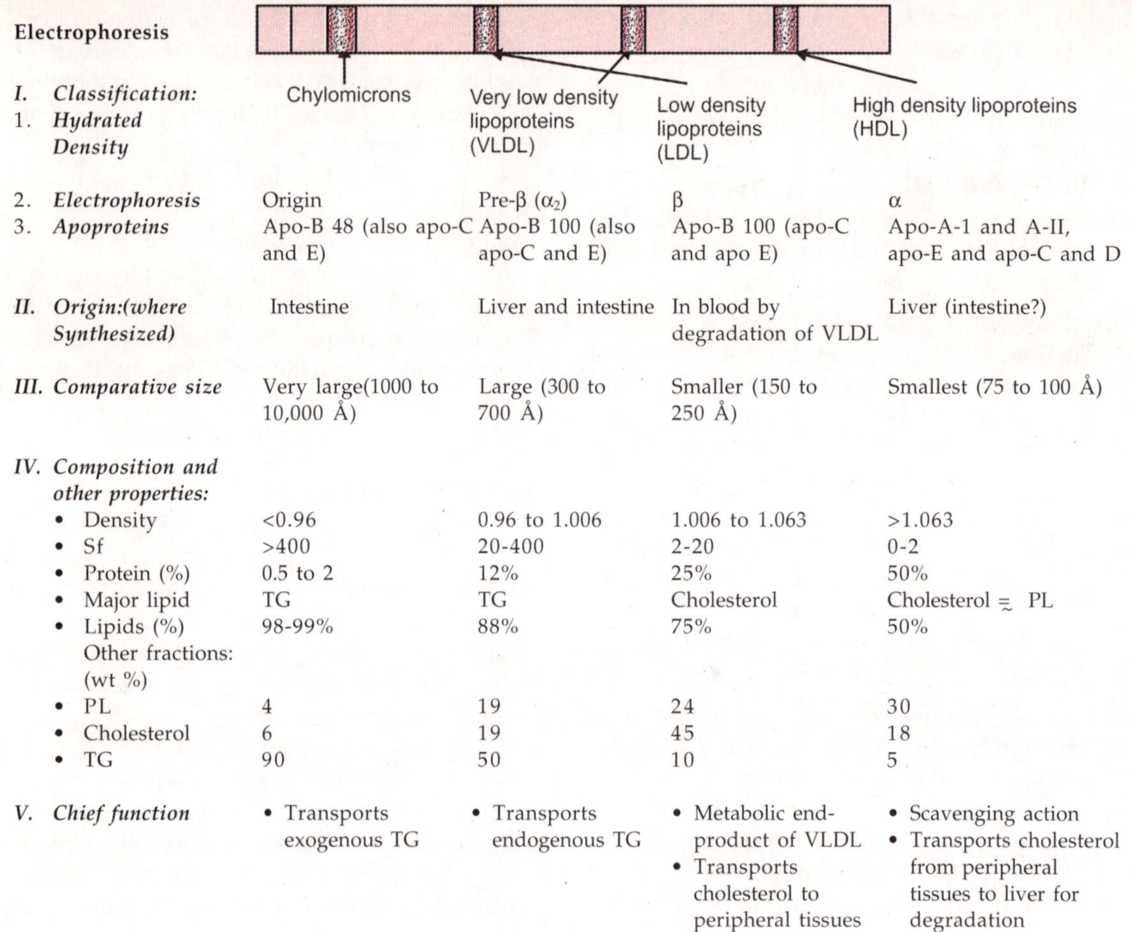

Electrophoresis				
I. *Classification:* 1. *Hydrated Density*	Chylomicrons	Very low density lipoproteins (VLDL)	Low density lipoproteins (LDL)	High density lipoproteins (HDL)
2. *Electrophoresis*	Origin	Pre-β (α_2)	β	α
3. *Apoproteins*	Apo-B 48 (also apo-C and E)	Apo-B 100 (also apo-C and E)	Apo-B 100 (apo-C and apo E)	Apo-A-1 and A-II, apo-E and apo-C and D
II. *Origin:(where Synthesized)*	Intestine	Liver and intestine	In blood by degradation of VLDL	Liver (intestine?)
III. *Comparative size*	Very large(1000 to 10,000 Å)	Large (300 to 700 Å)	Smaller (150 to 250 Å)	Smallest (75 to 100 Å)
IV. *Composition and other properties:*				
• Density	<0.96	0.96 to 1.006	1.006 to 1.063	>1.063
• Sf	>400	20-400	2-20	0-2
• Protein (%)	0.5 to 2	12%	25%	50%
• Major lipid	TG	TG	Cholesterol	Cholesterol ≅ PL
• Lipids (%)	98-99%	88%	75%	50%
Other fractions: (wt %)				
• PL	4	19	24	30
• Cholesterol	6	19	45	18
• TG	90	50	10	5
V. *Chief function*	• Transports exogenous TG	• Transports endogenous TG	• Metabolic end-product of VLDL • Transports cholesterol to peripheral tissues	• Scavenging action • Transports cholesterol from peripheral tissues to liver for degradation

Fig 13.16: Characteristics of human plasma lipoproteins

protein, PL and cholesterol esters to form the hydrophilic lipoprotein complex VLDL which is thrown to circulation.

- VLDL is the *carrier of endogenous TG*. Circulating VLDL is acted upon by *lipoprotein lipase*. ***Delipidation of VLDL produces smaller particle IDL (intermediate density lipoprotein).*** IDL thus represents the end of degradation of VLDL by lipoprotein lipase and thus corresponds to "chylomicrons remnants". ***Circulating IDL particles are converted to LDL (cholesterol-rich) particles.***

3. **LDL:** ***LDL is not synthesized/or secreted by liver or intestine. It is formed principally by degradation of circulating VLDL, which initially forms IDL.*** Most of IDL particles change into LDL particles, by losing their apo-E and some of TG. ***This makes LDL richer in cholesteryl esters, and cholesterol,*** and poorer in TG and total lipids. Thus, they become smaller in diameter and higher in density than IDL.

- Site of catabolism of LDL was initially thought to be solely by liver. But studies on partially hepatectomized dogs have indicated that catabolism of LDL, in addition to liver, principally occurs in peripheral tissues, viz:
  - ***Fibroblasts***

- *Lymphocytes*
- *Arterial smooth muscle cells.*
- Studies on cultured fibroblasts, lymphocytes and arterial smooth muscle cells have shown the existence of "specific LDL receptors" (B-100 receptors).

Lipoprotein (a) or LP (a): LP (a) is seen only in some persons. In 40% population, there is no detectable level of LP (a) in serum. Only in 20% of population the LP (a) concentration in blood is more than 30 mg/dl.

When present it is associated with LDL and attached to apo-B_{100} by S-S bond. It is *highly atherogenic and is associated with myocardial infarction in younger age group 30 to 40 years.*

4. HDL: *HDL is synthesized in liver cells and also in intestinal mucosal cells.*

Scavenging Action of HDL: **Glomset (1968)** has suggested that HDL plays a major role in the removal of cholesterol from peripheral extra-hepatic tissues and transport of this cholesterol to the liver where it is further metabolized. This has been called as *"scavenging action"* of HDL (*"reverse cholesterol transport".*)

Difference of nascent intestinal HDL from "nascent" hepatic HDL:

- Nascent intestinal HDL contains only apo-A, when it circulates, it acquires apo-C and Apo-E.
- Nascent hepatic HDL on the other hand contains both apo-A and apo-C.

Note: Apo-C and apo-E are only synthesized in liver and not intestinal mucosal cells.

- LDL formed in circulation from VLDL through IDL, contains 79 percent lipids with about 44 to 58 percent of cholesterol (very rich in cholesterol), LDL deposits cholesterol in blood vessel walls hence it is ***bad cholesterol.*** Increased LDL is harmful and increases "risk" of myocardial infarction.
- HDL also contains about 41 percent cholesterol, but this cholesterol is as a result of scavenging action (reverse cholesterol transport) which is carried to liver for degradation to bile acids. Thus, HDL cholesterol is *"good cholesterol"*. **High HDL is beneficial for health and reduces the 'risk' of myocardial infarction.**

HDL 2

Cholesterol released from chylomicrons and VLDL, during *"Lipoprotein Lipase" activity* is accepted by circulating HDL.

With HDL-bound LCAT, the *latter esterifies cholesterol into cholesteryl esters* in HDL and thus maintains a *low concentration of free cholesterol* in HDL particles enabling the transfer of more cholesterol into the latter.

The *HDL_3 is changed to HDL-2* which is richer in cholesteryl esters and very low in free cholesterol. *HDL-2 is thus good cholesterol.* It *contains Apo-A-I.*

It has been further fractionated to 2a and 2b. *HDL-2b is the main anti-atherogenic fraction.*

HDL 3

HDL_{-3} is the spherical HDL and contains Apo-D and Apo-A II.

- It *functions as the "Cholesteryl-ester transfer protein"* and transfers some cholesteryl esters from HDL to VLDL, LDL and Chylomicrons in the plasma. These lipoproteins then transfer these cholesteryl esters to liver for degradation.
- HDL_{-3} has been further fractionated into 3a, 3b and 3c.

HDLc:

HDLc has been recently described which is found in *the blood of diet-induced hypercholesterolaemia.*

- *HDLc is rich in cholesterol* and its *sole apoprotein is Apo-E.* It is taken up by the liver via the Apo-E "remnant" receptor and also by LDL-receptors.

MAJOR FUNCTIONS OF LIPOPROTEINS

- Chylomicrons transport mainly TG and smaller amounts of PL, cholesterol-esters and fat soluble vitamins from intestine to liver and adipose tissue. *The lipids carried by chylo-*

microns principally is dietary lipids (carrier of "exogenous" TG).

- ***VLDL transports mainly "endogenous TG" synthesized in hepatic cells from the liver*** to the extrahepatic tissues including adipose tissue for storage.
- High carbohydrate intake, high (insulin/glucagon) ratio, high plasma FFA, and alcohol intake increase the hepatic synthesis of both TG and VLDL so that the enhanced amounts of FA reaching the liver is speedily mobilized in VLDL to adipose tissue.
- LDL rich in cholesterol-esters transports cholesterol and its esters from hepatic cells to extrahepatic tissues ***(bad cholesterol).***
- HDL transports cholesterol and its esters from peripheral tissues to the liver for its catabolism ***"Scavenging" action](good cholesterol).***
- Apo-D-of HDL-3 functions as the cholesteryl-ester transfer protein.
- Albumin-FFA complexes transport mainly free FA, released by adipose tissue lipolysis and small amounts of lysophospholipids from extrahepatic tissues to the liver.
- Certain apoproteins can act as activators/inhibitors of specific enzymes.

CLINICAL DISORDERS ASSOCIATED LIPOPROTEIN METABOLISM

Clinical disorders may be:

- ***Hyperlipoproteinaemias***
- ***Hypolipoproteinaemias***

Hyperlipidaemias may be further divided into:

- ***Primary:*** They are genetic disorders characterized by distinct clinical syndromes.
- ***Secondary:*** Due to underlying disease process usually thyroid, liver and renal diseases.

INHERITED DISORDERS

A. Primary Hyperlipoproteinaemias: Fredrickson *et al* (1967) proposed **five types** based on changes in plasma lipoproteins. ***Table 13.11*** shows five types of hyperlipoproteinaemias.

B. Hypolipoproteinaemias

1. Abeta Lipoproteinaemia:

- A rare inherited disorder, the disease is characterized by decreased plasma cholesterol ↓ due to absence of β-lipoproteins (LDL).
- Most lipids are present in low concentration specially TG, which is virtually absent. No chylomicrons and/or pre-β lipoproteins (VLDL) are formed.
- ***Other clinical features associated*** with above lipid change are:
  - **Atypical retinitis pigmentosa.**
  - Red blood cell abnormalities like *"acanthosis"*.
  - Malabsorption of fats.
  - Both small intestine mucosal cells and in liver cells accumulation of fats occur (fatty infiltration).
- ***Metabolic defect:*** Principal metabolic defect is in "synthesis of apo-B" leading to gross deficiency of apo-B resulting in deficiency of lipoproteins containing apo-B, viz. chylomicrons, VLDL and LDL.
- Classic form of this disease is called as ***Bassen kornzweig syndrome***

2. Familial α-Lipoprotein Deficiency (Tangier's disease): This disease is characterized by deficiency of α-lipoprotein (HDL ↓). In homozygous patient, plasma HDL may be nearly completely absent.

- ***Inheritance:*** Autosomal recessive
- ***Metabolic defect***: Reduction in apo-A I and apo-A II, leading to accumulation of cholesteryl esters in different tissues.
- ***Clinical features:*** Clinically, cardinal feature of this disease is:
  - ***Hyperplastic orange yellow tonsils.***
  - ***Adenoids.***
- There is no impairment of chylomicrons formation or secretion of endogenous TG by the liver. However, on electrophoresis, there is no pre-β-lipoprotein, but a ***"broad β-band"*** is found containing the endogenous TG.

Note: The presence of low plasma cholesterol levels, associated with normal or elevated TG levels is often diagnostic of this disease. Due to HDL deficiency, clearance of TG from plasma is

Table 13.11: Five types of Hyperlipoproteinaemias

Type	Genetic classification	Electrophoretic classification	Inheritance	Plasma lipids	Plasma lipoproteins	Clinical features	Treatment
I.	**Familial lipoprotein lipase deficiency**	Hyperchylomicro-naemia	Autosomal recessive	TG ↑, may be cholesterol increased	Chylomicrons ++, Pre-β lipoproteins may be ↑ and α & β Lipoproteins ↓	Rare • Early childhood • Eruptive xanthomas, • Recurrent abdominal pain	• Fat induced, • Diet low in fat
Note: 1. Slow clearing of chylomicrons 2. Premature CV diseases does not occur.							
II.	**Familial hypercholestero-laemia (FHC)**	Hyper-β-lipoprotein aemia	Autosomal dominant	Total cholesterol ↑, TG ↑ or N	LDL ↑ VLDL may be ↑	Common occurrence, Associated with Xanthomas-tendinous and tuberous	• Reduction of dietary cholesterol and saturated fats
Note: 1. Increased incidence of premature CV diseases and atheroselerosis. 2. Metabolic defects: (a) Increased synthesis of apo-B ↑ (b) Defective catabolism of LDL (Defective LDL receptor)							
III.	**Familial dysbeta lipoproteinaemia (Broad β-disease) ('Remnant remnant' disease)**	Broad-β-lipo proteinaemia (floating β-band)	Autosomal dominant	Cholesterol ↑ TG ↑	VLDL ↑ IDL ↑ LDL↑	Rare, xanthomas-tuberous and palmer	• Weight reduction-Low carbohydrate diets. • Unsaturated fats with little cholesterol
Note: • Metabolic defects: Increased synthesis apo-B ↑. • Increased synthesis of apo-E ↑ • Premature CV disease and peripheral vascular disease.							
IV.	**Familial hyper triglyceridaemia (FHTG)**	Hyper pre-B-lipopro-teinemia	Autosomal dominant	TG and cholesterol ↑ or N	VLDL and α and β lipoproteins subnormal	• Present in early adulthood • Synthesis of lipids from carbohydrates↑	• Weight reduction • Replacement of much carbohydrates with unsaturated fats • Low cholesteol diet • Hypolipidaemic drugs.
Note: This lipoprotein pattern is associated with coronary heart disease, obesity, maturity onset DM Type-II, alcoholism and taking progesterone hormones							
V.	**Combined hyper-lipidaemias**	Variable	Autosomal dominant	Both TG and cholesterol ↑	Both VLDL and chylomicrons ↑ α and β lipoproteins ↑	• Uncommon occurrence • Xanthomas present • Abnormal glucose tolerance	• Weight reduction followed by a diet not too high either in carbohydrate or fats
Note: Associated with ketotic DM, incidence of atherosclerosis less							

slow tending to elevated TG levels (hypertriglyceridaemia), probably as a result of absence of apo-C-II which is an activator of *lipoprotein lipase.*

PLASMA LIPOPROTEINS AND ATHEROSCLEROSIS

- Over the last several years, an intensive investigations has focussed on the identification of "risk factors" for the development of premature atherosclerosis. The high incidence of cardiovascular diseases in the western world has necessitated a major scientific effort to elucidate the etiology of this disease.
- ***Hypercholesterolaemia or more accurately, hyper-β-lipoproteinaemia (LDL↑) has clearly been identified as a major risk factor.***
- Of recent interest, has been the retrospective analysis of epidemiological data which has suggested a ***negative correlation between HDL cholesterol in human plasma and risk of premature heart disease.***
- In a series of patient with any given LDL cholesterol level, the probability of CV disease increases as HDL-cholesterol level decreases. These studies are consistent with hypothesis that ***HDL-deficiency is an independent risk factor for premature CV disease.***
- Two separate mechanisms have been postulated to explain the role of HDL in the regulation of intracellular concentrations of cholesterol.

1. *Glomset (1968)* proposed that HDL played a role in cholesterol metabolism by facilitating removal of cholesterol from peripheral cells and transporting to liver for degradation. This has been termed as **"reverse cholesterol transport". (Scavenging action)** Hence, lowered levels of HDL in the plasma would be less effective in the removal of cholesterol from peripheral cells.
2. An additional mechanism has recently been proposed to explain the inter-relationship between LDL and HDL. In these studies, HDL was demonstrated to influence the binding and uptake of LDL by the peripheral cells. In *in vitro* experiments, in fibroblasts, endothelial cells, lymphocytes and arterial smooth muscle cells in tissue culture ***HDL was shown to competitively inhibit LDL binding and uptake.***

- Thus, ***decreased plasma levels of HDL could be postulated to increase LDL uptake, while increased HDL levels would decrease cellular uptake of LDL. A ratio of LDL cholesterol and HDL cholesterol is important.*** If it is high the risk is more and if the ratio is low risk is less.
- Recently, estimation of apolipoproteins are being done in clinical biochemistry. Apo-A-I apoprotein of HDL and apo-B apoprotein of LDL have been considered as the better determinants of the "risk" and are regarded as better indicators for myocardial infarction. They can be estimated by various immunoassay techniques, viz RIA, immunonephelometric, immunoturbidimetric, and radial immunodiffusion.

FATTY LIVER

The amount of lipids in the liver at any given time is the resultant of several influences, some acting in conjunction with and some in opposition to other. ***Normal liver contains about 4 percent as total lipids,*** three fourths of which is phospholipids (PL) and one-fourth as neutral fats (TG).

Factors that Regulate Fat Content of Liver *(Fig. 13.17)*

1. ***Factors that tend to increase ↑ the fat content of liver are:***
   - Influx of dietary lipids.
   - Synthesis of FA from carbohydrates and proteins.
   - Mobilization of FA from depots to liver.
2. ***Factors that tend to decrease ↓ the liver fats are:***
   - Mobilization of fats into the blood and then to the depots from the liver.
   - Degradation of FA within the liver itself.

Normal levels of lipids in the liver are the result of maintenance of a proper balance between the above mentioned factors. A relative increase or decrease in the rate of one or other of these processes can result in accumulation of abnormal quantity of lipids in the liver, producing fatty liver.

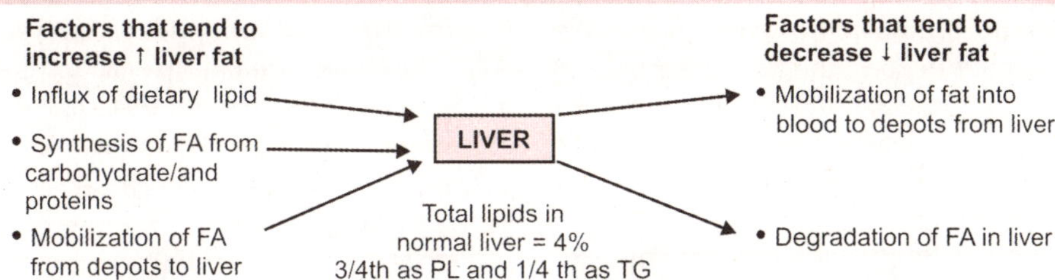

Fig. 13.17: Factors that tend to increase/decrease the liver fat

TYPES OF FATTY LIVER

Biochemically, theoretically fatty liver can be of **Five types:**

Type-1 Overfeeding of fat
Type-2 Oversynthesis of fats from carbohydrates
Type-3 Overmobilization from depots to liver
Type-4 Undermobilization from liver to depots
Type-5 Underutilization in the liver.

Type 1: Overfeeding of Fats: Overfeeding of fats produce increase in circulating chylomicrons.

- Liver can take up by pinocytosis, leading to increased TG in liver cells.
- Circulating chylomicrons are acted by *lipoprotein lipase,* which produces increase in FFA by hydrolysis of TG of chylomicrons. Leads to influx of FFA in liver, synthesis of TG is enhanced and formation and secretion of more VLDL.
  Lipids deposited in type-1, reflects the composition of dietary lipids.

Type 2: Oversynthesis of Fats from Carbohydrates: Ingestion of carbohydrates in excess of caloric requirement, overloads the capacity of the cells which normally store glycogen. Surplus carbohydrates are chanelled to synthesis of FA and TG (lipogenesis) in liver and adipose tissue.

Type 3: Overmobilization from Depots to Liver: This type of fatty liver is referred as ***physiological fatty liver.*** This represents an exaggeration of normal process, excessive mobilization of FFA from depot to liver. Liver responds to increased synthesis of TG and VLDL and increases the plasma level of LDL.

Causes: Fatty liver of this type develops in conditions involving greatly increased utilization of fats as "fuel" and where there is interference with oxidation of carbohydrates. (Non-utilization of carbohydrates for energy). Thus it ***occurs in:***

- ***Diabetes mellitus:*** human or experimental of the hypoinsulin, hyperpituitary or hyperadrenocortical type.
- ***Starvation.***
- ***Carbohydrate deprivation.***

Type 4: Undermobilization from Liver to Depot: Fatty liver of this type has been differentiated from the preceding type by being designated as ***pathological fatty liver.*** It is accompanied by a decrease ↓ in plasma lipids (hypolipaemia), which effects mainly PL and Cholesterol. The pattern of lipids is also abnormal, ***fatty livers of this type, if not treated, eventuates in cirrhosis liver,*** and there may be associated haemorrhagic lesions in the kidneys.

Causes: They appear to be caused by agents or conditions, which produce either absolute or a relative deficiency in certain of the ingredients used by the liver for synthesis of VLDL such as:

- ***Protein: apoprotein itself.***
- ***The building blocks of its structural lipid*** moieties, suh as cholesterol esters and PL, viz. inositol phosphatides, choline and the polyunsaturated FA.
- ***Factors interfering with secretory mechanism.***

Lipotropic Agents: Agents such as ***choline, methionine, betaine, inositol,*** etc. which have the apparent effect of facilitating the removal of fat from liver, and thus prevents accumulations of fat in liver cells. Such substances which prevent accumulations of fat in liver are said to be ***lipotropic (lipotropic agents or lipotropins). The phenomenon itself is called lipotropism.***

- Antagonistic agents and the converse condition are "anti lipotropic" and anti-lipoprotein respectively.

Type 5: Underutilization in the Liver: It is possible that the fatty livers of pantothenic acid deficiency are of this type, i.e. underutilization. Deficiency of pantothenic acid leads to decrease ↓ in availability of CoA-SH. Hence, activation of FA and its oxidation suffers.

- Poisoning by salts of rare earth elements (e.g. Cerium) also appears to cause underutilization, by inhibition of the mitochondrial system which oxidizes FA.

Note:
Though we have discussed above, 5 types of biochemical mechanisms which can cause fatty liver, in practice clinically type 1 and type 5 are rather rare.

Causes of fatty liver seen in clinical practice are:

- *Alcohol abuse:* most common cause in India (Mechanism of production of fatty liver by alcohol is discussed below).
- *Malnutrition-protein,* also deficiency of EFA and lipotropic agents.
- *Diabetes mellitus*
- *Obesity*
- *Hepatotoxins and Drugs*

Biochemical mechanisms for production of fatty liver by the following agents:

1. *Carbon tetrachloride (CCl_4):* CCl_4 produces the fatty liver by the following mechanisms:

- Interferes with synthesis of apo-protein required to be incorporated in lipoprotein complex in liver;
- Also affects the secretory mechanism itself;
- Or can interfere with conjugation of the lipid moiety with lipoprotein apoprotein;
- Also mobilizes FA through release of catecholamines.

2. *Ethionine:* Ethionine is chemically α-amino-γ-ethyl mercaptobutyric acid. Ethionine produces fatty liver, probably due to decline in m-RNA ↓ and protein synthesis caused by a reduction in availability of ATP.

Mechanism: The above happens when ethionine replacing methionine in "S-adenosyl methionine" ***traps available adenine and prevents synthesis of ATP.*** The above mechanism of action is supported by the fact that effect of ethionine may be reversed by administration of ATP or adenine.

3. *Orotic acid:* Administration of orotic acid causes fatty livers.

Mechanism of Action of Orotic Acid:

- Probably blocks specifically the synthesis of apo-VLDL (apo-B_{100}).
- Also probably interferes with inclusion of glucosamine in VLDL-apoprotein.

4. *Ethyl alcohol:* Chronic alcoholism leads to fat accumulation in liver which leads to cirrhosis liver. Plasma shows hyperlipidaemia.

Lipid Changes:

- Increased FFA level ↑. Extra FFA mobilization plays some part or not is not clear. Experimental studies in rats, after a single intoxicating dose of ethanol shows elevated level of FFA—(increased synthesis of FA?).
- Increased TG synthesis ↑ occurs.
- Decreased FA oxidation ↓ and inhibition of TCA cycle ↓.
- Increased cholesterol synthesis ↑.
- Depresses transport of fats from liver.

In chronic alcoholics, there is also associated nutritional deficiencies:

- Deficiency of vitamins.
- Deficiency of proteins/amino acids like threonine, isoleucine, glycine, tryptophan, etc.

The above occurs due to lack of appetite, and associated gastritis and thus can aggravate.

Metabolism of ethanol: Metabolism takes place exclusively in liver. Ethanol oxidation is catalyzed by the enzyme *"alcohol dehydrogenase"*, which is a zinc-containing metallo-enzyme and requires NAD^+ as acceptor of H^+ ***(Fig. 13.18).***

Biochemical mechanism: Due to ethanol oxidation, ratio of $\frac{NADH + H^+}{NAD^+}$ ↑.

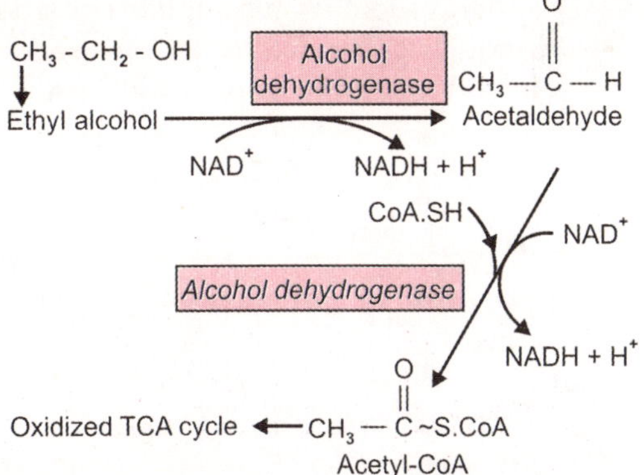

Fig.13.18: Steps in metabolism of ethanol

This leads to following alterations:

- ***Shifts to the right*** of the following reaction:

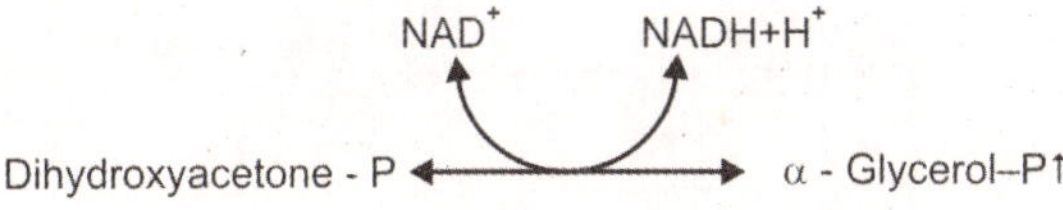

Increased α-glycero-(P) enhances esterification

- ***Shift to left*** of the following reaction:

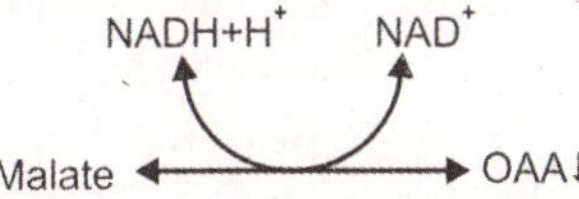

Produces relative deficiency of OAA and thus reduces activity of TCA cycle.

☞ SALIENT POINTS TO REMEMBER

- Lipoproteins are conjugated proteins containing lipids as prosthetic group.
- TG (Triacyl glycerol) is hydrophobic (water-insoluble). It is coated with more "polar" substances like PL, cholesterol and cholesterol esters and a specific apoprotein and forms hydrophilic (water soluble) complexes.
- Lipoprotein are separated by
  1. Ultra centrifugation - chylomicrons, very low density lipoproteins (VLDL), Low Density Lipoproteins (LDL) and high density lipoproteins (HDL).
  2. Electrophoresis-chylomicrons, β-Lipoproteins (LDL), Pre-β-lipoproteins (VLDL) and α-lipoproteins (HDL).
- Chylomicrons are formed in intestine, contain specific apoprotein apo-B_{48} and are carrier of exogenous dietary TG.
- VLDL are formed in liver principally (also small extent in intestine), contain specific apoprotein apo-B_{100}, and are carrier of endogenous T.G. synthesized in liver.
- HDL is synthesized in liver principally, to a small extent in small intestine, contains specific apo-protein apo-A.
- HDL in association with "lecithin-cholesterol acyl transferase (LCAT) are responsible for the elimination of cholesterol ***("Scavenging action")*** from tissues to liver for degradation ***("Good cholesterol").***
- Delipidation of TG of chylomicrons and VLDL takes place by an enzyme called *"Lipoprotein lipase"*, which requires PL and apo-CII as cofactors.
- Injection of heparin, stimulates release of ***"Lipoprotein lipase,"*** into the circulation and is accompanied by clearing of lipaemia, hence called as ***"clearing factor".***
- Dilipidation of VLDL produces smaller particle ***IDL (Intermediate density lipoprotein). Circulating IDL particles are converted to LDL (cholesterol-rich) particles which deposits cholesterol in blood vessel walls which produces atherosclerosis.*** **("Bad cholesterol").**
- Atherosclerosis and coronary heart disease (CHD) are directly correlated with LDL and inversely with HDL.
- Primary hyperlipoproteinaemias (five types) are a group of inherited disorders characterized by elevation of one or more plasma lipoprotein fractions.
- Normal liver contains about 4 percent as total lipids, 3/4 of which is PL and 1/4 is neutral fat (TG).
- Excessive accumulation of TG in liver cells causes fatty liver, which can often be prevented by the consumption of "Lipotropic factors", viz. choline, Betaine, methionine, inositol, etc.

- Chronic alcoholism is associated with fatty liver, hyperlipidaemia and atherosclerosis. Fatty liver, if untreated, can form cirrhosis liver.

MULTIPLE CHOICE QUESTIONS

Give one correct answer:

1. **In β-oxidation of fatty acids, which of the following are utilized as coenzymes?**
   (a) FAD and FMN
   (b) NAD^+ and $NADP^+$
   (c) FAD and $NADP^+$
   (d) NAD^+ and FAD^+
   (e) FAD H_2 and NADPH.
2. **The most important source of reducing equivalents for FA synthesis in the liver is:**
   (a) Glycolysis
   (b) TCA cycle
   (c) HMP shunt
   (d) Uronic acid pathway
   (e) Gluconeogenesis
3. **Which of the following cofactors or their derivatives must be present for the conversion of acetyl CoA to Malonyl CoA in extramitochondrial denovo F.A. synthesis?**
   (a) Pyridoxine (b) Biotin
   (c) TPP (d) NAD^+
   (e) FAD
4. **All statements regarding HMG-CoA are true, *except:***
   (a) Required in Ketogenesis
   (b) Involved in synthesis of FA
   (c) It is formed in cytosol
   (d) An intermediate in cholesterol biosynthesis
   (e) Enzyme involved is HMG-CoA synthase
5. **During each cycle of β-oxidation of F.A. all the following compounds are generated, *except:***
   (a) $FADH_2$ (b) $NADH + H^+$
   (c) Acyl CoA (d) CO_2
   (e) Acetyl CoA
6. **The energy yield from complete oxidation of products generated by second reaction cycle of β-oxidation of palmityl CoA will be**
   (a) 6 ATP (b) 14 ATP
   (c) 18 ATP (d) 34 ATP
   (e) 42 ATP
7. **β-oxidation of odd-carbon F.A. chain produces:**
   (a) Malonyl CoA (b) Acetyl CoA
   (c) Succinyl CoA (d) Acetoacetyl CoA
   (e) Propionyl CoA
8. **A metabolite which is common to pathways of cholesterol biosynthesis from acetyl CoA and cholecalciferol formation from cholesterol is:**
   (a) Lanosterol
   (b) 7-dehydrocholesterol
   (c) Zymosterol
   (d) Tachysterol
   (e) Ergosterol
9. **Acetyl CoA required for extra-mitochondrial de Novo FA synthesis is produced by:**
   (a) Thiolase (b) Citrate Lyase
   (c) PDH (d) Malic enzyme
   (e) Acetyl-CoA synthetase
10. **The rate limiting step in cholesterol biosynthesis is:**
    (a) Mevalonate kinase
    (b) Thiolase
    (c) HMG-CoA Lyase
    (d) HMG-CoA synthase
    (e) HMG-CoA reductase
11. **Ketone bodies are synthesized from FA oxidation, produces by which of the following organs:**
    (a) Erythrocytes (b) Skeletal muscles
    (c) Brain (d) Liver
    (e) Kidney
12. **LCAT activity is associated with which of the lipoprotein complex?**
    (a) LDL (b) VLDL
    (c) IDL (d) HDL
    (e) Chylomicrons

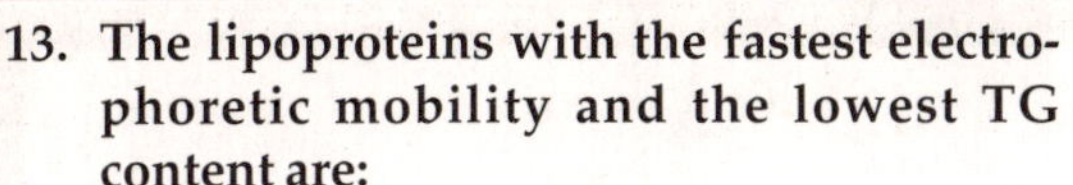

13. The lipoproteins with the fastest electrophoretic mobility and the lowest TG content are:
(a) LDL (b) HDL
(c) VLDL (d) IDL
(e) Chylomicrons

14. All of the following tissues are capable of utilizing ketone bodies as 'fuel', *except:*
(a) Erythrocytes (b) Cardiac muscle
(c) Skeletal muscle (d) Renal cortex
(e) Brain

15. The major source of cholesterol in arterial smooth muscle cells is from:
(a) HDL (b) VLDL
(c) LDL
(d) Chylomicrons
(e) All of the above

16. Triacylglycerol (TG) Present in VLDL is hydrolyzed by:
(a) Lipoprotein lipase
(b) Colipase
(c) Hormone sensitive TG lipase
(d) Intestinal lipase
(e) Pancreatic lipase

ANSWERS

1. (d)	2. (c)	3. (b)	4. (b)
5. (d)	6. (d)	7. (e)	8. (b)
9. (b)	10. (e)	11. (d)	12. (d)
13. (b)	14. (a)	15. (c)	16. (a)

Metabolism of Proteins and Amino Acids

AMINO ACIDS IN BLOOD AND TISSUES

1. Amino Acid Pool

- Amino acids, on absorption from intestine are carried to liver through portal blood. They are taken up by liver cells to some extent and remainder enters the systemic circulation and diffuse throughout the body fluids and taken up by tissue cells.
- At the same time, most of the tissue proteins both *"structural"* proteins and *"functional"* proteins, (including plasma proteins) are continually undergoing disintegration to release amino acids (except the "essential" amino acids).
- ***Amino acids from all these sources get mixed up*** to constitute what is known as general **"amino acid pool"** of the body.
- Amino acid pool has no anatomical reality but represents an availability of amino acid building units. ***No functional distinction can be drawn between the fate of the amino acids derived from the dietary source and those derived from the tissue breakdown.***
- All tissues including exocrine and endocrine glands draw freely from the amino acid pool to synthesize the tissue proteins, enzymes and protein hormones. ***Amino acid is taken up by each cell according to its own specific needs,*** to be built into the cell structure and materials as required.
- If a cell takes up as much amino acids as it loses, it is in a state of ***dynamic equilibrium,*** if the loss is greater, the cell wastes, and if the gain is greater the cell grows.
- ***In man, the protein turnover involves the breakdown and synthesis of 80 to 100 gm of tissue proteins perday,*** about half of it occurring in liver. On an average, plasma proteins are completely replaced every 15 days. the "pool" is constantly undergoing **depletion** because:
    - Large scale deamination of presumably surplus amino acids take place.
    - Amino acids and their derivatives, viz. urea, creatinine are lost in the urine and other excretions.
    - Amino acids are continually being built up into those proteins, e.g. hair, collagen proteins, which are not part of dynamic systems.
- On the other hand, amino acid pool is being always **re-established** by amino acids, derived from the following:
    - Re-amination of certain non-nitrogenous residues.
    - Amination of appropriate fragments which are present in the common metabolic pool (and therefore derived from carbohydrate and fat breakdown).
    - Amino acids split off from dietary proteins and absorbed from the intestine into the blood.

This state is called ***continuing metabolism*** of the amino acids.

2. Amino Acids in Blood

- All the amino acids occur in blood in varying concentration and make a total of 30 to 50 mg/ 100 ml in the "post-absorptive" state.
- In terms of amino acid N_2, it is 4 to 5 mg/100 ml.
- Following a protein containing meal, the amino acid levels rise to 45 to 100 mg per 100 ml (amino acid N_2 6 to 10 mg/100 ml).

3. "Circadian" Changes in Plasma Amino Acid Levels:

- The plasma levels of most amino acids do not remain constant throughout 24 hours period; but rather change by varying in ***circadian rhythm*** about a "mean" value. This was first noted for the amino acid "tyrosine" and later on confirmed for most other amino acids.
- In general, plasma amino acids levels are lowest at early morning (4 am) and rise 15 to 35 percent by noon to early afternoon.
- Amino acids present at the highest mean concentration, e.g. glycine, alanine, valine, serine, etc. change the least, whereas those present at a low mean concentration, e.g. trytophan, phenylalanine, methionine, cysteine, tyrosine, etc. show most striking changes in level. ***The exact physiological significance of the circadian changes occurring in plasma amino acids levels remain to be elucidated.***

4. Tissue Amino Acids:

The amino acids are transported into tissues **"actively"**. Pyridoxal-P (B_6-P) is one of the requirement for this active transport. ***Tissue uptake is also favoured by hormones.***

- ***Insulin, growth hormone*** and ***testosterone*** favour the uptake of amino acids by tissues ***("anabolic" hormones).***
- Oestradiol stimulates selectively their uptake by uterus.
- Epinephrine and glucocorticoids stimulate the uptake of amino acids by the liver.

Sources and utilization of blood amino acids are shown schematically in ***Fig. 14.1.***

NITROGEN BALANCE

In an adult healthy individual maintaining a constant weight, the amount of intake of N in food (mainly as dietary proteins) will be balanced by an excretion of an equal amount of N in urine (in the form of urea mainly, uric acid, creatinine/and creatine, and amino acids contribute to a minor extent) and in faeces (mainly as unabsorbed N.) The individual is then said to be in ***nitrogen balance*** or ***nitrogenous equilibrium.***

Experiments measuring N-intake and excretion under specified conditions are called ***nitrogen balance experiments studies.***

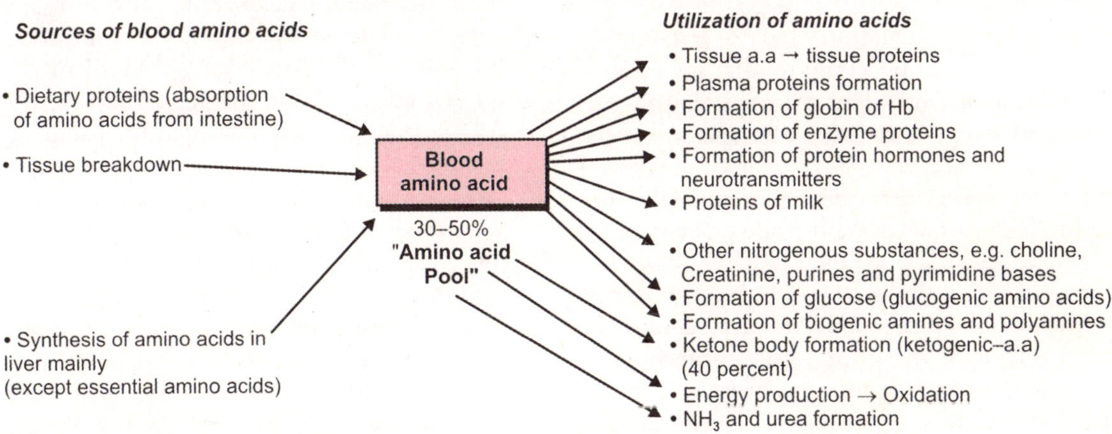

Fig. 14.1: Sources and utilization of amino acids

- A subject in nitrogenous equilibrium is said to be in **nitrogen balance,** i.e. intake of N equalizes the output.
- A subject whose intake of N is *greater* than the output, e.g. in growth, is said to have a ***positive nitrogen balance.*** In the growing period and also during covalescence from illness or when anabolic hormones are given, the body puts on weight and N-intake will be more than N-output, since some of the N is retained as tissue proteins.
- A subject whose intake of N is *less* than the output of N, (e.g. in losing weight), is said to have a ***negative nitrogen balance.*** In old age and during illness and starvation, weight is lost and results in negative nitrogen balance.

Lability of Proteins

There is no special storage form for proteins like glycogen for carbohydrates or fats in adipose tissue. Protein storage is always accompanied by tissue growth.

During starvation when protein is not available from the dietary sources, it is the liver, which loses the largest proportions of its proteins compared to other proteins. Additions of proteins in food similarly cause an appreciable increase in liver weight first. Thus, ***the liver proteins appear to be more labile*** than the proteins of other tissues. Kidney and blood proteins come next in degree of lability.

Types of Proteins Required for N-balance: To establish N-balance, certain minimum amounts of proteins or equivalent amino acids must be provided to replace the inevitable losses from the dynamic equilibrium and metabolic utilization of amino acids. This minimum replacement requires amino acids of specific type in adequate amounts and in appropriate ratios. They are ***"essential amino acids"*** which must be provided in the diet ***simultaneously together*** and they cannot be synthesized in the body. It is impossible to maintain N-equilibrium on diets which are deficient in any one or more of these essential amino acids, no matter how much protein is consumed. Examples of some incomplete proteins:

- **Gelatin:** lacks tryptophan
- **Zein** of corn/maize: low in both tryptophan and lysine.

ESSENTIAL AMINO ACIDS

Definition: An essential or indispensable amino acid is defined as one which cannot be synthesized by the organism from substances ordinarily present in the diet at a rate commensurate with certain physiological requirements and they must, therefore, be supplied in the diet usually combined in proteins.

Non-essential Amino Acids: The non-essential or dispensable amino acids can be synthesized in the body:

- By the amination of appropriate non-nitrogenous fragments derived from other sources.
- In special cases, directly from the essential amino acids, e.g. ***formation of tyrosine from phenylalanine or formation of cysteine from methionine.***
- But it should be emphasized that the body is "spared" the trouble of this synthesis if the dispensable amino acids are also available in the diet ***sparing effect.***

Features of Essential Amino Acids

- Animals given a basal diet which contains no proteins or amino acids, but which is otherwise complete in all respects, will rapidly die; if, however, right type of protein supplements are added, then normal health and reproductive power are maintained in adult animals and growth occurs in young animals.
- By measuring the N-balance on various amino acid supplements, it has been found that following ***eight amino acids*** are indispensable for human adults under normal conditions. ***Exclusion of any one of these essential amino acids leads to a negative N-balance*** manifesting as loss of weight, fatigue, loss of appetite and nervous irritability. When missing essential amino acid is supplemented in the diet, perfect health is promptly restored.

- The **eight** essential amino acids are: ***valine, leucine, isoleucine, threonine, methionine, phenylalanine, tryptophan, and lysine.***

Mattvilphly is used to remember eight essential aminoacids. The formula also contains two semi essential amino acids arginine and Histidine.

Note:
- Presence of tyrosine in the diet can spare 70 to 75% of the phenylalanine requirement in humans *(sparing action).*
- Similarly, presence of cystine/and cysteine in the diet can spare 80 to 90% of methionine requirement in humans.

Administration of "complete group": A curious fact concerning essential amino acids to be noted is that the ***complete group of eight amino acids must be administered to the organism simultaneously*** and ***together***. If a single essential amino acid is omitted from the group and fed separately several hours later, the nutritional effectiveness of the entire group is impaired. The ***"excess" amino acids, not utilized in absence of a missing one, are almost completely oxidized during the elapsed period and not utilized for tissue protein synthesis.***

Optimal ratio of essential amino acids in the diet should approximate that found in carcass of the animal concerned. ***Significant deviations from the "optimal ratio" result in certain adverse effects.*** True imbalance of amino acids can occur when the diet is marginal or suboptimal in one essential amino acid, whereupon increasing the dietary level of another essential amino acid sets up an imbalance and growth is decreased.

Quantitative aspect: How much to take? For normal adult, ***the minimum amount of each essential amino acid*** which must be supplied/ per day when all other amino acids are present, has been set as ***0.3 to 1.0 gm of the natural L-form.*** **Rose** after performing experiments on animals suggested that a "safe" intake would be double of the amount mentioned.

"Semi-essential" amino acids: In addition, animal growth experiments indicate that dietary supplies of two other amino acids ***histidine*** and ***arginine*** may be required under ***conditions of growth or equivalent physiological stress as pregnancy and lactation.*** The capacity of the body to synthesize histidine and arginine, though adequate for protein maintenance, may not suffice for the more extensive calls of protein accumulation.

DISSIMILATION OF AMINO ACIDS (N-Catabolism of Amino Acids)

$$R-\overset{\alpha}{C}H(NH_2)-COOH$$

Aminoacid

In mammalian tissues, α-NH_2 group of amino acids, derived either from the diet or breakdown of tissue proteins, ultimately is converted first to $\mathbf{NH_3}$ and then to **urea** and is excreted in the urine.

$$\alpha\text{-}NH_2 \text{ group} \rightarrow NH_3 \rightarrow \text{urea} \downarrow \text{excreted in urine}$$

The formation of urea involves the action of several enzymes. ***Formation of NH_3 and urea can be discussed under the following heads:***
- *Transamination*
- *Deamination* →
  - *Oxidative deamination*
  - *Non-oxidative deamination*
- *Transdeamination*
- *NH_3 transport*
- *Formation of urea*

Vertebrates other than mammals share all features of the above scheme except urea formation.

Urea is the characteristic end-product of amino acid N-catabolism in human beings and ***ureotelic*** organisms.

Urea synthesis is replaced by:
- Uric acid formation in ***uricotelic*** organism, e.g. reptiles and birds; and
- NH_3 in ***ammonotelic*** organism, e.g. bony fish.

TRANSAMINATION

It was first discovered by **Braunstein** and **Kritzmann** (1947). *It is a process of combined deamination and amination.*

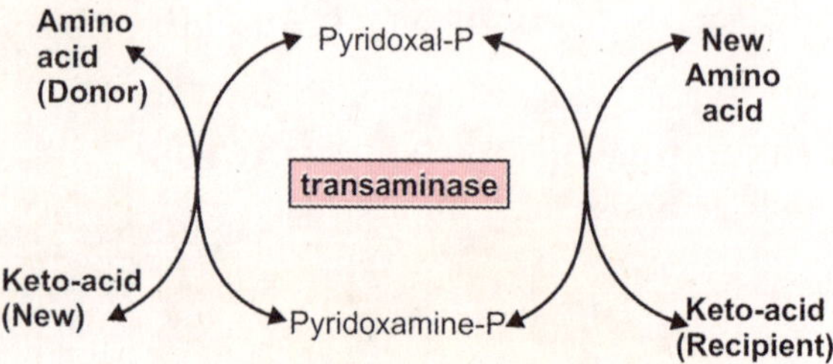

Definition: Transamination is a ***reversible*** reaction in which ***α-NH_2 group of one amino acid is transferred to a α-keto acid resulting in the formation of a new amino acid and a new keto acid.***

The general process of transamination may be represented as follows:

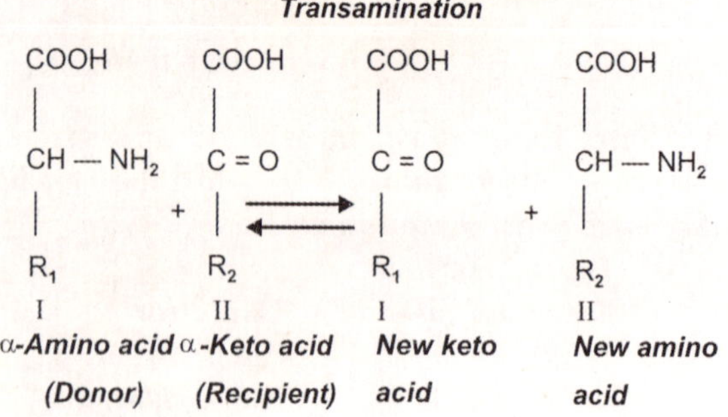

Donor amino acid (I) thus becomes a new keto acid (I) after losing the α-NH_2 group, and the recipient keto acid (II) becomes a new amino acid (II) after receiving the NH_2 group.

Note: The process ***represents only an inter-molecular transfer of NH_2 group*** without the splitting out of NH_3. ***NH_3 formation does not take place by transamination reaction.***

Salient Features:

- ***Reversible reaction:*** The reaction is reversible and is catalyzed by enzymes.
- ***Site of transmination:*** Transamination takes place principally in liver, kidney, heart and brain. But the enzyme is present in almost all mammalian tissues and transamination can be carried out in all tissues to some extent.
- ***Enzymes concerned:*** The enzymes concerned in transamination are called **transaminases** (better called as **amino-transferases.**
- ***Coenzyme for the reaction:*** The coenzyme required for the reaction is **pyridoxal-P** (B_6P). In the process of transamination, the amino acid reacts with enzyme-bound pyridoxal-P which then yields keto acid and pyridoxamine-P. The pyridoxamine-P then reacts with a second keto acid to produce a similar enzyme bound complex, which then decomposes forming a second new amino acid and regenerates the pyridoxal-P. The role of pyridoxal-P is shown above.

Specific transaminases**:** There are **two transaminases of clinical importance** in the body in that they use specific amino acid and specific keto acid. These **two specific transminases** are:

- ***Aspartate transaminase (or Aspartate amino transferase):*** Previously used to be called as S-GOT ***(serum glutamate oxaloacetate transaminase).***

  In this, aspartic acid is the donor amino acid and α-oxoglutarate is the recipient keto acid. New amino acid formed is always glutamic acid.

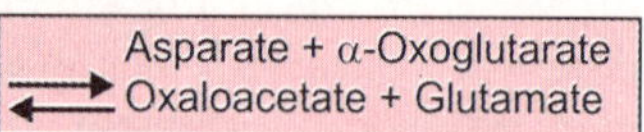

- ***Alanine transaminase (or Alanine amino-transferase):*** Previously used to be called as **S-*GPT (Serum glutamate pyruvate transaminase).***

  In this, alanine is the donor amino acid and α-oxoglutarate is the recipient keto acid. New amino acid formed is again always glutamic acid.

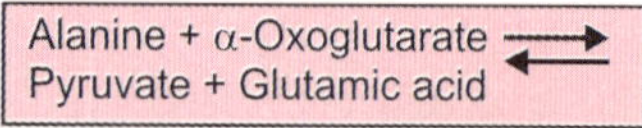

- ***Amino acids which do not take part in transamination:*** Though most of the amino acids can act as substrates for transamination, there are certain exceptions. ***Exceptions include:***

- **Lysine**
- **Threonine**
- **The cyclic imino acids, proline and OH-proline.**

- There are a few transaminases which do not utilize the three keto acid recipients men-tioned above.
- Transamination is not restricted to α-NH_2 groups. The δ-NH_2 group of ornithine is readily transaminated forming glutamate γ-semialdehyde.

Clinical Significance: As mentioned above two specific transaminases are of clinical importance.

1. ***Aspartate transaminase (Aspartate amino transferase or aminoferase): S-GOT (old nomenclature)***
   - Normal serum activity is 4 to 17 IU/L (7 to 35 Karmen units/ml).
   - ***Concentration of the enzyme is very high in myocardium and also in liver cells.*** The enzyme is also distributed in other tissues, viz. muscles, pancreas, kidney, etc. The enzyme is ***cytoplasmic*** and also ***mito-chondrial.***
   - Helpful in acute myocardial infarction, serum activity of the ***enzyme rises sharply within the first 12 hours, with a peak at 24 hours or over and returns to normal within 3 to 5 days.*** Level can be correlated with extent and size of the infarct.
   - Not increased in coronary insufficiency, and angina pectoris.
   - ***Other extra cardiac factors:***
     - Increases in ***liver diseases,*** but it is less than alanine transaminase (S-GPT).
     - Increase in ***muscular dystrophies:*** myositis. No increases in muscular disease of nervous origin.
     - Increased activity seen in ***acute pancreatitis, leukaemias and acute haemolytic anaemia.***
     - In normal persons, after prolonged severe exercise.
     - A rise has been seen in therapy with erythromycin.
2. ***Alanine transaminase (Alanine amino trans-feraseor aminoferase)-S-GPT (old nomencla-ture):***
   - The enzyme is found mainly in liver, liver cells are rich. It is entirely ***cytoplasmic*** (cf. S-GOT).
   - Normal enzyme activity is 3 to 15 IU/L (6-32 Karmen units/ml).
   - Most helpful in diagnosis of liver diseases. Increases in both transaminases are common finding in hepatic diseases but always S-GPT more than S-GOT, though in normal healthy persons, S-GOT is slightly more than S-GPT.
   - It is most useful in assessing severity and progress of the disease in ***acute viral hepatitis.*** Serial estimations are most useful. Highest values of enzyme activity seen in acute viral hepatitis, peak values 250 to 1500 IU/L or more seen at the time of maximum illness.
   - It is useful for 'screening' in outbreaks of acute viral hepatitis-useful for segregating the contacts.
   - Limited value in differential diagnosis of jaundice.
   - In other liver diseases: Less than 250 IU/L seen in uncomplicated portal cirrhosis, extrahepatic biliary obstruction and also in hepatic malignancy, primary/or second-ary.

DEAMINATION

Deamination is the process by which N of amino acid is removed as NH_3.

Types: It can be of **2 types:**

- ***Oxidative deamination***
- ***Non-oxidative deamination***

A. Oxidative Deamination

- ***Site of Oxidative Deamination:*** **Krebs (1935)** studied deamination of amino acids in various tissue slices and found **liver** and **kidney** to be very active.

- ***Enzymes:*** He also demonstrated the presence of ***D and L-amino acid oxidases*** in these tissues, which can act on D-and L-amino acids respectively, and can oxidatively liberate NH_3 from these amino acids. Essential differences between these two enzymes are tabulated below.
  Note: It is to be noted that it is rather peculiar that despite the absence of D-amino acids in tissues the activity of D-amino acid oxidases is generally much greater than that of the L-amino acid oxidases. The function of the D-amino acid oxidases is not clear.
- ***Nature of L-Amino Acid Oxidases:*** The amino acid oxidases are ***auto-oxidizable*** flavoproteins. The reduced flavoproteins are ***re-oxidized at substrate level directly by molecular O_2 forming H_2O_2*** without participation of cytochromes of electron transport chain or other electron carriers. The H_2O_2 formed is toxic to cells and is converted immediately to O_2 and H_2O by enzyme *catalase*.
  Note: It is to be noted, if catalase is absent genetically, the α-keto acid produced by oxidative deamination is decarboxylated non-enzymatically by H_2O_2 forming a carboxylic acid with one less carbon atom.
- ***Process of Oxidative Deamination:*** This takes place in two steps:
  - The amino acid is first dehydrogenated by the flavoprotein (FP) of the enzyme, *L-amino acid oxidase*, forming an ***"α-imino acid"***.
  - In the next step, water molecule is added spontaneously, and decomposes to the corresponding α-keto acid, with loss of the α-imino nitrogen as NH_3.

The process of oxidative deamination is shown schematically ***(Fig. 14.2)***.

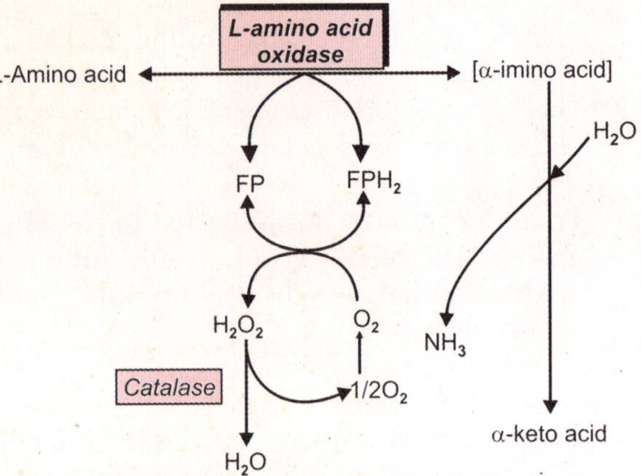

Fig. 14.2: Oxidative deamination

- ***Remarks and Conclusion***
  - Mammalian L-amino acid oxidase, an FMN-flavoprotein is restricted to liver and kidney only.
  - Activity of the enzyme in these tissues is quite low.
  - It does not have any effect on glycine, or the L-isomers of the dicarboxylic or β-OH-α-amino acids.

Hence, it is concluded that this enzyme does not fulfil a major role in mammalian amino acid catabolism and formation of NH_3.

B. Non-oxidative Deamination: There are certain amino acids, which can be non-oxidatively deaminated by specific enzymes, and can form NH_3. These reactions do contribute to NH_3 formation, but again they do not fulfil a major role in NH_3 formation.

D-amino acid oxidase	*L-amino acid oxidase*
• Can act on D-amino acids only	• Can act on L-amino acids only
• Can be readily extracted with water-'free' form	• Bound to tissue particles and not extractable with water
• Contains FP (FAD)	• Contains FP (FMN)

Examples of non-oxidative deamination are:

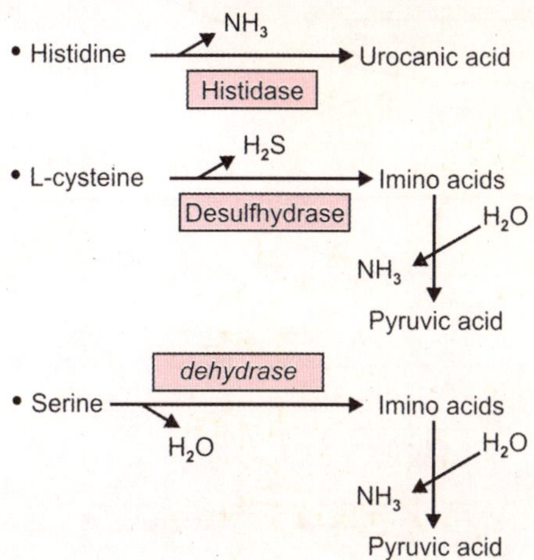

TRANSDEAMINATION (DEAMINATION OF L-GLUTAMIC ACID)

It is to be noted that L-glutamic acid is not deaminated by *L-amino acid oxidase* but by a specific enzyme called *L-glutamate dehydrogenase*. ***Characteristics of the enzyme L-glutamate dehydrogenase:***

- A Zn^{++} containing metalloenzyme, one atom of Zn^{++} present in each peptide chain.
- It is widely distributed in tissues in humans and has high activity.
- Specific for L-glutamate.
- It requires NAD^+ or $NADP^+$ as coenzyme.

Reaction: The enzyme *L-glutamate dehydrogenase* catalyzes the deamination of L-glutamate to form α-iminoglutaric acid, which on addition of a molecule of water forms NH_3 and α-ketoglutarate *(Fig. 14.3)*.

- It is to be noted that the ***reaction is reversible,*** and the equilibrium constant favours glutamate formation, but the quick removal of NH_3 to form urea in urea cycle and α-ketoglutarate to TCA cycle favours onward reaction, i.e. NH_3 formation.

Remarks and Conclusion: The amino groups of most amino acids are transferred to α-ketoglutarate by specific transaminases by the process of transamination forming L-glutamate as end-product. Release of this N_2 as NH_3 from

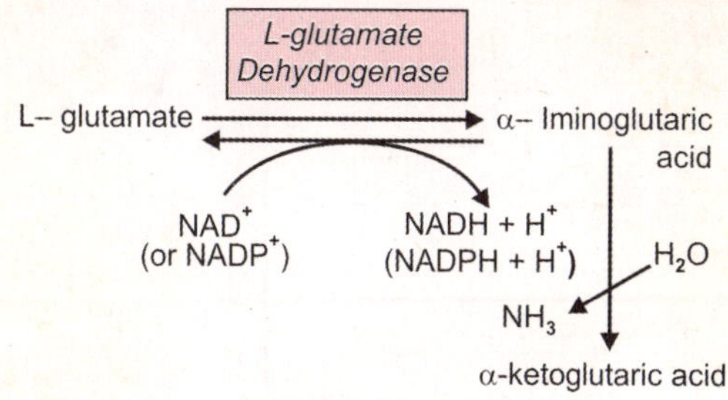

Fig.14.3: Deamination of glutamic acid

L-glutamate is catalyzed by *L-glutamate dehydrogenase*, an enzyme of high activity and wide distribution in mammalian tissues. It is suggested that the coupled action of an amino acid-α-oxoglutarate transaminase and L-glutamate dehydrogenase might explain the oxidative deamination of L-amino acids. As it involves first transamination and coupled with oxidative deamination, the process is called as **transdeamination.** This mechanism seems to be the major pathway for removal of NH_2 group from an L-amino acid and formation of NH_3.

Other sources of NH_3:

- From glutamine by hydrolysis by the enzyme *glutaminase.*
- Absorption from gut produced by intestinal bacteria, which can be a major source in intestinal obstruction.
- Pyrimidine catabolism.

NH_3 TRANSPORT

Formation of NH_3 has been discussed above and different sources from which NH_3 is formed are shown *Fig. 14.4.* It is stressed that in addition to NH_3 formed in the tissues, a considerable quantity of NH_3 is produced in the gut by intestinal bacterial flora, both.

- From dietary proteins; and
- From urea present in fluids secreted into the GI tract.

- This NH_3 is absorbed from the intestine into portal venous blood which contains relatively high concentration of NH_3 as compared to systemic blood.

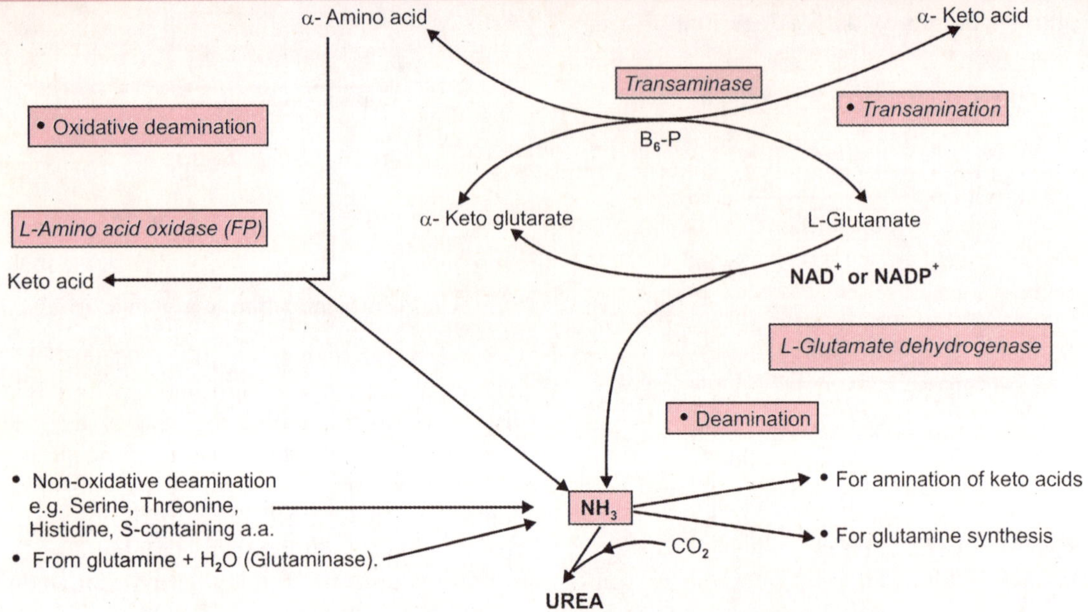

Fig. 14.4: Overall pattern of N-removal from an L-amino acid

- Under normal conditions of health, liver promptly removes NH_3 from the portal blood, so that blood leaving the liver is virtually NH_3-free. This is essential since even minute quantities of NH_3 are toxic to CNS.

Clinical Significance

- With severely impaired hepatic function or the development of collateral communications between portal and systemic veins as may occur in cirrhosis liver, the portal blood may bypass the liver.
- Surgically produced shunting procedures so called "Eck-fistula" or other forms of "portocaval shunts" are conducive to NH_3 intoxication, particularly after ingestion of large quantities of proteins or after haemorrhage in GI tract.

Normal Blood Ammonia Level: In man, normal blood level of NH_3 varies from 40 to 70 μg/100 ml.

- Free NH^+_4 (ammonium ion) concentration of fresh plasma is less than 20 μg per 100 ml.

Clinical Aspect

Hyperammonaemia: Hypermmonaemia is associated with comatose states such as may occur in hepatic failure. It may be **two types:**

- ***Acquired hyperammonaemia:*** Is usually the result of cirrhosis of the liver with the development of a collateral circulation, which shunts the portal blood around the organ, thereby severely reducing the synthesis of urea.
- ***Inherited hyperammonaemia:*** Results from genetic defects in the urea cycle enzymes.

Features of NH_3 Intoxication: The symptoms of NH_3 intoxication include:

- A peculiar flapping tremor;
- Slurring of speech;
- Blurring of vision; and
- In severe cases leads to coma and death.

These features resemble those of syndrome of hepatic coma where blood and brain NH_3 levels are elevated.

Why NH_3 is Toxic? The cause of NH_3 toxicity is not definitely known. Following associated biochemical changes are important.

- Increased NH_3 concentration enhances amination of α-ketoglutarate, an intermediate in TCA cycle to form glutamate in brain. ***This reduces mitochondrial pool of α-ketoglutarate consequently depressing the TCA cycle,*** affecting the cellular respiration.
- Increased NH_3 concentration enhances "glutamine" formation from glutamate and thus reduces 'brain-cell' pool of glutamic acid. Hence, there is ***decreased formation of inhibitory neurotransmitter "GABA" (γ-amino butyric acid) ↓.***
- Rise in brain glutamine level enhances the outflow of glutamine from brain cells. Glutamine is carried 'out' by the same "transporter" which allows the entry of 'tryptophan' into brain cells. Hence, 'tryptophan' concentration in brain cells increases which leads to abnormal increases in the synthesis of **"serotonin",** a neurotransmitter.

Metabolic fate of NH_3 in the body:

Three metabolic fates are:

- Mainly NH_3 is converted to urea (urea cycle).
- Formation of glutamine.
- Amination of α-keto acid to form α-amino acid.

UREA FORMATION (KREBS-HENSELEIT CYCLE)

The removal of excess of NH_3 derived from amino acid catabolism in the tissues or from bacterial action in the gut is accomplished by the production of urea which is excreted in the urine. Steps of urea synthesis have been elucidated by Krebs and Henseleit (1932) (see ***Fig. 14.5***)

Characteristic Features:

- It is a ***cyclic process:*** **Five reactions** which ***involve ornithine, citrulline, arginine*** and ***aspartic acid.***
- ***Site of synthesis:*** Urea formation takes place in **liver** in mammals and all of the enzymes involved have been isolated from liver tissue.

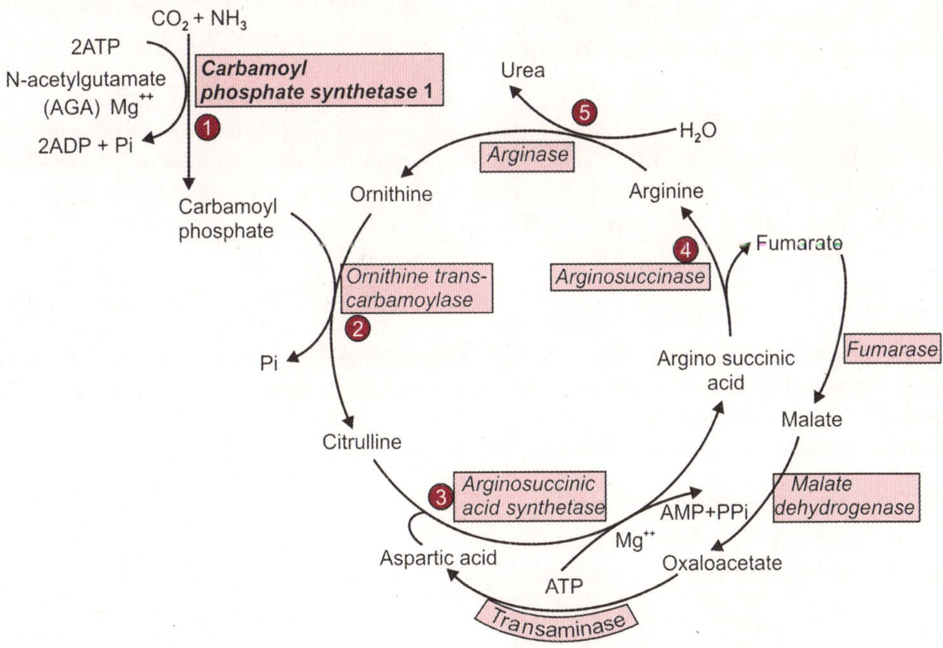

Fig. 14.5: **Biosynthesis of urea on ornithine-urea cycle**

- *Kidneys:* Urea cycle operates in a limited extent. ***Kidney can form up to arginine*** but cannot form urea, as enzyme *arginase* is absent in kidney tissues.
- ***Brain: Brain can synthesize urea from citrulline but lacks the enzyme*** for forming citrulline from ornithine.

  Thus, neither the kidneys nor the brain can form urea in significant amounts.
- *Location of enzymes:* Partly mitochondrial and partly cytosolic.
- One mol of NH_3 and one mol of CO_2 are converted to one mol of urea for each turn of the cycle and ***ornithine is regenerated at the end, which acts as a catalytic agent.***
- The overall process in each turn of cycle ***requires 3 mols of ATP.***

Stages: The reactions of urea cycle can be studied in **five** sequential enzymatic reactions.

Reaction 1. Synthesis of carbamoyl phosphate
Reaction 2. Synthesis of citrulline
Reaction 3. Synthesis of arginino-succinate
Reaction 4. Cleavage of arginino-succinate
Reaction 5. Cleavage of arginine to form ornithine and urea.

Reaction 1: Synthesis of Carbamoyl-P (Mitochondrial): In this reaction, HCO^-_3, NH^+_4 and phosphate derived from ATP reacts to form 'carbamoyl-P' (also called carbamoyl-P). The reaction is catalyzed by the *mitochondrial* enzyme *carbamoyl synthetase I.*

- **Role of N-Acetyl Glutamate (AGA):** Exact role of N-acetyl glutamate is not known. Its presence brings about some conformational changes in the enzyme molecule and affects the affinity of the enzyme for ATP.

Formation of Carbamoyl-P

Carbamoyl synthetase I

$HCO^-_3 + NH^+_4 \xrightarrow{Mg^{++}} {}^+H_3N—C(=O)—O—P(=O)(O)—O$

N-Acetyl glutamate (AGA)

2 ATP → 2 ADP + Pi

Carbamoyl-P

- **Role of Biotin:** Earlier it used to be thought that biotin is required for activation of CO_2 but now it is known that biotin does not take part.

Reaction 2: Synthesis of Citrulline (Mitochondrial):

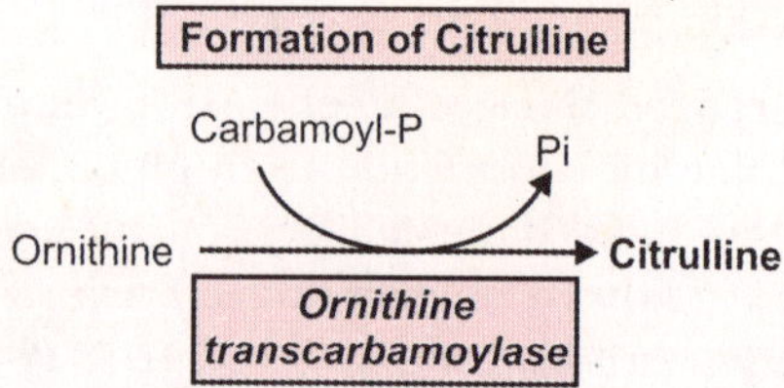

- Ornithine transcarbamoylase enzyme, also called as ornithine carbamoyl transferase is found associated with carbamoylphosphate synthetase I in the mitochondrial matrix. During this reaction, the δ-NH_2 group of orinithine attaches to the carbanyl group of carbamoyl-P and the phosphate group (Pi) is released.

Note:

- Ornithine which is regenerated in cytosol in the 5th reaction, is transported into the mitochondrial matrix by a ***specific "transport protein"*** in the inner mitochondrial membrane.
- Similarly, citrulline which is produced in mitochondrial matrix is transported across the inner mitochondrial membrane to the cytosol by a specific "transport protein".

Reaction 3: Synthesis of Argininosuccinate (Cytosolic):

- After citrulline has been transported to the cytosol, it condenses with Aspartate to form argininosuccinate in an ATP dependent reaction catalyzed by *arginino-succinate synthetase.*

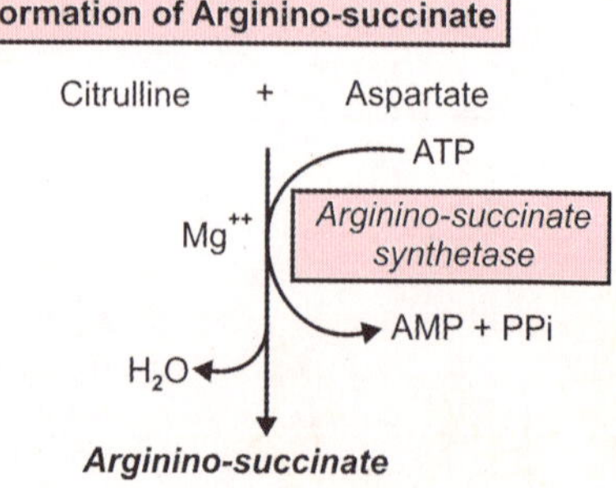

Reaction 4: Cleavage of Arginino-Succinate (Cytosolic):

Formation of Arginine

Arginino-succinate → **Arginine** + **Fumarate**

Arginino-succinase

- In this reaction of urea cycle, the enzyme ***arginino-succinase*** also known as ***arginino succinate lyase*** catalyzes conversion of arginino-succinate to arginine and fumarate. ***The urea cycle is linked to the TCA cycle through the production of fumarate.*** Amino acid catabolism is, therefore, directly coupled to energy production.
- *Arginino-succinase* is ***cold-labile enzyme*** of mammalian liver and kidney tissues. Loss of activity in the cold is associated with dissociation into two protein components. This dissociation is prevented by Pi, arginine, and arginino-succinate.

Fate of Fumarate: The fumarate is converted to oxaloacetate (OAA) via the *fumarase* and *malate dehydrogenase* reactions and then transaminated to regenerate aspartate to participate in the cycle.

Formation of Aspartate from Fumarate

Fumarate + H_2O → Malate (*Fumarase*)

Malate + NAD^+ → Oxaloacetate (OAA) + $NADH + H^+$ (*Malate dehydrogenase*)

Oxaloacetate (OAA) → **Aspartate** (*Transaminase*; from glutamate (NH_2))

Reaction 5: Cleavage of Arginine to Ornithine and Urea:

- The last reaction of the urea cycle which completes the cycle. It is catalyzed by the enzyme *arginase*, which is found only in the liver cells.
- Arginase catalyzes hydrolysis of the guanidine group of arginine, releasing urea and regenerating ornithine.
- Ornithine now enters mitochondrion through inner mitochondrial membrane by a specific receptor protein.

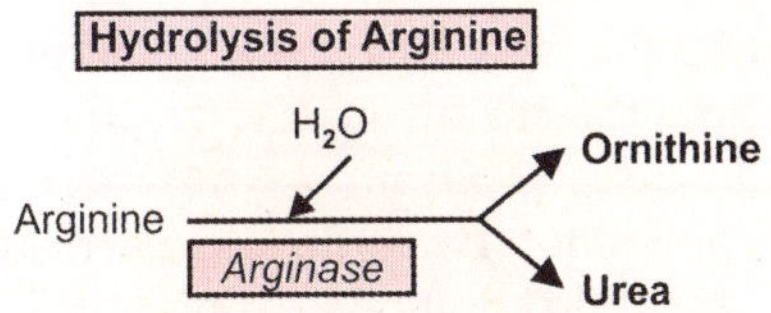

Significance of Urea Cycle

- ***Detoxification of NH_3:*** Major biological role in the pathway is the detoxication of NH_3, toxic ammonia is converted into a nontoxic substance urea and excreted in urine.
- ***Biosynthesis of Arginine:*** The urea cycle also serves for the biosynthesis of arginine from ornithine in liver, kidney and intestinal mucosa. Kidney and intestinal mucosa probably contribute most of the body arginine because they possess all the urea cycle enzymes ***except arginase.*** Hence they can form upto arginine and cannot form urea. ***The arginine is used for protein synthesis.***

Source of C and N of Urea

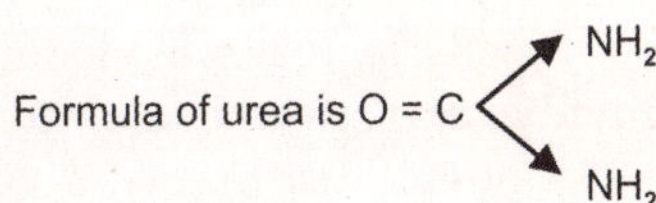

- One nitrogen of NH_2 group is derived from the NH^+_4 ion (Reaction 1).
- Other nitrogen of NH_2 group is provided by aspartate (Reaction 3).
- Bicarbonate, HCO^-_3 ion, provides the carbon atom of urea.

Regulation of Urea Synthesis

- Achieved by linkage of mitochondrial glutamate dehydrogenase with carbamoyl-P-synthetase-I.Carbamoyl-P-synthetase I is thought to act in conjunction with mitochondrial glutamate dehydrogenase to channelize nitrogen from glutamate and, therefore, from all amino acids as NH_3 and then through carbamoyl-P and thus finally to urea.

- Though the equilibrium constant of the glutamate dehydrogenase reaction favours glutamate formation rather than formation of NH_3, but removal of NH_3 by the carbamoyl-P-synthetase I reaction and oxidation of α-ketoglutarate by TCA cycle favours the glutamate catabolism.
- The above effect is favoured by the presence of ATP, which in addition to being a requirement for carbamoyl-P-synthetase I reaction, it also stimulates *glutamate dehydrogenase* activity unidirectionally in the direction of NH_3 formation ***(Fig. 14.6).***

CLINICAL SIGNIFICANCE OF UREA

A moderately active man consuming about 300 gm of carbohydrates, 100 gm of fat and 100 gm of proteins daily must excrete about 16.5 gm of N daily. Almost 95% is eliminated by the kidneys and the remaining 5%, for the most part as N, in the faeces.

I. Normal Level: The concentration of urea in normal blood plasma from a healthy fasting adult ranges from 20 to 40 mg%. Indians take less proteins hence normal level in Indians varies from 15 to 40 mg%.

II. Increased Levels: Increases in blood urea may occur in a number of diseases in addition to those in which the kidneys are primarily involved. The causes can be classified as:

• Prerenal • Renal and • Postrenal

1. Prerenal: Most important are conditions in which plasma vol/body fluids are reduced.

- Salt and water depletion.
- Severe and protracted vomiting as in pyloric and intestinal obstruction.
- Severe and prolonged diarrhoea.
- Pyloric stenosis with severe vomiting.
- Haematemesis.
- Haemorrhage and shock; shock due to severe burns.
- Ulcerative colitis with severe chloride loss.
- In crisis of Addison's disease (hypoadrenalism).

2. Renal: The blood urea can be increased in all forms of kidney diseases:

- In acute glomerulonephritis.
- In early stages of Type II nephritis (nephrosis) the blood urea may not be increased, but in later stages with renal failure, blood urea rises.
- Other conditions are malignant nephrosclerosis, chronic pyelonephritis and mercurial poisoning.
- In diseases such as hydronephrosis, renal tuberculosis; small increases are seen but depends on extent of kidney damage.

3. Postrenal Diseases: These lead to increase in blood urea, when there is obstruction to urine flow. This causes retention of urine and so reduces the effective filtration pressure at the glomeruli; when prolonged, produces irreversible kidney damage. Causes are:

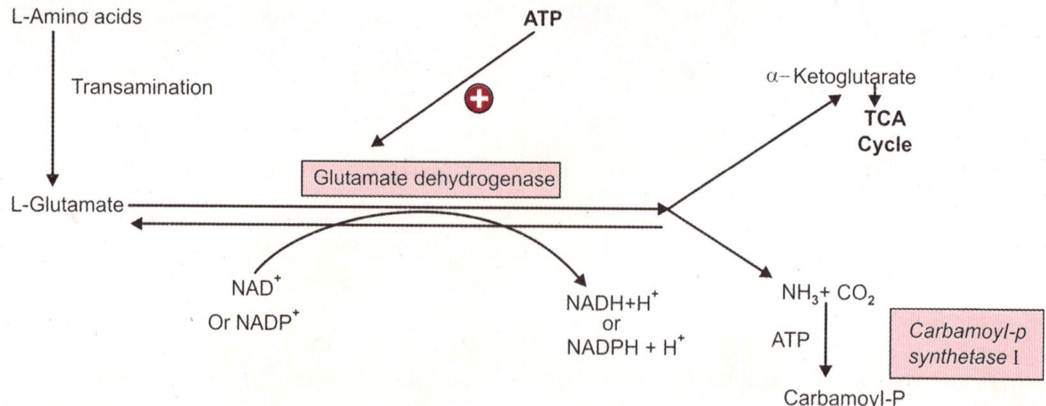

Fig. 14.6: Regulation of urea synthesis

- Enlargement of prostate.
- Stones in urinary tract.
- Stricture of the urethra.
- Tumors of the bladder affecting urinary flow.

Note: Increase in blood urea above normal is called ***'uraemia'***.

III. Decreased Levels:

Decreases in blood urea levels are rare and may be seen in:

- Some cases of severe liver damage.
- Physiological condition: blood urea has been seen to be lower in pregnancy than in normal non-pregnant women.

INHERITED DISORDERS ASSOCIATED WITH UREA CYCLE

Inherited disorders due to inherited deficiency of enzymes of urea cycle have been described.

1. **Hyperammonaemia Type I:**
   - A familial disorder.
   - Enzyme deficiency: *carbamoyl-P-synthetase I.*
   - Produces hyperammonaemia and symptoms of ammonia toxicity.
2. **Hyperammonaemia Type II:**
   (Also called "Ornithinaemia")
   - ***Inheritance.*** X-chromosome linked enzyme-*ornithine transcarbamoylase* deficiency.
   - Produces hyperammonaemia and symptoms of NH_3 toxicity.
   - ***Blood, urine and CS fluid:*** show characteristically increased level of glutamine - (glutamine synthesis is enhanced).
3. **Citrullinaemia:**
   - A rare disorder.
   - ***Inheritance:*** Autosomal recessive.
   - ***Enzyme deficiency:*** *Arginino-succinate synthetase.*
   - ***Clinically:*** It presents with hyperammonaemia and NH_3 toxicity, and mental retardation.
   - ***Biochemically:*** Blood and CSF shows increased level NH_3 and marked increase in citrulline. Large quantities of citrulline are excreted in urine (1 to 2 g/d).
4. **Arginino-succinic Aciduria:**

A rare inherited disorder, usually fatal. It manifests before 2 years of age and terminates fatally in early life.

- ***Inheritance:*** Autosomal recessive.
- ***Enzyme deficiency:*** *Argininosuccinase* (also called Arginino succinate lyase).

Clinically: Hyperammonaemia and NH_3 toxicity, Mental retardation, Occurrence of friable, tufted hairs called "tricorrhexis nodosa".

Biochemically:

- Blood and CS fluid show elevated levels of arginino-succinate.
- Increased excretion of arginino-succinate.
- The enzyme deficiency has been demonstrated in brain, liver, kidney and RB cells of the patient.

5. **Hyperargininaemia:**

- ***Enzyme deficiency:*** *Arginase,* deficient in liver and RB cells.
- ***Clinically:*** Manifests as hyperammonaemia.
- ***Biochemically:***
  - Blood and CSF show elevated levels of arginine.
  - Increased urinary excretion of lysine, cystine, ornithine and arginine.
  - Low protein diet resulted in lowering of plasma NH_3 levels and disappearance of urinary lysine-cystinuria pattern.

GLUTAMINE FORMATION AND FUNCTIONS

Chemically glutamine is *δ-amide of α-amino-glutaric acid.* ***Glutamine formation is a manoeuvre to remove NH_3 from blood,*** another mechanism of ammonia detoxication in many tissues. ***Glutamine serves as an important reservoir of NH_3 nitrogen in tissues which can be drawn upon for various synthetic processes.***

Synthesis of Glutamine:

- Glutamine is synthesized in tissues from glutamic acid and NH_3 by the action of the enzyme *glutamine synthetase*, a mitochondrial enzyme.

- The reaction is ***irreversible.***
- It requires ATP.
- **Site:** Synthesis takes place in tissues such as liver, kidney, brain and retina.

The reaction is shown below:

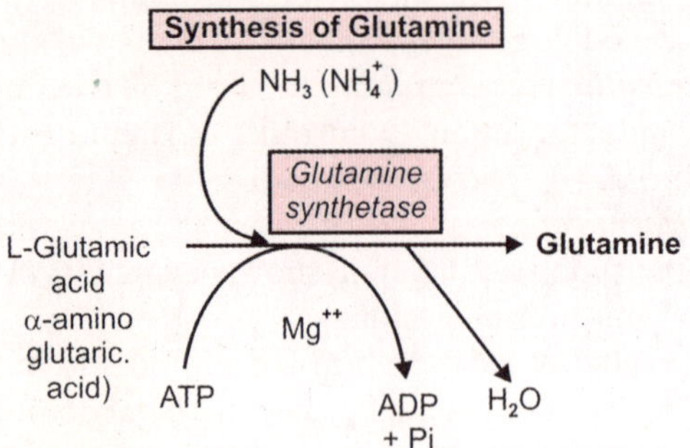

Blood Level of Glutamine: Blood glutamine is probably mostly synthesized in liver. Normal blood plasma level in humans ranges from 6 to 12 mg%. It represents approximately 18 to 25% of total free amino nitrogen of the plasma.

Hydrolysis of Glutamine:

- A ready source of NH_3.
- Glutamine is hydrolyzed by a specific enzyme *glutaminase.*
- The reaction is ***irreversible.*** The reaction can occur in various tissues specially liver, kidney, brain and retina.

Note: The reaction is specially important in renal distal tubular epithelial cells where it is a source of NH_3. Which is used for exchange of Na^+, thus conservation of base.

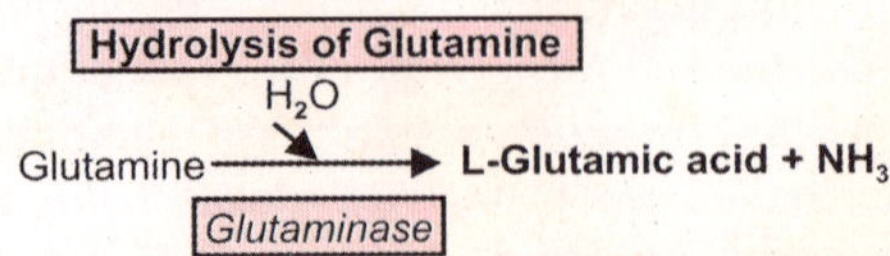

Functions of Glutamine:

1. ***Transamidation:*** Formation of glucosamine-6-P. The amide-N of glutamine can be transferred to a keto group.

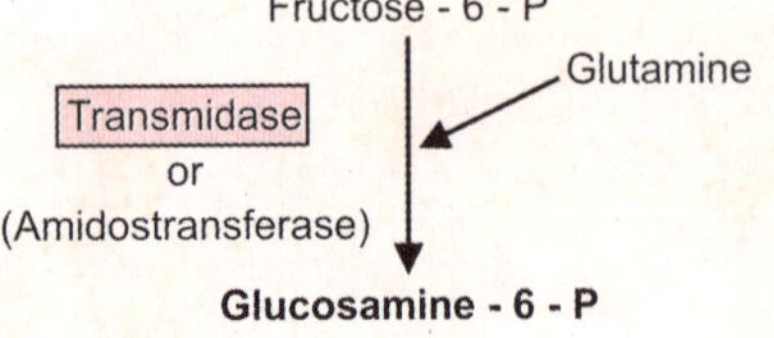

2. ***Formation of guanylate (GMP):*** The amide group of glutamine is transferred to C-2 of xanthylate (XMP), by the enzyme GMP *synthetase*, forming guanylate (GMP).

3. ***Role of glutamine in kidney: Conservation of Na^+:*** Glutamine is hydrolyzed to give NH_3 in kidney tubules. NH_3 combines with H^+ to form NH_4^+, and exchange with Na^+ in tubular lumen. Na^+ is reabsorbed to blood.

4. ***Role of glutamine in brain:*** The role of glutamate in detoxifying NH_3 in the brain by formation of glutamine is extremely important.
   - Glutamate is a major acceptor of NH_3 produced either in the metabolism or delivered to the brain when arterial blood NH_3 is elevated ↑. In this latter reaction, glutamic acid accepts one molecule of NH_3 and is thus converted to glutamine.
   - Formation of urea does not play a significant role in the removal of NH_3 in the brain.
   - When the levels of NH_3 in brain increases, as in hepatic failure, the supply of glutamic acid from the blood may be insufficient to form the additional amounts of glutamine required to detoxify the NH_3 in the brain. Under these circumstances, glutamic acid is synthesized in the brain by amination of α-ketoglutarate produced by TCA cycle within the brain itself. However, continuous utilization of α-ketoglutarate for this purpose would rapidly deplete the TCA cycle of its intermediates. Repletion is achieved by CO_2-fixation, involving PA to form OAA, which enters the TCA cycle and proceeds to the formation of α-ketoglutarate.

Clinical Aspect

Estimation of CS fluid glutamine level has been taken as ***indirect evidence of hepatic function test.***

- Normal range of CSF glutamine in health ranges from to 6 to 14 mg%.
- Studies have shown, ***in cirrhosis liver,*** CSF glutamine level is increased ↑ and ranges from 16 to 31 mg%.
- ***In hepatic failure and hepatic coma,*** very much increased values are obtained, ranging from 30 to 54 mg% or more.

- In *coma, due to various other causes, normal CSF glutamine level is obtained.*

It has been observed that high CSF glutamine level has a bad prognosis. The *dividing line 40 mg% has been kept.* Values greater than 40 mg% in hepatic failure cases usually show bad prognosis and ends fatally.

5. *Role of Glutamine in Conjugation Reaction:* In man and chimpanzee, phenyl acetic acid is conjugated with glutamine to form *"phenyl acetyl glutamine"*, which is excreted in urine.

Clinical Aspect

In inherited disorder "phenyl ketonuria", phenyl acetic acid is produced in increased amounts, which is conjugated with glutamine and *excreted in urine as phenyl acetyl glutamine.* It accounts for the *"mousy smell"* of urine in these patients.

6. **Role in cancer:** Recently *glutaminase* and *asparaginase* have both been investigated as "anti-tumour agents", since certain tumours exhibit abnormally high requirements for glutamine and asparagine for their growth.

AMINATION OF α-KETO ACIDS TO FORM AMINO ACIDS

NH_3 is also used to aminate certain α-keto acids to form corresponding α-amino acids.

Examples are:

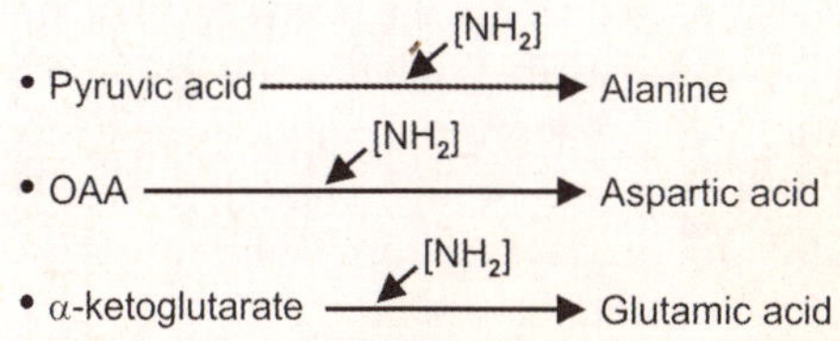

FATE OF C-SKELETONS

The fate of the keto acids yielded by removal of the-NH_2 group of the amino acids are now be considered. The keto acids formed after removal of NH_3 can undergo one of the following *3 fates.*

- *Reamination to form original amino acids.*
- *Formation of CO_2, H_2O and energy, after entering TCA cycle.*
- *Formation of glucose (glucogenic) or ketone bodies (ketogenic) or both.*

It has been shown about 60 gm (approx. 58 G.) of glucose are formed and excreted in the urine for 100 gm of proteins metabolized. In other words, **60% of protein is potentially glucogenic.**

- **"Glucogenic" (antiketogenic):** They form on deamination "amphibolic" intermediates, keto acids, which enter the TCA cycle and either can be oxidized to CO_2 and H_2O or they can go reverse pathway and form glucose or glycogen.
- **Ketogenic:** After deamination, they yield keto acids, which during subsequent oxidation to H_2O and CO_2, pass through the stage of "aceto acetate".
- **Both glucogenic and ketogenic:** The amino acids of this group give rise to both glucose and ketone bodies.

List of amino acids of the above three groups is given in *Table 14.1.*

Glucose: Nitrogen ratio (G : N ratio):

(Dextrose: Nitrogen ratio D : N ratio)

- It is ratio of glucose and nitrogen excreted in urine.
- G:N ratio (also called D : N ratio) is important, as it reflects the conversion of protein into glucose.

Table 14.1: Glucogenic, Ketogenic and Both Glucogenic and Ketogenic Amino Acids

Glycogen (Glucogenic amino acids)	*Fat (Ketogenic amino acids)*	*Both glycogen and fat (Glucogenic and ketogenic)*
• Alanine • Arginine • Aspartate • Cysteine/Cystine • Glycine • Glutamate • Histidine • OH-proline • Methionine • Proline • Serine • Threonine • Valine	• L-Leucine	• Isoleucine • Lysine • Phenylalanine • Tyrosine • Tryptophan

- It is experimentally proved by measuring the glucose and nitrogen excreted in urine in:
  - "Phloridzinized" animal (when glucose is not reabsorbed in renal tubules but are excreted).
  - "Starving" animal (as amino acids contribute to formation of glucose by gluconeogenesis, as glycogen store is depleted).
- The nitrogen excreted in such an animal comes from catabolism of proteins and the urinary glucose is thought to be formed from proteins. It is assumed that ***1 gm of urinary nitrogen represents 6.25 gm of proteins.***
- ***Normally, the G:N ratio = 3.65:1, i.e. 3.65 gm of glucose has come from 6.25 gm of proteins.***

  $\therefore \frac{3.65 \times 100}{6.25} = 58\%$ is the average conversion rate.

SALIENT POINTS TO REMEMBER

- The body proteins are not static, they are in dynamic state, body proteins undergo degradation and synthesis.
- Amino acids are absorbed from intestine after digestion of dietary proteins. At the sametime, body proteins undergo degradation liberating amino acids.
- Amino acids from these sources get mixed up to constitute the *general "amino acid pool".*
- ***Amino acid pool has no anatomical reality but represents an availability of amino acid building units.***
- If intake of N equalizes the output, the subject is said to be in nitrogen balance.
- A subject whose intake of N^- is greater than the output is said to be in positive nitrogen balance, e.g. in growth.
- A subject whose intake of N^- is less than the output of N^-, is said to be in Negative nitrogen balance, e.g. old age, illness, starvation.
- Nitrogen of α-NH_2 group of an amino acid is removed as NH_3 by a process of transamination and deamination, called transdeamination.
- As NH_3 is toxic, it is converted to urea in liver and excreted in urine.
- α-NH_2 gr of a.a. $\rightarrow NH_3 \rightarrow$ urea $\rightarrow$ excreted in urine.
- Transamination does not produce NH_3. It is a reversible reaction in which α-NH_2 group of one amino acid is transferred to a α-keto acid resulting in formation of a new amino acid and new keto acid.
- New amino acid produced by specific transaminases always form glutamic acid.
- Glutamic acid is deaminated by a specific enzyme ***"Glutamate dehydrogenase"*** of wide occurrence to form NH_3.
- Small amount of NH_3 is also formed to some extent by oxidative and non-oxidative deamination.
- NH_3 accumulation in blood is toxic to brain. Increased NH_3 concentration enhances amination of α-ketoglutarate to form glutamate in brain. This reduces mitochondrial pool of α-ketoglutarate resulting to depression of TCA cycle and cellular respiration.
- NH_3 toxicity is characterized by: slurring of speech, blurring of vision, a peculiar flapping tremor and in severe cases leads to coma and death.
- In mammals, NH_3 is converted to urea, a nontoxic excretory product, in liver and excreted in urine.
- Metabolic defects in urea cycle, due to inherited deficiency of enzymes, can produce hyperammonaemia.
- In mammals, in brain NH_3 is detoxicated by Glutamic acid which forms glutamine by the enzyme *"Glutamine synthetase"*.
- Glutamine is temporary store house of NH_3. Free NH_3 can be liberated from glutamine by hydrolysis by the enzyme *"Glutaminase"*.
- CS fluid glutamine level in normal ranges from 6 to 14 mg percent. In hepatic failure and hepatic coma it is very much increased ranging from 30 to 54 mg percent or above. It can be used as indirect hepatic function test.

- Urea has two NH_2 groups. One nitrogen of NH_2 group is derived from the NH_4^+ ion and the other nitrogen of NH_2 group is provided by the amino acid aspartic acid.
- Blood urea estimation is commonly used to assess renal function. Elevation of blood urea level above normal 15 to 40 mg percent is associated with several disorders which may be prerenal, renal and postrenal.
- The c-skeleton of an amino acid after removal of N as NH_3 can be:
  - reaminated to form original a.a.
  - formation of CO_2, H_2O and energy after entering TCA cycle (oxidized).
  - can form glucose (glucogenic amino acids or fats (ketogenic a.a.) or both glucogenic and ketogenic.

DECARBOXYLATION REACTIONS AND BIOGENIC AMINES

Decarboxylation: Decarboxylation is the reaction by which CO_2 is removed from the—COOH group of an amino acid as a result an amine is formed.

Formation of Biogenic Amine

$$\underset{\text{Amino acid}}{R-\underset{NH_2}{\underset{|}{CH}}-COOH} \xrightarrow[B_6-P]{CO_2} \underset{\textbf{Amine}}{R.\ CH_2-NH_2}$$

Decarboxylase

- The reaction is catalyzed by the enzyme *decarboxylase*, which requires pyridoxal-P (B_6-PO_4) as co-enzyme.
- Tissues like liver, kidney and brain and also microorganisms of intestinal tract possess the enzyme decarboxylase. The enzyme removes CO_2 from COOH group and converts the amino acid to corresponding amine. This is mostly a process confined to putrefaction in intestines and produces amines. Biogenic amines formed from various amino acids and their biologic importance are listed in ***Table 14.2.***

Table 14.2: Biogenic Amines and Their Functions

Amino acids	*Amine*	*Biologic importance*
• **Tyrosine**	Tyramine	• Increases blood pressure (vasoconstriction) • Contracts uterus
• **Trytophan**	Tryptamine	• Tissue hormone—a derivative 5-OH Tryptamine (serotonin) • Vasoconstriction • BP ↑
	5-Methoxy tryptamine (Melatonin)	• Hormone of pineal gland
• **Histidine**	Histamine	• Vasodilator, BP ↓ • HCl ↑ • Pepsin ↑
• **Serine**	Ethanolamine	• Forms choline by three methylations • Constituent of phospholipid like cephalin
• **Threonine**	Propanol amine	• Constituent of Vitamin B_{12}
• **Cysteine**	β-mercaptoethanolamine	• Constituent of coenzyme A.
• **Aspartic**	β-alanine	• Constituent of pantothenic acid (coenzyme A) • As a constituent of dipeptide carnosine and anserine
• **Glutamic acid**	γ-amino butyric acid (GABA)	• Presynaptic inhibitor in brain. • Forms a bypass in TCA cycle (GABA-shunt)
• **3,4, di-OH-phenylalanine (DOPA)**	Dopamine	• Precursor of epinephrine and nor-epinephrine
• **Cysteic acid**	Taurine	• Constituent of bile acid taurocholic acid
• **Lysine**	Cadaverine	• Product of Putrefaction
• **Ornithine**	Putrescine	• Product of Putrefaction
• **Arginine**	Agmatine	• Product of Putrefaction

SOME OF THE IMPORTANT BIOGENIC AMINES

1. Histamine: ***Histamine is formed by decarboxylation of amino acid "Histidine"*** by the enzyme *Histidine decarboxylase or aromatic L-amino acid decarboxylase* in presence of B_6-PO_4.

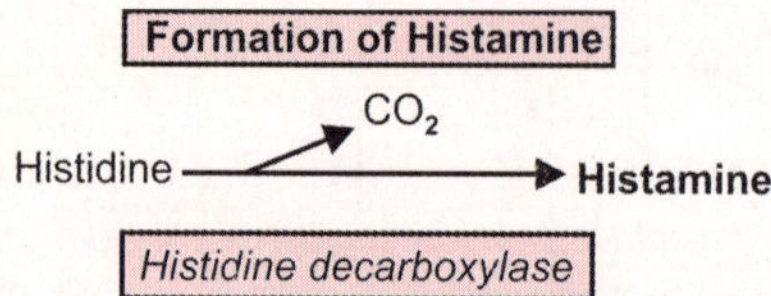

Site of formation: Mast cells are the chief source of histamine in the tissues and histamine constitutes about 10% of the weight of mast cell granules. Also produced by gastric mucosa cells and histaminergic neurones of the central nervous system.

- ***Basophils are the chief source of histamine in the circulating cells.***
- Also produced in the gut by bacterial decarboxylation of histidine.

Storage: Other than in the enterochromaffin cells of the gastric mucosa, virtually no histamine is stored in the tissues except for that found in mast cells.

Mechanism of Action and Effects

- Histamine acts as ***a neurotransmitter***, particularly in the hypothalamus.
- It acts as ***an anaphylactic and inflammatory*** agent on being released from mast cells in response to antigens.
- Effects of released histamine are mediated through 2 types of receptors designated as H_1 and H_2 receptors.
  Similarities and differences between H_1 and H_2 receptors action are given in Box, next page

Applied Clinical Aspect

Elevated plasma levels of histamine have been demonstrated in various clinical conditions.

- Patients with anaphylaxis, provoked by exercise or antigen. Such reactions are related to the explosive liberation of histamine caused by entrance of the sensitizing substances in the tissues.
- During spontaneous episodes of increased symptoms in patients with ***"mastocytosis"*** mast cell tumour.
- During experimentally induced angiooedema in patients with cold urticaria.
- In patients with antigen-induced bronchial asthma.

Actions through H_1 receptors	*Actions through H_2 receptors*
• Contracts smooth muscle including air ways and the GI tract	• Produces bronchodilation
• Increases venular permeability	• Increases vasopermeability dilatation
• Induces nasal mucus production	• Induces airway mucus production
• Causes pruritus with cutaneous vasodilation	• Also causes pruritus with H_2 receptor-stimulates gastric acid secretion- HCl ↑ and pepsin ↑

- Also formed in injured tissues. Excessive liberation of histamine may be related to traumatic shock. Histamine markedly depresses blood pressure ↓ and large doses may cause extreme vascular collapse.

Local Action of Histamine: Subcutaneous injection of histamine causes pruritus, erythema, circumferential flare and a central raised wheal (**"wheal and flare"**).

Blockers of Histamine (Antihistaminics):

- **Blockers of H_1 receptors:** The anaphylactic reactions can be minimized by pharmacological agents, e.g. Promethazine and Mepyramine which block H_1 receptors.
- **Blockers of H_2 receptors:** 'Cimetidine' is used to reduce the gastric acidity in peptic ulcer patients—it is blocker of H_2 receptor.

2. γ-Amino Butyric Acid (GABA): Decarboxylation of glutamic acid produces γ-amino butyric acid (GABA).

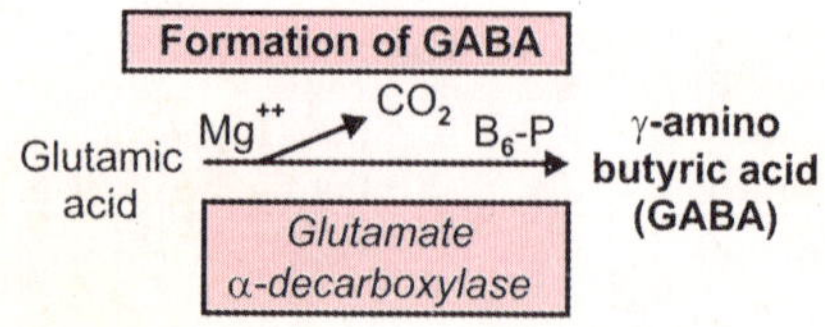

Characteristics of the Reaction:

- Reaction is ***irreversible.***
- *Glutamate α-decarboxylase* is the enzyme which catalyzes the reaction.
- It requires B_6-PO_4 as coenzyme and Mg^{++} as cofactor.

Site of Formation

- Principally formed in CN system in the grey matter. It is released partcularly in corpora quadrigemina and in diencephalon.
- Kidney also can produce but it possesses a different isoenzyme for the same reaction.

FUNCTIONS

- GABA is known to serve as a normal regulator of neuronal activity **being active as an inhibitor** (***Presynaptic inhibition***)
- It is released at the axon terminals of neurons in grey matter and acts as inhibitory neurotransmitter by enhancing K^+ permeability of postsynaptic membranes.

Clinical Aspect

Vitamin B_6 deficiency in child-ren may be responsible for some of the cases of infantile convulsions. B_6-deficiency causes less formation of GABA leading to neuronal hyperexcitability and convulsions (see vitamin B_6).

GABA Shunt: GABA by its conversion to succinic acid can form a "by-pass" in TCA cycle and this is called as GABA-Shunt ***(Fig. 14.7).***

3. Polyamines

- Polyamines are:
  - ***Spermidine***
  - ***Spermine***
- Ornithine in addition to its role in urea cycle, serves as the precursor of ubiquitous mammalian and bacterial polyamines-spermidine and spermine. Ir requires 'active' methionine.
- Normal human can synthesize approximately 0.5 n mol of spermine/day.

Structures of Natural Polyamines: Spermine and spermidine are polymers of diamino butane and diamino propane.

- **Putrescine** → 1,4-diamino butane (NH_2—$(CH_2)_4$—NH_2)
- **Spermidine** → Putrescine + 1,3-diamino propane (NH_2—$(CH_2)_3$—NH_2—$(CH_2)_4$—NH_2)
- **Spermine** → 1,3-diamino propane + Putrescine + 1,3-diamino propane. (NH_2—$(CH_2)_3$—NH—$(CH_2)_3$—NH_2)

FUNCTIONS OF POLYAMINES

- They have been implicated in diverse physiological processes and are involved in cell proliferations and growth. **Putrescine is best "marker" for cell proliferation.**
- They are ***required as 'growth factors'*** for cultured mammalian and bacterial cells.
- They have been implicated in the stabilization of intact cells, subcellular organelles and membranes.
- As polyamines have multiple +ve charges, they can associate readily with polyanions such as DNA and RNAs and have been implicated in such fundamental processes as stimulation of DNA and RNA biosynthesis, DNA stabilization and packaging of DNA in bacteriophages.

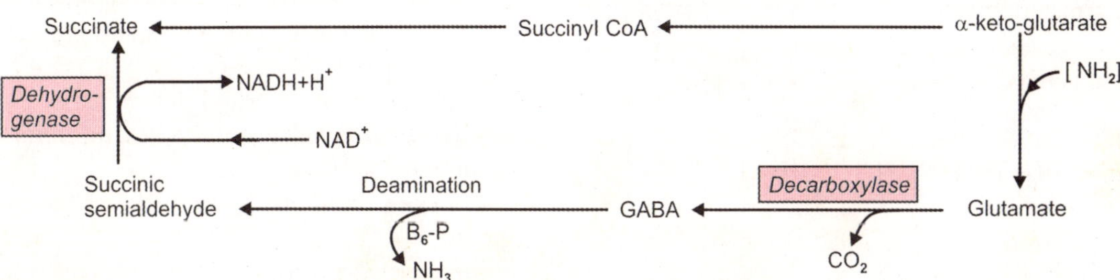

Fig. 14.7: GABA shunt

- Polyamines also exert diverse effects on protein synthesis.
- They act as inhibitor of enzymes that incluae *protein kinases.*
- Polyamines added to cultured cells induce synthesis of a *'protein antienzyme'* that binds to ornithine decarboxylase and inhibits putrescine formation.
- **Spermidine has been claimed to be best "marker" of tumour cell destruction.**
- In pharmacologic dosage polyamines have been found to be ***"hypothermic"*** and ***"hypotensive"***.

Ranges of Normal Excretion of Polyamines:

The polyamines are excreted normally in urine as conjugates. Normal values:

- Putrescine—2.7 ± 0.5 mg
- Spermine—3.4 ± 0.7 mg
- Spermidine—3.1 ± 0.6 mg

Clinical Significance

- ***Increased polyamine excretion has been claimed to be characteristic of malignant diseases.*** Thus, excretion has been reported to be increased in leukaemias, and in carcinoma of ovaries, lungs, colon, rectum, prostate, GI tract, kidney, bladder and testes.
- The urinary excretion is increased 5 to 10 times but the excretion fluctuates with the clinical state and response to treatment. Good correlation has been found between urinary excretion and clinical course.
- However, not all patients with malignant disease exhibit increased excretion of polyamines.
- **Russell et al** have postulated that ***spermidine is the best "marker" of tumor cell destruction, whereas putrescine is the best 'marker' for cell proliferation.***

METABOLISM OF INDIVIDUAL AMINO ACIDS

Two groups will be discussed in detail:

A. Metabolism of aromatic amino acids, viz. phenylalanine and tyrosine.

B. Metabolism of sulphur-containing amino acids, viz. methionine, cysteine.

The other amino acids will be discussed in brief but stress will be given on metabolic role in the body.

A. AROMATIC AMINO ACIDS

Structures of phenylalanine and tyrosine are given below.

Phenylalanine (Phe)

C_6H_5–CH_2-CH(NH_2)-COOH

α-Amino-β-phenyl propionic acid

Tyrosine (Tyr)

HO–C_6H_4–CH_2-CH(NH_2)-COOH

α-Amino-β (p-OH) phenyl propionic acid

Difference in structure: Tyrosine possesses an additional—OH group at para position of benzene ring.

Points to remember

- Phenylalanine is ***nutritionally an essential amino acid.*** It cannot be synthesized in humans, hence must be provided in diet
- Tyrosine is not essential, as it can be formed in the body from phenylalanine
- Phenylalanine is readily converted to tyrosine, but the reaction is **NOT reversible**
- The feeding of tyrosine decreases the need of phenylalanine in the diet ***("sparing action").***
- In phenyl ketonuric patient, where phenylalanine cannot be converted to tyrosine in the body due to inherited deficiency of the enzyme, ***tyrosine becomes essential amino acid to the patient***
- ***Both amino acids are 'glucogenic' and 'ketogenic'***
- Both can participate in transamination reaction

Metabolic Fate: This can be discussed as:
- Conversion of phenylalanine to tyrosine, and
- Metabolic fate of tyrosine.

1. Conversion of phenylalanine to Tyrosine: The reaction involves hydroxylation of phenylalanine at p-position in benzene ring.
- Enzyme *Phenylalanine hydroxylase* is present in liver. The conversion occurs in liver.
- ***Coenzymes and Cofactors:***

The enzyme requires the following for its activity.
- Molecular oxygen
- NADPH
- Fe^{++}
- Pteridine (folic acid) coenzyme, Tetrahydro biopterin-FH_4.

The reaction is complex and takes place in **two stages** as shown below:
- Reduction of O_2 to H_2O and conversion of phenylalanine to tyrosine, reduced form of pteridine, FH_4 acts as H-donor to the molecular O_2.
- Reduction of dihydrobiopterin, FH_2 by NADPH, catalyzed by the enzyme *dihydrobiopterin reductase.*

The overall reaction in stage I involves incorporation of one atom of molecular O_2 into the p-position of phenylalanine while the other atom of O_2 is reduced to form H_2O.

2. Metabolic Fate of Tyrosine:
- Tyrosine is degraded to produce as end products '**fumarate**' and '**acetoacetate**'.
- Fumarate is '**glucogenic**', whereas acetoacetate is '**ketogenic**'.
- Phenylalanine is catabolized via tyrosine. Hence **both phenylalanine and tyrosine are glucogenic and ketogenic.**

Reaction Sequences: Five sequential enzymatic reactions are necessary for complete degradation.

Formation of Tyrosine from Phenylalanine

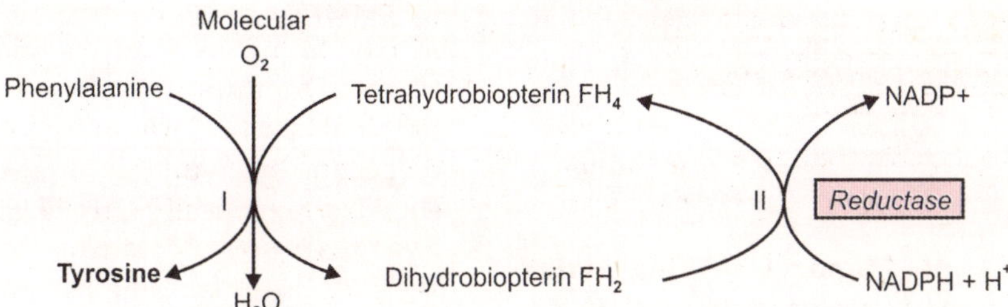

1. Conversion of Tyrosine to p-OH Phenyl Pyruvic Acid (PHPPA): Tyrosine undergoes transamination and forms p-OH-phenyl pyruvate. The reaction is catalyzed by the enzyme *tyrosine-α-ketoglutarate transaminase* which requires B_6-PO_4 and ascorbic acid.

Formation of PHPPA

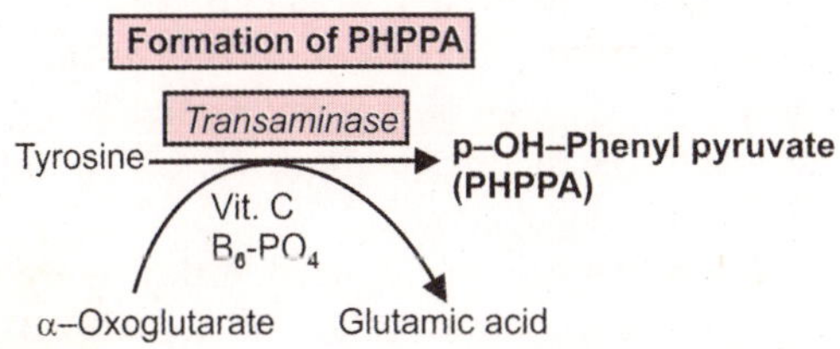

2. Conversion of p-OH-Phenyl Pyruvate to Homogentisic Acid: The reaction is catalyzed by the enzyme *p-OH-phenyl pyruvate oxidase,* which is a Cu-containing metalloenzyme. It requires ascorbic acid (vitamin C) and vitamin B_{12}.

Formation of Homogentisic Acid

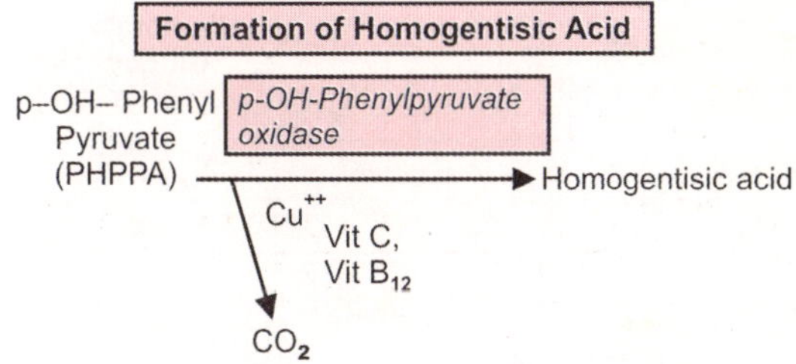

3. Conversion of Homogentisate to Maleyl Acetoacetate: The oxidative reaction is catalyzed by the enzyme *homogentisate oxidase,* an Fe-containing metalloenzyme present in liver. The benzene ring of homogentisic acid is ruptured forming "maleyl acetoacetate".

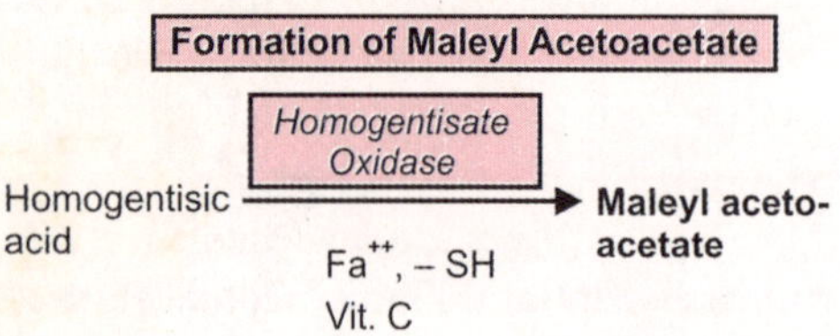

Inhibitor: ***α-α′-Dipyridil-a chelating agent can strongly bind to Fe^{++} of the enzyme and inhibits the reaction.*** Thus, homogentisic acid accumulates and appears in urine ***(experimental alkaptonuria).***

4. Conversion of Maleyl Acetoacetate to Fumaryl Acetoacetate: A cis-trans isomerization about the double bond, is catalyzed by *maleyl acetoacetate cis-trans isomerase,* a—SH enzyme present in liver.

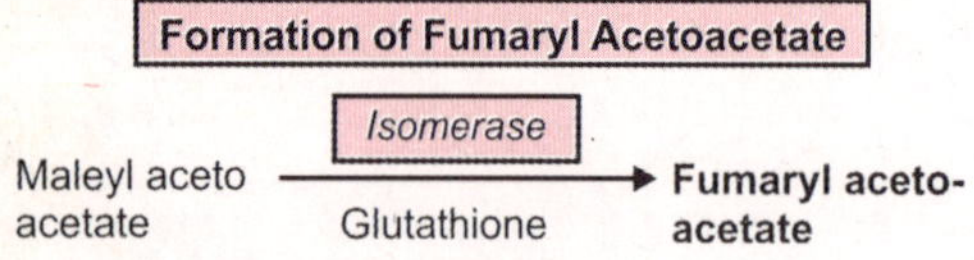

5. Hydrolysis of Fumaryl Acetoacetate: Hydrolysis of fumaryl acetoacetate is catalyzed by the enzyme *fumaryl acetoacetate hydrolase* and forms ***fumarate*** and ***acetoacetate***. Acetoacetate can then be converted to acetyl CoA and acetate by the β-ketothiolase reaction.

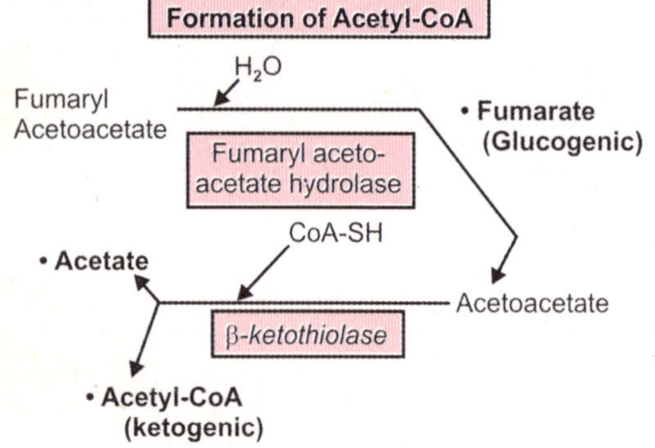

Metabolic Role of Tyrosine

Tyrosine, though 'dispensible' (non-essential amino acid), it is of great importance in human body. Many biological compounds of importance are synthesized from tyrosine. They are listed as:

- *Synthesis of thyroid hormones: Thyroxine (T_4) and tri-iodo thyronine (T_3)*
- *Synthesis of catecholamines*
- *Synthesis of melanin pigment*
- *Formation of tyramine*
- *Formation of phenol and cresol*
- *Formation of tyrosine-O-sulphate*

1. Synthesis of Thyroid Hormones

(See thyroid hormones)

2. Biosynthesis of Catecholamines: Catecholamines are ***epinephrine (adrenaline), norepinephrine (noradrenaline) and dopamine.*** All three are synthesized from tyrosine.

- Epinephrine and norepinephrine are hormones produced by adrenal medulla and dopamine is a precursor.
- *All three act as "neurotransmitters".*
- Epinephrine and norepinephrine are released at axon terminals of adrenergic sympathetic fibers. Dopamine is produced in nerve terminals particularly in hypothalamus and diencephalon. Synthesis of catecholamines is shown schematically ***(Fig. 14.9).***

3. Synthesis of Melanin: Melanins are synthesized from tyrosine in "melanosomes", membrane bound particles within melanocytes in skin which are cells of neural crest origin.

TYPES OF MELANINS

- **Eumelanins:** Are insoluble, heterogenous, high molecular weight, black to brown 'heteropolymers' of 5,6-dihydroxy indole and several of its biosynthetic precursor, viz. Leucodopachrome and dopachrome.
- **Pheomelanins:** Are yellow to reddish-brown polymers, though of high molecular weight, are soluble in dilute alkali. They contain sulfur.
- **Trichochromes:** Low molecular weight compounds, contain sulfur and are related to pheomelanins.

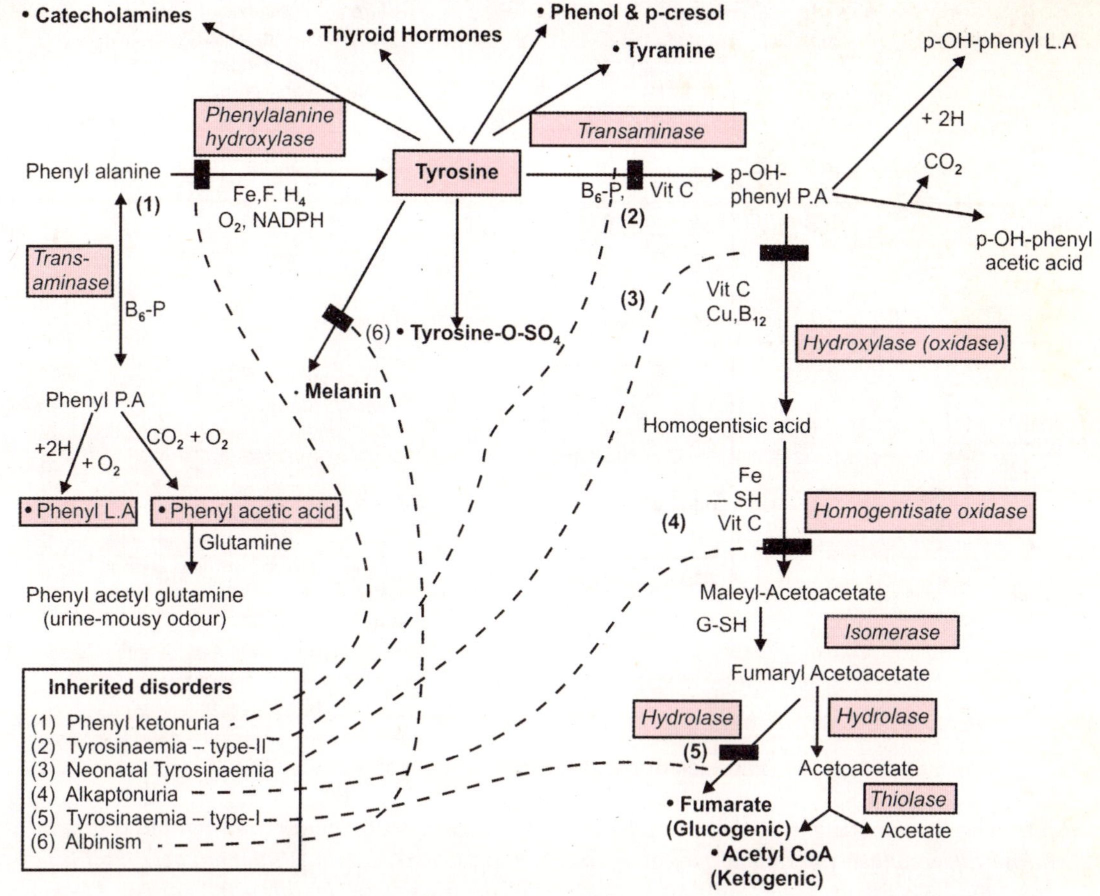

Fig. 14.8: Flow chart metabolic fate and metabolic role of phenyalanine and tyrosine

Biosynthesis is complex and not fully understood.

4. **Formation of Tyramine:** Tyramine is formed from tyrosine by decarboxylation.

5. **Formation of Phenol and Cresol:** Phenylalanine (through tyrosine) and tyrosine are acted upon by intestinal bacteria in the gut to form **p-cresol** and **phenol**. These are absorbed from the gut and conjugated in liver with H_2SO_4 and D-glucuronic acids and are excreted in urine.

6. **Formation of Tyrosine–O-Sulphate:** Tyrosine-O-sulphate is formed by sulphation by 'active' sulphate. This is present in fibrinogen molecule. During conversion of fibrinogen to fibrin two peptides are liberated, one of the peptides contains tyrosine-o-sulphate (see Plasma Protein Fibrinogen).

Metabolic fats and metabolic role of phenylalanine and tyrosine is shown schematically above refer *Fig. 14.8*.

INHERITED DISORDERS

Following disorders are associated with phenylalanine and tyrosine metabolism.

1. **Phenyl Ketonuria:** ***Classical type of phenyl ketonuria (PKU):***

- An inherited disorder with incidence of 1 in 10,000 liver births.
- ***Enzyme deficiency: Phenylalanine hydroxylase is absent.***

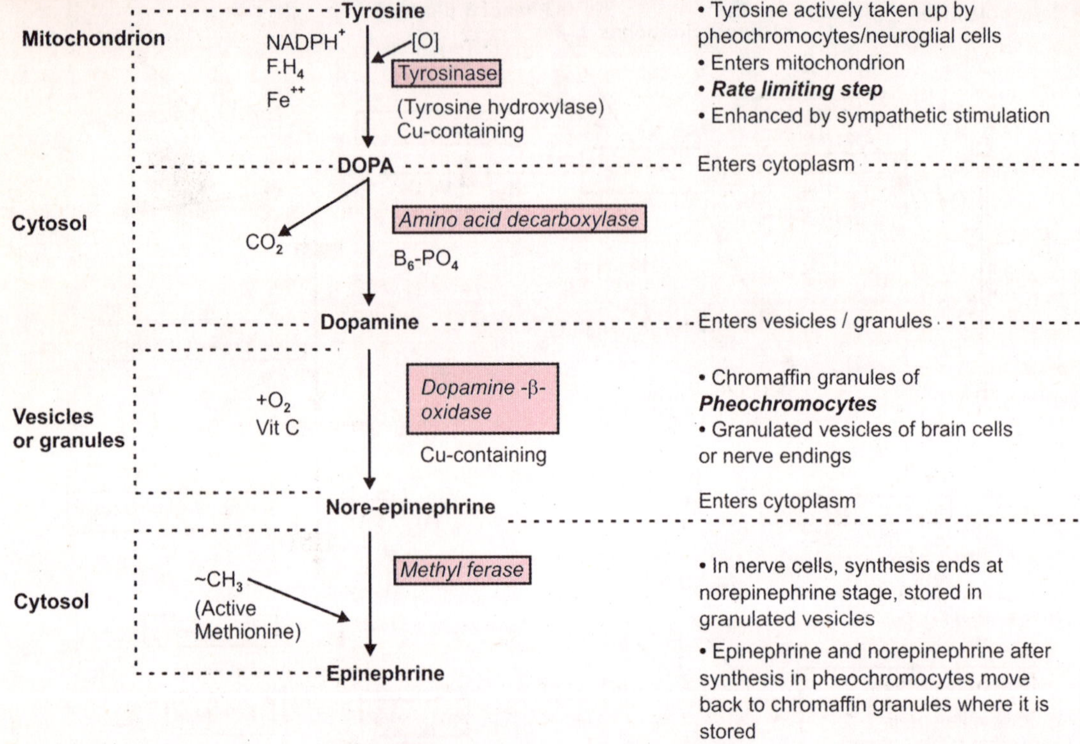

Fig. 14.9: Biosynthesis of catecholamines

Metabolic changes due to absence of *phenylalanine hydroxylase*, phenylalanine cannot be converted to tyrosine, as a result alternative catabolites are produced. Phenylalanine accumulates in the blood; Phenylalanine undergoes transamination to form phenyl pyruvic acid and its products as phenyl lactic acid and phenyl acetic acid are produced.

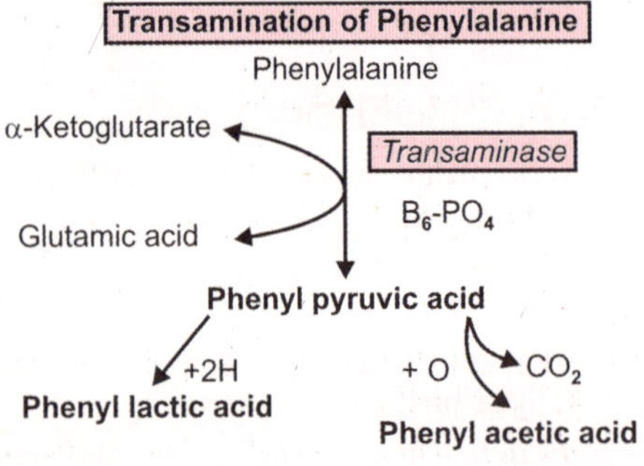

- *Phenyl acetic acid is conjugated with glutamine and excreted as phenyl acetyl glutamine in urine (responsible for "mousy odour"* of urine).
- Accumulation of phenylalanine leads to:
  - defective "serotonin" formation
  - impaired melanin synthesis. Children with the defect tend to have fair skin and fair hair; and
  - excretion of this amino acid into the intestine where it competes with tryptophan for absorption. Tryptophan becomes subject to action of intestinal bacteria resulting in formation of indole derivatives which are absorbed and excreted in urine.

Clinical features: Child is mentally retarded. Other features include seizures, psychoses and eczema.

Blood: Increased levels of phenylalanine. Normal level in blood is 1-2 mg%. It increases to 15 to 65 mg%.

Urine

- Excretion of phenylalanine, and its catabolites phenyl pyruvic acid, and phenyl lactic acid.
- Phenyl acetic acid excreted as phenyl acetyl glutamine which produces **'mousy odour'.**
- Also an abnormal O-hydroxy derivative is formed, whose ***metabolite*s** may also be found in urine.

Diagnosis:

- By estimation of plasma phenyl alanine level.
- "Screening test" for presence of phenyl pyruvate with $FeCl_3$ (in urine).
- Administration of phenylalanine to a phenylketonuric patient should result in prolonged elevation of the level of this amino acid in blood ("phenylalanine tolerance test).

Treatment: By giving diet having very low levels of phenylalanine. The diet can be terminated at 6 years of age, when high concentration of phenylalanine and its derivatives are no longer injurious to brain.

Note: In phenylketonurics, tyrosine constitutes as an essential amino acid and must be provided in the diet.

2. Alkaptonuria: A rare inborn error or hereditary defect in metabolism of phenylalanine and tyrosine. It is of historical interest that Garrod's ideas concerning heritable metabolic disorders were proposed.

- ***Inheritance:*** Autosomal recessive.
- ***Incidence:*** Estimated to be 2 to 5 per million live births. Over 600 cases have been reported in literature.
- ***Enzyme deficiency:*** Lack of the enzyme ***homogentisate oxidase.*** Homogentisic acid accumulates in the tissues and blood and appears in urine.

Clinical features:

- Most striking clinical manifestation is ***occurrence of dark urine on standing in air.*** Homogentisic acid like many derivatives of tyrosine is readily oxidized to black pigments **("alkapton").** ***Urine when exposed to air slowly turns black from top to bottom.***
- In long standing cases, deposition of homogentisic acid derivatives in cartilages of ears and other exposed places leading to generalized pigmentation of connective tissues and deposition in joints leading to arthritis, a condition called ***ochronosis. Mechanism of Ochronosis:*** The precise mechanism of ochronosis is not known. It probably involves oxidation of homogentisate by ***polyphenol oxidase, forming benzoquinone acetate; which polymerizes and binds to connective tissue macromolecules.***

Note:

- Alkaptonuria may also occur in premature infants on account of vitamin C deficiency. Condition is improved in premature infants by administration of this vitamin.
- Experimental alkaptonuria may be produced by "α-α'dipyridyl", a chelating agent of Fe.

3. Albinism: It includes a spectrum of clinical syndromes characterized by "hypomelanosis", arising from inheritred defects in the pigments cells (melanocytes) of eye and skin. There are various forms of the disease.

B. SULPHUR-CONTAINING AMINO ACIDS

- Sulphur containing amino acids are **three:**
  - *L-Methionine-Essential amino acid*
  - *L-Cysteine* } *Non-essential amino acid*
  - *L-Cystine* }
- Other sources of sulphur in the body are the sulphur-containing vitamins, thiamine vitamin β_1, lipoic acid and biotin.

Structure of S-containing Amino Acids:

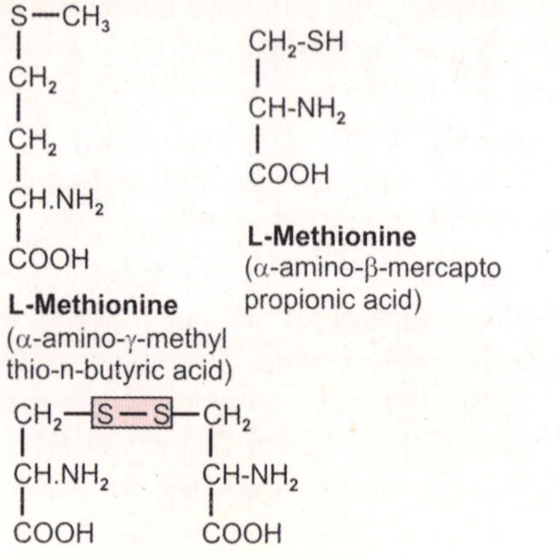

```
S—CH3
|
CH2
|
CH2
|
CH.NH2
|
COOH
```

L-Methionine
(α-amino-γ-methyl thio-n-butyric acid)

```
CH2-SH
|
CH-NH2
|
COOH
```

L-Methionine
(α-amino-β-mercapto propionic acid)

```
CH2—S—S—CH2
|          |
CH.NH2     CH-NH2
|          |
COOH       COOH
```

L-Cystine (β-β-dithio-α-amino propionic acid)

Note: The difference in structure of cysteine and cystine. Two molecules of cysteine are joined together by **S—S bond** to form one molecule of cystine.

Points to remember

- ***Methionine, cysteine and cystine are the principal sources of sulphur in the body.***
- Demethylation of methionine produces homocysteine which may be re-methylated to form methionine again.
- Cystine is reversibly convertible to cysteine and homocystine to homocysteine by oxidation reduction.
- Both methionine and cysteine can undergo transamination reaction.
- ***Methionine is an essential amino acid and has to be supplied in the diet.*** Cysteine is not essential and can be synthesized in the body from methionine.
- The presence of cysteine and cystine in the diet reduces the requirement of methionine *("sparing action".)*
- Methionine before being catabolized has to be activated first to *"active" methionine (S-adenosyl methionine)*, which can act as $-CH_3$ group donor in the body.

Metabolic Fate of L-Methionine

Metabolic fate of L-methionine can be discussed in **three stages.**

Stage 1: Activation of methionine and its demethylation to form L-homocysteine.
Stage 2: Conversion of L-homocysteine to L-homoserine.
Stage 3: Degradation of L-homoserine to end products L-propionyl-CoA and α-amino butyrate.

Stage 1: Activation of L-Methionine and its Demethylation to form L-Homoserine:

- L-methionine condenses with ATP in presence of an activating enzyme in liver to form **"active" methionine (S-adenosyl methionine).** It requires Mg^{++} and reduced glutathione.
- "Activated" S-methyl group may donate the CH_3 group to an "acceptor" forming S-adenosyl homocysteine.
- Hydrolysis of the S—C bond yields L-homocysteine and adenosine.

Stage 2: Conversion of L-Homocysteine to L-Homoserine.

- *L-homocysteine condenses with the amino acid serine* and forms **'cystathionine'** the reaction requires B_6-P and enzyme *cystathionine synthetase"*.
- Hydrolytic cleavage of cystathionine forms L-homoserine and one molecule of L-cysteine.

Note:

- Sulphur of methionine is directly transferred in formation of cysteine, the ***carbon-skeleton is derived from the amino acid serine.***
- Sulphur occurring in urine is derived almost entirely from oxidation of cystine. ***Methionine does not contribute directly to "SO_4^-pool" of the body.***

Stage 3: Degradation of L-Homoserine: Homoserine is converted to α-ketobutyrate by *homoserine deaminase* via formation of imino acid. α-ketobutyrate is converted to 'propionyl CoA' by oxidative decarboxylation or it can be aminated by transamination to α-amino butyrate.

End-products of methionine degradation are:

- **Propionyl CoA**
- **α-Amino butyrate**

Fate of End Products

- Propionyl CoA is converted to succinyl CoA through formation of methyl malonyl CoA and thus it is "**glucogenic**".
- α-Amino butyrate is excreted in urine.

Metabolic Role of Methionine

- *Methionine is "glucogenic":* Propionyl CoA the endproduct of catabolism is converted to succinyl CoA, an intermediate of TCA cycle.
- *Cysteine formation* (see above).
- *Lipotropic function:* "Active" methionine can donate "methyl group" and can from choline from ethanolamine. ***Choline is lipotropic and prevents accumulations of fat in liver.***
- *Polyamine synthesis:* 'Active' methionine after decarboxylation combines with putrescine to form first polyamine **"spermidine".**
- *Formation of methyl mercaptan and its clinical significance:* Patients with severe liver diseases, exhibit foul odour in breath called as *"Foetor hepaticus". It has been attributed to methyl mercaptan,* which appears to be formed from methionine. Methyl mercaptan has been found in urine of these patients.
- *Transmethylation:* Certain compounds of the body, with structures containing CH_3 group attached to an atom other than carbon can take part in enzymic reactions, whereby these-CH_3 groups are transferred to a suitable "acceptor", which have no CH_3-group. Such reactions are termed as transmethylation reaction", and the substrate, i.e. the —CH_3 donor is said to possess *biologically labile* —CH_3 groups". The most important compounds with biologically labile methyl group are given below:
- **"Active" methionine** containing

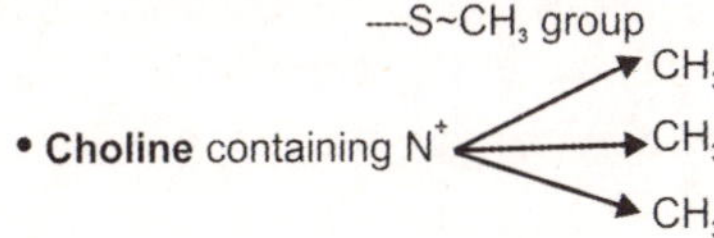

- **Betaine,** an oxidation derivative of choline.

"ACTIVE" METHIONINE

- Chemically called as **"S-adenosyl methionine".**
- Activation of methionine occurs in presence of ATP, catalyzed by an enzyme, called *L-methionine adenosyl transferase.* It requires presence of Mg^{++} and G-SH. In the process of activation, ATP donates the entire adenosine moiety to methionine and loses 3 molecules of PO_4, one as orthophosphate and two as pyrophosphate.
- CH_3 group forms a ***'high energy'*** bond with sulphur (-S~ CH_3), this attributes to lability of methyl group. Formation of 'active' methionine is shown ***(Fig. 14.10).***

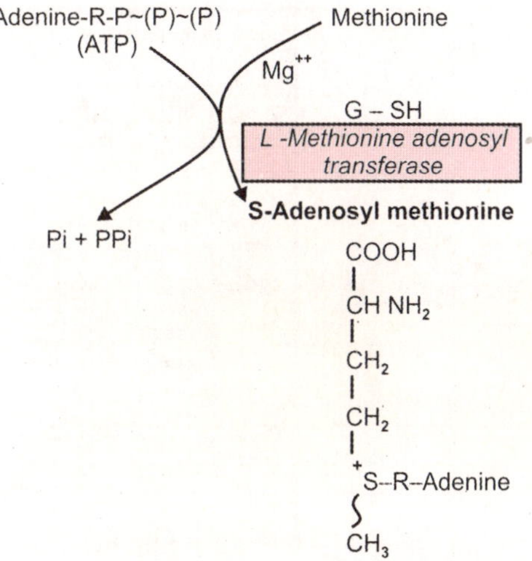

Fig. 14.10: Formation of active methionine

- Transmethylation reaction is ***highly "exergonic".*** In most cases, a hydrogen ion is released in the reaction, contributing to the liberation of free energy at physiological pH. The free energy of transmethylation approximates that of hydrolysis of a high energy bond.

Example of transmethylation reaction is shown schematically ***(Fig. 14.11).***

Other examples are:

- Homocysteine ⟶ L-Methionine
- Uracil ⟶ Thymine
- Orthomethylation of oestrogens.

Metabolism of Cystine: Cystine metabolism proceeds through cysteine, to which it is readily converted. The reaction is ***reversible*** and catalyzed by NADH-dependant *oxido-reductase.*

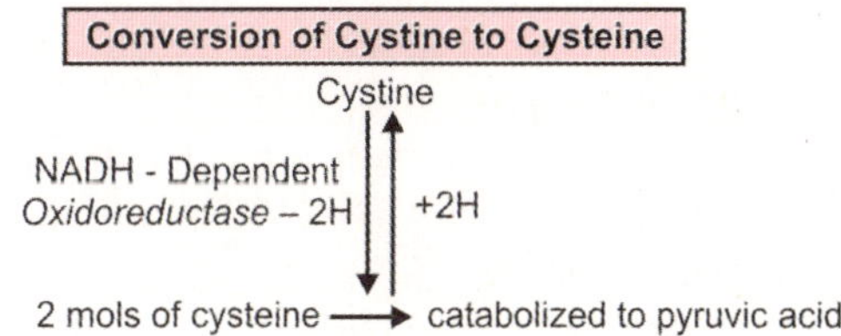

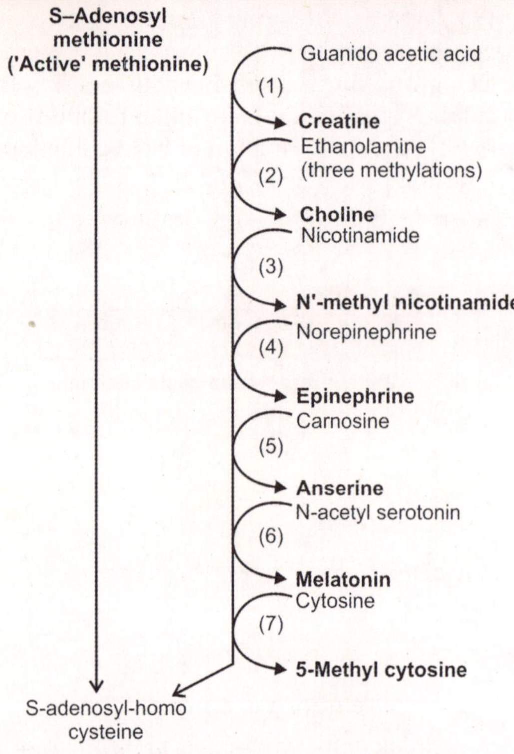

Fig. 14.11: Transmethylation

One molecule of cystine is reduced to form two molecules of cysteine and vice versa.

Metabolic Fate of Cysteine: Cysteine is catabolized to form pyruvic acid, which can be converted to glucose. *Thus cysteine is a glucogenic amino acid.*

- formed in pathway is oxidized to form catalyzed by *sulfite oxidase,* which requires lipoic acid and hypoxanthine for its activity.

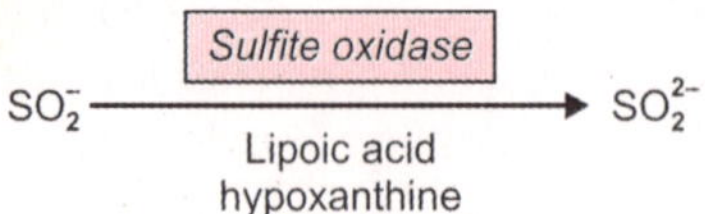

Metabolic Role of Cysteine

- *Glucogenic:* Cysteine is catabolized to Pyruvic acid which is glucogenic.
- *Formation of glutathione:* Cysteine is required for synthesis of glutathione. G-SH is the reduced form—active group is SH group. G-S-S-G is the oxidized form.
(Chemistry and functions of glutathione—see ahead).
- *Formation of taurine:* Cysteine is utilized in the formation of **'taurine',** which combines with cholic acid (obtained from degradation of cholesterol in liver), to form bile acid 'taurocholic acid'.

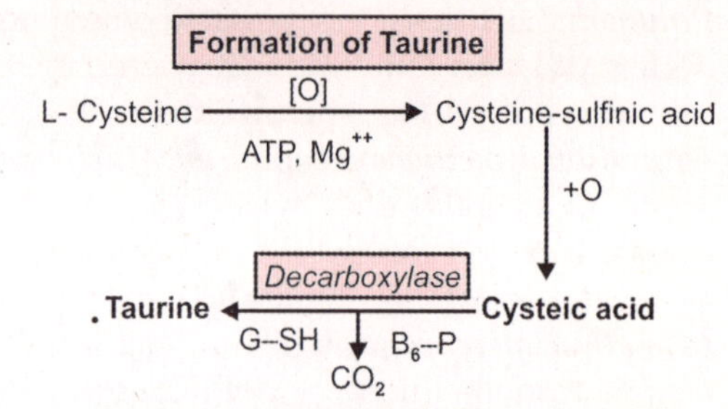

- *Formation of taurocholic acid:*

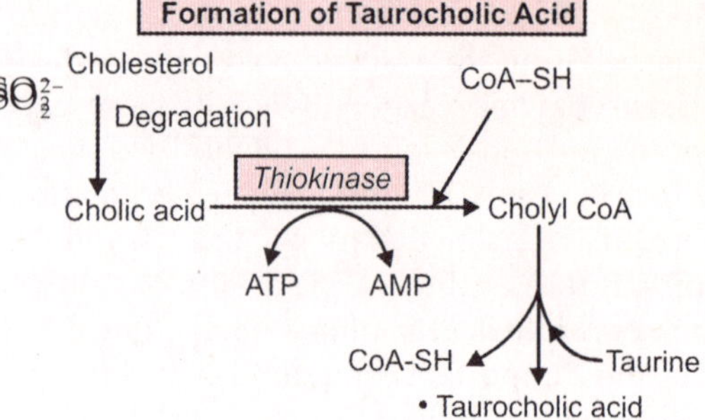

- *Formation of mercaptoethanolamine:* L-cysteine can undergo decarboxylation by a *decarboxylase* and forms mercaptoethanolamine, which is an important constituent of coenzyme A.

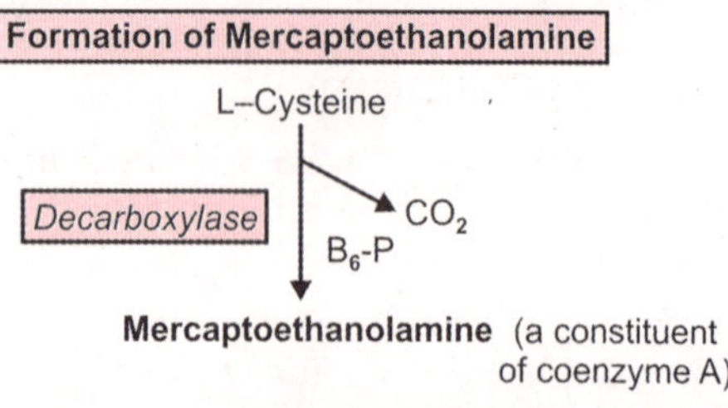

- Cysteine is a particularly prominent amino acid in the proteins of nails, hairs, hoofs and keratin of the skin *("sclero-protein")*

- Cysteine is also a constituent of many other proteins, including certain protein hormones like insulin, vasopressin, etc. where it is of great importance in maintaining secondary and tertiary structures of the proteins.
- ***Role of cysteine in detoxication:*** Cysteine is involved in detoxication reactions to a limited extent in man. It couples with certain aromatic compounds which then undergo acetylation to form ***"mercapturic acids"*** which are excreted in urine. The aromatic compounds are benzene, polycyclic hydrocarbons, e.g. naphthalene, and ring halogenated hydrocarbons, e.g. bromobenzene.

• Bromobezene + Cysteine + Acetic Acid

↓

Bromophenyl mercapturic acid

• Naphthalene + Cysteine + Acetic Acid

↓

Naphthyl mercapturic acid

INHERITED DISORDERS OF S-CONTAINING AMINO ACIDS

1. **Cystinuria:** An inherited disorder of cystine metabolism. Excretion of cystine in urine increases 20 to 30 times of normal. Also there occurs increased excretion of dibasic amino acids ***lysine, arginine*** and ***ornithine*** (specific dibasic aminoaciduria).

- ***Defect:*** It is considered to be ***due to a renal transport defect*** in that reabsorption of the above four amino acids do not occur—***a single reabsorptive site is involved.*** Evidences are there to indicate that there may be an intestinal transport defect of these amino acids as well.
- ***Complications:*** Cystine is ***relatively insoluble*** amino acid, which may precipitate in renal tubules, ureters and bladder to form ***cystine calculi,*** Cystine stones account for 1 to 2% of all urinary tract calculi. It forms a major complication of the disease.

Diagnosis

- ***Urine examination:*** Detection of hexagonal, flat crystals in urinary deposit in a patient who is not taking sulpha drugs is pathognomonic.
- ***Cyanide-Nitroprusside test (Lewis):*** It is a simple and valuable test. Urine sample is made alkaline with ammonium hydroxide and then sodium cyanide is added and mixed. Sodium cyanide reduces cystine, if any present, to cysteine. Cysteine forms magenta-red color, when sodium nitroprusside is added. The intensity of the color is proportional to free-SH content.
- ***Chromatography:*** Amino acids can be detected by chromatography.

2. **Cystinosis:** A second hereditary abnormality of cystine metabolism is "cystinosis", also called ***"cystine storage disease."***

- A rare familial disease characterized by widespread deposition of cystine, sometimes as distinct crystals in various tissues. Patients with cystinosis accumulate cystine in liver, spleen, bonemarrow, peripheral leucocytes, lymphnodes, kidney and cornea. Cystine accumulates with lysosomes of cells of RE system.
- ***Defect:*** The cause of the condition may be an impaired conversion of cystine to cysteine in the involved tissues due to deficiency of the enzyme *cystine reductase.*
- ***Clinical features:*** The condition may appear in children as well as in adults: **Three forms:**

a. ***In children (nephropathic):*** The diseases runs an ***acute course and leads to renal insufficiency.*** There may be associated amino aciduria, glycosuria, polyuria, chronic acidosis leading to uremia, and death.

b. ***Juvenile type:*** Renal features as stated above seen in second decade.

c. ***Adult type:*** Runs a benign clinical course. Cystine gets deposited in cornea but not in kidney.

Diagnosis

- Cystine crystals can be detected easily in cornea by silt lamp microscopy.
- Cystine crystals can be demonstrated in unstained preparation of peripheral blood or in biopsies of rectal mucosa.

- Confirmed by chemical determination of cystine content of peripheral leucocytes or cultured fibroblasts.

3. Homocystinuria: An inborn error of metabolism, which involves the catabolism of methionine or more specifically its metabolic intermediates, homocysteine/and homocystine.

- ***Enzyme deficiency:*** Genetic deficiency of the enzyme *cystathionine synthetase.* The enzyme defect leads to accumulation of homocystine. Plasma level of homocystine increases and excreted in urine ("overflow" amino aciduria), 50 to100 mg or more excreted in urine per day. In some cases, S-adenosyl methionine is also excreted.
- ***Incidence:*** 1 in 60,000 live births.

Clinical Features

- Mental retardation in children and surviving adults.
- Some affected individuals, are extraordinarily tall, with long extremities, frequently with flat feet with toes out (***Charlie-Chaplin gait).***
- Liver is enlarged (***hepatomegaly).***
- Skeletal deformities involving spine, (vertebrae), and thorax, resulting to kyphosis, scoliosis, arachnodactyly. May be premature osteoporosis which also accounts to above deformities. X-ray spine shows ***"cod fish"*** vertebrae.
- ***Ectopia lentis:*** Curious dislocation of lens of the eye. Not seen at birth, may show at the age of 2 to 3 years.
- ***Life-threatening arterial/venous thrombosis.***
- Most of the patients show abnormal EEG.
- ***Urine:*** Sodium cyanide-nitroprusside test is positive and helps in diagnosis.

Fig. 14.12 shows flow chart for metabolic fate and role of S-containing amino acids.

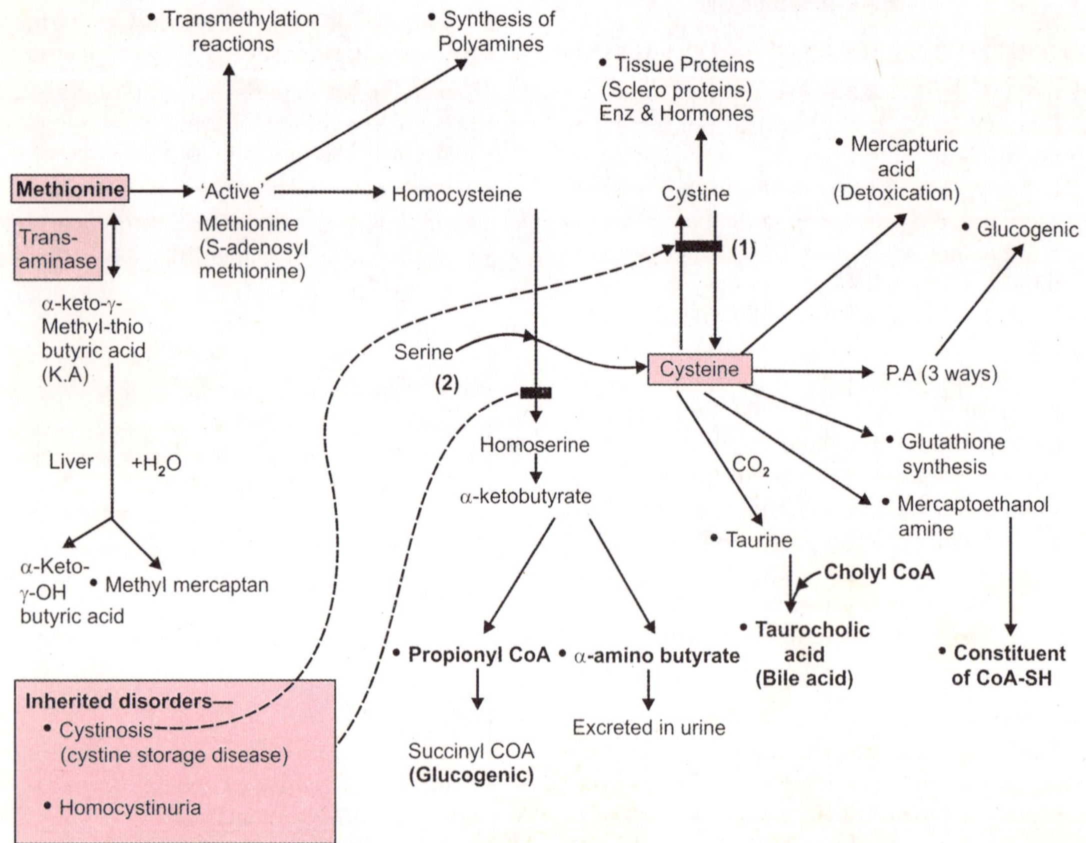

Fig. 14.12: Showing flow chart for metabolic fate and metabolic role of S-containing amino acids

GLUTATHIONE-CHEMISTRY AND FUNCTIONS

- Glutathione is a ***tri-peptide*** of three amino acids, ***glutamic acid, cysteine*** and ***glycine***. Chemically it is γ-L-glutamyl-cystinyl-glycine.

IMPORTANT FUNCTIONS

- Glutathione is an important ***reducing agent*** in the tissues.
- By donating H_2, it helps to ***destroy H_2O_2*** and other peroxides in cells. The reaction is catalyzed by the selenium-containing enzyme *glutathione peroxidase.*
- It acts as ***a coenzyme*** with liver enzyme *glutathione-insulin transhydrogenase* which helps in the catabolism and degradation of protein hormone insulin.
- Glutathione and the enzyme *glutathione transhydrogenase* help to cause reductive cleavage of S-S linkages in thyroglobulin, glycoprotein.
- Glutathione takes part in "***γ-glutamyl cycle***" for absorption of amino acids from gut.
- Oxidized glutathione is harmful for red cell

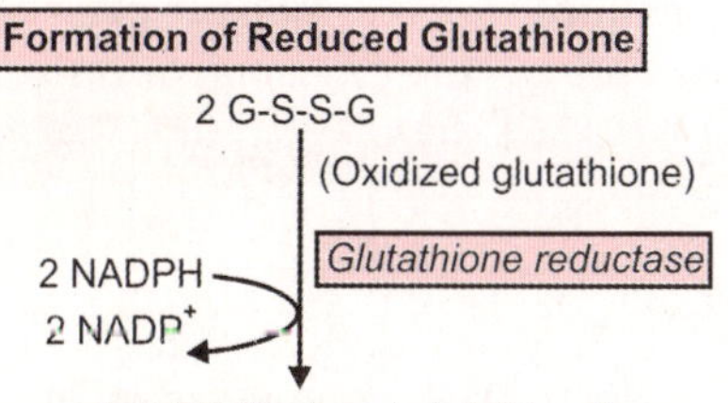

membrane and lens proteins. Oxidized glutathione formed during coenzyme actions is reduced back to glutathione by an NADPH-dependant flavoprotein called *glutathione reductase* which contains FAD as prosthetic group.

- G-SH is required as coenzyme/cofactor with PG-*synthetase System* (cyclo-oxygenase) required for formation of endoperoxides from arachidonate in PG synthesis.
- G-SH is required as a coenzyme for liver enzyme for activation of methionine to form "S-adenosyl methionine" ("active" methionine).

☞ SALIENT POINTS TO REMEMBER

- The amino acids are mainly utilized for protein biosynthesis, production of specialized products, viz. Biogenic amines, creatine, porphyrin, purines, pyrimidines, etc and generation of energy
- Removal of CO_2 from COOH group of an amino acid by an enzyme ***"Decarboxylase"*** produces a biogenic amine. The process is called decarboxylation
- Histamine is formed by decarboxylation of amino acid histidine. Histamine acts as a neurotransmitter, and acts as an anaphylatic and inflammatory agent on being released from mast cells in response to antigens
- Histamine is vasodilator, decreases B.P., increases HCl↑ and Pepsin↑ in stomach
- γ-amino butyric acid (GABA), produced from glutamic acid by decarboxylation, is an inhibitor neurotransmitter. Low levels of GABA results in convulsions
- Infantile convulsions due to deficiency of pyridoxal-P is due to low levels of GABA
- Polyamines (Putrescine, spermidine, and spermine) are involved in the synthesis of DNA, RNA and proteins and thus they are essential for cell growth and differentiation.
- Putrescine is considered as best 'marker' for cell proliferation and spermidine is held as the best 'marker' of tumour cell destruction
- Phenylalanine is nutritionally an essential amino acid. It cannot be synthesized in humans, hence must be provided in the diet.
- Tyrosine can be formed from phenylalanine in the body by the enzyme ***"phenylalanine hydroxylase"*** but is not essential. The reaction is irreversible.
- Both the amino acids, phenylalanine and tyrosine are glucogenic and ketogenic
- Tyrosine though a dispensible (non-essential amino acid), it is of great biological importance as it is a precursor for the formation of thyroid hormones (T_3 and T_4), synthesis of catecholamines (epinephrine, norepinephrine and Dopamine), synthesis of Melanin pigment in skin, formation of tyramine, phenol, cresol and tyrosine-o-SO_4

- Phenyl Ketonuria, an inherited disorder, due to deficiency of the enzyme ***"Phenylalanine hydroxylase"*** is characterized by failure of growth, seizures and mental retardation
- Tyrosine becomes essential amino acid in phenyl Ketonurics
- Alkaptonuria is another inherited disorder, due to deficiency of the enzyme ***"homogentisate oxidase"*** producing accumulation of homogentisic acid
- Homogentisic acid undergoes oxidation followed by polymerization to produce the pigment "alkapton". Urine on standing becomes black
- In longstanding cases, the pigment gets deposited in connective tissues, cartilages and joints producing arthritis. The condition is called ***"ochronosis"***
- Lack of melanin synthesis, mostly due to a deficiency of ***"tyrosinase"*** causes albinism
- Sulphur containing amino acids are: L- Methionine, L-cysteine and L-cystine.
- Methionine is an essential amino acid and must be supplied in the diet
- Cysteine is nonessential and dispensible amino acid and can be formed in the body from methionine
- One molecule of cystine can form two molecules of cysteine by reduction. The reaction is reversible
- Methionine is catabolized to form propionyl-CoA and α-amino butyrate. Propionyl-CoA is converted to succinyl CoA, thus methionine is glucogenic
- The "active methionine"–S-adenosyl methionine (SAM) is a donor of $-CH_3$ group, the process called transmethylation
- It is utilized for synthesis of many biological compounds in the body, viz. creatine, choline, epinephrine, melatonin, thymine, etc
- In formation of cysteine from methionine, sulphur of methionine is transferred directly, whereas C-skeleton is obtained from the amino acid serine
- Cysteine is catabolized to form pyruvic acid (P.A), thus it is glucogenic
- Cysteine though non-essential dispensible amino acid, it is of biological importance as many biologically important compounds are formed, viz. Glutathione, taurine, mercapto ethanolamine, etc
- Cysteine takes part in detoxication
- Inherited disorders associated with cysteine/cystine metabolism are cystinuria and cystinosis (cystine storage disease)
- Inherited disorder associated with Methionine metabolism is homocystinuria, due to deficiency of the enzyme ***"cystathionine synthetase"*** in which there is increased accumulation of homocysteine
- Increased homocysteine concentration has been recently implicated as a "risk" factor in the onset of coronary heart disease (CHD).

METABOLISM OF OTHER AMINO ACIDS

GLYCINE

- Glycine is the simplest of amino acids. Chemically it is ***'amino acetic acid'***
- ***It does not possess asymmetric carbon atom, hence does not exist in isomeric forms.***

$$H-\underset{\underset{NH_2}{|}}{CH}-COOH$$

Amino acetic acid (glycine)

- It is dispensible or non-essential amino acid and can be synthesized in animal tissues.
- ***Though it is non-essential it is an important amino acid as it forms many biologically important compounds in the body.***

METABOLIC FATE

Deamination: Glycine is deaminated by a specific enzyme ***glycine oxidase*** (a flavoprotein enzyme) present in liver and kidney to produce ***"glyoxylic acid" (glyoxylate).*** Glyoxylate can further be converted to either oxalic acid or formic acid and thus enters " one-carbon pool".

Note: ***Amino acid glycine is a source of oxalic acid in the body.***

Conversion to Serine: Glycine can be converted to serine which by non-oxidative deamination can form pyruvic acid, thus glycine may be ***glucogenic.***

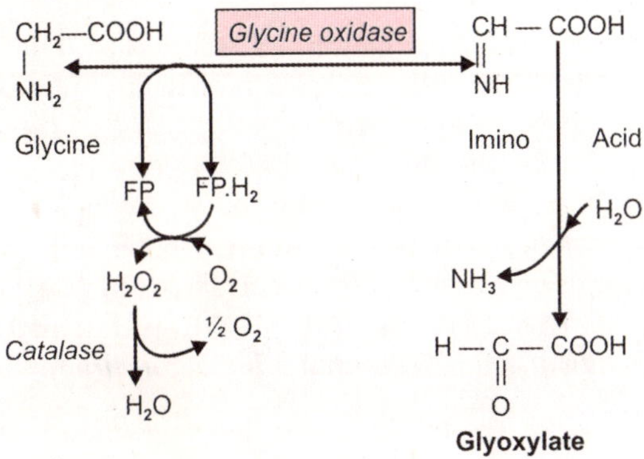

Metabolic Role

- ***Synthesis of Heme:*** Glycine is necessary in the first reaction of heme synthesis (see heme synthesis).
- ***Synthesis of Purine Nucleus:*** The entire glycine molecule is utilized to form C_4, C_5 and N_7 of Purine (see Purine synthesis).
- ***Synthesis of Glutathione:*** Glutathione is a tripeptide formed from three amino acids glutamic acid, cysteine and glycine.
- ***Synthesis of Creatine:*** Arginine and glycine, in presence of the enzyme *transamidinase* in kidney, reacts to form ***"glycocyamine"*** ***("guanido acetic acid")***, which is further converted to creatine (P) in liver (see biosynthesis of creatine).
- ***Conjugation:*** Glycine also acts as a conjugating agent (See detoxication).
- ***Glycine is Glucogenic:*** Glycine is converted to serine which is converted to PA (glucogenic) (see above).
- ***Source of Formate:*** Glycine produces formate and oxalate.

Fig. 14.13 is flow chart of glycine, showing metabolic fate and metabolic role.

SERINE

- Serine is hydroxy amino acid
- It is non-essential (dispensible) and can be synthesized in the body.
- Chemically it is ***"α-amino-β-OH-propionic acid"***.

$$\underset{\displaystyle OH}{\underset{|}{CH_2}} - \underset{\displaystyle NH_2}{\underset{|}{CH}} - COOH$$

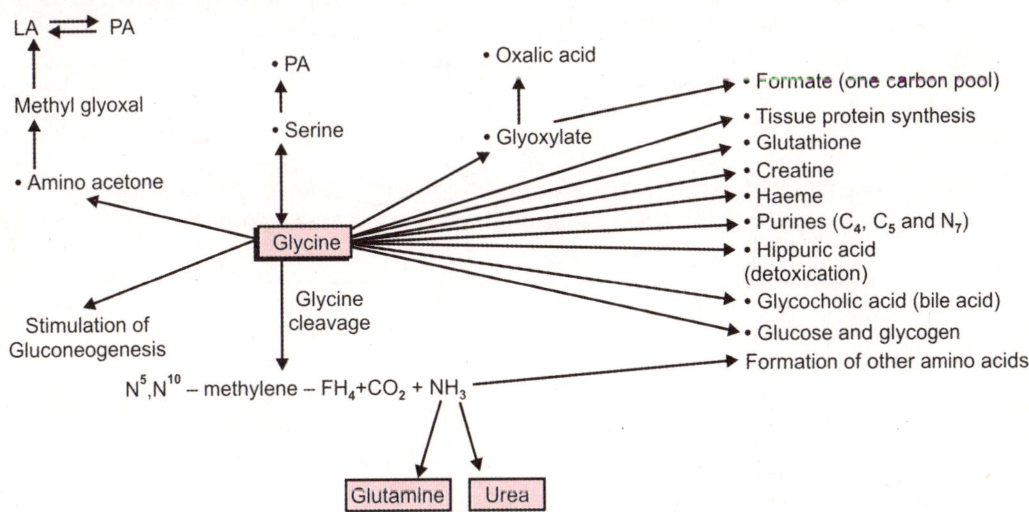

Fig.14.13: Flow chart for glycine showing metabolic fate and metabolic role

Metabolic Fate (*Fig. 14.14*)

It is deaminated by *L-serine-dehydrase* in liver to form pyruvic acid (non-oxidative deamination).

Metabolic Role

- As serine produces pyruvic acid, it is ***glucogenic.***
- Serine can be utilized, like all amino acids for the formation of tissue proteins.
- Serine is a "carrier" of PO_4 group in phosphoproteins.
- Serine contributes the carbon-skeleton to form cysteine. Sulphur of cysteine comes from methionine.
- Serine undergoes decarboxylation to form "ethanolamine" by the enzyme *decarboxylase* in presence of B_6-PO_4. This is very important reaction as 'ethanolamine' is the precursor for:
  - Formation of phosphatidyl ethanolamine (cephalin).
- Formation of 'choline' (a lipotropic factor) by three successive methylations, ~ CH_3 group is donated by S-adenosyl methionine ("active" methionine).

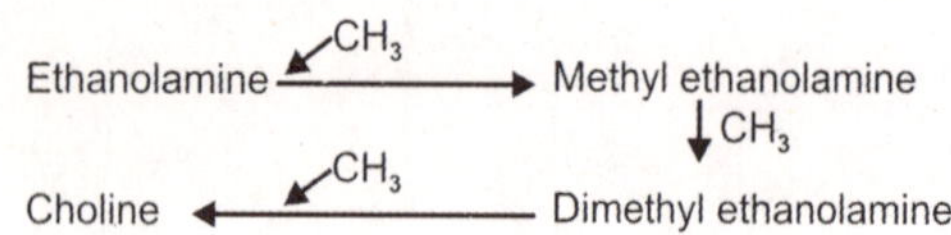

- Serine is used for synthesis of sphingol.
- β-carbon of serine used for thymine formation.
- Hydroxyl group of serine in an enzyme protein is phosphorylated/dephosphorylated to form active/inactive forms of the enzyme.

HISTIDINE

Nutritionally ***semi-essential*** amino acid. Histidine is required in the diet in growing animals and in pregnancy and lactation. Under these conditions, the amino acid becomes essential. An adult can withstand short term deprivation and still can maintain positive nitrogen balance. Long term deprivation in adults and short term deprivation in growing individuals is harmful. ***Chemically it is "α-amino β-imidazole propionic acid".***

Metabolic Fate

Histidine on deamination produces urocanic acid, which is converted to 4-imidazolone-5-propionate by the enzyme *urocanase.* This product on addition of water produces ***"formiminoglutamic acid"("Figlu"),*** which is converted to glutamate, the latter is transaminated to α–ketoglurate, which is an intermediate of TCA cycle. Metabolic fate is shown ahead *(Fig. 14.15).*

Metabolic Role

- It is ***Glucogenic*** through formation of glutamate to α-ketoglutarate.
- ***Histamine formation:*** Decarboxylation of histidine produces histamine (see biogenic amines).

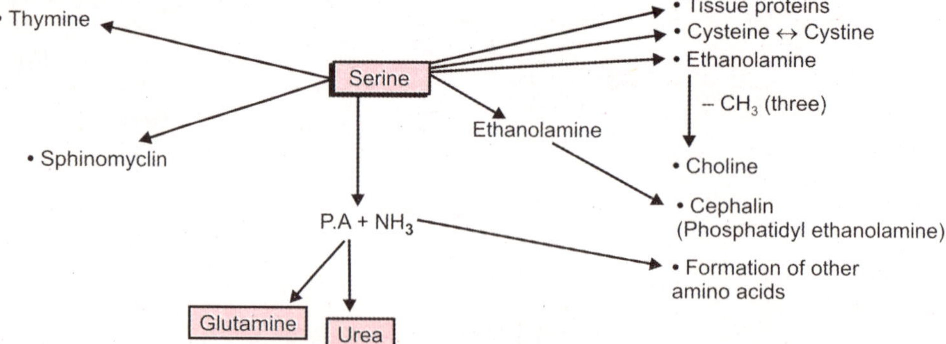

Fig. 14.14: Flow chart for serine showing metabolic fate and metabolic role

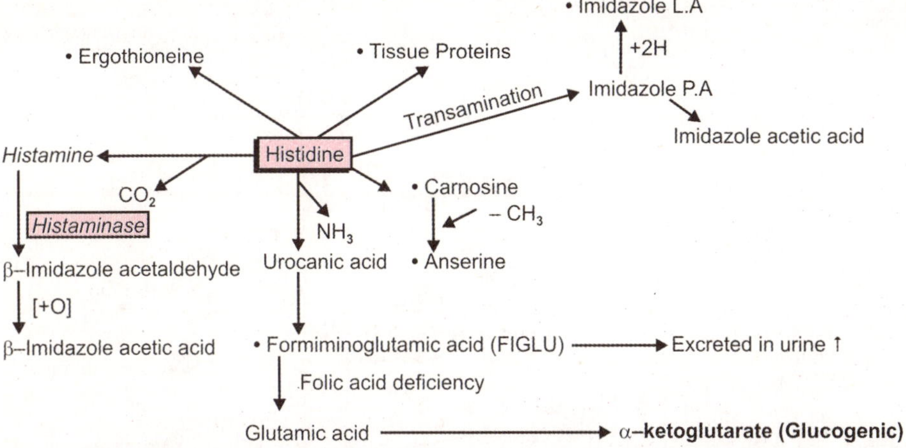

Fig. 14.15: Flow chart of histidine showing metabolic fate and role

- ***Formate can serve as one carbon moiety.*** The 'one-carbon' fragment of histidine is taken up by folic acid and metabolized by transformylation reaction normally. In deficiency of folic acid, the histidine derivative, formiminoglutamic acid, ("figlu") accumulates and excreted in urine, used as a test for folic acid deficiency ("figlu' test—see vitamins).
- **Other histidine compounds:**
  - *Ergothioneine:* Present in RB cells and liver. It is a reducing substance and reduces alkaline copper sulphate solution. Hence its liberation from hemolyzed red blood cells ***can give false high blood glucose*** when estimation of blood glucose is done by Folin and Wu's method.
  - *Carnosine:* A dipeptide of histidine with **β-alanine** (β-alanyl histidine).
  - *Anserine:* A methyl derivative of carnosine "***1-methyl carnosine***". It is formed by methylation of carnosine"; methyl group is donated by "active" methionine.

    Both carnosine and anserine occur in muscles. In myopathies, methyl derivatives of histidine is found in urine.

TRYPTOPHAN

- It is an ***essential amino acid.*** Omission of tryptophan in diet of man and animals is followed by tissue wasting and negative nitrogen balance.
- It is ***both glucogenic and ketogenic.***
- Tryptophan can ***synthesize niacin*** (nicotinic acid) a vitamin of B-complex group.
- It is a heterocyclic amino acid and chemically it is ***"α-amino-β-3-indole propionic acid". It is the only amino acid with an indole ring.***

Structure is shown below:

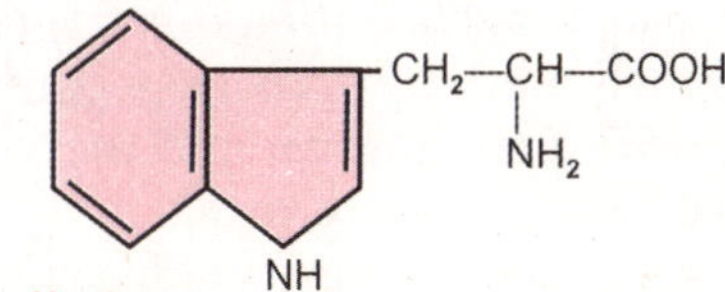

Metabolic Fate:

1. Main pathway ***(Fig. 14.16)*** of its catabolism is by way of anthranilic acid called as ***"kynurenine-anthranilate" pathway.*** In this pathway, tryptophan is finally converted to glutaric acid, which in turn gives two molecules of acetyl CoA (thus it is ***ketogenic*** from aceto acetyl CoA.
   - It also produces alanine which on transamination can form pyruvic acid (thus it is ***glucogenic.***

Metabolic Role

- The amino acid tryptophan is ***both glucogenic and ketogenic.***
- ***Nicotinic acid formation:*** Amino acid tryptophan has been shown to synthesize

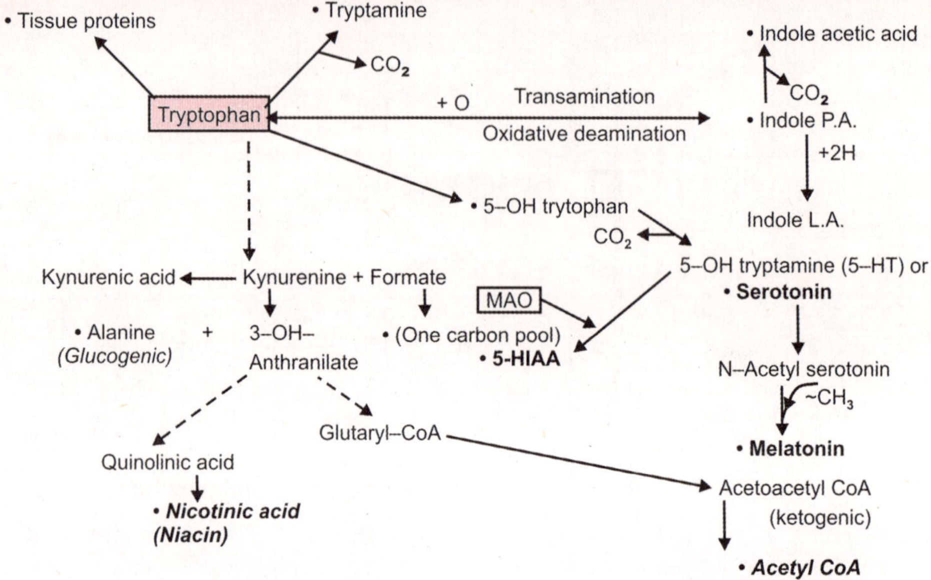

Fig. 14.16: Flow chart for tryptophan showing metabolic fate and metabolic role

nicotinic acid in the body and normally contributes the niacin supply of body.

- Many of the diets causing pellagra are low in good quality protein as well as vitamins. ***Staple maize eaters suffer from pellagra as maize protein is deficient/lacks in tryptophan.*** Pellagra is usually due to a combined deficiency of tryptophan and the vitamin niacin (See chapter on Vitamins).
- Tryptophan rich diet has "sparing effect" on niacin requirement in diet. ***60 mg of tryptophan can give rise to 1 mg of Niacin.***
- ***Formation of tryptamine:*** Decarboxylation of tryptophan in presence of B_6-PO_4 forms ***tryptamine*** (see Biogenic amines).

Tranasmination of Tryptophan

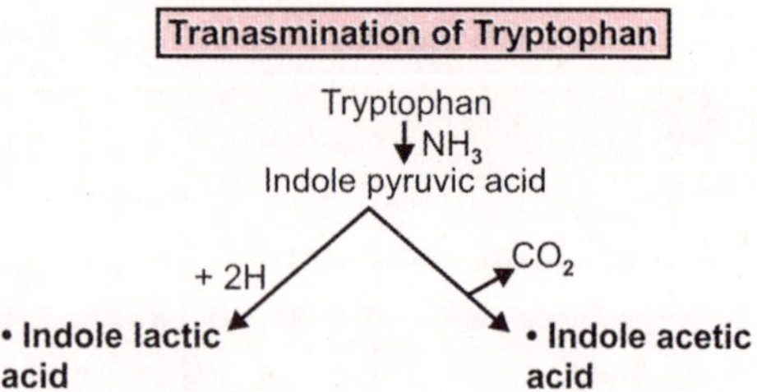

- ***Transamination:*** Tryptophan on transamination or oxidative deamination produces indole PA, which can be reduced to indole lactic acid or decarboxylated to indole acetic acid.
- ***Formation of xanthurenic acid:*** In B_6-deficiency, 3-OH Kynurenine cannot be converted to 3-OH-anthranilic acid. Hence, kynurenine and

Formation of Xanthurenic Acid

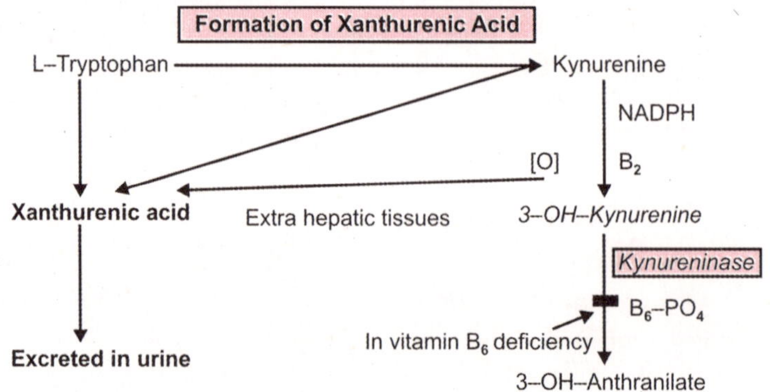

3-OH kynurenine accumulate, and they are converted to *"xanthurenic acid"* in extrahepatic tissues, which is excreted in urine. ***Xanthurenic acid excretion in urine is an index for B_6-deficiency (see Vitamin B_6).***

Clinical Interpretation

- Normal persons excrete only 1 to 3 mg of xanthurenic acid per day and 2 to 11 mg in 24 hours urine after taking a 2 gm "load" of tryptophan (loading test).
- In pyridoxine deficiency much greater amount of xanthurenic acid is excreted in urine. Following a "loading" test up to 60 mg is excreted in 24 hours urine.

SEROTONIN

Synonyms: enteramin, thrombocytin.

- ***Formation of serotonin:*** Serotonin is produced from tryptophan by another special major pathway. Chemically, it is 5-OH tryptamine (5-HT). Serotonin is a ***vasoconstrictor*** substance. It is present in the blood and is produced in tissues like gastric mucosa, intestine, brain, mast cells and platelets(?) —probabaly stored in platelets. It is produced by special cells called as ***"serotonin-producing"*** cells. These cells take up silver staining hence also called "**argentaffin"** cells. The cells are also known as **"Kultchitsky's cells".**

Synthesis of Serotonin

- Tryptophan is first hydroxylated to form 5-OH tryptophan in liver.
- In the next step, 5-OH tryptophan is decarboxylated, by the enzyme *5-OH tryptophan decarboxylase,* in presence of B_6-PO_4 to form 5-hydroxy tryptamine (5-HT), also called serotonin. The enzyme is present in kidney, liver and stomach.

Functions of Serotonin

- It is a ***potent vasoconstrictor.***
- Produces ***contraction of smooth muscles.***
- ***Stimulator of cerebral activity.***

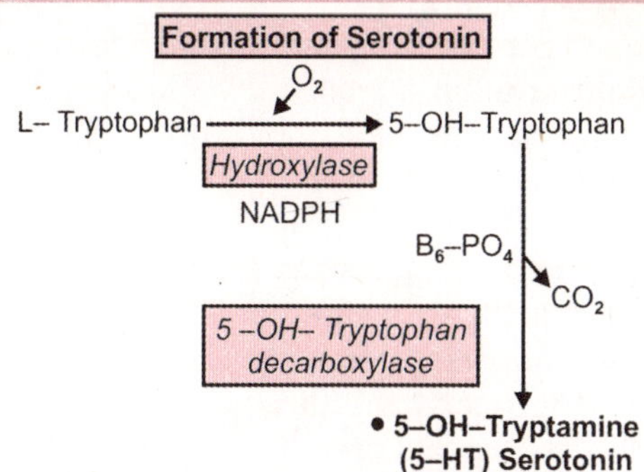

Note: Serotonin is actually synthesized in tissues where it is found rather than produced in one organ and carried by blood to other organs.

Effects of Serotonin on Brain: Serotonin does not pass *blood brain barrier* to any significant amount. For action, it has to be produced locally from the amino acid.

- Excess of serotonin in brain tissues produces ***stimulation of cerebral activity (excitation).***
- Deficiency of serotonin produces ***depressant effect.***

Catabolism of Serotonin

- The enzyme which catalyzes the conversion of serotonin to 5-HIAA (5-OH-indole acetic acid) is called ***monoamine oxidase*** (MAO).
- 5-HIAA is excreted in urine. Normal adults excrete about 7 mg HIAA per day.

Clinical Aspect

A malignant tumour of serotonin producing cells is called **"carcinoids" (or 'argentaffinoma')** and the clinical feature associated with is called as **'carcinoid syndrome'.**

Clinical Features

- Symptoms are mainly due to presence of excessive amount of serotonin produced by malignant cells.
- Normal person utilizes 1% of tryptophan in serotonin production; ***in this condition 60% of tryptophan is metabolized by serotonin pathway.*** Consequently symptoms of pellagra as well as negative N_2 balance can occur.

Effects of Serotonin: Symptoms are due to effects on smooth muscles:

- Cutaneous vasomotor episodes of *"flushing"*.
- Occasionally cyanotic appearance
- Chronic diarrhoea.
- Respiratory distress and bronchospasm.
- Some may have right sided heart failure. Serotonin passing through lungs is destroyed by MAO hence left side is not affected.

Urine: In malignant carcinoids, urinary excretion of 5-HIAA may increase to as much as 400 mg per day.

Formation of Melatonin from Serotonin

- Melatonin is a hormone of pineal body and peripheral nerves of man.
- The hormone is synthesized from serotonin.

Table 14.3 shows important metabolic role of other amino acids (see p. 331).

Role of Nitric Oxide in the Body

Nitric oxide (NO) is formed in the body from the amino acid arginine. It is a wonder molecule having diverse biological functions like PG's.

Formation:

Arginine is acted upon by a cytosolic enzyme called *"Nitrogen oxide synthase"*, which converts arginine to citrulline and Nitric oxide (NO).

Nitric oxide synthase is a very complex cytosolic enzyme which requires five redox cofactors: NADPH, FAD, FMN, haeme and tetrahydrobiopterin ($F.H_4$).

Nitric Oxide Synthase

$$\text{Arginine} \xrightarrow[\text{NADPH, FAD, FMN, Heme, } F.H_4]{} \text{Nitric oxide} + \text{citrulline}$$

FUNCTIONS OF NITRIC OXIDE

- ***Acts as a vasodilator*** and ***causes relaxation of smooth muscles.***
- Has important role in the regulation of blood flow and maintenance of B.P.
- ***Acts as a neurotransmitter*** in the brain and peripheral autonomic nervous system.
- Also produces relaxation of skeletal muscles.
- ***Inhibits adhesion, activation and aggregation of platelets.***
- May mediate bactericidal actions of macrophages.

METABOLISM OF CREATINE

Two closely related nitrogenous compounds which are connected with protein metabolism are—**creatine** and **creatinine**. Structure and relationship of these two compounds are shown below in the box:

Structure of Creatine and Creatinine

$$HN{=}C\begin{cases} NH\text{-}P \\ N(CH_3)\text{-}CH_2\text{-}COOH \end{cases} \xrightarrow{\text{non-enzymatic}} HN{=}C\begin{cases} NH\text{-}C{=}O \\ N(CH_3)\text{—}CH_2 \end{cases}$$

Creatine-P (methylguanido-acetic acid) → **Creatinine** (Anhydride of creatine)

Characteristics of the above reaction:

- Reaction is *irreversible*
- It is *non-enzymatic.*
- Creatinine has ring structure.

OCCURRENCE AND DISTRIBUTION

1. **Creatine:** It is a ***normal constituent of the body.*** It is present in muscle, brain, liver, testes and in blood. Can occur in ***'free' form*** and also as ***'phosphorylated' form.*** The phosphorylated form is called as **'creatine-PO_4'** or **'phosphocreatine'** or **"Phosphagen"**.

- Total amount in adult human body is approximately 120 gm. Of the total amount, 98% is present in muscles, of which 80% occurs in phosphorylated form, 1.3% in nervous system (brain) and 0.5 to 0.7% in tissues.
- ***Urinary excretion:*** Urinary excretion in normal health is in the form of creatinine and it is only 2% of the total. In males, it is 1.5 to 2.0 gm in 24 hours urine, and in females-varies from 0.8 to 1.5 gms.

Note:

- Only vertebrate muscles contain creatine.

Table 14.3: Showing Important Metabolic Role of Other Amino Acids

S.No	*Name of the Amino acid*	*Nature and properties*	*Metabolic role*
1.	**Arginine**	• Basic amino acid • Semi-essential • Becomes essential in growing children, in pregnancy and lactation	• Tissue protein formation • Required in creatine synthesis • Required in urea formation • Glucogenic amino acid • ***Nitric oxide (NO) formation***
2.	**Ornithine and citrulline**	• Both are basic amino acids • Both are non-essential	• Both are intermediates in formation of urea (urea cycle) • Ornithine is regenerated in urea cycle and acts as catalytic agent to continue the cycle • Ornithine is required for synthesis of polyamines • Ornithine is glucogenic
3.	**Threonine**	• Essential amino acid • Cannot be formed by transamination of the keto acids	• Glucogenic amino acid • By non-oxidative deamination forms α-keto butyric acid, which on oxidative decarboxylation gives Propionyl CoA (glucogenic) • Cleaved by the enzyme *threonine aldolase* to form glycine and acetaldehyde • Threonine can also be converted to Pyruvic acid (thus glucogenic) • Like serine, it is a hydroxy amino acid acts as PO_4 carrier
4.	**Glutamic acid and aspartic acid**	• Both are acidic amino acids • Both are non-essential • Both can participate in transamination reactions	• Both glucogenic—on deamination forms OAA and α-ketoglutarate (Intermediates of TCA cycle) • Glutamic acid on decarboxylation forms GABA • Glutamate is a constituent of glutathione • Aspartate participates in synthesis of purines and pyrimidines • Glutamate is a constituent of folic acid • ***Glutamine is formed from glutamate*** • Glutamic acid helps in transport of K^+ ions in brain tissue • N-acetyl glutamate (N-AGA) and asparate both take part in urea cycle • Proline and OH-proline can be formed from glutamic acid • Amide of glutamic acid, glutamine takes part in conjugation reactions • Amide of aspartic acid, asparagine, is an important NH_3 donor
5.	**Proline and OH-proline**	• Both are non-essential amino acids	• OH-proline forms structural part of collagen tissues and elastin • OH-proline is synthesized in collagen tissue from proline for which vitamin C is required

Contd...

Contd...

S.No	Name of the Amino acid	Nature and properties	Metabolic role
			• OH-proline is catabolized to form pyruvic acid and glyoxylate (glucogenic)
6.	**Lysine**	• Essential amino acid	• It is both glucogenic and ketogenic • Cannot take part in transamination reactions • OH-lysine, like OH-proline is required for collagen tissues • OH-lysine is synthesized in collagen tissues from lysine for which vitamin C is required.
	Note: This amino acid is not present in adequate amounts in cereal proteins. Hence its deficiency may occur in strict vegetarians		
7.	**Branched-chain amino acids valine, leucine and isoleucine**	• All the three amino acids are essential	• Valine is glucogenic. On deamination forms methyl malonyl CoA which is converted to succinyl CoA (glucogenic) • Leucine is potent ketogenic amino acid • Isoleucine, after oxidative removal of one carbon forms propionyl CoA (glucogenic) and one molecule of acetate (ketogenic).

- Creatine concentration is higher in striated muscles as compared to smooth muscles and also in rapidly contracting muscles as compared to pale muscles. Total is 300 to 500 mg/100gm.
- In invertebrates, arginine replaces creatine in muscles.

Blood and plasma level:

- In whole blood, creatine level varies from 2 to 7 mg%.
- In plasma it is less than 1 mg%.
- In males, it varies from 0.2 to 0.6 mg%.
- In females, 0.35 to 0.9 mg%.

2. Creatinine: Creatinine is the anhydride of creatine, and it is in this form that creatine is excreted in normal health.

- Removal of one molecule of H_2O is ***non enzymatic and irreversible.***
- Formation of creatinine is a preliminary step and prerequisite for excretion of most of creatine. Total creatinine in muscle is only 0.01% (10 mg).
- ***Blood:*** Whole blood creatinine level varies from 1.0 to 2.0 mg%. Creatinine is evenly distributed in between plasma and RB cells.

	Whole blood	*Muscles*
• **Creatine:**	2.0 to 7.0 mg%	300 to 500 mg
• **Creatinine:**	1.0 to 2.0 mg%	0.01% (10 mg)

Urinary excretion

- **Creatinine** In males: 1.5 to 2.0 gm in 24 hrs.
  In females: 0.8 to 1.5 gm in 24 hrs.

Biosynthesis of Creatine: *Three amino acids* are required in biosynthesis of creatine. They are:

- ***Glycine***
- ***Arginine***
- ***Methionine***

- Substrates to start synthesis are: glycine and arginine
- ***Site of synthesis:***
  - Kidney
  - Liver

1. Reaction I: Formation of "Guanidoacetic acid": It is called 'glycocyamine'. *Takes place* in **kidney.**

Formation of Guanidoacetic Acid

(In Kidney)

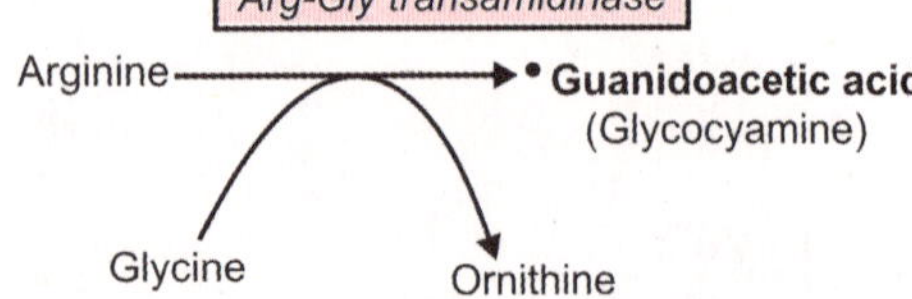

Transfer of an "amidine Group" (HN = C(–NH_2)) from arginine to glycine, under the influence of the enzyme *arginine-glycine transamidinase* takes place. The process is called as *"transamidination"*.

2. **Reaction II: Formation of Creatine-(P):** Enzyme catalyzing the reaction is *guanidoacetate methylferase.* S-adenosyl methionine ('active' methionine) is the "methyl" donor, for methylation.

- ATP is required for the synthesis which donates the PO_4.
- O_2 is required for the reaction ***(aerobic),*** Reaction is ***irreversible***, and ***occurs in liver.***
- Once creatine –(P) is formed in liver, it goes to muscles, and stored. Creatinine is formed from creatine-(P) in muscles by non-enzymatic and irreversible reaction.

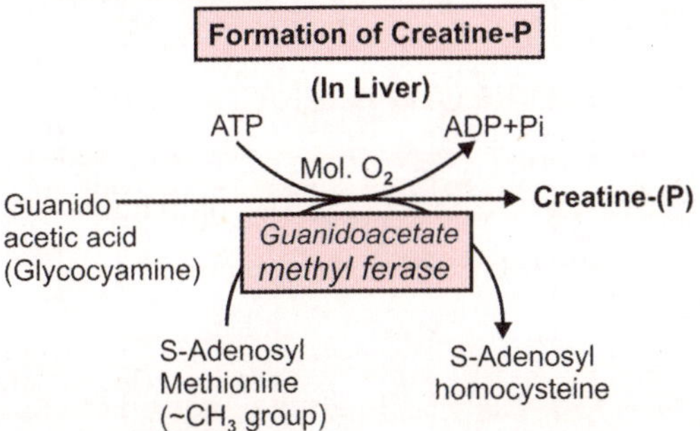

Other Methyl Donors: Betaine and choline (after oxidation to betaine) may also serve indirectly by producing methionine through the methylation of homocysteine.

Other Sites of Creatine Synthesis: Recently it has been shown that ***pancreas can synthesize glycocyamine and creatine-(P).*** It has been concluded that pancreas singly may play a unique role in the synthesis of creatine within the body of mammals.

REGULATION OF CREATINE SYNTHESIS

- Dietary creatine has effect on creatine synthesis. In rats, fed a complete diet containing 3% creatine, *transmidinase* activity of the kidney was markedly lower as compared to control animals.
- But dietary creatine or a high blood creatine has no effect on rate of synthesis of creatine in liver.
- It is also shown that hepatic synthesis of creatine is related to the blood glycocyamine levels and that this compound is produced in kidney, suggests that the rate of creatine biosynthesis is actually dependant on kidney transmidinase activity.
- Thus, ***the activity of transamidinase activity in kidney is the key regulating enzyme for creatine biosynthesis*** and is affected by creatine level as a "feedback" mechanism.

Excretion

- When creatinine is ingested, most of it is rapidly eliminated in urine. It can be quantitatively recovered.
- But when creatine is taken, some is retained in the body, whose fate is not known definitely. It has been seen by giving labelled creatine that 20 to 30% is excreted as creatine and some is retained in the body whose fate is not known.
- Urine of normal healthy adult male ***contains creatinine but no creatine.*** Amount of creatinine excreted as discussed above is approxi-mately 1.0 to 1.5 gm/day and this is:
  - Independent of amount of proteins taken in the diet.
  - Greater in muscular persons and appears to be related to muscular development and muscular activity.
  - After severe exercise, may increase but total amount remains constant from day to day.

Creatinuria: ***Excretion of creatine in urine is called creatinuria.*** Creatine excretion occurs in:

- ***children:*** Probably due to the lack of ability to convert creatine to creatinine;
- ***adult females:*** In pregnancy and maximum after parturition (2 to 3 weeks);
- ***febrile conditions;***
- ***thyrotoxicosis:*** Probably due to associated myopathies;
- ***muscular dystrophies,*** Myositis, and myasthenia gravis;

- *subjects lacking carbohydrate in diets and in diabetic;*
- *wasting diseases,* e.g. in malignancies; and starvation.

ROLE OF CREATINE IN MUSCLES

- Creatine is the reservoir of energy in muscles
- When muscles contract, energy is derived from breakdown of ATP to ADP and Pi.
- ATP must be reformed quickly to supply the energy, which initially comes from creatine – (P), subsequently from glycolysis (contracting muscle).

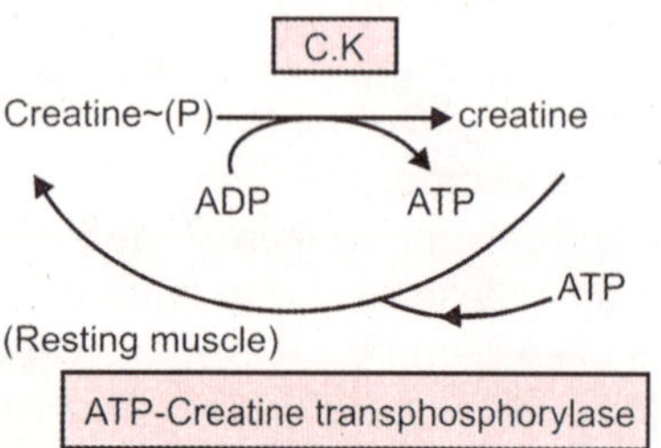

- From the above reaction, ATP is formed from creatine~(P). The high energy phosphate is transferred to ADP and ATP is formed. This reaction is called **Löhman reaction** and it takes place during activity of the muscles. In the resting condition, creatine~(P) is reformed, the enzyme that catalyzes the reaction is *ATP creatine transphosphorylase.*
- Another source of ATP in muscle is the **Myokinase reaction.** Two ADP molecules react to produce one molecule each of ATP and AMP, the reaction is catalyzed by the enzyme *myokinase (adenylate kinase).*

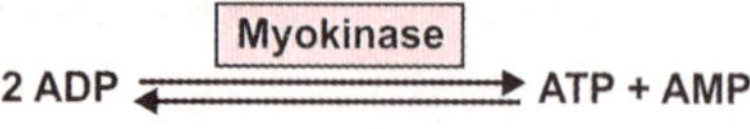

In this reaction, one high energy phosphate is transferred from one ADP to another ADP molecule to form one ATP.

Estimation of Creatinine

- Serum is treated with alkaline picrate solution when a red colour develops ***(Jaffe's reaction).***
- The colour is read against a 'standard' similarly treated in a colorimeter

ESTIMATION OF CREATINE

- When heated with acid solution, creatine is converted to creatinine, which can be measured in a similar way as stated above.
- Value after boiling with acid solution-value before boiling =gives creatine content.
- One gm of creatinine is formed from 1.16 gm of creatine.
- Hence, subtract the preformed creatinine from the total creatinine and multiply by 1.16.

"True" Creatinine: Serum creatinine estimation by Jaffe's reaction does not give "true" creatinine. It measures also certain non-creatinine chromogens, upto 20% in blood and upto 5% in urine. For excluding the chromogens and to get 'true' creatinine after precipitating the proteins, creatinine is absorbed on the Lloyd's reagent (Fuller's earth), a hydrated aluminium silicate, and then colour developed with alkaline picrate.

CREATININE COEFFICIENT

It is the ratio of total urine creatinine in 24 hours urine in mg and total body weight in kg

$$= \frac{\text{Mg of creatinine in urine in 24 hours}}{\text{body wt. in kg.}}$$

The value is 20 to 26 for males and 14 to 22 in females.

Significance

- It depends on muscular development and remains fairly constant.
- As the rate is so constant in a given individual, the creatinine coefficient may serve as a reliable index of the adequacy of a 24-hours urine collection.

Creatinine Clearance: Endogenous creatinine clearance is used as renal function test. At normal levels of creatinine in the blood, this metabolite is filtered at the glomerulus but ***neither secreted non reabsorbed by the tubules.*** Hence, its clearance measures the glomerular filtrate rate (GFR).

- It is a convenient and easy method for estimation of GFR,
  - As it is totally filtered by glomeruli and neither reabsorbed nor secreted by tubules; and

- Since it does not require the IV administration of a test substance as is the case with an exogenous clearance study with inulin. For calculation and value –see Chapter on Renal Function Test.

☞ SALIENT POINTS TO REMEMBER

- Glycine (Aminoacetic acid) is the simplest of amino acids. It is dispensible (non essential) amino acid.
- Though Glycine is non-essential but it is an important amino acid as it forms many biological important compounds in the body, viz. synthesis of haeme, creatine, purine nucleus, glutathione and in detoxication.
- Glycine is glucogenic and produces formate and oxalate.
- Histidine loading test, characterized by elevated excretion of N-formimino-glutamic acid (FIGLU) is employed to assess the deficiency of folic acid.
- Tryptophan is both glucogenic and ketogenic.
- Nicotinic acid (Niacin) can be synthesized in the body from amino acid tryptophan, ***60 mg. of tryptophan can give rise to 1 mg of Niacin.***
- In B_6 - deficiency, the metabolism of Tryptophan suffers. 3-OH kynurenine cannot be converted to 3-OH anthranilic acid. Hence, ***Kynurenine and 3-OH kynurenine accumulate and they are converted to "xanthurenic acid" in extrahepatic tissues which is excreted in urine.***
- ***Xanthurenic acid excretion in urine is an index for vitamin*** B_6 ***deficiency.***
- Serotonin (5-OH tryptamine), a vasoconstrictor, is produced from tryptophan.
- Excess of serotonin in brain tissues produces stimulation of cerebral activity (excitation) and deficiency of serotonin produces depressant effects.
- Serotonin is produced by special cells called serotonin-producing cells or argentaffin cells or also called as Kultchitsky's cells.
- A malignant tumour of serotonin producing cells of GI tract is called "**carcinoids**" (or argentaffinoma) and the clinical feature associated with is called as "carcinoid syndrome".
- The disease is characterized biochemically by excessive production of serotonin. The disease can be diagnosed by the elevated levels of 5-OH-indole acetic acid (5-HIAA) in urine.
- Melatonin is a hormone of pineal body and peripheral nerves. It is synthesized from serotonin.
- Melatonin is involved in circadian rhythms or diurnal variations, i.e. maintenance of body's biological clock.
- ***Nitric oxide (NO),*** is synthesized from the amino acid arginine. It has been incriminated recently to be involved in several biological functions, viz. vasodilation, neurotransmission, platelet aggregation and bactericidal action.
- Two closely related nitrogenous compounds related with protein metabolism are creatine and creatinine.
- Creatine is synthesized in the body in kidney and liver from three amino acids: Glycine, Arginine and Methionine.
- Creatinine is anhydride of creatine. Removal of one molecule of H_2O is non-enzymatic and irreversible.
- In normal health, creatine is excreted in urine as creatinine.
- Excretion of creatine in urine is called creatinuria and occurs in thyrotoxicosis, muscular dystrophies, wasting diseases, starvation, febrile conditions, etc.
- The high energy phosphate of creatine ~P is transferred to ADP to form ATP in muscles. This is called as **Löhman reaction.**
- Another source of ATP in muscle is Myokinase reaction. Two ADP molecules react to produce one molecule each of ATP and AMP, catalyzed by the enzyme *myokinase (adenylate kinase).*
- Estimation of serum creatinine (normal 1.0 to 2.0 mg/dl) is considered to be a more reliable indicator for the evaluation of kidney function.

MULTIPLE CHOICE QUESTIONS

Give one correct answer:

1. **Which of the following compounds serve as a priamry link between the TCA cycle and the urea cycle?**
   (a) Citrate (b) Fumarate
   (c) Malate (d) Oxaloacetate
   (e) Succinate
2. **The two nitrogen atoms in urea arise from:**
   (a) Ammonia and aspartic acid,
   (b) Ammonia and glutamine
   (c) Glutamine and aspartic acid
   (d) Glutamine and glutamic acid
   (e) Aspartic acid and alanine
3. **Quantitatively the most important enzyme involved in formation of NH_3 from amino acids in humans is:**
   (a) Histidase
   (b) L-amino acid oxidase
   (c) Glutamate dehydrogenase
   (d) Serine dehydratase
   (e) Desulfhydrase
4. **Which of the following amino acids produce a vasodilator on decarboxylation?**
   (a) Glutamic acid
   (b) Arginine
   (c) Ornithine
   (d) Proline
   (e) Histidine
5. **Which of the following amino acids on degradation produces a glucogenic intermediate of TCA cycle and a ketone body?**
   (a) Cysteine
   (b) Glycine
   (c) Serine
   (d) Phenylalanine
   (e) Alanine
6. **Phenyl ketonuria is an inherited disorder due to deficiency of the enzyme:**
   (a) Transaminase
   (b) Dehydrogenase
   (c) Phenylalanine hydroxylase
   (d) Homogentisate oxidase
   (e) Isomerase
7. **Ochronosis is a feature of:**
   (a) Phenylketonuria (b) Cystinosis
   (c) Albinism (d) Tyrosinaemia
   (e) Alkaptonuria
8. **Epinephrine is formed from nor-epinephrine by:**
   (a) O-methylation
   (b) N- methylation
   (c) Hydroxylation
   (d) Oxidative deamination
   (e) Decarboxylation
9. **Tryptophan is best described by which of the following statement?**
   (a) A precursor of melanin
   (b) A precursor of pineal hormone melatonin
   (c) Produces thyroid hormones
   (d) It is glucogenic only
   (e) Produces catecholamines
10. **Niacin is produced in the body from which of the following amino acid?**
    (a) Tyrosine (b) Tryptophan
    (c) Glycine (d) Histidine
    (e) Serine
11. **The rate limiting step in the biosynthetic pathway of catecholamines is:**
    (a) Hydroxylation of phenylalanines
    (b) Hydroxylation of tyrosine
    (c) Decarboxylation of tyrosine
    (d) The reduction of biopterin
    (e) Transamination of tyrosine
12. **Which of the following amino acids are required for synthesis of creatine?**
    (a) Arginine, glutamic acid, active methionine
    (b) Arginine, aspartic acid, active methionine
    (c) Arginine, glycine, active methionine
    (d) Lysine, active methionine, arginine
    (e) Glycine, aspartic acid, arginine
13. **Deficiency of which of the following vitamins cause creatinuria?**
    (a) Vit A (b) Vit D
    (c) Vit B_{12} (d) Vit K
    (e) Vit E

14. Which of the following amino acid provides C-skeleton of cysteine?

(a) Histidine (b) Glycine
(c) Methionine (d) Serine
(e) Tyrosine

15. Depletion of α-ketoglutarate during increased NH_3 influx leads to the formation of:

(a) Histamine (b) Serotonin
(c) Proline (d) Serine
(e) Glutamine

ANSWERS

1. (b)	2. (a)	3. (c)
4. (e)	5. (d)	6. (c)
7. (e)	8. (b)	9. (b)
10. (b)	11. (b)	12. (c)
13. (e)	14. (d)	15. (e)

15 Integration of Metabolism of Carbohydrates, Lipids and Proteins

INTRODUCTION

Though metabolism of each of major food nutrients, viz. carbohydrates, lipids and proteins have been considered separately for the sake of convenience, it actually takes place simultaneously in the intact animal and are closely interrelated to one another. The metabolic processes involving these three major food nutrients and their interrelationship can be broadly divided into *three stages (Refer Fig. 15.1):*

1st stage: **Stage of hydrolysis to simpler units**
2nd stage: **Preparatory stage**
3rd stage: **Oxidative stage: Aerobic final (TCA cycle).**

1st Stage: Stage of Hydrolysis to Simpler Units

- The complex polysaccharides, starch/glycogen are broken down to glucose; and disaccharides are hydrolyzed to monosaccharides in GI tract by various carbohydrate-splitting enzymes present in digestive juices.
- Similarly, principle lipids, triacylglycerol (TG) is hydrolyzed to form FFA and glycerol.
- Proteins are hydrolyzed by proteolytic enzymes to amino acids.

The above is the prelude to either further synthesis of new substances or for their oxidation.

Very little of energy is produced in this hydrolytic phase and it is dissipated away as heat. There is no storage of energy at this stge.

2nd Stage: Preparatory Stage:

- The monosaccharide glucose runs through the glycolytic reactions to produce the 3-C keto acid pyruvic acid (PA) in the cytosol, which, in turn, is transported to mitochondrion where it undergoes oxidative decarboxylation to produce 2-C compound ***"acetyl- CoA" ("active" acetate).***
- The glycerol of fat, either goes into formation of glucose (gluconeogenesis) or by entering the same glycolytic pathway through the triose-P, forms PA and then finally 2-C compound "acetyl-CoA.
- The fatty acids undergo principally b-oxidation and form several molecules of "acetyl-CoA"
- The amino acids are deaminated/and/or transaminated first and the C-skeleton is metabolized differently in different amino acids.
  - In the case of amino acids, viz. alanine, serine, cysteine/cystine, when catabolized form pyruvic acid (PA), similar to carbohydrates and is finally converted to "acetyl-CoA".
  - In the case of amino acids, viz. glutamic acid, histidine, proline and OH-proline, arginine and ornithine produces α-keto glutaric acid when catabolized and thus they enter the TCA cycle.
  - Yet a few others like leucine, phenylalanine, tyrosine and isoleucine yield acetate or acetoacetate, the latter can be converted to "acetyl-CoA".

During the second stage (glycolysis, β-oxidation, etc.) also ***relatively small amount of energy is produced and this is stored as ATP.***

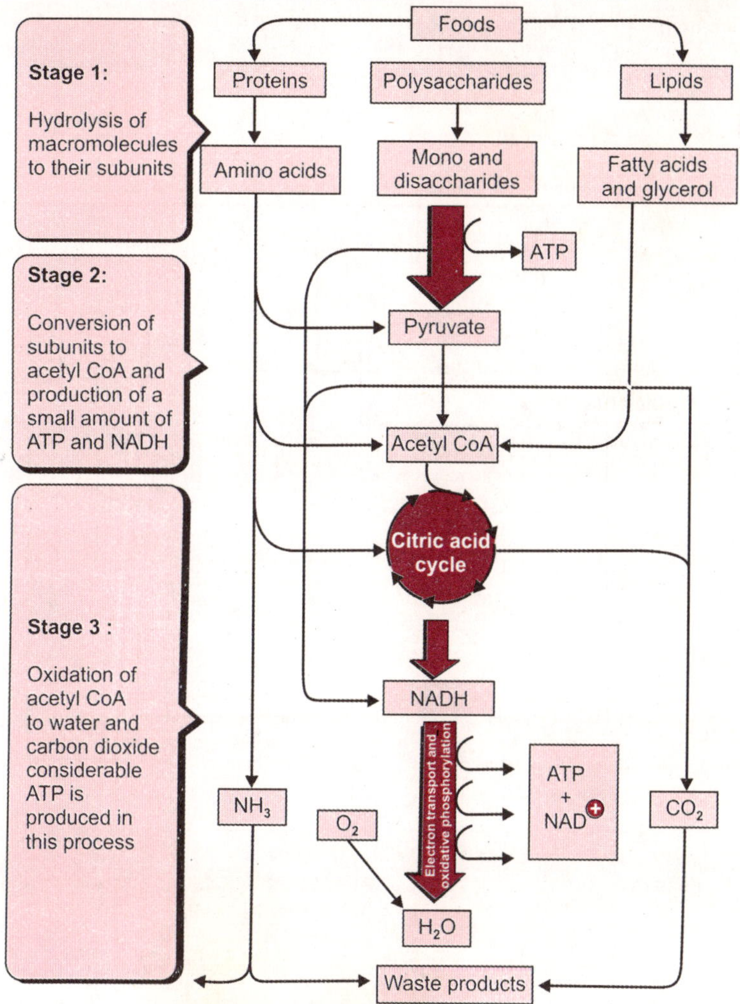

Fig. 15.1: Three stages of metabolism

3rd Stage: Oxidative Stage: Aerobic Final (TCA Cycle)

- In the presence of oxygen, acetyl CoA is oxidized to CO_2 and H_2O by common final pathway, TCA cycle.
- The carbohydrates, lipids and proteins all form acetate or some other intermediates like oxaloacetate (OAA), α-ketoglutarate, succinyl CoA, or fumarate, which are all intermediates of TCA cycle.
- Having gained entry into the TCA cycle at any site, two of the carbons of "citrate" constituting an acetate moiety are oxidized finally to CO_2 and H_2O and the energy of oxidation by the electron transport chain is captured as energy-rich PO_4, ATP mostly.

This stage yields the largest amount of energy of all three stages. Thus, the pathways are similar to a large extent and identical in the final stage of oxidation of the metabolites, whether derived from carbohydrates, lipids or proteins. This is schematically represented in ***Figure 15.2.***

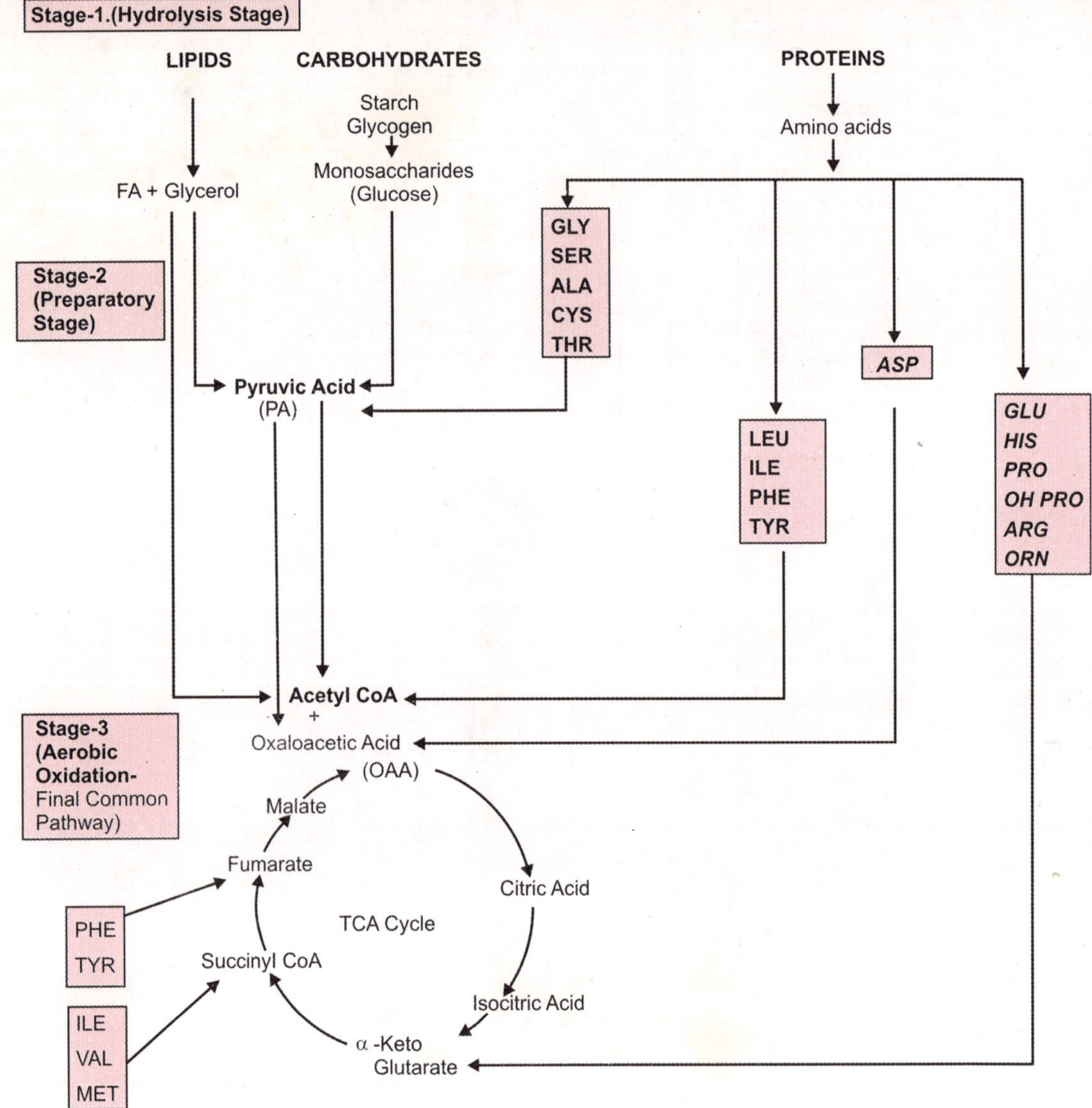

Fig. 15.2: Schematic representation of the three stages and their relationship

INTERCONVERSION BETWEEN THE THREE PRINCIPAL COMPONENTS

I. *Carbohydrates can form lipids through formation of:*

- α-glycero-P from glycerol or dihydroxy acetone-P (from glycolysis) which is necessary for triacyl glycerol (TG) and
- FA from acetyl CoA (extramitochondrial *de novo* synthesis).
- *Carbohydrates can form nonessential amino acids* through amination of α-keto acids. Viz. pyruvic acid (PA), oxaloacetic acid (OAA) and α-ketoglutarate to form amino acids alanine, aspartate and glutamate respectively.

II. *Fatty acids can be converted to some amino acids* by forming the dicarboxylic acids like malic acid, oxaloacetic acid and α-keto-glutarate.

- Fatty acid carbon may theoretically be incorporated into carbohydrates by the acetate running through TCA cycle. But there is no net gain in carbohydrates, since two carbons, equivalent of acetate are oxidized in the cycle.
- However, acetate can form glucose by running through the glyoxylate cycle.
- Acetone, one of the ketone bodies may be glucogenic. Acetone can be converted to acetol-P which, in turn, can produce propanediol-P. ***Propanediol-(P) is glucogenic.***

III. ***Proteins can form both carbohydrates and lipids*** through the glucogenic and ketogenic amino acids.

REGULATION AND CONTROL OF THE REACTIONS

The ratio of ATP/AMP of the cells/or tissues seems to decide the extent of its aerobic metabolism.

1. ***Inhibition:*** If the ratio is high (low AMP or ADP level), this will have certain inhibitory effects of certain enzymes of glycolytic-TCA cycle.
   - A high level of ATP and low level of AMP will inhibit the enzyme *phosphofructokinase* of glycolytic pathway and thereby inhibit glycolysis.
   - As a result, there is accumulation of hexose-P which interacts with UTP to form UDP-G and proceeds to increase glycogen synthesis.
   - G-6-P will also be channelized to HMP shunt leading to increased formation of NADPH which will participate in reductive synthesis, like FA synthesis which will be increased. The converse happens with low ATP and high AMP levels.
   - ***Increased ATP/ADP ratio will stimulate PDH-kinase*** which in turn converts dephosphorylated *'active' PDH (pyruvate dehydrogenase* complex) to 'inactive' phosphorylated PDH inhibiting the oxidative decarboxylation of pyruvic acid (PA).
   - *High ATP/AMP ratio,* also lowers the activity of the enzyme *isocitrate dehydrogenase* (ICD) of TCA cycle resulting in accumulation of citrate. The oxidation in TCA cycle decreases and ATP production falls.
2. ***Stimulation:*** Increased citric acid levels stimulate the enzyme *acetyl-CoA carboxylase.* Increased activity of acetyl CoA carboxylase converts acetyl-CoA to malonyl CoA, the first step in extramitochondrial *de novo* FA synthesis. Thus, the acetyl-CoA, in the presence of adequate stores of ATP and low AMP levels, is diverted to the synthesis of fats.

☞ SALIENT POINTS TO REMEMBER

- For our convenience, we learn the chemical processes occurring in the body in terms of individual metabolic reactions and pathways of each biomolecules.
- But in body thousands of such reactions occur in a living cell simultaneously.
- The metabolism of carbohydrates, lipids and proteins is integrated to meet the energy and metabolic demands of the individual.
- The metabolic pathways, viz. glycolysis, FA oxidation, citric acid cycle and oxidative phosphorylation, are directly concerned with the generation of ATP.
- The metabolic pathways are arbitrarily divided into 3 stages.
- ***First stage:*** Stage of hydrolysis of the complex biomolecules to simpler units. Thus complex carbohydrates are converted to simpler monosaccharide units, TG is hydrolyzed to form FFA and Glycerol, and proteins are degraded to amino acids. Very little of energy is produced at this stage and is dissipated as heat. There is no storage of energy at this stage.
- ***2nd stage is the preparatory stage:*** Glucose is degraded to form pyruvic acid which in presence of O_2 is converted to acetyl-CoA. Similarly, FA undergoes β-oxidation to form acetyl-CoA.

  In the case of amino acids, viz. alanine, serine, cysteine/cystine, etc. are converted to acetyl-CoA. Few others like leucine, phenylalanine/tyrosine and isoleucine yield acetate or acetoacetate which is converted to acetyl-CoA. In this stage, relatively small amount of energy is produced which is stored as ATP.

- ***Third stage constitutes oxidative stage aerobic final:*** In this stage, in presence of O_2, the acetyl-CoA obtained from carbohydrates, fats and proteins are oxidized to CO_2 and H_2O by final common pathway of TCA cycle. This stage yield the largest amount of energy which is stored as ATP.
- Interconversions of carbohydrates, lipids and proteins can occur:
  - Carbohydrates can form lipids through formation of α-Glycero-P from di-OH-acetone (P).
  - Glycerol part of TG can form glucose by gluconeogenesis.
  - Carbohydrates can form non-essential amino acid by amination of various α-ketoacids.
  - Acetate can form glucose by running through the glyoxylate cycle.
  - Acetone can be converted to 1, 2 propane-diol-P by propanediol pathway which is glucogenic.
  - Proteins can form both carbohydrates and lipids through the glucogenic and keto-genic amino acids.

MULTIPLE CHOICE QUESTIONS

Give one correct answer:

1. **Increased citric acid levels in the blood will stimulate which of the enzyme?**
   (a) Enolase
   (b) Transaldolase
   (c) Pyruvate carboxylase
   (d) Acetyl-CoA carboxylase
   (e) Transketolase
2. **Leucine enters the TCA cycle, the third stage of metabolism at the level of:**
   (a) Fumarate
   (b) Succinyl CoA
   (c) α-Ketoglutarate
   (d) Oxaloacetate
   (e) Acetyl-CoA
3. **Histidine enters the TCA cycle at the level of:**
   (a) Oxaloacetate
   (b) Acetyl-CoA
   (c) α-ketoglutarate
   (d) Fumarate
   (e) Malate
4. **Which of the following dicarboxylic acids is not a member of the TCA Cycle?**
   (a) Maleic acid
   (b) Fumarate
   (c) Succinate
   (d) Oxaloacetate
   (e) None of the above
5. **Valine enters the TCA cycle at the level of:**
   (a) α-ketoglutarate
   (b) Succinyl CoA
   (c) Fumarate
   (d) Oxaloacetate
   (e) Acetyl-CoA
6. **A high ATP/AMP ratio will inhibit which of the following enzyme?**
   (a) Pyruvate kinase
   (b) Phospho-fructokinase
   (c) Enolase
   (d) G-6-PD
   (e) Glyceraldehyde-3-P dehydrogenase

ANSWERS

1. (d)	2. (e)	3. (c)
4. (a)	5. (b)	6. (b)

Metabolism of Purines and Pyrimidines

INTRODUCTION

Mammals and most of the lower vertebrates can synthesize purines and pyrimidines and are said to be prototrophic.

SOURCES OF C AND N IN PYRIMIDINE RING

Pyrimidine is a heterocyclic ring.

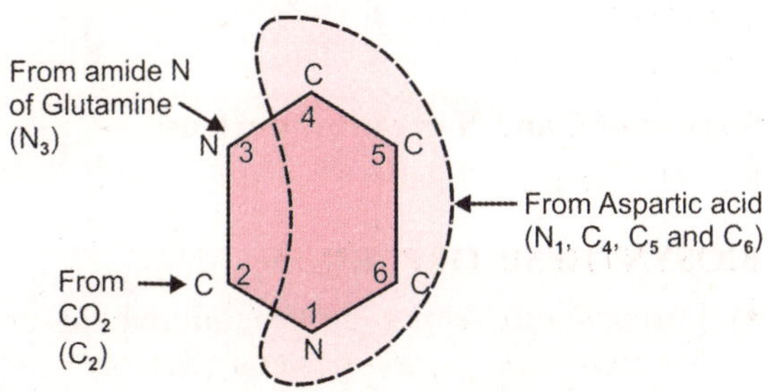

METABOLISM OF PYRIMIDINES

Synthesis of Pyrimidines

- A complex pathway, ingredients required are:
  - Glutamine
  - CO_2
  - ATP
  - Aspartic acid
  - PRPP (Phosphoribosyl pyrophosphate)
  - Certain enzymes and coenzymes
- ***First pyrimidine nucleotide formed is uridine-5′- monophosphate (UMP)*** which is further converted to other pyrimidine nucleotides, viz. CTP, TMP.

Catabolism of Pyrimidines: Overall reactions for catabolism of pyrimidines are given on next page ***(Fig. 16.1).***

Formation of Cytidine Nucleotides (CTP)

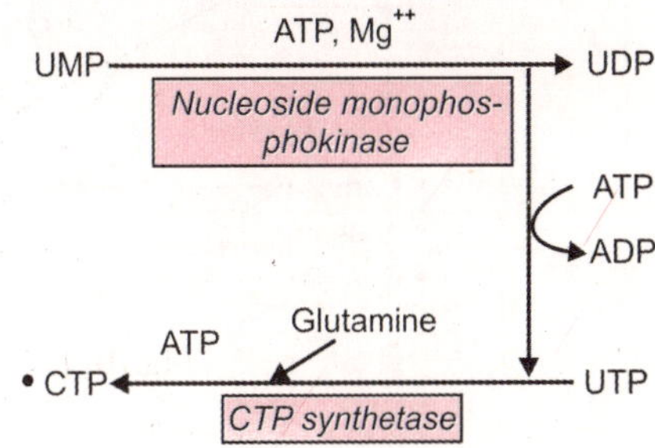

Note:

- Liver is the main site for catabolism of pyrimidines.
- ***CO_2 and NH_3 formed as end-products.***
- Side product from cytosine and uracil is β-alanine.
- β-alanine can be utilized for synthesis of carnosine, anserine and CoA-SH.
- Alternatively, it can be oxidized to acetate, NH_3 and CO_2.
- β-amino isobutyric acid is formed from catabolism of thymine.

Clinical Significance

- β-amino isobutyric acid is excreted in large quantities in leukaemias and when body is subjected to X-ray irradiation (***β-amino isobutyric aciduria***).
- β-amino isobutyrate can be converted to methylmalonic semi-aldehyde which, in turn, can form propionic acid which is converted → to succinate (thus can be "glucogenic").

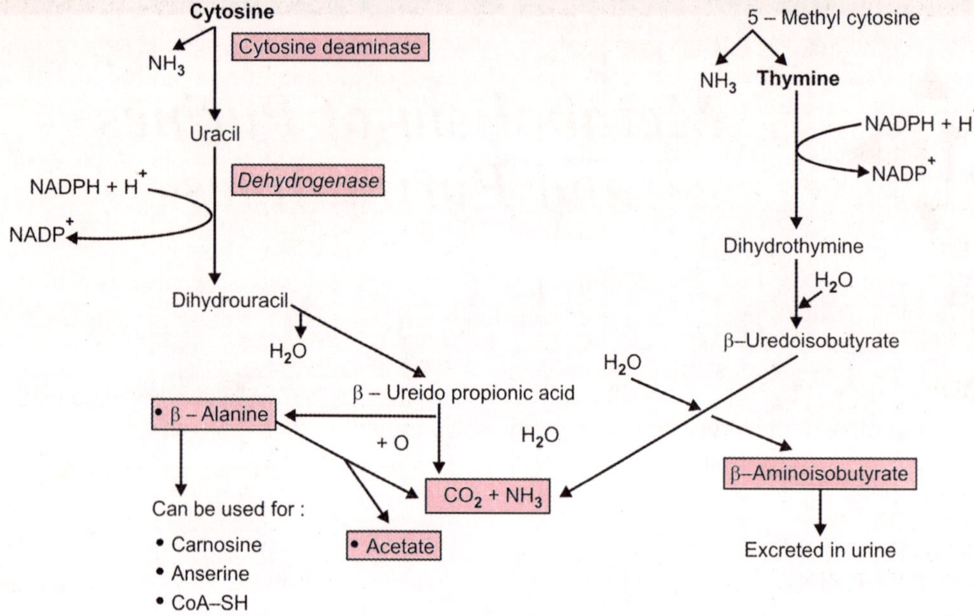

Fig. 16.1: Catabolism of pyrimidines

METABOLISM OF PURINES

Adenine and guanine are the two purines either with a ribose or deoxyribose sugar, found in living organisms.

Points to remember

- ***Purines are built up as nucleotides.***
- There is ***no dietary requirement of purines. Body can synthesize them.***
- Various enzymes that catalyze specific reactions in the synthetic pathway have been studied.
- The pathway of synthesis is essentially the same in all the living organisms.
- ***Synthesis takes place in the liver.***
- Purines are first synthesized as nucleotide, ***inosinic acid (hypoxanthine ribose 5'—phosphate)*** which is then converted into the adenine and guanine nucleotides.
- Purine ring is built on ribose-5'-P.

Sources of C and N in purine nucleus:

Refer *Fig. 16.2.*

BIOSYNTHESIS OF PURINES:

- Purine synthesis is complex and involves at least ten steps (Details of steps given on next page)
- Purine ring is built upon a molecule of PRPP (5'—phosphoribosyl-1-pyrophosphate).

Ingredients required are:

- PRPP
- Glutamine-amide N_2
- Glycine
- CO_2
- Aspartic acid
- Two one—carbon fragments from the one-carbon "folate pool".
- ATP, Mg^{++}, and various enzymes.

- ***First purine nucleotide formed is inosine monophosphate (IMP).***

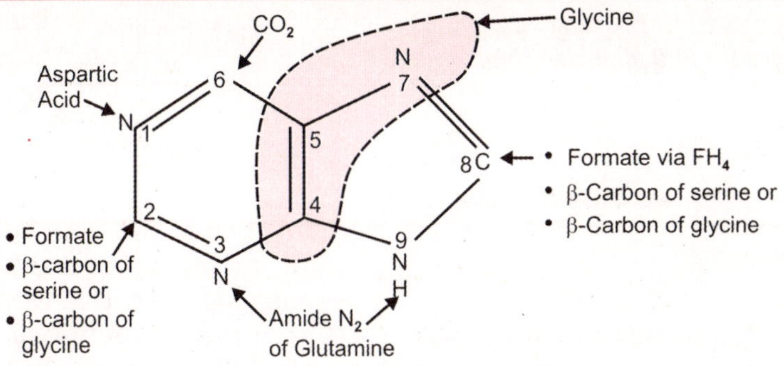

Fig. 16.2: Sources of C and N of Purine

- ***Expenditure of six high energy phosphate bonds, hence, it is energetically expensive process.***

Formation of PRPP:

- PRPP is formed from ribose-5-P and ATP.
  Ribose-5-P+ATP → PRPP + AMP.
- Enzyme *"PRPP synthetase"* is an allosteric enzyme.
- **Uses of PRPP.** PRPP is required for:
  - Synthesis of both purine and pyrimidine nucleotides.
  - Salvage pathways for both purine and pyrimidine bases.
  - Biosynthesis of nucleotide coenzyme.

Once IMP is formed, it can form other purine nucleotides, viz. AMP, GMP.

1. Formation of AMP from IMP:

It occurs in **two steps:**

- Aspartic acid condenses with IMP to form adenylosuccinate.

IMP —(Aspartic acid, Mg^{++})→ **Adenylosuccinate**

Enzyme: *"Adenylosuccinate synthetase".*
GTP: It provides the energy.

- Adenylosuccinate is then cleaved to form fumaric acid and **AMP.**

Adenylosuccinate → • **AMP** (↘ Fumarate)

Enzyme: *"Adenylosuccinate lyase".*

2. Formation of GMP from IMP: It occurs in **two steps.**

- IMP is first oxidized to xanthylic acid (xanthine monophosphate, XMP).

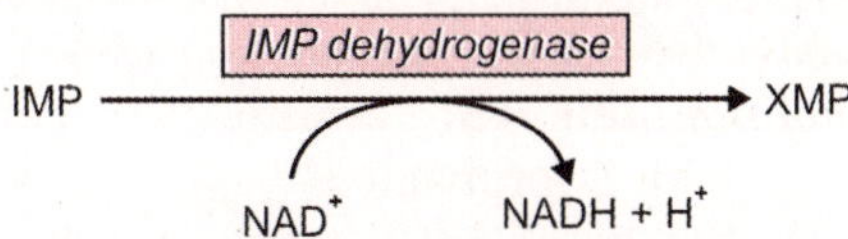

- Glutamine gives the amide group to C_2 of XMP to form GMP

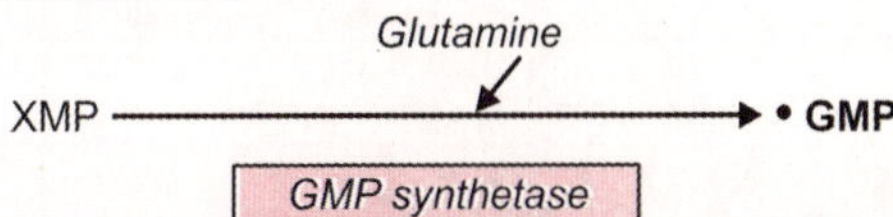

STEPS OF BIOSYNTHESIS:

1. **Formation of PRPP:** Synthesis begins with D-Ribose-5'-P obtained from HMP-shunt pathway. PRPP is synthesized by the enzyme ***"PRPP synthase"*** from D'-ribose-5'-P and ATP.

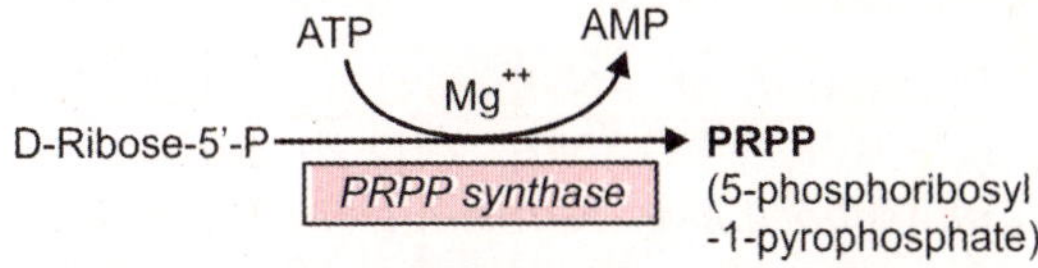

2. **Formation of 5'-Phospho-ribosyl-1 Amine (PRA):** Amide group of glutamine is transferred to ***C1 of PRPP*** by the enzyme ***"Glutamine PRPP amidotransferase".***

Phosphate group is replaced by –NH2 group. *This gives the N-9 of purine ring.*

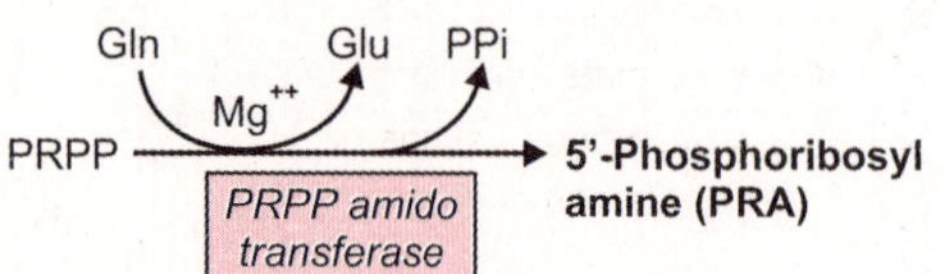

3. **Formation of Glycinamide Ribotide, GAR** *(also called 5'-Phosphoribosyl-glycinamide):* Glycine condenses with PRA using ATP as energy source to form glycinamide ribotide (GAR), the reaction is catalyzed by the enzyme *"Glycinamide kinosynthase". This provides C-4, C-5 and N-7 of the Purine ring.*

4. **Formation of Formyl glycinamide ribotide, FGAR** *(also called 5'-phosphoribosyl-N-formyl glycinamide):* The amino nitrogen of glycinamide is formylated by N10-formyl H4-folate catalyzed by the enzyme "formyl transferase". *The formyl carbon becomes C-8 of the purine ring.*

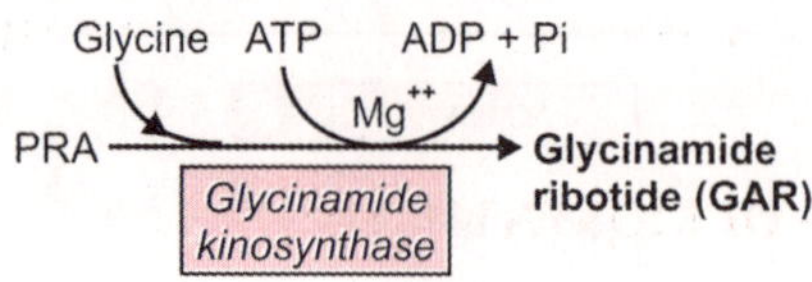

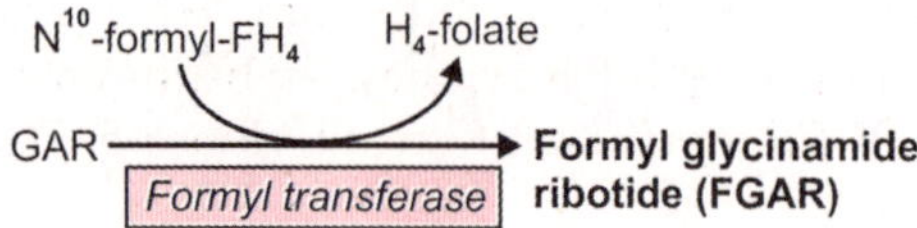

5. **Formation of a-N-formyl glycinamidine ribotide, FGAM:** *(also called 5'-phosphoribosyl-N-formyl glycinamidine):* Another of amide group of glutamine is transferred to FGAR to form FGAM. *"Phosphoribosyl glycinamidine synthase"* is the enzyme that catalyzes the reaction and ATP provides the energy. The *reaction contributes N-3 of Purine ring.*

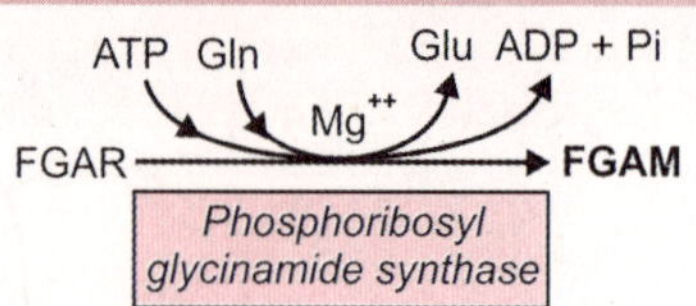

6. **Formation of 5-Amino-imidazole riboside, AIR** *(also called 5'-phosphoribosyl-5-aminoimidazole):* This reaction is catalyzed by the enzyme *"amino imidazole ribosyl phosphate synthetase" (AIR-Psynthetase),* which brings about the dehydratative closure of the ring, by removal of a molecule of H_2O. ATP is required for the reaction.

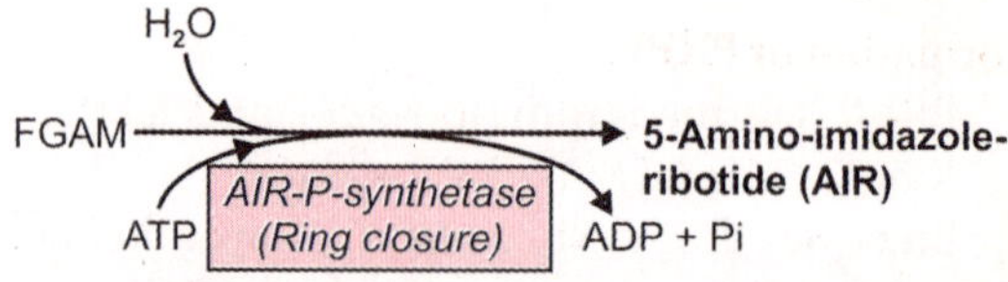

7. **Formation of 5-Amino-Imidazole-4-carboxylic acid ribotide, C-AIR** *(also called 5'-phosphoribosyl-5-amino imidazole-4 carboxylate):* This reaction uses CO_2 to carboxylate AIR. *It contributes to C-6 of the purine nucleus. This reaction is somewhat unusual since neither Biotin nor ATP is required for carboxylation.*

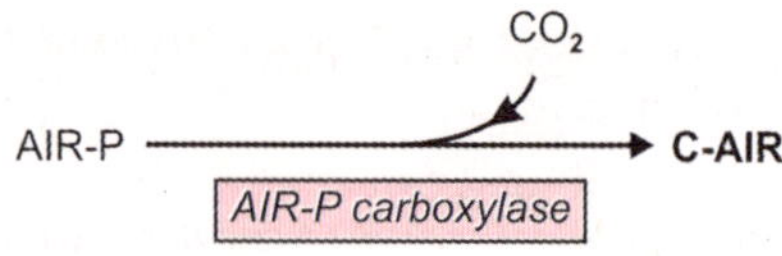

Mechanism: *The imidazole ring acts as a nucleophile in this reaction. The atoms from C-4 to the aminogroup at C-5 constitutes an "enamine". Since enamines are already activated nucleophiles, hence no further activation is necessary. The reaction occurs by attack of the nucleophilic C-4 atom of the enamine upon the electrophilic carbon of carbon dioxide (CO_2).*

8. **Formation of 5-amino-imidazole-N-succinyl carboxamide ribotide, 5-AISCR.** *(Also called 5'phosphoribosyl-5-aminoimidazole-4-N succino carboxamide):* This reaction is catalyzed by the enzyme ***"succinyl carboxamide synthetase".*** This uses ATP to condense Aspartic acid with amino-imidazole carboxylate-5-P. ***This contributes to N-1 of the purine nucleus.***

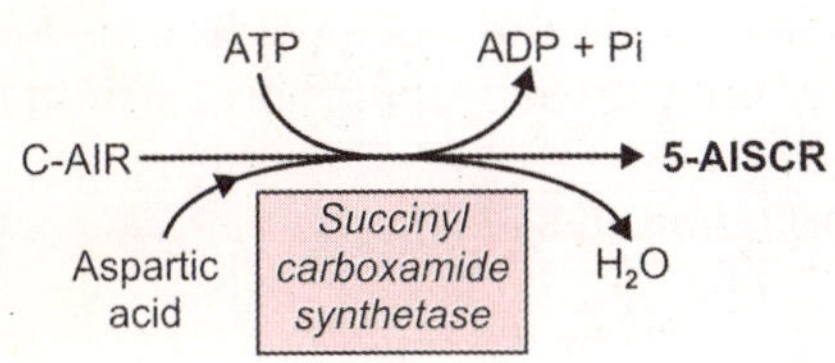

9. **Formation of 5-Amino-imidazole-4-Carboxamide ribotide, 5-AICAR.** *(Also called 5'-Phosphoribosyl-5-amino-imidazole-4-carboxamide):* 5-AISCR undergoes cleavage by the cleaving enzyme ***"adenylo-succinate lyase"*** to form 5-AICAR and fumarate.

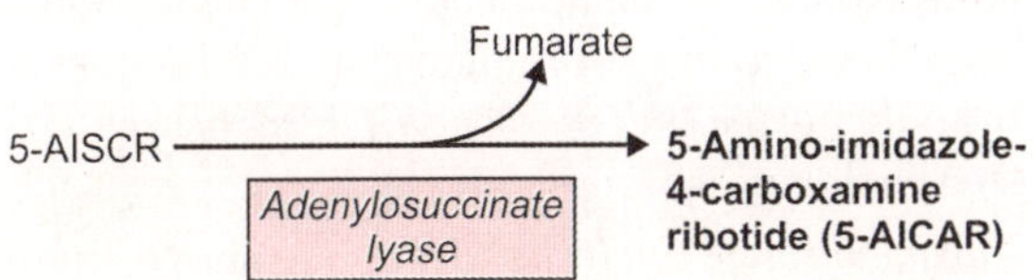

10. **Formation of 5-formamido imidazole-4-Carboxyamide ribotide, 5-FICR.** *(Also called 5'-phosphoribosyl-5-formamido imidazole-4-carboxamide): Carbon-2 (C-2) the final carbon of the Purine ring* is donated by N10-formyl F.H4 in a reaction catalyzed by the enzyme ***"formyl transferase"*** and forms 5-FICR.

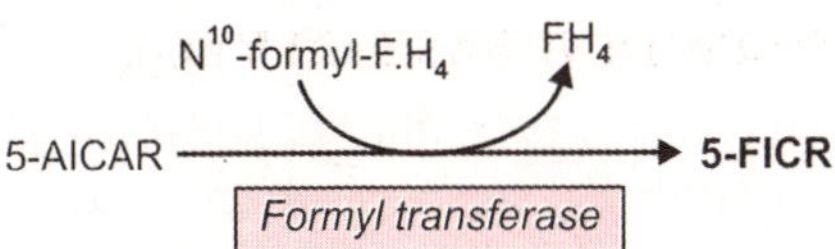

11. **Formation of Inosinic acid (IMP):** 5-FICR undergoes a ***dehydrative ring closure,*** by elimination of one molecule of H2O. The reaction is catalyzed by the enzyme ***"IMP cyclohydrolase"*** to form Inosinic acid (IMP).
Note: ***Hypoxanthine nucleotide (inosinic acid) is the first purine that is synthesized in the body.*** Adenine and guanine nucleotides are then synthesized from the hypoxanthine or xanthine nucleotides respectively by amination.

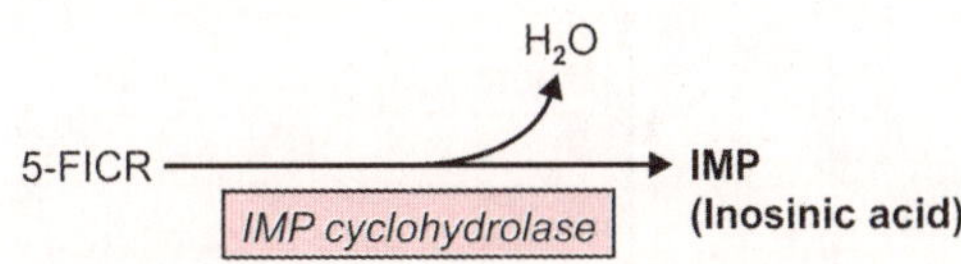

SALVAGE PATHWAYS FOR PURINES AND PYRIMIDINE BASES

General Remarks: Points to note:

- The *"de novo"* synthesis of nucleotides is ***expensive*** in terms of the use of high energy phosphate bonds specially for the purine biosynthesis.
- Many cells have pathways that ***"salvage"*** purine and pyrimidine bases for the corresponding nucleotides.
- All tissues are not capable of *"de novo"* synthesis of purine nucleotides, e.g. ***erythrocytes, Neutrophils*** and the ***brain cells***. These cells lack the enzyme *"PRPP-amido transferase"*.
- Nucleotides do not enter cells directly but are converted to *"nucleosides"* by cell membrane *"nucleosidases"*.
  - After entering the cells the nucleoside is either
    - converted to the nucleotide again by a *"kinase"* enzyme or
    - degraded to corresponding base by the enzyme *"nucleoside phosphorylase"*.

A. PURINE SALVAGE PATHWAYS

Two pathways are available.

1. One-step Synthesis

- *Formation of GMP and IMP: "Hypoxanthine-guanine phosphoribosyl transferase"* (HGPRTase) catalyzes the one-step formation of the nucleotides from either guanine or hypoxanthine, using PRPP as the donor of the ribosyl moiety.

Thus,

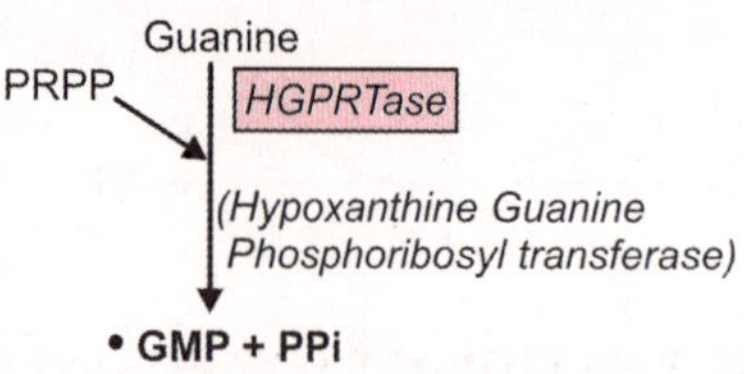

Similarly,

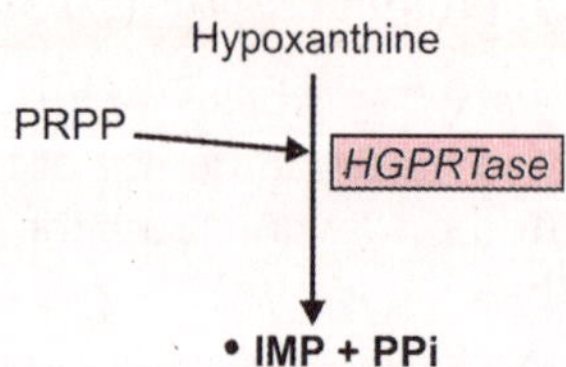

Regulation: The enzyme HGPRTase is regulated by the competitive inhibition of GMP and IMP respectively.

- ***Formation of AMP:*** The enzyme *"Adenine phosphoribosyl transferase"* (APRTase) in a similar way catalyzes the formation of AMP from Adenine, ribosyl moiety is donated by PRPP.

Thus,

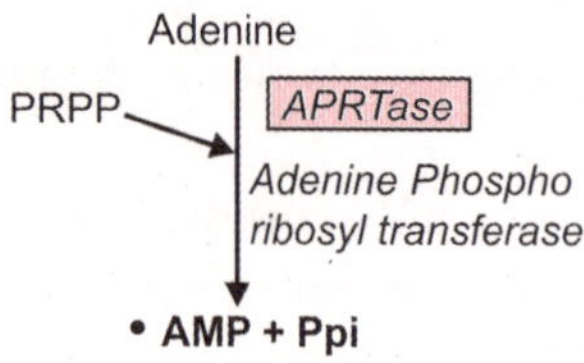

Regulation: The enzyme APRTase is regulated by the competitive inhibition of AMP.

2. Two-Step Synthesis

(Nucleoside Phosphorylase-nucleoside Kinase Pathway)

Under some conditions, it is possible for purine bases to be salvaged by a two-step process as under:

"Nucleoside Phosphorylase" is an enzyme that brings about nucleoside breakdown. But the reaction is readily ***"reversible"*** and can form back 'nucleoside' which is rather a **favourable** pathway. Once the nucleoside is formed, a *"kinase"* enzyme may phosphorylate it to the 5'-nucleotide.

- *Formation of AMP:*

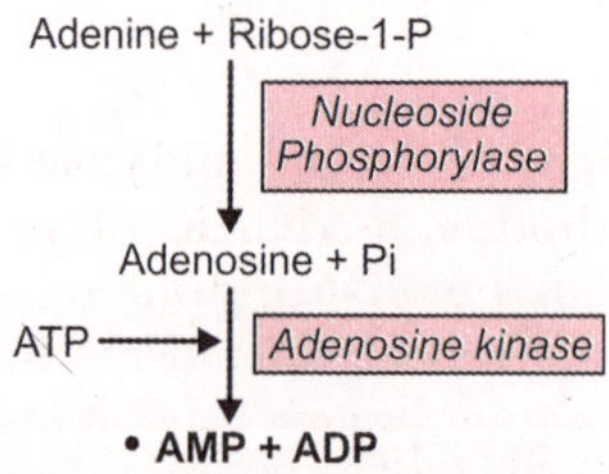

Note: Neither *"Guanosine nor Inosine Kinases"* have been detected in mammalian cells. ***So Adenine is the only purine that may be salvaged by the two-step pathway.***

Purine Salvage Cycle: In addition to above, there is a cycle in which GMP and IMP as well as their deoxyribonucleotides are converted into their respective 'nucleosides' by a *"purine 5'-nucleotidase"* enzyme. The nucleosides so formed can be hydrolytically cleaved producing the corresponding sugar phosphates and setting free the N-bases. The guanine and hypoxanthine then can be phosphoribosylated again to complete the cycle, called ***"Purine salvage cycle" (Figure 16.3).***

B. PYRIMIDINE BASE SALVAGE

The enzyme *"Pyrimidine Phosphoribosyl transferase"* catalyzes the formation of pyrimidine nucleotide, using PRPP as the donor of the ribosyl moiety.

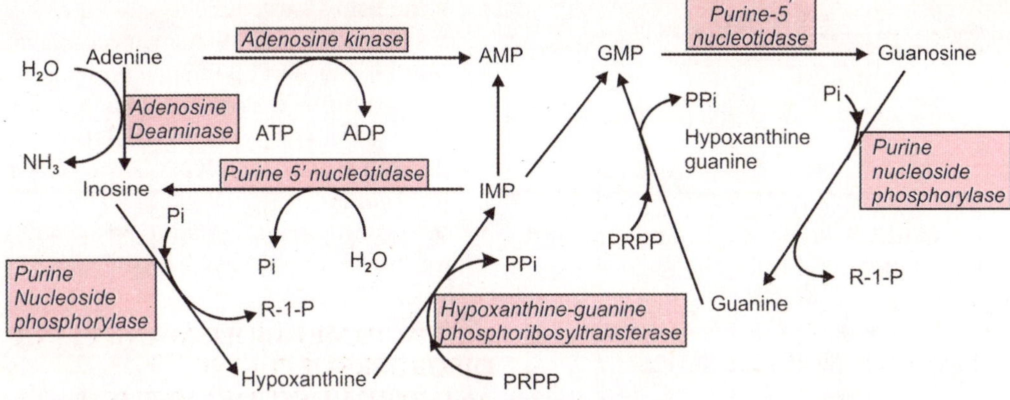

Fig. 16.3: Purine-salvage cycle

Thus,

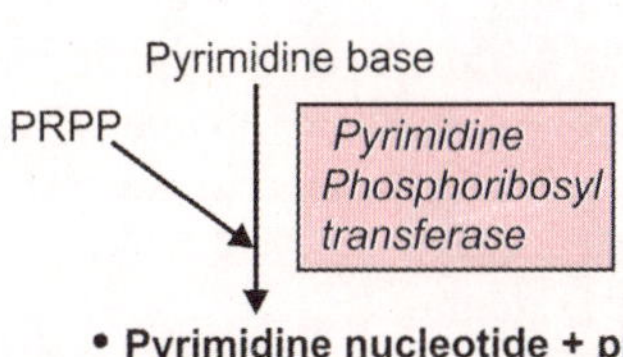

Note: The enzyme obtained from human red cells can use orotate, uracil and thymine as substrates.

Regulation of Purine Synthesis

- *PRPP synthetase* is an important enzyme that regulates purine synthesis. ***It is allosterically inhibited by the feedback effects of PRPP** and **number of purine nucleotides such as AMP, GMP, ADP, GDP, NAD** and **FAD.***
- *Glutamine PRPP amidotransferase* is the enzyme for the rate-limiting step of purine synthesis. It is regulated by feedback inhibitory effects of AMP and GMP.
- A proper balance between the adenine and guanine concentration is maintained by adenylosuccinate synthetase and IMP dehydrogenase, respectively.

CATABOLISM OF PURINES (Formation of Uric Acid)

Uric acid is the chief end-product of purine catabolism in humans and primates.

- Organisms that form uric acid are said to be *"uricotelic".*
- An average of 600 to 800 mg of uric acid is excreted by human beings, most of it is found in urine.

Steps of Degradation of Purine Bases ***(Refer Fig. 16.5):*** Degradation of purine bases consists of following **six steps:**

1. AMP is hydrolyzed to adenosine by *nucleotidase"* or deaminated to IMP by *"AMP deaminase".*
   $AMP + H_2O \rightarrow Adenosine + Pi$
   $AMP + H_2O \rightarrow IMP + NH_3$
2. Adenosine is then converted to inosine by *"Adenosine deaminase",* and *"nucleotidases"* convert IMP to inosine.
   $Adenosine + H_2O \rightarrow Inosine + NH_3$
   $IMP + H_2O \rightarrow Inosine + Pi$
3. Inosine undergoes phosphorolysis by *"purine nucleoside phosphorylase"* to give hypoxanthine
   $Inosine + Pi \rightarrow Hypoxanthine + Ribose\text{-}1\text{-}P$
4. Similarly, guanine nucleotides are converted to guanine by sequential action of *"nucleotidases"* and *"purine nucleoside phosphorylase"*
   $GMP + H_2O \rightarrow Guanosine + Pi$
   $Guanosine + Pi \rightarrow Guanine + Ribose\text{-}1\text{-}P$
5. Guanine is then deaminated to xanthine by the enzyme *"guanase"*
   $Guanine + H_2O \rightarrow Xanthine + NH_3$
6. The final steps of purine degradation in humans are carried out by the enzyme ***"xanthine Oxidase"***. *"Xanthine oxidase"* oxidizes hypoxanthine to xanthine and xanthine to uric acid.

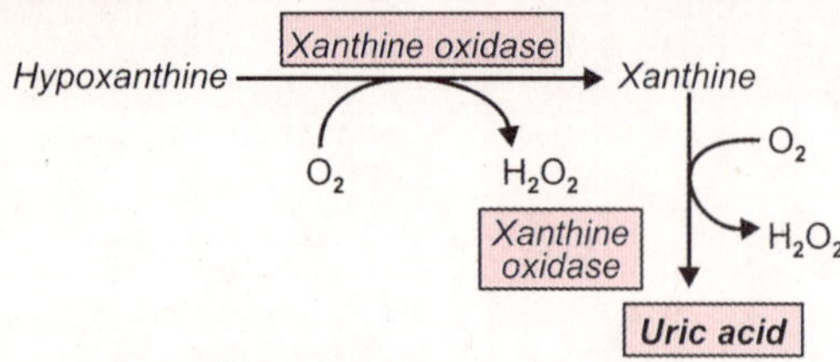

Xanthine oxidase is a metalloenzyme and contains 'molybdenum' (Mo), the trace element and also Fe^{3+}.

It requires • *FAD,* • *Molecular O_2*
Produces H_2O_2 at substrate level.

Clinical Significance

- *Allo-Purinol:* Resembles structurally hypoxanthine. When administered, it inhibits the enzyme *"xanthine oxidase"* by competitive inhibition and thus, inhibits uric acid formation. Hence, the drug has been used for lowering blood uric acid level in ***GOUT.***

Purine catabolism is shown schematically in (Fig. 16.4)

Further Catabolism of Uric Acid: Non-primates (Refer reaction in the next page)

- In many non-primate animals uric acid may be oxidized and decarboxylated by *uricase,* a hepatic copper containing enzyme to ***allantoin.***

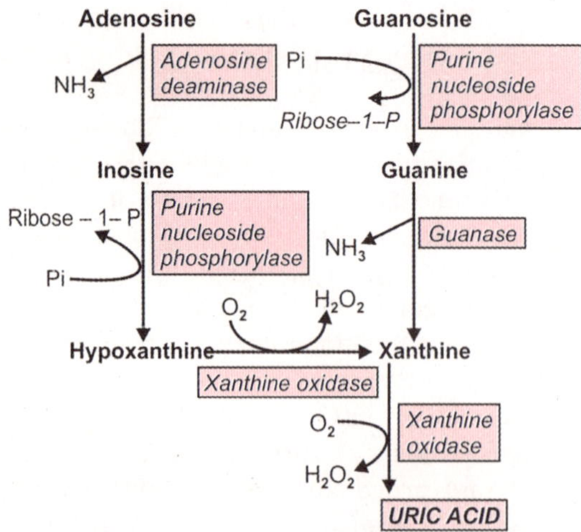

Fig.16.4: Purine catabolism

- Some fishes carry *uricase* as well as *allantoinase.* This converts allantoin into *allantonic acid.*
- Amphibians and other such animals contain allantoicase which converts allantoic acid into ureidoglycolate. Ureidoglycolate is further cleaved by *ureidoglycolase* into ***urea*** and ***glyoxylate.***
- Urea is further converted to NH_3 and CO_2 in crustaceans by an enzyme urease found in their liver.

URIC ACID METABOLISM AND CLINICAL DISORDERS OF PURINE AND PYRIMIDINE METABOLISM

- The main site of uric acid formation is liver from where it is carried to kidneys.
- *Miscible pool:* It is the quantity of uric acid present in body water. In normal subjects an average of 1130 mg of uric acid is present. Plasma contains higher concentration of uric acid compared to other body compartments containing water.
- *Turn over:* This is the rate at which the uric acid is synthesized and lost from the body. Normally, 500-600 mg of uric acid is synthesized. Not all is excreted in urine, further some uric acid is excreted in bile. Some is converted to urea and ammonia by the intestinal bacteria.
- *Distribution:* It is very irregularly distributed in the body. Serum contains 3-7 mg/dl. Average values are slightly higher in males. Red cells contain half as much uric acid as serum. Muscles also contain less amount compared to blood.
- *Dietary effects:* Uric acid excretion continues at a rather steady rate during starvation and during a purine-free diet owing to the so-called endogenous purine metabolism. The ingestion of foods high in nucleoproteins such as glandular organs produces a marked increase in urinary uric acid. Diets like milk, eggs and cheese, with low purine contents causes practically no increase in urinary uric acid.
- *Effect of hormones:* Administration of the glucocorticoid hormones and ACTH increases the excretion of uric acid in urine.

- *Excretion of uric acid:* Uric acid in the plasma is filtered by the glomeruli but is later partially reabsorbed by the renal tubules; ***glycine is believed to compete with uric acid for tubular reabsorption.*** Certain uricosuric drugs such as salicylates, block reabsorption of uric acid. There is now conclusive evidence for tubular secretion of uric acid by kidney. Thus, uric acid is cleared both by:
  - ***Glomerular filtration;*** and
  - ***Tubular secretion.***

Lactic acid also competes with uric acid excretion.

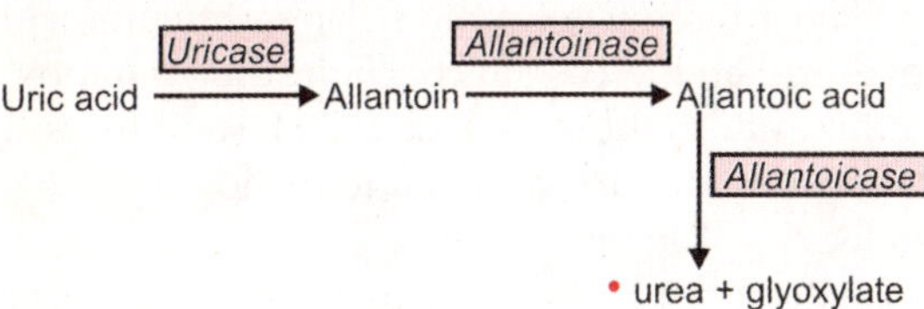

CLINICAL DISORDERS

I. Gout:

Gout is a chronic disorder characterized by:

- Excess of uric acid in blood ***(Hyperuricaemia)***
- Deposition of sodium monourate in alveolar and non-alveolar structures producing so called ***tophi.***
- ***Recurring attacks of acute arthritis.*** These are due to deposition of monosodium urate in and around the structures of the affected joints.

Types: There are **two main types** of gout:

- **Primary gout,**
- **Secondary gout.**

1. *Primary Gout:* Here the hyperuricaemia is not due to increased destruction of nucleic acid. ***The essential abnormality is increased formation of uric acid*** from simple carbon and nitrogen compounds without intermediary incorporation into nucleic acids.
   a. ***Primary metabolic gout:*** It is due to inherited metabolic defect in purine metabolism leading to excessive rate of conversion of glycine to uric acid. X-linked recessive defects enhancing the *de novo* synthesis of purines and their catabolism can also lead to hyperuricemia. For example, such defects of PRPP synthetase may make it feedback resistant. X-linked recessive defects of *hypoxanthineguanine phosphoribosyl transferase* may reduce utilization of PRPP in the salvage pathway. Increased intracellular PRPP enhances *de novo* purine synthesis.
   b. ***Primary renal gout:*** It is due to failure in uric acid excretion.
2. *Secondary gout:*
   a. ***Secondary metabolic gout:*** It is due to secondary increase in purine catabolism in conditions like leukemia, prolonged fasting and polycythemia.
   b. ***Secondary renal gout:*** Due to defective glomerular filtration of urate due to generalized renal failure.
   c. ***In von Gierke's disease:*** Deficiency of G-6 *phosphatase* leads to elevated rate of pentose formation in HMP. This acts as a good substrate for *PRPP synthetase* and enhances the synthesis of purines followed by their catabolism to uric acid. ***Increase lactic acid competes with uric acid excretion resulting to retention of uric acid*** (Refer, Glycogen Storage Diseases).

Treatment of Gout: Consist of:

- ***Palliative treatment***
- ***Specific treatment***

  (a) Palliative treatment:
  - Bed rest in acute stage
  - Diet-Purine free diet
  - Restricting alcohol consumption
- ***Antiinflammatory Drugs:***
  1. ***Colchicine:*** One of the nonspecific anti-inflammatory drug. It has no effect on urate metabolism or excretion. Colchicine therapy is instituted during acute attack.

     Mechanism: Suppresses the synthesis and secretion of the chemotactic factor that is produced in urate crystal-induced inflammation.

     Dosage: Available as 0.5 mg tablet. In acute gout: one tablet hourly till symptoms are relieved or diarrhoea occurs.

Long-term management: one tab 3 to 4 times a week.

2. *NSAIDs:* Drugs like:
   - Indomethacin,
   - Diclofenac,
   - Naproxen,
   - Piroxicam,
   - Fenoprofen
   - Elurbiprofen
   - Ibuprofen, Refecoxabin etc.

These drugs inhibit the synthesis of PGs which are important mediator of the inflammatory response. These drugs have been found effective in treating patients having recurrent attacks of acute gout and also for terminating acute attack of gout.

(b) Specific Treatment

Aim: to lower the uric acid level of blood.

Methods: The above can be achieved in ***three ways:***

- ***By increasing the renal excretion of uric acid (uricosuric drugs).***
- ***By decreasing the synthesis of uric acid using enzyme inhibitor***
- ***By increasing oxidation of uric acid.***

1. Uricosuric Drugs:

Definition: An uricosuric agent is one that enhances the renal excretion of uric acid probably by specific inhibition of its tubular reabsorption or secretion.

Drugs used are:

- ***Salicylates:*** Effects vary with dosage. In low dosage of 1 to 2 gm/day, salicylates cause uric acid retention but in higher dosage 5 to 6 gm/day it has uricosuric effect. Long-term therapy with high dosage is not desirable due to the side effects.
- ***Probenecid (Benemide):***
  - It is an efficient and harmless uricosuric drug.
  - Lowers the uric acid level-fall is immediate and sustained.

Dose: Available as 500 mg tablet. ½ tablet twice daily for the first week and then one tablet twice daily. Not recommended for children. Therapy is continued for 10 to 12 weeks and patients can return to normal activities.

- ***Halofenate:*** The drug has good uricosuric effect. Also has a hypolipaemic effect. It liberates urates from urate binding sites of proteins of plasma and removes uric acid by normal excretion. The drug can be safely used for short-term and long-term therapy.

Note: ***Uricosuric drugs are effective provided renal function is normal.***

2. Enzyme Inhibitor:

- ***Allopurinol (Zyloprin): Drug of choice.*** It has similar structure like hypoxanthine. ***Acts by competitive inhibition on "xanthine oxidase" and thus uric acid synthesis is impaired.***

The drug causes a rapid fall in serum uric acid level and an increase in concentration of hypoxanthine and xanthine in blood. Both xanthine and hypoxanthine are more soluble and so are excreted easily in urine.

Allopurinol is acted upon by *"Xanthine oxidase"* and converted to *'alloxanthine'*.

Dosage: Available as 100 mg tablet. Initially 100 to 200 mg daily. ***Maintenance:*** 200 to 600 mg daily. Not recommended in children.

Note:

- In addition to gout, the drug can be used in secondary hyperuricaemia.
- Allopurinol also has an inhibitory action on the enzyme ***"tryptophan pyrrolase"***.

3. Drugs Increasing Uric Acid Oxidation:

- ***Urate oxidase:*** The drug can be used in lowering uric acid level by oxidizing uric acid.

Dosage: 10,000 IU daily for 10 days. It shows a significant decrease in uric acid level. Can be used in severe gout with renal involvement and secondary hyperuricaemia.

II. Lesch-Nyhan Syndrome: Only males are affected by this. It is X-linked recessive defect of *hypoxanthine-guanine phosphoribosyl transferase*. The enzyme is almost absent and leads to increased purine salvage pathway from PRPP. This can result in severe gout, renal failure, poor growth, spasticity and ***tendency for self-mutilation.***

III. Orotic Aciduria: It is of **2 types**

- ***Type I Orotic aciduria:*** It is an autosomal recessive genetic disorder of a protein, acting as both *orotate phosphoribosyl transferase* and *OMP decarboxylase.* Orotate fails to be converted to uridylate. This results in accumulation of orotate in blood elevating its level, growth retardation and megaloblastic anaemia.

- ***Type II Orotic aciduria:*** It is autosomal recessive affecting *OMP decarboxylase* and is characterized by megaloblastic anaemia and the urinary excretion of orotic acid.

☞ SALIENT POINTS TO REMEMBERS

- Pyrimidine nucleotides are synthesized from the precursors aspartate, glutamine and CO_2. In addition it requires PRPP (Phosphoribosyl) Pyrophosphate, ATP and certain enzymes and coenzymes.
- First Pyrimidine nucleotide synthesized is uridine-5′-monophosphate (UMP). UMP is further converted to CTP and TMP.
- Pyrimidines are degraded to amino acids, namely β-alanine, and β-amino isobutyrate, the latter is excreted in urine.
- β-amino isobutyrate is excreted in large quantities in Leukaemias and when body is subjected to X-ray irradiation (β-amino isobutyric aciduria)
- β-amino isobutyric acid can be converted to methyl malonic semi aldehyde, which in turn can form propionic acid which is glucogenic.
- Orotic aciduria is a defect in pyrimidine synthesis caused by the deficiency of orotate phosphoribosyl transferase and OMP decarboxylate. Diet rich in uridine and cystidine is an effective treatment for orotic aciduria.
- Purine nucleotides are synthesized by a series of complex reactions using PRPP as a starting material. Glycine, glutamine-amide N_2, aspartic acid, formate and CO_2 contribute to the synthesis of purine ring. In additions, it requires ATP, Mg^{++} and various enzymes.
- ***The first purine nucleotide formed is inosine monophosphate (IMP).***
- From IMP other purine nucleotides, viz. AMP and GMP are formed.
- Purine nucleotides can also be synthesized from free purines by a "Salvage Pathway".
- Lesch-Nyhan syndrome is an X-linked recessive defect, only affects males, in which enzyme HGPRTase is absent.
- The Syndrome is characterized by severe gout, renal failure, poor growth, spasticity and tendency for self-mutilation.
- Purine nucleotides are degraded in the body to form uric acid.
- Uric acid in many animal species, other than primates, is converted to more soluble forms such as allantoin, allantoic acid, etc. and excreted.
- Gout is a metabolic disease characterized by overproduction of uric acid. It leads to the accumulation of sodium urate crystals in the joints, producing painful gouty arthritis.
- ***Allopurinol, an inhibitor of xanthine oxidase, is the drug of choice for the treatment of gout.*** By inhibiting the enzyme the drug decreases the production of uric acid in the body.
- Uricosuric drugs are those which decreases uric acid level in the blood by enhancing the excretion of uric acid probably by specific inhibition of its tubular reabsorption or secretion, viz. salicylates, probenecid (Benemide, Halofenate.

MULTIPLE CHOICE QUESTIONS

Give one correct answer:

1. **Glycine contributes to the following C and N of purine nucleus:**
   (a) C_1, C_2 and N-7
   (b) C_3, C_4 and N_1
   (c) C_4, C_5 and N_9
   (d) C_4, C_5 and N_7
   (e) C_6, C_8 and N_9
2. **Two nitrogen of the pyrimidine ring are obtained from:**
   (a) Aspartate and carbamoyl-P
   (b) Aspartate and NH_3
   (c) Glutamine and NH_3
   (d) Glutamine and carbamoyl-P
   (e) Glutamic acid and NH_3

3. **In humans, the principal catabolic product of pyrimidines is:**
   (a) Uric acid (b) β-alanine
   (c) Hypoxanthine (d) Allantoin
   (e) Urea
4. **The probable metabolic defect in gout is:**
   (a) An under production of purines,
   (b) An over production of pyrimidines
   (c) An over production of uric acid
   (d) A defect in excretion of uric acid by kidneys
   (e) Increase in calcium leading to deposition of calcium urate.
5. **In most mammals, *except* primates, uric acid is metabolized by:**
   (a) Reduction to NH_3
   (b) Oxidation to allantoin
   (c) Hydrolysis to form NH_3
   (d) Isomerization to form urea
   (e) None of the above
6. **In humans, the principal breakdown product of purines is:**
   (a) Allantoin (b) Ammonia
   (c) β-alanine (d) Uric acid
   (e) Urea
7. **A drug which inhibits the enzyme xanthine oxidase thus decreasing the uric acid synthesis:**
   (a) Colchicine (b) Allopurinol
   (c) Probenecid (d) Halofenate
   (e) Aspirin
8. **The four nitrogen atoms of purines are derived from:**
   (a) Aspartate, NH_3 and Glutamate
   (b) Aspartate, Glutamine and glycine
   (c) Glycine, NH_3 and aspartate
   (d) NH_3, Glycine and Glutamate
   (e) NH_3 Glutamic acid and formate
9. **Synthesis of GMP from AMP requires the following:**
   (a) Glutamine, NAD^+, ATP
   (b) Glutamine, $NADP^+$, GTP
   (c) Glutamine, NAD^+, CTP
   (d) NH_3, NAD^+, ATP
   (e) NH_3, NAD^+, GTP
10. **All are true about Lesch-Nyhan syndrome *except:***
   (a) Inherited deficiency of the enzyme HGPRT
   (b) Hyperuricaemia
   (c) Mental retardation
   (d) Produces self-mutilation
   (e) inheritance is autosomal recessive.
11. **Which of the following amino acids is required for both purine and pyrimidine synthesis?**
   (a) Alanine
   (b) Aspartate
   (c) Glycine
   (d) Glutamate
   (e) None of the above
12. **Increased uric acid level (hyper-uricaemia) is observed in all the following diseases *except:***
   (a) Xanthine oxidase deficiency
   (b) Lesch-Nyhan syndrome
   (c) von Gierke's disease
   (d) Acute leukaemia
   (e) Glutathione reductase deficiency

ANSWERS

1. (d)	2. (a)	3. (b)
4. (c)	5. (b)	6. (d)
7. (b)	8. (b)	9. (a)
10. (e)	11. (b)	12. (a)

Protein Synthesis

INTRODUCTION

The central dogma defines the most important basis of molecular biology that genes are units perpetuating themselves and functioning through their expression in the form of proteins. ***Genetic information is carried by the sequence of DNA.*** The information is perpetuated by replication. This information is then expressed by a two step process:

- ***Transcription:*** Generates a single stranded RNA identical in sequence with one of the strands of duplex DNA
- ***Translation:*** Converts the nucleotide sequence of the RNA into the sequence of amino acids comprising a protein.

TRANSCRIPTION

Transcription is the process by which the synthesis of RNA molecules is initiated and terminated representing one strand of DNA duplex. By 'representing' we mean that the RNA is ***Identical in sequence*** with one strand of the DNA, it is complementary to the other strand, which provides the ***template for its synthesis.*** It takes place by the usual process of complementary base pairing; catalyzed by the enzyme *RNA polymerase.*

RNA Polymerase: RNA polymerase being the key enzyme in transcription. A single type of RNA polymerase is responsible for synthesis of m-RNA, r-RNA and t-RNA in bacteria. However, in eukaryotes, several different enzymes are required to synthesize the different types of RNA. They are called as *RNA polymerase I, RNA polymerase II* and *RNA polymerase III.*

Post-transcriptional Modification of RNA: All RNAs, i.e. m-RNA, r-RNA and t-RNA are obtained by transcription. However, the required modifications take place after they are released from polysomes.

- ***Modification in nucleoside:*** *Methylferases, deaminases and dehydrogenases* may methylate, deaminate or reduce the bases into the 'minor' bases, e.g. 5 methycytosine, N^6-methyladenine, hypoxanthine, dihydrouracil, etc. Uridine may be converted into pseudouridine
- ***Ligations and cleavages of nucleotides:*** The gene contains *exons* and *introns*. The *introns* need to be separated out and *exons* must be joined as they are actual amino acid coding sequences, specific *nucleases* and *ligases* bring about this function. These change an RNA into functional mRNA
- Additional nucleotides may be added at the end of RNA transcript, e.g. 7 methyl GTP cap is added at 5′-end while poly A-tail is added at the 3′-end
- Different subspecies of r-RNA such as 5.8s, 18s, 28s r-RNA are made after transcription from a precursor RNA.

Inhibitors of Transcription: Several antibiotics have been found to inhibit the process of transcription.

- ***Rifamycin:*** Rifampicin and streptovaricin bind with β-subunit of the polymerase to block the intiation of transcription
- ***Actinomycin D:*** It forms a complex with double stranded DNA and prevents the movement of core enzyme and as a result inhibits the process of chain elongation

- ***Streptoglydigin:*** If blinds with the β-subunit of prokaryotic polymerase and thus inhibits the elongation
- ***Heparin:*** It is a polyanion that binds to the β′ subunit and inhibits transcription *in vitro.* The γ-subunit has no known role in the process.

Stages of Transcription:

The process of transcription can be divided into four stages:

- ***Formation of transcription complex (of DNA and RNA polymerase)***
- ***Initiation***
- ***Elongation and***
- ***Termination.***

1. ***Formation of Transcription Complex:*** The enzyme RNA polymerase needs to bind with specific sequences on a DNA. These sequences recognized by RNA polymerase are called as promoter. The size of the promoter region is variable. In prokaryotes, it varies from 20-200 bases. As already mentioned core enzyme cannot recognize the promoter region, sigma factor is required for recognition and formation of the complex. Following four steps occur:

- Sigma factor recognizes the promoter sequences.
- RNA polymerase attaches to promoter region.
- RNA polymerase melts the helical structure and separates 2 strands of DNA locally.
- RNA polymerase initiates RNA synthesis. The site at which the first nucleotide is incorporated is called the ***start site or start point.***

Characteristics of Promoter sequence: There are few specific characteristics of promoter sequence:

- The Pribnow box is a sequence contained with the promoter region. It is located 5-10 bases to the left, i.e. upstream the first four bases that will be copied into RNA. It orients RNA polymerase as to the direction and start of synthesis.
- All Pribnow boxes are variants of TATAATG sequences and sometimes referred to as **TATA box.**
- The T at position 6 (conserved T) is present in every promoter region of box.
- The –"35" sequence is a second recognition site in many promoter regions upstream from Pribnow box. It is thought to be the initial site of s subunit binding. Typically it contains nine bases.
- Since the RNA polymerase has a huge size, it comes into contact with Pribnow box.
- Once bound to the Pribnow box, RNA polymerase dissociates from the initial recognition site.
- This complex is active intermediate in RNA chain initiation. ***The important event is the melting of DNA duplex*** that takes place about 10 base pairs upstream of Pribnow box and extending to the first transcribed base at the start point ***(Fig. 17.1).***

2. ***Initiation:***

- Core enzyme starts transcription at the separated DNA strands of an initiation complex. As the enzyme moves along, the unwound region moves with it.
- The first base copied is always within six to nine bases of the conserved T of the Pribnow box on the unwound portion of 3′-5′ strand of DNA.

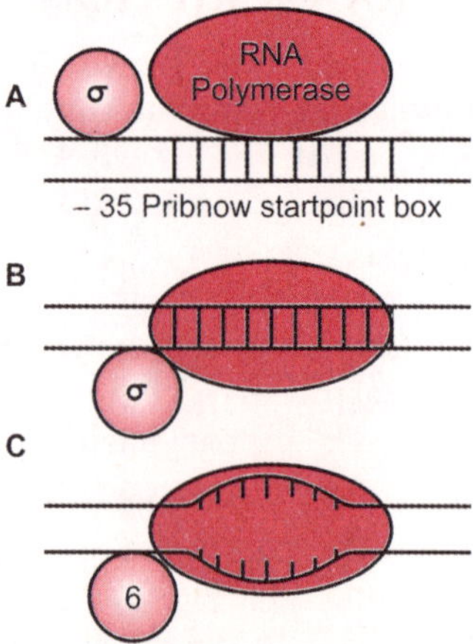

Fig. 17.1: Formation of initiation-complex: (A) Template binding, (B) Dissociation of s subunit, (C) Unwinding of duplex-open complex formation

- It is observed that the subunit of RNA polymerase has two specific binding sites for the binding of nucleotide triphosphates (NTP).
- Formation of hydrogen bonds is always as per the base-pairing rules. The first incoming NTP binds to RNA polymerase at the start point of initiation site and H-bonds to the complementary base on the DNA within the complex. This site binds only purine NTP- either A or G. ***The binding is with 3′ end of the NTP leaving 5′ end to be free.***
- The second incoming NTP ***binds to the elongation site on the polymerase.*** The NTP is selected as per base-pair rule which can H-bond with complementary base on DNA. This dinucleoside tetraphosphate has either PPPA or PPPG as the 5′ terminal nucleotide. After this phosphodiester bond formation the s factor is released.
- First base is then dissociated from initiation site and that marks the completion of initiation.

3. *Elongation:*

- The core enzyme polymerase moves in 3′-5′ direction of the coding strand and it adds successive NTPs at the 3′-OH end of the ribonucleotide chain already laid down in 5′-3′ direction.
- The incoming NTP forms a phosphodiester bond with 3′-OH end of the preceding ribonucleotide.
- The bases are determined by the sense strand by base-pair rules.
- The DNA helix recloses after RNA polymerase transcribes through it and growing RNA chain dissociates from the DNA *(Fig. 17.2).*

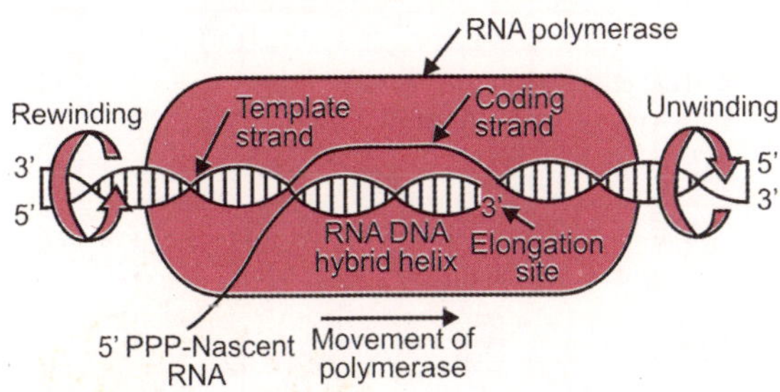

Fig. 17.2: Model of transcription bubble

4. *Termination:* Specific sequences on the DNA molecule function as the signal for termination of the transcription process.

- The signal could be two inverted GC rich regions separated by intervening region followed by AT rich sequences.
- A sequence of Adenine that codes for 6 to 8 Uracil residues. The Uracil residues are followed by one Adenine.
- There is no unique base for the termination of transcription e.g., for a given promoter, RNA might end with 5 U's or 6 U's + 1 A.
- Rho (r) protein and the sequences mentioned, together bring about termination. At specific termination sites the new RNA chain may be released. The rho protein binds very tightly to the RNA (not to polymerase) and in this bound state it acts like ATPase.
- Rho factor then dissociates RNA and RNA polymerase from the DNA.

Summary of the transcription is given in *Fig. 17.3.*

GENETIC CODE

Transcription makes the base sequence in the form of m-RNA available to be translated into specific proteins. There are four kinds of base (A, U,G,C) present in RNA while there are 20 different kinds of amino acids found in proteins. Therefore neither one nor two bases can specify all amino acids. However, 64 kinds of amino acids can be

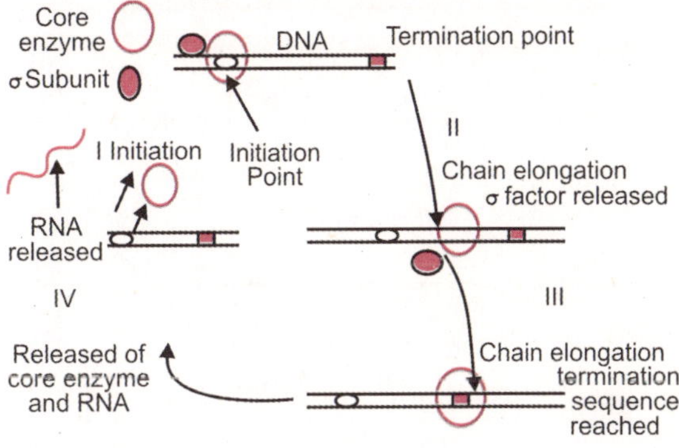

Fig. 17.3: Summary of transcription

specified by a three base code. ***Genetic experiments have proved that an amino acid is coded by a group of three bases called as codon.*** The 64 combinations of three bases responsible for coding amino acids, initiating protein synthesis and stopping the protein synthesis are arranged in the form of table which generally known as ***Genetic code.*** Determination of all sequence of bases in codons was carried out by ***H.G. Khorana*** and ***Marshall Nirenberg.*** Later experiments by Francis Cricks, S. Brenner and others fully uncovered the meaning of 64 codons of the genetic code. The sequence of coding strand of DNA, read in the direction from 5′ to 3′, consists of triplets corresponding to the amino acid sequence of the protein read from N-terminus to C-terminus. The genetic code is summarized in ***Fig. 17.4.***

CHARACTERISTICS OF GENETIC CODE

1. ***Degeneracy:*** The striking feature is the degeneracy of the code. 61 codons represent 20 amino acids.
   - Every amino acid except methionine is represented by several codons
   - Codons that represent same amino acid are called as synonyms
   - Codons tend to be clustered in groups representing a single amino acid
   - Often the base of the third position is insignificant, because the four codons differing only in the third base represent the same amino acid. Sometimes distinction is made only between a purine versus a pyrimidine in this position.
   - ***The reduced specificity at the last position is known as third base degeneracy*** or ***Wobbling phenomenon***
   - This feature, together with a tendency for similar amino acids to be represented by related codons, minimizes the effects of mutations. It increases the probability that a single random base change will result in no amino acid substitution or in one involving amino acids of similar character.
2. ***Unambiguity:*** A given codon designates only one single specific amino acid and does not incorporate any unspecified amino acid into the peptide chain.
3. ***Universality:*** In all the living organisms the genetic code is the same. This phenomenon is called as ***universality of the code.***
   - The exception to universality is found in mitochondrial genome where AUA codes for methionine and UGA for tryptophan instead of isoleucine and termination or stop respectively

				Second Base					
First Base	U		C		A		G		*Third Base*
U	UUU	Phe	UCU	Ser	UAU	Tyr	UGU	Cys	U
	UUC	Phe	UCC	Ser	UAC	Tyr	UGC	Cys	C
	UUA	Leu	UCA	Ser	**UAA**	**Stop**	**UGA**	**Stop**	A
	UUG	Leu	UCG	Ser	**UAG**	**Stop**	UGG	Tyr	G
C	CUU	Leu	CCU	Pro	CAU	His	CGU	Arg	U
	CUC	Leu	CCC	Pro	CAC	His	CGC	Arg	C
	CUA	Leu	CCA	Pro	CAA	Gln	CGA	Arg	A
	CUG	Leu	CCG	Pro	CAG	Gln	CGG	Arg	G
A	AUU	Ile	ACU	Thr	AAU	Asn	AGU	Ser	U
	AUC	Ile	ACC	Thr	AAC	Asn	AGC	Ser	C
	AUA	Ile	ACA	Thr	AAA	Lys	AGA	Arg	A
	AUG	Met	ACG	Thr	AAG	Lys	AGG	Arg	G
G	GUU	Val	GCU	Ala	GAU	Asp	GGU	Gly	U
	GUC	Val	GCC	Ala	GAC	Asp	GGC	Gly	C
	GUA	Val	GCA	Ala	GAA	Glu	GGA	Gly	A
	GUG	Val	GCG	Ala	GAG	Glu	GGG	Gly	G

Fig. 17.4: The genetic code

- AGA and AGG code for arginine in normal condition but in mitochondria it terminates protein synthesis
- Studies of mutations in viruses, bacteria and higher organisms have established the universality of the genetic code
- Most of the amino acid substitutions in proteins can be accounted for by a change of a single DNA base

4. *Colinearity of Gene and Product:* The product of the gene is a protein specified by base sequences. High resolution genetic mapping techniques have established that there is a linear correspondence in base sequence in gene and amino acid sequence in protein.

5. *Non-overlapping:* All codons are independent sets of three bases. There is no overlapping, i.e. no base functions as a common member of two consecutive codons.

6. *Commalessness*

- Codons are arranged as continuous structure. There is not one or more nucleotides between consecutive codons
- The last nucleotide of preceding codon is immediately followed by the first nucleotide of succeeding nucleotide.

Note: All the 64 codons are grouped in 16 families each characterized by first two bases. A mixed codon family codes for more than one amino acid, depending on the third base in its codons. Unmixed codon family codes for the same amino acid irrespective of the third base.

- When the first base in the anticodon is C or A, the pairing with the third base in codon is regular (i.e. G or A)
- When the first base in the anticodon is U then the third base in the codon can be either of the purines (i.e. G or A)
- When the first base in the anticodon is G, then the third base in the codon can be either of the pyrimidines
- When the first base in the anticodon is inosine (I), the third base in the codon can be A, C or U.

TRANSLATION OF m-RNA (PROTEIN SYNTHESIS)

Protein is a polymer of amino acids joined together by peptide bonds. In the process of protein synthesis also known as translation of m-RNA, the amino acids are added sequentially in a specific number and sequence, determined by the sequence of codons in the genetic code of the relevant m-RNA.

Materials Required for Protein Synthesis are:

- Amino acids—at least 20 amino acids
- DNA and three RNAs—m-RNA, t-RNA and γ-RNA
- Polyribosomes (Polysomes)
- ***Enzymes:***
  - *Amino-acyl-t-RNA synthetase*: enzyme required for activation of amino acids.
  - *Peptide synthetase* (Peptidyl transferase)
- ***Factors***
  - Initiation factors— elF-1, elF-2, elF-3, elF-4A, elF-4B, elF-4G, elF-4E, elF-5
  - Elongation factors—EF_1 and EF_2
  - Release factors R_1 and R_2
- ***Coenzymes and Cofactors:***
  - $F.H_4$-required in prokaryotes only for formylation of methionine
  - Mg^{++}
- ***Energy:*** ATP and GTP.

RIBOSOMES

- Protein synthesis takes place on *ribosomes* which is a nucleoprotein and contains 65% r-RNA and 35% proteins. It is a large particle and in prokaryotes it has 70s as its sedimentation coefficient while **80s in eukaryotes.**
- It can be split into two unequal portions by EDTA which decreases the conc. of Mg^{++} by chelate formation. Mg^{++} is required to hold the two subunits together

- The two subunits in prokaryotes are 50s large subunit and 30s small subunit while **in eukaryotes they are 60s and 40s**
- The 50s subunit has been found to contain about 34 proteins (L-proteins) and 2 moles of 23s and 5s r-RNA
- The 30s subunit contains about 21 proteins (S-proteins) and a 16s RNA molecule
- Most of the ribosomal proteins (L- and S-) are low molecular weight basic proteins. Due to their basic charge they can easily interact with RNA which is negatively charged
- The RNAs in ribosomal subunits have a specific well defined secondary structure and they interact with ribosomal proteins in a well defined manner
- The eukaryotic 60s subunit of ribosome has 45 proteins and 28s, 5.8s and 5s r-RNA and 40s subunit contains 30 proteins and 18s RNA
- The mitochondrial ribosomes are similar to those of prokaryotes
- A polysome or polyribosome is a beaded string-like linear cluster of 5 to 8 ribosomes on a m-RNA
- *Each ribosome has peptidyl (P) and aminoacyl (A) site.*

STEPS OF PROTEIN SYNTHESIS

The process of protein synthesis (after transcription has taken place) can be divided in **following steps:**

- *Activation of amino acids*
- *Initiation*
- *Elongation, and*
- *Termination.*

1. Activation of amino acids: ***(Formation of Aminoacyl t-RNA):*** The amino acids need to be activated before they can be incorporated into the peptide chain. ***The key enzyme in this process is aminoacyl t-RNA synthetase.*** These are specific for a particular L-amino acid and also for t-RNA. Obviously there are at least 20 different t-RNAs and 20 different *aminoacyl t-RNA synthetases* in a protein synthesizing system. The enzymes vary in molecular size, subunit and amino acid composition. There is at least one and sometimes two specific enzymes for each amino acid. Very high specificity is the most significant feature, because once amino acid is attached to t-RNA, recognition of a specific codon on m-RNA is due entirely to the t-RNA, not to the amino acid. This very high specificity of aminoacyl t-RNA synthetases is due to:

- High selectivity in terms of the acceptance of the amino acid to be activated
- High selectivity toward the t-RNA to which the activated amino acid will be transferred. Incorrectly activated amino acids are hydrolyzed and do not get incorporated

Steps of Activation of Amino Acids

- The reaction requires amino acid, t-RNA and ATP. First an intermediate is formed.

$$\text{Amino acid} + \text{ATP} \xrightarrow{Mg^{+2}/Mn^{+2}} \text{(Aminoacyl AMP)} + \text{PPi}$$

Aminoacyl-adenylate complex

- Transfer of aminoacyl group to t-RNA constitutes the next step.

$$\text{Aminoacyl–AMP} + \text{t-RNA} \rightarrow \text{Aminoacyl t-RNA} + \text{AMP}$$

- **Overall reaction is:**

$$\text{Amino acid} + \text{ATP} + \text{t-RNA} \quad \text{Aminoacyl t-RNA} + \text{AMP} + \text{PPi}$$

In the aminoacyl t-RNA, the α-carboxyl group of the amino acid remains esterified with the 3′-OH of the 3′-terminal adenosine on acceptor arm of t-RNA. The hydrolysis of pyrophosphate which renders the reaction virtually ***irreversible,*** drives the reaction to completion. ***Thus 2 high energy bonds of ATP are used in the formation of an aminoacyl t-RNA.***

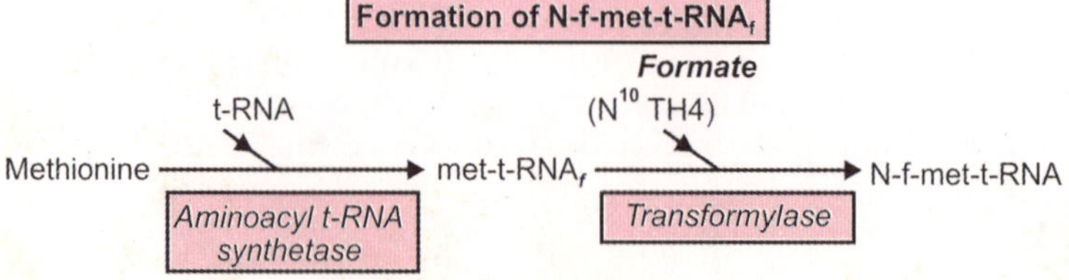

As each t-RNA forms an aminoacyl t-RNA with specific amino acid, the codon-anticodon reactions bring the amino acid to ribosomes (or polysomes) in a particular sequence depending on the codon sequence in m-RNA.

2. Initiation: The initiation may be divided arbitrarily into following **4 steps:**

1. ***Dissociation of the ribosome 80s into 60s and 40s subunits.***
2. ***Formation of 43s pre-initiation complex.***
3. ***Formation of initiation complex.***
4. ***Formation of 80s initiation complex.***

A. *Dissociation of Ribosome*

Before initiation process starts, **80s** ribosome **dissociates** into **40s** and **60s** subunits. Two initiation factors, **elF-3** and **elF-1A** binds to the newly dissociated 40s subunit.

FUNCTION

- This binding of initiation factors prevent reassociation of 60s and 40s.
- It allows the other translation initiation factors to associate with 40s subunit and prepares it for formation of 80s initiation complex ***(Refer Fig. 17.5).***

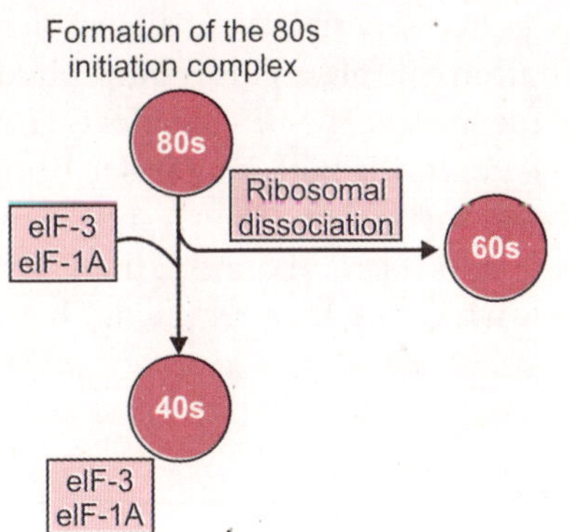

Fig. 17.5: Dissociation of 80s ribosome

B. *Formation of the 43s Pre-initiation complex*

The process involves the **binding of GTP** with **elF-2**, and forms a binary complex, which then binds to met-RNA, and forms a ternary complex. Methionine having anticodon UAC is the first amino acid required to be involved in the binding to the initiation codon AUG on m-RNA.

This ternary complex binds to 40s ribosomal subunit and forms the **43s pre-initiation complex**. This complex is stabilized by association with **elF-3** and **elF-1A** ***(Refer Fig. 17.6).***

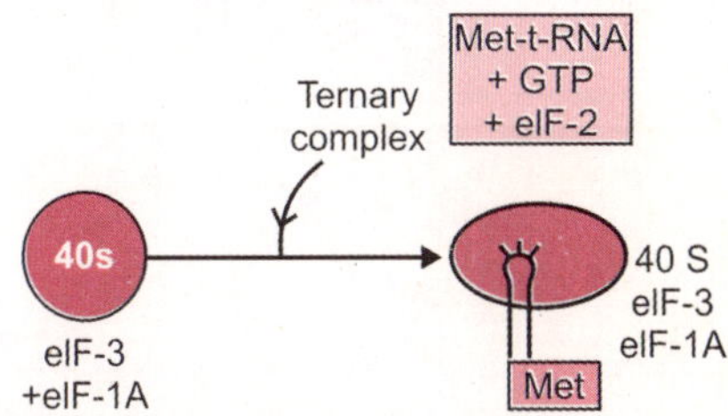

Fig. 17.6: Formation of 43s pre-initiation complex

In eukaryotes, the **elF-2 is the controlling factor in protein synthesis** initiation. Structurally elF-2 is a heterotrimer and consists of 3 subunits α, β, and γ. ***Subunit α is important***, elF-2α is phosphorylated by at least four different **protein kinases** (**HCR**, **PKR**, **PERK**, and **GCN2**). The kinases are activated when a cell is under stress, e.g. virus infection, heat shock, carbohydrate and protein deprivation, etc.

Clinical Importance

PKR protein kinase is important. The kinase is activated by viruses and provides a host defense mechanism that decreases protein synthesis, thereby inhibiting viral replication.

C. *Formation of Initiation Complex (Refer Fig. 17.7)*

Binding of m-RNA with pre-initiation complex is necessary to form the '***Initiation complex***'. In all eukaryotic cells, 5′ terminals of m-RNA are "**capped** which is methyl guanosyl triphosphate (Refer structure of RNAs). The binding is facilitated by 5′ methylated cap, which needs a "**cap binding protein complex**" consisting of, **elF-4F = elF-4E** and **elF-4G + elF-4A**. This complex binds to the cap through elF-4E protein.

Then elF-4A and elF-4B bind and reduce the complex secondary structure of the 5′-end of m-RNA through hydrolysis of **ATP** by ***helicase activities*** providing energy. ***The association of m-RNA with the 43s pre-initiation complex produces the 48s initiation complex.*** After formation of 48s

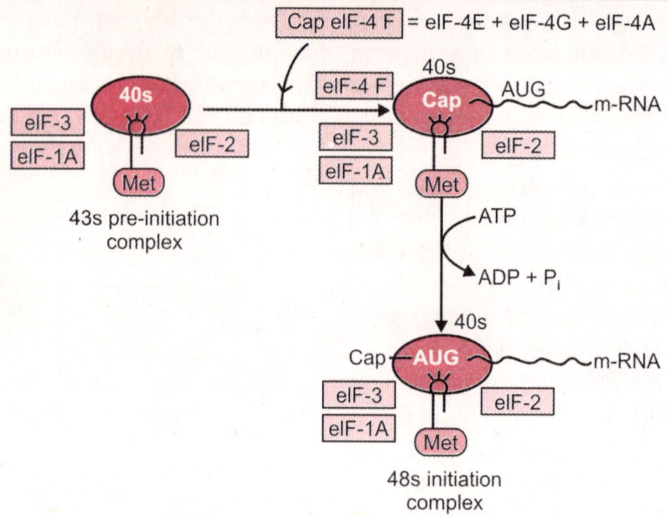

Fig. 17.7: Showing formation of initiation complex

initiation complex, it searches for precise **initiation codon AUG** for methionine. This is determined by "**Kozak consensus sequence**" in eukaryotes and in bacteria, it is **"Shine-Dalgarno" sequence**.

elF-4E is the most important factor because it recognizes the cap of 5′-methylated end of m-RNA and is the **rate limiting step** in protein synthesis. **Insulin** and **mitogenic factors**, e.g. IGF-1, PDGF, inter-leukin-2 and angiotensin II, phosphorylate elF-4E and increases protein synthesis.

Role of 3′-Poly(A) Tail in Initiation

3′-Poly (A) tail has a ***binding protein.* "Pablp"** This complex helps in the initiation acting synergistically with 'cap'.

Pablp bound to the poly (A) tail interacts with **elF-4G**, which in turn binds to **elF-4E** that is bound to the 'cap' structure, which probably **help to direct the 40s ribosomal subunit** to the 5′-end of the m-RNA.

D. *Formation of 80s initiation complex (Fig. 17.8):* The 48s initiation complex now binds to 60s which was free after ribosomal dissociation, forms **80s initiation complex. This requires hydrolysis of GTP for energy.** The ***elF-2 carries GTP and elF-5 GTP-ase activity,*** both interacts to bring about hydrolysis. This reaction then results in release of all the initiation factors bound to the 48s initiation complex, which are then recycled. There occurs

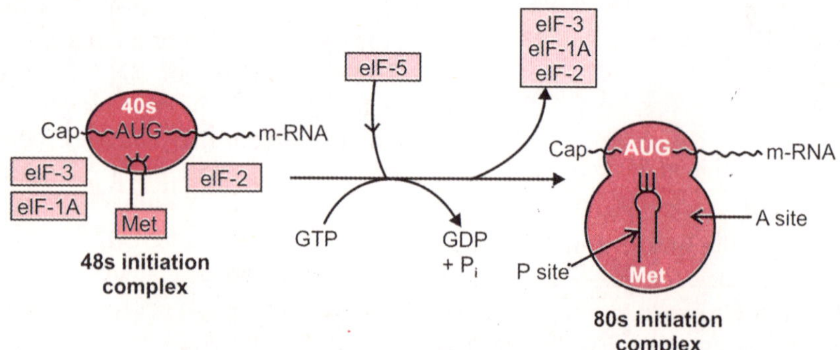

Fig. 17.8: Formation of 80s ribosomal initiation complex

rapid association of 40s and 60s sub units to **form the 80s ribosomal complex ready for protein synthesis.**

The 80s complex has *two receptor sites:*

- **'P' site or peptidyl site:** At this point the met-t-RNA is on the 'P' site. **On this site the growing peptide chain will grow.**
  'A' site or **aminoacyl site:** At this point it is free, the new incoming t-RNA with the amino acid to be added next is taken up, at this site.

The **t-RNA binds with ribosome through the pseudo uridine arm.**

3. Elongation

- Elongation is a **cyclic process** on the ribosome in which one amino acid is added to the nascent peptide chain
- The peptide sequence is determined by the **codons** present in the m-RNA
- It requires *elongation factors*-**EF-IA, EF-2.**

Steps Involved in Elongation

The steps are mainly **three:**

- The binding of new aminoacyl-tRNA to 'A' site
- Peptide bond formation
- Translocation process.

A. Binding of aminoacyl-t-RNA to the A site (Fig. 17.9)

In the 80s ribosomal initiation complex, the 'P' site is occupied by met-t-RNA and **'A' site is free.** The fidelity of protein synthesis depends on having correct aminoacyl-t-RNA in the 'A' site as per codon reading.

Elongation factor EF-IA forms a ternary complex with **GTP** and the entering aminoacyl-t-RNA (A_1). This complex allows the amino acyl-t-RNA to enter the 'A' site. GTP is hydrolyzed to give energy and this is catalyzed by an active site on the ribosome. This releases the EF-IA-GDP and Pi. The EF-IA-GDP is converted again to EF-IA-GTP by other soluble protein factors and GTP. It is further recycled.

B. ***Peptide bond formation (Fig. 17.10):*** The α-NH_2 group of the new aminoacyl-t-RNA (A_1) in the 'A' site combines with the –COOH group of Met-t-RNA (m) occupying the 'P' site. The reaction is catalyzed by the enzyme ***Peptidyl transferase***, a component of the 28s RNA of the 60s ribosomal subunit. ***Because the amino acid on the aminoacyl-t-RNA is already "activated" the reaction does not require any further energy.*** The reaction results in formation of a peptide to the t-RNA in the 'A' site. Now the growing peptide chain is occupying 'A' site and naked free t-RNA at 'P' site.

Note: Peptidyl transferase is an example of a ribozyme where RNA acts as the enzyme (direct role of RNA in protein synthesis).

C. Translocation:

The t-RNA is fixed at the 'P' site, attached by its anticodon and having no amino acid (free and naked t-RNA) ***by the open CCA tail*** it is bound to an exit site (E site) on the large ribosomal subunit.

At this point ***elongation factor 2 (EF-2)*** binds to and displaces the peptide-tRNA from the 'A' site to the 'P' site and at the same time the deacylated free ***t-RNA*** is on the 'E' site from which the ***t-RNA leaves the ribo-some.***

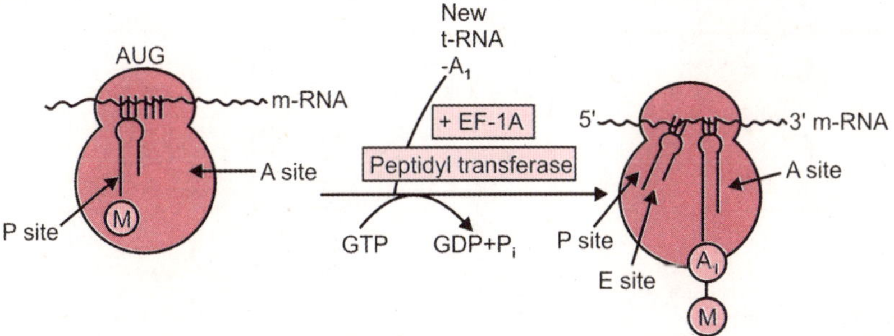

Fig. 17.9: Showing binding of aminoacyl-t-RNA to 'A' site and peptide bond formation

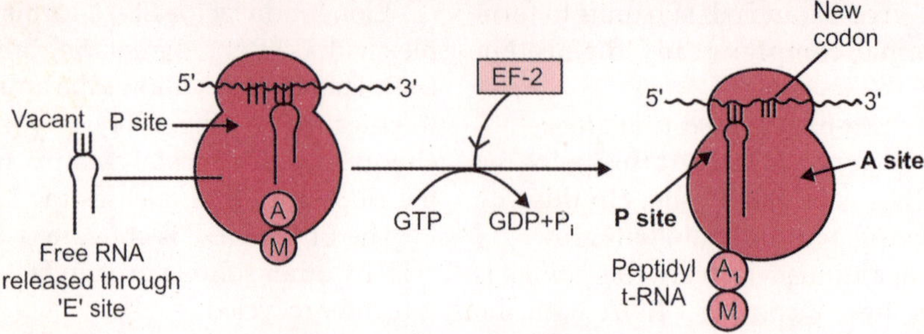

Fig. 17.10: Showing elongation

Now, **EF-2-GTP complex** is hydrolyzed to **EF-2-GDP**, the energy from hydrolysis ***moves the m-RNA forward by one codon, leaving the 'A' site free to receive another ternary complex of a new amino acid as per codon and repeat the cycle of elongation.***

D. *Termination process (Fig. 17.11)*

After multiple cycles of elongation process, it results to formation of polypeptide chain. When the desired protein molecule is synthesized, a **'stop codon'** or **'terminating codon'** appears in the **A site** of m-RNA. The stop codons are**: UAB, UAG,** or **UGA**. There is no t-RNA with an anticodon capable of recognizing such a termination signal.

Releasing factor RF-1 recognizes that a stop codon has come in the 'A' site. This ***protein factor RF-1 is a complex consisting of another releasing factor RF-3 with bound GTP.*** This complex with the help of "peptidyl transferase" brings about hydrolysis of the bond between the peptide and the t-RNA occupying the 'P' site. The energy is provided by GTP → GDP + Pi conversion. The hydrolysis releases the synthesized peptide chain, m-RNA and t-RNA from the 'P' site.

The 80s ribosome now dissociates into 60s and 40s subunits which are then recycled.

POLYRIBOSOMES

In eukaryotic cell, a single ribosome is capable of synthesizing 400 peptide bonds each minute. Many ribosomes can work on the same m-RNA molecule simultaneously and these aggregate are called **polyribosomes** or **polysomes.** In such cases, each ribosome may be 80 to 100 nucleotides apart on the m-RNA (minimum 35 nucleotides).

Polyribosomes actively synthesizing proteins can exist as:

- ***Free cellular particles in cytoplasm*** or
- ***May be attached to the endoplasmic reticulum (ER)***

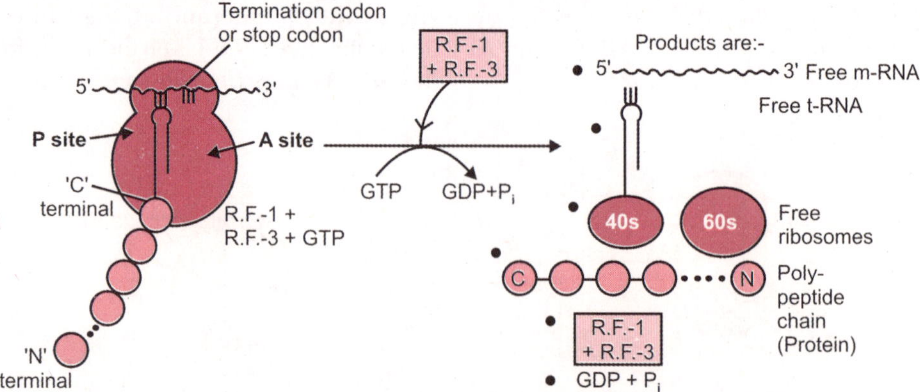

Fig. 17.11: Showing termination process

Attachment of the particular polyribosomes to the ER makes the

- **Rough** appearance viewed by electron microscopy and called **Rough endoplasmic reticulum**
- **Free ribosomes in cytoplasm synthesizes cytoplasmic proteins** required for cellular function
- **Bound polyribosomes** of ER synthesize proteins that are transported through cisternal space to Golgi apparatus, where it is packaged and **stored** for eventual export.

Energy requirements in protein synthesis

Mainly

- ATP and
- GTP are used

- **ATP:** is required for the activation of amino acids and formation of t-RNA-amino acid complex. In this reaction, as one molecule of ATP is converted to AMP, it can be considered equivalent to utilization of 2 ATPs (two high energy PO_4 bonds used).
- One ATP is required for formation of initiation complex.
- One ATP required in formation of 48s initiation complex. The hydrolysis of ATP by *"helicase"* activity for associating 5′-end of m-RNA, with binding of eIF-4A and eIF-4B.
- **GTP:** is required for the following:
  - GTP is required for ***binding with eIF-2*** for forming a binary complex required in formation of 43s pre-initiation complex.
  - GTP hydrolysis provides energy ***for formation of 80s initiation complex***. eIF-2 carries GTP and eIF-5 GTP-ase activity.
  - GTP is required in binding of amino acyl-tRNA to 'A' site.
  - EF-2 (elongation factor)—GTP complex is hydrolyzed to give energy—***for translocation***, movement of m-RNA forward by one codon.
  - RF-3 with bound GTP is required for *termination process*.

Note: *Total energy requirement:*

- ATP = 4
- GTP = 5.

CHAPERONES: PROTEINS THAT PREVENT FAULTY FOLDING

The exit of a protein after synthesis from the endoplasmic reticulum may be the ***rate-limiting step***. Certain proteins called chaperones have been found to play a role in the assembly and proper folding of the synthesized proteins so that it has biological activity. The word chaperones as per dictionary literally means "older woman in charge of young unmarried woman on certain social occasions".

Heat shock proteins (HSPs): The chaperones belong to a large family of proteins called ***"heat shock proteins"* (HSPs)** which were first identified in response to heat shock. Any stress to the cell like radiations, heavy metals, free radicals, toxins, etc would cause increased production of HSPs and hence also called as ***"stress proteins"***.

Mechanism of Action:

- Most chaperones exhibit ATPase activity and bind ADP and ATP. This activity is important in their effect on folding of proteins
- The ADP-chaperone complex has a high affinity for the unfolded protein which when bound stimulates release of ADP with replacement of ATP
- The ATP-chaperone complex in turn, releases segments of the protein that have folded properly, and the cycle involving ADP and ATP binding is repeated until the folded protein is released.

Properties of chaperone proteins: Some properties of chaperone proteins are listed in the box below.

Properties of Chaperones

- Present in a wide range of species from bacteria to humans.
- Also called as heat shock proteins (HSPs) as stated above.

- Inducible by conditions that cause unfolding of newly synthesized proteins, e.g. elevated temperature, exposure to various chemicals ("stress proteins").
- They bind unfolded and aggregated proteins.
- Show ATPase activity and ADP and ATP which has important role in effecting folding (see mechanism of action above).
- Found in various cellular compartments, e.g. cytosol, mitochondria and the lumen of endoplasmic reticulum.

Examples of Chaperones:

- **Bip** ***(immunoglobulin heavy chain binding protein):*** Located in the lumen of the endoplasmic reticulum.

  Function: Chaperone Bip binds to abnormally folded immunoglobulin heavy chains and prevent them from the endoplasmic reticulum in which they are degraded.
- **Calnexin**: Located in the endoplasmic reticulum membrane.

  Function: It binds the monoglucosylated species of glycoproteins that occur during processing of glycoproteins, retaining them in the endoplasmic reticulum until the glycoprotein has folded properly
- **PDI** ***(Protein disulfide isomerase):*** An enzyme chaperone which promotes rapid reshuffling of disulfide (-S-S-) bonds until the correct folding is achieved
- **PPI** ***(Peptidyl prolyl cis-trans-isomerase):*** Another enzyme chaperone which accelerates folding of proline containing proteins.

Clinical Aspect

Abnormal folding of proteins, unassisted by chaperones may lead to Alzheimer's disease.

ALZHEIMER'S DISEASE

Alzheimer's disease occurs in old age and it is the fourth leading cause of death among aged peoples after myocardial infarction, stroke and cancer.

Clinical features: The disease is characterized by slow progression of memory loss, hallucinations, personality changes, confusion, dementia and finally the patient enters into a vegetative state with no comprehension of outside world.

Pathological changes: The disease is characterized pathologically:

- By neurofibril tangles in CNS,
- Formation of senile neuritic plaques and cerebral amyloid deposits.

Biochemical alterations: The biochemical changes include:

- The neurofibrillary tangles are paired helical filaments made up of abnormal **"Tau"** proteins. Normal "Tau" is soluble and catabolized easily but abnormal "Tau" protein found in this condition is insoluble and cannot be degraded by tissue cathepsins and are deposited around neurons

- *Role of Chaperone Enzyme*

  Pin I: Recently an enzyme ***"Pin I"*** has been found which is necessary for formation of normal ***"Tau"*** protein. Absence of ***"Pin I"*** in this condition produces the abnormal "Tau" protein
- Deposition of abnormal insoluble "Tau" leads to loss of microtubule, thus damaging the communication channels in nerve fibres. The ***synthesis of acetylcholine is reduced leading to memory loss***
- Neuritic plaques have been found to be due to deposition of an abnormal amyloid protein β-***APP.*** This is derived from normal APP (Amyloid Precursor Protein). Mutation in APP gene leads to formation of β-APP from wrong cleavage of APP. ***β-APP is precipitated around neurons as β-amyloid.***

INHIBITORS OF PROTEIN SYNTHESIS

Many antibiotics inhibit the protein synthesis at some specific steps:

- ***Streptomycin:*** It is a highly basic trisaccharide.
  - It interferes with the binding of f-met t-RNA to ribosomes and thereby inhibits the initiation process.
  - It also leads to misreading of m-RNA.

- ***Puromycin:*** This inhibits protein synthesis by releasing nascent polypeptide chains before their synthesis is complete. It binds to the A site on ribosome and inhibits the entry of aminoacyl-t-RNA. It acts both in bacterial and mammalian cells.
- ***Tetracycline:*** It binds to the 30s subunit and inhibits binding of aminoacyl t-RNA, thus inhibits the initiation process.
- ***Chloramphenicol:*** It inhibits the ***peptidyl transferase*** activity of 50s subunit. Thus it inhibits the process of elongation.
- ***Cycloheximide:*** This inhibits ***peptidyl transferase*** activity of 60s ribosomal subunit in eukaryotes. It also inhibits elongation.
- ***Erythromycin:*** It binds to the 50s subunit and inhibits translocation.
- ***Diphtheria toxin:*** *Corynebacterium diphtheriae* produces a lethal protein toxin. It binds with EF-2 in eukaryotes and blocks its capacity to carry out translocation.
- ***Ricin and abrin:*** These are toxic lectins. They inhibit protein synthesis by unknown mechanisms, preventing aminoacyl t-RNA from binding to the A site. This operates in eukaryotes, inactivates eukaryotic 28s ribosomal RNA.
- ***Sparsomycin:*** This inhibits ***peptidyl transferase*** and release factor-dependent termination. It does not prevent termination codon-dependent binding of release factor to the ribosome.
- ***a-Sarcin:*** It is a toxic RNAse that prevents aminoacyl-t-RNA binding by cleaving a single phosphodiester bond in 28s r-RNA.

☞ SALIENT POINTS TO REMEMBER

- Genetic information is carried by the sequence of DNA, the information is perpetuated by replication
- The information is expressed through formation of m-RNA, which carry the message to cytosol to protein synthesizing machinery
- m-RNA is formed in the nucleus by the process of transcription from one strand of duplox DNA. RNA polymerase being the key enzyme in transcription
- Initially bigger molecular size RNA is formed called "hn RNA" which first forms "Pre-m-RNA"
- Pre-m-RNA has two regions called (i) Exons - active region used for coding and (ii) Introns - intervening regions not required for coding
- Pre-m-RNA is pruned in that the 'introns' transcripts are excised and 'extrons' transcripts are spliced together to give the proper m-RNA-required for translation, i.e. protein synthesis
- Several antibiotics like Rifampicin, Actinomycin D, etc. have been found to inhibit the process of transcription.
- m-RNA comes to cytosol and attaches to the ribosomes where the protein synthesis occurs.
- In eukaryotes, it is a combination of ribosomes (polysomes) and each ribosome is 80s made of two portions one 40s and other 60s, which are separate in the begining of synthesis
- The 60s piece of ribosome has got two sites: one called aminoacyl site (A site) and the other peptidyl site (P site)
- Stages in translation (protein synthesis) are - (i) Activation of amino acids (ii) initiation (iii) elongation and (iv) termination
- The required amino acid is first activated and the key enzyme is "***amino acid t-RNA synthetase,***" which are specific for a particular amino acid and for particular t-RNA
- Two high energy bonds of ATP are used in the formation of an aminoacyl-t-RNA.
- The 60s piece of eukaryote ribosome and 40s ribosome are separate at the beginning of protein synthesis. The 60s piece has 2 sites- 'A' site (aminoacyl site) and 'P' site peptidyl site
- In euokaryotes, the first codon is AUG which codes for methionine, the first amino acid to be taken up. (e.f. in prokaryote) it is formylated derivative of methionine
- In initiation process, the 60s ribosome fuses with 40s and with t-RNA methionine forms

the complex "m-RNA-80s-t-RNA methionine" complex which occupies the `P' site

- Energy for fusion of 60s and 40s is given by hydrolysis of GTP. During initiation 'A' site remains vacant
- Then elongation takes place. The codon present in vacant 'A' site signals to the t-RNA to bring the particular amino acid
- The activated "t-RNA-AA" now combines with GTP and EF-1 and enters the `A' site. Energy being provided by hydrolysis of GTP.
- The two amino acids now interact and form a peptide bond, catalyzed by the enzyme "peptidyl transferase".
- 'P' site becomes vacant after naked t-RNA leaves the site and 'A' site is occupied by "t-RNA-dipeptide"
- Now translocation takes place, GTP and EF-2 ("translocase") react, GTP undergoes hydrolysis and the energy makes the ribosome move along the m-RNA from 5'- to 3'-end
- By the movement, 't-RNA-peptide' which was in the 'A' site and now occupies the 'P'site and 'A' site falls vacant
- The third codon in 'A' site now directs the t-RNA to bring the specific amino acid required
- Above processes continue till the polypeptide required to be synthesized is grown to the desired length. When termination occurs
- Termination takes place by the appearance of a "chain terminating codon" or called "nonsense codon" at the `A' site
- They are 3 types - UAA, UGA or UAG. They are recognized by "Release factors" with high specificity
- RF-1 recognizes UAA or UAG, while RF-2 recognizes UAA or UGA
- RF-1 or RF-2 binds with chain terminating codon on the 'A' site and activate ***"Peptidyl" transferase"*** which hydrolyzes the bond between polypeptide and t-RNA at 'P' site
- Polypeptide chain leaves the ribosome alongwith the 't-RNA' from the 'P' site.
- The 80s ribosome now dissociates into 60s and 40s subunits which are then ready to restart the cycle
- Energy requirement in protein synthesis is provided by ATP and GTP
- ATP provides two high energy bonds and GTP five high energy bonds
- Chaperones: Certain proteins called chaperones have been recently found which play a role in the assembly and proper folding of the synthesized proteins so that it has biological activity
- A number of inhibitors of protein synthesis have been described which have been found to inhibit protein synthesis by acting on some specific sites, viz. puromycin, streptomycin, tetracyclins, erythromycin, chloramphenicol, diphtheria toxin, etc.

MULTIPLE CHOICE QUESTIONS

Give one correct answer:

1. **In the process of transcription, the flow of genetic information is from:**
   (a) DNA to DNA
   (b) RNA to Protein
   (c) DNA to protein
   (d) DNA to RNA
   (e) Protein to RNA
2. **The anticodon region is an important part of the structure of:**
   (a) DNA (b) m-RNA
   (c) hn-RNA (d) r-RNA
   (e) t-RNA
3. **Polysomes do not contain:**
   (a) Protein (b) DNA
   (c) m-RNA (d) t-RNA
   (e) r-RNA
4. **The formation of a peptide bond during the elongation step of protein synthesis results in the splitting of how many high energy bonds?**
   (a) 1 (b) 2
   (c) 3 (d) 4
   (e) 5

5. **During protein synthesis the amino acid sequence is specified by:**
   (a) Soluble RNA
   (b) Ribosomal RNA
   (c) Messenger RNA
   (d) Transfer RNA
   (e) None of the above
6. **Polypeptide synthesis requires all of the following *except:***
   (a) Primer (b) Ribosome
   (c) m-RNA (d) t-RNA
   (e) GTP
7. **Translocase is an enzyme required in the process of:**
   (a) Transcription
   (b) DNA replication
   (c) Initiation of Protein synthesis
   (d) Elongation of peptides
   (e) Termination of protein synthesis
8. **Elongation of polypeptide chain requires all the following proteins, *except:***
   (a) Peptidyl transferase
   (b) Translocase
   (c) Rho factor
   (d) GTP
   (e) Eongation factors
9. **Nonsense codons bring about**
   (a) Amino acid activation
   (b) Initiation of protein synthesis
   (c) Elongation of peptide chains
   (d) Post translational modification of proteins
   (e) Termination of proteins
10. **In prokaryotes, the chain initiating amino-acid in protein synthesis is:**
   (a) N-formyl methionine
   (b) Methionine
   (c) Glycine
   (d) Threonine
   (e) Phanyl alanine

ANSWERS

1. (d)	2. (e)	3. (b)	4. (b)
5. (c)	6. (a)	7. (d)	8. (c)
9. (e)	10. (a)		

18 Recombinant DNA Technology

Recombinant DNA technology is genetic engineering which effects artificial modification of the genetic constitution of a living cell by introduction of foreign DNA through experimental techniques. The technique involves the splicing of DNA by restriction endonucleases, preparation of chimeric DNA molecule, followed by cloning for the production of large number of identical target DNA molecules.

TOOLS OF RECOMBINANT DNA TECHNOLOGY

The various **"biological tools"** used to bring about genetic manipulations are:

A. Enzymes
B. *Passenger DNA:* Foreign DNA (insert DNA fragment) which is passively transferred from one cell to another cell or organ is known as **passenger DNA (Foreign DNA).**
C. *Vector or vehicle DNA:* The DNA which acts as the carrier is known as the vector or vehicle DNA.

A. Enzymes: The various enzymes which may be required to be used are:

- ***Restriction endonucleases:*** To cut DNA chains at specific locations (called as "chemical knife")
- ***Exonucleases:*** To cut DNA at 5' terminus
- ***Endonucleases:*** To cut in the interior to produce "nicks"
- ***Reverse transcriptase***
- ***DNA polymerases***
- ***DNA ligase (T_4 ligase)***
- ***S_1 nuclease*** and
- ***Alkaline phosphatase*** (Refer: ***Table 18.1***).

B. Passenger DNA (foreign DNA): DNA insert to be introduced into the vector DNA. They are:

a. cDNA (complementary DNA)
b. Synthetic DNA
c. Random DNA

a. ***Synthesis of cDNA:*** An enzyme called ***"reverse transcriptase"*** is used for this purpose. A double stranded DNA molecule, comple-

Table 18.1: Showing some enzymes used in recombinant DNA technology with their functions other than restriction endonucleases

Name	*Reaction*	*Function*
• *Reverse transcriptase*	Synthesizes DNA from RNA template	Synthesis of cDNA from m-RNA
• *S_1 nuclease*	Degrades single stranded DNA	Removal of "hairpin" in synthesis of cDNA
• *DNA ligase*	Catalyzes bonds between DNA molecules	Joining DNA molecules
• *DNA polymerase I*	Synthesizes double stranded DNA from single stranded DNA	Synthesis of double stranded cDNA, 'nick' translation
• *BAL3 1 nuclease*	Degrades, both 3' and 5' ends of DNA	Progressive shortening of DNA molecule
• *Alkaline phosphatase*	Dephosphorylates 5'-ends of RNA and DNA	Removal of 5'-PO_4 groups prior to kinase labelling to prevent self ligation

mentary in base sequence to a m-RNA molecule, can be prepared by using this enzyme.

It is prepared from RNA tumour viruses, can use RNA as a template to synthesize on RNA-DNA hybrid molecule. It requires a "primer" which is provided by hybridizing a short chain of oligo dT to the 3'-Poly-A tail of m-RNA.

Under *"in vitro"* conditions, the ***"reverse transcriptase"*** appears to turn the corner at the end of the newly formed DNA chain and starts to form a complementary strand. This forms the **"hairpin-bend".** The 3′-end of the hairpin-bend forms a "Primer" for ***"DNA polymerase I"*** to complete the synthesis of the complementary strand.

The hairpin-bend is then removed by the action of the enzyme ***"S_1 nuclease"*** which is specific for single stranded DNA.

The cDNA does not contain 'introns', which are present in the genomic DNA sequence, as these have been spliced out during m-RNA processing as explained in the process of transcription.

It is important to note that the source of m-RNA is quite critical. The tissue that is extracted to obtain the m-RNA strand should express adequately the gene that is required to be expressed.

b. ***Synthetic DNA:*** Synthetic DNA can be produced purely by chemical means. Short segments (10 to 15 nucleotides) with sticky ends are synthesized chemically, with ***"T_4 ligases"***. These are connected to give synthetic DNA with "Sticky" ends.

c. ***Random DNA:*** If it is not possible to use the cDNA or synthetic DNA, a shot-gun experiment is carried out to produce random pieces of DNA ("insert DNA") using the enzyme restriction endonucleases.

C. Vector or Vehicle DNA: Following types of DNA may be used as vector or vehicle DNA

1. ***Bacterial plasmids***
2. ***Bacteriophages***
3. ***Cosmids.***

1. ***Bacterial plasmids:*** They are small circular, duplex DNA molecules whose natural function is to confer antibiotic resistance to the host cell.

Plasmid DNAs replicate independently and they can be easily separated from host bacteria. The DNA sequences and restriction maps of many plasmids are known, hence the precise location of restriction enzyme cleavage sites for inserting the foreign DNA (insert DNA) is available.

The plasmids are the most commonly used vectors and ***can accept short DNA pieces about 6 to 10 kb long.***

Type of plasmids: ***Three main types*** of plasmids have been studied. However, many have been found in a variety of strains of *E. coli.*

- ***F plasmids (Sex plasmids):*** This plasmid transfers a replica of the plasmid from a donor (F^+) cell to a recipient (F^-) cell without the F^+ cell losing its plasmid. The F plasmid DNA can integrate into the chromosome of the recipient cell to produce Hfr cell. When an imperfect excision of F occurs, it produces a plasmid containing chromosomal gene. This is called F′-plasmid.
- ***R plasmids, drug resistance plasmids:*** These plasmids carry genes conferring resistance to one or more antibiotics and usually can transfer this resistance to an R-free recipient cell.
- ***Col plasmids or colicinogenic factor plasmids:*** They carry genes for the synthesis of a protein known as ***colicins***. These proteins can kill related strains of bacteria that lack the *col* plasmid. The *col plasmids* are non-self-transmissible. They can prepare their DNA for transfer but do not have the genes necessary for determining effective contact between donor and recipient cells.
- ***Ent Plasmids:*** Plasmids called *Ent* are responsible for traveller's diarrhoea and some types of dysentery. These plasmids contain genes that code for *enterotoxin* which is an intestinal irritant. Some strains of *Bacillus*

thuringiensis, which has genes that code for a product that is toxic to gypsy moths and tentworms.

Note: ***Plasmid vector PBR 322*** has both tetracycline *(tet)* and ampicillin *(amp)* resistance genes. A single Pst I site within the ampicillin resistance gene is commonly used as the insertion site for a piece of foreign DNA. In addition to having sticky ends, the DNA inserted at this site disrupts the ampicillin resistance gene and makes the bacterium carrying this plasmid ampicillin-sensitive.

2. *Bacteriophages:* They usually have linear DNA molecules into which foreign DNA can be inserted at several restriction enzyme sites.

   The chimeric or hybrid DNA is collected after the phage proceeds through its lytic cycle and produces mature, infective phage particles.

   A major advantage of phage vector is that ***they can accept DNA fragments 10 to 20 kb long*** (one kb = 1000 nucleotide long base sequence).

3. *Cosmids:* These are specialized plasmids that contain DNA sequences, so-called **"COS sites"** required for packaging λ (lambda) DNA into the phage particle.

Larger fragments of DNA can be inserted in cosmids which combine with best features of plasmids and phages. ***Cosmids can accept very large DNA fragments 35 to 50 kb.***

Table 18.2 shows the common vectors and DNA insert size.

Table 18.2: Common vectors and DNA insert size

Vector	*DNA insert size*
• Plasmid PBR 322	0.01 to 10 kb
• Bacteriophage (Lambda charon 4A)	10 to 20 kb
• Cosmids	35 to 50 kb

STAGES

I. Isolation of specific DNA (insert DNA):

The genomic DNA is very large in size. Isolation of a specific fragment of DNA can be achieved by splicing or cleaving brought about by a group of key enzymes called ***"restriction endonucleases"***.

Restriction endonucleases: (They are compared to ***chemical knife***). Certain endonucleases, enzymes that cut DNA at specific DNA sequences within the molecule (cf. exonucleases which digest from the ends of DNA molecules), are a key biological tool in recombinant DNA technology (Genetic engineering). These enzymes were originally called *"restriction enzymes"* because their presence in a given bacterium restricted the growth of certain bacterial viruses called bacteriophages.

Restriction enzymes cut DNA of any source into short pieces in a sequence-specific manner in contrast to other methods, e.g. enzymatic, physical or chemical that break DNA in a random fashion.

Nomenclature of restriction enzymes: Large number of restriction enzymes have been found. They have named after the bacterium from which they are isolated.

Examples:

- **Eco R I and Eco R II** isolated from *Escherichia coli*,
- **Bam HI** is from Bacillus amyloliquifaciens.

  The first three letters of the restriction enzymes name consist of the first letter of the genus (E) and the first two letters of the species (Co). These may be followed by a strain designation (R) and a Roman numeral I or II to indicate the order of discovery, e.g. Eco R I, Eco R II, etc.

Table 18.3 shows a few selected restriction endonuclease and their sequence specificities.

Mechanism of action: Each restriction endonuclease enzyme recognizes and cleaves a specific double stranded DNA sequence that is 4 to 7 bp long. These DNA cuts result in:

- *Blunt ends (by Hpa I)*
- *Sticky ends (also called staggered or cohesive ends)* by Bam HI or Eco R I.

Sticky ends are particularly useful in preparation of chimeric or hybrid DNA molecule.

By using different restriction endonucleases for the digestion of a particular DNA, a *"restriction map"* with characteristic sites of action can be prepared ***(Table 18.4)***.

Table 18.3: A few selected restriction endonuclease and their sequence specificities

Endonuclease	*Sequence cleaved*	*Bacterial source*
• Eco R I	G|A A T T C C T T A A|G	Escherichia coli Ry 13
• Bam H I	G|G A T C C C C T A G|G	Bacillus amyloliquifaciens H
• Eco R II	|C C T G G G G A C C|	Escherichia coli R 245
• H Pa I	G T T|A A C C A A|T T G	Haemophilus parainfluenzae
• Pst I	C T G C A|G G|A C G T C	Providencia stuartii 164

Table 18.4: Shows DNA splicing by restriction endonucleases

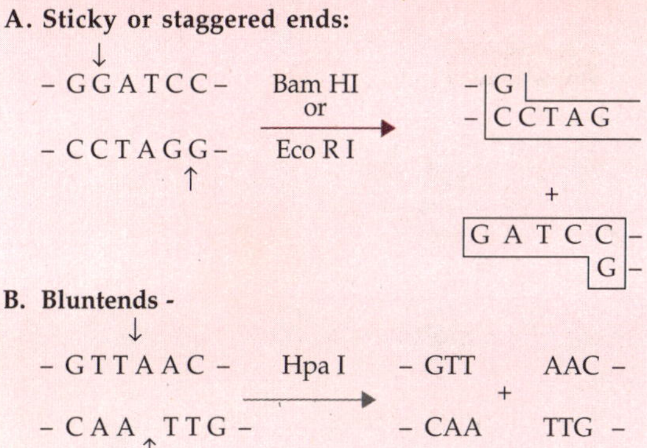

When DNA is digested with a given enzyme, the ends of all the fragments would have the same DNA sequence. The fragments produced can be isolated by agarose electrophoresis or polyacrylamide gel electrophoresis. This is an essential step in cloning and a major use of these enzymes.

II. Chimeric or Hybrid DNA:

The main aim of genetic engineering is to insert a DNA of interest (foreign DNA) into a vector DNA so that the DNA fragment replicates along with the vector after annealing. This hybrid combination of two fragments of DNA is referred to as chimeric DNA or hybrid DNA or recombinant DNA.

STEPS OF PREPARATION

- A circular plasmid vector DNA is first cut with a specific ***"restriction endonuclease"***. If Eco R I is used, sticky ends with TTAA sequence on one DNA strand and AATT sequence on the other strand are produced.
- The human DNA (foreign or insert DNA) is also cut with the same ***restriction endonuclease,*** so that the same sequences are produced on the sticky ends of the cut piece.
- Next, the vector DNA and human cut piece DNA are incubated together so that ***"annealing"*** occurs. The sticky ends of both vector and human DNA have complementary sequences hence they come into contact with each other.
- The enzyme ***"DNA Ligase"*** is allowed to act on the hybrid or chimeric DNA molecule. The enzyme joins the two fragments by covalent phosphodiester linkages between the vector and insert molecules and finally the chimeric DNA molecule is produced ***(Refer Fig. 18.1).***

Problems in Preparation of Chimeric DNA:

Although sticky ends ligation is technically easy, but sometimes problems may come up as follows and some special techniques are required to overcome these:

a. Sticky ends of a vector may recombine with themselves without taking up the "insert" molecule.
b. Sticky ends of insert fragments similarly also can anneal without joining the vector.
c. Lastly, sometimes sticky end sites may not be available.

HOMOPOLYMER TAILING

To circumvent the above mentioned problems, a reaction enzyme like Hpa I can be used. ***It produces "blunt ends".*** The new ends are joined using the enzyme terminal ***"transferase".*** If poly d (G) is added to the 3'-ends of the vector and poly d (C) is added to the 3'-ends of the insert foreign DNA molecule, the two molecules can only anneal to each other circumventing the problems mentioned above. This procedure is called ***"homopolymer tailing"***.

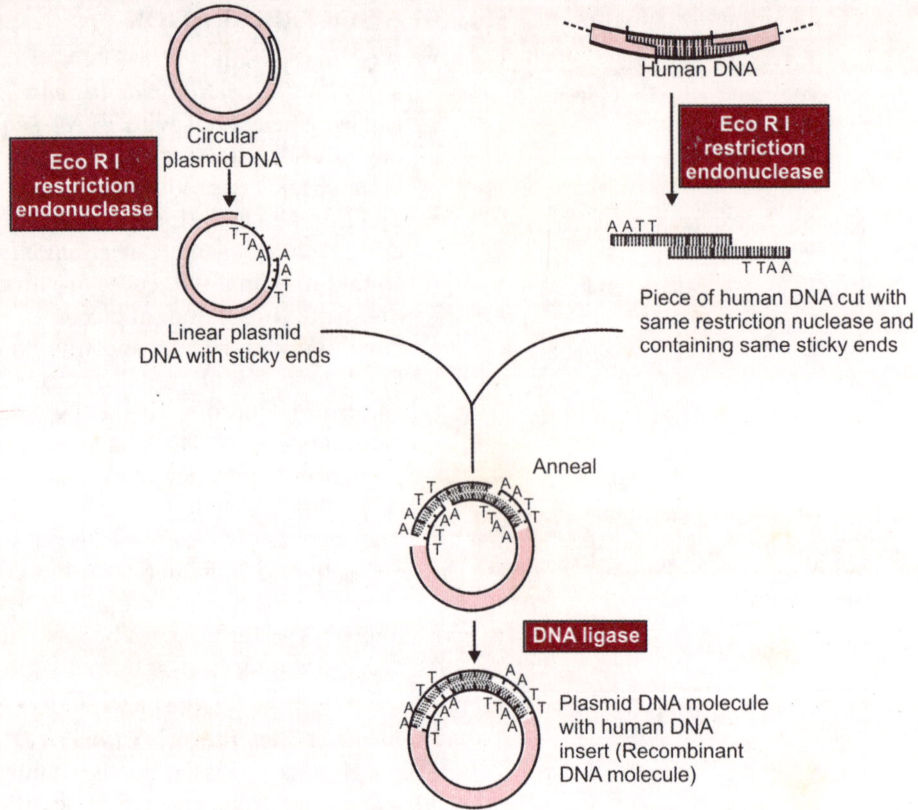

Fig. 18.1: Preparation of chimeric DNA molecule

Other Methods:

1. ***Use of synthetic DNA "Linker":*** Sometimes a synthetic DNA called a **"linker"** is used. The linker helps for the recognition of sequence and effective binding between the human DNA (insert DNA) and vector DNA having "blunt ends".
2. ***Use of T_4 DNA ligase:*** Direct blunt end ligation can be done by using the enzyme bacteriophage *"T_4 DNA ligase"*. This technique though more difficult than sticky ends ligation has the advantage of joining together any pairs of "blunt ends".

III. Cloning of Chimeric DNA:

What is a clone?

A clone is a large population of identical molecules, bacteria or cells that arise from a common ancestor.

This cloning allows for the production of a large number of identical DNA molecules which can then be characterized or used for various purposes.

The chimeric DNA contained in a plasmid vector or phages or cosmids can be introduced into bacterial cells *E. coli* strain C 101 by a process called ***transfection.*** The replicating bacterial cell (host cell) permits the amplification of the chimeric DNA of the vector.

In this way, cloning results in the production of large number of identical target DNA molecules. The cloned target DNA is released from its vector by cleavage using appropriate restriction endonucleases, isolated, characterized and used for various purposes.

GENE LIBRARY

By the combination of restriction enzymes and various cloning vectors the entire DNA of an organism can be packed into a suitable vector.

A collection of these recombinant clones is called a gene library. **A DNA gene library can be of two types:**

a. **Genomic library**
b. **cDNA library**

a. *Genomic Library:*
- A genomic library is prepared from the total DNA of a cell line or tissue.
- It is prepared by performing partial digestion of total DNA with restriction enzyme, e.g. Saul III A that cuts the DNA frequently to produce larger fragments so that intact genes can be obtained.
- ***Phage vectors are ideal and preferred*** for this as they accept large pieces of DNA up to 20 kb.

b. *cDNA Library:*
- A cDNA library represents the population of m-RNAs in a tissue.
- cDNA libraries are prepared by first isolating all the m-RNAs in a tissue.
- m-RNA serves as a template to prepare the cDNA using the enzymes ***"reverse transcriptase"*** and ***"DNA polymerase"***. Full length cDNA copies are usually not obtained and smaller DNA fragments are cloned.
- ***Plasmids are the ideal and preferred vectors for*** cDNA libraries as they are workable with smaller fragments.
- cDNA libraries contain relatively smaller DNA fragments compared to genomic libraries.

DNA Probes

Probes are used to search libraries for specific genes or cDNA molecules. Gene libraries contain large numbers of DNA fragments and it is extremely difficult to find out or choose a specific DNA sequence of interest from these.

- A variety of molecules can be used to "Probe" libraries to search for specific genes or cDNAs
- Probes are generally pieces of DNA or RNA labelled with ^{32}P-containing nucleotide. To be effective, the probes must recognize a complementary sequence
- A cDNA synthesized from a specific m-RNA can be used to screen either a cDNA library for a longer cDNA or a genomic library for a complementary sequence in the coding region of a gene.
- cDNA probes are used to detect DNA fragments on Southern Blot transfers and to detect and quantitate RNA on Northern Blot transfers (See below).
- Specific antibodies can also be used as probes.

Blotting and Hybridization

Visualization and identification of a specific DNA or RNA fragment or protein among the many thousands of molecules requires the convergence of a number of techniques which are called collectively as ***Blot transfer techniques.***

ANALYSIS OF DNA, RNA AND PROTEINST

1. **Analysis of Chromosomal DNA (Southern Blot):** Following are the steps that are normally employed in Southern Blot Analysis of DNA.
   - ***Cleavage:*** DNA is cleaved with the help of ***restriction endonuclease*** at specific sites
   - ***Electrophoresis:*** The DNA thus obtained will be in fragments. These DNA fragments are separated by agarose gel electrophoresis or polyacrylamide gel (Slab) electrophoresis
   - ***Blotting:*** The separated DNA fragments are transferred to a sheet of nitrocellulose by a flow of buffer. These fragments bind to the nitrocellulose, creating a replica of the pattern of DNA fragments
   - ***Hybridization:*** The next step is the hybridization of fragments with a labelled probe. This probe has a homology with the gene of interest. The probe is hybridized to filter. The probe can be
     - Purified RNA
     - c-DNA
     - A segment of cloned DNA.

- *Autoradiography:* This is the final step. The pattern of bands that contain the DNA fragments, or fragments that contain the gene are visualized by virtue of radiation from the probe.

2. **Analysis of RNA (Northern Blot):**
   - *Electrophoresis:* Total cellular RNA, or isolated m-RNA is subjected to agarose gel electrophoresis in the presence of a denaturing agent to remove secondary structure constraints
   - *Blotting:* The gel is blotted as above with the difference that, paper has been treated chemically so that it will covalently bind RNA.
   - *Hybridization:* A labelled probe is used. This allows visualization of the RNA species that are complementary to the probe.
3. **Analysis of Proteins (Western Blot):** By Western blot test, proteins are identified. Proteins are first isolated from the tissues.
   - *Electrophoresis and fixation:* Electrophoresis of the whole protein is done and transferred on to a nitrocellulose membrane and fixed.
   - *Probing:* After fixation, the protein is probed with radioactive antibody.
   - *Autoradiography:* This is the final step. The pattern of bands that contain protein are visualized by virtue of radiation from the probe.

   Note: The Western blot is very useful to identify the production of a specific protein in a tissue ***(Refer Fig. 18.2)***.

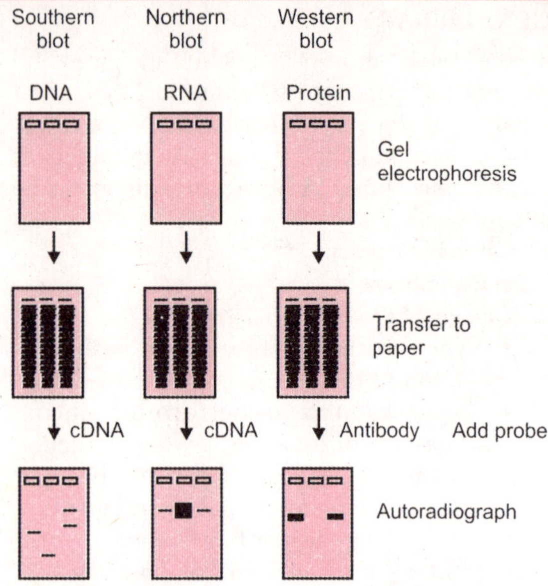

Fig. 18.2: Blot transfer techniques

POLYMERASE CHAIN REACTION (PCR):

Principle: Polymerase chain reaction (PCR) is a method of amplifying a target sequence of DNA. It provides a ***sensitive***, ***selective*** and extremely ***rapid*** means of amplifying a desired sequence of DNA.

Specificity is based on the use of two oligonucleotides ***"primers"*** that hybridize to complementary sequences on opposite strands of DNA and flank the target sequence (flanking sequence).

PROCEDURE

1. *Denaturation of DNA:* The double stranded DNA is first heated to separate the two strands into single strand.
2. *Annealing with "primers":* The single DNA strand obtained as above is cooled and allowed to bind (or anneal) with the two 'primers' (one for each strand) complementary to the flanking sequences.
3. *Amplification of DNA:* In presence of ***"DNA polymerase"*** and the substrates "deoxyribonucleotide triphosphates", the synthesis of new DNA strands take place. These strands are complementary to the target DNA.

As the first cycle is over, the double stranded DNAs are again denatured by heating, each strand is allowed to bind to the complementary "Primers" and DNA amplification with *'DNA polymerase"* is repeated again and again which result in the amplification of DNA segments of defined length.

Magnitude of amplification:

DNA sequences as short as 50 to 100 bp and as long as 2.5 kbp can be amplified. Twenty cycles provide an amplification of target DNA by about

10^6 times with high specificity and 30 cycles provide amplification of 10^9.

Difficulties: Early PCR used an *E. coli 'DNA polymerase'* that was destroyed by each heat generation cycle. This difficulty was later on circumvented by using a heat-stable *"DNA polymerase"* from "Thermus aquaticus", which can withstand 70° to 80°C.

CLINICAL APPLICATIONS OF PCR

1. ***Application in forensic medicine:*** PCR allows DNA in a single cell, hair follicle or sperm to be amplified enormously and analyzed.
2. ***In detection of infectious agents:*** Specially used to detect latent viruses in tissues.
3. ***In diagnosis of inherited disorders:*** PCR technology is being widely used to amplify gene segments that contain known mutations for diagnosis of inherited diseases viz. sickle cell disease, β-thalassaemia, cystic fibrosis, etc.
4. ***In prenatal diagnosis:*** PCR is especially useful for prenatal diagnosis of inherited diseases, where cells obtained from foetus by amniocentesis are few.
5. ***In transplantation:*** PCR has been used to establish precise tissue types for transplants.
6. ***In cancer detection:*** Specific chromosomal translocation, e.g. chronic myeloid leukaemia (CML) could be identified by PCR.
7. ***To study evolution:*** Using DNA from archaeological samples.

APPLICATIONS OF RECOMBINANT DNA TECHNOLOGY:

Recombinant DNA technology (genetic engineering) has revolutionized the application of molecular biology to medical/agricultural sciences that has immensely benefitted the mankind.

A few of the useful practical applications of recombinant DNA technology are listed below:

1. ***Manufacture of proteins/hormones:*** A practical goal of recombinant DNA research is the production of materials for biomedical application. This technology has two distinct merits:
   i. It can supply large amounts of materials that could not be obtained by conventional purification methods, e.g. interferon, plasminogen activating factor, other blood clotting factors.
   ii. It can provide human materials, e.g. insulin (refer Chapter on Hormones), growth hormone, etc.
2. ***AIDS Test:*** By using recombinant DNA techniques, the diagnosis of diseases like AIDS by laboratory has become simple and rapid.
3. ***Diagnosis of molecular diseases:*** Many genetic diseases that yield developmental abnormalities can be detected by characteristic patterns in DNA primary structure. Such mutational changes in DNA sequences are identified by restriction fragments analysis and southern blotting, using appropriate DNA probes. Analysis of this type could be done in understanding the molecular basis of diseases like sickle cell anaemia, thalassaemias, familial hypercholesterolaemia, cystic fibrosis, etc.
4. ***Prenatal diagnosis:*** If the genetic lesion is understood and a specific probe is available prenatal diagnosis is possible. DNA from cells collected from as little as 10 ml of amniotic fluid or by chorionic villi biopsy can be analyzed by Southern blot transfer.
5. ***Gene therapy:*** Diseases caused by deficiency of a gene product are amenable to replacement therapy. The strategy is to clone a gene into a vector that will readily be taken up and incorporated into genome of a host cell. In 1990, a patient with ***"adenosine deaminase"*** deficiency was treated successfully with gene replacement therapy. In future, probably many inherited disorders like sickle cell anaemia, thalassaemias, various enzyme deficiencies, etc. may be treated by gene replacement therapy.
6. ***Applications in agriculture:*** Genetically engineered plants have been developed to resist draught and diseases. Good quality of food and increased yield of crops could be possible by applying this technology. Incorporation of ***"nif genes"*** to cereals has given higher yield of the crops.

7. ***Industrial application:*** Enzymes synthesized by this technology are in use to produce sugars, cheese and detergents. Certain protein products produced by this technology are used as *food additives* to increase the nutritive value, besides imparting flavour. Ethylene glycol is in great demand for industry. Preparation of ethylene glycol from ethylene is made possible by this technology.
8. ***Application in forensic medicine:*** Advances in genetic engineering have greatly helped to specifically identify criminals and settle the disputes of parenthood of children. The restriction analysis pattern of DNA of one individual will be very specific (DNA finger printing), but the pattern will be different from person-to-person.
9. ***Transgenesis:*** The somatic gene replacement therapy will not pass on to the offspring. Transgenesis refers to the transfer of genes into fertilized ovum which will be found in somatic as well as germ cells and passed on to the successive generations.

Note: The above depicts the brighter aspects of genetic engineering. But it is to be remembered that there are likely "hazards" also e.g. by any chance, in the course of cloning using bacterial vectors, some drug-resistant or harmful bacteria are produced and released, the new varieties may cause incurable diseases to the humanity and the live stock. Scientists should use the technology for useful purposes only like atomic energy and not for harmful purposes to humanity.

19 Detoxication

INTRODUCTION

The term "detoxication" includes all the biochemical processes, whereby ***noxious substances are rendered less harmful and are more easily excreted in urine.***

DEFINITION

The term detoxication covers all those biochemical changes proceeding in the body, which convert foreign molecules, generally toxic, but not always so, to generally non-toxic or less toxic but not always so and more soluble so that they can be easily excreted.

- Foreign molecules may be ***exogenous,*** which include those substances which are not ordinarily ingested or utilized by the organism. Those may enter the body through the dietary foodstuffs or in the form of certain medicines/ or drugs which are administered to the body.
- Some of them be ***endogenous*** and may be produced in the body by synthesis or as metabolites of various processes in the body.

XENOBIOTICS

Foreign molecules, which enter the body are called ***xenobiotics.*** Humans are now subjected increasingly to exposure to various foreign chemicals (xenobiotics) whether they may be ***drugs, food additives or pollutants or carcinogens.*** In some cases, the reactions to which xenobiotics are subjected may increase their biologic activity and even toxicity, instead of making less toxic.

MECHANISM OF DETOXICATION

The mechanism of detoxication involves reactions mainly of **four** types: **A:** Oxidation **B:** Reduction, **C:** Hydrolysis, and **D:** Conjugation

Sometimes these reactions may occur independently and at others there may be a combination of these processes operating together. In many cases among human beings, oxidation and other reactions may be followed by conjugation. ***In man, detoxication is principally carried out in liver,*** but to some extent it can be carried out in kidneys also. Present concept is that the reactions of xenobiotics occur in ***two phases:***

Phase 1: This phase involves the hydroxylation, the major reaction, catalyzed by ***mono-oxygenases*** **or** ***cytochrome*** P_{450} species. Other types of reactions in Phase 1 include oxidation, reduction and hydroxylation.

Phase 2: The hydroxylated or other compounds produced in phase 1 are ***converted by specific enzymes to various water soluble polar metabolites by conjugation with various conjugating agents,*** viz. glucuronic acid, "active" sulfate, methylation, acetylation, etc.

The overall purpose of these two phases is to increase their water solubility and thus facilitate their excretion from the body.

A. OXIDATION

A large number of foreign substances are destroyed in the body by oxidation. Aliphatic as well as aromatic alcohols may be oxidized to corresponding acids, probably via aldehyde formation. In addition, certain amines, anilides and drugs also can undergo oxidation.

Examples of oxidation

1. *Methyl Groups:* These groups can be oxidized to form –COOH group through formation of aldehyde.

$$—CH_3 \rightarrow —CH_2OH \rightarrow —CHO \rightarrow —COOH$$

2. *Primary Aliphatic and Aromatic Alcohols:* These are oxidized to corresponding acids, e.g.

- **Methanol** ⟶ Formic acid
- **Benzyl alcohol** ⟶ Benzoic acid ↓ Conjugated with glycine to form Hippuric acid ↙ excreted in urine

3. *Aromatic Hydrocarbons:* Aromatic hydrocarbons are oxidized to phenol and other phenolic compounds. Again they are conjugated with glucuronic acid or sulphuric acid and excreted as corresponding glucuronides and sulphates.

- **Benzene** ⟶ Phenol ⟶ Catechol

In rare cases, aromatic ring may open, but only to a slight extent, for example:

- **Catechol** ⟶ Muconic acid

4. *Aldehydes:* Aldehydes are oxidized to form the corresponding acids.

- **Benzaldehyde** ⟶ Benzoic acid ↓ conjugated with glycine ↓ Hippuric acid (excreted)

5. *Anilides:* Anilides are oxidized to the corresponding phenols, e.g. acetanilide is present as a constituent of analgesic drugs, which relieves pain. It is oxidized in the body to form p-acetyl amino phenol.

- **Acetanilide** ⟶ p-acetyl amino phenol

6. **Amines:**

- Many primary aliphatic amines undergo oxidation to the corresponding acids and N is converted to urea.
- **Benzylamine** ⟶ Benzoic acid+urea.
- Aromatic amines like aniline is oxidized to corresponding phenol.
- **Aniline** ⟶ p-amino phenol

7. *Sulphur Compounds:* The sulphur present in organic sulphur compounds is oxidized to $SO^{=}_4$ which in turn may be excreted in inorganic or organic form or as neutral (unoxidized) sulphur.

8. *Drugs:* Certain drugs can be oxidized in the body and are excreted as hydroxy derivatives or salts. *Examples* are:

- *Meprobamate:* A tranquilizer used in psychiatric disorders is excreted largely as the oxidation product hydroxy meprobamate.

  Meprobamate ⟶ OH –Meprobamate
- *Chloral:* It is used as a hypnotic. Most of the chloral undergoes reduction and conjugation; but partly it can be oxidized to form trichloroacetic acid which is excreted as its salt.

  Chloral: ⟶ Trichloroacetic acid

  (See hydroxylation of drugs and role of cyt. P_{450} species below)

B. REDUCTION

Reduction usually does not occur extensively in man. Some of the reduced metabolites are less toxic, some of them are more toxic *Examples* are:

1. *Certain aldehydes,* e.g. chloral, a hypnotic, principally undergoes reduction in the body to form corresponding alcohol, which is then conjugated with D-glucuronic acid and excreted as corresponding glucuronides.

- **Chloral** ⟶ Trichlorethanol ↓ + D-glucuronic acid excreted as corresponding glucuronides

2. *Aromatic nitro-compounds,* e.g. p-nitrobenzaldehyde is reduced to corresponding amines and excreted after conjugation.

CHO → (+O, +2H) → COOH / NHOH → (+2H) → COOH / NH_2

NO_2 (*p*-nitro-benzaldehyde) — NHOH — NH_2 (*p*-amino benzoic acid (excreted after conjugation.))

C. HYDROLYSIS

There are quite a number of therapeutic compounds, used as drugs, which undergo hydrolysis, usually in liver. ***Example are:***

- **Acetyl salicylic acid** → Salicylic acid
  (Aspirin) + Acetic acid
  Salicylic acid can reduce Benedict's qualitative reagent.
- **Atropine** → Tropic acid
  (Tropyl tropate) + Tropine
- **Digitalis** → Sugar + Aglycone
  (a cardiac glycoside) (Non sugar component)
- **Procaine** → p-amino benzoic acid
  + Diethylamino ethanol

D. CONJUGATION

Definition: A process by which the foreign molecules or its metabolites are coupled with a conjugating agent and converted to soluble, nontoxic derivatives which are easily excreted in urine.

Features

- Various conjugating agents are available in the body and some of them are synthesized in the body, e.g. *D-glucuronic acid* formed from glucose by uronic acid pathway. Certain amino acids such as ***glycine, cysteine*** can be available from dietary proteins/or breakdown of tissue proteins or synthesized.
- ***Conjugation reaction principally occurs in liver*** and to some extent it can occur in kidneys also.
- Conjugation produces less toxic, more soluble compounds which are excreted.
- Conjugation can occur independently or it can follow oxidation, reduction or hydroxy-lation of a compound.

Types of Conjugation

1. *Methylation*

Methylation as a detoxication process though limited in the body, is quite important. Usual methyl donor is **"S-adenosyl methionine" ("active" methionine).**

- Methylation of heterocyclic N-atom of compounds of the pyrimidine and quinoline types e.g. Nicotinamide.

$\swarrow$ ~CH_3

- **Nicotinamide** → N′-methyl nicotinamide

This occurs also with other heterocyclic aromatic compounds, e.g. Histamine.

- Methylation of **p-aminomethyl amino azo benzene** to p-dimethyl amino azo benzene (butter yellow), a potential hepatic carcinogen.
- O-methylation of certain naturally occurring amines (with phenolic hydroxyl group), e.g. epinephrine and nor-epinephrine and their metabolites are methylated at the phenolic hydroxyl group.
- O-methylation of natural estrogens.

2. *Acetylation Reactions*

In detoxication reactions, conjugation with acetic acid occurs only with aromatic NH_2 group.

- Acetic acid helps in conjugation of **aromatic compounds** alongwith cysteine to form corresponding ***mercapturic acids*** (see below-conjugation with cysteine).
- In humans, certain drugs, e.g. **sulpha drugs** are conjugated by acetylation. As much as 50% of excreted sulpha drugs my be acetylated and excreted as acetylated derivatives.

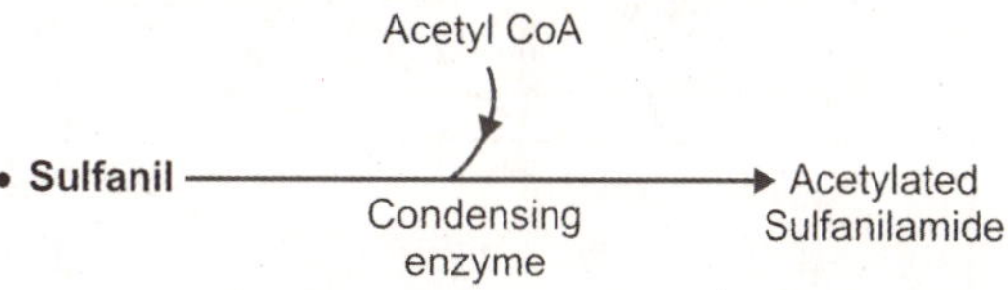

- Similarly, like sulphonamide drugs, **PABA** is also acetylated and excreted as acetyl derivative.

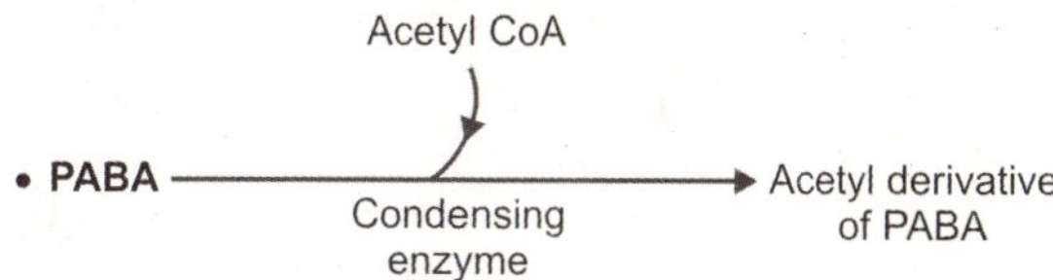

Acetylation is done by active acetate (Acetyl-CoA): It is catalyzed by the enzyme *acetyl transferase* present in the cytosol of various tissues.

BIOMEDICAL IMPORTANCE

The drug **"Isoniazid"**, used in treatment of TB is detoxicated by acetylation.

Polymorphic types of ***acetyl transferases*** exist, resulting in individuals who are classified as: (1) ***'Slow'*** acetylator and (2) ***'fast"*** acetylator.

- **'Slow' acetylators:** are more prone to certain toxic effects of isoniazid because the drug persists longer in these individuals due to slow acetylation.
- **'Fast' acetylators**- removes the drug by acetylation in a faster rate.

3. *Conjugation with Sulfuric Acid:*

Sulfuric acid is used by human beings for detoxication of various compounds having phenolic or hydroxyl groups.

- Substances like ***Phenol, Cresol, Indole and Skatole*** formed in the gut by the action of intestinal bacteria are absorbed and transported to liver, to be conjugated with sulphate to form ***"Ethereal sulfates"***, which are excreted in urine, being less toxic and more acidic.
- ***"Active" sulphate acts as the donor. Chemically it is "3'-phospho adenosine-5'-phospho sulphate" (PAPS).***
- Other compounds which are conjugated in the body to form corresponding esters are ***tyrosine to form tyrosine-O-SO_4 required for fibrinogen molecule, the amino sugars, certain hormones like oestrogens and androgens.***

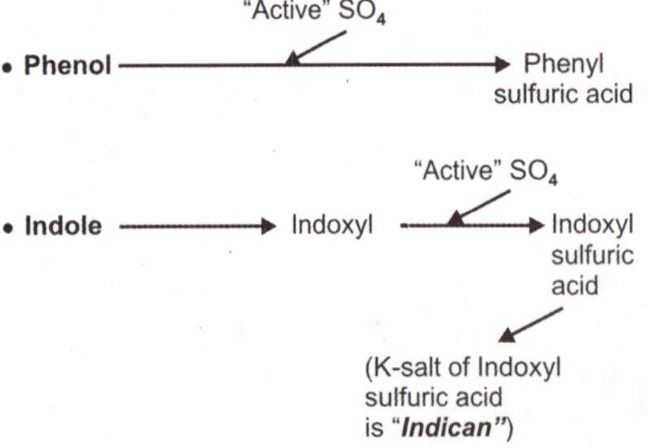

4. *Conjugation with D-glucuronic Acid*

Most important and commonest detoxication reaction. Participates in its detoxication reaction as its active form ***"UDP-glucuronic acid"*** which is formed in "uronic acid" pathway of glucose oxidation. Enzyme required is ***Glucuronyl transferase.***

Various compounds that are conjugated with glucuronic acid:

- Bilirubin to form Bilirubin diglucuronide
- Aromatic acids, e.g. benzoic acid
- Phenols and other secondary and tertiary aliphatic alcohols
- Certain drugs like morphine, menthol, pyramidon, acetanilide, sulfpyridine, etc.
- Antibiotics like chloramphenicol
- Hormones like thyroid hormones, derivatives of steroids, e.g. tetrahydroderivatives of cortisol. Sex hormones-metabolites.

Thus, formation of glucuronides plays an important role in detoxication mechanisms of exogenous and endogenous compounds and their excretion as corresponding glucuronides.

5. *Conjugation with Amino Acids:*

a. Glycine: Glycine combines with potentially harmful substances, mainly aromatic carboxylic acids in the body to form harmless derivatives which are excreted in urine. ***Examples are:***

- Reaction with "Nuclear" carboxyl group *(Fig.19.1).*
- Reaction with aromatic-COOH group separated from the aromatic ring by a "Vinyl" group, e.g. Cinnamic acid.
- Other aromatic carboxylic acids that can be conjugated with glycine and excreted are—naphthoic acid, furoic acid, thiophene carboxylic acid, etc.
- Aliphatic carboxyl group does not combine as a rule except endogenous cholic acids produced in the liver by catabolism of cholesterol. Thus cholic acid and deoxycholic acid are conjugated with glycine to form glycocholic acid and glyco deoxy cholic acid.

(b) L-cysteine: In man, few aromatic compounds are conjugated with L-cysteine in presence of acetic acid to form ***"mercapturic acids".***

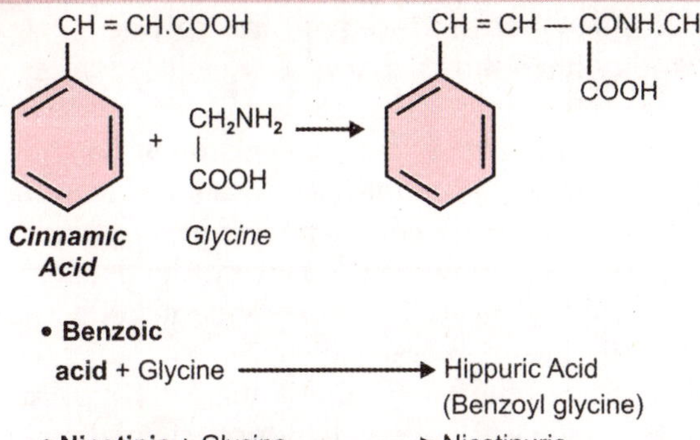

- **Benzoic acid** + Glycine ⟶ Hippuric Acid (Benzoyl glycine)
- **Nicotinic acid** + Glycine ⟶ Nicotinuric acid

Fig. 19.1: Conjugation with glycine (reaction with nuclear-COOH gr.)

Coupling of cysteine with aromatic compounds is linked with acetylation reaction ***(Fig. 19.2)***.

- **Bromobenzene** + L-cysteine + Acetic acid → Bromophenyl mercapturic acid
- **Naphthalene** + L-cysteine + Acetic acid→ Naphthyl mercapturic acid

Fig. 19.2: Conjugation with cysteine

6. ***Conjugation with Glutamine:***

In man and in primates (chimpanzee), glutamine conjugates phenyl acetic acid to form ***'phenyl-acetyl glutamine'*** and excreted in urine. This accounts for ***"mousy"*** odour of urine in phenyl ketonurics ***(Fig. 19.3)***.

- **Phenyl acetic acid** + glutamine ⟶ Phenyl acetyl glutamin (mousy smell)

Fig. 19.3: Conjugation with glutamine

7. ***Conjugation with Thiosulfates (thiocyanate formation):***

Animal organism normally excretes thiocyanates which is non-toxic. Human saliva contains an average of 0.01%. Normal human blood contains about 1.31 mg KCNS (potassium thiocyanates) per 100 ml. Highly toxic cyanides are derived in body in small amounts from fruits, proteins and tobacco smoke. Cyanides are conjugated by ***"thiosulfates"*** or even in presence of colloidal sulphur. The reaction takes place in the liver and is catalyzed by the enzyme ***thiosulfate cyanide sulfur transferase*** (also called ***Rhodanase)***. Formerly *Rhodanase* used to be called "Rhodanese".

$$HCN + S \xrightarrow{\text{Rhodanase}} HCNS + Na_2SO_3$$

8. ***Conjugation with Glutathione:***

A number of potentially toxic electrophilic xenobiotics, e.g. certain carcinogens are conjugated to the nucleophilic G-SH, in reactions that can be represented as follows:

$$R + G\text{–}SH \longrightarrow R - S - G$$

Where R represents an electrophilic xenobiotic.

- The reaction is catalyzed by the enzyme ***glutathione-S-transferases.*** The enzyme is present in high amounts in liver cytosol and in lower amounts in other tissues.

Note: If the potentially toxic xenobiotics are not conjugated with G-SH, they would be free to combine covalently with DNA, RNA or cell proteins and can produce serious cell damage. ***G-SH is thus an important defence mechanism*** against certain toxic compounds, such as some drugs and carcinogens.

Detoxication of Drugs:

Most of the drugs, more than 50% are detoxicated by hydroxylation. Enzymes concerned are ***monooxygenases* or *cytochrome P_{450}*** species. The reaction can be represented as follows:

$$AH + O_2 + NADPH + H^+ \longrightarrow A - OH + H_2O + NADP^+$$

AH represents the drugs, which can be of wide variety, carcinogens, chemicals, pollutants, and certain endogenous compounds, such as steroids or its metabolites.

Characteristic features of cytochrome P_{450} system

- Present in endoplasmic reticulum (ER), microsomal fraction of liver (highest concentration)
- At least six closely related species of cytochrome-P_{450} in ER of liver described
- Chemically they are "haemo proteins."
- Enzyme is **"NADPH-cyt. *P_{450} reductase*"**
- The enzyme requires NADPH

- Cytochrome-P_{450} system contains lipids and most common lipid is phosphatidyl choline (lecithin)
- It is an inducible enzyme.

SELENIUM POISONING

Selenium poisoning develops due to high feeding of products obtained from the soil having high contents of selenium.

Reason for Toxicity: Selenium replaces sulphur in cysteine and methionine in body tissues and interferes with the availability of these S-containing amino acids.

Detoxication: The above can be cured by administering p-bromobenzene. Selenium containing species now forms mercapturic acid type of compound with p-bromobenzene and thus excreted in urine.

Dithio Propanol:

It is known as **2, 3-mercaptopropanol or "BAL" (British antilewesite).** 'BAL' was used as a detoxicant for certain war poisons (chemical warfare). It is now known that "BAL" is valuable for removal of a number of toxic materials, e.g. arsenic (As), gold (Au), mercury (Hg), cadmium (Cd).

Mechanism of Action: Exact mechanism of action is not known. Toxic metal ions combine with –SH groups of body enzymes or other important –SH groups containing molecules and thus inactivate them. 'BAL' having a greater affinity for certain metals, when administered pulls the metal ions from their enzyme combinations and forms a similar complex which is rather readily excreted.

Biochemical Importance of Mono-oxygenases: Cytochrome-P_{450} System

Recently another *cytochrome P_{450}* species has been found, called as ***cytochrome P_{448}***. This species has been found to be ***specific for metabolism of polycyclic aromatic hydrocarbons (PAHS).*** Hence this species has also been named as ***aromatic hydrocarbon hydroxylase (AHH).***

Importance: It has been found to be very important enzyme for metabolism of PAHS and in carcinogenesis produced by these agents. Studies have shown that:

- In the lungs of cigarette smokers the ***enzyme may be involved in conversion of inactive PAHS (procarcinogens) present in cigarette smoke to active carcinogens by hydroxylation reactions.*** Smokers were found to have higher levels of this enzyme in cells and tissues than nonsmokers.
- Some reports have shown that activity of this enzyme is increased (induced) in placentae of pregnant women who are cigarette smokers and thus foetus is exposed to potentially harmful metabolites (carcinogens?).

☞ SALIENT POINTS TO REMEMBER

- Detoxication deals with the series of biochemical reactions occurring in the body to convert the foreign (often toxic) compounds to non-toxic or less toxic and more soluble and easily excretable forms
- Liver is the major site of all forms of detoxication processes
- The term metabolism of xenobiotics or biotransformation are better terms than detoxication
- Detoxication may be divided into phase I (oxidation, reduction, hydroxylation) and phase II (conjugation)
- Oxidation is a major process of detoxication involving the microsomal enzyme cytochrome P_{450} which is inducible NADPH dependent haemoprotein.
- Reduction usually does not occur extensively in man. Certain aldehydes, e.g. chloral (a hypnotic) and aromatic p-nitrobenzaldehyde undergo reduction
- A number of therapeutic compounds used as drugs undergo hydrolysis in the liver, e.g. Acetyl salicylic acid (aspirin), Atropine, Digitalis, Procaine
- Conjugation is another major and frequent common process in which a foreign compound combines with a substance produced in the body
- The process of conjugation may occur either directly or after phase I reactions

- At least eight different conjugating agents have been identified in the body, viz. D-Glucuronic acid, glycine, cysteine, glutamine, methylation, acetylation, sulfation, thiosulfates and glutathione.
- D-Glucuronic acid is the most common and important detoxicating agent. Formed in the body by uronic acid pathway. Substance is converted to corresponding glucuronide which is soluble and easily excretable, by active form UDP-Glucuronic acid in presence of the enzyme glucuronyl transferase.
- In man and in primates, glutamine conjugates phenyl acetic acid to form phenyl acetyl glutamine and excreted in urine which gives "mousy" odour of urine in phenylketonurics.

MULTIPLE CHOICE QUESTIONS

Give one correct answer:

1. **The water soluble vitamin Nicotinic acid is detoxicated in the body with:**
   (a) Glucuronic acid
   (b) Glutamine
   (c) Cysteine
   (d) Glycine
   (e) 'Active' sulphate
2. **Ingestion of sodium benzoate in man results in an increase in urinary excretion of:**
   (a) Glyoxalic acid
   (b) Oxalic acid
   (c) Hippuric acid
   (d) Phenyl Pyruvic acid
   (e) Ethereal sulphates
3. **In Phenylketonurics, the phenyl acetic acid is conjugated with:**
   (a) Glycine (b) Glutamine
   (c) Glutathione (d) Glucuronic acid
   (e) Acetylation
4. **The drug 'isoniazid' (isonicotinic acid hydrazide) used in the treatment of tuberculosis is detoxicated by:**
   (a) Acetylation (b) Methylation
   (c) Glutathione (d) Cytochrome P-450
   (e) Hydroxylation
5. **Nicotinamide is detoxicated in the body by:**
   (a) Acetylation (b) Methylation
   (c) Hydroxylation (d) Glucuronic acid
   (e) Glycine
6. **Indican exereted in urine is formed from detoxication of indoxyl in liver by:**
   (a) Glutathione (b) Acetylation
   (c) Methylation (d) SAM
   (e) PAPS
7. **Selenium poisoning can be cured by the administration of:**
   (a) Aniline
   (b) P-nitrobenzaldehyde
   (c) Benzyl amine
   (d) p-bromo-benzene
   (e) Acetanilid
8. **The enzyme "cytochrome P-450 reductase" which catalyzes hydroxylation of drugs requires the coenzyme:**
   (a) $NADP^+$ (b) $NADPH + H^+$
   (c) NAD^+ (d) $NADH + H^+$
   (e) FMN

ANSWERS

1. (d)	2. (c)	3. (b)
4. (a)	5. (b)	6. (e)
7. (d)	8. (b)	

Free Radicals: Chemistry and Functions

Oxygen is required for all living organisms for their survival. But, at the same time, one has to remember that *oxygen is potentially toxic.* **Salvemini** has *described oxygen as a double-edged sword: it is vital to life but leads to formation of byproducts that are toxic such as formation of superoxide (O_2^-) anions.* Dissolved oxygen at high concentration is toxic to animals. Rats when subjected to breathe pure oxygen at 2 atmospheric pressure, undergo convulsions in 5 to 6 hours and may die.

Formation of "Free" Radicals:

The univalent reduction of molecular oxygen in tissues gives rise to so-called *"superoxide radical"* O_2^-. It is one of the "free radicals" produced in the body.

Why oxygen is more prone to produce superoxide radical O_2^-?: Molecular oxygen is *paramagnetic* and contains two unpaired electrons with parallel spins. These unpaired electrons reside in separate orbitals unless their spins are opposed. Reduction of O_2 by direct insertion of a pair of electrons, e^-, into its partially filled orbitals is not possible without inversion of one electronic spin and such an inversion of spin is a slow change. Hence electrons are added to molecular oxygen as single electron successively.

When oxygen molecule takes up one electron, by univalent reduction, it becomes *"Superoxide"* anion O_2^-. Thus,

$$O_2 + e^- \longrightarrow O_2^-$$

Superoxide anion is highly reactive and toxic to cell membranes.

Other "Free Radicals" in the Body:

Sequence of events that can occur in formation of other 'free' radicals are:

1. Superoxide anion can capture further electrons to form *"hydrogen peroxide"*, H_2O_2, which is toxic and injurious.

$$O_2 \xrightarrow{e^-,\ 2H^+} \underset{\text{(Hydrogen peroxide)}}{H_2O_2} \xrightarrow{2e^-,\ 2H^+} 2\,H_2O$$

2. H_2O_2 can further react with "Superoxide" anion, in presence of Fe^{++} (ferrous) to form *"Hydroxyl"* radical, and *"Singlet oxygen"*.

$$O_2^- + H_2O_2 \xrightarrow{Fe^{++}} \underset{\text{(Free hydroxy radical)}}{OH^{\bullet}} + \underset{\text{(Singlet oxygen)}}{O_2} + OH^-$$

The above reaction is called **"Haber's reaction"** (or **Haber-Weiss-Fenten's reaction**).

Role of Caeruloplasmin:

Caeruloplasmin, which acts as *"ferroxidase"*, can serve as antioxidant. It can convert $Fe^{++} \rightarrow Fe^{+++}$ (ferric) and thus it can halt the "Haber's reaction" preventing further formation of highly reactive hydroxyl free radicals.

3. Superoxide anion can accept a H^+ and form **"hydroperoxy"** radical.

$$O_2^- \xrightarrow{H^+} \underset{\text{Hydroperoxy radical}}{HOO^{\bullet}} \xrightarrow{HOO^{\bullet}} H_2O_2 + O_2$$

Note: Whenever superoxide anion, , is formed in tissues, it will lead to the formation of other **"free radicals"** like hydroperoxy radical, hydroxyl free radical and hydrogen peroxide. ***All these free radicals are very reactive and toxic to biological membranes.***

4. Nitric oxide produced in the body from Arginine by the action of **"Nitrogen oxide synthase"** has a short half-life 3 to 4 seconds because it reacts with oxygen and superoxide anion (O_2^-). The reaction with superoxide produces ***"peroxynitrite" ($ONOO^-$), which decomposes to form the highly reactive $OH^•$ radical.***

5. Other toxic 'free' radicals produced in the body are 'free' radical CCl_3^- and 'free' halogen radical like Cl^- formed from CCl_4.

Formation of Superoxide Anion in Metabolic Pathways (Cytosolic Oxidations):

1. Cytosolic oxidations by autooxidizable FP dependent enzymes, e.g
   - ***Xanthine oxidase***
   - ***Aldehyde dehydrogenase***
   - ***Oxidative deamination by L-amino acid oxidase***

   Superoxide anion, O_2^-, may be formed when reduced flavins are reoxidized univalently by molecular O_2.x
2. It is also formed during univalent oxidations with molecular oxygen in the respiratory chain.

$$EnZ.\ H_2 + O_2 \longrightarrow EnZ.\ H + O_2^- + H^+$$

3. Superoxide anion, O_2^-, can be formed during methaemoglobin formation.

$$\underset{Fe^{++} + O_2}{\overset{Hb}{|}} \longrightarrow \underset{Fe^{++},\ O_2}{\overset{Hb}{|}} \longrightarrow \underset{Fe^{3+}.\ O_2}{\overset{Hb}{|}}$$

4. Superoxide anion, O_2^-, may also be formed during cytosolic hydroxylations of steroids, drugs, and xenobiotics, by Cyt P_{450} or Cyt P_{448} system. The hydrogens for these hydroxylations are donated by NADH (or NADPH) routed through Fp and Cyt P_{450}.

$$Cyt\ P_{450} + Subs + Fe^{2+} + O_2$$
$$\downarrow$$
$$Cyt\ P_{450} - Subs - Fe^{2+} + O_2^-$$
$$\downarrow$$
$$Cyt\ P_{450}\ .\ Fe^{3+}\ Subs - OH + H_2$$

5. Free radicals are also produced in tissues when exposed to ionizing radiations.

SCAVENGERS OF FREE RADICALS

- **Superoxide Dismutase:** In ***both cytosol and in mitochondria*** an enzyme is present called ***"superoxide dismutase"*** which can destroy the superoxide anion, O_2^-.

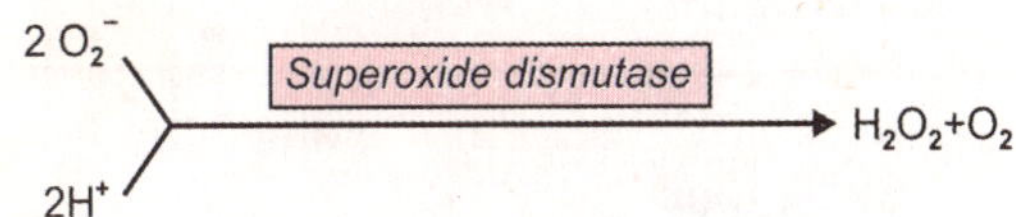

The enzyme is present in all major aerobic tissues. The function of the enzyme seems to be that of protecting aerobic organisms against the potential deleterious effects of superoxide anion, O_2^-.

- **Catalase:** ***Catalase*** having high Km value which is situated close to aerobic dehydrogenases, like liver peroxisomes, can destroy H_2O_2 formed in the tissues to O_2.

$$H_2O_2 + H_2O_2 \xrightarrow{\text{Catalase}} 2\ H_2O + O_2$$

Glutathione Peroxidase: If the concentration of H_2O_2 is less than the optimum required for hydroperoxidation by catalase, then the selenium-containing enzyme ***"glutathione peroxidase"*** can destroy H_2O_2 with the help of reduced glutathione (G-SH), having low Km. It is present in cytosol and mitochondria.

$$\underset{\textit{(Reduced Glutathione)}}{H_2O_2 + 2G\text{-}SH} \xrightarrow[\text{(Se-containing)}]{\text{Glutathione Peroxidase}} \underset{\textit{(Oxidized Glutathione)}}{G\text{-}S\text{-}S\text{-}G + 2\ H_2O}$$

- **Ferricytochrome:** Superoxide anion, can also be oxidized to O_2 by ferricytochrome.

$$O_2^- + \underset{Cyt\ c}{\overset{Fe^{3+}+}{|}} \longrightarrow \underset{Cyt\ c}{\overset{Fe^{2+}+}{|}} + O_2^-$$

- ***Endogenous Caeruloplasmin can halt Haber's Reaction (see above)***

EFFECT OF 'FREE' RADICALS ON BIOMEMBRANES

1. Free radicals are highly reactive so can initiate chain reaction and brings about lipid peroxidation producing lipid peroxides and

lipoxides. These radicals constitute a threat to the integrity of biomembranes which could be oxidized. ***The 'free hydroxyl' radical is most reactive and can also be mutagenic. It is an extraordinarily potent oxidant.***

2. ***These oxidants can oxidize***
   - —SH groups containing membrane proteins in the cells and biomembranes to S—S group.
   - Methionine sulphur is oxidized to its sulphoxide, and
   - Membrane lipids, unsaturated FA to lipid peroxides and lipoxides, called lipid peroxidation. The above will affect the optimum fluidity of the membrane causing *membranopathy.*

3. ***Lipid peroxidation:*** It is a chain reaction initiated by 'free' radicals which provides a continuous supply of other 'free' radicals formed from unsaturated FA which initiate further peroxidation.

Stages of Lipid Peroxidation

Whole process consists of **three stages:**

- **Initiation:** Production of R^- from a precursor

$$ROOH + metal^{(n)+} \longrightarrow ROO^{\bullet} + metal^{(n-1)+} + H^+$$
$$X^{\bullet} + RH \longrightarrow R^{\bullet} + XH$$

- **Propagation:**

$$R^{\bullet} + O_2 \longrightarrow ROO^{\bullet}$$
$$ROO^{\bullet} + RH \longrightarrow ROOH + R^{\bullet} \text{ and so on.}$$

- **Termination:**

$$ROO^{\bullet} + ROO^{\bullet} \longrightarrow ROOR + O_2$$
$$ROO^{\bullet} + R \longrightarrow ROOR$$
$$R^{\bullet} + R^{\bullet} \longrightarrow RR$$

Since the molecular precursor for the initiation process is generally the hydroperoxide product ROOH, ***lipid peroxidation is a branching chain reaction with potentially devastating effects.***

4. ***Effect on Biomembranes: $OH^{\bullet}$ free radical is very reactive. O_2^- and $OH^{\bullet}$ can initiate chain reaction and bring about oxidation of polyunsaturated FA of membranes.*** A "free" radical with unpaired electrons may take away hydrogen from "methylene group" of polyunsaturated FA and convert it into a free FA radical, which binds with O_2 to give FA "Peroxy radical", the latter then changes to FA "hydroperoxide" by accepting hydrogen of the methylene group of another polyunsaturated FA and converting into another free FA radical and so on.

ANTI-OXIDANTS

To control and reduce lipid peroxidation both in humans and in nature, anti-oxidants are used.

A. ***Anti-oxidants used "in vitro":*** These are used to prevent lipid peroxidation in foods, examples are:
   - Propyl gallate (PG)
   - Butylated hydroxy anisole (BHA)
   - Butylated hydroxy toluene (BHT)

B. ***Naturally occurring anti-oxidants:*** They include:

   (a) Lipid soluble:
   - Vit E (tocopherols)
   - β-carotene: is an anti-oxidant at low pO_2
   - Lycopene

   (b) Water soluble:
   - Vitamin C (Ascorbic acid)
   - Urates

Anti-oxidants can be classified into **two classes according to their mode of action.**

1. **Preventive anti-oxidants:** These reduce the rate of chain initiation, e.g.
   - Catalases
   - Other peroxidases that react with R OOH
   - Natural endogenous caeruloplasmin, and
   - Chelators of metal ions such as:
     - DTPA (diethylene triamine penta acetate), and
     - EDTA (Ethylene diamine tetra acetate)

2. **Chain breaking anti oxidants:** which interfere with chain propagation, examples are:
   - Phenols or aromatic amines.
   - *In vivo* the principal chain breaking antioxidants are:
     - ***Superoxide dismutase*** both cytosolic and mitochondrial
     - Vitamin E and selenium-containing ***glutathione peroxidase***
     - Urates
   - Peroxidation is also catalyzed ***in vivo*** by haeme-containing compounds and by lipooxygenases found in platelets and leucocytes.

Vitamin E action as anti-oxidants (Refer chapter on Vitamins). Role of selenium and relation with vitamin E (Refer chapter on Mineral Metabolism).

Synzyme: Recently researchers have prepared a synthetic enzyme that works just like the body's own scavengers like superoxide dismutase (SOD), to mop up "free" radicals.

They have named it as "synzyme" and one of its first user may be in treating stroke. The enzyme goes by the experimental name of M40403, based on the metal manganese. The compound is more powerful than traditional anti-oxidants such as vitamin E or C.

CLINICAL SIGNIFICANCE

1. ***Role in Ageing:*** Free radicals play an important role in ageing and aggravate certain disease processes like diabetes mellitus, atherosclerosis, cancer, etc.
2. ***Neonatal Oxygen Radical Diseases:*** The preterm baby may be specially vulnerable to 'free' oxygen radicals, because it is exposed more liberally to oxygen radical generation and its defence against oxygen radicals is low. It has, therefore, been postulated that a "**neonatal oxygen radical disease**" does exist. Diseases like:
   - Bronchopulmonary dysplasia
   - Retinopathy of prematurity
   - Necrotizing enterocolitis
   - Periventricular leukomalacia
   - Patent ductus arteriosus, and
   - Perhaps intracranial haemorrhage represent different facets of this syndrome. The symptoms are determined by which organs are principally affected, but basic pathogenetic mechanisms may be identical.
3. ***Rheumatoid Arthritis:*** Diseases like rheumatoid arthritis is self-propagated by the "free radicals" released by the neutrophils. This is further accentuated by decrease of 'scavengers' in joint cavity which mop up the "free radicals." Drugs like corticosteroids and NSAIDs interfere with the formation of "free radicals" and thus provides relief.
4. ***Atherosclerosis Vs Thrombosis—Role of 'free radicals':*** 'Free radicals' released by the endothelial cells of blood vessels oxidizes the LDL deposited under the endothelial cells increasing the level of lipid hydroperoxides which in turn increases the 'thromboxane' production. This decreases the prostacyclin/thromboxane ratio and leads to thrombosis.
5. ***Chronic Granulomatous Diseases:*** In patients with ***chronic granulomatous diseases,*** phagocytic function of macrophages have been found to be defective and there is increased susceptibility to microbial and fungal infections.
6. ***Role in Phagocytosis:*** H_2O_2 is used in killing micro-organisms in phagocytosis. In this process, O_2 uptake is increased greatly and production and utilization of H_2O_2 occurs as early event in phagocytosis. A characteristic feature of phagocytosis by macrophages is increased utilization of glucose by HMP-shunt. There is also tremendous increase in O_2 uptake. NADPH produced by this pathway can react with O_2 to produce superoxide anion O_2^- which can subsequently produce H_2O_2 also.

$$\text{NADPH} + 2O_2 \longrightarrow \text{NADPH} + 2O_2^- + H$$

$$2O_2^- + H^+ \longrightarrow H_2O_2 + O_2$$

7. ***Role in Malaria:*** G-6-PD deficient patients are more resistant to infection with *Plasmodium falciparum*. Normally, the parasite generates H_2O_2 by oxidizing NADPH, produced by HMP-shunt pathway, by a plasma membrane bound oxidase for their survival. In G-6-PD deficiency, the parasites fail to thrive as they cannot produce H_2O_2 for their survival as NADPH production is lacking.

Bile Pigments: Metabolism

INTRODUCTION

Under physiological conditions in the human adult 1 to 2 × 10^8 erythrocytes are destroyed per hour, ***thus in one day, a 70 kg man turns over approximately 6.0 gm of haemoglobin.***

When haemoglobin is destroyed:

- Protein portion globin or constituent amino acids, are reutilized after proteolysis.
- Fe^{++} of haeme enters "***iron pool***" for—reutilization or stored as "***ferritin***", and
- Fe-free porphyrin portion of haeme is degraded to bile pigments, ***Biliverdin and Bilirubin,*** in reticuloendothelial cells.

The formation of bilirubin, the chief bile pigment in humans, and its elimination from the body as a waste product of haeme catabolism requires a series of metabolic alterations and transport processes. ***Partial or complete failure at any point in this sequence can result in clinical condition Jaundice (See Fig. 21.1).***

SOURCES OF BILIRUBIN

Mainly two:

- ***From 'haeme' of "effete" erythrocytes and***
- ***From sources other than effete erythrocytes.***

1. From 'Haeme' of Erythrocytes: Approximately ***85% of bilirubin is derived from senescent erythrocytes*** by conversion of 'haeme' of Hb to biliverdin within reticuloendothelial cells.

Site: The principal sites are ***bone marrow, spleen*** and ***liver***—the bone marrow appears to be the most active site.

Amount: Approximately 210 to 250 mg of bile pigments are excreted daily by the liver in the bile.

One gram of Hb yields approximately 35 mg bilirubin.

Nature of Bile Pigments: Principal bile pigments are ***"biliverdin"*** and ***"bilirubin".*** The colour of the bile is due primarily to these and to derivatives of them. Normally, there are only traces of biliverdin in human bile, ***bilirubin is the principal bile pigment.*** Biliverdin is the chief pigment of the bile in birds.

Formation of Bile Pigments from "Haeme": Precise steps are not clear, controversy has centred largely on the question whether the ***α-methane bridge*** of the protoporphyrin ring of haeme is split before or after the removal of globin and Fe moieties from Hb. Accordingly, there are two views, which are shown schematically in ***(Fig. 21.2).*** Oxidative scission of the iron-porphyrin ring takes place in presence of the enzyme ***haeme α-methenyl oxygenase,*** occurs in microsomal fractions of RE cells. The opening of the porphyrin ring in some way labilizes the removal of Fe. Whether the globin is separated first or after ring opening, the bile pigment first formed is ***Biliverdin.*** Site of oxidative scission is at the α-methane bridge, between pyrrole rings I and II—this results in ***loss of one carbon as CO.***

Clinical Importance

Rate of elimination of CO in expired air has been used clinically as ***an index of rate of haeme catabolism.***

Formation of Bilirubin from Biliverdin: Biliverdin is converted to bilirubin in RE cells. Conversion occurs in presence of a specific enzyme, *Bilirubin*

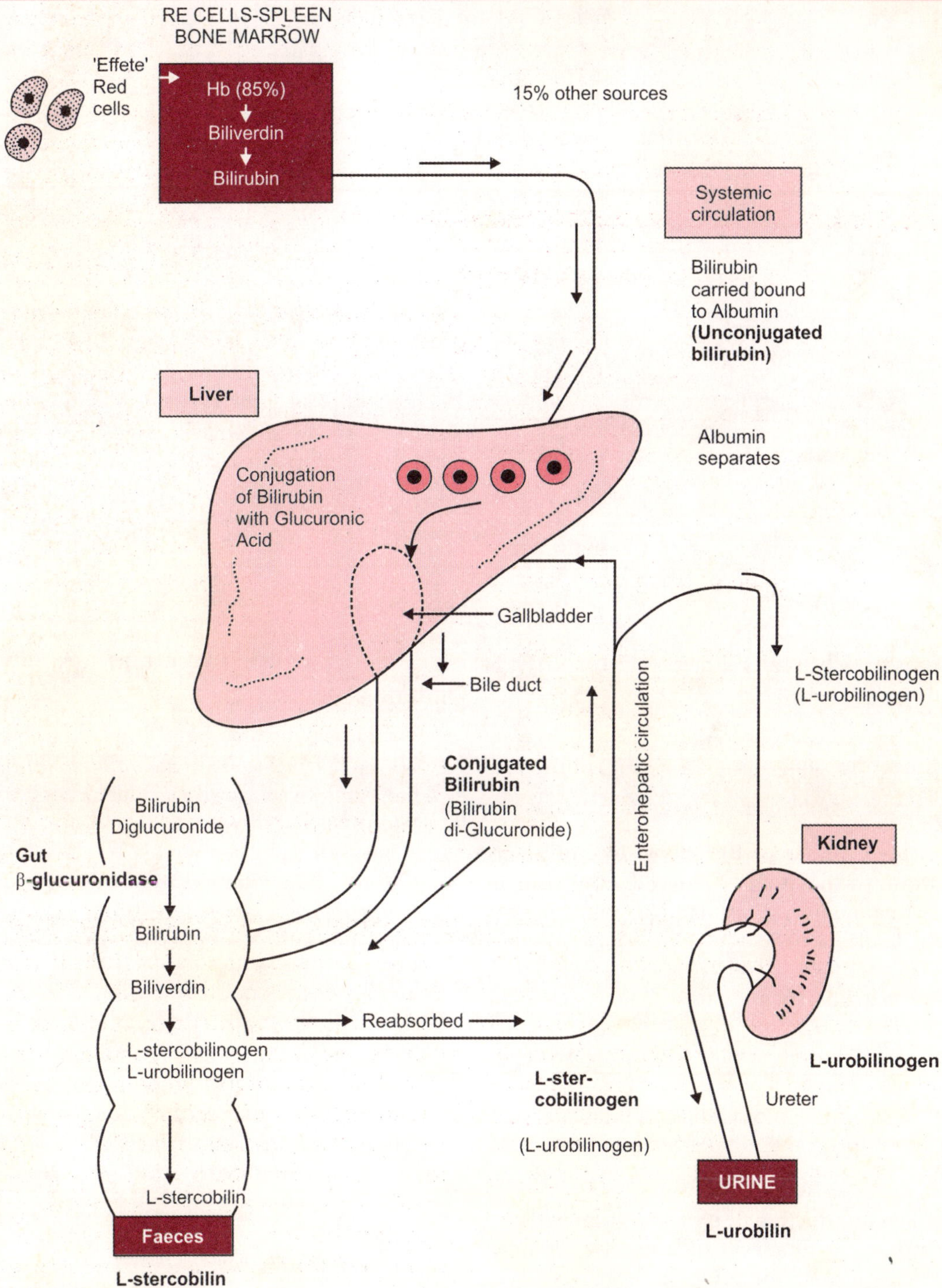

Fig. 21.1: Diagrammatic representation of bile pigment metabolism

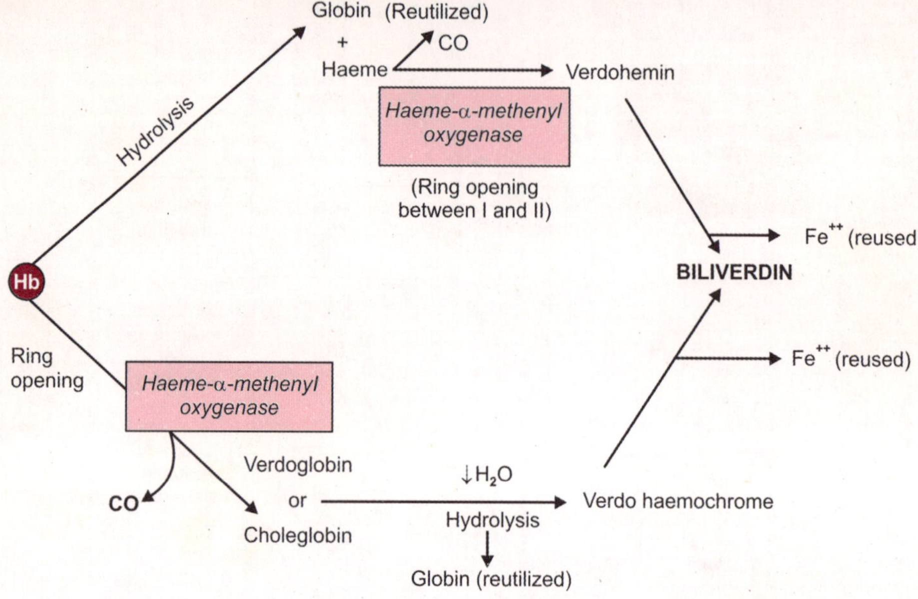

Fig. 21.2: Breakdown of Hb

reductase which utilizes either NADH or NADPH as hydrogen donor.

$$\text{Biliverdin} \xrightarrow[\textit{Bilirubin reductase}]{\text{NADH or NADPH}} \textbf{Bilirubin}$$

2. Other Sources of Bilirubin: 15% of newly synthesized bilirubin is derived from sources other than maturing circulating erythrocytes.

Possible origins are:
- Haeme formed from Hb-synthesis,
- Destruction of immature erythrocytes in the bonemarrow,
- Degradation of Hb, within erythrocyte precursors,
- Breakdown of other haeme pigments such as cytochromes, myoglobin and *catalase.*

Clinical Importance

Excessive production of bilirubin from heme or erythrocyte precursors in bone-marrow, or direct synthesis in marrow, gives rise to increased, bilirubin level in blood, producing jaundice. Such a condition is called as ***"shunt hyper-bilirubinaemia".***

TRANSPORT OF BILIRUBIN

Bilirubin-Albumin Binding:

- The bilirubin formed in RE cells from breakdown of Hb is called ***"unconjugated bilirubin"***, which is highly lipid soluble, has limited aqueous solubility from 0.1 to 5 mg/100 ml at physiologic pH and tonicity. ***Binding of bilirubin by albumin increases its solubility in plasma.***
- Each molecule of albumin appears to have
  - One "high-affinity" site and
  - One "low-affinity" site for bilirubin.
- Normally in 100 ml of plasma , approximately 25 mg of bilirubin can be tightly bound to albumin to its high affinity site. ***Bilirubin in excess of this quantity can be bound only loosely and can thus be easily detached and can diffuse into the tissues.***

Clinical Importance

Clinical interest in binding of bilirubin by albumin has primarily related to the development of ***"bilirubin encephalopathy", ("Kernicterus").*** In this condition, seen only rarely outside the new-born period, unconjugated bilirubin ***enters the neurons*** *of the basal ganglia, hippocampus, cerebellum, and medulla, causing necrosis of nerve cells,* probably by interfering with cellular respiration.

Alterations of Albumin-Bilirubin Binding and its Biomedical Significance:

The *binding capacity of albumin for bilirubin can be modified by a variety of physical and chemical alterations:*

- Several "anionic drugs" such as *sulphonamides: Administration of sulphonamides to pregnant women and neonates increases the risk of kernicterus in the jaundiced infants.*
- Increased free fatty acids behave similarly.
- Asphyxia, hypoxia and acidosis are also associated with increased risks,
  - By interfering with bilirubin-albumin binding, and
  - May also increase the permeability of brain for unconjugated bilirubin.

Transfer of Bilirubin from Plasma to Liver Cells:

Liver appears to have a *selective affinity to remove unconjugated bilirubin.*

Two views are prevalent in this regard:

- Lateral extension of plasma membrane of liver cells facing hepatic sinusoids has specific "*receptors sites"* for bilirubin.
- Plasma membrane is permeable to "non-polar molecules" like dissociated unconjugated bilirubin and an "intracellular" protein (or proteins) which acts as an acceptor and facilitates the transfer of bilirubin to liver cells. Earlier *two 'non-albumin' proteins, designated as 'Y' and 'Z' have been isolated from liver cytoplasm and account for most of intracellular binding of bilirubin. Recent studies have shown that the protein are same single one and has been named as* **ligandins.**

CONJUGATION OF BILIRUBIN WITH D-GLUCURONIC ACID IN LIVER CELLS

- Mammalian liver cells contain an enzyme referred to as *glucuronyl transferase.* The enzyme catalyzes the transfer of glucuronic acid from UDP-GA to various phenolic, carboxylic and amine receptors.
- The process is called **"Conjugation"** reaction and it is carried out in the smooth endoplasmic reticulum of liver cells.
- Two glucuronyl groups are transferred from *"active-glucuronide"* (UDP-GA) by the catalytic action of *glucuronyl transferase.* In the conjugation reaction, *"monoglucuronide"* is formed first, followed by formation of *"bilirubin diglucuronide" (See Fig. 21.3).*
- Two bilirubin monoglucuronides can form one molecule of bilirubin diglucuronide and one molecule of free 'bilirubin' by the action of the enzyme *dismutase Mono and diglucuronides of bilirubin are called as "conjugated bilirubins".*
- Conjugated bilirubins, unlike unconjugated bilirubins are:
  - Water soluble and
  - Smaller in molecular size as they are not bound to albumin. Hence, *conjugated bilirubin can pass through glomerular filter and can appear in urine (bilirubinuria). Unconjugated bilirubin cannot pass through glomerular filter and does not appear in urine.*

BIOMEDICAL IMPORTANCE

A. *Inhibition of Glucuronyl Transferase Activity:*

Glucuronyl transferase activity may be *inhibited by certain drugs,* viz. *novobiocin, dyes and steroidal derivatives,* e.g. *Pregnane-3α-20β-diol. The latter is an unusual isomer of pregnanediol which can form due to inherited defect* in steroid metabolism. This isomer may be excreted in the breast milk by a small portion of nursing mothers. The isomer can inhibit the glucuronyl transferase activity and *produce prolonged non-haemolytic unconjugated hyperbilirubinaemia* leading to jaundice in infants. On stopping breast milk feeding jaundice disappears.

1. Lucey-Driscoll Syndrome: This is a transient *familial neonatal nonhaemolytic unconjugated hyperbilirubinaemia.* Healthy looking women can give birth to infants with severe nonhae-molytic

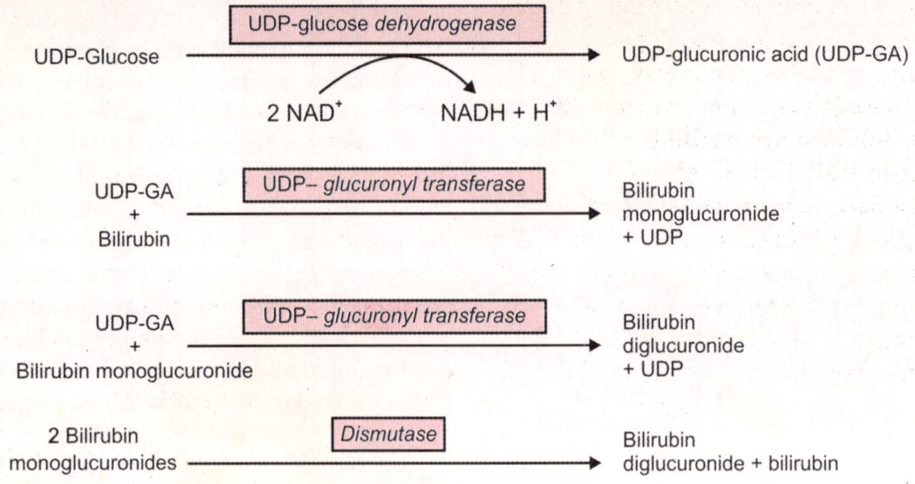

Fig. 21.3: Steps of conjugation of bilirubin in liver cells

unconjugated hyperbilirubinaemia with risk of kernicterus. ***An unidentified factor, probably progestational steroid, has been isolated from serum of the mother, which inhibits the glucuronyl transferase activity producing the condition.***

2. Transient Neonatal "Physiological" Jaundice: Most common cause of ***neonatal unconjugated hyperbilirubinaemia.*** It results from an accelerated haemolysis and due to an immature hepatic system for uptake, conjugation and secretion of bilirubin. Glucuronyl transferase activity is delayed and reduced. Probably also reduced synthesis of substrate, i.e. UDP-glucuronic acid. Risk of kernicterus is present.

Treatment:

- Administration of ***phenobarbital,*** which stimulates the enzyme activity is useful
- Exposure to visible light **(phototherapy)** is helpful, it promotes hepatic excretion of unconjugated bilirubin by converting some of the bilirubin to other derivatives: ***Maleimide fragments*** and ***Geometric isomers,*** which are excreted in bile.

3. Crigler-Najjar Syndrome:

Type I :

- A rare autosomal recessive disorder.
- Primary metabolic defect is inherited absence of ***glucuronyl transferase*** activity
- Characterized by severe ***congenital nonhaemolytic unconjugated hyperbilirubinaemia and jaundice.***
- Usually fatal within the first 15 months of life. When untreated serum bilirubin usually exceeds 20 mg/dl leading to risk of kernicterus.
- **Phototherapy has been found to be useful.**

Type II:

- A rare inherited disorder.
- Milder defect in the bilirubin conjugating system and has a more benign course.
- Unconjugated hyperbilirubinaemia, serum bilirubin usually do not exceed 20 mg/dl. ***No risk of kernicterus.***
- Bile of these patients have been found to contain ***"bilirubin monoglucuronide"*** only.
- Proposed ***genetic defect lies in the inability to add second glucuronyl group to bilirubin monoglucuronide.***
- Patients respond to treatment with large doses of phenobarbitone.

4. Gilbert's Syndrome: A heterogenous group of diseases, many of which are now recognized to be:

  - due to a compensated haemolysis associated with ***unconjugated hyperbilirubinaemia.***
  - due to a defect in hepatic clearance of bilirubin, possibly due to defect in uptake of bilirubin by liver cells,

- due to reduced *glucuronyl transferase* activity.
- *Gilbert and his colleagues* described the syndrome to be characterized by *low grade chronic unconjugated hyperbilirubinaemia and jaundice.*
- Bilirubin level in 85% cases usually less < 3 mg/dl.
- *Age:* 18 to 25 yrs, detected suddenly during examination—a mild icterus of sclera of eye.
- Patient usually complaints of fatigue, weakness, and an abdominal pain.

5. Dubin-Johnson Syndrome:

- An autosomal recessive disorder.
- Characterized by *conjugated hyperbilirubinaemia* and jaundice in childhood and during adult life.
- *Defect* in hepatic secretion of conjugated bilirubin in bile.
- *BSP test* when performed *shows a secondary rise in plasma concentration due to reflux of the conjugated BSP (pathognomonic).* Dyes, viz. indocyanine Green and Rose Bengal, do not require conjugation hence secondary rise do not occur.
- Another interesting feature is that 80 to 90% of coproporphyrins excreted in urine are of type 1, reasons not known. No abnormalities in porphyrin synthesis seen.
- Hepatocytes in centrilobular area have been found to contain *an abnormal pigment* in this disease that has not been identified.

B. *Increased Activity of Glucuronyl Transferase:*
Hepatic glucuronyl transferase activity is increased after administration of certain drugs viz. Benzpyrene, aminoquinolines, chlorcyclizine and phenobarbitones to normal adults and neonates. ***Administration of these drugs results in proliferation of smooth endoplasmic reticulum and increase the synthesis of the enzyme.***

EXCRETION OF BILE PIGMENTS

Conjugated bilirubins are secreted in the GI tract in bile. In the lower portion of the intestinal tract, specially in the caecum and the colon, the bilirubin is released from the glucuronides with the help of the enzyme **β-*glucuronidase*** produced by bacteria, and then the released bilirubin is subjected to series of reductive action of enzyme system present in the intestinal tract, mainly derived from the anaerobic bacteria in the caecum. The series of reductive changes that take place are shown in ***Fig. 21.4.***

In the intestine, progressive hydrogenation (reduction) occurs, to produce a series of intermediary compounds which beginning with ***"meso-bilirubinogen"*** comprise a number of colourless uroblinoids, which may be oxidized, with loss of hydrogen, to coloured compounds. The end product is colourless ***"L-stercobilinogen" (L-urobilinogen).*** Auto-oxidation in the presence of air, produces ***"L-stercobilin" (L-urobilin),*** an orange-yellow pigment which contributes to the normal colour of the faeces and urine. Stercobilin is strongly ***Laevo-rotatory.***

Urobilin IX (D-(1) urobilin or inactive (1) urobilin), is an optically inactive urobilinoid that has been identified in the faeces. It is less stable than stercobilin, is oxidized in air to form violet or blue-green pigments.

Entero-Hepatic Circulation of Bile Pigments:

The various products derived from the progressive reduction of bilirubin may in part be absorbed from the intestine and returned to the liver for its re-excretion, called as ***'entero-hepatic circulation"*** of bile pigments. A small part escapes enterohepatic circulation and excreted in urine, which normally contain traces of "urobilinogen" and urobilin as well as meso-bilirubinogen and perhaps other intermediary products. The great majority of the metabolites of bilirubin are, however, excreted with faeces.

Clinical Significance of Alteration of Intestinal Flora with Bile Pigments Metabolism:

If the intestinal flora are modified or diminished, as by the administration of orally effective broad spectrum antibiotics, which are capable of producing partial sterilization of the intestinal tract, bilirubin may not be further reduced and may later be auto-oxidized, in contact with air, to ***"biliverdin".*** Thus, ***the faeces acquire a greenish tinge*** under the above circumstances.

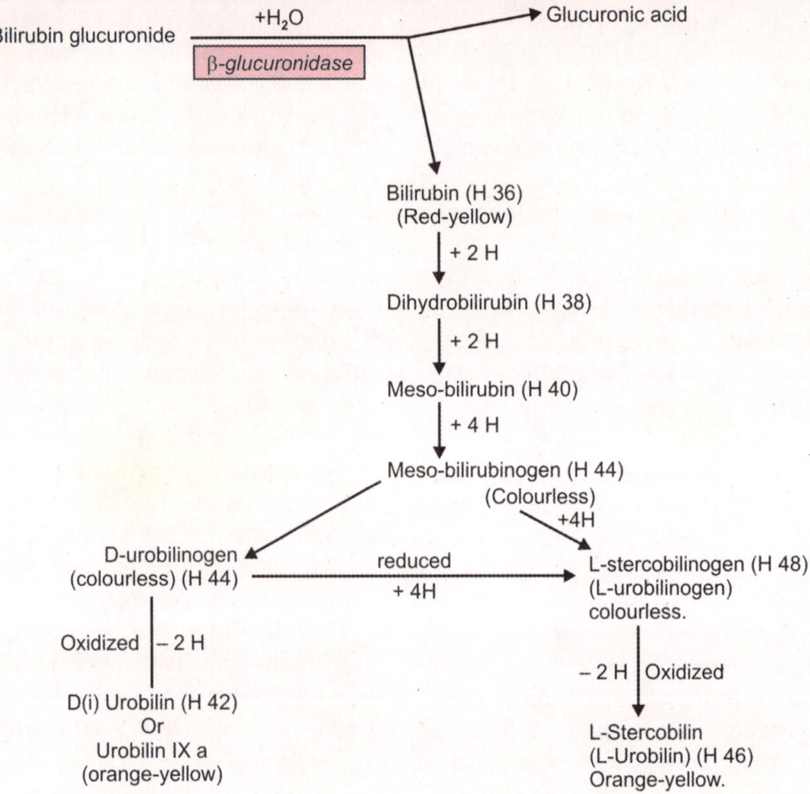

Fig. 21.4: Reductive changes of bilirubin in intestine

Similar condition may develop in premature babies/or in infants where the bacterial flora develop late.

In the patients whose intestinal flora are altered by oral administration of oxy-tetracyclines/or chlortetracyclines, as stated above, a dextrorotatory urobilinoid, **"D-urobilin"**, has been identified. It is believed to be derived from dihydrobilirubin by way of *D*-urobilinogen.

☞ SALIENT POINTS TO REMEMBER

- Hb is broken down in the body to form: Globin, Fe and Haeme.
- Globin after proteolysis produces amino-acids which are reutilized. Fe enters "iron pool" for reutilization or stored as ferritin.
- Haeme is broken down to form the bile pigments Biliverdin and Bilirubin. ***The first bile pigment formed is biliverdin.***
- Principal sites for degradation of haeme are bonemarrow, spleen and liver. ***Bone marrow appears to be the most active site.***
- Approximately 210 to 250 mg of bile pigments are formed and excreted in the bile daily. ***One gram of Hb yields approximately 35 mg of bilirubin.***
- Bilirubin is the principal bile pigment in humans. Normally there are only traces of biliverdin in human bile. Biliverdin is the principal bile pigment in bile of birds.
- Principal enzyme which brings out oxidative scission of haeme is "haeme-α-methenyl oxygenase".
- Biliverdin is first formed which is converted to Bilirubin in R.E. cells. The conversion occurs in presence of the enzyme ***"Bilirubin reductase"*** which uses either NADH or NADPH.

- Bilirubin thus formed is highly lipid soluble and it is carried in the blood in combination with albumin. This bilirubin is called "*unconjugated bilirubin*" or `*Indirect Bilirubin*."
- In cases of excessive bilirubin formation like haemolytic jaundice, bilirubin exceeds the binding capacity of albumin, is deposited in basal ganglia, hippocampus, cerebellum and Medulla being lipid soluble producing '*bilirubin encephalopathy ("Kernicterus")*.
- Unconjugated bilirubin is taken up by liver cells, where it is conjugated with UDP-Glucuronic acid in presence of the enzyme "***Glucuronyl transferase***" forming water soluble "***conjugated bilirubin***" ***(Bilirubin diglucuronide)***.
- Glucuronyl transferase enzyme may be inhibited by drugs, and an unusual isomer of pregnanediol due to inherited defect in steroid metabolism or there can be reduced glucuronyl transferase activity.
- These may lead to development of "non-haemolytic unconjugated hyperbilirubinaemia", viz. Transient neonatal "Physiological" jaundice, Lucey-Driscoll syndrome, Gilbert's syndromes, Crigler-Najjar syndrome type I and II.
- Dubin-Johnson syndrome is an autosomal recessive disorder characterized by 'Conjugated hyperbilirubinaemia and jaundice in childhood and adult life.
- Defect in Dubin-Johnson syndrome is a defect in hepatic secretion of conjugated bilirubin in bile.
- A pathognomic test is BSP test which shows a secondary rise in plasma concentration of BSP due to reflux of the conjugated BSP.
- Normally after conjugation, the conjugated bilirubin is secreted in G.I. tract through bile.
- In lower part of G.I. tract it is converted to L-stercobilinogen which is excreted in the faeces. A part of L-stercobilinogen is absorbed and excreted as L-urobilinogen in urine.
- Auto oxidation in presence of air produces L-stercobilirubin in faeces and L-urobilin in urine, orange-yellow pigment which contributes to normal colour to faeces and urine respectively.

MULTIPLE CHOICE QUESTIONS

Give one correct answer:

1. **Bile Pigments are:**
   (a) Cholic acid
   (b) Deoxycholic acid
   (c) Lithocholic acid
   (d) Bilirubin
   (e) All of the above
2. **In haeme catabolism, the first bile pigment formed is:**
   (a) Cholic acid
   (b) Bilirubin
   (c) Biliverdin
   (d) Deoxy cholic acid
   (e) Lithocholic acid
3. **Biliverdin is converted to Bilirubin in R.E. cells by the process of:**
   (a) Oxidation
   (b) Reduction
   (c) Hydroxylation
   (d) Decarboxylation
   (e) Conjugation
4. **Bilirubin is derived from all of the following *except:***
   (a) Haemoglobin
   (b) Destroyed 'effete' R.B. Cells
   (c) Catalase
   (d) Coenzyme
   (e) Cytochromes
5. **Bilirubin formed in R.E. Cells is transported in blood to liver in combination with:**
   (a) Haptoglobin (b) Albumin
   (c) Globulin (d) Transferrin
   (e) Caeruloplasmin
6. **Bilirubin is conjugated in Liver cells with:**
   (a) Glutathione
   (b) Glycine
   (c) Cysteine
   (d) Iduronic acid
   (e) UDP-Glucuronic acid

7. **Oxidative scission of haeme by the enzyme "heme-α-methenyl oxygenase" releases one molecule of:**
   (a) Nitrogen dioxide
   (b) Carbon dioxide
   (c) Carbon monoxide
   (d) NH_3
   (e) Water
8. **The enzyme responsible for conjugation of bilirubin in liver is:**
   (a) UDP-Glucuronyl transferase
   (b) Bilirubin reductase
   (c) Haeme oxygenase
   (d) Bilirubin esterase
   (e) Ferrochelatase
9. **Following are the example of unconjugated non-haemolytic hyperbilirubinaemia *except:***
   (a) Gilbert's syndrome
   (b) Dubin-Johnson syndrome
   (c) Transient neonatal hyperbilirubinaemia
   (d) Lucey-Driseoll syndrome
   (e) Criglar-Najjar syndrome
10. **All are true about Gilbert's syndrome *except:***
   (a) Serum bilirubin is usually < 5 mg/dl
   (b) Liver function tests are normal
   (c) Sclera of the eye shows mild icterus
   (d) Liver biopsy shows dark pigmentation of hepatic cells
   (e) There is unconjugated hyperbilirubinaemia
11. **All the following are produced from degradation of haeme, *except:***
   (a) Urobilinogen
   (b) Stercobilinogen
   (c) Porphobilinogen
   (d) Biliverdin
   (e) Bilirubin

ANSWERS

1. (d)	2. (c)	3. (b)
4. (d)	5. (b)	6. (e)
7. (c)	8. (a)	9. (b)
10. (d)	11. (c)	

22 Hormones: Chemistry and Functions

INTRODUCTION

Most glands of the body deliver their secretions by means of ducts. These are called *exocrine glands.* There are few other glands that produce chemical substances that they directly secrete into the blood stream for transmission to various target tissues. These are ***ductless or endocrine glands.*** The secretions of endocrine glands are called as **hormones.**

Definition of Hormone: It is a chemical substance which is produced in one part of the body, enters the circulation and is carried to distant target organs and tissues to modify their structures and functions. Hormones are, strictly speaking, stimulating substances and act as body catalysts. The word hormone is derived from Greek word *hormacin* meaning to excite.

Similarities with Enzymes:

- They act as body catalysts resembling enzymes in some aspect
- They are required only in small quantities
- They are not used up during the reaction

Differences from Enzymes:

- They are produced in an organ other than that in which they ultimately perform their action.
- They are secreted in blood prior to use. Thus the circulating levels of hormones can give some indication of endocrine gland activity and target organ exposure. Because of the small amounts of the hormones required, blood levels of the hormones are extremely low. In many cases it is ng/μg or mIU, etc
- Structurally they are not always proteins. Few hormones are protein in nature, few are small peptides. Some hormones are derived from amino acids while some are steroid in nature.

Major hormone secreting glands are:
Pituitary, thyroid, parathyroid, adrenal, pancreas, ovaries, and testes.

Several other glandular tissues are also considered to secrete hormones, viz,

- *JG cells of kidney:* May produce the hormone *erythropoietin* which regulates erythrocyte maturation (erythropoiesis.).
- *Thymus:* Produces a hormone that circulates from this organ to stem cells in lymphoid organ inducing them to become immunologically competent lymphocytes.
- *Pineal gland:* It produces a hormone that antagonizes the secretion or effects of ACTH. It also produces factor called *glomerulotrophins* that regulates the adrenal secretion of aldosterone.
- *GI tract:* Few hormones are also produced by certain specialized cells of GI tract and they are called GI hormones.

Classification of Hormones

According to **Li** the hormones can be classified chemically into *three major groups:*

- *Steroid Hormones:* These are steroid in nature such as adrenocorticosteroid hormones, androgens, estrogens and progesterone.
- *Amino acid derivatives:* These are derived from amino acid tyrosine, e.g. epinephrine, norepinephrine and thyroid hormones.
- *Peptide/Protein hormones:* These are either large proteins or small or medium size peptides, e.g. insulin, glucagon, parathormone, calcitonin, pituitary hormones, etc.

Factors Regulating Hormone Action: Action of a hormone at a target organ is regulated by ***four factors:***

- Rate of synthesis and secretion of hormone
- In some cases specific transport system in plasma
- Hormone-specific receptors in target cell membranes which differ from tissue-to-tissue and
- Ultimate degradation of the hormone usually by the liver or kidneys.

Variations in any of these factors can result in a rapid change in the amount or activity of a hormone at a given tissue site.

MECHANISM OF ACTION OF HORMONES

Although the exact site of action of any hormone is still not well established. ***5 general sites*** have been proposed.

1. Interaction with Nuclear Chromatin:

- Steroid hormones act mostly by changing the transcription rate of specific genes in the nuclear DNA.
- The steroid hormone has a ***specific soluble, oligomeric receptor protein (mobile receptor)*** either in the cytosol and/or inside the nucleus. This brings about conformational changes and also changes in the surface charge of the receptor protein to favour its binding to the nuclear chromatin attached to nuclear matrix.
- **The *receptor-steroid complex is translocated to the nuclear chromatin and binds to a steroid recognizing acceptor site called the hormone responsive element (HRE) of a DNA strand on*** the upstream side of the promoter site for a specific steroid responsive gene.
- The consequent change in the intracellular concentration of m-RNA alters the rate of synthesis of a structural, enzymatic, carrier or receptor protein coded by it. This results in ultimate cellular effects.

2. Membrane receptors:

- As per the suggestion of **Heller,** certain molecules cannot enter target cells through the membrane lipid bilayer. This is achieved by the ***specific receptor molecules present on the surface of the plasma membrane***
- Many hormones seen specifically involved in the transport of a variety of substances across cells membrane. In general, these hormones specifically bind to the receptors on cell membrane. They cause rapid secondary metabolic changes in the tissue but have little effect on metabolic activity of membrane-free preparations
- Most protein hormones and catecholamines activate transport of membrane enzyme systems by direct binding to specific receptors on the membrane.

3. Stimulation of Enzyme Synthesis at the Ribosomal Level:

- Activity at the level of translation of information is carried by the m-RNA on the ribosomes for the production of enzyme. Ribosomes taken from growth hormone treated animal have a modified capacity to synthesize protein in the presence of normal m-RNA. Thus, in this case ***either increased production of new ribosomes or to create new population of more active or more selective ribosomes might be taking place.***

4. Direct Activation at the Enzyme Level: Although the direct effect of a hormone on a pure enzyme is difficult to demonstrate, treatment of the intact animal or of isolated tissue with some hormones results in a change of enzyme activity, not related to *de novo* synthesis. These hormonal effects are usually extremely rapid. Since cell membranes are usually required, it is probable that the initiating hormonal event is activation of membrane receptor.

5. c-AMP and Hormone Action

- 3′-5′ c-AMP plays a unique role in the action of many protein hormones. Its level may be decreased or increased by hormonal action as the effect varies depending on the tissue.
- The hormones such as glucagon, catecholamines, PTH, etc. act by influencing a change in intracellular c-AMP concentration through the adenylate cyclase c-AMP system.
- The ***hormone binds to a specific membrane receptor. Formation of the receptor-hormone complex promotes the binding of GTP which in turn through α_s GTP stimulates adenylate cyclase***

located on the cytoplasmic surface of the membrane and changes its conformation to activate it.

- *Adenylate cyclase* catalyzes the conversion of ATP to c-AMP thus increasing the intracellular concentration.
- On the other hand α_i-GTP inhibits *adenylate cyclase* by binding with it. This lowers the intracellular concentration of c-AMP.

6. Role of polyphosphoinositol and Diacylglycerol in Hormone Action:

- Just like c-AMP, other compounds such as 1, 4, 5 inositol triphosphate (ITP) and diacylglycerol (DAG) act as second messengers
- This is specially found in case of vasopressin, TRH, GnRH, etc. These hormones activate the phospholipase C polyphosphoinositol system to produce ITP and DAG.
- ***Inositol triphosphate enhances the mobilization of Ca^{++} into the cytosol from intracellular Ca^{++} pool from mitochondria, calcium ions then act as tertiary messenger.***

7. Role of Calcium in Hormone Action: The action of most protein hormones is inhibited in absence of calcium even though ability to increase or decrease c-AMP is comparatively unimpaired. Thus calcium may be more terminal signal for hormone action than c-AMP ***It is suggested that ionized calcium of the cytosol is the important signal.*** The source of this calcium may be extracellular fluid or it may arise from mobilization of intracellular tissue bound calcium.

REGULATION OF HORMONE SECRETION

Hormone secretion is strictly under control of several mechanisms.

A. Neuroendocrinal Control Mechanism:

Nerve impulses control some endocrine secretions. Cholinergic sympathetic fibres stimulate catecholamine secretion from adrenal medulla. ***Centres in the midbrain, brainstem, hippocampus, etc. can send nerve impulses which react the hypothalamus through cholinergic and bioaminergic neurons. At the terminations of these neurons they release acetylcholine and biogenic amines to regulate the secretions of hypophysiotropic peptide hormones from Hypothalamic peptidergic neurons.***

B. Feedback Control Mechanism:

- It is due mainly to negative feedback that control is brought about. When there is a high blood level of a target gland hormone, it may inhibit the secretion of the tropic hormone stimulating that gland.
- Adrenal cortex secretes a hormone called cortisol which bring about the inhibition of secretion of corticotrophin from anterior pituitary and corticotrophin releasing hormone from the hypothalamus by a long-loop feedback. This leads reduction in cortisol secretion.
- It is sometimes due to positive feedback effect of another hormone or of a metabolite. For example, there is a steep rise in LH (pre-ovulatory) from the stimulation of anterior pituitary by the blood glucose level or plasma calcium level due to secretion of insulin and calcium respectively.

PITUITARY HORMONES

Pituitary Gland: Anatomical Review

The human pituitary gland is reddish-grey, oval structure, about 10 mm in diameter located in the brain just behind the optic chiasma as an extension from the floor of the hypothalamus. Average weight of the gland in females is 0.5-0.6 gm and in males is 0.6-0.7 gm. Embryonically, the ***pituitary tissue is derived from two sources:***

- ***a neural component*** originating from the infundibulum. It is called **neurohypophysis.**
- ***A buccal component,*** which develops upwards from the ectoderm of the primitive oral cavity (stomoderm) to meet and surround the infundibular rudiment, adenohypophysis.

Pituitary gland is made of 3 lobes namely, anterior pituitary lobe (largest of all), middle lobe and posterior pituitary lobe.

Control of Secretion: Secretions of hormones from anterior pituitary are ***controlled by two mechanisms:***

- ***Nervous mechanism:*** By release of regulatory factors from hypothalamus.
- ***Hormonal mechanism:*** By feedback inhibition.

Hypothalamic Releasing Factors: Control of hormone secretion from the pituitary is in part modulated by regulating factors or hormones from the hypothalamus. At present ***10 discrete regulatory factors*** have been described that may affect the synthesis as well as secretion of specific pituitary hormone. They are listed as under:

Hypothalamic Hormone or Factor	*Abbreviation*
• Corticotropin (ACTH) releasing hormone	CRH or CRF
• Thyrotropin (TSH) releasing hormone	TRH or TRF
• Follicle stimulating hormone (FSH) releasing hormone	FSH-RH or FSH-RF
• Luteinizing Hormone (LH) releasing hormone	LH-RH or LH-RF
• Growth-hormone (GH) releasing hormone	GH-RH or GH-RF
• Growth-hormone release inhibiting hormone	GH-RIH or GIF
• Prolactin (PL) release inhibiting hormone	PL-RIH or PL-RIF
• Prolactin (PL) releasing hormone	PRH or PRF
• Melanocyte stimulating hormone (MSH) release inhibiting hormone	MSH-RIH or MSH-RIF
• Melanocyte stimulating hormone (MSH) releasing hormone	MSH-RH or MSH-RF

HORMONES OF THE ANTERIOR PITUITARY

The hormones secreted by the anterior lobe of the pituitary gland are:

- **Growth hormone,** and
- **Pituitary** ***tropic hormones,*** e.g. prolactin, (PRL), thyrotropic hormone (TSH), adreno-corticotropic hormone (ACTH), gonadotropin (FSH) and (LH).

Growth Hormone (Somatotropin)

Chemistry:

- Growth hormone from all mammalian species consists of ***a single polypeptide*** with a molecular weight of about 21500. ***It consists of 191 amino acids.***
- Although there is a high degree of similarity in the amino acid sequences of human, bovine and porcine **GH;** only human GH or that of other primates is active in man.
- GH can bring about some of the actions of prolactin and human placental lactogen (HPL) due to amino acid sequence homology.

Functions:

Growth hormone has a variety of effects on different tissues. The hormone ***acts slowly*** requiring from 1-2 hours to several days before its biological effects are detectable. This slow action and its stimulatory effects on RNA synthesis suggest that ***it is involved in protein synthesis.*** The hormone acts by binding to specific membrane receptors on its target cells.

1. ***Protein synthesis:*** Growth hormone brings about ***positive nitrogen balance*** by retaining nitrogen. ***It stimulates over all protein synthesis.***

- It facilitates the entry of amino acids into the cell.
- Growth hormone increases DNA and RNA synthesis. It increases the synthesis of collagen.

2. ***Lipid metabolism:*** Growth hormone brings about ***lipolysis*** in a mild way by mobilizing fatty acids from adipose tissue by ***activating the hormone sensitive triacylglycerol lipase. Thus it increases circulating free fatty acids in the liver.***

3. ***Carbohydrate metabolism:*** Growth hormone is a ***dibetogenic hormone,*** i.e. it antagonizes the effect of insulin by reducing insulin sensitivity and thereby decreasing the hypoglycemic effect of insulin. Hypersecretion of GH can result in ***hyperglycaemia by increasing gluconeogenesis, poor sugar tolerance and glycosuria.*** Growth hormone brings about glycostatic effect, i.e. increases liver glycogen. It can also increase muscle and cardiac glycogen level probably by reducing glycolysis.

4. ***Effect on growth of bones and cartilages:***

- The effect of growth hormone partly depends upon its ***calcium anabolic action.*** It promotes the retention of calcium and phosphate which helps in ossification and osteogenesis
- It ***enhances the incorporation and hydroxylation of proline*** in the matrix collagen
- ***Incorporation of amines into glycosoamino-glycans of cartilage***
- Incorporation of sulphate into matrix proteo-glycans like chondroitin sulphates, the synthesis of DNA and RNA in chondrocytes.

5. ***Ion or mineral metabolism:*** It is observed that the intestinal absorption of calcium is increased by GH, since the bone growth and development is stimulated by growth hormone. Growth hormone retains Na, Ca, K, Mg and PO_4^{-3}.

Regulation of Growth Hormone Secretion

Hypothalamic growth hormone releasing hormone or GHRH stimulates release while somatostatin inhibits the release of growth hormone. Factors such as stress, emotions, exercise, etc. promote GH secretion by stimulating GHRH release. However, beta-adrenergic effects inhibits GHRH release.

GH itself may reduce GH secretion by a short loop feedback inhibition of the hypothalamic GHRH release.

PITUITARY TROPIC HORMONES

In addition to GH, anterior pituitary gland secretes some tropic hormones usually called as *pituitary tropins.*

What are Tropins?

A tropin or tropic hormone is the one which influences the activities of other endocrine gland, principally those involved in stress and repro-duction. These are carried by the blood to other (target) gland. The pituitary tropins are under the positive and negative control of peptide factors from hypothalamus. Further the tropic hormones are usually subject to feedback inhibition at the pituitary or hypothalamic level by hormone product of the final target gland.

The **tropic hormones secreted by the pituitary gland:**

- *Prolactin (mammotropin)*
- *TSH (thyrotropin)*
- *FSH* } *(gonadotropins)*
- *LH* }
- *ACTH (corticotropin).*

A. Prolactin (PRL) or Leuteotropic Hormone (LTH)

This is a monomeric simple protein (MW 23,000). It contains 199 amino acids with three-S-S linkages. It is secreted by lactotroph α-cells of anterior pituitary and has sequence homology with growth hormone.

FUNCTIONS OF PRL

- ***The main function of PRL is to stimulate mammary growth and the secretion of milk.*** By acting through specific glycoprotein receptors on plasma membrane of mammary gland cells, it stimulates mRNA synthesis. This ultimately leads to enlargement of breasts during pregnancy. This is called as ***mammotropic action.***
- The synthesis of milk proteins such as lactalbumin, and casein takes place after parturition. This effect is called as ***lactogenic action.***
- Estrogens, thyroid hormones and glucocorticoids increase the number of prolactin receptors on the mammary cell membrane.
- Progesterone has the opposite effect.

2. Thyrotropic Hormone or Thyroid Stimulating Hormone (TSH)

This is ***produced by basophil cells*** of anterior pituitary and is ***glycoprotein*** in nature. Its molecular weight is approximately 30,000. ***This consists of α and β subunits. The α-subunit of TSH, LH, HCG and FSH are nearly identical.*** The ***biological specificity of thyrotropin must, therefore, be in β-subunit.*** The α-subunit consists of 92 amino acids while β-subunit has 112 amino acids. Both α and β have several disulphide bridges. Its carbohydrate content is 21%.

FUNCTIONS OF TSH

There are ***glycoprotein receptors on the thyroid cell membrane*** which bind to the receptor binding site on ***β-subunit of TSH.*** The complex then activates ***adenylate cyclase*** which ***catalyzes the formation of c-AMP*** which ***acts as the second messenger*** for most TSH actions as follows:

- The ***TSH stimulates the synthesis of thyroid hormones at all stages*** such as iodine uptake, organification and coupling.
- It enhances the release of stored thyroid hormones.
- It increases DNA content, RNA and translation of proteins, cell size.
- It stimulates glycolysis, TCA cycle, PPP and phospholipid synthesis. Stimulation of last two does not involve c-AMP.

- It activates adipose tissue *lipase* to enhance the release of fatty acids (lipolysis).

Control of Secretion:

The main controlling mechanism is carried out by thyrotropin releasing hormone (TRH) secreted by hypothalamus. ***TRH is a tripeptide consisting of pyroglutamic acid, histidine and prolinamide.*** It causes an increase in c-AMP and thyrotropin release within 1 minute. Regulation scheme is as shown in Box.

C. Adrenocorticotropic Hormone (ACTH) or Corticotropin:

It is a ***single polypeptide*** containing ***39 amino acids*** in its structure with a molecular weight of 4500. Two forms have been isolated, ***α-corticotropin*** and ***β-corticotropin. Biological activity of ACTH resides in the first 23 amino acids from N-terminal end.*** ACTH is synthesized as a part of precursor peptide of mol. wt. of 31500 with 260 amino acids. The precursor molecule is synthesized as a glycoprotein called ***Propiomelanocortin POMC.*** Various proteolytic enzymes hydrolyze POMC to give different peptides. Thus, ***POMC is broken down into ACTH, β-lipotropin (LPH). β-LPH is further cleaved into γ LPH and endorphins***

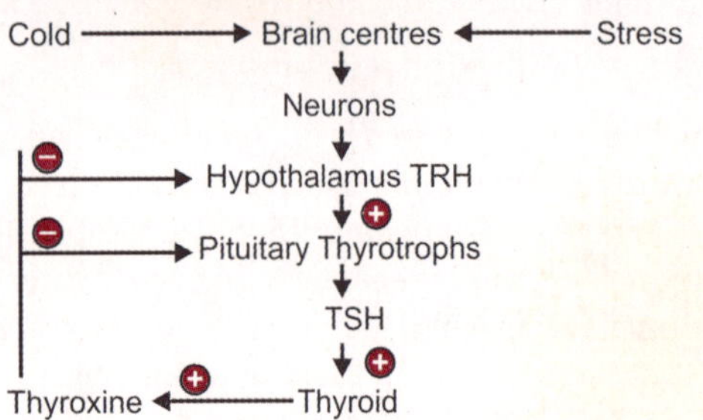

FUNCTIONS OF ACTH

- The principal actions of corticotropin are exerted on the adrenal cortex and extra-adrenal tissue. ***ACTH increases the synthesis of corticosteroids by the adrenal cortex and also stimulates their release from the gland.***
- ACTH also stimulates the synthesis and secretion of glucocorticoids.
- ***By activating adenylate cyclase*** of adipose tissue, it increases intracellular c-AMP which in turn activates hormone sensitive lipase, involved in lipolysis which ***increases the level of free fatty acids.***
- It leads to increased ketogenesis and decreased R.Q.
- It has MSH activity due to homology in amino acid sequence.

The circulating concentration of ACTH in normal plasma is 0.1 to 2.0 mg/dl. The pituitary stores 5-10 mg.

Control of Secretion: Corticotropin secretion has a peak and nadir normally in the morning and at midnight respectively. Corticotropin releasing hormone (CRH) stimulates the synthesis of precursor (POMC) of β-LPH and ACTH. The CRH is increased under stress such as cold and hypoglycemia. The secretion is also done by the feedback effects of glucocorticoids like cortisol and ACTH itself. The figure summarizes the regulatory mechanisms (Box below).

Clinical Importance

Cushing's Disease: Results due to overproduction of corticotropin because of tumour or hyperplasia of β-cells of the anterior pituitary. This leads to hypersecretion of corticosteroids specially glucocorticoids. This produces symptoms like hyperglycaemia, glycosuria, muscle wasting, atrophy of skin, high urinary NPN (negative N_2 balance), high level of free fatty acids, abnormal retention of fats giving moon shape face appearance, retention of Na^+ and water and hypertension.

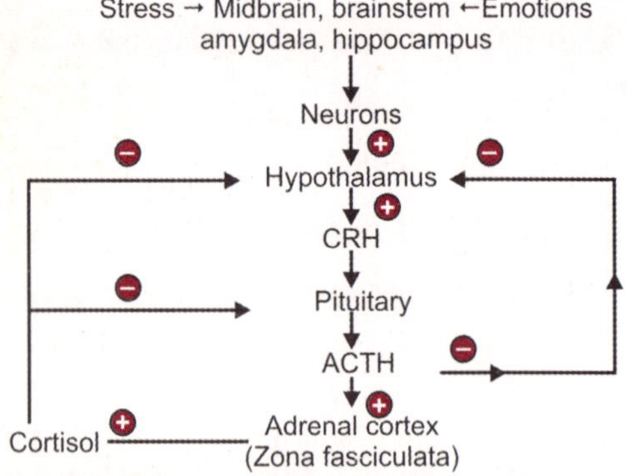

D. Pituitary Gonadotropins:

These ***influence the function and maturation of the testes and ovary*** and are of ***two types:***

- ***Follicle Stimulating Hormone (FSH)***
- ***Luteinizing Hormone (LH)***

Both of them are glycoproteins with sialic acid, hexose and hexosamine as the carbohydrate moiety (16%). Molecular weight of FSH is 25000 and that of LH is 40000. As already mentioned FSH, LH are dimers of α- and β-chains linked noncovalently. The α-chain is identical for TSH, FSH and LH of the same species. The β-chain of human FSH and LH have respectively 118 and 112 amino acid residues. Each chain has several disuphide bridges.

FUNCTIONS OF FSH

It brings about its action by specific receptor binding and c-AMP.

In females:

- It promotes follicular growth
- Prepares the graafian follicle for the action of LH and
- Enhances the release of estrogen induced by LH.

In males:

- It stimulates seminal tubule and testicular growth, and
- Plays an important role in maturation of spermatozoa.

Role of FSH in Spermatogenesis: The conversion of primary spermatocytes into secondary spermatocytes in the seminiferous tubules is stimulated by FSH. ***In absence of FSH spermatogenesis cannot proceed.*** However, FSH by itself cannot cause complete formation of spermatozoon. For its completion testosterone is also required.

FUNCTIONS OF LH

This hormone is also known as ***interstitial cells stimulating hormone (ICSH).***

In females:

- It ***causes the final maturation of graafian follicle and stimulates ovulation.***
- Stimulates secretion of estrogen by the theca and granulosa cells.
- It helps in the formation and development of corpus luteum for luteinization of cells.
- In conjunction with leuteotropic hormone (LTH), it is concerned with the production of estrogen and progesterone by the corpus luteum.
- ***In the ovary it can stimulate the nongerminal elements, which contain the interstitial cells to produce the androgens, androstenedione, DHEA and testosterone.***

Action of LH in Ovulation: Ovulatory surge for LH: It is necessary for final follicular growth and ovulation. Without this hormone, even though large quantities of FSH are available, the follicle will not progress to the stage of ovulation. It is worth noting that especially large amount of LH called ***ovulatory surge*** is secreted by the pituitary during the day immediately preceding ovulation.

Regulation of Testosterone Secretion by LH: Testosterone is produced by the Interstitial cells of Leydig only when the testes are stimulated by LH from the pituitary gland, and the quantity of testosterone secreted varies approximately in proportion to the amount of LH available.

Control of Secretion of Gonadotropins: Gonadotropin releasing hormone (Gn RH) is the regulatory factor in FSH and LH secretions. Gn RH activates the phosphatidylinositol, Ca^{2+}-dependent mechanism in the pituitary gonadotroph cells. It is suggested that the negative feedback effect of ovarian steroids on short axon neurons, located near the arcuate nucleus, maintains the basal levels of gonadotropin secretions.

Endorphins and Encephalins:
Endorphins and Encephalins are a group of polypeptides which influence the transmission of nerve impulses. They are also known as **"opioides"** because they bind to those receptors which bind opiates like morphine and plays a role in pain perception.

The opioids first discovered were two pentapeptides in the brain and were named **"encephalins"**. They are ***Methionine-encephalin*** and ***Leucine encephalin.***

Endorphins: There are **3 types** of endorphins, α, β and γ. The sequence of 31 aminoacids at the C-terminus of β-LPH (obtained from POMC) i.e. a.a 104 to 134 gives **"β-endorphin."**

"α-endorphin (104 to 117) containing 17 a.a less than the β-form from the C-tenminal and

"γ-endorphin" (104 to 118) containing 16 a.a less than the β form from C-terminal end.

Function: Endorphins and encephalins bind to the same CNS receptors like the morphine opiates and they ***play a role in the endogenous control of pain perception. They have higher analgesic potency than morphine.***

HORMONE OF MIDDLE LOBE OF PITUITARY

Melanocyte Stimulating Hormones (MSH): The hormones secreted by intermediate lobe or middle lobe of pituitary gland are called melanocyte-stimulating hormones or MSH. The ACTH is cleaved to β-MSH which has 13 amino acids. There is also α-MSH which is present in larger quantities. Amino acids 11-17 of β-MSH are common to both α-MSH and ACTH.

Functions: MSH darkens the skin and is involved in skin pigmentation by deposition of melanin by melanocytes.

Clinical Importance

Hydrocortisone and cortisone inhibit the secretion of MSH. Epinephrine and norepinephrine inhibit the action of MSH. Thus, ***when production of corticosteroids is less, MSH is in excess which increases the synthesis of melanin resulting in brown pigmentation of skin.*** Such a condition occurs in **Addison's disease.**

HORMONES OF POSTERIOR PITUITARY LOBE

The hormones have been isolated and characterized from extracts of posterior pituitary gland.

They are:

- ***Vasopressin (Pitressin or Arginine Vasopressin (ADH)*** and
- ***Oxytocin.***

- Both are small peptides containing nine (9) amino acids. Oxytocin differs from vasopressin with respect to 3rd and 8th amino acid residues.
- Posterior pituitary hormones are synthesized in neurosecretory neurons. They are stored in the pituitary in association with two proteins ***neurophysin I and II*** with molecular weights of 19000 and 21000 respectively. The release of these two hormones is independent of each other.

FUNCTIONS OF VASOPRESSIN

- This ***is antidiuretic hormone (ADH) and antidiuretic effect is its main function.*** It reabsorbs water from the kidneys by distal tubules and collecting ducts. It is found to be mediated through formation of cAMP. It is released due to rise in plasma osmolarity.
- ***Urea-retention effect:*** Permeability of medullary collecting ducts to urea is increased by vasopressin. This leads to retention of urea and subsequently contributes to hypertonicity of the medullary interstitium. Urea retention effect can be reversed by phloretin.
- ***Pressor effect:*** It stimulates the contraction of smooth muscles and thus causes vasoconstriction by increasing cytosolic Ca^{+2} concentration.
- ***Glycogenolytic effect:*** By increasing intracellular calcium concentration.

Clinical Importance

Condition of **Diabetes insipidus** is described due to failure in secretion or action of vasopressin. It is characterized by very high volumes of urine output, up to 20-30 litres per day with a low specific gravity and excessive thirst.

- In primary, central or neurohypophyseal diabetes insipidus, vasopressin secretion is poor.
- In nephrogenic diabetes insipidus, kidneys cannot respond to vasopressin due to renal damage. The damage is common in psychiatric patients of Lithium therapy.

FUNCTIONS OF OXYTOCIN

Contraction of smooth muscle is the primary function of oxytocin. There are basically two effects: one on mammary glands called as **galactabolic effect** and

The other on uterus called as **uterine effect.**

- ***Galactobolic effect:*** This is released due to neuroendocrinal reflex such as sucking of nipples. By doing so it causes the contraction of myoepithelial cells around mammary alveoli and ducts and the smooth muscles surrounding the mammary milk sinuses; estrogen increases the number of oxytocin receptors during pregnancy while progesterone decreases the same and also inhibits the secretion of oxytocin.

- ***Uterine effect:*** It is found to be elevated at full term pregnancy. It ***causes contraction of uterine muscle for child birth.*** Estrogens enhance while progesterone decreases oxytocin receptors as well as its secretion.

ABNORMALITIES OF PITUITARY FUNCTION

Principal abnormalities are listed below:

1. *Hyperpituitarism:*
- Excess production of growth hormone (eosinophilic adenoma),
  - *Gigantism*
  - *Acromegaly.*
- Excess production of ACTH (Basophilic adenoma).
  - *Cushing's disease*

2. *Hypopituitarism:*
  - *Dwarfism*
  - *Pituitary myxedema*
  - *Panhypopituitarism*

1. Hyperpituitarism

- **Gigantism:** Gigantism results from hyperactivity of the gland during childhood or adolescence, i.e. before closure of the epiphysis, long bones increase in length and the patient reaches an abnormal height. There are also associated metabolic changes attributed to a generalized pituitary hyperfunction. There is an increase in size of all viscera.
- **Acromegaly:** This is due to ***hyperactivity that begins after epiphyseal growth has been completed and growth has ceased.*** The patient exhibits characteristic facial changes, an increase in size of skull, prominent cheek bones, large protruding jaw and frontal bossing. There is an enlargement of nose and enlargement of hands, feet and viscera as well as thickening of the skin.
- **Cushing' s Disease:** This is pituitary in origin. Cushing's syndrome denotes adrenocortical hyperfunction directly involving the adrenal gland. (Details already discussed above, p. 400).

2. Hypopituitarism: It occurs as a result of certain types of pituitary tumours, or infarct or atrophy of the gland.

- **Dwarfism:** It is due to hypoactivity of the gland sometimes caused by chromophobe tumours or craniopharyngioma. In either case, the underactivity is due to pressure of the tumour on the remainder of the gland.

  When hypopituitarism develops in childhood, it may assume the following forms:
  - **Frohlich's syndrome: *(Adipose genital dystrophy):*** Several pituitary functions are disturbed. The children become stunted and idiotic. The genitals are hypoplastic and there are diffuse deposits of fats.
  - **Lorain-levy type:** Mentally these patients are normal, general metabolism is unaffected. But skeletal growth ceases and the secondary sexual characters do not appear.
- **Pituitary Myxedema:** It is due to lack of TSH. It produces the symptoms similar to those described for primary hypothyroidism.
- **Panhypopituitarism:** This condition refers to a deficiency of function of the pituitary which involves all of the hormonal functions of the gland. This ***can result from destruction of the gland because of age or infarct. Milder forms*** of longstanding panhypopituitarism may result from the ***pressure of a tumour on the pituitary.*** In this condition, there is a tendency to hypoglycaemia with increased sensitivity to insulin. The excretion of sex hormone products (17-ketosteroids) in urine is much reduced in panhypopituitarism.
- **Hypophyseal Cachexia (Simmond's Disease):** This disorder occurring at any age is more frequent in adults and has a 2 to 1 preponderance in females. It is quite remarkable that most patients survive many years with an average duration of disease of 30-40 years. Systemic manifestations reflect a pluriglandular deficiency. Insufficiency of adrenals, thyroid and gonads secondary to the loss of this tropic hormones. Addison's disease must be separated into these types resulting from primary

adrenal insufficiency and those resulting from pituitary disease. The ***Addisonian pattern of pituitary origin differs from that of patient with panhypopituitarism do not have the abnormal pigmentation of the skin.***

☞ SALIENT POINT TO REMEMBER

- Hormones are the organic chemical substances, produced in minute quantities by specific tissues or glands called endocrine-glands or ductless glands and secreted directly in the blood stream and carried to target tissues or organs to modify their structures and functions.
- They act as body catalysts and regarded as chemical messengers involved in the regulation and coordination of body functions.
- Major hormone secreting glands are pituitary, thyroid, parathyroids, pancreas (Islets of Langerhans), adrenal cortex and medulla, testes and ovaries.
- Hormones are classified into three major groups according to their chemical nature-
  (a) Steroid hormones like glucocorticoids, mineralocorticoids and sex hormones.
  (b) Protein or peptide hormones like insulins glucagon, Parathormone, calcitonin, etc.
  (c) Amino acid derivatives like thyroid hormones, epinephrine, norepinephrine, etc.
- Hormones can also be classified according to function—group I hormones bind to the intracellular receptors like glucocorticoids, estrogens, calcitriol, etc and group II hormones bind to the cell surface receptors and act through the second messengers like LH, ACTH, etc.
- Cyclic AMP is an intracellular second messenger for a majority of polypeptide or protein hormones. Membrane bound adenylate cyclase enzyme, through the mediation of G-proteins, is responsible for the synthesis of c-AMP, which acts through protein kinases that phosphorylate specific enzyme proteins which ultimately produces biological response.
- Phosphatidyl inositol and calcium system also functions as second messenger for certain hormones.
- Hypothalamus is the master coordinator of hormonal action as it liberates certain releasing factors or hormones like CRH, TRH, GHRH, etc. that stimulate or inhibit the corresponding trophic hormones (also called 'Tropins') from the anterior pituitary gland.
- Anterior pituitary gland is the master gland which produces:
  (a) Growth hormone which acts directly on the target tissues.
  (b) Topic hormones (tropins), e.g. TSH, ACTH, FSH, LH, etc.
- A 'tropin' or tropic hormone is the one which influences the activities of other endocrine glands, which in turn produces their hormones which act on target glands or tissues.
- Growth hormone is a polypeptide containing 191 amino acids. It is ***anabolic hormone*** and is directly involved in growth promoting processes like protein synthesis.
- Tropic hormones like TSH, FSH, LH, ACTH respectively influence thyroid gland, gonads and adrenal cortex to synthesize their hormones respectively which are secreted directly into blood to have their effects on target organs.
- Hormones isolated from posterior lobe of Pituitary gland are
  (a) Vasopressin (ADH) (b) Oxytocin
- They are synthesized in neurosecretory neurons and are stored in the pituitary in association with two proteins neurophysin I and II.
- Both are peptides containing 9 amino acids, oxytocin differs from vasopressin with respect to 3rd and 8th amino acid residues.
- Vasopressin is called antidiuretic hormone (ADH), it reabsorbs water from the kidneys by distal tubules and collecting tubules - Action is mediated through c-AMP.
- Oxytocin has uterine effect and increases contraction of uterine muscle during child birth.

THYROID GLAND AND ITS HORMONES

Anatomy: The normal adult thyroid gland weighs about 20 gram. The gland consists of two lobes, which are connected in humans, by a bridge of tissue the thyroid *'isthmus'* and the gland is closely attached to the anterior and lateral aspects of the upper part of trachea. There is sometimes a "pyramidal lobe" in front of the larynx.

Light microscopy: It shows the gland to consist of numerous 'acini' or 'follicles' about 200 μ in diameter. Each spherical follicle is lined by cuboidal epithelium, ***whose height varies with the degree of glandular activity (stimulation).*** Each follicle contains a clear, viscid, proteinaceous ambercoloured ***colloid,*** which normally comprises iodinated ***'thyroglobulin'***

When the gland is inactive:

- The colloid is abundant
- The follicles are large,
- The cells lining the follicles are flat and squamous type.

When the gland is active:

- The follicles are smaller in size.
- ***The cells lining them are cuboidal or columnar epithelia,***
- ***The edge of the colloid is "scalloped" (eaten-away), forming many small "resorption lacunae".***

C-cells: Between the follicles there are 'Parafollicular' cells (called as 'C-cells') which are derived from the ultimobranchial bodies (formed from the hinder part of the pharyngeal entoderm).

Hormones Produced:

- ***Follicular cells Produces***—T_3, T_4 and "reverse" T_3.
- ***Parafollicular cells (C-cells)*** Produces calcitonin.

THYROID HORMONES

The principal hormones secreted by the follicular cells of thyroid are:

Structure of Thyroid Hormones

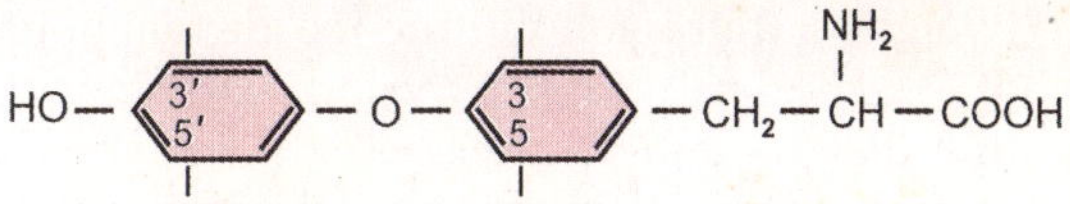

HO— [ring 3′,5′ with I, I] —O— [ring 3,5 with I, I] —CH_2—CH(NH_2)—COOH

3,5,3′,5′,– tetraiodothyronine (Thyroxine, T_4)

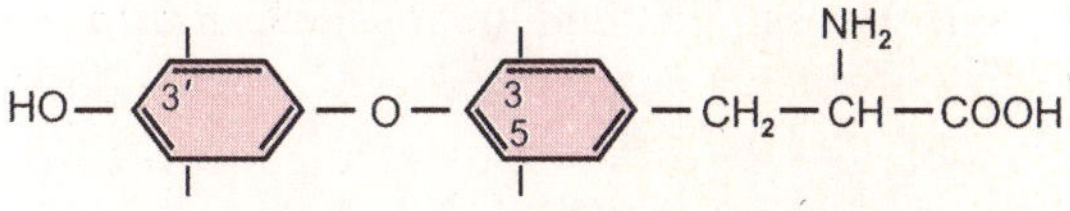

HO— [ring 3′ with I] —O— [ring 3,5 with I, I] —CH_2—CH(NH_2)—COOH

3,5,3′– Tri-iodothyronine (T_3)

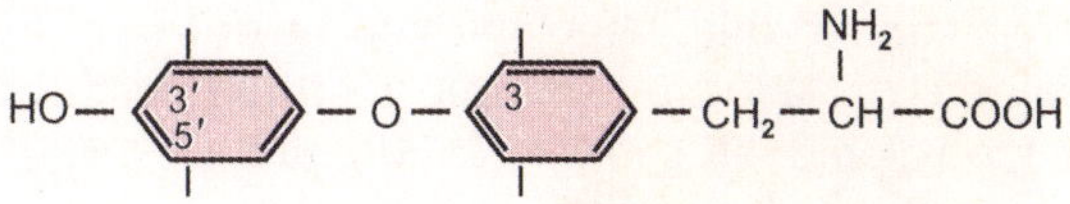

HO— [ring 3′,5′ with I, I] —O— [ring 3 with I] —CH_2—CH(NH_2)—COOH

3,3′,5′– tri-iodothyronine ("Reverse" T_3)

- *Thyroxine (T_4)*
- *Tri-iodothyronine (T_3)*
- *'Reverse' T_3*

Chemistry of Thyroid Hormones: The hormones T_4, T_3 and "reverse" T_3 are iodinated amino acid tyrosine. The iodine in thyroxine accounts for 80% of the organically bound iodine in thyroid venous blood. Small amounts of 'reverse' triiodothyronine, monoiodotyrosine (MIT) and other compounds are also liberated. The chemical name and structures of thyroid hormones are shown above in the box.

Biosynthesis of Thyroid Hormones: Two raw materials (substrates) are required by thyroid gland to synthesize the thyroid hormones.

- *Thyroglobulin*
- *Iodine*

1. ***Thyroglobulin:*** Thyroid hormones are synthesized by the iodination of tyrosine residues of a large protein called ***"thyroglobulin".***

Chemistry of Thyroglobulin:

- Thyroglobulin is a ***glycoprotein,*** 19s in type (a macroglobulin) with a molecular weight of 660,000.
- The receptor tyrosine molecules are present in this macroglobulin protein—***each molecule containing 115 tyrosine residues.***

- Carbohydrates accounts for 8 to 10% of the weight of thyroglobulin and iodide for about 0.2 to 1%, depending on the iodine content of the diet. T_3 and T_4 after being synthesized, remains in the bound form until it is secreted. ***When they are secreted, the peptide bonds are hydrolyzed and free T_3 and T_4 enter the thyroid cells, cross them and are discharged into the capillaries.***

2. ***Iodine:*** The other substrate required for thyroid hormone synthesis is iodine.

Iodine metabolism: Vegetables and fruits grown and obtained from sea-shore and also sea fishes are rich in iodine. Vegetables and fruits in hilly regions lack iodine (people residing in hilly regions table salt should be iodinated).

- Ingested dietary iodine is converted to iodide and absorbed from the gut. Of a total of 50 mg of iodine in the body about 10 to 15 mg are in thyroids.
- The normal daily intake of iodide is 100 to 200 μg. Minimum requirement is 25 μg. This iodide is absorbed mainly from small intestine and is transported in plasma in loose attachment to protein; can also be absorbed from Lungs, other mucous membranes and skin.
- Small amount of iodide are secreted by the salivary glands, stomach, and small intestine and traces in milk.
- About 2/3 (40-80%) of the ingested iodide is excreted by the kidneys, the remaining 1/3 is taken up by the thyroid glands for synthesis of thyroid hormones.
- Thyroid-stimulating hormone (TSH) of anterior pituitary gland stimulates iodide uptake by the thyroid gland.
- Inorganic iodide in plasma and cells varies from 0.3 to 1.0 μg%. Part of the "circulating pool" is iodide liberated from thyroid hormones broken down in the tissues and to a minor extent in the thyroid itself.
- In the kidneys, 97% of the filtered iodide is reabsorbed, so that the loss from the body by this route, at normal plasma iodide levels is about 15 μg/day.

Synthesis of Thyroid Hormones

1. ***Iodine trapping:*** The thyroid concentrates iodide by ***"actively"*** and ***"selectively"*** transporting it form the circulation to the colloid. The transport mechanism is called as ***"iodide-trapping"*** mechanism or ***"iodide-pump"***.

The I_2 trapping is done:

- ***Against electrical gradient,***
- ***Against concentration gradient.***
- ***As it is 'actively' taken in against electrochemical gradient, it is energy dependent and requires energy.***

The iodide "transporter" (pump) is located in the basal plasma membrane in ***association with Na^+- K^+ dependent ATPase"*** and requires a simultaneous activity of the "sodium-pump" (Na^+ pump). The iodide-pump requires ATP and show substrate specificity for iodides (I^-).

2. ***Oxidation of iodide:*** Oxidation of iodide and other steps as mentioned below in thyroid hormone synthesis are catalyzed by a ***"haeme-containing", particulate–bound "peroxidase", called thyroperoxidase which requires*** H_2O_2 for its activity. Thyroperoxidase is a tetramer, having a molecular weight = 90,000. H_2O_2 is produced by an NADPH-dependent enzyme system similar to cytochromic-c-reductase.

At the colloid-membrane interface, ***"thyroperoxidase" binds iodide (I^-) and thyroglobulin*** at distinct sites of its molecules and then in presence of H_2O_2, the ***enzyme oxidizes the enzyme bound I to form "active" iodine,*** which may be, **"iodinium"** ion (I^+) or **"hypoiodite"** (HIO) or both or **"free"** iodine radical (I)

$$I_2 + H_2O \rightleftharpoons HIO + I^- + H^+$$

Note: ***TSH is active in stimulating this process.***

3. ***Iodination of tyrosine:*** 'Active' Iodine transfers iodine from its iodidebinding site to a tyrosine residue of the enzyme bound thyro-globulin under the influence of ***thyroperoxidase*** enzyme.

- ***Iodination*** of the tyrosine residues in thyroglobulin ***occurs first in "3 position"*** of the aromatic nucleus forming ***"mono-iodotyrosine"*** (MIT).
- Monoiodotyrosine is ***next iodinated in the "position 5"*** to form ***"Diiodotyrosine"*** (DIT)

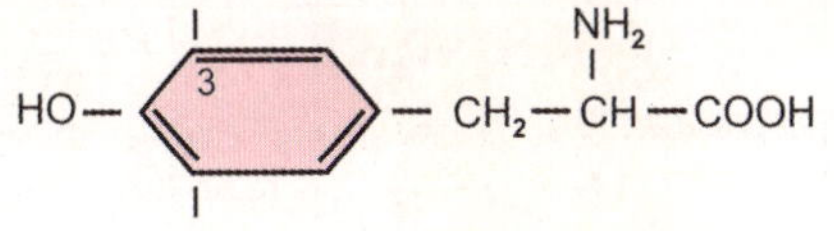

HO— (ring with I at 3) — CH_2—CH(NH_2)—COOH

3-mono-iodotyrosine (MIT)

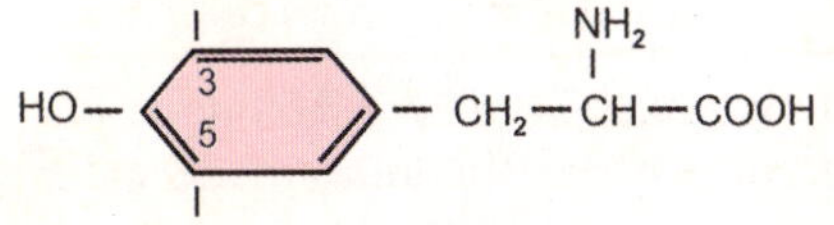

HO— (ring with I at 3, 5) — CH_2—CH(NH_2)—COOH

3-5 -Di- iodotyrosine (DIT)

- This process of iodination, also called as ***"organification"***, occurs whithin seconds in luminal thyroglobulin. Once iodination occurs, the iodine does not readily leave the thyroid.

4. ***Coupling of Iodotyrosines:*** Two molecules of DIT when undergo an oxidative condensation, under the influence of the enzyme ***thyroperoxi dase,*** forms thyroxine (T_4) molecule still in peptide linkage. In the process an "alanine" residue is liberated, which ultimately forms pyruvate and NH_3.

$$\text{DIT + DIT} \xrightarrow{\text{Thyroperoxidase}} \text{Thyroxine } (T_4) + \text{Alanine} \rightarrow \text{PA} + NH_3$$

- Similarly, tri-iodothyronine (T_3) is probably formed by condensation of MIT with a molecule of DIT and **'reverse' triiodothyronine (*'reverse'* T_3)** by condensation of DIT with MIT.

$$\text{MIT + DIT} \longrightarrow T_3 + \text{Alanine} \rightarrow \text{PA} + NH_3$$

$$\text{DIT + MIT} \longrightarrow \text{"Reverse" } T_3 + \text{Alanine} \rightarrow \text{P.A.} + NH_3$$

The condensation reaction is an ***aerobic*** and ***energy requiring*** reaction.

- ***TSH stimulates the synthesis of thyroglobulin and all the steps from oxidation to coupling reactions for forming thyroid hormones.***

Secretion: About 80-95 µg of thyroxine is secreted daily under normal physiological conditions. It is not definitely known where the peptide bond linking thyroxine to thyroglobulin in the colloid is hydrolyzed.

Recycling of Iodine in the Gland:

- The hydrolysis of thyroglobulin also liberate MIT and DIT. If these iodotyrosines are lost from the gland, considerable amounts of iodide would be biologically unavailable for the synthesis of active hormones.
- Thyroid cells have microsomal enzyme ***de-iodinase (dehalo-genase),*** which uses NADPH, and they rapidly de-iodinate the iodotyrosines, and the removed iodides are recycled in the gland and utilized for tyroid hormones synthesis.
- ***Approximately 1/3 of the total iodides in the thyroid gland is recycled in this manner.***

Transport: Within the plasma, T_4 and T_3 are mostly transported almost entirely ***in association with two proteins,*** the so-called ***"thyroxine-binding proteins"*** which act as specific carrier agents for the hormones.

Two main carrier proteins are:

- ***Thyroxin binding globulin (TBG)***
- ***Thyroxine binding prealbumin (TBPA)***

- When large amounts of T_4 and T_3 are present and the binding capacities of the above two specific carrier proteins are saturated, the hormones can be bound to "serum albumin".
- Approximately, 0.05% of the circulating thyroxine is in the 'free', unbound form ***"Free" T_3 and T_4 are the metabolically "active" hormones in the plasma.***

Abnormal TBG Level:

In certain circumstances, TBG levels may become abnormal and it may affect binding of hormones.

- ***An increase occurs:*** Pregnancy, after administration of estrogens, women taking contraceptive pills.
- ***Decrease levels are seen:*** In nephrosis, after treatment with androgenic or anabolic steroids, Hypoproteinaemic states, viz. liver diseases, cirrhosis liver.

T_3 Versus T_4: Although the circulating level of T_3 are much lower than the corresponding T_4 levels, ***T_3 appears to be the major thyroid hormone metabolically.***

Characteristics of T_3:

- Extrathyroidal de-iodination converts T_4 to T_3

- *T_3 binds to the "thyroid receptor" in target cells* with 10 times the affinity of T_4
- About 80% of circulating T_4 is converted to T_3 or reverse T_3 (r T_3) in the periphery
- T_3 is loosely bound to serum proteins
- T_3 is 3 to 5 times more active than T_4
- Has a more rapid onset of action
- It is also more rapidly degraded in the body.

Chemical Hyperthyroidism:

In rare subjects with chemical hyperthyroidism, in whom circulating level of bound and free T_4 is normal, the T_3 concentration is elevated and accounts for the thyrotoxic state. In these patients, significant amount of T_3 probably arises by deiodination of T_4 at peripheral level.

ACTIONS OF THYROID HORMONES

Metabolic Actions

1. *Effects on Protein Metabolism:*

- In *hypothyroid children and in physiological doses, thyroid hormones when given in small doses, favour protein anabolism* leading to N-retention (+ve N-balance), because they stimulate growth. Thyroxine promotes incorporation of amino acids into proteins, which is depressed after thyroidectomy and may be restored to normal by appropriate replacement therapy.
- *Large, unphysiological doses of thyroxine cause protein catabolism,* leading to –ve N-balance.

Clinical Significance

The catabolic response in skeletal muscle, in cases of hyperthyroidism, is sometimes so severe that muscle weakness is a prominent symptom and creatinuria is marked, called *thyrotoxic myopathy.* The K^+ liberated during protein catabolism appears in urine and there is an increase in urinary hexosamine and uric acid excretion.

Effects on Bone Proteins: Mobilization of bone proteins leads to hypercalcaemia and hypercalciuria, with some degree of osteoporosis.

Effect on Skin: The skin normally contains a variety of proteins combined with polysaccharides, hyaluronic acid and chondrotin sulphuric acid.

Clinical Significance

In *hypothyroidism, these complexes accumulate promoting water retention, which produces characteristic puffiness of the skin;* when thyroxine is administered, the proteins are mobilized and diuresis continues until the puffiness (myxoedema) is cleared.

2. *Effect on Carbohydrate Metabolism:*

- *Net effect on carbohydrate metabolism, increase in blood sugar ↑ (hyperglycaemia),* glycosuria, increase glucose utilization and decreased glucose tolerance. Thyroid hormones are, therefore, antagonistic to insulin. Thyroid hormones increases the rate of absorption of glucose from intestine.
- *Diabetes mellitus is aggravated by co-existing thyrotoxicosis or by administration of thyroid hormones.* In addition there is increased sensitivity to catecholamines, they potentiate the glycogenolytic effect of epinephrine by increasing the β-adrenergic receptors on hepatic cell membrane.

3. *Effect on Lipid Metabolism:*

- *Increases lipolysis* ↑ in adipose tissue thus increasing plasma FFA ↑.
- *Cholesterol:* The concentration of cholesterol and to a lesser extent PL in plasma is increased in hypothyroidism and decreased in hyperthyroidism.

Decreased value in hyperthyroidism is explained as follows: Although thyroid hormones increase the rate of biosynthesis of cholesterol, they increase

- The rate of degradation
- Increases the formation of bile acids (cholic acid/ deoxycholic acid) and
- Increases biliary excretion, to a greater extent accounting for the lowered blood concentration.
- *Lipoproteins:* The concentration of plasma lipoproteins of Sf 10 to 20 class, (LDL) is frequently increased in hypothyroidism and decreased in thyrotoxicosis, or following administration of thyroid hormones to normal subjects.

4. *Calorigenic Action:* Thyroid hormones increases considerably O_2 consumption and oxygen co-efficient of almost all metabolically active tissues. Exceptions are brain, testes, uterus,

lymphnodes, spleen and anterior pituitary. There is increase in heat production and BMR.

5. *Effects on Growth and Development:* Thyroxine is one of the factors essential for normal growth and skeletal maturation. In hypothyroid children, bone growth is slowed, and epiphyseal closure delayed. In the absence of thyroxine, pituitary GH content and secretion are depressed. ***Thyroxine also potentiates the action of GH on tissues.***

6. *Vitamins:* Administration of large amounts of thyroid hormones increase the requirement of certain members of vitamin B-complex (thiamine, pyridoxine, pantothenic acid) and for vitamin C. These are presumably related to the stimulation of oxidative and catabolic processes.

Regulation:

- TSH of anterior pituitary stimulates the growth of the thyroid tissue, iodide uptake and oxidation, iodination of tyrosine residues of thyroglobulin, coupling and release of thyroid hormones by the thyroid gland.
- The secretion of TSH is in turn largely stimulated by hypothalamic TRH and inhibited by the negative feedback (short loop and long loop) of high blood levels of thyroid hormones.
- *Effect of "Stress".* 'Stress' inhibits thyroid secretion. The mechanisms responsible for this inhibition are complex. ***Fig. 22.1*** shows the regulation diagrammatically.

Antithyroid Drugs: Most of the drugs which inhibit thyroid function act either by:

- ***Interferring with 'iodide trapping'***
- ***Inhibiting iodination and coupling***
- ***Inhibiting hormone release***
- ***By inhibiting conversion of T_4 to T_3 at target*** tissues. Refer box in the next page.

Iodide excess—its effects: Another substance which inhibits thyroid functions under certain conditions is "iodide" itself. The position of iodide in thyroid physiology is unique in that a minimal amount is necessary for functioning of thyroid normally, while a large amount is inhibitory, when the gland is hyperplastic. At high serum concentrations, exceeding 30 μg/dl, iodide exerts antithyroid effects and sometimes produces even a transient goitre. This is called as ***Wolff- Chaikoff effect.***

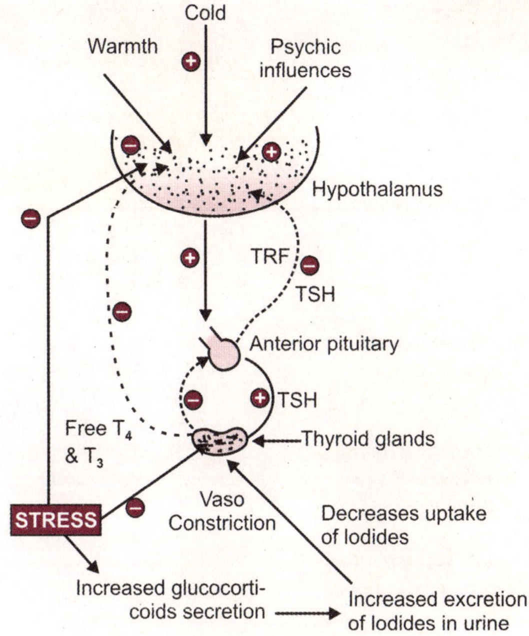

Fig. 21.1: Control of release of thyroid hormones and effects of 'stress'

Clinical Importance

Iodide therapy is sometimes done by surgeons to hyperthyroid patients for a short interval to prepare the patient for surgery (subtotal thyroidectomy).

Advantages:

- Colloid accumulates and enhances firmness to the gland.
- Vascularity of the gland is decreased.
- Decreases the blood thyroid hormone level
- Reduces the chance of acute postoperative hyperthyroidism.

Naturally Occurring Goitrogens:

- Thiocyanates are sometimes ingested with foods.
- Vegetables of the 'Brassicasae' family, particularly rutabagas, cabbage, mustard seeds, tunips, etc. contain thioglycosides called as ***"pro-goitrin".***

  Pro-goitrin can be converted to ***'goitrin'*** an active antithyroid agent.

Important antithyroid drugs

	Type of drug	*Examples*	*Mechanism of action*
1.	**Monovalent anions**	Chlorate, hypochlorite, periodate, nitrate, perchlorate pertechnate, etc.	• Compete with iodide for transport into thyroid and inhibit iodine uptake (Iodine trapping)
2.	**Thiocarbamides**	Thiourea, thiouracil, Propyl thiouracil, Methimazole (tapazole), carbimazole, etc.	• Block oxidation of iodide to active iodine • Inhibits iodination of MIT • Block the coupling reaction • May inhibit synthesis of thyroglobulin
3.	**Aminobenzenes**	Sulfonamides, PABA, Sulfonyl urea, tolbutamide, carbutamide, etc.	• Inhibit the conversion of iodide to "active" iodine • Inhibit *thyroperoxidase* • Reduces iodination and coupling reactions
4.	**Drugs that inhibit release of thyroid hormones**	Colchicine, vinblastin, vincristine, cytochalasin	• Inhibit the formation of microtubules and microfilaments in apical thyroidal cells, which are required for pinocytosis of colloid droplets
5.	**Drugs that inhibit $T_4 \rightarrow T_3$ conversion**	Propylthiouracil Propanolol	• Inhibit conversion of $T_4 \rightarrow T_3$ in target cells

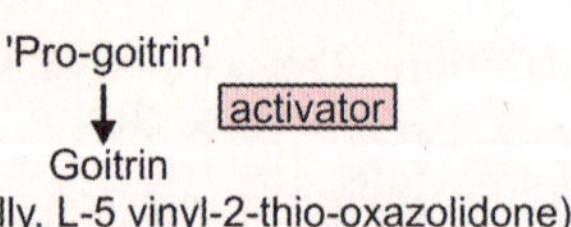

- Pro-goitrin 'activator' present in vegetables is "heat-labile", but their activators present in intestine (colonic bacteria), goitrin is formed in the intestine by bacterial action even if the vegetables are cooked.
- The "goitrin"intake on a normal mixed diet is uaually not great enough to be harmful, but in vegetarians and in food faddists "cabbage goitres" may occur.

ABNORMAL PHYSIOLOGY

This can be classified under following **three groups:**

I. *Hypothyroidism:* Resulting from lack or deficiency of thyroid hormones secretion. The main clinical conditions are:

- ***Myxoedema in adults***
- ***Cretinism in children***

II. *Hyperthyroidism:* Resulting from excessive secretion and over action of thyroid hormones. The main clinical conditions being:

- ***Exophthalmic goitre (Grave's disease)***
- ***Toxic nodular goitre.***

III. *Simple goitres:* Compensatory enlargement of thyroid glandular tissue, owing to I_2 deficiency, with normal thyroid functions.

IV. ***Goitre due to inherited metabolic defects:*** Goitre is produced by inherited defects like

- I^- transport defect
- Iodination defect
- Coupling defect
- ***De-iodinase*** deficiency and
- Production of abnormal iodinated proteins.

I. Hypothyroidism: The syndrome of adult hypothyroidism is generally called **'myxoedema'** although the term myxoedema is also used to refer specifically to skin changes in this syndrome.

Causes: Hypothyroidism may be:

- The end result of a number of diseases of thyroid gland including chronic thyroiditis and ***"auto-immune thyroiditis'***.
- It may be secondary to pituitary failure, ***'Pituitary hypothyroidism'***, or
- Hypothalamic failure-***Hypothalamic hypothyroidism***

In the latter two conditions, unlike the first, the thyroid gland responds to a test dose of TSH, and hypothalamic hypothyroidism can be distinguished from pituitary hypothyroidism by the presence in the former of a rise in plasma TSH following a test dose of TRF.

1. **Myxoedema:** Myxoedema is caused by hypothyroidism in adults (adult analogue of 'cretinism').

Clinical features and biochemical findings: The patient ***complaints of undue sensitivity to cold, mentation is slow,*** body temperature lowered↓. ***Other characteristic findings*** *include:*

- Puffiness of face and extremities
- Thickening and drying of skin
- Skin shows yellowish tinge (due to carote naemia)
- Falling of hairs, specially from eyebrows,
- In some patients obesity
- Anaemia usually develops
- BMR is lowered to 40%
- ***Blood cholesterol level is usually high (hypercholesterolaemia)***

Note: Slowing of physical and mental reactions are present- Mentation is slow, and memory is poor and in some patients mental symptoms may develop **(*"myxoedema madness"*).**

Spontaneous adult myxoedema is now considered as an auto-immune disease.

2. **Cretinism:**

- Results from incomplete development or congenital absence of thyroid.
- Children who are hypothyroid from birth are called cretins.
- The children are dwarfed, mentally retarded, and have enlarged protruding tongue and pot bellies.

3. **Childhood Myxoedema: (Juvenile Myxoedema):** It appears later in life than cretinism. It is generally less severe, and some of the typical cretinoid symptoms are absent.

The most important signs of Juvenile myxoedema are:

- Stunted growth (due to lack of bone growth)
- Cessation of mental development, and
- In some cases, changes in the skin are observed.

II. Hyperthyroidism (Or Thyrotoxicosis): It is characterized by nervousness, weight loss, hyperphagia, heat intolerance, increased pulse pressure, a fine tremor of the outstretched fingers, a warm and soft skin and a high BMR from +10 to +80 or more. ***Blood cholesterol is usually low ↓ (hypocholesterolaemia),*** increased serum PBI.

Cause: It may be caused by a variety of thyroid disorders, including in rare instances benign and malignant tumours including toxic nodular goitres and cases due to TSH- secreting pituitary tumours have been reported. The most common form of hyperthyroidism is **"Grave's disease"** (or exophthalmic goiture). In Grave's disease, the thyroid is diffusely enlarged and hyperplastic and there is portrusion of the eyeballs called ***"exophthalmos".*** Plasma TSH levels are actually subnormal in this disease.

Pathogenesis: In this disease, auto-immunization against thyroid components, probably a low molecular weight 4s compound in thyroid cell sap, produces ***"Thyroid stimulating antibody",*** an IgG immunoglobulin. Its effects on the thyroid are of much longer duration, hence it is also called as ***"Long-acting thyroid stimulator" (LATS).*** It binds to TSH "receptors" on thyroid cell membrane and ***simulates the action of TSH*** in stimulating the thyroid gland. But, unlike TSH, its action is not inhibited by feedback of thyroid hormones. So its prolonged continued action produces an over-active enlarged thyroid (*"Thyrotoxic goitre"*) and thyroid hormone over secretion producing hyperthyroidism.

Exophthalmos: A protrusion of eyeballs results from mucoprotein deposition and oedema in the retrobular tissue due to probably production of an ***"exophthalmos producing IgG".***

Complications: Two important complications are:

- ***Cardiac failure***
- ***Hepatic failure***

III. Iodine Deficiency Simple Goitres: When the dietary iodine intake falls below 10 μg/day thyroid hormone synthesis is inadequate and secretion declines. As a result of increased TSH secretion ↑, the thyroid hypertrophies, producing an iodine deficient simple goitre, which may become very large.

Precaution: In endemic area where soil is deficient in I_2 it is advisable to add KI or NaI in common salt in proportions of one part of KI to 100,000 parts of common salt thus providing daily intake of 200 μg of I_2 (such iodized salts are available in market).

PARATHYROID GLANDS AND THEIR HORMONES

Anatomy and Physiology of Parathyroid Glands: In humans, there are usually four parathyroid glands, two embedded in superior poles and two in inferior poles of thyroid gland. Four glands together weigh 0.05 to 0.3 gm. Each parathyroid gland is a richly vascularized disk, about 3x 6x 2 mm.

The gland contains *two distinct type of cells:*

- *Chief cells:* Abundant, polyhedral, has clear cytoplasm, nongranular, contains glycogen. They ***secrete the parathyroid hormone, parathormone (PTH).***
- *Oxyphil cells:* Less frequent larger cells with granules, contain large number of mitochondria but no glycogen. Their function is unknown.

  The microscopic section of the gland appears as solid mass of epithelial cells in between which lie sinusoids.

INTRODUCTION

The parathyroid glands are intimately concerned with regulation of the concentration of Ca and PO_4 ions in the blood plasma. This is accomplished by secretion of a hormone, **parathormone (PTH)** by the chief cells, the net effect of which is:

- ***To increase the concentration of Ca ↑ and***
- ***To decrease the PO_4 ↓.***

In addition to its effects on plasma ionized Ca via its action on bone, parathormone controls renal excretion of Ca and PO_4.

PARATHORMONE (PTH)

Chemistry: Parathormone is a linear polypeptide consisting of 84 amino acids. PTH has molecular weight of 9500. Parathormone from different species differ only slightly in structure.

Core of Activity: Studies on the synthetic PTH indicate that the ***amino acid sequence 1 to 29 or possibly 1 to 34 from N-terminal end is essential*** for the physiologic actions of this hormone on both skeletal and renal tissues. ***Methionine is important amino acid and necessary for calcium-mobilizing effect.*** The N-terminal end upto 34 amino acids possesses the "receptor-binding" ability.

Biosynthesis

PTH is intially synthesized in chief cells as a pro-hormone. Formation of PTH from prohormone is shown below. PTH thus formed is packaged and stored in secretory vesicles. ***Increased c-AMP concentration and a low Ca^{++} level stimulates its release from secretory vesicles.*** On the other hand, a high concentration of Ca^{++} stimulates the degradation of the stored PTH in secretory vesicles instead of its release.

Metabolism: PTH secreted in the body is degraded very rapidly in the circulation to smaller fragments, ½ life approximately 18 minutes.

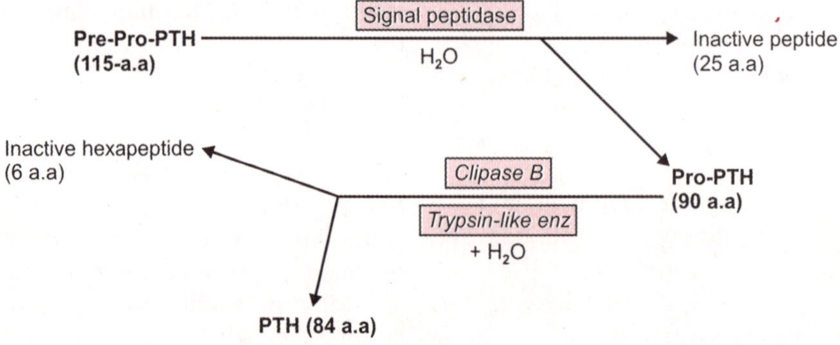

Mechanism of Action:

- PTH increases serum Ca^{++} level by acting on bones, kidney and intestines.
- PTH binds to "specific receptor" on the plasma membrane of bone cells, it activates the *adenyl cyclase* to form c-AMP in the cells. c-AMP acts as the "second messenger" which activates specific cAMP dependent protein kinases, which phosphorylate and thereby modulate the activities of specific proteins in the bone cells and kidney cells.
- c-AMP also increases the Ca^{++} concentration in these cells, which in turn may act as a "messenger" to modulate the activities of some intracellular proteins.

ACTIONS OF PTH

The action of PTH are reflected in the consequences of:

- Its administration
- Removal of the parathyroid glands

The most conspicuous metabolic consequences of adminstration of PTH are:

- ***Increase in serum Ca^{++} concentration*** ↑
- ***Decrease in serum inorganic PO_4 ↓ concentration.***
- Increased urinary Ca^{++} ↑ following an initial decrease.
- Increased urinary PO_4↑.
- Removes Ca from bones, particularly if dietary intake of Ca is inadequate.
- Increases serum *alkaline phosphatase* ↑ if changes in bone have been produced activity at higher levels of physiological concentrations.
- Increase in ***'Citrate'*** ↑ content of blood plasma, kidney and bones.
- Activates vitamin D in renal tissue by increasing the rate of conversion of 25-OH-cholecalciferol to 1,25-di-OH-cholecalciferol, by stimulating *α-I-hydroxylase* enzyme.
- *Effect on Mg metabolism:* PTH has been reported to exert an influence on Mg metabolism. Primary hyperparathyroidism has been found to be associated with excessive urinary excretion of Mg and –ve Mg balance.

Regulation of PTH Release

- ***PTH is not stored in the gland; it is thus synthesized and secreted continually.***
- *Negative-feedback mechanism:* Its secretion is mainly under the "feedback" control of serum Ca^{2+} level. A rise in serum Ca^{++} level inhibits and a fall in serum Ca^{++} stimulates PTH secretion.
- *Mg. level:* Serum Mg^{++} has similar effects like calcium but the effects are weaker.
- *Cyclic AMP:* Cyclic AMP is a mediator of the action of serum Ca^{2+} on PTH secretion. A positive linear correlation has been found with c-AMP level. Rise in serum Ca^{2+} increases intracellular Ca^{++} which lowers the cyclic AMP in cells by inhibiting *adenyl cyclase/or* activating *phosphodiesterase,* the ***fall in c-AMP level decreases the PTH secretion.*** The reverse effect is seen by lowering of serum Ca^{2+} level.
- *Other agents:* Substances like PGE_1 and hormones like catecholamines (β-effects) and dopamine increase PTH secretion by increasing the concentration of c-AMP in parathyroid cells.

ABNORMALITIES OF PARATHYROID FUNCTION

1. Hyperparathyroidism: In hyperparathyroidism there is oversecretion of PTH.

Causes

- *Primary hyperparathyroidism:* May be hyperplasia or a tumor, (usually a parathyroid adenoma).
- *Secondary hyperparathyroidism:* Seen in chronic renal disease with renal failure due to tubular damage, formation of 1,25-$(OH)_2$ cholecalciferol (calcitriol)does not take place.

Clinical effects: These are seen on bones and kidneys

- *Bones:* Show increased osteoclastic activity resulting to resorption of bones. It gives to *osteitis fibrosa cystica* **(Von Reckling Houssen's disease).**
- *Kidneys:* Kidney functions are impaired along with a tendency to recurring formation

of *"renal calculi"* (with calcium phosphate stones), which is due to hypercalciuria.

- There is urinary loss of Mg^{2+}, and also loss of K^+ and Na^+
- The effective action of ADH on kidneys is much reduced, and symptoms of thirst and polyuria are apparent.

Blood Changes:

- *Hypercalcaemia:* Serum Ca^{++} may reach up to 20 to 30 mg% particularly increase in ionic Ca^{++}.
- *Hypophosphataemia:* Lowering of serum inorganic PO_4 (Pi).
- *Mg^{++}:* Serum Mg^{++} may be low, in cases of prolonged hyperparathyroidism.
- *Alkaline phosphatase:* Serum alkaline phosphatase (ALP), usually elevated.

Note: Recently some extra-parathyroid tumours associated with hyperparathyroidism have been described. An active material isolated in such cases, which is immunologically indistinguishable from PTH, is called **PTHrP** (refer to calcium metabolism).

2. Hypoparathyroidism: There is diminished secretion of PTH.

Causes:

- *Primary hypoparathyroidism:* Usually due to auto-immune destruction of the gland.
- *Secondary hypoparathyroidism:* Most common cause is accidental removal of parathyroid while performing total or partial thyroidectomy.
- *Idiopathic hypoparathyroidism:* Failure of parathyroid to function due to unknown causes.

Clinical effects: Bone changes are as follows:

- Reduced osteoclastic activity
- Enhanced tendency to calcification process of bones.

X-ray examination of skull may reveal calcification of basal ganglia and bones may be more dense than normal.

Other findings include:

- *Tendency to cataracts*-early cataract may be detected
- Under developed teeth and brittleness of nails.
- Dryness of skin
- ***If hypoparathyroidism begins in early childhood-stunting of growth, defective teeth development and mental retardation.***

Blood Changes

- *Hypocalcaemia:* Serum calcium level falls characteristically to 6 to 7 mg%.
- *Hyperphosphataemia:* Serum inorganic PO_4 (pi) level rises to 8 to 10 mg%.
- *Serum Mg^{++}* and hydroxy-proline levels are reduced.
- *Increase of blood pH:* The blood reaction is more alkaline owing to excessive loss of CO_2.

Urinary changes:

- Urinary Ca is low ↓ or absent
- Urinary PO_4 is low ↓ in absence of renal failure (increases renal tubular resorption of PO_4)

Tetany: Most characteristic feature seen in hypoparathyroidism. Neuromuscular hyper excitability is observed which leads to tetany (parathyroid tetany).

Clinical features: In tetany, there is hypocalcaemia, hyperexcitability of muscular apparatus, fibrillation and twiching of muscles, generalized clonic and tonic muscular spasms resulting in epileptiform convulsions. The spasms of laryngeal muscles may cause asphyxia and death.

Signs:

- *Trousseau's sign (Carpopedal spasm):* Application of pressure over arm with blood pressure Cuff results in muscular spasm causing what is called as *"accoucheur hand"*—the hand gets flexed at wrist, fingers are flexed at metacarpophalangeal joints, with extension of interphalangeal joints. The fingers are drawn together with thumb abducted from palm.
- *Chvostek's sign:* If the skin in front of ear (site of facial nerve course) is tapped there is twitching or spasm of facial nerves.

Mechanism of tetany: Tetany is due to hyper-irritability of the tissues, which is caused by increase of Na^+ and K^+ and decrease Ca^{2+} and Mg^{2+} in the tissue fluid. However, ***it is mainly the decrease of ionic Ca in the fluid which is immediate factor in causation of neuromuscular hyperexcitability.***

3. Pseudo-hypoparathyroidism: A congenital disorder. ***PTH secretion is not reduced.*** Probably the defect is that the bones and kidneys are resistant to PTH action.

- ***Biochemical defect*** is an ***inherited deficiency of the GTP-dependant regulatory protein (Gs or Ns) which is necessary for activation of adenyl cyclase at target cell membrane.***
- Though PTH is available it cannot act on target cells, thus c-AMP is not increased to duplicate the function of PTH.

Clinically:

- Neuromuscular hyperexcitability
- Stunted growth and may be mental retardation.
- Short metacarpals and metatarsals.

Blood changes:

- ***Hypocalcaemia:*** Serum Ca is low ↓.
- ***Hyperphosphataemia:*** Serum inorganic PO_4 (Pi) is high ↑
- ***Serum PTH:*** Normal or high, usually rises as hypocalcaemia stimulates parathyroids to secrete more PTH.

CALCITONIN

Calcitonin is a calcium regulating hormone. **Copp and his associates** (1962) first postulated the existence of a specific plasma calcium-lowering hormone and they termed it as ***'calcitonin'.***

Hirsch *et al* (1963) while confirming the existence of such a calcium-lowering hormone, indicated that it is probably derived from the thyroid gland. The term ***thyrocalcitonin*** was given by them.

Site of Formation: It is finally proved that the hormone originates from special cells, called **"C-cells"**-parafollicular cells. ***C-cells constitute an endocrine system.*** These cells are derived from ***"neural crest"*** and are found in thyroid, parathyroids and in thymus. Anatomically, the "C-cells" in thyroid gland are usually situated near the basement membrane of the thyroid follicles but not in contact with the colloids.

Chemistry: Calcitonin is a single chain lipophilic polypeptide, having a mol wt of 3600. As many as four separate active fractions have been isolated and they have been designated as α, β, γ and δ-calcitonin. It contains 32 amino acids, an interchain disulfide bridge joins two cysteine residues between position 1 and 7.

Mechanism of Action: Calcitonin binds to specific calcitonin receptors on the plasma membrane of bone osteoclasts and renal tubular epithelial cells, activates *adenyl cyclase* which increases c-AMP level ↑ which mediates the cellular effects of the hormone.

ACTIONS

Calcitonin acts both on (a) bone and (b) kidneys indirectly, the effects of these two organ systems account for:

- ***Hypocalcaemia*** and
- ***Hypophosphataemia*** produced by the hormone.

1. ***Action on Bones:***

- Calcitonin inhibits the resorption of bones by osteoclasts and thereby reduces mobilization of Ca and inorganic PO_4 from bones into the blood.
- It also stimulates influx of phosphates in bones.
- Decrease in collagen metabolism and decreased excretion of urinary OH-proline.
- Whether or not calcitonin promotes bone formation is uncertain and controversial. But it has been established that the hormone in addition to causing a decrease in number of osteoclasts, increases osteoblasts cells, which are thought to be involved in bone laying.

2. ***Action on kidneys:*** The hormone acts on the distal tubule and ascending limb of Loop of Henle and decreases tubular reabsorption of both calcium and inorganic PO_4 thus *producing*

calcinuria and phosphaturia. The hormone inhibits *α-1-hydroxylase* and inhibits synthesis of 1,25-di-OH-D_3 thus decreasing calcium absorption from intestine. Both the above effects account also for hypocalcaemia.

Regulation of Secretion

1. ***Serum Ca level:***

- Like PTH, calcitonin also is secreted continuously under normal conditions.
- Secretion of calcitonin is controlled and regulated by level of blood calcium.
- Rise in serum calcium level stimulate the secretion of calcitonin, on the other hand, fall in serum calcium decreases its concentration.

2. ***Other agents:*** Secretion or release is increased by specific cations, e.g. Ca^{++}/and Mg^{++} infusions.

3. ***Hormones:***

a. ***Stimulation:***

- Glucagon and catecholamines (β-effects) stimulate calcitonin secretion by activating the *adenylcyclase* and increasing cyclic AMP level.
- G.I. hormones: Gastrin and CCK-PZ also stimulate calcitonin secretion.

b. ***Inhibition:*** Somatostatin inhibits calcitonin.

Clinical Aspect

- Abnormal calcitonin secretion is now proved in case of **"medullary carcinoma of thyroid"**, this tumour arises from parafollicular C-cells of thyroid.
- Frequently patient with this tumour has been found to have associated:
  - Cutaneous neuromas,
  - Adrenal tumours, and
  - Parathyroid enlargement.
- Patient also suffers from severe diarrhoea.

Therapeutic Uses of Calcitonin

Calcitonin has been used in the following disorders:

- ***In Paget's disease***
- ***Idiopathic hypercalcaemia of infancy.***
- ***Hypercalcaemia secondary to malignancies, hyperparathyroidism and vitamin D intoxication.***

☞ SALIENT POINTS TO REMEMBER

- Thyroid gland produces the hormones - Thyroxine (T_4), Triiodothyronine (T_3) and "reverse" T_3.
- Two raw materials are required by thyroid gland to synthesize thyroid hormones. They are iodine and thyroglobulin, a protein.
- Two main carrier proteins for thyroid hormones are: Thyroxine binding globulin (TBG) and thyroxine binding prealbumin (TBPA). When these are saturated, excess hormone can be bound to serum albumin.
- "Free" (unbound) T_3 and T_4 are the metabolically "active" hormones in the plasma.
- In physiological doses and in hypothyroid children, thyroid hormones favour protein anabolism. Large unphysiological doses, cause protein catabolism.
- In hyperthyroidism, catabolic effect on muscle is seen as thyrotoxic myopathy.
- Net effect of thyroid hormones on carbohydrate metabolism produces increase blood sugar level ↑ (hyperglycaemia).
- In adipose tissue, produces increased lipolysis with increased plasma FFA.
- Goitre is a disorder caused by enlargement of thyroid gland and is mainly due to iodine deficiency in the diet. This can be prevented by using iodised salt.
- Parathyroid glands produce the hormone parathormone (PTH), a linear polypeptide consisting of 84 amino acids.
- Initially it is synthesized in chief cells as a prohormone. Pre-prohormone (115 a.a) is converted to pro-PTH (90 a.a) by "signal peptidase", which is converted to PTH (84 a.a) by "clipase B".
- Methionine is important amino acid and necessary for Ca-mobilising effects.
- Main effects of PTH are increase in serum Ca^{++} ↑ concentration and decrease in serum inorganic PO_4 ↓.
- Calcitonin is a hormone, a polypeptide consisting of 32 amino acids.

- It is produced by "C-cells," parafollicular cells of thyroids chiefly. C-cells are also found in parathyroids and thymus.
- *C-cells constitute an endocrine system.* Calcitonin produced by C-cells has opposite action of PTH on calcium metabolism. It produces hypocalcaemia and hypophosphataemia.
- Abnormal calcitonin secretion is produced by medullary carcinoma of thyroid which is a tumour produced from C-cells of thyroid.
- Calcitonin has been used in the following disorders: In paget's disease, idiopathic hypocalcaemia of infancy, hypercalcaemia secondary to malignancies, hyperparathyroidism and vitamin D intoxication.

PANCREAS AND ITS HORMONES

Anatomy: The endocrine function of pancreas is localized in ***"Islet of Langerhans"***. They are ovoid, 75 x 175 μm collections of epithelial cells, scattered throughout the pancreas. They are more plentiful in tail of pancreas than in the body and head. They make up 1 to 2% of the weight of the pancreas. In humans, there are 1-2 million of islets. In humans and all mammals studied, except guinea pig, there are **three types of cells**. In humans,

- *α-cells:* Approximately 20% contain granules. They secrete the hormone ***"glucagon"***.
- *β-cells:* Approximately 75%, contain granules. These cells secrete the hormone, ***"Insulin"*** In the β-cells, the insulin molecule forms 'polymers' and also complexes with Zn^{++}.
- *δ-cells:* Constitute to 1 to 8% of the cells. Recently, it has been reported they are responsible for secretion of ***"somatostatin"*** and a pancreatic polypeptide.

INSULIN

- *Insulin is a protein hormone, secreted by **β-cells of Islets of Langerhans of pancreas.*** It plays an important role in metabolism causing increased carbohydrate metabolism, glycogenesis/and glycogen storage; FA synthesis/TG storage and amino acid uptake/protein synthesis. ***Thus Insulin is an important anabolic hormone*** which acts on variety of tissues.
- Major target tissues of insulin are the muscles, liver, adipose tissue and heart.

  Note: RB cells, GI tract epithelial cells and renal tubular epithelial cells are rather generally unresponsive to insulin.

Chemistry:

- Insulin is a protein; has been isolated from pancreas and prepared in crystalline form. ***For crystallization, it requires*** Zn^{++}. Zinc is also a constituent of stored insulin and normal pancreatic tissue is relatively rich in Zn.
- ***Insulin molecule is composed of two polypeptide chains, called 'A'-chain and 'B'-chain containing total 51 amino acids.***
- A-chain contains 21 amino acids and B-chain contains 30 amino acids.
- ***Disulphide bridges:*** Both the chains are held together by two S-S linkages—Cys 7 and Cys 20 of 'A' chain are joined to Cys 7 and Cys 19 of B chain respectively.
- In addition, the 'A' chain carries an "intra-chain" S-S linkage between Cys 6 and Cys 11 ***(see Fig. 22.2)***.

Molecular Weight of Insulin: Minimum calculated molecular weight is 5734. Most estimates of molecular weight by physical measurements range from 12,000 to 48,000. Insulin can exist in different 'polymeric' forms (dimers, trimers, etc). depending on pH, temperature and concentration.

Biosynthesis of Insulin: In biosynthesis of insulin, first ***"prepro-insulin"*** is formed, which is converted to **pro-insulin**. The latter is finally converted to insulin, as shown in the next page:

Note:

- Pro-insulin is comparatively inactive biologically, but it can cross-react with antisera prepared against insulin.
- Plasma pro-insulin is not elevated in human diabetes or in normals after glucose stimulation, but it may be the predominant

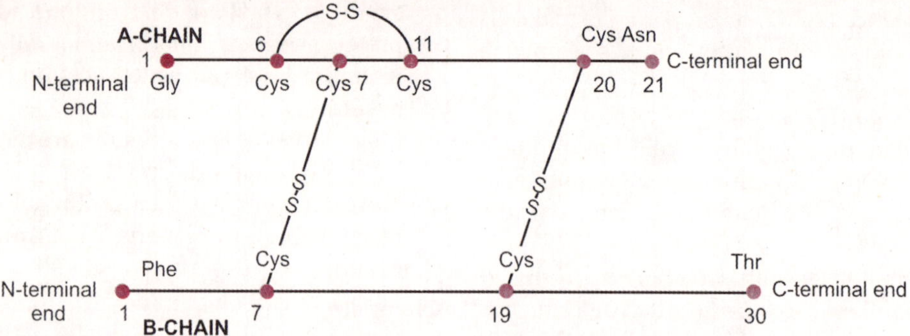

Fig. 22.2: Shows structure of insulin schematically

circulating form in some subjects with islet-cell tumours.

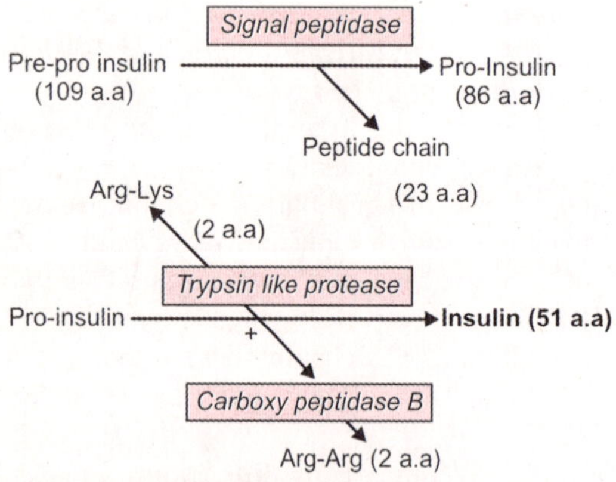

Factors Affecting Secretion of Insulin (Regulation of Secretion)

1. *Nervous:* Stimulation of right vagus causes secretion of insulin and a fall in blood glucose.
2. *Blood Glucose:* This is single most important factor in the control of insulin secretion. During intestinal absorption or infusion of glucose producing increased blood glucose level or hyperglycaemia, directly stimulate β-cells for synthesis and release of insulin.
3. *Effect of Other Sugars:* Other readily metabolizable sugars, e.g. fructose, mannose can also stimulate insulin release.
4. *Glucagon:* It is a potent stimulant of insulin secretion. It acts directly on the β-cells, since the plasma insulin rises before there is any increase in blood glucose, and it is possible that the glucagon is released from α-cells to pass directly into the adjacent β-cells. In addition, the hyperglycaemia induced by glucagon will enhance insulin secretion still further.
5. *Fatty Acids:* FA such as octanoate stimulate β-cells to secrete insulin, but the role of higher FA in physiological concentrations is not established.
6. *GI hormones:* GI hormones, viz. Gastrin, CCK-PZ and secretin can directly stimulate insulin secretion both *in vivo* and *in vitro*. GIP stimulates insulin secretion in presence of hyperglycaemia, but not at normal blood glucose levels.
7. *Amino acids:* Leucine and Arginine can stimulate the pancreas to produce insulin. They act in presence of glucose.

Note: In children with spontaneous hypoglycaemic episodes and in subjects with functioning islet cell tumours, leucine is particularly effective in causing a rise in circulating insulin and hypoglycaemia ***("leucine-sensitive hypoglycaemia" in children).***

8. *Hormones:*
   - *GH and Gluco-corticoids:* Both can produce an increase in circulating insulin (not *in vitro*). Since these agents cause hyperglycaemia, it is possible that they act on the pancreas primarily by way of increasing stimulation by glucose rather than by a direct effect.
   - *Epinephrine:* Both *in vivo* and *in vitro* is a potent and highly effective inhibitor of insulin secretion regardless of blood glucose concentration.

TRANSPORT AND METABOLISM

Insulin is very rapidly metabolized. Its plasma ½ life is < 3 to 5 minutes under normal conditions. Major organs where insulin is catabolized are liver, kidneys and placenta. About 50% of insulin is degraded in its single passage through the liver.

- *Enzyme responsible:* The enzyme is ***glutathione-insulin transhydrogenase (also called insulinase)***, found in highest concentration in Liver and Kidneys, also present in skeletal muscles and placenta. This brings about reductive cleavage of the "S-S bond" which connects the A and B-chains of insulin molecule. ***Reduced glutathione (G-SH), acting as coenzyme for the transhydrogenase, donates the H-atoms for the reduction and is itself thus converted to oxidized glutathione (G-S-S-G).***
- After insulin is reductively cleaved, the A-chains and B-chains are further hydrolyzed by *proteolysis*.

INSULIN RECEPTORS

Insulin acts on target tissues by binding to specific "insulin receptor", which are 'glycoproteins'.

Regulation: A high blood insulin level decreases the number of insulin receptors on target cell membrane, probably through internalization of the insulin receptor complex into the cell and thus decreases the insulin-sensitivity of the target tissues.

Metabolic Role and Functions of Insulin

1. Action on Carbohydrate Metabolism

Net effect is lowering of blood glucose ↓ level and increase glycogen store ↑. The above is achieved by several mechanisms:

- *Increases glucose uptake:* Insulin increases glucose uptake from E.C. fluid by the various tissues, viz. muscles, adipose tissue, mammary glands, lens, etc. Also in hepatocytes, insulin increases hepatic uptake of glucose (freely permeable to liver cells). It induces the synthesis of the enzyme *glucokinase*, which simultaneously phosphorylates glucose, thereby lower intracellular concentration.
- *Increases glycolysis:* Increases utilization of glucose for providing energy which takes place in muscles, liver and many other tissues.
- *Increases conversion of pyruvate to acetyl-CoA:* Insulin increases aerobic oxidative decarboxylation of pyruvate to acetyl CoA ↑.
- *Stimulates glycogenesis:* Insulin stimulates glycogenesis ↑ in the liver and muscles.
- *Decreases Gluconeogenesis:* Insulin reduces gluconeogenesis ↓ by repressing the synthesis of the key rate limiting enzyme PEP-carboxy-kinase.
- *Decreases glycogenolysis:* Insulin decreases glycogenolysis ↓.
- *Increasing HMP-shunt:* Insulin stimulates HMP shunt producing more NADPH (required for FA synthesis), by inducing the synthesis of *glucose-6-P-dehydrogenase (G-6-PD)* and 6 *phosphogluconate dehydrogenase.*

2. Action on Lipid Metabolism

Net effect is lowering of FFA level ↓ and increase in TG store ↑. This is achieved as insulin affects the following reactions:

- *Decreases lipolysis:* Insulin decreases lipolysis ↓ in adipose tissue cells and consequently lowers plasma FFA ↓.
- *Increases FA synthesis:* Insulin increases the extramitochondrial *de novo* FA synthesis ↑, by making available of more substrate acetyl CoA and also increasing the activity of *acetyl-CoA carboxylase.*
- *Increases synthesis of TG:* Insulin enhances TG synthesis ↑ in adipose tissue by providing more α-glycero-p, as glucose uptake and utilization is enhanced in adipocytes.
- *Decreases ketogenesis:* As plasma FFA level is decreased, less is oxidized by β-oxidation and less acetyl-CoA will be available for cholesterol synthesis and ketogenesis.

3. Action on Protein Metabolism

Net effect is insulin promotes protein synthesis↑. This is achieved as described below:

- ***Insulin increases amino acids uptake by the tissues,*** by enhancing the rate of synthesis of membrane 'transporters' for amino acids.

- Adequate supply of insulin is necessary for protein anabolic effect of GH *permissive effect.*
- In most of the tissues, insulin affects the synthesis of many enzymes, structural proteins, carrier proteins, secretory proteins, etc.

4. Action on Mineral Metabolism

Decrease in concentration of $K^+\downarrow$ and inorganic P↓ in blood due to enhanced glycogenesis and phosphorylation of glucose.

Insulin-Like Growth Factors

- Two insulin like growth factors, IGF-I and IGF-II have recently been found.
- They are not of pancreatic origin but produced by liver and other tissues.
- It is difficult to separate the effects of insulin on cell growth and replication from similar actions exerted by IGF-I and IGF-II. ***Insulin and IGFs may interact in this process.***
- Insulin is more potent metabolic hormone and IGFs are involved more in stimulating growth.
- Each hormone has unique receptor to act.

INSULIN PREPARATIONS

- ***Soluble insulin:*** Aqueous solution of crystalline "acts quickly, duration of action is approximately 6 hours only."
- ***Lente insulin:*** Insulin-Zinc-suspension, slow absorption, hence action is prolonged. One injection is effective for 24 hours.
- ***Protamine insulin:*** Insulin chemically united to simple protein protamine (extracted from nuclei and contains Arg/Lys), slow absorption and has prolonged action.
- ***Zinc and protamine insulin combined (PZI):*** Protamine insulin combined with $ZnCl_2$. Remains stable for months. Action starts within 6 to 8 hours and lasts for 48 to 72 hours.
  Note: Serial Nos, 2, 3 and 4 are also called "***Retard insulin***" due to their prolonged action.
- ***Regular insulin + "Retard" insulin:*** Double advantage of both quick and prolonged action.
- ***Globin insulin:*** Combination of insulin with globin obtained from Hb and a small proportion of $ZnCl_2$. It has a delayed action intermediate between regular and PZI.

INSULIN ANALOGUES

Recently major breakthrough of synthesizing insulin analogues with pharmacologic advantages have been made possible by ***"computer modelling"***. The programme furnishes appropriate modifications in the molecular structure necessary for altering the stability, self association and pharmacologic activity of insulin. Synthesis of these altered molecules is then done by ***"Re-combinant DNA technology"***. Using technique, **three types** of insulin analogues have been prepared. They are:

- ***Short (fast) acting analogues: monomeric insulins***
- ***Intermediate acting analogues and***
- ***Long acting analogues***

Note: It is not possible to discuss all the analogues, a few prototype examples are given:

1. Short (Fast) acting analogues:

- ***B 9 Asp B 27 Glu:*** In normal subjects this analogue is absorbed 2 to 3 times faster than soluble human insulin after S.C. injection and it is accompanied by more rapid rise in plasma insulin and more rapid onset of hypoglycaemia.
- ***Lys (B 28). Pro (B 29): (Lispro Insulin):*** Studies have shown onset of hypoglycaemic activity seen within 15 minutes of administration, Peak serum insulin reached in approx. one hour, and duration of action was shorter (3.5 to 4.5 hrs).

2. Intermediate acting Insulin analogues:

- ***Diarginyl insulin:*** This is an interesting product of recombinant DNA technology, an intermediary metabolite in the bioconversion of proinsulin to insulin. It behaves like an intermediate acting insulin preparation.
- ***DES 64, 65 HPI (D PRO):*** This is a normal metabolite of pro-insulin formed by split between positions 65 and 66 and removal of Arg and Lys at position 64 and 65 of human proinsulin. Data generated in humans are very preliminary.

3. **Long acting insulin analogues:**
   - *Novosol basal:* In this, substitution of threonine in position B 27 with arginine, and amidation of the 'C' terminal of the B chain adds two positive charges and increases the isoelectric point (pI) from 5.4 to 6.8. A further substitution of asparagine in A 21 with glycine renders the molecule stable in acid solution. This preparation is soluble in its formulation of pH 3.0. After injection, when the pH rises to about 7.4, it crystallizes (crystal less than < 5.0 micrometers in diameter) ***acts as a subcutaneous depot*** from which insulin is slowly absorbed, thus acts as long acting insulin analogue.

Abnormal Physiology

Absolute or relative deficiency of insulin produces the metabolic disease called ***Diabetes mellitus.***

GLUCAGON [HYPERGLYCAEMIC-GLYCOGENOLYTIC FACTOR (HGF)]

Glucagon is a hormone produced by α-cells of Islet of Langerhans of pancreas and is an important hormone involved in:

- ***Rapid mobilization of hepatic glycogen to give glucose by glycogenolysis, and***
- ***To a lesser extent FA from adipose tissue.***

Thus, ***it acts as a hormone required to mobilize metabolic substrates from storage depots.***

Chemistry:

- It is a polypeptide containing 29 amino acids. There are only 15 different amino acids in the molecule.
- Amino acid sequence has been determined, histidine is the N-terminal amino acid and threonine is the C-terminal.
- Molecular weight is approximately 3485.
- Unlike insulin:
  - It does not require Zinc or other metals for its crystallization.
  - Glucagon contains no cystine, proline or isoleucine, but contains Tyrosine, methionine and tryptophan.

Synthesis

It is synthesized first as a **pro-hormone *"proglucagon"*** in α-cells. Lysosomal enzymes peptidases like *carboxy-peptidase B* and *trypsin-like peptidases* in α-cells hydrolyze pro-glucagon from both its N-terminal end and C-terminal end to yield glucagon and inactive peptides.

Note:

Entero-glucagon or glucagon-like immune reactive factor (GLI):

- Recently a glucagon like immuno reactive factor (GLI) has also been identified in gastric and duodenal mucosa.
- GLI is immunologically similar though not identical to the pancreatic hormone. Moreover, it is less active than pancreatic glucagon in stimulating *adenyl cyclase* and therefore, cannot duplicate many of the functions of pancreatic hormone.
- GLI if stimulated by absorbed glucose causing an apparent elevation of circulating pancreatic glucagon.

Mechanism of Action: Glucagon binds to specific receptors on the plasma membranes of hepatocytes and adipocytes and activates *adenyl cyclase* to produce c-AMP in these cells, which is the principal "second messenger" and duplicates the functions of the hormone.

Factors Controlling Glucagon Secretion—(Regulation)

- *Glucose:* In contrast to Insulin, ***secretion of pancreatic glucagon increases with low blood glucose (hypoglycaemia)*** whether induced by starvation, insulin or sulphonyl ureas. ***Glucagon secretion is directly inhibited by glucose.***
- *Fatty acids:* FA also inhibits glucagon release whereas exercise stimulates it.
- ***Amino acids:*** Most amino acids, particularly arginine and alanine cause a rapid secretion of glucagon from the pancreas.
- ***Growth hormone and CCK-PZ:*** They also stimulate the secretion.

- *Calcium:* Rise in serum calcium concentration is a potent stimulus for glucagon secretion.

ACTIONS

1. On Carbohydrate Metabolism:

Net effect of the hormone is to increase the blood sugar level (hyperglycaemia). Hyperglycaemic effect is due to various causes:

- ***Glycogenolysis***: Glucagon increases glycogenolysis in liver. In muscles, it cannot bring about glycogenolysis, ***as muscle cell membrane lacks the glucagon specific receptors.***
- ***By increasing Gluconeogenesis in liver.*** Glucagon stimulates the conversion of LA and glucogenic amino acids to form glucose.

2. On Lipid Metabolism:

Lipolysis: In adipose tissue and also possibly in liver, glucagon increases the breakdown of TG to produce FFA ↑ and glycerol ↑. FA undergo β-oxidation, increased breakdown may lead to ketone bodies formation and ketosis.

- *Thyroid hormones help in the lipolytic action of* glucagon, probably the hormones increase the number of glucagon-specific receptors on adipocytes.
- *Anti-lipogenic Action:* Glucagon reduces FA synthesis. This is achieved by increased lipolysis which raises the concentration of FFA in blood. Long-chain acyl CoA inhibits the rate-limiting enzyme *acetyl-CoA carboxylase.*

3. On Protein Metabolism:

Glucagon reduces protein synthesis by depressing incorporation of amino acids into peptide chains. Glucagon also stimulates protein catabolism ↑ specially in liver thus increases the hepatic amino acid pool which is utilized for gluconeogenesis.

4. Action on Heart

Glucagon exerts a +ve ionotropic effect on heart without producing increased myocardial irritability. Hence, ***Use of glucagon in treatment of heart disease, cardiac failure and cardiogenic shock, has been advocated.***

Advantage over nor-epinephrine: Glucagon increases the force of contraction, but does not produce any arrythmias, tachycardia or increase in O_2 consumption.

5. Calorigenic Action:

Glucagon increases heat production and rise in BMR. ***The calorigenic action requires the presence of thyroid and adrenocortical hormones and fails to occur in their absence.***

6. On Mineral Metabolism:

- ***Potassium:*** Glucagon increases K^+ release from the liver, an action which may be related to its glycogenolytic activity.
- ***Calcium:*** Recently it has been shown that glucagon can increase the release of calcitonin from the thyroid, thus have calcium lowering effect.

Clinical and Therapeutic Uses

- Most important use is in ***treatment of severe insulin-induced hypoglycaemia.***
- Long acting Zinc—glucagon has been used in inoperable pancreatic cell tumours.
- Has been used in ***heart failure*** and ***cardiogenic shock*** due to its direct ionotropic effect on cardiac muscle.
- Recently it has also been used in treatment of ***acute pancreatitis*** due to inhibitory effect on exocrine secretion of pancreas.

SOMATOSTATIN

The peptide somatostatin (also called as "GH release inhibiting factor") was first isolated from the hypothalamus and was ***implicated as a regulator of GH secretion.***

Chemistry: It is a peptide consisting of 14 amino acids. There is an intrachain S-S linkage joining cycteine 3 and cysteine at position 14.

```
            3                      14
H-Ala-Gly-Cys                  Cys-OH
            |                      |
            |_______ S-S __________|
```

Source: There are three sources of somatostatin

- *Hypothalamus:* As stated above.
- *Pancreas:* Somatostatin is also ***secreted by δ-cells of islet of Langerhans*** of pancreas.
- *GI tract:* It is ***also produced by D-cells of antral mucosa of stomach*** and also duodenal mucosa.

The above suggest that the hypothalamic releasing hormones may actually be more widely distributed.

Functions: In contrast to 'telecrine' action of hypothalamic somatostatin on anterior pituitary, the GI somatostatin has local "paracrine" actions limited to GI mucosa and pancreas.

1. *Hypothalamic Somatostatin:*
   - Acts as a regulator of Growth hormone secretion.
   - *It inhibits GH release*
   - It may also serve as a neurotransmitter substance in the brain.
2. *Pancreatic Somatostatin*

It ***inhibits both insulin and glucagon secretion and thus may serve as an "intraislet" (paracrine) regulator of secretion of these hormones.*** Thus acts as intraorgan "synaptic transmitters" or neuromodulators.

- Somatostatin is secreted into the portal vein blood as a result of glucose or amino acid stimulus indicating extraislet role.
- Also directly inhibits secretion of both HCO_3^- and enzymes in pancreatic juice.

3. *GI Somatostatin:*

- It ***inhibits the secretions of gastrin, CCK, GIP and motilin.***
- It also inhibits gastric acid secretion, secretion of Brunner's glands, pancreatic HCO_3^- and enzyme secretions, gastric emptying and gallbladder contraction.

☞ SALIENT POINTS TO REMEMBER

- The endocrine function of Pancreas is located in ***"islet of Langerhans."***
- β-cells of islet of Langerhans produces the hormone Insulin. It is a protein hormone, consists of two Polypeptide chains 'A' chain (21 a.a) and 'B'-chain (30 a.a) joined by disulphide bridges.
- It is an anabolic hormone and plays an important role in metabolism causing increased carbohydrate metabolism viz. increased glucose utilization by tissues, glycogenesis and glycogen storage, increased FA synthesis and TG storage and increased amino acid uptake and protein synthesis.
- Insulin is produced in β-cells as pre-pro-hormone (109 a.a) which is converted to pro-insulin (86 a.a) by signal peptidase and then to Insulin (51 a.a) by protease enzyme.
- Insulin is degraded by the enzyme ***"glutathione-insulin transhydrogenase" (insulinase)*** which brings about reductive cleavage of S-S bond.
- α - cells of islets of Langerhans produces the hormone ***'Glucagon'***, a polypeptide containing 29 aminoacids.
- Glucagon has opposite effect of Insulin-it increases blood sugar level (hyperglycaemia) by glycogenolysis in liver and increasing gluconeogenesis.
- Glucagon produces lipolysis in adipose tissue increasing FFA ↑. The hormone decreases protein synthesis.
- Glucagon ***exerts a +ve ionotropic effect on heart without producing increased myocardial irritability.*** Hence glucagon has been used in treatment of heart disease, cardiac failure and cardiogenic shock.
- Recently glucagon has also been used in treatment of acute pancreatitis due to inhibitory effect on exocrine secretions of pancreas.

ADRENAL GLANDS AND ITS HORMONES

Anatomy: Adrenal glands are two semilunar/ or pyramidal structures lying one each on upper pole of both the kidneys. Also called as 'suprarenal glands'. ***Each gland consists of two developmentally and physiologically separate parts:***

- ***Adrenal cortex***
- ***Adrenal medulla consisting 10 percent of the whole gland.***

ADRENAL CORTEX AND STEROID HORMONES

Adrenal cortex occupies outer peripheral portion and is yellowish in colour.

Histologically **three layers or zones** can be differentiated:

- ***Zona glomerulosa:*** Outer most layer consisting whorls of columnar cells,
- ***Zona fasciculata:*** Middle layer-large cuboidal cells arranged in columns separated by venous sinuses. Cells of this layer are very rich in lipids and vitamin C.
- ***Zona reticularis:*** Innermost layer, cells are interlaced to form a network. Poor in lipids and has R.E. cells.
- Cells of all three layers can form the steroid hormone 'corticosterone'. Cells of inner two zones can form 'cortisol' and sex hormones. On the other hand, ***Cells of zona glomeru-losa can synthesize aldosterone only.***

Steroid Hormones Produced by Adrenal Cortex: About 50 steroids have been isolated from the adrenal cortex. But out of them only 7 (seven) are important and known to possess physiologic activity. They are all derived from cholesterol which can be synthesized from "active" acetate, and they contain the steroid nucleus, called ***"cyclo-pentano perhydro phenanthrene" nucleus.*** (Refer to chemistry of cholesterol).

Seven important hormones are given below:

- 11-Dehydrocorticosterone (DOC)—(Earlier called as compound A)
- Corticosterone (Compound B)
- Cortisone (Compound E)
- Cortisol (17-OH corticosterone) (Compound F)
- Aldosterone (mineralo-corticoid)
- Androstenedione } Two androgens
- Dehydroepiandrosterone (DHE) } Two androgens

Cortisol is the major free-circulating adrenocortical hormone (glucocorticoid) in human plasma.

Functional classification: Steroids are divided into ***three types according to function (using Seyle's terminology)***

- ***Gluco-corticoids:*** Which primarily affect metabolism of carbohydrates, proteins and lipids and relatively minor effects on electrolytes and water metabolism, e.g. ***cortisol, cortisone*** and ***corticosterone.***
- ***Mineralocorticoids:*** These primarily affect the reabsorption of Na^+ and excretion of K^+ (Mineral metabolism) and distribution of water in tissues, e.g. ***Aldosterone*** (chief mineralocorticoid). Others are corticosterone, 11-deoxy cortisol and 11-deoxycorticosterone (DOC).

Corticosterone (Compound B) **Cortisol (Compound F)**

- ***Cortical sex hormones:*** (Androgens and estrogens): These primarily affect secondary sex characters.

GLUCOCORTICOIDS

Biosynthesis of Glucocorticoids:

I. ***Common Pathway for all Cortico-steroids:*** Corticosteroids are synthesized by a common pathway from cholesterol in the adrenal cortex. In all the three zones of adrenal cortex,

1. ***Cholesterol is first changed to form pregnenolone (common pathway);***

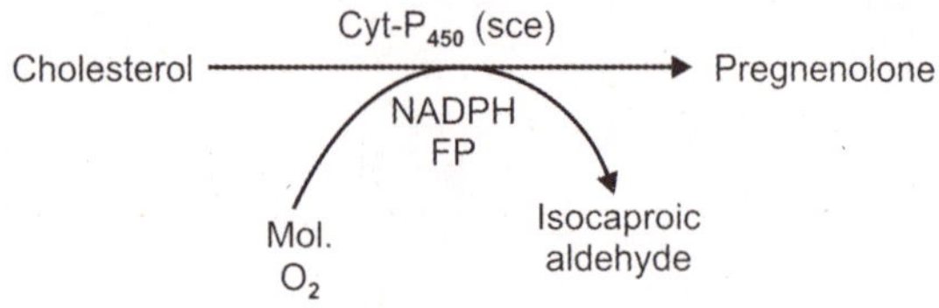

2. *Glucocorticoid synthesis* Glucocorticoids, as mentioned above are synthesized in zona fasciculata cells. Steps are:

- ***Pregnenolone is converted to 17-OH pregnenolone.***
- Conversion of 17-OH pregnenolone to 17 OH progesterone.

- In the next step, 17-OH progesterone is converted to 11-deoxycortisol, catalyzed by the enzyme ***21-hydroxylase*** present in endoplasmic reticulum (E.R).
- Finally, 11-deoxycortisol is acted by the enzyme ***11-β hydroxylase*** and is converted to **'cortisol'**.

Regulation of Glucocorticoids Secretion:

- Cortisol secretion has a ***diurnal rhythm.*** Peak secretion occurs in early morning 4 to 6 AM and decreases at night.
- During a 24-hour period, a normal adult human secretes about 5 to 30 mg of cortisol and 1 to 6 mg of corticosterone.
- Glucocorticoid secretion is stimulated by pituitary corticotropin ACTH which is in turn, regulated by hypothalamic ***"corticotropin-releasing hormone" (CRH)*** and negative "feedback inhibition" by the high blood cortisol ***(See Fig. 22.3).***

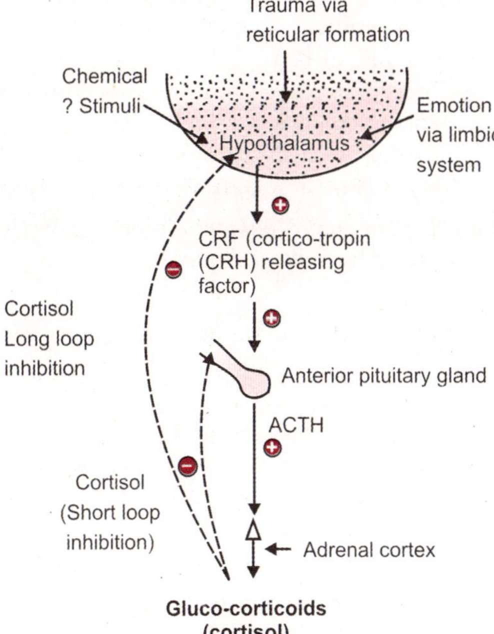

Fig. 22.3: Regulation of secretion of cortisol

Action of ACTH on Steroidogenesis:

- ACTH acts through cyclic AMP. It ***binds to "specific receptors"*** on plasma membrane of fasciculata cells, ***stimulate adenyl cyclase and increases c-AMP level;*** for this action it requires the presence of Ca^+
- ***c-AMP acts as 'second messenger"*** to modify activities of many enzymes including some ***protein kinases,*** leading to increase in DNA, increases transcription of RNA and protein synthesis in cells.
- ACTH stimulates the synthesis and secretion of glucocorticoids.
- ACTH increases the conversion of cholesterol to pregnenolone, the ***"rate-limiting" step.***

Mechanism of Action:

- All of the steroids act primarily at the level of cell nucleus ('nuclear' action) to increase mRNA synthesis and increased protein synthesis.
- The first step occurs within minutes, which involves the binding of the steroids to a corresponding specific *"receptor protein"* present in cytosol.
- Gluco-corticoid binds to the 'specific' receptor in cytosol to 'steroid binding site'. This changes the conformation of receptor/ protein and exposes the "DNA-binding domain".
- The steroid-receptor complex now enters the nucleus, and binds by DNA-binding site to the ***"Hormone-responsive element (HRE)*** of specific nuclear genes. This modulates the transcription rate of the those genes, leading to increased synthesis of many proteins and enzymes and also to decreased synthesis of some proteins like corticotrophin.

Plasma Level: In the resting state: Plasma contains 5 to 15 μg/100 ml of cortisol (average 12 μg%) There is a marked 'diurnal' variation. In humans, the level of plasma cortisol is highest in early morning at 4 AM and lowest in the night. This is related with cyclic variations in secretions of ACTH. Plasma corticosterone level varies from 0.04 to 2.0 μg/100 ml (average =1.0 μg%).

Transport: Under conditions of normal plasma cortisol concentration, only about 10% (approx. 0.5 to 0.8 μg) is in 'free' active state and 90% being bound to proteins. Out of protein bound, 30% is bound to albumin and 60% (approx. 10 to 15 µg) is bound to a specific cortisol-binding protein, an α_2 globulin, called ***"Transcortin"***. Transcortin also carries corticosterone and de-oxycorticosterone as well. At concentrations, exceeding the binding capacity of transcortin (approx. 20 µg/100 ml), the proportions bound to albumin and 'free' state increases.

Catabolism:

- *Inactivated in liver*
- *Converted to tetrahydroderivatives,* which are conjugated with glucuronic acid and excreted as soluble glucuronides in urine.

Adrenal Androgens

Main hormones are:

- *Dehydro epiandrosterone (DHEA)*
- *DHEA-SO_4*
- *Δ^4-Androstenedione*
- *11-β-OH-Androstenedione*

Note: Salient Points—regarding adrenal androgens are:

- DHEA and DHEA-SO_4 are freely interconvertible.
- Δ^4-Androstenedione is derived from DHEA.
- *Androstenedione is the precursor of testosterone,* more potent male hormone.
- A proportion of androstenedione may be converted to 11-β-OH androstenedione, a much weaker androgen.
- *In Plasma: 5% occur in 'free' form, which is nonprotein bound and freely diffusible.*
- 95% is reversibly bound to plasma albumin.
- Inactivation takes place in Liver.

Actions of Glucocorticoids

I. Metabolic Actions

Points to note:

- In general, glucocorticoids have ***antiinsulin effect.***
- *Glucocorticoids are catabolic to peripheral tissues and anabolic to liver.*

1. *Effects on carbohydrate metabolism*

Overall effect: increases blood glucose ↑ level (Hyperglycaemia)

Mechanism of hyperglycaemia:

- Decreases glucose uptake ↓ and utilization in muscles, and other tissues.
- Enhancing gluconeogenesis ↑ in liver.
- Decreases glycolysis ↓ in peripheral tissues.

In liver: Glucocorticoids are anabolic. It increases the glycogen store ↑ in liver.

2. *Effects on Lipid metabolism*

Net effect increases FFA ↑ in plasma and also glycerol.

Glycerol is utilized for gluconeogenesis in liver.

- ***In adipocytes:*** Glucocorticoids increases 'Lipolysis' and liberates FFA and glycerol by activating ***hormone sensitive TG Lipase.***

3. *Effects on Protein metabolism*

In peripheral extrahepatic tissues,cortisol is catabolic and increases protein breakdown, leading to increased 'amino acids' availability in plasma.

- ***In liver: Cortisol is anabolic,*** it increases protein synthesis ↑. It increases:
  - Hepatic uptake of amino acids ↑.
  - Incorporation of amino acids into ribosomal proteins.
  - Increased mRNA formation and synthesis of protein including plasma proteins.

Overall effect on protein metabolism by cortisol is "Negative Nitrogen balance".

Summary:

1. Action on 'Peripheral' tissues like muscles, adipose tissue and Lymphoid tissue is **'catabolic'** ("spares" glucose)
   - Glucose uptake ↓ and glycolysis ↓
   - Lipolysis ↑, FFA in plasma ↑, glycerol in plasma ↑, esterification, i.e. T.G. formation ↓, a-Glycero-p ↓
   - Protein synthesis ↓, protein breakdown ↑, plasma aminoacids ↑.
2. Action on Liver. is **anabolic**
   - Gluconeogenesis ↑, from amino acids and glycerol. Glycogen in Liver ↑ increased.
   - Protein synthesis in Liver cells ↑ enhanced.

II. Other Actions

1. *Permissive Action:* Small amount of glucocorticoid is required for a number of metabolic reactions to occur.
    - Required for adipokinetic activity of G.H.
    - Required for calorigenic action of glucagon and catecholamines.

2. *Anti-inflammatory Action:* Normal cortisol level does not affect; but therapeutic doses exert an anti-inflammatory effect.

Three basic mechanisms by which glucocorticoids exert anti-inflammatory effects are:

- ***Action on Lysosomes:*** Stabilizes cell membrane of lysosomes and thus blocks the release of lysosomal hydrolases.
- ***Action on Kinin formation:*** Prevents formation of bradykinin which is produced by action of Kallikrein, a proteolytic enzyme on α-globulin.
- ***Action on Capillaries:*** Decreases permeability of capillary walls and prevent protein leakage.

Clinical Aspect

Based on above, ***steroids have been used as anti-inflammatory drugs in treatment of Rheumatoid arthritis,*** Rheumatic fever and acute glomerulo nephritis.

3. *Immunosuppressive Effect:* Cortisol decreases immune response associated with infections and allergic states.

Clinical Aspect

Based on above, glucocorticoids have been ***used in organ transplantation*** as it prevents graft rejection. Being anti-allergic, it is also ***used for treatment of bronchial asthma and status asthmaticus.***

4. *Effect on Exocrine Secretion:* Chronic and prolonged treatment with glucocorticoids causes:
    - Increased secretion of HCl ↑,
    - Increased secretion of pepsinogen ↑ in stomach, and
    - Also increases trypsinogen ↑ secretion in pancreatic juice.

Clinical Aspect

In prolonged treatment with glucocorticoids the patient ***may develop GI ulcers.***

5. *Effect on Bones:* Glucocorticoids reduce the osteoid matrix of bone, thus favouring ***osteoporosis*** and there may be excessive loss of calcium from the body.

Clinical Aspect

Osteoporosis is a major complication of prolonged glucocorticoid therapy.

6. *Haematological Changes:* Large doses of glucocorticoids and in hypertrophy of adrenal cortex, the hormone brings about destruction of "Lymphocytes" and also shift to lymphocytes to lymphoid tissues producing ***"Lymphopenia".*** Also there is ***reduction in circulating monocytes and eosinophils.***

ABNORMAL PHYSIOLOGY OF ADRENAL CORTEX

1. **Hypoadrenocorticism:** It produces **Addison's disease.**

Causes: Results from failure of adrenal cortices to produce adrenocortical hormones, and this is caused by:

- Primary atrophy of adrenal cortex, so called ***Idiopathic (auto-immune disorder),*** >53% show circulating auto-antibodies.
- ***Tuberculosis:*** Tuberculous destruction of gland.
- ***Malignancy:*** Invasion of adrenal cortices by cancer cells.

Other rarer causes are:

- Amyloidosis
- Fungus infection (Torulosis and coccidiomycosis)
- Haemosiderosis and
- Leukaemic infiltrations.

Clinical Features and Biochemical Changes:

1. ***Due to mineralocorticoid deficiency:*** Lack of aldosterone secretion causes:
    - Decreases Na^+ reabsorption. As a result Na^+ ions, Cl^- and water are lost in urine in greater amounts.
    - The above leads to greatly decreased ECF volume ↓.

- The individual develops *acidosis* because of failure of H^+ ions to be secreted in exchange for Na^+ reabsorption.
- As the ECF volume becomes depleted,
  - Plasma volume falls ↓.
  - RB cells concentration increases ↑ leading to haemoconcentration.
  - And cardiac output decreases ↓
- Reduced urinary NPN ↓ and K^+ ↓
- **Blood:** Hyponatraemia and hyperkalaemia.

If mineralocorticoid is not replaced, the patient dies from shock. Death usually occurring 4 to 7 days after complete cessation of mineralocorticoid activity.

2. *Due to Glucocorticoid Deficiency:*

- Loss of cortisol secretion makes it impossible to maintain normal blood glucose concentration in between meals, because the patient cannot synthesize significant quantities of glucose by "gluconeogenesis" which is hampered. The above contributes to *"hypoglycaemia"* tendency.
- Lack of cortisol reduces the mobilization of both proteins and fats from peripheral tissues, thereby depressing many other metabolic functions in the body.

  Note: Lack of adequate glucocorticoid secretion also makes the patient highly susceptible to the deteriorating effects of 'stress' and even mild respiratory infection can assume severe and can sometimes cause death.
- *Melanin Pigmentation:* A characteristic feature, patients develop abnormal bronze pigmentation of skin and mucous membranes.

II. Hyperadrenocorticism: Increased secretion of corticoids.

Causes: Adrenocortical hyperfunction may be caused by:

- Benign or malignant tumors of the adrenal cortex, or
- Adrenocortical hyperplasia initiated by increased production of ACTH.

Types:

- Congenital
- Acquired

1. *Congenital Form:* ***Congenital forms are always due to hyperplasia,*** termed as ***"congenital virilizing hyperplasia'*** when it is present at birth, and ***"Adrenogenital syndrome"***, when it occurs in postnatal period. Under the influence of excess androgens, females assume male secondary sex characteristics. When it occurs in males, there is excessive masculinization. Ferminizing adrenal tumours may rarely occur in males.

2. *Acquired:* ***Cushing's Disease and Cushing's Syndrome:***

Causes: Adreno cortical hyperfuntion may be caused:

- Benign or malignant tumours of the cortex, and
- Adrenocortical hyperplasia initiated by increased production of ACTH.

To distinguish between the two etiologic forms of the disease, pituitary and adrenal the following terms are used.

- The term ***Cushing's disease*** has been restricted to those cases which are of **pituitary origin,** i.e. due to pituitary basophilism.
- The term ***Cushing's Syndrome:*** Denotes adrenal cortical hyperfunction directly ***in volving the adrenal gland.***
- *"Cushingoid state":* Both cortisol and ACTH when adminstered for prolonged periods due to treatment induce **"Cushingoid state"**, which is reversible when these agents are discontinued.

Clinical features and biochemical findings:

- *Adiposity:* Rapidly increasing adiposity of the face, neck and trunk-plethoric ***'Moon' face*** and ***Buffalo-fat distribution.***
- ***Purple striae on abdomen,*** atrophic and cracking skin (due to excessive protein breakdown and its Loss).
- Mascular Wasting and asthenia.
- Impaired carbohydrate metabolism and excessive gluconeogenesis ↑, leading to ***hyperglycaemia*** and glycosuria (Insulin resistance and Non-ketotic D.M.).
- ***Osteoporosis*** due to decalcification and protein loss.

- ***Hypertension:*** Increased BP ↑
- ***Blood:*** Shows polycythaemia, eosinopenia, and lymphocytopenia. Tendency to develop purpura.
- Sodium level ↑ is increased, while K^+ ↓ is lowered, leading to ***alkalosis.***
- Increased protein catabolism and –ve nitrogen balance
- In females, there is amenorrhoea and sometimes signs of hirsutism, i.e. appearance of beard and moustache.
- Sex functions-depressed with impotence in males and sterility in females.
- Urinary excretion of 17-oxosteroids ↑ and 17-OH-steroids ↑ is increased.

MINERALOCORTICOIDS

Mineralocorticoids are C_{21} steroids, which influence mainly the metabolism of Na^+ and K^+. the chief mineralocorticoid is ***Aldosterone. It is produced by Zona glomerulosa of the adrenal cortex.*** Structurally, it bears a-OH gr. at C-11 and an aldehyde (-CHO) group at C-18.

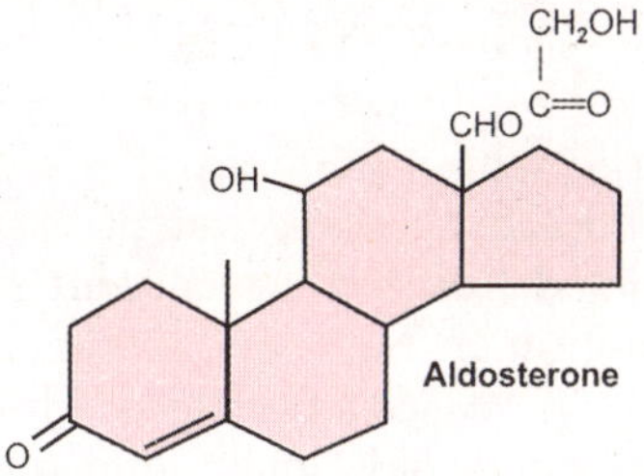

CH_2OH | C=O, CHO, OH, O

Aldosterone

Other corticosteroids which have mineralocorticoid activity are:

- Corticosterone
- 11-Deoxycortisol
- 11-Deoxy corticosterone (DOC) is secreted in minute quantities and has almost the same effects as aldosterone, but a potency only 1/30th that of aldosterone.

Biosynthesis: ***Mineralcorticoids are synthesized in Zonaglomerulosa cells only.*** They cannot be synthesized in other two layers of adrenal cortex. ***Only Zonaglomerulosa cells have the enzymes 18 hydroxylase and 18-hydroxysteroid dehydrogenase, which are lacking in other layers.***

Steps in Synthesis:

- Cholesterol is converted to pregnenolone. Pregnenolone is then converted to progesterone in smooth ER catalyzed by the enzymes ***3-β-OH-steroid dehydrogenase and $\Delta^{4,5}$-isomerase.***
- Progesterone is then directly hydroxylated by the enzyme ***21-hydroxylase*** and forms 11-deoxy-corticosterone (DOC).
- 11-deoxycorticosterone is next ***translocated to mitochondrion*** where it is converted to corticosterone, the reaction is catalyzed by the enzyme ***11-β-hydroxylase.***
- In the next step, by the enzyme ***18-hydroxylase,*** corticosterone is converted to 18-OH corticosterone, which is then acted upon by a dehydrogenase.

Secretion and Transport: Human adrenal cortex secretes approximately 30 to 75 µg of aldosterone per 24 hours. A diurnal variation is seen-its secretion rises in day hours with activity and erect posture as compared to night when rate of secretion decreases.

Plasma level: 0.03 to 0.08 µg of aldosterone/100 ml of plasma (average 0.05 µg%). It is carried weakly bound to serum albumin.

Mechanism of Action: ***Nuclear action:*** Similar ***to glucocorticoids.***

ACTIONS

1. **Renal Effects of Aldosterone:**

- ***Effect on Tubular Reabsorption of Sodium:*** By far the ***most important effect of aldosterone and other mineralcorticoids is to increase the rate of tubular reabsorption of Na.***
- ***Effect on tubular reabsorption of chlorides:*** Aldosterone also increases the reabsorption of Cl^- ions from the tubules. This probably occurs secondarily to the increased Na reabsorption.
- ***Increased renal excretion of K^+:*** It ***increases loss of K^+ in the urine by the renal distal tubules and collecting ducts.*** This may result from the elimination of K^+ in exchange of the reabsorbed Na^+ due to the adlosterone stimulated activity of the 'sodium pump'.

Clinical Significance

Hypokalaemia and muscle paralysis-The loss of K^+ in urine decreases K^+ in ECF resulting in ***hypokalaemia.*** Thus at the same time that Na^+ and Cl^- ions become increased in ECF, there will be gross decrease in K^+ ions. The low K^+ concentration sometimes leads to ***muscle paralysis***-this is caused by hyperpolarization of the nerve and muscle fibre membrane which prevents transmission of action potentials.

- *Effect on acid-base balance* **(Alkalosis):** A large proportion of Na^+ reabsorption from the tubules results from an exchange reaction in which H^+ ions are secreted into the tubules to take the place of Na^+ that is reabsorbed. Hence, when the rate of Na^+ reabsorption is enhanced, in response to aldosterone, the H^+ concentration in the body fluids is reduced. ***For each Na^+ ion reabsorption by H^+ exchange, one HCO_3^- ion enters the ECF which shifts the reaction to alkaline side.*** Thus, ***increased secretion of aldosterone promotes alkalosis. Whereas decreased secretion produces acidosis.***

2. Effects of Aldosterone on Fluid Volume and CV Dynamics

- *Effect on ECF volume:* Mineralocorticoids greatly increase the quantities of Na^+, Cl^-, and HCO_3^- ions in the ECF. This in turn increases water reabsorption from the tubules by:
  - Stimulating the hypothalamic ADH system, and
  - Creating an osmotic gradient across the tubular membrane. When the electrolytes are absorbed, carries water through the membrane in the wake of electrolytes absorption.

Also increased electrolyte concentration of ECF causes thirst, thereby making the person to drink excessive amount of water. *Hence, the final result is an increase in ECF volume* ↑, sometimes enough to cause generalized oedema.

Note: *ECF volume must increase about 30% before frank oedema appears.*

Effect on blood volume: The plasma volume ↑ increases almost proportionally during the early part of increase in ECF volume.

- *Effect on cardiac output.* When aldosterone secretion is excessive, the resultant increase in ECF volume and blood volume tends to increase the cardiac output. The cardiac output rarely rises more than 10 to 20%.
- *Effect on arterial blood pressure:* Excess secretion of aldosterone usually causes moderate to marked hypertension.

3. Effects of Aldosterone on Sweat Glands, Salivary Glands and Gastric Mucosa: The mineralocorticoids have almost the same effect on the sweat glands, salivary glands, intestinal glands as on the renal tubules, greatly reducing the loss of Na^+ and Cl^- in the glandular secretions.

Regulation of Aldosterone Secretion

Primary Factors that Stimulate Aldosterone Secretion: In normal person the rate of aldosterone secretion is automatically regulated to the level required to maintain normal Na^+ concentration in the ECF and normal ECF volume. To perform these functions, the rate of aldosterone secretion is responsive to the following changes:

1. *Increased K^+ concentration of Plasma:* A 10% change in K^+ (about 0.5 mEq/l) is required to effect a 2-fold change in secretion.
2. *Decreased Sodium concentration:* Only 10% reduction in Na^+ concentration (about 14 mEq/I) increases the rate of aldosterone secretion about 2-fold almost immediately and perhaps much more than this if the stimulus is continued for several days.

Note: It is the ratio of Na: K that regulates aldosterone secretion.

3. *Decreased ECF volume, Hypovolaemia, and hypotension:* These act in a similar manner like Na^+ depletion, increases the rate of aldosterone synthesis. This effect is also mediated through angiotensin II.

Basic Mechanisms

Three theories have been put forward.

- *Direct stimulation*, of the adrenal cortex to regulate its output.

- ***Renin-angiotensin system:*** Regulation by angiotensin II.
- ***Neuro secretory regulation*** of adrenocortical output ***(Refer Fig. 22.4).***

1. Renin-Angiotensin System:

JG Cells: Afferent arteriole of nephron (vascular Pole?) show cytoplasmic granules which contain an enzyme called ***Renin*** (granules are secretory vesicles for renin).

Factors for Release of Renin:

- A fall in sodium concentration, hypovolaemia, hypotension and a fall in intracellular Ca^{++} stimulate release of "renin" from JG cells to blood.
- Bradykinin and glucagon also stimulate release of renin.

Chemistry: Renin is a proteolytic enzyme, Mol. Weight=35,000.

Action of Renin

(a) Formation of Angiotensin I:

- Renin acts on a plasma substrate, an α_2-globulin, called ***'angiotensinogen'*** or ***'hypertenstinogen'***, which is produced by liver.
- The enzyme cleaves the "Leucyl-Leucyl" bond between 10 and 11 position from N-terminal end to produce ***"Angiotensin I"*** a decapeptide and a polypeptide having >400 amino acids ('inactive').

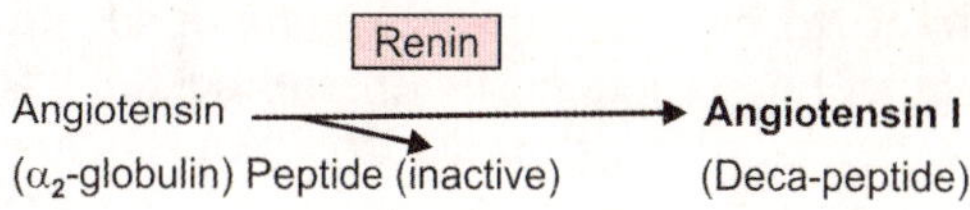

This is the ***'rate-limiting'*** step. Cortisol and β-estradiol enhances this reaction, ***probably by increasing hepatic synthesis of "angiotensinogen".***

(b) Formation of Angiotensin II:

- ***Angiotensin I, a decapeptide,*** having a molecular weight of 1296, while circulating, is acted upon by another enzyme, called ***converting enzyme (a protease)*** which occurs on the walls of small vessels of lung.
- ***The enzyme is Ca^{++} dependent,*** and ***it removes terminal Histidyl-Leucyl" dipeptide,*** in pulmonary circulation, forming ***'Angiotensin II',*** an octapeptide, molecular weight=1046 and an inactive dipeptide.
- ***Angiotensin II is the "active" component which acts on Zona glomerulosa cells to increase synthesis of aldosterone*** and increases rate of release of the hormone.
- ***Inactivation of angiotensin II:*** An enzyme ***angiotensinase,*** an amino-peptidase, present in kidney, intestine and blood inactivates angiotensin II by hydrolysis.

c. ***Angiotensin III.*** Recently in rats, heptapeptide angiotensin III has been isolated. It is

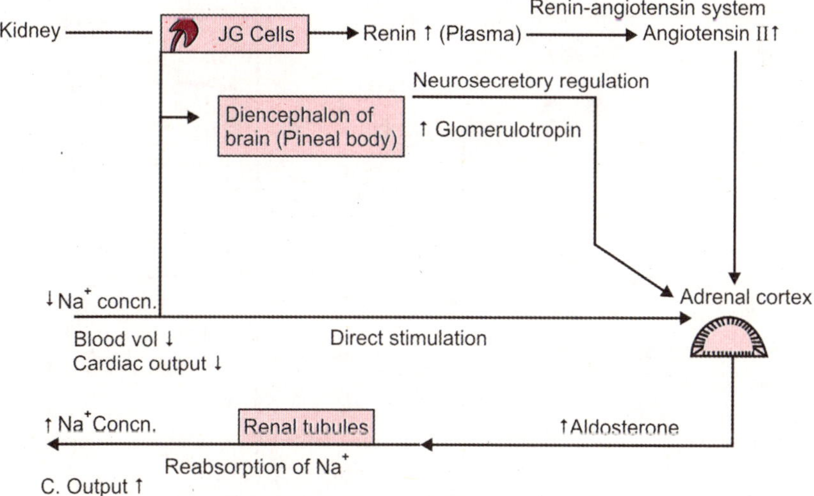

Fig. 22.4: Mechanisms of aldosterone secretion

claimed to be present in humans also. Both heptapeptide (angiotensin III) and octa peptide (angiotensin II) are claimed to be equipotent in stimulating aldosterone secretion. *(See Fig. 22.5)*.

Feedback inhibition of renin: ***Aldosterone can 'inhibit' the enzyme 'renin' by "feed-back" inhibition*** so that angiotensin II formation is decreased.

Inactivation of Renin: In addition to "feedback" inhibition by aldosterone

- Renin is also destroyed by cephalin derivative in plasma and
- Also inhibited by a lysophospholipid, liberated by the action of *phospholipase* A_2.

Action of Angiotensin II: Principal action is angiotensin II stimulates aldosterone synthesis in Zona glomerulosa cells and increases rate of secretion of aldosterone.

Mechanism of action and effects: Angiotensin II binds with specific "receptor" on membrane of Zona glomerulosa cells and

- Enhances cytosolic concentration of Ca^{++} ions ↑ in cells, and
- Formation of "inositol-1,4,5-triphosphate".

The above act as 'second messenger" and in turn,

- Enhances conversion of cholesterol to Pregnenolone,
- And corticosterone to aldosterone by increasing the activity of *18-hydroxylase.*

Aldosterone thus formed and secreted:

- Increases the active tubular reabsorption of Na^+, and
- Consequently, 'Passive' reabsorption of Cl^- and water.

Renal retention of water restores the falling ECF volume and helps in long-term increase of arterial BP.

ABNORMAL PHYSIOLOGY-ALDOSTERONISM

Increased secretion of aldosterone.

Type: **Two types:**

- ***Primary aldosteronism***
- ***Secondary aldosteronism.***

1. Primary Aldosteronism (Conn's Syndrome):

This results from tumours of adrenals, an adenoma, called ***"aldosteronoma"***—hyperactivity of adrenal cortex is confined to excess production of aldosterone.

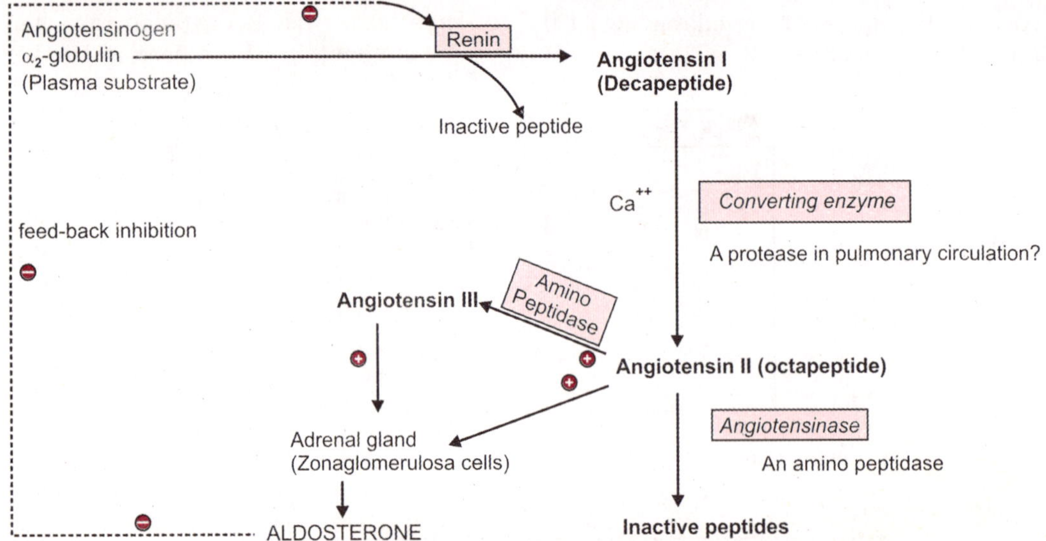

Fig. 22.5: Showing formation of angiotensin II

Clinical Features and Biochemical Findings:

- Salient changes in the blood are:
  - Increased Na^+ retention,
  - Severe K^+ depletion, and
  - Alkalosis
- Na^+ retention causes:
  - Hypertension which may result in congestive cardic failure without oedema.
- K^+ depletion and
- Alkalosis gives rise to periodic muscle weakness and intermittent 'tetany'.

Failure of renal tubules to respond to ADH causes polyuria and polydypsia.

Diagnosis:

- Aldosterone excretion in urine, particularly after Na^+ loading is helpful in establishing the diagnosis.
- A consistently low level of K^+ in the serum is a characteristic finding in primary hyperaldosteronism.
- The administration of aldosterone antagonist *'spironolactone'* (Aldactone) restores serum K^+ to normal levels.

2. Secondary Hyperaldosteronism: In this condition adrenal cortex is not affected, but the hypersecretion of aldosterone is due to other factors, like conditions associated with excessive Na^+ and water loss such as:

- *Congestive heart failure*
- *Cirrhosis liver, and*
- *Nephrotic syndrome.*

In such situations there may be hyperactivity of renin-angiotensin system due to low Na^+ concentration.

ADRENAL MEDULLARY HORMONES

Anatomy and Physiology:

- The cells of adrenal medulla are large, ovoid and columnar in type and called as ***pheochromocytes.*** The cells are grouped in clumps around the blood vessels.
- The adrenal medulla is derived from the primitive cells of the neural crest, which migrate into the centre of foetal adrenal cortex forming medulla.
- Most of the cells contain fine granules which are coloured brown by chrome salts, giving so called ***"chromaffin reaction"*** which is due to oxidation of the hormones and their precursors in granules.
- Active principles of adrenal medulla are ***'catecholamines'.***
  - *Adrenaline (Epinephrine)* and
  - *Noradrenaline (Nor-epinephrine)*
- In humans, adrenal medulla contains 80% of epinephrine and 20% norepinephrine. In early foetal life, only norepinephrine is produced (epinephrine cannot be produced due to absence of enzyme *methyl transferase).* The proportion of epinephrine steadily increases after birth and norepinephrine declines.

Chemistry: ***Two biologically active compounds*** have been isolated from the adrenal medulla and synthesized. They are:

- ***Epinephrine (Adrenaline or Adrenine)***
- ***Norepinephrine (Noradrenaline or Arterenol)***

- The above two hormones are called catecholamines and are closely related to tyrosine and ***synthesized in body from tyrosine.***
- Their structures are shown below:

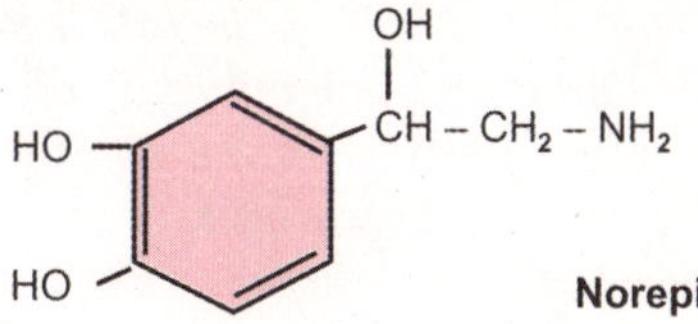

Norepinephrine

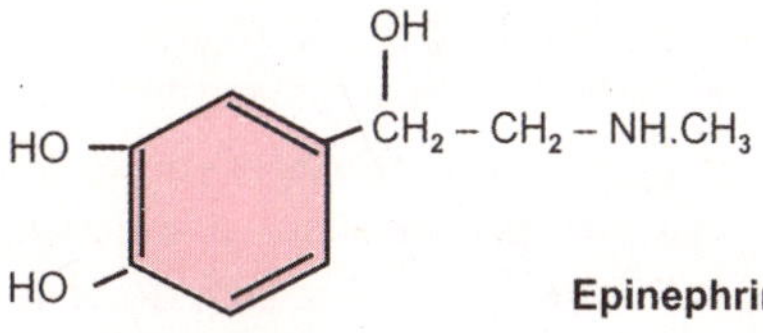

Epinephrine

Epinephrine differs from tyrosine in following respects:

- Contains an additional phenolic-OH gr. in meta-position to benzene ring.

- Additional-OH gr. attached to β-carbon of the sidechain
- Has no-COOH gr.
- Has a-CH_3 gr. attached to N-atom in side chain.

- Epinephrine is primarily synthesized and stored in adrenal medulla. Norepinephrine is primarily synthesized in sympathetic nervous system and acts locally as a 'neurotransmitter' at the postsynaptic cell. Norepinephrine is also synthesized and stored in adrenal medulla.

Biosynthesis: In adrenal pheochromocytes and neuronal cells, the synthesis of catecholamines is essentially same. Both are produced from the amino acid tyrosine.

(For details of synthesis see Metabolic role of tyrosine in protein metabolism)

Storage:

- Epinephrine, norepinephrine and Dopamine are stored in the form of granules, 0.1 to 0.5 μ in diameter, in the pheochromocytes of adrenal medulla.
- Norepinephrine only occurs in adrenergic nerve terminals as granules/or vesicles 400 to 500 Å in diameter, and some is probably free in the cytoplasm.

Both the hormones are stored in the granules in the adrenal medulla and in adrenergic neurones ***as a complex containing ATP in the ratio, about 4 molecules of hormones: one molecule of ATP*** and in combination with several incompletely characterized proteins like ***chromogenin A*** and ***chromomembrin B.***

Release: The release of catecholamines from the cells of the adrenal medulla is brought about by the action of acetylcholine released by stimulation of the preganglionic fibres of the splanchnic nerve. ***Acetylcholine acts by promoting the entry of Ca^{2+} ions (influx) which then release catecholamines from granules.***

Transport: Epinephrine and norepinephrine are present in the blood plasma both in free and conjugated (sulfate or glucuronides) forms. Epinephrine is almost completely bound to plasma proteins chiefly albumin and norepinephrine is to a lesser extent. ***Catecholomines do not cross the blood-brain barrier.***

Clinical Importance

As catecholamines cannot penetrate blood-brain barrier, the norepineph-rine in the brain must be synthesized within that tissue. 'L-DOPA', the precursor of catecholamines does penetrate the barrier. It is, hence, ***used to increase brain catecholamine synthesis in Parkinson's disease.***

Adrenergic Receptors:

Site of action of catecholamines on postsynaptic membrane: The catecholamines released from the adrenal medulla enter the blood stream and carried long distances to the target cells on which they act.

The norepinephrine released at presynaptic adrenergic nerve terminals has only to pass across a gap 200 to 1000 Å before making contact with postsynaptic membranes of the innervated cells.

On the membranes of the smooth muscle and cardiac muscle which are innervated by sympathetic there are two kinds of adrenergic receptors:

- *α-receptor:* ***Being concerned mainly with excitatory effects.***
- *β-receptors:* ***Which have inhibitory effects on smooth muscles*** and ***excitatory effects on heart muscle.***

At physiological concentrations:

- *Norepinephrine:* Combines with and acts more on α-receptors than β-receptors.
- *Epinephrine:* Can combine and act on both α and β receptors equally. Typical norepinephrine stimulated responses such as a vascular venous constriction are denoted as α-adrenergic. Typical epinephrine effects such as increased heart rate ↑ and atrial contractility are β-phenomenon (β-effect)

α Blockers: α-adrenergic receptors are blocked by phentolamine and ergot alkaloids competitively and by phenoxy benzamine-non-competitively. Of α-adrenoreceptors, α_1 and α_2 receptors are blocked selectively by Prazosin and Yohimbine respectively.

β-Blockers: β-adrenergic receptors are blocked by β-blockers such as propanolol, pronethalol. β_1 receptor is selectively blocked by practolol and β_2 receptor by butoxamine.

Metabolism

The secreted catecholamines are metabolized in the target tissue or the liver.

1. ***Re-uptake Mechanism for Norepinephrine:*** Norepinephrine can be taken up again into the vesicles of neuronal cells by ***an energy-dependant process.*** This ***re-uptake into the neurones converts norepinephrine to the inactive storage form*** and ***constitutes an important mechanism for quickly terminating hormonal/or neurotransmitter activity.*** This process accounts for inactivation of about 85% of released norepinephrine. This reuptake is performed, against a ***concentration gradient*** of 10,000 to 1 and is affected by an active membrane transport mechanism in the oxonal membrane.

2. ***Fate of Circulating Catecholamines***

- When radio-tagged epinephrine is injected into animals, only about 5% is excreted in urine as such (unchanged).
- Remaining part of hormones are mostly metabolized in tissues by either
  - ***Methylations of phenolic group*** or
  - ***Oxidations on the amino side chains.***

Two enzymes are involved in above reactions:

1. ***Mono-amine oxidase (MAO):*** For ***oxidation reactions.***
   - It is a ***mitochondrial enzyme*** (probably a series of isoenzymes).
   - Has broad specificity of action and capable of catalyzing oxidation of side chains on a large variety of catechols.

2. ***Catechol-O-methyl transferase (COMT):*** Brings about methylation of phenolic-OH gr. at 3-position.
   - It is a Mg^{2+} dependant enzyme and is ***cytosolic***
   - This enzyme capable of methoxylating a variety of catecholamines intermediates with the help of "Active" methionine which acts as a CH_3 group donor.

Although MAO and COMT are found in most tissues, their activity is particularly high in the liver, where most of the circulating catecholamines are degraded.

The ***first step in catabolism can be either,***

- ***Methoxylation*** or
- ***Oxidation of the side chain.***

The preferred step varies with the circumstances not yet delineated.

Norepinephrine which is tightly bound to tissues is initially acted upon by mitochondrial MAO, whereas the less tightly bound component is intially methoxylated by COMT. ***Degradation products are e xcreted in urine.***

Metabolites in Urine: One of the principal metabolites of epinephrine and norepinephrine which occurs in the urine is ***"4-OH-3-methoxy mandelic acid" [also called as vanil mandelic acid (VMA)].***

Percentage of excretory products in urine are as follows:

• Unchanged catecholamines	= 5 to 6%
• ***3-Methoxy epinephrine (Metanephrine)***	= **40%**
• ***VMA (4-OH-3-methoxy Mandelic acid)***	= **41%**
• 4-OH-3-methoxy phenyl glycol	= 7%
• Miscellaneous	= 6%

The urinary metabolites are excreted mostly as conjugated with sulphates or glucuronides; sulphate being preferred conjugated in humans.

Normal Values:

1. *Urine*

- **Epinephrine:** 3 to 35 μg (average 16) daily
- **Norepinephrine:** 25 to 135 μg (average 55) daily
- **Metanephrine and Metanorepinephrine:** Daily excretion in normal persons is less than 1.0 mg.
- **VMA** = 1.8 to 7.1 mg daily.

Note: In pheochromocytomas:

- VMA: Much increased values up to 530 mg per day may be observed.

- Metanephrine and Metanorepinephrine: 3 to 112 mg daily.

2. *Blood:* Varies with methods used,
   - Ethylene diamine method:
     Epinephrine = o to 0.6 μg/litre
     Norepinephrine = 0.5 to 6.5 μg/litre
   - Trihydroxy indole method:
     Epinephrine: 0.05 to 0.2 μg/litre
     Norepinephrine: 0.09 to 0.5 μg/litre

ACTIONS

Metabolic Effects:

1. *Glycogenolysis:*

Liver: Epinephrine stimulates rapid breakdown of glycogen liver (glycogenolysis) producing hyperglycaemia. ***Action is mediated by the following two ways:***

- ***Its binding to β_2 receptors on hepatic cell membrane by increasing cyclic AMP level.***
- ***Also exerts its effect by binding to α_1 receptors on hepatic cell membrane, which increases intracellular Ca^{++} level which acts as second messenger.***

- ***Muscle:*** In muscle, epinephrine also causes breakdown of glycogen (glycogenolysis) by increasing cyclic AMP level (β-effect), but in this tissue it is more active than glucagon. ***Glucagon has very little effect or no effect due to lack of specific receptors.*** In exercising muscle, this can result in increased LA formation, which passes to blood.
- ***Heart muscle:*** increases in cyclic AMP after epinephrine administration is seen in 2 to 4 seconds, the effect of epinephrine on cardiac output (ionotropic effect) is seen shortly afterwards, whereas activation of phosphorylase is not detectable for 45 seconds.

2. *Lipolytic Action:* Both epinephrine and norepinephrine ***increases breakdown of TG in adipose tissue by increasing cyclic-AMP level (β_1 effect). Net effect of lipolysis is rapid release of FFA and glycerol from adipose tissue to blood.***

3. *Gluconeogenic Action:*

- ***Epinephrine increases hepatic gluconeogenesis (β_2 effect).*** Epinephrine increases cyclic AMP which induces the synthesis of key enzymes.
- Increased FFA level in blood produced by lipolytic action can also activate hepatic gluconeogenesis.

4. *Action on Glycolysis:* Epinephrine increases blood LA level by promoting muscle glycolysis, nor-epinephrine has very little effect on blood lactic acid (LA).

5. *Action on Insulin Release:* ***Epinephrine has a direct inhibitory action on insulin release from β-cells of pancreas (α_2 effect).*** Thus, in pancreas, the α-adrenergic response to epinephrine predominates, cyclic-AMP decreases and insulin release is inhibited. However, ***in the presence of an α-blocker, such as "phentolamine" (Regitine), the β-effect predominates and epinephrine causes increased cyclic AMP and increased insulin release.***

ABNORMAL PHYSIOLOGY

Clinical Aspect

No clinical state directly attributable to a deficiency of the adrenal medulla is known. But tumour of the medullary chromaffin cells in adrenal medulla or elsewhere can produce symptoms which simulate those of hyperactivity of adrenal medulla. The tumour is called **'pheochromocytoma'.**

It is characterized by:

- *Abnormal rise in blood pressure,* the hypertension due to pheochromocytoma may be *'Paroxysmal' or sustained.*
- if paroxysmal, in between paroxysms the blood pressure may not be raised.
- *The features of a paroxysm:*
  - Headache, severe palpitations, sweating, nausea and vomiting,
  - Increased depth and rate of breathing, anxiety, weakness and substernal pain,
  - On physical examination, patient looks anxious, skin is pale, cool and moist,
  - Pupils are dilated,
  - Heart rate is usually increased, but in some patients there is bradycardia, extrasystoles may occur,
  - Arterial BP rises considerably-occasionally to 300 and above/200 mm Hg.

- Body temperature is raised.
- There is hyperglycaemia, increased plasma FFA
- BMR is increased.

- The sweating which may be profuse, is due to:
  - Raised body temperature,
  - Central action on the hypothalamic temperature regulating centre, and
  - Possibly due to direct stimulation of sweat glands, by catecholamines.

Nonepinephrine content of adrenal medullary tumors is usually much higher than that of epinephrine.

Laboratory Tests

These include chemical analysis for increased catecholamines in the blood and urine, in particular for urinary VMA the principal metabolite in urine of catecholamines.

Urine: Urinary examination may show presence of glucose (glycosuria).

Difficulty arises in diagnosis in between paroxysms.

The following additional tests can be used.

- ***Phentolamine (Regitine) test:*** Phentolamine is a specific antagonist to norepinephrine. In the presence of sustained hypertension due to pheochromocytoma, the rapid IV injection of phentolamine should produce a sustained fall of BP within 2 to 5 minutes. This test is useful for diagnosis of pheochromocytoma.
- ***Histamine test:*** This is used in paroxysmal hypertension. If hypertension is paroxysmal, attack can be induced artificially by histamine-25 to 50 μg IV, which in normal persons and in essential hypertension produces small fall in BP. But in patients with pheochromocytoma, with the sme dose, marked rise in systolic and diastolic pressure, e.g. 250/170 mm. Hg can occur. The rise can be rapidly reversed by α-adrenergic antagonists.

GONADAL HORMONES

The sex hormones or the gonadal hormones are elaborated by the testes, ovary and corpus luteum mostly, and also in small quantities by the placenta and adrenal cortex. They are all steroid compounds related to cholesterol and are synthesized from that precursor.

Types: **Sex hormones are 3 *types***

- *Androgens or male hormones*
- *Oestrogens or female hormones*
- *Gestogens or progestational hormones*

ANDROGENS

Androgens are hormones capable of producing certain chracteristic musculinizing effects, i.e. they maintain the normal structure and function of the prostate and seminal vesicles and influence the development of secondary male sex characteristics, such as hair distribution and voice.

Chemistry: The naturally occurring androgens in man are:

- *Testosterone*
- *Epiandrosterone (3 β-androsterone)*
- *Androsterone*
- *Dehydroepiandrosterone (DHEA)*

Biosynthesis:

- Androgens are produced in testes (Leydig cells), adrenal cortex, ovary and placenta?
- They may be formed from either acetate ('active' acetate) or cholesterol and pregnenolone being an important intermediate.

Steps of synthesis:

- Cholesterol is converted to pregnenolone in the Leydig cells mitochondria (pathway similar to adrenal cortex). This is the ***'rate limiting'*** step.
- Next pregnenolone is translocated to smooth endoplasmic reticulum where testosterone is synthesized. (Shown in box in next page).

Note: ***Androstenedione is the immediate precursor of testosterone.***

Structure of Testosterone

OH

O

Testosterone

Structure of immediate precursor Androstenedione

Note:

- Circulating DHEA-SO_4 from the adrenal cortex can be converted in the testes to form "free DHEA" by a *sulfatase* enzyme and thus provide an additional source of testosterone precursor.
- ***Active form:*** Testosterone is converted to more "active" and potent form, called ***'Dihydrotestosterone' (DHT)*** in the testes and extratesticular tissues like prostate, seminal vesicles and target tissues. This is achieved by reduction of Δ5- double bond by a *reductase* and NADPH. ***Approximately 0.4 mg of testosterone is reduced daily to 'dihydrotestosterone' (DHT) in testes and extratesticular tissues.***

Plasma Level:

- In normal male, approximately 4 to 12 mg of testosterone is secreted per day.
- Direct measurement of testosterone by isotope dilution and RIA methods:
  Plasma level in males= approx. 0.6 μg %
  and females = approx. 0.03 μg %
- The small amount of testosterone in females, results mainly from peripheral conversion of androstenedione to testosterone by the ovary.
- DHEA is secreted in greater amounts than testosterone in normal men = 10 to 15 mg per day.

Transport: The hormone is transported as follows:

- About 10% bound specially and more tightly to a β-globulin called ***"sex hormone binding globulin" (SHBG) (also called as "Testosterone-estrogen binding globulin", TEBG).***
- About 87 to 89% is transported bound non-specifically to serum albumin.
- Remaining approximately ***1 to 3% circulates in 'active' free form*** which is in equilibrium with the protein-bound form.

Metabolism:

- Testosterone is normally not found in the urine. Following its injection, 15 to 60% (average 35%) of the amount is recovered in urine chiefly as two ***'17-oxosteroids'.***
  - ***Androsterone*** and
  - ***Etiocholanolone,*** with small amounts of Epiandrosterone.
- These metabolites are conjugated in liver and excreted as water-soluble conjugates of sulphates and glucuronides. In addition, DHEA-SO_4 occurs normally in urine in small amounts.

Note:

17-Ketosteroids (17-oxo-steroids): The androgens excreted in urine are classed as ***17-keto-***

Δ^4 Pathway for synthesis of Testosterone

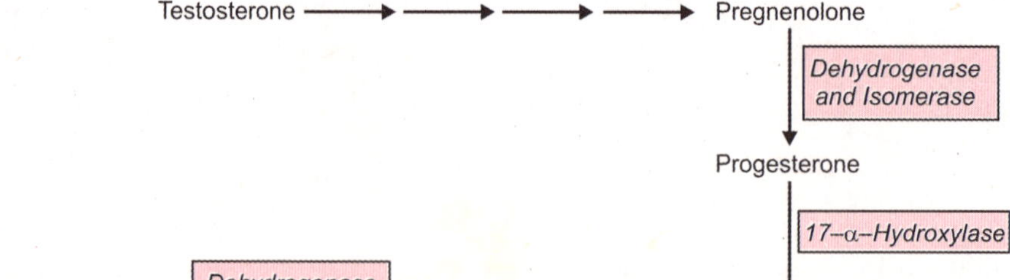

steroids (17-oxo-steroids). In the case of females, it gives an idea about the condition of the adrenal cortex and its functions.

- ***In males:*** 17-ketosteroids arise from testes (1/3 of the total), while the major amount arises from the adrenal cortex (2/3 of total).
- ***In females:*** The 17-ketosteroids are almost entirely from adrenal cortical origin.
- ***Normal value:*** In 24 hours excretion of urine, normal adult males excrete 9 to 24 mg of neutral 17-ketosteroids. Normal adult females excrete 5 to 17 mg.

Metabolic Actions

Both testosterone and dihydrotestosterone are ***protein anabolic and growth promoting hormones.***

1. ***Protein Metabolism:*** Dominant general metabolic effect is stimulation of protein anabolism. This is reflected in:

- A decrease in urinar N_2 (urea) ↓ without an increase in blood NPN.
- ***Creatine metabolism:*** Creatine is virtually absent from the urine of normal men, increases after castration. This increase is abolished by administration of testosterone, owing to increased storage of creatine in the muscles.
- There is ***increase in body weight, due chiefly to an increase in skeletal muscle.***

2. **Protein Synthesis**

- Androgens promote protein synthesis in male accessory glands.
- Androgens also act at the mitochondrial level to increase the respiratory rate, the number of mitochondria and the synthesis of mitochondrial membrane.

3. ***Carbohydrate metabolism: Androgens increase the fructose production*** ↑ by seminal vesicles and utilization of this sugar by the seminal plasma.

4. ***Skeletal growth:*** In the growing organism, a growth spurt is induced with increase in bone matrix and skeletal length. Androgens stimulate the growth of bones before the closure of epiphyseal cartilage. Mineralization of added skeletal tissue is accompained by decreased excretion of Ca and PO_4 i.e. a more +ve balance in respect of these.

5. ***Renotrophic action:*** Androgens cause a rather selective increase in size and weight of the kidneys, ("renotrophic" action).

6. ***Mineral metabolism:*** The decreased excretion of urinary N_2 (chiefly urea) that follows administration of adrogens is accompanied by a lower urine volume and diminished excretion of Na, Cl, K, SO_4 and PO_4, with no increase in their concentration in blood plasma.

- The tissue retention of K, SO_4, PO_4 is probably related to the increased storage of proteins. The retention of Na, CI and water due to increased tubular reabsorption.

Regulation: ***Testosterone secretion is regulated by LH of the anterior pituitary.*** A high blood level of testosterone exert "feedback" inhibition of LH secretion.

FEMALE SEX HORMONES

Two main types of female hormones are secreted by the ovary:

- ***the follicular or estrogenic hormones:*** produced by cells of developing graffian follicles, and
- ***the progestational hormone***-derived from the corpus luteum that is formed in the ovary from the ruptured follicles.

ESTROGENS

Estrogens are hormones capable of producing certain biological effects. The most characteristics of which are the changes which occur in mammals of estrus. They include:

- growth of female genital organs.
- the appearance of female secondary sex characteristics.
- growth of the mammary duct system and numerous other phenomena which vary somewhat in different species.

Structures of Estrogens

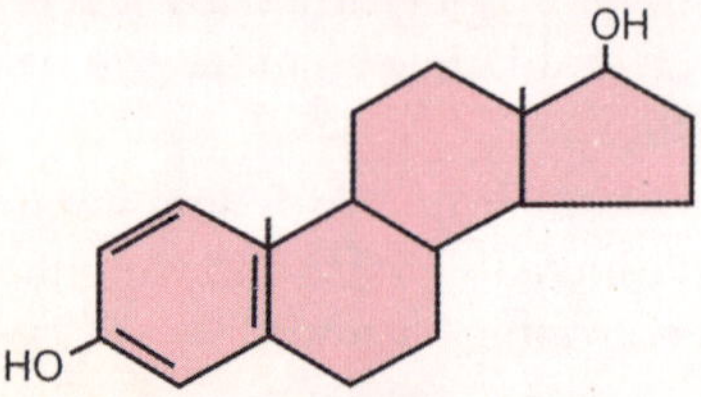

OH

HO

β- Estradiol

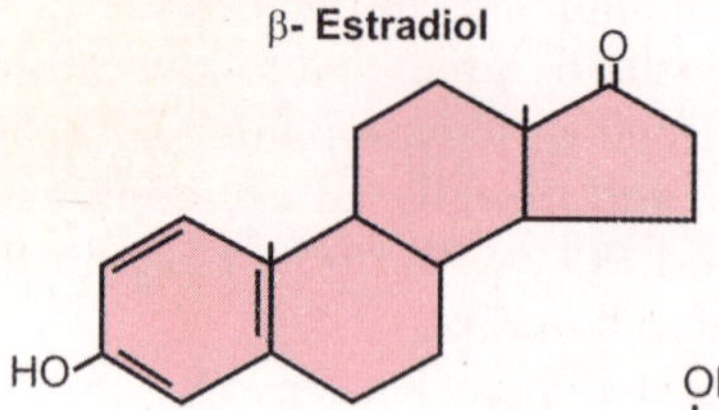

O

HO

Estrone

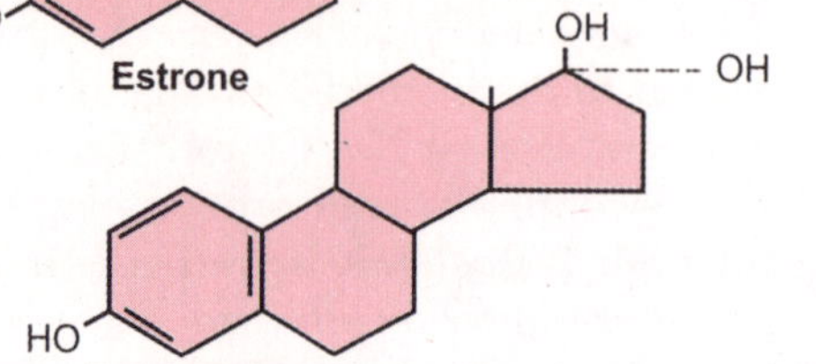

OH

OH

HO

Estriol

Chemistry: The ***naturally occurring estrogens in humans:***

- ***β-Estradiol***
- ***Estrone and***
- ***Estriol***

- The principal estrogenic hormone in circulation and ***the most active form of the estrogen is β-estradiol,*** which is in metabolic equilibrium with estrone,
- Estriol is the principal estrogens found in the urine of pregnant women and in the placenta. Estriol is produced from estrone by hydroxylation of estrone at C_{16} and reduction of the ketone group at C_{17}.
- ***Estrone is the hormone produced in the follicles but released into the blood as β-estradiol. In the liver, it is converted to Estriol. β-Estradiol and Estrone are interconvertivle.***
- β-Estradiol is 10 times more potent than estrone and 300 times more potent than estriol.

Site of Formation:

- In the ovary, estrogens are produced by the maturing graffian follicles, both thecal cells and granulosa cells are involved, and also in corpus luteum.
- All the three pituitary gonadotropins, FSH, LH and LTH are involved in stimulation of estrogen secretion.
- Estrogens are also formed in the adrenal cortex, placenta and testes in small amounts.

Biosynthesis

Androgenic steroids testosterone and androstenedione are precursors for the synthesis of estrogens in testes, ovaries, adrenal cortex and placenta.

Steps of Synthesis:

- Cholesterol is converted to pregnenolone and progesterone by the ovarian steroidogenic cells.
- Theca interna cells of graafian follicles convert both pregnenolone and progesterone to testosterone and androstenedione, which are the precursors.
- In granulosa cells of the follicle → testosterone is converted to β-estradiol.
- ***β-Estradiol and estrone are interconvertible by the enzyme β-estradiol dehydrogenase.***

Metabolism:

Role of Liver: Liver plays an important role in the metabolism of estrogens.

- It effectively removes estrogens from the systemic circulation by:
  - Biliary excretion, and
  - Metabolic degradation to less active and inactive compounds.
- It conjugates estrogens and their metabolites with glucuronic acid and sulphates, converting them to water soluble forms which return to systemic circulation and are excreted in urine.

Transport and Plasma Level: Approximately 0.1 to 0.2 mg of estrogens are secreted daily in adult females; secretion increases during ovulation, up to 0.5 mg/day.

- Plasma level varies according to menstrual cycle:
  - first 10 days of cycle: 20 to 70 pg/ml
  - Next 8 days of cycle: 50 to 290 pg/ml and
  - Last 10 days of cycle: 70 to 140 pg/ml.

Hormones are transported as follows:

- Large amounts of estrogens about 50 to 65% are carried tightly bound to a 'specific' carrier protein, a β-globulin, called ***"sex-steroid binding protein" (SBT),*** which also transports androgens.
- ***Another major portion is carried by serum albumin*** less tightly bound and non-specific.
- Around 1 to 3% of β-estradiol and estrone circulate as ***"free" active forms*** which are in equilibrium with protein bound forms.

Metabolic Actions

1. ***After Administration of Estrogens:*** The following biochemical changes are observed to occur:

- Proliferation of vaginal epithelium and endometrium, an ***increase in glycogen ↑ in the cells,*** and increase in alkaline phosphatase activity ↑ in endometrium. Glycogen also increases in vaginal epithelial cells.
- There is ***increased rate of glycolysis with accumulation of lactic acid (LA).*** The vaginal glycogen is probably the source of LA, which, by increasing the acidity of the vaginal secretion (pH 4.0 to 5.0), favours a homogenous flora of acid bacteria.
- Acceleration of incorporation of amino acids into proteins of uterus, ***increased protein synthesis*** ↑.
- Favours retention and elevation of Ca and P and skeletal deposition of Ca producing hypercalcaemia and hyperphosphatemia and calcification and ossification of bones.

  Note:
  - Estrogens also stimulate the closure of bone epiphyses.
  - ***β-Estradiol prevents osteoporosis.*** Menopausal women are liable to get fracture due to weakness of bones from osteoporosis.
- An increase in O_2-consumption in endometrium, placenta, mammary gland and adenohypophysis.
- Estrogens also produce an effect on mineral metabolism. β-estradiol particularly causes a slight retention of Na, CI and water.
- In certain mammalian species, estrogens may exert a ***'lipotropic effect',*** i.e. tendency to prevent accumulation of fats in the Liver.
- Estrogens also have ***a cholesterol lowering effect*** ↓ and reduces plasma cholesterol level and a fall in the level of β-lipoproteins ↓ (LDL)

Clinical Aspect

Young women are protected against myocardial infarction whereas women in menopause, with decline in estrogenic activity are more susceptible to myocardial infarction. Estrogenic activity in pre-menopause is associated with increased HDL.

II. ***Transhydrogenation Reaction:*** Estrogens may also act as cofactor in transhydrogenation reaction in which H^+ ions and electrons are transferred from reduced $NADP^+$ to NAD^+.

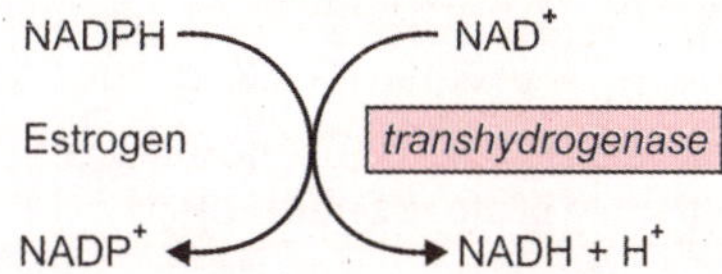

Synthetic Estrogens: A number of synthetic estrogens have been produced. The following are clinically valuable.

- ***Ethinyl estradiol:*** A synthetic estrogen which when given orally is 50 times as effective as water soluble estrogenic preparations or 30 times as effective as estradiol benzoate injected IM.
- ***Diethyl stilbestrol:*** An example of a group of p-OH-phenyl derivatives, which though not steroidal (non-steroid) in structure, exerts potent estrogenic effects.

PROGESTATIONAL HORMONES (LUTEAL HORMONES)

PROGESTERONE

Progesterone is the hormone of the corpus luteum, the structure which develops in the ovary from the ruputured graffian follicle.

- It is also formed by the placenta, which secretes progesterone, during the later part of pregnancy. Progesterone is also formed in the adrenal cortex, as a precursor of both C_{19} and C_{21} corticosteroids. It is also formed in the testes.

- It is secreted by the corpus luteum of the ovary during the period of its functional activity. It appears suddenly on the day of ovulation or perhaps a day or two earlier. It is concerned in the latter half of the menstrual cycle, mainly with preparing the endometrium for the nidation of the fertilized ovum, if conception has occurred.
- During early pregnancy, it is produced by corpus luteum of pregnancy (stimulated by Leutenizing hormone and Lactogenic hormone) and perhaps by other ovarian leuteinized cells and later mainly by the syncytial cells of the palcenta.

Chemistry: Progesterone may be regarded as a derivative of "pregnane" and is designated chemically as "4-pregnane-3,20-dione". It is a C_{21} steroid and has a—CH_3 group at C_{10} and C_{13}.

Structure of progesterone CH_3

C = O

O

Progesterone (4-Pregnane-3,20-dione)

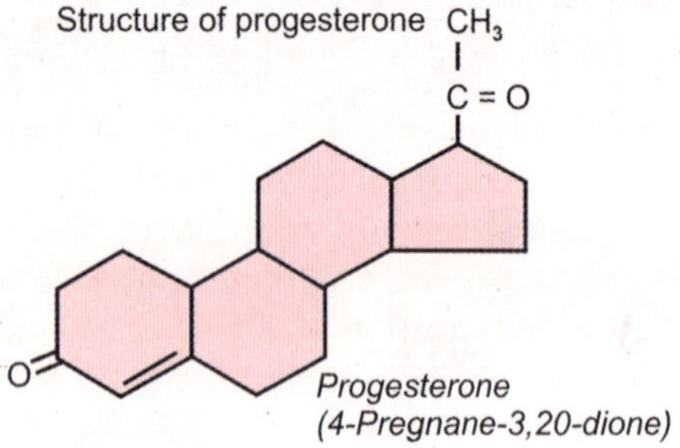

Biosynthesis

- Progesterone has a role as an intermediate in the biogenesis of adrenocortical hormones and of androgens. Indirectly via androstenedione and testosterone it also serves as precursors for estrogens also.
    - Progesterone is formed from acetate via cholesterol, *'Pregnenolone' is the immediate precursor.*

Secretion and Transport: Progesterone is secreted at the rate of about 2 mg/day in follicular phase, and increases to approximately 25 mg/day in luteal phase.

Plasma Level: It is 0.2 to 1.5 mg/dl in follicular phase and increases to 6.5 ng/dl in luteal phase.

Transport:

- In contrast to estrogens/and androgens, about 40% of progesterone is carried by ***"corticosteroid binding globulin"***, β-globulin, being tightly bound.
- About 1 to 5% of total progesterone is transported in active ***'free' form***.
- Remaining is carried being loosely bound principally to albumin and also to a small extent other plasma proteins and ***orosomucoid.***

Metabolism: Liver is the principal organ involved in removal of this hormone from the circulation and in its degradation. Chief metabolite is ***"pregnanediol"*** which is biologically inactive and is excreted in urine as glucuronides. By injection of C^{14}-labelled hormone, it has been observed that about 75% of injected progesterone/and its metabolites are transported to intestine by way of bile and elminated in faeces.

Actions: In humans, progesterone produces characteristic changes (progestational) in the estrogen-primed endometrium. This hormone appears after ovulation and causes,

- Extensive development of the endometrium preparing the uterus for the embedding of the embryo and for its nutrition.
- It causes an increase in glycogen ↑, mucin ↑ and fat ↑ in the lining epithelial cells. Alkaline phosphatase ↓ decreases in activity.
- The hormone also suppresses estrus, ovulation and the production of pituitary leuteinizing hormone (LH). Progesterone modifies the action of estrogen on the vaginal epithelium during the menstrual cycle, causing desquamation and basophilia of the superficial layer of cells and leucocytic infiltration.
- Hormone also stimulates the mammary glands. In conjunction with estrogen, progesterone causes development of the alveolar system of the breasts and sensitizes them for the action of lactogenic hormone.
- Progesterone is responsible for the rise in basal temperature ↑, which occurs during the corpus luteum phase of the normal menstrual cycle. This is due to increase in basal metabolic rate (BMR↑).

- In large doses, progesterone exerts androgenic effects, perhaps by conversion to androgenic metabolites.
- The normal effects on electrolyte and water metabolism vary in different species. In dogs and rodents, it appears to favour retention of Na, CI and water. In humans, there is evidence that it exerts an opposite effect.

Synthetic Analogues

(Orally effective progestational agents)

Progesterone is relatively ineffective when taken orally. Recently several synthetically produced progestational agents have been made available which are much more effective biologically than progesterone when taken orally.

Two such compounds are:

- *Norethindrone (Norlutin)*
- *Norethynodrel (Enovid)*

Note: Like progesterone these compounds are able to suppress *ovulation*, and hence they have found application in association with estrogens as oral contraceptives.

PLACENTAL HORMONES

Pregnancy activates the placental hormones. The implanted blastocyst forms the trophoblast which is subsequently organized into the placenta. The placenta provides the nutritional connection between the embryo and the maternal circulation.

Human placenta produces and secretes following hormones:

1. **Peptide hormones**
   - ***Human chorionic gonadotropin hormone (hCG)***
   - ***Chorionic somatomammotropin (CS) (also called placental lactogen)***
2. **Ovarian steroid hormones:**
   - ***Progestins***
   - ***Estrogens chiefly Estriol***

1. Human Chorionic Gonadotropin (HCG)

Chemistry: It is a glycoprotein, a heterodimer consisting of two subunits α and β. **α-chain** is made up of 92 amino acids and is ***identical to human FSH, LH and TSH. β-chain is*** made up of 145 amino acids.

Carbohydrate moieties present are as follows:

- ***α-Chain*** carries two asparagine linked oligosaccharides,
- ***β-Chain*** has more carbohydrate and contains two asparagine-linked oligosaccharides and four serine linked oligosaccharides.

Origin: It is ***formed by the syncytiotrophoblast of chorionic villi within 12 to 14 days of fertilization.***

Blood and Urinary Levels: Levels of HCG in blood and urine rises rapidly in first few weeks. Maximum peak level is reached by 12th week of pregnancy, then it declines slowly, 1/5th of peak by the end of 20th week and then continues at low level for a few days even after parturition.

Actions

- ***Luteotrophic effect:*** The hormone produces enlargement of corpus luteum and stimulates its secretion. It maintains a secretory corpus luteum in first three months of pregnancy.
- ***Testosterone secretion:*** Like LH, the hormone stimulates the growth of interstitial cells (Leydig cells) of embryonic testes and produces testosterone. This helps in virilization of the reproductive system of male embryo.

2. Chorionic Somatomammotropin (Placental Lactogen)

- The hormone has biologic properties of prolactin and growth hormone of anterior pituitary.
- It is a ***peptide hormone*** and amino acid sequences are similar to GH and prolactin (85% homology).
- The hormone is secreted by the syncytiotrophoblasts from about the second week of pregnancy, rises slowly and reaches a peak approximately by 36 weeks of pregnancy.

Actions: The exact physiologic function of this hormone is not clear, because pregnant women lacking this hormone have normal pregnancies and deliver normal babies. But as the hormone has similar structure to anterior pituitary GH and prolactin, it exerts similar effects. The hormone shows following effects:

- *Somatotrophic effect:* May promote growth of maternal tissues.
- *Luteotrophic effect:* Stimulates the enlargement, growth and secretion of corpus luteum and helps to maintain a secretory corpus luteum.
- *Mammotrophic effect:* Stimulates alveolar growth of mammary glands during pregnancy.
- *Lactogenic effect:* Stimulates lactation.
- *Anabolic effect:* Stimulates foetal and maternal tissue growth. Promotes retention of N, Ca^{2+} and inorganic P.
- *Anti-insulin effect:* May decrease glucose utilization, decreased carbohydrate tolerance and hyperglycaemic effect.

3. Ovarian Steroids

(a) Progestins: The corpus luteum is the major source of progesterone for the first 6 to 8 weeks of pregnancy and then placenta takes over the function. The corpus luteum though continues to function, but in third trimester onwards, the plcenta produces 30 to 40 times more progesterone than the corpus luteum.***Placenta cannot synthesize cholesterol from 'active' acetate, hence for cholesterol it has to depend on maternal supply.***

(b) Estrogens: Plasma concentrations of estradiol, estrone and estriol gradually increase throughout pregnancy. Estriol is produced in the largest amount. Adrenal cortex of foetus produces DHEA and DHEA SO_4 which are converted to 16 α-OH dervatives by the foetal liver, and these are subsequently converted to estriol by the placenta. After its formation, travels via the placental circulation to the maternal liver, where they are conjugated to glucuronides, and then are excreted in the urine.

Clinical Significance

1. Feto-placental function: As estriol is formed by placenta, ***the measurement of urinary estriol levels has been used as a test of feto-placental function.*** Failure of urinary estriol or total estrogens to rise in late pregnancy reflects the integrity of the fetoplacental unit and may indicate imminent fetal death or placental insufficiency, e.g. pre-eclamptic toxaemia.

Note: Urinary pregnanediol (or plasma progesterone) reflects placental function only as does estimation of plasma placental lactogen. ***A falling titre of urinary estrogen or plasma placental lactogen is serious.***

2. Pregnancy tests: Increased urinary excretion of HCG which occurs in early pregnancy (as early as 10th day of gestation) forms the basis for pregnancy tests. The classical biological tests, e.g. Ascheim-Zondek test, Friedman test, etc. depend on the hCG stimulation of the sex glands of a test animal, rats or mice and observing the changes in ovaries have become obsolete now and have been replaced completely by immunological tests.

a. Immunological Test

Anti-HCG serum slide test: Kits are available in the market.

Steps:

- Patient's urine is mixed on a slide (provided with the kit) with anti-HCG serum from sensitized rabbits (Provided in the kit).
- HCG-coated latex particles (provided in the kit) are then mixed with the above
- The final mixture is allowed to react for two minutes and then examined for any agglutination present or not.
- A positive and a negative control should be put.

Interpretation:

- ***Absence of agglutination indicates pregnancy (+ve),*** because HCG present in pregnant patient's urine binds the HCG antibodies of the anti-HCG serum, leaving no antibody for agglutination of HCG-coated latex particles to take place.
- Presence of agglutination indicates no pregnancy (-ve).

  Note: If the urine of a patient who is thought to be in early pregnancy gives a –ve result, the test should be repeated two weeks later.

- *False+ve result:* Hydatidiform mole, chorion carcinoma or testicular teratoma contain chorionic tissues and produce HCG to give strongly +ve results with pregnancy diagnosis tests.
- At the peak of HCG excretion in pregnancy, a +ve reaction is usually given by urine diluted 1 in 20, whilst in late pregnancy the test may be positive only on undiluted urine.
- Urine from a patient suffering from hydatidiform mole may give a+ve reaction at a dilution of 1 to 100 or more.

b. Biological Test

Ascheim-Zondek test: The urine of the patient is injected into immature female rats or mice. Subsequent appearance of haemorrhagic spots in their ovaries (seen after dissection of the animals) indicates the presence of HCG in the urine indicating pregnancy.

GI HORMONES

INTRODUCTION

GI tract secretes many hormones, perhaps more than other single organ.

Purpose of GI tract is:

- to propel food stuff to sites of digestion,
- to provide the proper milieu (enzyme, pH, salt, etc.) for the digestive processes,
- to move the digested products across the intestinal mucosa through the mucosal cells and into the EC space,
- to move these products to distant cells via the circulation, and
- to expel waste products.

The GI hormones assist in all these functions.

BIOMEDICAL IMPORTANCE

- Disease syndromes due to excessive production of several of these hormones have been described. Signs and symptoms often involve many organ systems and accurate diagnosis can be difficult unless the physician is aware of these syndromes.
- GI hormones are of interest also because of their close link to the neuropeptides.

Characteristics of GI Hormones

1. *Diversity: Examples of GI hormones*:

(a) *"True" hormones*

- Gastrin
- Secretin
- GIP (Gastric inhibitory peptides) and Possibly
- CCK (cholecystokinin)
- Motilin
- PP (Pancreatic polypeptide), and
- Enteroglucagon

(b) *Other GI Peptides* These can have:

- Paracrine functions
- Neurocrine functions.

The above is based on the observation that although these substances are found in high concentration in neurons or in various cells in GI tract, they either are not found in circulation under normal conditions or have such short plasma half life that would not be effective.

Peptides with neurocrine action:

- VIP (vasoactive intestinal peptide)
- Somatostatin
- Substance-P
- Eucephalins
- Bombesin like peptide (BLI)
- Neurotensin

Note: Many of these have Paracrine action *in vivo* because they affect various cells when added to tissues or organ cultures.

2. *Location of GI Peptide Producing Cells:* A unique feature of GI endocrine system is that the cells are scattered throughout the GI tract rather than collected in discrete organs as in more typical endocrine glands. Since many of the GI peptides are found in the nerves of GI tissues, it is not surprising that most of them are also present in the CNS.

3. *Precursors and Multiple Forms:* Of the major GI hormones, only secretin exists in a single form in tissues and in the circulation, viz. Gastrin, CCK, etc.

4. *Overlapping Structure and Function of GI Peptides:* The amino acids sequences of GI peptides have been determined. Many of these hormones can be placed in one of the 2 families based on sequence and functional similarity.

These are:

1. *Gastrin family:*
   - Gastrin
   - CCK
2. *Secretin family:*
   - Secretin
   - Glucagon including Glicentin
   - GIP
   - VIP
3. *Neurocrine peptides;*
   - Neurotensin
   - Bombesin like peptides (BLI)
   - Substance-P
   - Somatostatin

They bear no structural similarity to any other GI peptide. They have very short half lives in plasma and may play no physiologic role in plasma.

INDIVIDUAL GI HORMONES

A. SECRETIN FAMILY

1. Secretin: Jorpes *et al.* anouced isolation of secretin from hog duodenal mucosa. ***Bodansky et al*** 1966 synthesized the hormone.

Chemistry: A basic peptide having 27 amino acids. Out of 27 amino acids, 14 occupy the same position as of glucagen. Also similar in structure to GIP and VIP. All the 27 amino acids are required for activity.

Distribution and site: Highest concentration found in duodenum, restricted more to villous layer in villous epithelium. Cells are called ***'S' cell;*** they are numerous in duodenum and upper jejunum.

Release of secretin: Stimuli required are not known definitely.

- ***Duodenal acidification*** is the most potent stimulus, pH threshold for secretin release is pH 4.5
- FA and amino acids → 50% stimulation.

Actions

1. *In Low doses:*
   - Stimulates secretion of water ↑ and electrolytes (bicarbonate) ↑ from pancreas
   - Stimulates secretion of water ↑ and electrolytes ↑ by Liver (Bile),
   - Inhibits lower oesophageal (Cardiac) sphincter,
   - Inhibit gastric emptying (gastric motility)↓,
   - Inhibits gastric H^+ acid ↓ secretion,
   - Stimulates gastric pepsin ↑ secretion,
   - Decreases duodenal motility.
2. *In High Doses:*
   - Releases Insulin ↑,
   - Stimulates Brunner's glands (duodenum) in cats/and dogs,
   - Stimulates renal excretion of water ↑, Na^+↑ and K^+ ↑ in dogs (renal function),
   - Stimulates lipolysis ↑ in fat cells

2. GIP (Gastric Inhibitory Peptide): First extracted from duodenal mucosa and isolated in 1970.

- A polypeptide having 43 amino acids, calculated MW=5105
- Released from the duodenal and jejunal mucosa in response to glucose,
- Endocrine cells are ***"K-cells".*** Not localized in gut nerves.

Actions

- Inhibits gastric acid H^+ ↓ secretion.
- Inhibtis gastric motility.
- ***Major action is to stimulate insulin ↑ release.***

3. VIP (Vasoactive Intestinal Polypeptide): ***Isolated from upper intestinal wall.*** It is a basic peptide having 28 amino acids, calculated MW=3100. It has been synthesized recently. Endocrine cell of origin are ***"D_1 cells".*** Localized in pancreas. Also mainly localized in gut-nerves. It is present in the nerves of submucosal plexus, the myenteric plexus, and blood vessels. Exact physiological role not well defined, it may be involved in gut motility and sphincter relaxation and blood flow.

Actions

- A weak stimulation of pancreatic volume ↑ flow but not enzyme secretion.
- Inhibits gastric H^+ ↓ and pepsin ↓.

- Stimulation of intestinal secretion ↑.
- ***Inhibits gastric and gall bladder motility.***
- Relaxation of tracheal, gastric and gallbladder musculature.
- *Glycogenolysis* ("glucagon" like activity).

VIP is destroyed while passing through the lungs.

Clinical Significance

VIP omas: Tumors of D_1 cells, produces peptide syndrome:

- Watery diarrhoea,
- Achlorhydria and
- Hypokalaemia.

4. Glucagon: ***Enteroglucagon:*** A peptide extracted from duodenal mucosa. It is made by ***gastric and duodenal 'A' cells and pancreatic "α-cells".*** It is thought to contribute to the metabolic action of pancreatic glucagon.

GLI (Glucagon-like immunoreactivity): Other peptides with glucagon-like immunoreactivity (GLI) have been ***isolated from "L" cells of the ileum and colon.*** The major component of GLI is a large 100 amino acids peptide called ***"Glicentin"***, which contains the exact sequence of pancreatic glucagon. ***Glicentin may mimic the actions of glucagon.***

B. GASTRIN FAMILY

1. Gastrin: A linear polypeptide with 17 amino acids, a heptadecapeptide. → Previously called as ***"Little" Gastrin, LG (now called as G-17).***

Two forms:

- ***Gastrin I-*** without SO_4 esterification
- ***Gastrin II-*** with SO_4 esterification

SO_4 esterification occurs with phenolic-OH gr. of tyrosine at 12 position. Both terminal groups are blocked thus protected from digestion by amino peptidases/and carboxypeptidases. ***Both Gastrins I and II are equally active.***

Core of Activity: All the diverse actions were reproduced by one small fragment → ***the C-terminal "tetrapeptide amide"***, which is:

Trp—Met—Asp—Phe—NH_2.

Smaller fragments had no activity. Hence the above is called as ***"minimal fragment".***

Penta-gastrin: Is a synthetic product, C-terminal tetrapeptide with substituted β-alanine. It possesses all the physiological properties of natural gastrin and is used in man to test gastric secretory capacity.

Source and Distribution:

- ***Major source: Antral mucosa of stomach.***
- Small amounts of immunoreactive gastrin have been demostrated in the duodenal mucosa.
- ***δ-cells*** of pancreatic islets?

Location: By histochemistry, electron microscopy and immunofluorescence studies, special types of endocrine cells called ***'G-cells'*** located in deeper portion of pyloric glands, have been found.

Release of Gastrin: ***Controlled by two main stimulatory mechanisms:***

- ***Intake of food:*** Produces "Cephalic stimulation by vagal reflexes ***("Long reflex").***
- By chemical and mechanical stimulation of the antral mucosa, by food and digestion products ***("short reflexes").***

Short reflexes occur in response to stimuli acting in the stomach like,

- Distension
- Chemical agents: Bathing the mucosa.

Gastrin release is ***"auto-regulatory"*** (high acidity within the antrum inhibits the mechanism of gastrin release).

Chemical stimulation: Most active gastrin releasing agents are found to be "small molecules" such as:

- ***Amino acids***
- ***Lower aliphatic alcohols***
- ***Choline***

"Feedback" Control: The release of gastrin is subject to strong "feedback control" → acid bathing antral mucosa inhibits all mechanisms of release. Optimum pH for release → pH 5 to 7; Below pH 5 → release inhibited.

Other Modulating factors:

- ***Secretin:*** IV administration of secretin has been found to lower the plasma gastrin ↓ level.
- ***Ca^{++}:*** IV infusion of Ca^{++} increases ↑ plasma gastrin level.

Nature of Tissues and Circulating Gastrins

In tissues		*In Plasma*
Large Precursors:		
34 aa	G-34	G-34
17 aa	G-17	G-17
14 aa	G-14	G-14

- ***"Little" Gastrin (LG) (now called as G-17):***
  - 50% of total reactivity
  - A Hepta decapeptide
  - MW-2100
  - half life = 3.2 minutes.
- ***Big Gastrin (BG):*** Now called as *G-34.*
  - 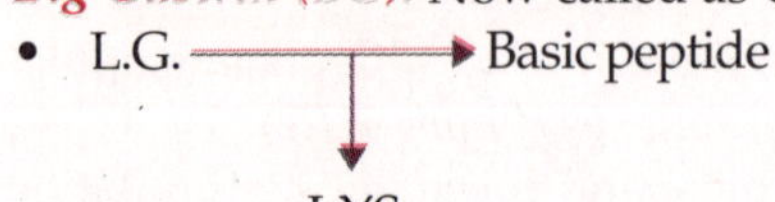

  - MW=3870
  - ½ life 15.8 minutes.

G-34 is more 'abundant' in the circulation than G-17, probably because its plasma ½ life (15.8 min) is five times that of G-17.

- ***'Big' 'Big' Gastrin (BBG).*** Large precursor molecule, constitutes a minor fraction. MW= 20,000
- ***Mini Gastrin (MG):*** Now called as G-14

The carboxy-terminal 14a a of G-34, G-17 and G-14 are identical. All the above can occur as I and II.

Actions of Gastrin

Gastrin has effects on all major GI activites including:

- Secretion
- Motility
- Absorption

1. *In physiological doses:*

- Gastric motility ↑.
- Secretion of water ↑, and electrolytes ↑ by stomach, pancreas, liver and Brünner's gland.
- Inhibits absorption of water and electrolytes from ↓ Ileum.
- Stimulates secretion of ↑ enzymes from stomach and pancreas.
- Causes contraction of smooth muscle of lower oesophageal sphincter (cardiac) and stomach.
- Inhibits contraction of sphincter of Oddi.
- Increases gastric mucosal blood flow ↑.
- Releases histamine ↑.
- Stimulates incorporation of amino acids into proteins in gastric mucosa (protein synthesis ↑).

2. *In large doses:*
   - Stimulation of growth ↑ of gastric mucosa ***("trophic action").***
   - Stimulation of release of insulin ↑.
   - Stimulation of smooth muscles of gut, gallbladder and uterus.

CCK: It belongs to "gastrin family". This hormone was discovered twice. ***Ivy and Oldberg*** (1928) discovered CCK, demonstrated liberation of the hormone from duodenal mucosa by food specially fat and caused contraction and emptying of gallbladder. ***Harper and Raper*** (1943) extracted a substance from duodenal mucosa, which stimulate secretion of pancreatic enzyme called **PZ** (Pancreozymin) later established → ***it is one single polypeptide possessing both the activities and called CCK-PZ (now called only CCK).***

Chemistry: ***Exists at least in five (5) molecular forms:***

In tissues	In Plasma
CCK—Large precursor	
• CCK-39	
• CCK-33	
• CCK-12	• CCK-12
• CCK-8	• CCK-8
• CCK-4	

CCK 8 appears to be the most abundant and potent form in circulation. CCk 8 is also found in brain.

Core of activity: In CCK → a methionine residue is interposed between tyrosine and glycine, which is responsible for characteristic powerful effect on gallbladder.

Site and distribution: Maximum output from duodenojejunal portion, form distal jejunum less.

Cells of origin: Found special endocrine cells called *"I-cells:*

Release:

- Most potent stimulus is peptone, Amino acids and FA less potent.
- HCl, produced 50% response, produced by peptone.
- Among amino acids, Phe, Tryp are most active. In man essential amino acids release CCK.
- Ca^{2+}

Actions:

- Produces contraction of gallbladder.
- Secretion of enzyme rich pancreatic juice.
- Stimulation of release of insulin ↑ and Glucagon.
- Increased intestinal ↑ motility. Like all GI hormones, it has numerous secondary actions.

OTHER GI PEPTIDES

Several other peptides have been isolated from GI tract and appear to be involved in the regulation of digestion, probably by paracrine or neurocrine mechanisms, since appreciable concentrations are not found in the circulation. It is emphasized that no certain physiologic role has been assigned to any of these molecules.

1. Substance-P: First peptide found in both gut and brain. A peptide containing 11 amino acids, 5-carboxy terminal aa are required for its action.

Action: Produces smooth muscle contraction in the intestine.

2. Bombesin: Found in frog's skin. A similar peptide, called as gastrin-releasing peptide (GRP) has been isolated from endocrine cells in the gut, gut neurons and brain. The amino acids at positions 5 to 14 of Bombesin are identical to those at positions 18 to 27 of GRP except at one residue.

Actions:

- Bombesin stimulates gastric ↑ and pancreatic ↑ secretion.
- Increases motility of the gallbladder and intestine.
- This *peptide may have a "growth promoting" autocrine action in small cell carcinoma of lungs*

3. Motillin: A polypeptide isolated from small intestinal mucosa of Hog by *Brown et al 1972. Contains 22 amino acids, Calculated MW = 2700*

Actions:

- It stimulates acid ↑ and pepsin ↑ secretion by gastric mucosa.
- A stimulator of intestinal smooth muscle ↑ contraction.

4. Somatostatin: ***First isolated from the hypothalamus as the factor that inhibited growth hormone secretion.*** Hence the name.

- It is a cyclic peptide.
- It is synthesized as large somatostatin precursor a prohormone MW ~ 11,500, in the δ-cells of pancreatic islet of Langerhans.
- Rate of transcription of the "Prohormone" gene is markedly enhanced by cyclic AMP.
- Prohormone contains 28 amino acids.
- Finally hormone is produced, a peptide with 14 aa (MW 1640).
- All forms have biologic activity.

In addition to its presence in the hypothalamus and pancreatic islets, somatostatin is found in many GI tissues, where it is thought to regulate variety of functions and in multiple sites in CN system, where it may be a "neurotransmitter". In GI tract → it is produced by *gastric 'δ' cells* and inhibits, by paracrine action, the release of gastrin, secretin, CCK, motilin and GIP.

It decreases the delivery of nutrients from the GI tract into the circulation, because it:

- Prolongs gastric emptying,
- Decreases gastrin ↓ secretion therefore gastric acid production,
- Decreases pancreatic exocrine (digestive enzyme) Secretion ↓,
- Decreases ↓ splanchnic blood flow, and
- Slows ↓ sugar absorption.

5. Pancreatic Polypeptide (PP):

- 36 aa peptide
- MW=4200
- Recently discovered product of *pancreatic 'F' cells.* Its secretion in humans is,

- Increased by a protein meal, fasting, exercise, and acute hypoglycaemia and is
- Decreased by Somatostatin and IV glucose

Actions: The function of PP is unknown, but its
- Effect on Hepatic glycogen levels and
- GI secretions have been suggested.

It inhibits pancreatic ↓ bicarbonate and protein enzyme secretion.

6. Chymodenin:
- Produced in mucosa of small intestine.
- Polypeptide containing 43 aa, MW=4900
- Stimulus for release → fat in the intestine.

Action

Specific stimulation of chymotrypsin ↑ secretion of the pancreas.

7. Neurotensin: It is a 13 aa Peptide; Met and Leu-enkephalins and serotonin are found in intestinal cells and may be active in these tissues.

☞ SALIENT POINTS TO REMEMBER

- Adrenal glands consist of two parts adrenal medulla in the centre and adrenal cortex is periphery.
- Adrenal cortex produces two types of steroid hormones—(a) Glucocorticoids—chief hormone is cortisol and (b) Mineralocorticoids, chief hormone is aldosterone.
- Cortisol is synthesized in all the three layers of cortex. But aldosterone is synthesized only by zonaglomerulosa as it contains the enzyme '18-hydroxylase'.
- Cortisol has castabolic effect on periphoral tissues but it is anabotic to liver.
- ***Action on peripheral tissues*** like muscles, adipose tissue and Lymphoid tissue is ***'catabolic'*** (spares glucose), viz. Glucose uptake ↓ and glycolysis ↓, increased lipolysis producing increase FFA ↑ in plasma, T.G. formation ↓. Protein synthesis ↓, protein breakdown is increased leading to increased plasma aminoacids ↑.
- ***Action on liver is 'anabolic',*** viz gluconeogenesis ↑ from aminoacids and glycerol, liver glycogen is increased ↑, protein synthesis in liver cells ↑ is enhanced.
- Adrenal cortex also produces small amounts of sex hormones androgens. Main adrenal androgens are Dehydroepiandrosterone (DHEA), DHEA-SO_4, Δ^4 - Androstenedione and 11-β-OH-androstenedione.
- ***Androstenedione is the precursor of teststerone,*** more potent male hormone.
- Chief mineralocorticoid is Aldosterone. It is produced by Zonaglomerulosa only.
- It influences mainly the metabolism of of Na^+ and K^+. It increases the rate of tubular reabsorption of Na^+ and also Cl^-.
- It increases renal excretion of K^+ in the urine by the renal distal tubules and collecting ducts.
- Increased secretion of aldosterone promotes alkalosis, whereas decreased secretion produces acidosis.
- Conn's syndrome, primary aldosteronism is produced by a tumor adenoma called "**aldosteronoma**" which produces excess amount of aldosterone.
- Adrenal medulla produces two important hormones, viz. epinephrine (adrenalin) and norepinephrine (Noradrenaline).
- They influence diverse biochemical functions with an ultimate goal to mobilize energy resources and prepare the individual to fight 'stress'.
- Pheochromacytomas are the tumors of adrenal medulla, characterized by excessive production of epinephrine and norepinephrine (catecholamines) associated with hypertension which may be severe and paroxysmal.
- Two enzymes Monoamino Oxidase (MAO) and Catechol-o-melthyl transferase (COMT) are involved in catabolism of catecholamines.
- Chief metabolite exereted in urine is 4-OH-3-methoxy mandelic acid, also called vanyl mandelic acid (VMA).
- The steroid hormones, primarily androgens in males and oestrogens in females are respectively synthesized by testes and ovaries respectively.

- These hormones are responsible for growth, development, maintenance and regulation of reproductive system in either sex.
- Oestrogen is required as a cofactor in trans-hydrogenation reaction in which $NADP^+$ can be converted to NAD^+.
- Several gastrointestinal hormones e.g. gastrin, secretin, CCK–PZ, etc. are produced in the G.I. tract by specialized cells and are closely involved in the regulation of digestion and absorption of food stuffs.

MULTIPLE CHOICE QUESTIONS

Give one correct answer:

1. **One of the following hormones are produced by anterior pituitary gland, *except:***
   (a) Growth hormone
   (b) MSH
   (c) TSH
   (d) Prolactin
   (e) FSH
2. **Which of the following hormone is involved in increased reabsorption of water from renal tubular epithelial cells?**
   (a) Insulin (b) Glucagon
   (c) Vasopressin (d) Oxytocin
   (e) Epinephrine
3. **Which of the following is required for crystallization and storage of the hormone Insulin?**
   (a) Mn^{++} (b) Zn^{++}
   (c) Mg^{++} (d) Ca^{++}
   (e) Fe
4. **Which of the following hormone does not produce lipolysis?**
   (a) Insulin (b) Glucagon
   (c) Cortisol (d) Epinephrine
   (e) Thyroxine
5. **All of the following hormones use cyclic AMP as a second messenger *except:***
   (a) Glucagon (b) FSH
   (c) LH (d) Epinephrine
   (e) Estrogen
6. **The rate limiting step in the biosynthetic pathway of catecholamines is:**
   (a) The hydroxylation of Phenylalanine to tyrosine
   (b) The decarboxylation of DOPA
   (c) The reduction of biopterin
   (d) The hydroxylation of tyrosine
   (e) Methylation of norepinephrine.
7. **Epincphrine is formed from Nor-epinephrine by:**
   (a) N-methylation
   (b) O-methylation
   (c) Decarboxylation
   (d) Hydroxylation
   (e) Transamination
8. **All of the following may act as second messenger, *except:***
   (a) Cyclic AMP
   (b) Ca^{++} ions
   (c) 1, 2-diacylglycerol
   (d) 2, 3-diphosphoglycerol
   (e) Inositol triphosphate
9. **Which of the following substances is present in high concentration in the urine of patients with pheochromocytomas?**
   (a) Metanephrine
   (b) 3-methoxy-4-OH mandelic acid
   (c) Epinephrine
   (d) Dopamine
   (e) Norepinephrine
10. **Insulin causes all of the following *except:***
    (a) Increased ketogenesis
    (b) Increased glycogenesis
    (c) Shift of K^+ from E.C.F. to cells
    (d) Increased Lipogenesis
    (e) Increased aminoacid uptake
11. **Hypothyroidism is characteristically associated with high serum:**
    (a) Calcium
    (b) Phosphate
    (c) Cholesterol
    (d) Glucose
    (e) Uric acid

12. **Hyperthyroidism is characteristically associated with:**
    (a) High serum glucose
    (b) High serum calcium
    (c) High serum cholesterol
    (d) Low serum phosphate
    (e) High serum creatine

ANSWERS

1. (b)	2. (c)	3. (b)
4. (a)	5. (e)	6. (d)
7. (a)	8. (d)	9. (b)
10. (a)	11. (c)	12. (e)

23 Metabolism of Minerals and Trace Elements

INTRODUCTION

It is observed that there are at least 29 different types of element in our body. Organic components such as carbohydrates, proteins, and lipids form about 90% of the solid matter and mainly consists of C, H, O and N. The elements of the body are divided in ***five major groups:***

Gr.I: → C, H, O, N. Components of macromolecules such as carbohydrates, proteins, lipids, etc.

Gr. II: → Nutritionally important minerals or principal elements. The daily requirement of these is >100 mg. The deficiency of these can prove fatal. These include, Na, K, Cl, Ca, P, Mg, and S. They are also called **macroelements**.

Gr. III: → **Trace elements** which are essential. The requirement is less than 100 mg per day. Deficiency can lead to serious disorders. These include Cr, Co, Cu, I, Fe, Mn, Mo, Se,Zn.

Gr. IV: → These are additional trace-elements which may be possibly essential. The exact role is not known. These include Cd, Ni, Si, Sn, Vn.

Gr. V: → These are not essential element and may be toxic. They have no known function in the body and may enter the body through polluted air, water, soil or food substances, e.g. As, CN^-, Hg, etc.

SODIUM

Body water is found mainly in intracellular and extracellular compartments with a small amount in interstitial fluid compartment. Sodium is the electrolyte which is found in large concentrations in extracellular fluid compartment. Approximate body distribution of sodium is as follows:

	Total m Mol	*Conc. m Mol/l*
Total body	3150	–
Intracellular	250	10
Extracellular	2900	140
Plasma	400	140

Sodium is found in the body mainly associated with chloride as NaCl and $NaHCO_3$.

Sources: Sodium is widely distributed in food material; more in animal sources than plants. However, major source is table-salt used in cooking or seasoning. It is also found in cheese, butter, khoa.

Daily Requirement: Adults require 1-3.5 g of Na daily. Infants need 0.1-0.5 g and children 0.3-2.5g daily.

Absorption of Sodium: Sodium is absorbed by sodium pump situated in basal and lateral plasma membrane of intestinal and renal cells. Na-pump actively transports Na into extracellular fluid.

Sodium Pump: This is also called as ***Na^+-K^+-ATPase.*** It requires ATP and Mg^{++}. Intracellular Na^+ concentration is arround 10 mM/L while that of extracellular is 150 mM/L. Na pump is an enzyme, *Na^+-K^+-ATPase*. It is a glycoprotein composed of 2 α and 2 β chains. Its activity depends on presence of *Na^+*and *K^+*and requires *ATP* and Mg^{++} ions as cofactor. The enzyme hydrolyzes a high energy phosphate bond of ATP and uses the energy thus released to transport three Na^+ ions outside and simultaneously two K^+ ions inside across the cell membrane.

Inhibitors: Oubain, a glycoside of a steroid and digitalis is the cardiotonic drug which inhibits the Na^+-K^+ pump.

Excretion of Na: Every 24 hours approximately 25000 mmol of sodium are filtered by the kidneys. However, due to tubular reabsorption, less than 1% of this sodium appears in the urine (100-200 mM/day). Approximately 70% of the filtered sodium is reabsorbed in proximal tubule. Further 20-30% of filtered Na is reasorbed by ascending loop of Henle.

FUNCTIONS OF SODIUM

- ***Fluid balance:*** Sodium maintains crystalloid osmotic pressure of extracellular fluids and helps in retaining water in ECF
- ***Neuromuscular excitability:*** Alongwith other cations Na^+ is also involved in neuromuscular irritability which is given as: Neuromuscular irritability

$$\alpha = \frac{[K^+][Na^+]}{[Ca^{++}] + [Mg^{++}] + [H^+]}$$

- ***Acid base blance:*** Na^+-H^+ exchange in renal tubule to acidify urine. (See chapter on Acid Base balance for details).
- ***Maintenance of viscosity of blood:*** The salts of Na with globulins are soluble and further Na^+ and K^+ both regulate in maintaining the degree of hydration of the plasma proteins.
- ***Role in resting membrane potential:*** Plasma membrane has a poor Na^+ permeability and passive Na^+ inflow through it. Na Pump keeps Na^+ concentration far higher outside than inside. This separation of charges is called ***polarization*** of the membrane. ***It creates a potential difference of -70 to -95 millivolts across the membrane and is called as resting membrane potential.***
- ***Role in action potential:*** A local depolarization of nerve or muscle fibre is observed in stimulation. This rapidly increases its permeability to Na^+ causing considerable transmembrane influx of Na^+ down its inward concentration gradient.

Clinical conditions

Clinical conditions are of two major types–Hypernatremia and Hyponatremia.

1. Hypernatremia: A high plasma sodium concentration does not necessarily mean that the total body sodium content is increased, but infers that the extracellular sodium is excessive relative to water. The general scheme to evaluate hypernatremia is given at next page in box.

Decrease in body water and increase in body sodium. Specific conditions in which hypernatremia occurs are as follows:

- ***Simple dehydration:*** This occurs as a result of excessive sweating with inadequate or no water replacement. (Refer chapter on Water and Electrolyte Balance).
- ***Diabetes insipidus:*** A special type of water loss occurs in D.I. The disease is characterized by lack of antidiuretic hormone (ADH) or failure of the hormone to act on its target cells. It occurs usually as a complication of pituitary surgery, when hormone is not produced in adequate amount. In nephrogenic *Diabetes insipidus,* the kidney cells are unable to respond to the hormone.
- ***Osmotic loading:*** If the kidney is required to excrete large quantities of very soluble substances such as glucose, urea, amino acids, osmotic effect of these substances on the urine causes the co-excretion of large amounts of water. Relatively little sodium is excreted and hence the plasma level rises.
- ***Excess sodium intake:*** Normally in clinical medicine, 0.9% NaCl is administered intravenously—154 mEq/L. Excessive use of isotonic saline particularly in children leads to hypernatremia. Hypernatremia may also occur following the administration of $NaHCO_3$ in treatment of acidosis.
- ***Steroid therapy:*** Certain adrenal steroids, the mineralocorticoids, control the metabolism of

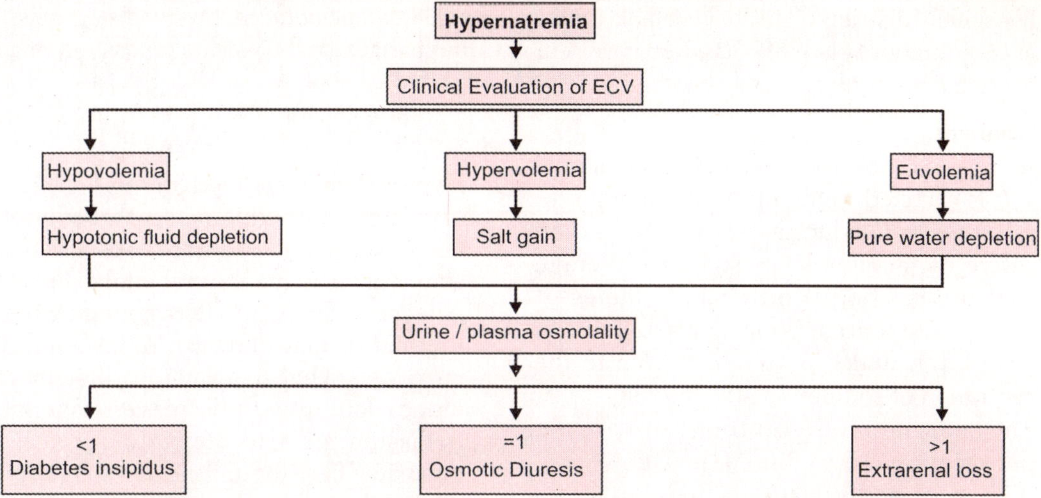

sodium. Among other effects, mineralocorticoids cause the kidney to absorb sodium from the glomerular filtrate, which results in increased plasma concentration. In certain tumours of adrenal gland large amounts of most potent mineralocorticoid-aldosterone is produced ***(Conn's syndrome)***

2. Hyponatremia:

- ***Diuretic medication:*** One of the most commonly encountered causes of hyponatremia today is due to the use of diuretics. Many of the standard diuretic medications act by promoting excretion of Na by kidney. The object is to lower the total body sodium and thus reduce the total extracellular water. There are many diseases in which this objective is desired—congestive heart failure, chronic kidney disease and hypertension. Reduced total body sodium is achieved but as the extracellular volume reaches critical dimension, there is a counter effort to retain water which then dilutes the sodium and hyponatremia results.
- ***Sweating***: Heavy sweating with adequate replacement of water but no salt is common cause of hyponatremia.
- ***Kidney disease***: Kidneys are impaired, glomerulus is the one in which blood is filtered and Na is reabsorbed by the renal tubules. Due to kidney dysfunction Na^+ is not reabsorbed and is thus excreted in the urine. There is also a progressive failure to excrete water.
- ***Congestive heart failure***: Hyponatremia is common in heart failure for two reasons: (1) Diuretics. (2) In advance stages congestive heart failure cause low Na^+ conc. It is because the low cardiac output is sensed incorrectly by the brain as low blood volume, calling for the increased secretion of ADH.
- ***Gastrointestinal loss***: Diarrhoea, particularly if prolonged and severe results in reduced sodium/chloride levels in plasma and extracellular fluid. Greater loss is observed in patients with enteritis in patients with ileostomy. Intestinal fistula causes number of bowel disorders. Prolonged vomiting will also produce some loss of electrolytes, however, the chloride lost in vomiting is much more and dominates the clinical picture.

POTASSIUM

Potassium is the ***major intracellular cation.*** It is widely distributed in the body fluids and tissues as follows.

- Whole blood 200 mg/dl
- Plasma 20 mg/dl
- Cells 440 mg/100g
- Muscle tissue 250-400 mg/100g
- Nerve-tissue 530 mg/100 g.

It is widely distributed in the vegetable foods. An average amount of 4 g of potassium is present in the diet. Potassium is easily absorbed.

Metabolism

As soon as it is absorbed, potassium enters the cells. It is excreted in the urine. The amount of potassium excretion increases, when there is an excessive dietary intake of sodium. Average normal human body contains 3.6 moles of potassium. The concentration of intracellular K^+ is 150 mEq/L which is roughly equal to the concentration of sodium outside the cell.

- The normal concentration of plasma potassium is 3.5 to 5 mEq/L. The *Na^+-K^+-ATPase* or sodium pump maintains this concentration gradient. Potassium is also excreted in gastrointestinal tract, saliva, gastric juice, bile, pancreatic and intestinal juices. This fact becomes clinically important if these secretions are lost in large amounts. Potassium is continuously filtered by the glomeruli of the kidney and reabsorbed by the cells of proximal convoluted tubules. Potassium (and hydrogen) ions are also secreted in distal tubule in exchange for sodium.

FUNCTIONS OF POTASSIUM

Many functions of potassium and sodium are carried out in coordination with each other and are common. These functions have already been described under sodium. Some other functions of potassium are given below:

- It influences the muscular activity.
- Involved in acid-base balance.
- It has an important role in cardiac function.
- Certain enzymes such as *pyruvate kinase* require K^+ as cofactor.
- Involved in neuromuscular irritability and nerve conduction process

Clinical Importance

Extracellular levels of potassium are measured on a sample of serum. Since RBCs contain a large amount of potassium, ***care must be taken that sample is not hemolyzed.*** On standing, potassium value changes, so the plasma potassium must be measured as soon as possible on fresh sample. Both high values and low values are clinically important.

1. **Hyperkalemia:** The mechanisms for excretion of potassium in normal persons are so effective that it is difficult to produce hyperkalemia by simply increassing the oral intake. Increases, however, may occur after rapid intravenous infusion of potassium salts. In clinical practice, most cases of hyperkalemia are due either to • kidney failure with decreased excretion of potassium or • to the sudden release of potassium from the intracellular compartment which may happen in a variety of diseases.

- ***Anuria:*** Complete shut-down of kidney function regardless of cause results in increasing concentration of K^+. the rise may be particularly rapid if the kidney failure is associated with sudden release of intracellular potassium from any organ.
- ***Tissue damage:*** Damage to body cells from any cause results in release of cell contents including K^+ into ECF. Crush injuries, with damages to large volumes of muscle tissue, massive hemolysis are examples. In both of these conditions, there is often reduced kidney function which adds to the hyperkalemia.
- ***Violent muscle contraction*:** Vigorous exercise produces a release of potassium from muscle cells into the extracellular space and may cause a temporary elevation in plasma potassium. The same mechanism is responsible for the increase seen in status epilepticus.
- ***Addison's disease:*** Primary adrenal insufficiency. In the absence of aldosterone the exchange of Na^+ for potassium in the kidney is reduced, with increased loss of sodium and retention of K^+ in body. ***Low serum Na^+ and high serum K^+ are characteristics of this disease.***
- ***Diabetes mellitus:*** In ketoacidosis there is substantial loss of intracellular K^+ to the ECF. This is partly due to increased activity of *Na^+-K^+-ATPase* which results from impaired glucose metabolism. If ketoacidosis presents

for a long time, there will be major depletion of total body K^+. Treatment with insulin allows resumption of sodium pump activity and movement of K^+ back into the cells. This, in turn, causes an abrupt fall in plasma K^+. This must be treated by administration of K^+ to restore that which has been lost in the urine during the period of acidosis. ***Frequent monitoring of K^+ is vital to DM with ketoacidosis.***

3. Hypokalemia: Low serum K^+ usually results from the depletion of total body K^+. Since nearly all food contains large quantities of K^+, dietary deficiency by itself is uncommon. Dietary supplements of K^+ are required only in patients with some disease or drug use which causes potassium depletion. Some of the more common causes of hypokalemia are described here.

a. ***Loss of K^+ in GI. Secretions:***
   - Both prolonged vomiting and severe diarrhoea cause depletion of total body potassium and causes hypokalemia.
   - The intestinal fluid which drains from a recent ileostomy is rich in K^+. Excessive loss of fluid from this site may rapidly produce hypokalemia.
   - Habitual users of laxative eventually develop a state of chronic mild diarrhoea which may cause low K^+ levels.
   - A special instance of K^+ loss through GIT is a mucous secreting tumour called as **cillous adenoma.** This tumour secretes large amounts of K^+ into lumen of colon.

b. ***Loss of K^+ in urine:***
   - Many medications which are used to decrease total body sodium such as some diuretics also cause loss of K^+. This is especially true of thiazides, acetazolamide, and the organic mecurical diuretics. In clinical practice, the use of ***thiazide diuretics*** is one of the most common causes of low plasma K^+. The degree of hypokalemia is usually not severe. It can be corrected by increasing K^+ intake.
   - Rarely a tumour (**Conn's tumour)** develops in the adrenal gland which produces excess amounts of aldosterone. The resulting syndrome of primary hyperaldosteronism is characterized by increased loss of K^+ in urine.
   - A compound found in ***licorice*** glycyrrhizinic acid has aldosterone like activity and people who eat large amounts of licorice may develop hypokalemia.
   - ***In Cushing's syndrome*** (adrenocortical hyperfunction), hypokalemia is the rule. It is particularly severe if the process is due to production of ACTH by an ectopic tumour.

c. ***Loss of extracellular potassium into the intracellular space:*** As already mentioned above, treatment of diabetes ketoacidosis causes rapid fall in plasma K^+ from a state of hyperkalemia to normal and then to hypokalaemia as the acidosis is brought under control.

d. ***Other causes of hypokalemia:***
   - There is an inherited disorder called **familial periodic paralysis** in which there is sudden shift of K^+ into ICF causing parlysis.
   - ***In thyrotoxic periodic paralysis (TPP)*** similar thing happens. In both cases, it normally happens after heavy exercise or large carbohydrate meal. Thyroid hormone excess is also observed in TPP patients.
   - ***Renal tubular acidosis:*** Low serum K^+ is seen in renal tubular acidosis, in ***Bartter's syndrome*** and after administration of steroids such as deoxycorticosterone, cortisone and tetosterone.

CHLORINE

Chloride is taken in diet as sodium chloride. Many vegetables and meats have small proportions of chloride. It is also available in the 'chlorinated water' which is normally supplied as a process of purification of water for drinking purpose.

Daily Requirment: About 100-200 mMol is taken in diet as sodium chloride (table salt).

Distribution:

- Whole blood 250 mg/dl
- Plasma 375 mg/dl
- CSF 440 mg/dl
- Cells 190 mg/100 g
- Muscles 40 mg/100 g

Absorption and Excretion

Absorption: It takes place in small intestine. The mechanism of chloride uptake is unclear, but it appears to depend on an exchange process with the HCO^-_3, whilst the accompanying sodium exchange for a hydrogen ion.

Excretion:

- ***Sweat:*** 5 mM/day depends on weather
- ***Faeces:*** 5 mM/day
- ***Renal:*** 100-200 mM/day. 99% of the Cl^- in the glomerular filtrate is reabsorbed by renal tubules mainly in proximal tubule (60-70%) and then in ascending loop of Henle (20-25%) followed by distal tubule, collecting duct (10-15%).

Regulations: Control of absorption and excretion of chloride appears to be similar to that of sodium. Increase in blood volume decreases reabsorption of chloride and vice-versa. Plasma levels of chloride vary with and to, a great extent depend on, the plasma concentration of Na^+ and HCO_3^-.

↓ Na^+ associated with Cl^- ↓
↑ Na^+ usually associated with Cl^- ↑
↑ HCO_3^- associated with Cl^- ↓
↓ HCO_3^- associated with Cl^- ↑

FUNCTIONS

- It is important in the production of HCl in the gastric juice.
- It is important in *chloride shift*.

Clinical Importance

'Spot' urinary chloride concentration is useful in classifying metabolic alkalosis into the saline responsive and saline unresponsive types.

- Urine Cl^- < 10 mM/L: *Saline responsive metabolic alkalosis*—vomiting, previous diuretic therapy, chloride diarrhoea, ingestion of alkali.
- Urine Cl^- > 20 mM/L: *Saline unresponsive metabolic alkalosis*—mineralocorticoid excess, Barter's syndrome, severe K^+ deficiency, current diuretic therapy.

CALCIUM

Calcium is an important mineral mainly found in bone and teeth.

Dietary sources: it is widely distributed in food substances such as milk, cheese, egg-yolk, beans, lentils, nuts, figs, cabbage.

Body distribution: the total calcium of the body is 25-35 mols(100-170g). About 99% of it is found in bones. It exists as carbonate or phosphate of calcium. About 0.5% in soft tissue and 0.1% in ECF. ***The normal level of plasma calcium is 9-11 mg/dl. The calcium in plasma is of 3 types, namely: • ionized calcium (diffusible); • protein bound calcium and • complexed calcium,*** it is probably complexed with organic acids. About 40% of total calcium is in ionized form. Albumin is the major protein with which calcium is bound. All the three forms of calcium in plasma remain in equilibrium with each other. Ionized calcium is physiologically active form of calcium (also called 'free' form).

Absorption: Calcium is taken in the diet principally as calcium phosphate, carbonate and tartarate. Unlike Na and K which are readily absorbed, the absorption of Ca is rather incomplete. About 40% of average daily dietary intake of Ca is absorbed from the gut. Calcium is absorbed mainly from the duodenum and first half of jejunum against electrical and concentration gradients.

Mechanism: Two mechanisms have been proposed for absorption of calcium by gut mucosa,

- Simple diffusion
- An ***"active"*** transport process involving energy and ***Ca^{++} Pump***. Both the processes

require, 1,25-di hydroxy-D_3 (Calcitriol) which regulates the synthesis of Ca-binding proteins and transport and also a Ca^{++}-dependant ATPase.

Factors Affecting Absorption:

Various factor which influence the absorption of calcium are discussed below:

1. ***pH of intestinal milieu:***

- An acidic pH favours calcium absorption because the Ca-salts, particularly PO_4 and carbonates are quite soluble in acid solutions.
- In an alkaline medium, the absorption of calcium is lowered due to the formation of insoluble tricalcium PO_4.

2. ***Composition of the diet:***

- ***High protein diet:*** A high protein diet favours absorption, 15% of dietary Ca is absorbed. If the protein content is low, only 5% may be absorbed.

  Reason: Amino acids increases the solubility of Ca-salts and thus its absorption. ***Lysine*** and ***Arginine*** obtained from basic proteins cause maximal absorption of Ca.
- ***Fatty acids:*** In malasorption syndrome, fatty acids are not absorbed properly. Fatty acids produce insoluble calcium soaps which are excreted in faeces, thus decreasing the Ca-absorption.
- ***Sugars and organic acids:*** Organic acids produced by microbial fermentation of sugars in the gut, increases the solubility of Ca-salts and increases their absorption. Citric acid also may increase the absorption of calcium.
- ***Phytic acid:*** Cereals contain phytic acid (inositol hexaphosphate), which forms insoluble Ca-salts and decreases the absorption of Ca.
- ***Oxalates:*** Oxalates present in vegetable like cabbage and spinach forms insoluble calcium oxalates which are excreted in the faeces, thus lowering the calcium absorption.
- ***Fibres:*** Presence of excess of fibres in the diet interferes with the absorption of calcium.
- ***Minerals:***
  - ***Phosphates:*** Excess of phosphates lower calcium absorption.
  - ***Magnesium:*** High contents of magnesium in the diet decreases absorption of calcium.
  - ***Ca: P ratio:*** A ratio of food Ca to P not more than 1:2 and not less than 1:2 (ideal 1:1) is necessary for optimal absorption of calcium.
  - ***Fe in diet:*** Food Fe may form insoluble ferric phosphates. These indirectly increases the Ca: P ratio in the gut beyond the range of optimal absorption.
  - ***Vitamin D:*** Promotes Ca absorption.

3. ***State of health of the individual and aging:***

- A healthy adult absorbs about 40% of dietary calcium.
- Above the age of 60 years, there is a gradual decline in the intestinal absorption of Ca.
- In sprue syndrome, the intestinal absorption of calcium suffers due to formation of Ca-soaps with FA which are excreted in faeces.

4. ***Hormonal:***

- ***PTH (Parathormone):*** PTH directly cannot increase the calcium absorption. But PTH stimulates *"1-α-hydroxylase"* enzyme in the kidney and increases the synthesis of 1, 25-$(OH)_2$-D_3 (calcitriol) which enhances calcium absorption. (Refer to vitamin D)
- ***Calcitonin:*** Calcitonin directly cannot affect Ca-absorption. Increased calcitonin level inhibits *"1-α-hydroxylase"* enzyme, thus decreasing synthesis of calcitriol and Ca-absorption.
- ***Glucocorticoids:*** Diminishes intestinal transport of calcium.

Regulation: Kidneys filter about 250 mMol of Ca^{2+} every day, some 95% of which is reabsorbed by the tubules. The major portion of this filtered Ca^{2+} is taken up by proximal tubule without hormonal regulation. A fine adjustment to the amount reabsorbed occurs in distal tubules under the influence of PTH (PTH-uptake). Plasma level of ionized calcium concentration is the principal regulator of PTH secretion by a simple negative feedback mechanism. A threshold level of magnesium is required for PTH release.

Hypermagnesemia inhibits PTH secretion. PTH secretion is also subject to negative feedback by the vitamin D metabolite 1,25$(OH)_2D_3$. PTH rapidly stimulates osteoclast activity, the increased bone resorption causing an increase in plasma Ca^{2+} and PO_4, Vitamin D_3 plays a permissive role for this effect. PTH stimulates more slowly (days) osteoblast activity. PTH via cAMP increases the distal nephron reabsorption of calcium and decreases that of PO_4 in the proximal tubule. In doing so, PTH increases the tubular synthesis and excretion of cAMP. PTH also stimulates the enzyme *1-α-hydroxylase* that converts 25, OH D_3 to 1, 25$(OH)_2D_3$, thereby increasing calcium uptake from the gut.

Hypercalcemia stimulates calcitonin release while hypocalcemia has inhibitory effect. Calcitonin strongly inhibits osteoclastic bone resorption.

Thyroid hormones, ACTH, prostaglandins have some effect on Ca level of plasma. General scheme of control is shown in *Fig. 23.1.*

FUNCTIONS OF CALCIUM

- *Calcification of Bones and Teeth:* The process of bone formation and teeth formation is known as calcification which is a continuous process for bones. Osteoblasts secrete an enzyme *alkaline phosphatase* which can hydrolyze certain phosphoric esters.
- Calcium plays a role in blood coagulation by producing substances for thromboblastic activity of blood.
- Calcium has a role in neuromuscular transmission.
- Calcium ions are needed for excitability of nerves.
- Calcium plays role in muscle contraction.
- Normal excitability of heart is Ca ion dependent
- It plays role as secondary or tertiary messenger in hormone action.
- It plays role in permeability of gap junctions.

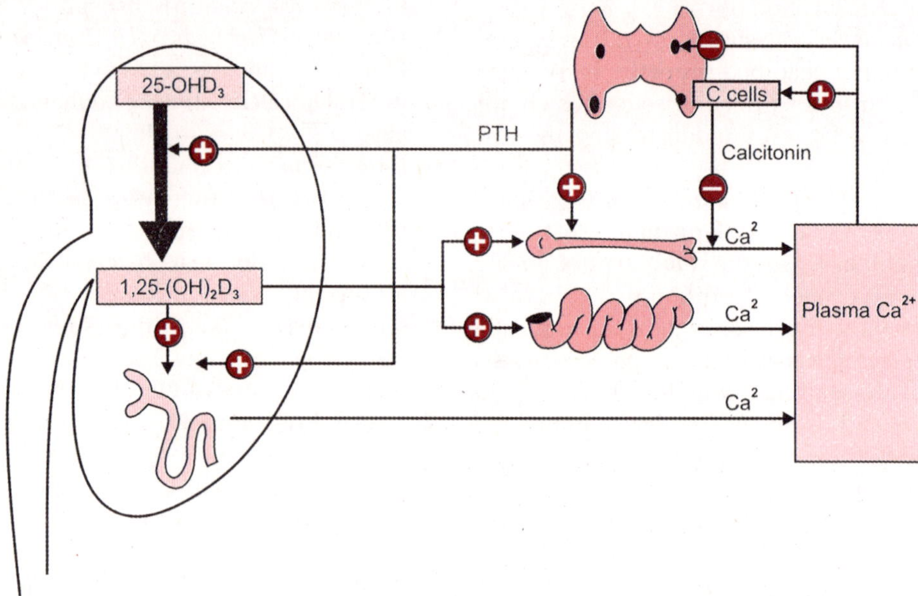

Fig. 23.1: Major hormone control mechanisms of plasma Ca^{2+} homeostasis

Clinical Importance

The two conditions namely Hyper and Hypocalcemia occur.

I. Hypercalcemia: Causes of hypercalcaemia are multiple. They are as follows:

1. ***Malignancy:*** Most important cause for hospital in-patients. Hypercalcaemia in malignancy may be due to:

a. ***Humoral factor:*** No direct skeletal involvement (HMM-Humoral hypercalcaemia of Malignancy).

- PTH-related protein (PTHrP)
- Growth factors: Tumour growth factor (TGF), Epidermal growth factor (EGF), Platelet derived growth factor (PDGF).

b. Direct skeletal involvement by tumours:
  - Direct erosion of bone by tumour
  - Production of PGE-2 by the tumour which can produce bone resorption.

c. Haematological malignancies: Production of
  - Cytokinase-Interleukin-1; tumour-necrosis factor (TNF); lymphotoxin.
  - 1,25-di (OH)-D_3 production by lymphomas.

2. ***Primary hyperparthyroidism:*** Most common cause for out-patients (OPD cases).

May be—
- Familial
- Hyperplasia of parathyroids
- Tumour like adenoma or multiple adenomas
- "Ectopic" hyperparathyroidisms:
  - ***Multiple endocrine neoplasia-Type-I (Men I)*** with pituitary and pancreatic tumours
  - ***Multiple endocrine neoplasia: Type II (Men II):*** medullary carcinoma of thyroid and pheochromocytoma.

3. ***Other endocrine causes:*** Hyperthyroidism, Hypothyroidism, Acromegaly, Acute adrenal insufficiency.

4. ***Granulomatous diseases:*** Tuberculosis, Sarcoidosis, Berrylliosis, Coccidiomycosis.

5. ***Overdosage of vitamins***: Vitamin A intoxication, Hypervitaminosis D.

6. ***Drug-induced hypercalcaemia (Iatrogenic):*** Thiazide diuretics, Spironolactone, Milk-alkali syndrome

7. ***Miscellaneous other causes***:
   - Idiopathic hypercalcaemia of infancy ***(William syndrome)***
   - Familal hypocalcinuric hypercalcaemia
   - Prolonged immobilization
   - Increased serum proteins
     - Hyperalbuminaemia-haemo concentration
     - Hyperglobulimaemia—due to multiple myeloma
   - Renal failure: Acute renal failure—Diuretic phase, Chronic renal failure, Post renal transplantation

II. Hypocalcaemia: The commonest cause of hypocalcaemia is hypolbuminaemia, closely followed by renal failure. The other most common cause of hypocalcaemia is surgically-induced hypoparathyroidism. Hence, if a thyroidectomy scar is present the cause becomes quite apparent.

However, causes of hypocalcaemia are multiple and they are as follows:

1. ***Reduction in serum albumin (Hypoalbuminaemia):*** Malnutrition, malabsorption states, nephrotic syndrome

- Chronic liver diseases and liver failure

2. ***Hypoparathyroidism:***
   - May be surgically-induced-Partial or complete
   - Idiopathic-may be auto-immune
   - Bio-inactive paraahtyroid hormone (PTH)
   - Transient hypoparathyroidism of infancy —may be partial

3. ***Renal disease and renal failure:*** Renal tubular dysfunction, Acute tubular necrosis, Chronic renal failure

4. ***Pseudo-hypoparathyroidism:***

5. ***Hypoparathyroidism in association with other disease states,*** which may be familial:
   - Addison's disease
   - Pernicious anaemia
   - Fungal disease like candidiasis

6. *Other miscellaneous causes:*

- Acute pancreatitis—haemorrhagic or oedematous.
- Osteomalacia and rickets due to vitamin D deficiency or resistnce
- Medullary carcinoma of thyroid, with or without associated endocrinopathies.
- "Healing Phase" of bone disease of treated hyperparathyroidism, hyperthyroidism and haematological malignancies *("Hungry bone" syndrome)*
- Magnesium deficiency

7. ***Iatrogenic (Drug-induced):*** Asministration of *Foscarnate*—given for therapy of cytomegalo virus retinitis in patients with Acquired Immune Deficiency Syndrome (AIDS), has been reported to produce hypocalcaemia.

PHOSPHORUS

Food Sources: Foods rich in phosphorus content are cheese, milk, nuts, organ meats, egg.

Body distribution: Total body phosphate is about 25 mol (700 gm). More than 85% (600 gm) is found in bones, 15% in soft tissues and 1% is found in ECF, about 5 gm in brain and 2 gm in blood. About 1.5 gm of phosphate is required to be taken in the diet daily.

Absorption: A Major part (90%) of daily dietary phosphate is absorbed. The absorption is stimulated by both PTH and Vitamin D_3. The Ca:P ratio in diet affects the absorption and excretion of phosphorus. If one is in excess in diet, the excretion of the other is increased.

Regulation: Regulation of Ca and P is under the similar control mechanisms by kidney with respect to PTH and vitamin D.

Role of Kidneys:

- Phosphate uptake is sodium dependent, about 85% of filtered PO_4 is reabsorbed by the proximal tubules. Phosphate reabsorption is increased when dietary intake is reduced by a PTH-dependent mechamism.
- Plasma inorganic phosphate is a major regulator of 25-OH-D_3. Increase ↑ of 1,25$(OH)_2$-D_3 activity increases ↑ PO_4 absorption. Decreases ↓ of 1,25 $(OH)_2$-D_3 decreases ↓ PO_4 absorption.

FUNCTIONS OF PHOSPHORUS

- Phosphate is the constituent of bone and teeth.
- ***Energy transfer:*** The free energy produced by metabolic reactions may be stored as high energy phosphate—ATP, creatine phosphate.
- ***Acid-base balance:*** The buffer which is effectively handled by kidneys is a phosphate buffer. It is a mixture of dibasic and monobasic phosphates.
- Phosphorylation and phosphorolysis reactions involve phosphate.
- ***Enzyme action:*** Phosphate of several coenzymes such as NADP, TPP, PLP is involved in enzymatic reactions.
- Constituent of phospholopids, nucleotides/nucleic acids, lipoproteins phosphoproteins is phosphate.

Clinical Importance

Rickets and Osteomalacia are important dietary deficiency disorders of calcium, phosphorous or vitamin D.

Plasma levels of adult 0.6-1.2 mMol/L are lower compared to childhood 1.3-2.8 mMol/L. There is often a slight fall in PO_4 after a meal rich in carbohydrates. Plasma Ca and phosphate together are normally measured.

↑ Ca + ↓ PO_4	Primary hyperparathyroidism
↑ Ca + ↑ PO_4	Malignancy (1° or 2°) tumour deposits is done, post dialysis in rental failure.
↓ Ca + ↑ PO_4	hypoparthyroidism
↓ Ca + ↓ PO_4	Vitamin D deficiency

1. **Hypophosphatemia:** It may be due to following:

- ***Decreased intake may be due to:***
  - Starvation, Malabsorption, Vomiting
- ***Increased cell uptake:***
  - High dietary carbohydrate, liver disease.
- ***Increased Excretion:***
  - Diuretics, hypomagnesaemia, ↑ PTH.

2. **Hyperphosphataemia:** It may occur due to the following:

- Factitious hemolysis, prolonged contact of plasma with red cells 7 to 8 hours.
- ***Increased intake:*** Diet, Vitamin D.
- ***Increased release from cells:*** Diabetes mellitus, Acidaemia, Starvation.
- ***Increased release from bone:***
- Malignancy, Renal failure — ↑ PTH
- ***Decreased excretion:*** Renal failure, Hypoparathyroidsm, ↑ Growth hormone.

SULPHUR

Sources: Sulphur is an essential element. The sulphur is made available to the body by the proteins ***containing methionine, cystine or cysteine***. These amino acids contain sulfur. Certain ***sulpholipids*** and ***glycoproteins*** (***mucoitin and chondroitin sulfuric acid***) also provide sulphur. (Sulphur as free element cannot be utlized) sulphur is thus available in meat, fish, legumes, egg, liver, cereals. Adequate protein in diet fulfils sulphur requirement.

Absorption: Sulphur is ingested as organic sulphates as in proteins or as inorganic sulphate. Inorganic sulphate is absorbed as such from the intestines, while sulphur containing amino acids are absorbed by active transport.

Distribution: About 0.25% (150-200 gm) of the total body weight is sulphur. It is mainly found as organic compounds such as, Met, Cys, heparin, glutathione, thiamine, biotin, CoA, lipoic acid, taurocholic acid, etc. Many proteins, hormones, keratin of hair contain sulphur. Small amounts of inorganic sulphates occur in tissues and body fluids. Hundred ml of blood contains 0.1 to 1.0 mg sulphur as organic compounds.

Fate: Catabolism of S-containing amino acids yields inorganic sulphates. Liver converts inorganic sulphate to ethereal sulphate by conjugation.]

FUNCTIONS OF SULPHUR

- Formations of 'active sulphate' (PAPS) is already mentioned in chapter on Nucleotides. Active sulphate participates in several transulfuration reactions.
- Sulphur is involved in the formation of proteins such as keratin, chondroproteins, sulfolipids.
- It is also involved in the formation of –SH groups which act as active centres of enzymes such as Acyl carrier protein (ACP) and multienzyme complex of fatty acid synthesis.
- It forms-S—S linkages between two-'SH' groups of cysteine to form a secondary and tertiary structure of proteins.
- Iron-sulphur proteins are found in electron transport chain.
- S-Adenosylmethionine is a co-substrate for methylferases.
- S-Adenosylmethionine also acts as the initiator in initiation process of protein synthesis.
- Sulphur containing vitamin such as biotin, pantothenic acid, thiamine, lipoic acid are involved as coenzymes.
- Sulphates, hexosamines and hexuronic acids are important constituents of mucopolysaccharides, sulphated galactose occurs in sulpholipids.
- Phenol, skatole, indole and steroids may be detoxicated in the liver with sulphate ions.
- Acyl complexes of CoA, S-adenosyl methionine, 'active' sulphate are high energy sulphur compounds.

IRON

Iron is one of the most essential trace element in the body. In spite of the fact that iron is the fourth most abundant element in the earth's crust, iron deficiency is one of the most important prevalent nutritional deficiencies in India. The reasons for this are numerous and, in many cases, not well understood. Total iron content in a human of 70 kg body weight varies approximately from 2.3 gm to 3.8 gm. Average iron content of adult males is about 3.8 gm and of females about 2.3.gm.

Types of Iron Present in Body

There are *two broad categories* that are used to describe iron in the body. They are:

- *Essential (or functional) iron*
- *Storage iron*

A. Essential Iron: Essential or functional iron is one which is involved in the normal metabolism of the cells.

They are mainly divided into *three groups:-*

(a) *Heme-Proteins:*

- ***Haemoglobin and Myoglobin:*** These are heme proteins, which are proteins with an iron-porphyrin prosthetic group attached to the protein globin. They are most abundant of the essential (or functional) iron compounds in the body.
- ***Catalases:*** It is a heme containing enzyme. It destroys hydrogen peroxide, H_2O_2, formed in the tissues and molecular O_2 is evolved in the reaction.

$$2\,H_2O_2 \xrightarrow{\text{catalase}} 2\,H_2O + O_2$$

- ***Peroxidases:*** It is typically a plant enzyme, but it is also found in milk, erythrocytes, leucocytes and lens fibres. Its molecular weight is 44,100 and its prosthetic group is protoheme which is only loosely bound to apoprotein.

Example: Typical example is ***glutathione peroxidase*** which also catalyzes destruction of H_2O_2, but it works in conjunction with reduced glutathione, G-SH

$$\underset{\textbf{(reduced glutathione)}}{H_2O_2 + 2\,G.SH} \xrightarrow[\text{(se-containing)}]{\text{Glutathione peroxidase}} \underset{\textbf{(oxidized glutathione)}}{H_2O + G\text{-}S\text{-}S\text{-}G}$$

Note:

- Both catalase and glutathione peroxidase catalyzes the destruction of H_2O_2 and forms H_2O and O_2.
- Catalase can directly act on H_2O_2, but glutathione peroxidase cannot, it requires reduced glutathione. The reason is ***Km of catalase of H_2O_2 is much greater than that of glutathione peroxidase.***
- To scavenge small amounts of H_2O_2 formed in cells like RB cells and lens fibres, glutathione peroxidase becomes the active enzyme.

(b) ***Cytochromes:*** A second group of organo-iron compounds in the body are the cytochromes. (Refer Biologic Oxidation).

(c) ***Iron Requiring Enzymes:*** A third group of iron containing compounds is the iron-requiring enzymes.

a. This group contains enzymes that also use riboflavin as coenzyme.

Examples:

- *Xanthine oxidase*
- *Cytochrome C reductase*
- *Acyl CoA dehydrogenase*
- *NADH-reductase*

b. Other enzymes in this group that require the metal only as cofactor

- *Succinate dehydrogenase*
- *Aconitase*
- *Ribonucleotide reductase*

c. Fe^{++} is required for conversion O_2^-, superoxide radical to free $OH^{\bullet}$ radical. This is called as ***Haber's reaction.***

B. Storage Iron: Storage iron is present in ***two major compounds***. They are:

- ***Ferritin***
- ***Haemosiderin***

1. *Ferritin:* ***Free iron is toxic and catalyzes the conversion of O_2^- to hydroxy $OH^{\bullet}$ oxy radicals. Iron bound to ferritin is non-toxic.*** It is the storage protein of iron and found in ***blood, liver, spleen, bonemarrow*** and ***intestine (mucosal cells).***

- Apoferritin is the apoprotein with a molecular weight of 550,000. Apoferritin is an interesting compound in that it is ***composed of 24 monomeric units,*** each having molecular weight of 18,000, that form a spherical shell. There are ***six pores in the shell*** that allow molecules of a certain size to enter and exit the shell. The pores have been shown to have catalytic activity, most notably the binding of ferrous iron (Fe^{2+}) and its subsequent oxidation to "ferric oxy hydroxide" (FeOOH)

- Bound form of iron with ferritin is more soluble and iron is present as "ferric oxyhydroxy phosphate" complex in ferritin and it is reddish-brown in colour. Up to 4500 Fe^{3+} atoms are found stored in a ferritin complex.

2. ***Haemosiderin:*** ***Evidence suggests that haemosiderin is derived from ferritin and is ferritin with partially stripped shell.*** Haemosiderin contains a larger fraction of its mass as Fe than does ferritin and exists as microscopically visible Fe-staining particles. ***Haemosiderin is usually seen in states of iron overload or when Fe is in excess,*** when the synthesis of apoferritin and its uptake of Fe are maximum. Haemosiderin is rather insoluble, Fe in haemosiderin is available for formation of Hb, but mobilization of iron is much slower from haemosiderin than ferritin. Distribution of iron in the body is shown in the ***Table 23.1.***

Table 23.1

Protein/Enzyme	*Iron content (in mg)*	*% of total*
• **Haemoproteins**		
Haemoglobin	2500	60-70
Myoglobin	400	5-10
Heme enzymes		
Catalase and peroxidase	2-3	1
• **Organo-iron compounds**		
Cytochromes	4-5	1
• **Storage iron**		
Ferritin, haemosiderin (Non-heme protein)	300-700	10-15
• **Transferrin** (Non-heme protein)	6-8	1
• **Iron requiring enzymes**		
Fp, Fe-s Non-heme enzymes	–	1
Other-dehydrogenases non-heme enzymes	–	1

c. **Transferrin:** transferrin is a ***non-heme iron binding glycoproteins.*** Apotransferrin is the apoenzyme and Fe is its prosthetic group. It has a molecular weight of 70,000 and ***it can bind with two atoms of iron in the ferric state (Fe^{3+})*** synergistically in presence of HCO_3^- ion. It exists in plasma as β_1 globulin and is the ***true carrier of iron.*** In plasma, transferrin is saturated only to the extent of 30% to 33% with iron. Prior to binding to transferrin, Fe^{2+} (ous) iron has to be oxidized to Fe^{3+} (ic) form. ***Caeruloplasmin and ferroxidase II are required for this conversion.***

Note: In copper deficiency, this conversion cannot occur and haemopoietic system will not be getting required amount of Fe for inclusion in Hb sysnthesis.

FUNCTION OF TRANSFERRIN

Major function of transferrin is the transport of iron to RE cells, bonemarrow to reach the immature red blood cells. Specific receptors are available on cells surface. Transferrin is internalized by receptor mediated endocytosis. Within the target cells, iron is released and apotransferrin is recycled to form new transferrin molecules ***(Fig. 23.2).***

Dietary Sources of Iron

1. *Exogenous:* Foods rich in iron include:
- *Animal Sources:* Meat, fish, liver, spleen, red marrow are very rich sources (2.0-6.0 mg/100 gm) Also found in shellfish.
- *Vegetable Sources:* Cereals (2.0-8.0 mg/100 gm) are the major rich source. Legumes, molasses, nuts, amaranth leaves. Dates are other good sources, Apple also a good source.

II. *Endogenous:* Fe is utilized from ferritin of RE system and intestinal mucosal cells. Fe obtained from "effete" red cells are also reutilized.

Absorption of Iron and factors Regulating Absorption

Normally, the loss of iron from the body of a man is limited to 1 mg per day. Menstruating women lose iron with menstrual blood. Around 10 to 20 mg of Fe is taken in the diet and only about 10% is absorbed. The greatest need of iron is during infancy and adolescence. The only mechanism by which total body stores of iron is regulated is at the level of absorption. **Garnick** prposed a ***"mucosal block theory"*** for iron absorption.

Mucosal Block Theory

- Soluble inorganic salts of iron are easily absorbed from the small intestine. HCl present in gastric juice liberates free Fe^{3+} from non-heme proteins, vitamin C and glutathione in diet reduce Fe^{3+} to Fe^{2+}, which is less

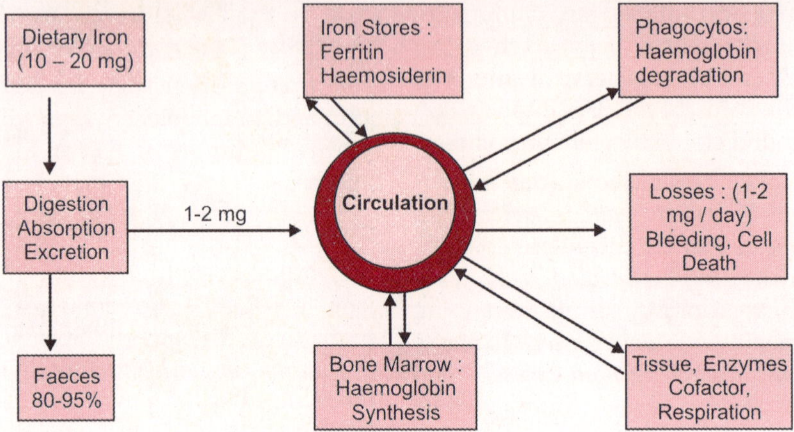

Fig. 23.2: Iron distribution and transport in humans

polymerizable and more soluble form of iron. Vitamin C and amino acids can form iron ascorbate and iron-amino acid chelates which are readily absorbed. Heme is abosrbed as such.

- *Gastroferrin*, a glycoprotein in gastric juice is believed to bind iron and facilitate its uptake in duodenum and jejunum. The absorption of iron from intestinal lumen into mucosal cells takes place as Fe^{2+}.

Events in intestinal mucosal cells: In the mucosal cell cytoplasm, there is a carrier called ***intracellular iron carrier (I. I. C)*** Fe^{2+} iron is oxidized again in mucosal cells to Fe^{3+} form principally by caeruloplasmin (Ferroxidase I) and also to some extent by ferroxidase II. Both are Cu-containing enzymes

- Intracellular iron carrier delivers a fixed amount of iron to mitochondria. It also transfers certain amount of Fe^{3+} to "apoferritin", which is synthesized by mucosal cells, to form the storage form "ferritin".
- I.I.C. transfers some iron across the serosal cell membrane to a plasma β_1-globulin, called 'apotransferrin' to form transferrin. Iron is carried in transferrin as Fe^{3+}.
- The I.I.C. holds Fe^{3+} in either protein bound or chelated forms which represent the *"carrier-iron pool"* in the intestinal mucosal cells. Presence of sufficient amount of Fe in *"carrier-iron pool"*, keeps the I.I.C. nearly or totally saturated and consequently reduces further iron absorption. This theory advanced by **Granick** is known as **"mucosal block theory"**, which regulates the iron absorption from the gut.

Other factors:

1. *Source of Fe has marked effect on absorption.*

- ***Heme iron*** which comes mainly from animal products and is from Hb and myoglobin, is efficiently absorbed (about 20 to 30%).
- ***Non-heme iron***, which is present in plants, though ingested in larger amount than heme iron, are inefficiently absorbed (only 1 to 5%).

2. The absorption of non-heme iron is influenced by the:
   - **Composition of the diet**
   - **pH of the intestinal milieu, and**
   - **State of health of the individual.**

1. Composition of the Diet: The composition of the diet exerts a profound effect on non-heme iron absorption.

- Dietary factors that increase iron absorption are the presence of vitamin C (ascorbic acid), glutathione, and some form of meat, fish or poultry ***(all contain an unknown "meat factor")***
- Foods that inhibit non-heme iron absorption to some extent are:
  - Tea (diminishes absorption by >60%),
  - Coffee (reduced absorption by > 35%),

- Phytates, found in corn, soya products, grains, and bran (producing insoluble complex)
- Oxalates found in spinach and chocolates.
- Some dietary fibres may also bind the iron or decrease gastrointestinal transit time.

2. **pH of Intestinal Milieu:**

- HCl secreted in gastric juice liberates Fe^{3+} from non-heme iron and serves to increase solubility of dietary non-heme iron.
- pH of duodenum is most conductive for absorption. Rate of absorption further decreases down the intestines as the pH becomes more alkaline.
- At high alkaline pH, the ingested iron is precipitated.

3. **State of Health of the Individual:**

- Healthy adults absorb about 5 to 10% of dietary iron, which is approximately 1 to 2 mg of iron.
- Iron-deficient adults absorb 10 to 20% of the dietary iron equivalent to 3 to 6 mg of Fe.

Note:

- Individuals having achlorhydria or achylia gastrica and in persons having resection of gut, partial or total gastrectomies iron absorption is diminished and they are at risk of iron deficiency.
- Intestinal epithelia normally are desquamated and again regenerated. Significant quantity of iron as ferritin is lost during desquamation.
- Parasitic infection, viz. ***Ankylostoma duodenale*** produces Fe loss as the parasites suck blood and thrive on it.

Iron Transport and Utilization

- Transport of Fe throughout the body is accomplished with a specific protein called ***transferrin*** (See above).
- Transferrin transports Fe from the GI tract to the bone-marrow for Hb synthesis and to all other cells as required. Transferrin can transport a maximum of two atoms of iron as Fe^{3+} per molecule. ***Normally, in plasma/serum transferrin is about 33% saturated with Fe.***
- As discussed above, cell surfce specific receptors are available for the iron-transferrin complex. Tissues having high uptake, e.g. liver, have a larger number of receptors present. ***The number of receptors decreases when a person is replete with iron and increases with depletion.***
- Iron is transported to bone marrow where it is required for Hb synthesis. Fe^{2+} is incorporated in protoporphyrin IX with the help of the enzyme *"ferrochelatase"*.
- Iron is also transported into cells where it is used for both oxidative phosphorylation and as an enzyme cofactor.
- A small amount of Fe is released each day from 'effete' red cells, which are destroyed by phagocytes, but this released Fe^{2+} is recycled into new Hb in the erythroblasts. A small amount of released Fe is also stored as ferritin. ***The turnover of iron in an adult in 24 hours has been calculated to be 35 to 40 mg.***
- Plasma "trasferrin iron pool" is in equilibrium with the iron in storage forms: ferrtin and haemosiderin. ***Ferritin in storage form of Fe occur in reticuloendothelial system (RES),*** viz liver, spleen and bone marrow and also in intestinal mucosal cells.
- When Fe is mobilized from ferritin, the storage form, the sequence is as follows:
  - ***First call:*** From ferritin of RE system (Liver, spleen and bone marrow):
  - ***Second call:*** From ferritin of intestinal mucosal cells.
  - ***Thirdly:*** Absorbed iron from intestines.
- Before Fe is released from ferritin to blood, Fe^{3+} of ferritin is first reduced to Fe^{2+}.

Iron Requirement and Clinical Significane

Requirement of iron varies according to age, sex, weight and state of health. An adult male requires approximately 10 mg/day and adult female 20 mg/day. Pregnancy and lactation demands more. Pregnant women require 10 mg/day and lactating mother 25-30 mg/day. Children require 10 to 15 mg/day.

- Adult women faces the risk of iron deficiency due to pregnancies. ***Each pregnancy extracts about 1000 mg of iron which exceeds the normal iron stores.***
  Menorrhagia can occur in approx. 10% of all women and entails extra loss of Fe. Hence iron must be supplemented in such cases to avoid iron deficiency anaemia.
- Iron status of adult males and postmenopausal women tends to increase throughout life and normally iron deficiency should not be a problem.

But certain chronic diseases at this age group, if not treated, can lead to iron deficiency. They are

- Chronic infections incl. Tuberculosis
- Malignancies
- Chronic aspirin ingestion
- Peptic ulcers
- Rheumatoid arthritis
- and parasitic infections, etc.

A. Iron deficiency: Three stages of iron deficiency are:

- **Iron storage depletion**
- **Iron deficiency**
- **Iron deficiency anaemia**

1. *Iron Storage Depletion:* This phase is not usually recognizable by the patient and normally does not elicit a medical examination. ***Serum ferritin decreases during this phase and is the only good indication of possible iron deficiency.*** Many women of child bearing age remain in this phase for years without being identified.

2. *Iron Deficiency:* In this phase iron stores are almost exhausted.

- ***Biochemically*** the serum ferritin is low ↓ and transferrin saturation is low ↓.
- Erythrocyte protoporphyrin increases, as erythropoiesis is slowed down due to non availability of Fe which cannot be incorporated in protoporphyrin IX.
- Haemoglobin concentration falls to the lowest limit of normal.

3. *Iron Deficiency Anaemia:* Iron deficiency anaemia is manifested as ***hypochromic microcytic anaemia.*** At this phase

- Hb concentration continues to fall ↓
- Serum ferritin level shows slow decline ↓
- Transferrin saturation continues to fall ↓
- and erythrocyte protoporphyrin increases to upper limit of normal ↑.

To classify as iron deficiency anaemia a low Hb plus a documented abnormal serum ferritin or other iron test must be present.

Note: It is imperative to determine iron levels in all patients with anaemias, since there are disorders such as thalassaemias that may be present and misdiagnosed as iron deficiency.

B. Iron Overload: Iron overload can also be an important clinical concern. Iron stores may increase due to:

- ***excessive absorption, or***
- ***parental iron therapy or***
- ***repeated transfusions***

Cells start to fill with excess of haemosiderin ↑ both reticuloendothelial cells and parenchymal cells sequester iron.

Types: ***Two broad types*** of iron overload seen

- ***Haemochromatosis:*** When iron overload is ***associated with injury to cells.***
- ***Haemosiderosis:*** When iron overload ***without cell damage*** is called haemosiderosis.

1. Haemochromatosis:

Haemochromatosis can be of ***two types:***

- ***Primary*** Hereditary haemochromatosis (Idiopathic)
- ***Secondary*** haemochromatosis

Note: Early diagnosis of haemochromatosis is essential. Untreated haemochromatosis can lead to, liver, pancreatic, and cardiac impairment, diabetes mellitus, and hepatic carcinoma. A helpful screening test is: serum trasferrin saturation. ***Patients with serum transferrin saturation >62% may have haemochromatosis.***

a. **Primary (Idiopathic) Haemochromatosis**

- Inherited disorder: Autosomal recessive
- Haemochromatosis "gene" is linked to HLA-A_3, with a frequency of 1:200.
- Massive accumulation of iron, mainly as ferritin and haemosiderin, in visceral organs, principally liver and skin.

Classic "triad" for diagnosis:

- Micronodular cirrhosis with marked brown pigmentation.
- Diabetes mellitus.
- Skin pigmentation called as ***"Bronze diabetes"***

- Deposition of iron in myocardium can cause ***cardiomyopathy*** and ***heart failure.*** Excess iron accumulates in the cytoplasm of parenchymal cells with possible "free" radical generation, leading to lysosomal disruption and cell damage.
- ***Increased risk of hepato-cellular carcinoma***

Postulated Mechnisms for the Disease:

The following mechanisms suggested:

- Hereditary defect in regulation of iron absorption by the duodenum and jejunum.
- A defect in immediate post-absorptive excretion of iron.
- A genetic inability of phagocytes to take up iron with loss of their regulatory control signals over iron absorption.

b. Secondary Haemochromatosis:

- Due to ineffective erythropoiesis as in thalassaemia, erythrogenesis imperfecta
  - with repeated blood transfusion/trans–fusion overload
  - patients with haemodialysis.

It exhibits more even distribution of iron between macrophages and hepatocytes leads to hepatocellular necrosis and secondary scarring and rarely a micronodular cirrhosis develops.

2. Siderosis or Haemosiderosis:

- ***Bantu siderosis:*** Bantus in Africa cook their food in iron pots. This causes enhanced absorption of Fe leading to Bantu siderosis. Their PO_4 intake is usually low as they consume plenty of corn. Low PO_4 aggravates increased Fe absorption.
  Note: Fe deficiency anaemia is not found in pregnant Bantu women.
- Repeated blood transfusions, thalassaemia and hereditary haemolytic anamias may also result in this condition
- ***Idiopathic pulmonary haemosiderosis:*** Chronic episodic haemorrhages of the lungs of unknown aetiology result in prominent haemosiderin deposition and fibrosis.

COPPER

Adult humans contain 100 to 150 mg of copper, out of which approximately 65 mg is found in muscles, 23 mg in bones and 18 mg in liver. Foetal liver contains aprroximately ten times more copper than adult liver.

It occurs as:

- ***Erythrocuprein*** (in red blood cells),
- ***Hepatocuprein*** (in liver) and
- ***Cerebrocuprein*** (in brain).

Erythrocuprein is a colourless protein containing 2 atoms of Cu per molecule. Molecular weight approximately 33,000.

Source: Average diet provides 2 to 4 mg/day in the form of meat, shellfish, legumes, nuts and cereals ***Milk and milk-products are poor sources.***

Absorption: Primarily absorbed from the duodenum. About 32% of the dietary Cu can be absorbed. Phytates, Zinc, Mo, Cd, Ag, Hg and high amount of Vitamin C inhibit Cu absorption. Absorption of Cu from GI tract requires a specific mechanism because of highly insoluble nature of Cu^{2+} ions. ***An unidentified low molecular weight substance from human saliva and gastric juice*** complexes with Cu^{++} to keep it soluble at pH of intestinal fluid. In the intestinal mucosal cells, Cu is associated with low molecular weight metal binding protein called as ***metallo-thionein.***

Plasma: After absorption Cu enters plasma, where it is bound to amino acids, particularly histidine and to serum albumin at a single strong binding site. In less than an hour, the recently absorbed Cu is removed from the circulation by liver.

Role of Liver: Liver processes absorbed Cu through ***two routes:***

- Cu is excreted in the bile into the GI tract from which it is not reabsorbed. In fact, copper homeostasis is maintained almost exclusively by biliary excretion, the higher the dose of the Cu more it is excreted in faeces. Normally, human urine contains only traces of Cu.

- ***Second route:*** Incorporation as an integral part of ***Caeruloplasmin,*** a glycoprotein synthesized exclusively by liver. (For details of ceruloplasmin and functions—see chapter on "Plasma proteins—Chemistry and Functions).

Serum Copper: Serum Cu level is approximately 90 µg % (average). In red blood cells: 93 to 115 µg/100 ml.

Serum Cu is present in two distinct forms:

- ***Direct reacting Cu:*** Which is loosely bound to albumin. Approximately 4% present in this form. So-called as it reacts directly with diethyl dithiocarbamate.
- ***Bound form:*** Which remains bound to α-globulin fraction of the serum, called "Caeruloplasmin" (as stated above). About 96% of serum Cu is found in combination with caeruloplasmin.

Excretion: Under normal conditions, 85 to 99% of the ingested Cu is excreted in the faeces via the bile, and remaining 1 to 15% in the urine.

Requirements:

- Infants and children: 0.05 mg Cu/kg body wt. per day
- Adult requirements is approximately 2.5 mg/day.
- Ordinary diets consumed daily contain about 2.5 to 5.0 mg Cu.

FUNCTIONS OF COPPER

- ***Role in Enzyme Action:*** Cu forms intergral part of certain enzymes, e.g. some of Cytochromes (*Cytochrome oxidase*), *Tyrosinase, Monoamine oxidase (MAO), Lysyl oxidase, Catalase, Ascorbic acid oxidase, Uricase* and *Superoxide dismutase.*

Superoxide dismutase: A colourless dimeric enzyme, having MW= 32,000, present in cytosol of mammalian liver, nerve and red cells and contain 2 Cu^{2+} and 2Zn^{2+} per molecule.

Functions of superoxide dismutase: Changes superoxide radicals, formed by univalent reduction of O_2 in tissues, to hydrogen peroxide (H_2O_2)

$$O_2' + O_2' + 2H^+ \rightarrow O_2 + H_2O_2$$

There is another "mitochondrial" form of *'superoxide dismutase'* enzyme which is a different protein with Mn^{2+} instead of Cu^{2+} and Zn^{2+} as its prosthetic group.

- ***Role of Cu^{++} in Fe Metabolism:***
  - Cu helps in the utilization of Fe for Hb synthesis in the body. (Refer caerulo plasmin)
  - Facilitatory role of Cu^{++} in iron absorption.
  - A yellow copper-protein called serum *Ferroxidase II* or non-caeruloplasmin ferroxidase may also participate in the oxidation of Fe^{2+} in human plasma.
- ***Role in Maturation of Elastin:*** Copper helps to form insoluble elastin fibres by cross-linking soluble pro-elastin chains.
- ***Role in Bone and Myelin Sheath of Nerves:*** Copper has been reported to help in the formation of bones and maintenance of myelin sheaths of nerve-fibres.

Copper-Deficiency Manifestations:

- ***Loss of weight***
- ***Bone disorder:*** A bone disorder has been reported; characterized by abnormally thin cortices, deficient trabeculae, and wide epiphyses.
- ***Anaemia:*** Copper deficiency produces microcytic hypochromic anaemia, due to impairment of erythropoiesis.
- Copper deficiency ***turns hair grey,*** which however, can be controlled by administration of Cu.
- Copper deficiency has been reported to involve ***atrophy of myocardium.***
- Depletion of brain Cu stores has been observed to cause non-coordinated movements and ***demyelination*** of the nerves in the animals.

Inherited Disorders

1. **Wilson's Disease**
   (Hepatolenticular degeneration)

- *Inheritence:* It is inherited as autosomal recessive.
- *Metabolic defects:* Mainly there are *two defects:*
  - Defect in incorporation of Cu into newly synthesized "apo-caeruloplasmin" to form caeruloplasmin.
  - In addition to above, the patients have impaired ability of the liver to excrete Cu into bile.
- *Clinical features:* Total body retention of Cu is increased particularly in organs like liver, brain, kidney and cornea.
  - *Liver:* Produces progressive hepatic cirrhosis of a coarse nodular type which leads to hepatic failure.
  - *Brain:* There is dysfunction of lenticular region of the brain, necrosis and sclerosis occurs.
  - *Kidneys:* Defects in renal tubular reabsorption producing aminoaciduria.
  - *Eyes:* Copper deposition in "Descemet's membrane" of the eye causes a golden brown, yellow or green ring round the cornea, called as ***Kayserfleischerring.***
- *Blood:* The serum Cu is low, as ceruloplasmin in patient's plasma contains no Cu.
- *Urine:* Urinary excretion of Cu is markedly increased ↑.
- *Treatment:* Improvement can be achieved by removing the excess of tissue Cu by administering Cu-chelating agent like ***"penicillamine".***

2. **Menke's Disease**

- ***Synonym: Kinky or Steel hair syndrome***
- *Inheritance:* It is an X–linked disorder of intestinal copper absorption.
- *Metabolic defect:* The first phase of Cu absorption is its uptake into the mucosal cells and the second phase of its intracellular transport within the mucosal cells are both normal in patients with Menke's disease. ***The third phase transport across the serosal aspect of the mucosal cell membrane is defective.***
- *Clinical Features:* IV administered Cu is handled normally by these children but unless therapy is commenced promptly at birth, many of severe signs of this disease like mental retardation, temperature instability, abnormal bone formation and susceptibility to infection are not prevented.

MAGNESIUM

Magnesium is the fourth most abundant and important cation in humans. It is extremely essential for life and is ***present as intracellular ion*** in all living cells and tissues.

Source: Magnesium is widely distributed in vegetables, found in porphyrin group of chlorophyll of vegetable cells and also found in almost all animal tissues. Other important sources are cereals, beans, green vegetables, potatoes, almonds and dairy products, e.g. cheese.

Distribution: Total body magnesium is approximately 2400 mEq. Approximately 2/3 occurs in bones, 1% in EC fluid and remainder in soft tissues.

Plasma level: Normal plasma levels of Mg is 1.5 to 1.8 mEq/L, which is rigorously maintained within normal limits.

Blood: Magnesium exists in blood partly bound to proteins. Under conditions of physiological pH roughly 1/3 is 'protein-bound', the remainder 2/3 is ionic.

CS Fluid: Concentration of Mg in CS fluid is ½ as high as in plasma.

Absorption: Average daily intake in humans is 250-300 mg, much of which is obtained from green vegetables where Mg is found in porphyrin group of chlorophyll. Roughly 1/3 of dietary Mg is absorbed; the remainder is passively excreted in faeces. Absorption takes place primarily in small bowel, beginning within hour after ingestion and continues at a steady rate for 2 to 8 hours, by that time 80% of total absorption has taken place.

Factors Affecting Absorption

- *Size of Mg load:* Absorption is doubled when normal dietary Mg requirement is doubled and vice versa.
- *Dietary calcium:* Increased absorption in calcium deficienct diets and vice versa.
- *Motility and mucosal state:* In hurried bowel absorption is decreased. Absorption decreases in damaged mucosal state.
- *Vitamin D:* Helps in increased absorption.
- *Parathormone:* Increases absorption.
- *Growth hormone:* Increases absorption.
- *Other factors:*
  - High protein intake and Neomycin therapy increases absorption.
  - Fatty acids phytates and phosphates decrease absorption.

Excretion: Magnesium is lost from the body in faeces, sweat and urine. Most (60 to 80%) of the orally taken Mg is lost in faeces.

Urine: Regulation of Mg balance is principally dependant on renal handling of the ion. In a normal healthy adult with normal diet, 3 to 17 mEq are excreted daily.

Factors Affecting Renal Excretion

- *Calcium intake:* Increased dietary calcium produced, increased excretion of Mg.
- *Parathormone (PTH):* Diminishes excretion.
- *Antidiuretic hormone (ADH):* Increases Mg excretion
- *Growth hormone (GH):* Also increases excretion of Mg.
- *Aldosterone:* Increases excretion
- *Thyroid hormones.* 80% greater excretion in hyperthyroidism.
- *Alcohol ingestion:* Oral ingestion of as little as 1.0 ml of 95% alcohol per Kg, increases urinary excretion 2 to 3 fold.

Note: The increased excretion partially accounts for Mg-deficiency in chronic alcoholics with Delirium tremens.

FUNCTIONS OF MAGNESIUM

- *Role in Enzyme Action:* Mg is involved as a cofactor and as an activator to wide spectrum of enzyme actions. It is essential for *peptidases, ribonucleases, glycolytic enzymes* and co-carboxylation reactions.
- *Neuromuscular Irritability:* Mg exerts an effect on neuromuscular irritability similar to that of Ca^{++}, high levels depress nerve conduction and low levels may produce tetany **(hypomagnaesemic tetany)**
- *As Constituent of Bones and Teeth:* About 70% of body magnesium is present as apatites in bones, dental enamel and dentin.

Plasma Mg in Diseases

1. **Hypermagnaesemia:** Raised values have been reported in: uncontrolled *Diabetes mellitus, Adrenocortical insufficiency, Hypothyrroidism, Advanced renal failure and Acute renal failure.*

2. **Hypomagnaesemia:** Low values are observed in:

- Malabsorption syndrome, Kwashiorkor, Prolonged gastric suction, Hyperthyroidism, Portal cirrhosis, Prolonged use of diuretics, Chronic alcoholism, Renal diseases, Primary aldosteronism, Delirium tremens, etc.

Magnesium Deficiency: In man, 'overt' magnesium deficiency rarely occurs. Experimentally induced prolonged Mg-depletion reported in two patients (reported by **Shils**). Both were fed Mg-deficient synthetic diets—one for 274 days and another for 414 days. In both, plasma Mg fell slowly over several months.

Clinical features: Personality changes, GI disturbances, gross tremors, hyporeflexia, abnormal electromyograph, +ve Chvostek's sign, epileptiform convulsions. Both cases, despite adequate Ca and K intake, developed hypocalcaemia and hypokalemia.

FLUORINE

Source:

- Fluoride is ***solely derived in human from drinking water.***
- **Other sources:** Tea, salmon, sardine and Mackerel contain small amounts of Fluoride.

Requirements: About one part of fluorine in one million parts of drinking water (one PPM) seems to serve the daily requirements of fluorine in human adults and children. ***Daily intake of fluoride should not exceed 3 mg as it is a toxic element.*** For an adult individual, the lethal dose is 2.5 gm.

Absorption and Excretion

- Dietary soluble fluorides are absorbed by diffusion from the intestine. About 10 to 20 μg of fluoride, mostly ionized are present in 100 ml of blood.
- Fluorides are present in significant amounts in calcified tissues like bones and teeth.
- Fluorides excreted mainly in the urine.

FUNCTIONS OF FLUORINE

1. *Role in Tooth Development and Dental Health:*
   - Fluorine is present in human tooth in trace amounts and helps in tooth development, normal maintenance and hardening of dental enamel and prevention of ***"dental caries".***
   - Destruction of dental enamel and incidence of dental caries are widespread among both adults and children in areas where drinking water contains less than 0.5 PPM of fluorine.
   - Cariostatic effect of fluorine is due to its entry into the apatite salts of dental enamel.
   - Greater than 1.2 PPM of fluorine in drinking water of infants/children may increase fluoride contents of the enamel and dentine, may reduce Ca deposition in those tissues and may cause ***mottling of enamel,*** in newly erupted permanent teeth-discoloration, corrosion and stratification of enamel including formation of pits are observed.
2. *Role in Bone Development:*
   - Fluorine is present in human bones in trace amounts.
   - Very small amount of fluorine in food and drinking water promote normal bone development, increases retention of Ca^{++} and PO_4 and prevent old age osteoporosis.
   - High fluoride intakes may raise the fluoride content of bone, stimulate osteoblast activity and cause an abnormal rise in calcium deposition and increased density of bone.
   - Catalytic amounts of fluorine are required for the conversion of the phosphates of calcium to 'apatite salts' of bones and teeth—these may be the basis of role of fluorine in teeth and bone development.

Fluoride Toxicity

Fluorosis: Excess of fluoride in water or diet or its inhalation is harmful and is considered to be the main cause of the crippling disease known as ***'fluorosis'.*** There is still dearth of information on the precise manner in which fluoride ions act upon the body tissues which cause such a derangement. The fluoride levels in GI tract, blood and urine have been reported to be high in fluoride toxicity.

Biochemical Changes in Fluorosis:

- ***Mitochondrial damage***: Administration of sodium fluoride in dosage of 50 mg/kg body weight for 45 days in rabbits resulted in mitochondrial damage and release of CPK. The fluoride ions adversely affect the sarcolemma by enhancing its permeability ↑ and CPK level in blood was raised.
- ***Action on enzymes:*** High fluoride concentration inhibits particularly Mg^{++} dependant enzymes. High fluoride consumption led to reduction in *succinic dehydrogenase* activity of rabbit diaphragm as well as reduction in the diameter of the fibres. The structural and biochemical changes led to muscle wasting and impairment of energy metabolism.
- ***Effects of protein synthesis:*** Fluoride intake in higher amounts resulted in 10 to 46% reduction, in protein contents of various organs, e.g. adrenal gland, cardiac muscles, kidneys, lungs, pancreas, skeletal muscles, spleen, stomach, testes and spinal cord, ***suggestive of inhibition of protein synthesis by fluorides.***

- ***Steroid synthesis: Steroid production was impaired*** because of depletion of *δ-5-3-β hydroxysteroid dehydrogenase* enzyme.
- ***Effect on collegen synthesis: Collagen content is found to be reduced*** and its biosynthesis adversely affected due to reduced proline uptake↓. Formation of deficient collagen fibres with abnormal biochemical sites, provide an impetus for pathological calcification which occurs during fluoride intoxication.

ZINC

Source:

- ***Animal sources:*** Good sources of zinc are liver, milk and dairy products, eggs.
- ***Vegetable Sources:*** Good vegetable sources are unmilled cereals, legumes, pulses, oil seeds, yeast cells, and vegetables (spinach, lettuce).

Distribution: An adult man weighing 70 kg contains approximately 1.4 to 2.3 gm of zinc in the body. It is distributed in different parts of the body as follows:

- High (70 to 86 mg/100 gm) in skin, and prostate
- Average (15 to 25 mg per 100 gm) in bones and teeth
- Low (2.3 to 5.5 mg/100 gm) in kidneys, muscles, heart, pancreas and spleen
- Very low (1.4 to 1.5 mg/100 gm) in brain and lungs.

Absorption:

- Only a small percentage of dietary Zinc is absorbed and the absorption occurs mainly from duodenum and ileum.
- ***Zinc binding factor:*** It has been reported and claimed that a ***low molecular weight zinc binding factor is secreted by the pancreas,*** which forms complex with zinc and helps in its absorption.
- High amounts of dietary calcium, phosphates and phytic acid have been found to interfere with zinc absorption.

Plasma: Plasma contains approximately 120 to 140 μg/100 ml of plasma, mostly in combination with serum albumin.

Requirments: The requirement for normal health has been recommended as 0.3 mg zinc/per kg body wt. Adult men and women require about 15 to 20 mg. For pregnant and lactating women the requirement is 25 mg and for infants and children, it is 3 to 15 mg.

FUNCTIONS OF ZINC

- ***Role in enzyme Action:*** Zinc forms an integral part of several enzymes (metallo-enzymes) in the body.

Important zinc containing enzymes are:

- ***Superoxide dismutase***
- ***carbonic anhydrase***: It is present in red blood cells, parietal cells and renal tubular epithelial cells and contains one Zn^{++} per molecule of the enzyme.
- ***Leucine amino peptidase*** (LAP) of intestinal juice.
- ***Carboxy peptidase*** *'A'* of pancreatic juice.

Examples of other zinc containing enzymes are: *Alcohol dehydrogenase* of mammalian liver and yeast cells, *retinine reductase of retina, Alkaline phsophatase* enzyme, *Glutamate dehydrogenase* involved in transdeamination, *Lactate dehydrogenase* which brings about reversible reaction PA to L.A, *DNA and RNA polymerase, δ-ALA dehydratase*

- ***Role in Vitamin A Metabolism:*** Zn^{++} has been claimed to stimulate the release of vitamin A from liver into the blood and thus increases its plasma level and its utilization in *rhodopsin synthesis.*
- ***Role in Insulin Secretion:*** Protamine zinc-insulin and globin zinc-insulin contain Zn^{++} for their functioning. Zinc is involved in storage and secretion of Insulin.
- ***Role in Growth and Reproduction:*** **Prasad *et al.*** have showed that zinc deficiency, may lead to ***dwarfism*** and ***'hypogonadism'.*** In such dwarfs-zinc concentration in plasma, red blood cells, hairs, urine and faeces was found to be less than control subjects. Zinc deficiency also lowers spermatogenesis in males and menstrual cycles are disturbed in females.
- ***Role in Wound Healing: Zinc is necessary for wound healing.*** Zinc has been found to

accumulate in granulation tissues and in and around the healing wounds. ***Zinc deficiency delays wound healing. Thus, zinc plays a vital role in wound healing.***

Zinc Deficiency Disease—Acrodermatitis Enteropathica: A rare inherited disorder in which primary defect is in zinc absorption.

Inheritance: Autosomal recessive.

Clinically: The disease is characterized by dermatologic, ophthalmologic, gastro-intestinal and neuro-psychiatric features alongwith growth retardation and hypogonadism.

Clinical Significance

- ***In diabetes mellitus:*** Total amount of zinc in pancreas has been reported to be reduced to half. ***Deficiency of zinc may interfere with storage and secretion of insulin.***
- ***Leukaemias:*** Normally leucocytes also contain zinc. In Leukaemias, zinc content is almost reduced to 10% of the normal amount.
- ***Malignancies:*** It has been reported that the liver zinc concentration is significantly higher in subjects dying due to malignant disease than in subjects who are non-malignant. It has been suggested that the liver zinc concentration rises probably as a part of the normal tissue biochemical defence reaction against invasion by the malignant cells.
- ***Atherosclerosis:*** Zinc therapy has been found to be useful in some cases of atherosclerosis. It also prevents platelet adhesiveness and increases the fibrinolytic activity.
- ***Wound healing***—(See above)
- ***Hepatic Diseases:*** Serum zinc level decreases in cirrhosis liver. Low plasma level of zinc has been noted in acute viral hepatitis which returns to normal with recovery.
- ***Acute myocardial infarction:*** Decreased plasma zinc level has been observed in acute myocardial infarction. Maximum fall found on 3rd day after the attack. It has been suggested the decrease in serum zinc in acute myocardial infarction may be mediated by a humoral factor released from polymorpho nuclear leucocytes called ***"Leucocytes endogenous mediator*** **(LEM).**
- ***Sickle cell anaemia:*** Recently in sickle cell anaemia decrease zinc level (hypozincaemia) with hyperzincuria have been noted.
- ***Dermatitis:*** Zinc deficiency produces skin lesions-scaly parakeratotic plaques with acanthosis. Zinc therapy is found to help healing intractable chronic leg ulcers.

COBALT

Cobalt forms an integral part of vitamin B_{12} and is required as a consitituent of this vitamin.

Sources and Requirements: Normal average diet contains about 5 to 8 mg of cobalt which is far more than the recommended daily allowence (1 to 2 μg of vitamin B_{12} contains approximately 0.045 to 0.09 μg of cobalt).

Main source: Foods from animal source. ***Not present in vegetables.***

Absorption and Excretion: About 70 to 80% of the dietary cobalt is absorbed readily from the intestine. About 65% of the ingested cobalt is excreted almost completely through the kidney Cobalt is stored mainly in the liver.

FUNCTIONS OF COBALT

1. ***Role in Formation of Cobamide Coenzyme:*** In formation of *cobamide coemzyme (Adenosyl coenzyme)*, cobalt of B_{12} undergoes successive reduction in a series of steps catalyzed by the enzyme *"B_{12a} reductatse"*, which requires NADH and FAD:
   - **B_{12} a**—Red coloured (Co^{+++})
     ↓
   - **B_{12} γ**—Orange coloured (Co^{++})
     ↓
   - **B_{12} γ**—Gray –Green (Co^{+})
     ↓

   B_{12} γ (Co^{+}) reacts with ATP to form the adenosyl coenzyme.
2. ***Bone-marrow Function:*** Cobalt is required to maintain normal bone marrow function and

required for development and maturation of red cells. ***Excess of cobalt results in overproduction of red blood cells causing polycythaemia.***
3. ***Role as cofactor:*** Cobalt may ***act as a cofactor for enzyme*** like ***"glycyl-glycine dipetidase"*** of intestinal juice.

Cobalt Deficiency: In ruminants, but not in other species, cobalt deficiency results in anorexia, fatty liver, macrocytic anaemia, wasting and haemosiderosis of spleen.

SELENIUM

Current evidences indicate selenium as an ***essential trace element for all species including humans.*** A positive role of selenium in human health has been suggested. On the other hand, excess selenium is harmful and produces toxic manifestations.

Occurrence and Distribution

- ***Biological forms*** of selenium which occur in animal body are selenium analogues of S-containing amino acids, viz. ***selenomethionine, selenocysteine*** and ***selenocystine***, found at a mean concentration of 0.2 μg/gm. It is widely distributed in all the tissues, highest concentration are found in liver, kidneys and finger-nails. Muscles, bones, blood and adipose tissues show a low concentration of selenium.
- Selenium in cereal ranges from less than 0.1 μg/gm to 1.0 μg/gm wet weight; whereas dairy products, fruits and vegetables are relatively poor sources of selenium. Principal source of selenium for the food is plant material, selenium uptake in plant tissue is passive and is influenced by its concentrations in soil.

Absorption and Excretion: Food constitutes the major route of human exposure to environmental selenium. ***Intake*** is in the range of 20 to 300 μg/day. Infants get their selenium through breast milk. Total body selenium has been estimated to be approximately 4 to 10 mg (average 6 mg).

- Selenium is absorbed mainly from the duodenum and is transported actively across the intestinal brush border particularly in the form of methionine analogue. Selenium after absorption is transported bound to plasma proteins particularly β-lipoproteins in humans.
- Main route of excretion of selenium appears to be through urine. Also small amount is excreted through faeces and expired air.

Blood and tissue levels: Selenium levels in blood and tissues are very much influenced by dietary selenium intake. Blood level varies 0.05 to 0.34 μg/ml.

Metabolic Role and Function of Selenium

The only metabolic role of selenium which has been established is as the prosthetic group of selenium enzyme ***Glutathione peroxidase*** which is present in cell cytosol and mitochondria and ***functions to reduce hydroperoxide:***

$$R.OOH + 2\,GSH \xrightarrow[\text{(Se – containing)}]{\text{Glutathione peroxidase}} R\text{–}OH + H_2O + G\text{-}S\text{-}S\text{-}G$$

The reaction has special significance in the protection of polyunsaturated fatty acids located within the cell membranes, where the enzyme functions in the cytosol as part of a multi-component antioxidant defence system within the cell.

Relation with Vitamin E: Selenium has sparing effect on vitamin E and it reduces the vitamin E requirements at least in 3 ways:

- Selenium is required for normal pancreatic function and thus the digestion and absorption of lipids including Vitamin E.
- As a component of *glutathione peroxidase,* selenium helps to destroy peroxides and thereby reduces the peroxidation of polyunsaturated acids of lipids membranes (discussed above). This diminished peroxidation greatly reduces the vitamin E requirement for the maintenance of membrane integrity.
- In some unknown way, selenium helps in retention of vitamin E in the blood plasma lipoproteins.

Selenium Toxicity: Numerous reports on toxicity in animal are on record. Ruminant farm animals grazing on soils which are selenium rich or high levels of selenium in plants develop toxicity.

1. ***Acute poisoning:*** Manifests as diarrhoea, elevated pulse rate and temperature, tetanic spasms, laboured breathing and respiratory failure.
   - ***Pathological changes include*** haemorrhage, necrosis, congestion and oedema of various tissues. However, such acute poisoning is rare, as plants containing high selenium are not palatable.

2. ***Chronic Poisoning:*** Occurs when plants containing selenium are consumed over long periods. The animals develop impaired vision and movement disorders ***(Blind staggers)***, which ultimately result in paralysis and death.

Toxicity in Humans: Reports of toxicity in humans are available, which manifests chronic dermatitis, loss of hair and, brittle nails, No hepatoxicity has been observed in humans. An early hallmark of selenium toxicity is a ***garlicky breath, caused by exhalation* of *dimethyl selenide.*** Likely cause is occupation exposure in electronics glass and paint industries.

Selenium Deficiency: Specific features of severe selenium deficiency have been reported in a number of species. These are: Liver cell necrosis, exudative diathesis, pancreatic degeneration, muscular dystrophies, myopathy, infertility, failure of growth and dilatation of the heart resulting in congestive cardiac failure.

Naturally occurring selenium deficiency in humans:

- ***Keshan disease:*** It manifests principally as ***cardiomyopathy*** and has been reported from Keshan country of north eastern China. Affects mainly children and younger women.
- ***Kaschinbeck disease:*** It manifests as ***endemic human osteopathy*** (as osteoarthritis). Seen in several parts of the eastern Asia and is characterized by degenerative osteoarthrosis particularly affecting children between 5 and 13 years of age.

Recommended Dietary Allowances:

- For an adult of 70 kg, the required daily selenium is approximately 50 to 100 μg.
- For children it is between 20 to 120 μg.

Clinical Significance

- ***Parenteral nutrition:*** Several reports have linked total parenteral nutrition to selenium deficiency. Selenium responsive muscular discomfort and cardiomyopathy have been reported.
- Low levels of selenium have been reported in the blood of ***Kwashiorkor*** children and selenium supplementation in Kwashiorkor children has been documented to stimulate growth.
- Low selenium levels are observed in cancer patients specially those with GI cancers, specially ***oesophageal cancer*** and ***oropharyngeal cancers***.
- ***Cardiovascular disorders:*** Recently selenium has been implicated in cardiovascular disorders also.
- ***Thrombosis:*** Low selenium intakes have been found to increase the risk of thrombotic episodes.
- ***Role of Selenium in Cancer:***
  - Evidences have shown that selenium may be a ***cancer protective agent.***
  - Areas having high selenium content in foods and high selenium levels in blood have lower incidence of cencers.
  - In a recent study it has been shown that ***with low selenium intakes the risk of human cencer is higher.***

Mechanism of Anti-cancer Activity: Several mechanisms are considered for antitumour activity:

- Probably selenium brings about changes in carcinogen metabolism.
- Protects from carcinogen induced oxidant damage.
- Toxicity of selenium metabolites to tumour cells.

☞ SALIENT POINTS TO REMEMBER

- The minerals or inorganic elements are required for normal growth and maintenance of the body.
- According to clinical importance they are divided into mainly two classes: Principal elements (also called ***macroelements***) and ***'trace' elements.***
- Principal elements are nutritionally important, daily requirement > 100 mg and deficiency of these can prove fatal. They are Na, K, Cl, Ca, P, Mg and S.
- Trace elements are essential, daily requirement < than 100 mg and deficiency can lead to serious disorders. They are Fe, Cu, Zn, I, Mn, Mo, Co, F, Cr and Se.
- Sodium, potassium and chlorine are involved in the regulation of acid-base equilibrium, fluid balance and osmotic pressure in the body.
- Sodium is the principal cation in E.C. fluid (serum level 135-145 m Eq/L), while potassium is the principal cation of intracellular fluid. (Serum level 3.5 - 5.0 mEq/L)
- Calcium is required for the development of bones and teeth, blood coagulation, Nerve transmission, muscle contraction, etc.
- The normal serum calcium level is 9-11 mg/dl, which is regulated by parathormone (PTH), calcitriol (1, 25-$(OH)_2$ D_3) and calcitonin.
- Absorption of Ca from the duodenum is promoted by vitamin D, PTH and acidity, while it is inhibited by phytate, oxalate, free fatty acid, fibres, etc.
- Increased level of serum Ca above normal is called hypercalcaemia. ***Most common cause of hypercalcaemia for out patient's (OPD) cases is primary hyperparathyroidism. Most important cause of hypercalcaemia in hospital in patients is malignancy.***
- Decreased level of serum Ca below normal is called hypocalcaemia. Hypocalcaemia causes ***tetany,*** the symptoms of which include neuromuscular irritability, spasm and convulsions.
- Osteoporosis is bone disorder of the elderly, characterized by demineralization resulting in a progressive loss of bonemass. It is the major cause of bone fractures in elderly people.
- Phosphorus besides being necessary for the development of bones and teeth alongwith Ca, is a constituent of high energy phosphate compounds like ATP, GTP, etc. and nucleotide coenzymes (NAD^+, $NADP^+$).
- Phosphorylation and Dephosphorylation are the principal method for activation and inactivation of enzymes.
- Copper is an essential constituent of several enzymes like cytochrome oxidase, catalase, tyrosinases, Monoamine oxidase (MAO), etc.
- ***Caeruloplasmin is a copper containing protein required for the transpot of iron (Fe^{3+}) in the plasma.***
- Wilson's disease is due to abnormality in copper metabolism. It is characterized by abnormal deposition of Cu in liver, brain and kidneys, besides the low level of plasma Cu and caeruloplasmin.
- Copper deposition in "Descemet's membrane" of the eye causes a golden brown yellow or green ring round the cornea called as ***"Kayserfleischer ring".***
- Iron is trace element and is mainly required for O_2 transport and cellular respiration.
- Absorptron of iron is increased by ascorbic acid, acidity, cysteine and small peptides while it is inhibited by phytates, oxalates and high phosphate.
- Certain enzymes require iron as integral part for activity or as cofactor: Examples of former cytochromes, catalase, peroxidase, xanthine oxidase, etc. and examples of latter are aconitase, succinate dehydrogenase, etc.
- Iron (Fe^{3+}) is transported in the plasma in a bound form to transferrin and it is stored as ferritin in liver, spleen and bonemarrow.
- Deficiency of iron causes Hypochromic microcytic anaemia. Excessive intake or administration of iron results in haemosiderosis which is due to tissue deposition of haemosiderin.

- Iodine is important as a component of thyroid hormones - T_3, T_4 and "reverse" T_3.
- Dietary iodine deficiency produces endemic goitre which is very common. Consumption of iodised salt is useful to overcome this disorder.
- Zinc is necessary for the storage and secretion of insulin hormone and maintenance of normal vitamin A levels in serum. It helps wound healing.
- Zinc forms an integral part of several enzymes and necessary for their activity, viz. ***carbonic anhydrase, alcohol dehydrogenase superoxide dismutase, lactate dehydrogenese (LDH), alkaline phosphatase (ALP),*** etc.
- Cobalt is an important constituent of vitamin B_{12}.
- Fluorine in trace amounts < 2 ppm prevents dental caries while its higher intake leads to fluorosis.
- The manifestations of fluorosis include mottling of enamal and discoloration of teeth. In advanced stages produces hypercalcification of limb bones and ligaments of spine producing crippling disease.
- Fluoride as sodium fluoride is used "*in vitro*" as anticoagulant in blood sugar bottle. It prevents `*in vitro*' glycolysis of glucose by, inhibiting the enzyme "**enolase**".
- Selenium is important as an anti-oxidant and anticancer activity. The enzyme "***glutathione peroxidase***" contains Selenium.
- Selenium toxicity can be seen as occupational hazard in people working in electronics, glass and paint industries.
- An early hallmark of selenium toxicity is a garlicky smell in breath, caused by exhalation of dimethyl selenide.

MULTIPLE CHOICE QUESTIONS

Give one answer:

1. **Iron is absorbed from:**
   (a) Stomach
   (b) Duotenum and Jejunum
   (c) Ileum
   (d) Caecum (e) Colon
2. **The normal route of calcium excretion is:**
   (a) Kidney
   (b) Liver
   (c) Kidney and Liver
   (d) Kidney and intestine
   (e) Kidney, Liver and Pancreas
3. **Molecular iron (Fe) is:**
   (a) Stored primarily in spleen,
   (b) Absorbed in the ferric (Fe^{3+}) form
   (c) Stored in the body in combination with ferritin
   (d) Excreted in the urine as Fe^{++}
   (e) Absorbed in the intestine by transferrin
4. **A hypochromic microcytic anaemia with increase Fe stores in the bone marrow may be:**
   (a) Pyridoxine responsive
   (b) Iron responsive
   (c) Vit B_{12} responsive
   (d) Vit C responsive
   (e) Folic acid responsive
5. **Transferrin is a type of:**
   (a) α - globulin (b) β_1 globulin
   (c) γ-globulin (d) Albumin
   (e) Microglobulin
6. **In case of Wilson's disease, the features include all of the following, *except:***
   (a) Aminoaciduria
   (b) Low levels of caeruloplasmin
   (c) Progressive hepatic cirrhosis
   (d) Keyser-fleischer ring
   (e) Urinary excretion of Cu is decreased
7. **Zinc is a constitutent of the enzyme:**
   (a) Aldolase
   (b) Mitochondrial superoxide dismutase
   (c) Carbonic anhydrase
   (d) Succinate dehydrogenase
   (e) Hexokinase
8. **Cytosolic superoxide dismutase contains:**
   (a) Zn only (b) Cu only
   (c) Zn and Mn (d) Zn and Cu
   (e) Manganese only
9. **Caeruloplasmin shows the activity of:**
   (a) As ferroxidase (b) As reductase
   (c) As hydrolase (d) As transferase
   (e) As lyase

10. In haemochromatosis, the liver is infiltrated with:
(a) Copper (b) Manganese
(c) Iron (d) Zinc
(e) Chromium

11. All of the following are true of Wilson's disease, *except:*
(a) Aminoaciduria
(b) Arthritis
(c) Low total plasma Cu
(d) Elevated urinary Cu
(e) Low Caeruloplasmin

12. Which of the following minerals is not likely to produce toxicity:
(a) Selenium (b) Sodium
(c) Iron (d) Fluoride
(e) Iodine

13. Iron is notoriously deficiant in:
(a) Milk (b) Egg
(c) Cereals (d) Pulses
(e) Maize

14. Which of the fillowing is not-present as a prosthetic group of enzymes?
(a) Copper (b) Iron
(c) Zinc (d) Nickel
(e) Molybdenum

ANSWERS

1. (b)	2. (d)	3. (c)
4. (b)	5. (a)	6. (e)
7. (c)	8. (d)	9. (a)
10. (c)	11. (b)	12. (b)
13. (a)	14. (d)	

Diet and Nutrition: Energy Metabolism

INTRODUCTION

Throughout the discussions of the metabolism of organic food stuffs, attention has been focussed particularly on the mechanisms and nature of their chemical transformations, various components of the body tissues that are undergoing degradation ***catabolism*** and resynthesis ***anabolism*** continually. Certain of the chemical reactions involved in these metabolic processes are ***exergonic***, i.e. they are accompanied by liberation of energy, whereas others are ***endergonic***, i.e. they require the introduction of energy. The manner in which energy is produced, stored, transferred and utilized has already been considered.

Energy expenditure by the body consists of two parts:

- Energy utilized for doing physical works and exercises,
- Energy utilized for doing involuntary works.

1. ***First category*** includes expenditure of energy in movement of body, lifting of any object, doing day to day works and muscular exercises. The extent of energy expenditure depends upon the extent of physical work done.

2. ***Second category*** includes the energy expenditure in doing osmotic work, absorption, transport of food materials, excretion, contraction of involuntary muscles, active transports, etc. Energy is continuously expended in such involuntary work throughout the life period for which we are not conscious. This part of expenditure is relatively constant and expenditure in such involuntary works occurs at a basal rate.

CALORIC VALUE OF FOODS

Different food stuffs on burning give different amount of energy. How much heat will be obtained by burning a particular food stuff is expressed by the term ***"caloric value"***

Definition: Caloric value is defined as amount of heat-energy obtained by burning 1.0 gm of the food stuff completely in the presence of O_2. Caloric value of different food stuffs is determined *in vitro* in a special apparatus called ***"bomb calorimeter"***.

Principle:

- A weighed amount of sample is burnt in an atmosphere of O_2 by an electrically heated platinum wire.
- The heat evolved is absorbed in a weighed amount of water which surrounds the burning chamber.
- The rise of temperature is recorded with the help of a sensitive thermometer.

Calculation: From the above data heat evolved by 1.0 gm of food can be calculated with the following formula:

$$H = \frac{W(T_2 - T_1)}{M(1000)} \text{ K cals/gm,}$$

Where,

W = Water equivalent of calorimeter and its water.

$T_2 - T_1$ = Rise in temperature in centrigrade

M = Amount of food burnt in gm.

Unit of Energy: The unit of energy is a calorie (c).

Definition: It is defined as the amount of heat required to raise the temperature of 1.0 gm of water by 1°C (specifically from 15 to 16°C). This is the ordinary calorie and is found too small a unit for measuring the energy value of foods.

A unit thousand times of the ordinary calorie is called **"kilo-calorie"** or simply **Calorie** (by capital 'C') is used for this purpose. ***Calorie in biological science always means a "kilocalorie" ("C").***

- Food materials undergo combustion in the animal body and liberate energy in the same way as in bomb calorimeter, ***but in a graded and continuous stepwise manner*** instead of in an explosive way.
- Taking into consideration, the variations in caloric value of individual carbohydrate/fat/protein, their average energy value when metabolized may be represented as follows in C/gm:

Carbohydrates	**= 4.1**
Fats	**= 9.3**
Proteins	**= 4.3**

- On accounts of losses in digestion and absorption and other unaccountable factors, the caloric value are usually rounded off and said to be 4.0 calories/gm of carbohydrates and proteins and 9.0 calories/ gm for fats.

HEAT PRODUCTION

The heat produced by the animal body can be directly measured by placing the animal in a calorimeter. The direct method is accurate but entails the construction of complicated and costly apparatus, such an apparatus is ***"At water-Rosa-Benedict calorimeter".*** In such apparatus not only is the heat measured, but the O_2 absorption and CO_2 output can also be determined.

BASAL METABOLISM AND BMR

The amount of energy required for any individual varies directly with the degree of activity and environmental conditions, but the rate of energy production in an individual by its over-all cellular metabolism is more or less constant under some standard conditions ***"basal conditions:*** and is known as ***"basal metabolism".***

The basal conditions are as follows:

- Person should be awake but at complete rest both physical and mental.
- Person should be without food for at least 12 to 18 hrs, i.e. in the "postabsorptive state". ***Postabsorptive state*** is allowed to pass for avoiding,
  - Effects of digestion and absorption,
  - The effects of SDA of food stuffs and
  - Also to prevent any chance of starvation.
- Should be in recumbent/reclining position in bed.
- Person should remain in normal condition of environment, i.e. at normal temeperature, pressure and humidity (environmental temeprature of between 20°C to 25°C).

Under these conditions energy output of the individual is to maintain respiration, circulation, muscle tone (skeletal and smooth muscles), functions of visceras like the kidney, liver and brain for the maintenance of the body temperature. ***The rate of energy production under such basal conditions per unit time (one hour) and per sq meter of body surface is known as "basal metabolic rate" (BMR).***

Definition of BMR: BMR may be defined as the amount of heat given out by a subject who though awake is lying in a state of maximum physical and mental rest under comfortable conditions of temperature, pressure and humidity, 12 to 18 hours (postabsorptive) after meal.

A constant ratio of endogenous carbohydrates, lipids and proteins are metabolized under such basal conditions. ***Under such conditions RQ is 0.82 and each litre of O_2 consumed represents 4.825 C of energy output.***

Determination of BMR: BMR can be determined by the following methods:

1. ***Open-circuit system:*** In which both O_2 consumption and CO_2 output are measured. It requires a high degree of technical skill and more cumbersome apparatus and is less rapid but is more accurate. ***Tissot method*** and ***Douglas method*** are both open-circuit methods.

2. ***Closed circuit method:*** In clinical practice, the BMR is estimated with sufficient accuracy merely by measuring O_2 consumption of the patient for 2.to 6 minutes period under "basal" conditions. The O_2 consumption is measured in a "closed circuit system". The apparatus commonly used is the ***"Benedict-Roth metabolism apparatus" (Fig. 24.1).***

The construction of apparatus is described below:

- A cylindrical spirometer vessel closed at upper end and
- Floating on water-jacket below, to make an air-tight water-seal,
- The spirometer is filled with O_2 and is connected by passages regulated by valves. The outlet passage directly to the mouth piece and the inlet passage through a sodalime container, to absorb the CO_2 of the expired air.
- The subject kept under basal conditions will be made to breathe by mouth by closing the nostrils and inserting the mouth piece into his mouth.
- The respiratory excursions are transmitted to the floating respirometer which moves up and down in the water jacket surrounding its lower portion.
- The movements of the respirometer, in turn, are transmitted to a pen connected to the top of the respirometer by a pulley and chain. The movements are recorded by the pen on a recording drum which is rotated by a mechanical or electrical clock work. The test is usually run for ***a period of 6 minutes*** and

Table 24.1: Caloric value, O_2 and CO_2 equivalents of Carbohydrate, Fats and Proteins

	Calories per gm	*Litres of CO_2/gm*	*Litres of O_2 per gm*	*RQ*	*Caloric value per litre O_2*
• *Cabohydrate*	3.7-4.3 (4.1)	0.75-0.83 (0.8)	0.75-0.83 (0.8)	1.0	5.0
• *Fats*	9.5	1.43	2.03	0.707	4.7
• *Proteins*	4.3	0.78	0.97	0.801	4.5

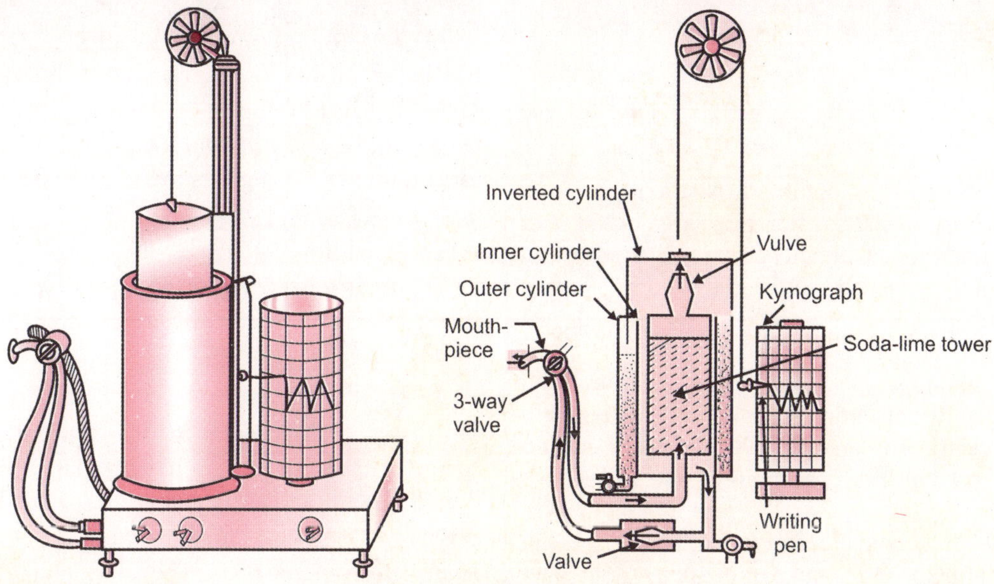

Fig. 24.1: Benedict-Roth spirometer

the volume of O_2 consumed in that period is obtained from the tracing on the recording drum. This is corrected to standard conditions of temperature and barometric pressure.

Calculation: The average O_2 consumption for the two periods is multiplied by 10 to convert it hourly basis, and then multiplied by 4.825 C, the heat production represented by each litre of O_2 consumed. This gives the heat production in C/hour.

Since BMR is to be expressed as C/sq. meter/hour, the energy output per hour obtained above has to be divided by the surface area of the individual.

Calculation of Surface area: The surface area of an average adult is about 1.8 square meteres.

1. ***A simple formula*** for calculating the surface area is as follows:

O^{ee} of mid-thigh × 2 × Height = Surface Area
(in cm) (in cm) (in sq. cm)

2. The classical formula is that of ***Du Bois***, as follows:

Du Bois' surface area formula:

$$A = H^{0.725} \times W^{0.425} \times 71.84$$

Where,

A = Surface area in sq cm
H = Height in cm
and W = Weight in Kg

Surface area thus obtained in sq cm has to be divided by 10,000 to get surface area in sq meter. To have the value directly in sq meter, the formula can be modified as:

$$A \text{ (in sq meter)} = H^{0.725} \times W^{0.425} \times 0.007184$$

*3. **By using Nomogram:*** More conveniently, in practice, the nomogram prepared by **Boothby** and **Sandiford** can be used for finding surface area for an individual if heights and weights are known.

Height: Given in feet/cm
Surface area: In square metres
Weight: Given in pounds/kg.

Example of calculation of BMR:

- The normal BMR for an individual of the patient's age and sex is obtained from standard tables.
- The patient's actual rate is expressed as + or-% of the normal.

A male aged 35 years, Height = 170 cm and weight = 70 kg, consumed an average of 1.2 litres of O_2 (corrected to normal temperature and pressure: O°C, 760 mm Hg) in a 6-minute period.

$\therefore$ O_2 consumption per hour = 1.2 × 10 = 12 litre.
$\therefore$ 12 × 4.825 = 58 C/hour

(one litre of O_2 consumed represents 4.825 C of energy output). Surface area from nomogram in this case is = 1.8 sq metre

$$\therefore \text{BMR} = \frac{58\text{C}}{1.8} = 32 \text{ C/sq m/hr.}$$

The normal BMR for this patient by reference to standard table is 39.5 C/sq m/hr. Hence the patient's BMR which is below normal is presented as:

$$\frac{39.5 - 32}{39.5} \times 100 = -18.98\%$$

A BMR between—15 to + 20% is considered normal.

Normal BMR values: A healthy adult male has a BMR of about 40 C/sq m/hour and adult female about 37 C/sq m/hour.

Determination of BMR by Read's formula: This formula gives a rough estimate of BMR and is often used at the bedside.

The formula given is as follows:

$$\textbf{BMR} = 0.75 (\text{PR} + 0.74 \times \text{PP}) - 72$$

Where
PR = Pulse rate
PP = Pulse pressure

The result obtained as the % of the normal and is correct within a range of ± 10% viz. if above 10%, the BMR is higher, and if below 10%, the BMR is lower than normal.

Factors Influencing BMR: The rate of metabolism at "basal" conditions has been found to vary in different individuals and therefore BMR varies with different factors.

- *Age: **The BMR of children is much higher than the adults.*** Roughly speaking it is inversely proportional to the age.
  - At the age of 6, it is 57.5 C,
  - At 12 it is 50.4 C,
  - Between 20 to 30 yrs it is 40 C and
  - Between 40 to 70 yrs, it varies between 38.5 and 35.5 C

In other words, with advancing age, BMR gradually falls. This is ***due to the fact that children possess a greater surface area in proportion to their body weight.*** (Exception, in newly born babies it is low, about 25 C/sq m/hr. In premature infants, it is still lower).

- *Sex:* Women normally have a lower BMR than men. The BMR of females decline between the ages of 5 to 17 more rapidly than those of males.
- *Surface area:* Since much of the basal metabolism is for the maintenance of body temperature and since heat loss is proportional to the surface area of the body, ***the BMR is directly proportional to the body surface.*** Hence it is customary to express BMR as C/sq. m/hr. When expressed in terms of surface area, the BMR of different individuals are remarkably constant.
- *Climate:* In colder climates, the BMR is high and in tropical climates the BMR is proportionally low.
- *Racial variations:* When the BMR of different racial groups is compared, certain variations are noted.

  Examples:
  - BMR of adult Chinese are equal to or below the lower limit of normal for occidentals (westerns).
  - BMR of oriental (Eastern countries) female students living in USA is average 10% below the standard—BMR for American women of the same age-groups.
  - High values 33% above normal have been reported in Eskimos.
- *State of nutrition:* BMR is lowered in conditions of malnutrition, starvation and wasting diseases.
- *Body temperature:* The BMR increases by about 12% with the rise of 1°C. This is due to the fact that increased temperature stimulates the chemical processes of the body and thereby increases the BMR.
- *Barometric pressure:* Moderate reduction of atoms. pr. does not affect the BMR, but a fall of pressure to ½ an atmosphere (viz. O_2 tension 75 mm Hg) as occurs in mountain climbing increases BMR, but increased pressure of O_2 does not raise BMR.
- *Habits:* Trained athelets and manual workers have a slightly higher BMR than persons leading a sedentary life.
- *Drugs:* Quite a number of drugs like Caffeine, Benzedrine, epinephrine, Nicotine, Alcohol, etc. increase the BMR. On the other hand, reverse is observed with most of the anaes-thetics.
- *Hormones :* Circulating levels of hormones secreted by thyroid, adrenal medulla and anterior pituitary increase BMR. One mg of thyroxine increases BMR by about 1000 calories (1 C).
  - *In thyrotoxicosis:* BMR may increase by 50 to 100% above normal, but RQ remains unaltered since both O_2 consumption and CO_2 production increase proportionately in such cases.
  - *In Myxoedema:* BMR is diminished to 30% or even 45% below normal. Anterior pituitary through its TSH affects BMR;
  - GH also causes about 20% rise in BMR, Catecholamines increase BMR by about 20% of the resting value.
  - Male sex hormones cause a 10% increase in BMR.
- *Pregnancy:* The BMR of pregnant mother after six months of gestation rises. It may be noted in pregnancy, the BMR of the mother is the sum total of:
  - Her own metabolism as in her nonpregnant state and
  - Combined with that of the foetus.

Hence, ***pregnancy exerts no specific effect upon BMR.***

Clinical Aspect

Pathological Variations in BMR

- ***Fever:*** Infections and febrile diseases elevate the BMR, usually in proportion to the increase in temperature.
- ***Diseases:*** Which are characterized by increased activity of cells also increase heat production due to increased cellular activity. Thus, BMR may increase in such diseases as:
  - Leukaemias (21 to 80%)
  - Polycythemia (10 to 40%)
  - Sometypes of anaemias, cardiac failure, hypertension and dyspnoea (25-80%)

  All of which involve increased cellular activity.
- ***Perforation of an eardrum:*** This causes falsely high readings.
- ***Endocrine diseases:***
  - The most important factor which alters BMR is the state of function of thyroid. In fact, ***determination of BMR is mainly used for the assessment of thyroid function.***
  - In hyperthyroidism: BMR is increased to + 75% or more. In hypothyroidism (myxoedema): BMR is reduced to –40% or more.
  - BMR is also increased in Cushing's disease and Cushing's syndrome and also in acromegaly.
  - BMR is decreased in ***Addison's disease*** (hypofunction of adrenal cortex).

Importance of BMR:

- **As a diagnostic aid:** For the diagnosis of various pathological conditions specially assessing the thyroid function (specially useful where hormone assays and isotope laboratory are not available).
- ***For calculation of caloric requirements:*** Essential in the calculation of caloric requirements of an individual for prescribing a diet of adequate calorific value and planning nutrition for individuals as well as communities and populations at large.
- ***Effects of foods and drugs:*** To note the effect of different types of foods and drugs on basal metabolic rate.

RESPIRATORY QUOTIENT (RQ)

Definition: RQ is the ratio of the volume of CO_2 produced by the volume of O_2 consumed (i.e. CO_2/O_2) during a given time.

Note:

- ***RQ is simply a ratio,*** it gives no idea as to the absolute quantity of gaseous exchange.
- Proportional increase or diminution of CO_2 produced and O_2 utilized, will keep the ratio unchanged. But any disproportionate variation will be reflected by a corresponding change in the RQ.

Normal RQ: In a healthy adult, ***on a mixed diet, it is 0.85.***

Method of Determination: It is done by measuring the volume of O_2 consumed and CO_2 produced during a given time with the help of Douglas bag and other similar instruments.

Factors Affecting RQ

- ***Role of Diet:***

1. ***Carbohydrate: In case of carbohydrate diet RQ is 1 (one),*** Because in carbohydrate diet the volume of CO_2 produced is the same as the volume of O_2 consumed.

Explanation: This is due to the fact that in carbohydrate molecule, the amount of O_2 present is just sufficient to oxidize the H present in the same molecule. Hence, external O_2 is necessary only to convert the C of the molecule to CO_2 so that the volume of O_2 consumed and the volume of CO_2 produced will be same.

$$C_6H_{12}O_6 + 6\,O_2 = 6\,CO_2 + 6\,H_2O$$

∴ RQ for carbohydrate =

$$\frac{CO_2 \text{ produced}}{O_2 \text{consumed}} = \frac{6}{6} = 1$$

2. ***Fats: In case of fats the RQ will be lowest and is about 0.7,*** because fat is an oxygen poor compound. The oxygen present in it cannot fully oxidize the H of the molecule so that O_2 consumed from outside is used for two purposes:

- Firstly, for oxidizing C and producing CO_2 and
- Secondly, for oxidizing H and giving H_2O.

Consequently, ***the volume of CO_2 produced will be less than the volume O_2 consumed.*** Hence, RQ will be low.

Example: Oxidation of tristearin will be used to exemplify the RQ for fats

$$2C_{15}H_{110}O_6 + 163\,O_2 \rightarrow 114\,CO_2 + 110\,H_2O$$

$$\therefore \text{ RQ for tristearin } \frac{114}{163} = 0.70$$

3. ***Proteins:*** The oxidation of proteins cannot be so readily expressed. By indirect methods the ***RQ for proteins has been calculated to be about 0.8.***

Example: Alanine

$$2\,C_3H_7O_2N + 6\,O_2 \rightarrow (NH_2)_2.\,CO + 5\,CO_2 + 5\,H_2O$$

$$\therefore \quad RQ = \frac{5}{6} = 0.8$$

4. ***RQ of mixed diets under varying conditions:*** In mixed diets, containing varying proportions of proteins, fats and carbohydrates, ***the RQ is about 0.85.*** As the proportion of carbohydrates metabolized is increased, the RQ approaches closer to 1.

Effects of Interconversion in the Body: When carbohydrates are converted into fats in the body, RQ will rise.

Explanation: In this process, an O_2-rich substance is converted into an O_2-poor compound, so that some amount of O_2 liberated from carbohydrates will be utilized for purposes of oxidation. Consequently, less O_2 will be needed from outside. Hence, the amount of CO_2 produced will be more than the amount of O_2 consumed. So that RQ will rise, and will be considerably elevated.

A reversal of the above process, i.e. conversion of fats to carbohydrate, would lower the RQ below 0.7. This has been reported but has not been generally confirmed.

It is therefore, evident that RQ value will indicate the following:

- The type of food stuffs burning in the body, or
- The nature of conversion of one food stuff into another in the body.

Muscular Exercise:

- ***With moderate exercise:*** (with a normal mixed diet) The RQ remains almost unaltered. Because in exercise, the body uses different food stuffs in the same proportion as at rest.
- ***With violent exercise:*** Lactic acid enters blood and produces acidosis, as a result pulmonary ventilation will be increased washing out more CO_2. Consequently, RQ rises, and may go even above 2.
- ***During recovery from violent exercise:*** RQ falls, because less CO_2 is evolved. Gradually it goes back to normal.

Clinical Aspect

- ***In acidosis:*** During acidosis CO_2 output is greater than O_2 consumption, hence RQ increases in acidosis.
- ***In alkalosis:*** In this RQ will fall, because respiration is depressed and CO_2 will be retained in the body, i.e. less CO_2 is produced.
- ***In febrile conditions:*** Such conditions may increase RQ. Rise of body temperature such as in high fever, will cause increased breathing and thereby will wash out more CO_2, hence CO_2 production increases.
- ***In Diabetes mellitus:***
  - In advanced cases of Diabetes mellitus, when little carbohydrate is burning, energy is supplied mainly by oxidation of fats. Hence RQ will fall.
  - In such cases, when insulin is administered, carbohydrates will start burning and RQ will rise.
- ***In Starvation:*** Here the subject has to live on its own body tissues.
  - In the early stages (initial 1 to 2 days) energy is derived mainly from the stored glycogen so that the RQ, although it falls below normal 0.85, is proportionately high 0.78.
  - But later on, when energy is derived chiefly from the combustion of fats, RQ will fall still further, and will be about 0.7.

Value and Significance of Determination of RQ:

- RQ acts as a guide as to the type of food burning or to the nature of synthesis taking place in the whole body as well as in a particular organ.
- RQ is very helpful in determining metabolic rate.
- Nonprotein RQ can be used (indirect method) for calculating the total energy output and the proportions of various food stuffs being burnt.
- Determination of RQ helps in the diagnosis of various pathological conditions such as acidosis, alkalosis, diabetes mellitus, etc.

CALORIC REQUIREMENTS

To maintain caloric balance in an adult, it is necessary to supply enough foods to replace the calories expended per day.

These include the following:

- A supply of "basal" requirements (BMR)
- Supplies of calories to meet the extra requirement caused by ***"specific dynamic action" (SDA)***, also called "calorigenic action" of foods.
- Supply for physical activity over and above the basal requirements (most 'Variable' under normal conditions).
- During periods of growth and/or convalascence, extra provision has to be made to meet the synthesis of tissues and weight gain.

1. BMR (See BMR for details): It is quite constant in health, for any given individual and is influenced by various factors. For an adult man of 70 kg body wt and surface area 1.7 square metre, the basal requirement will be @ 40 C/sq. metre/hr

= 1.7 × 40 × 24 = 1632 C (approx 1600 C/day)

2. Specific Dynamic Action (SDA): In an adult individual, whose BMR is 1600 C, is fed with just enough food to provide 1600 C and is kept under basal conditions, (except that he is not under post absorptive state), it is found that his energy output has increased beyond the basal output of 1600. The increase varies with the type of food that has supplied the calories. This stimulant action of foods on the metabolism is known as the ***"specific dynamic action" (SDA) or calorigenic action of food.***

Definition: SDA may be defined as "extra heat" production, over and above the actual heat ought to be produced outside from a given amount of food, when this food is metabolized inside the body. The mechanism of stimulation is not clear.

- Proteins have the greatest SDA, amounting to about 30% above its caloric value.
- Carbohydrates cause an increase of about 5% or 6% and
- Fats cause about 4%

Ordinarily the ***SDA of all together amounts to about 6% of the BMR.***

Explanation:

- The explanation for SDA is not clear. It cannot be due to a production of heat as a result of digestion as used to be thought earlier, because feeding of the products of digestion is as effective as undigested substances. Infact, intravenous administration of amino acids or glucose give rise to a SDA of the same order as results from feeding.
- Several studies indicate that the SDA of the various amino acids is best correlated with the metabolizable energy of the individual amino acid, i.e. it is not related to the N_2 but rather to the non-nitrogenous fraction. This fraction undergoes oxidative and synthetic changes that liberate heat. In other words, heat is evolved during the intermediary metabolism of carbon chains.
- ***The SDA of glucose is increased if thiamine is administered at the same time.*** Since thiamine stimulates the formation of fat from glucose, the SDA of glucose has been suggested as being due to the energy required to prepare it for deposition of fat.
- Possibly this is the explanation for the SDA of all foodstuffs, ***i.e. the energy required to prepare the non-nitrogenous parts of the molecule for storage.***

- To provide for this increase in metabolism, an extra provision 5 to 10% of basal requirement (usually take 6%) has to be made. Thus for a 70 kg man with BMR of 1600 C, another 80 to 160 C (96 C) have to be added on this account.

3. Physical Activity: Most variable element in the calculation of energy requirements.

- ***Influence of Muscular Work on Total Metabolism:*** Muscular work is accomplished by the body at the expense of increased metabolism. The potential energy of the food stuffs is transformed to the free energy of work and the energy of heat.
- A man sitting quietly has a total metabolism, on the average, of about 100 C/hr.
- When he stands up, his metabolism increases by about 10% because of the greater tonus of the muscles.
- If he engages in active works, it may increase 300 C or more/hr. The type of work or exercise influences the total amount of energy output, heavy work requiring more energy than light works. Many tables are available which give the total energy expenditure of various types of activity.
- ***Influence of Mental Work on Total Metabolism:*** Mental work results in very little increase in total metabolism. ***Benedict*** found, that the effort involved in solving mathematical problems increases metabolism by only 3% or 4%. Brain tissue has a high "basal" metabolism, amounting to about 1/10th of that for the entire body but the additional work it performs in thinking does not result in much of an increase over this high basal figure.
- ***Influence of Sleep:*** During normal sleep the muscles are relaxed and the metabolism is correspondingly low. It is usually 10% below the BMR.

Measurement of total heat production:

Example:

A carpenter of 70 kg body wt. having 1.7 sq m of body surface. He does carpentary works for 8 hours, and 8 hours he does sedentary works and sleeps for 8 hours.

Calculation

BMR for 24 hrs	= 1600 C
8 hrs sleep	= – 53 C
8 hrs carpentary (164 C extra/hr)	= 1312 C
8 hrs. sedentary (74 extra C/hr)	= 592 C
SDA	= 96 C
Total	= 3547 C

Table 24.2. Energy expenditure per hour under different conditions of muscular activity (includes BMR)

Forms of physical activity	*C/hour per 70 kg*	*Per kg*
Sleeping	65	0.93
Awake but lying still	77	1.10
Siting at rest	100	1.43
Standing relaxed	105	1.50
Singing	122	1.74
Tailoring	135	1.93
Carpentry	240	3,43
Typerwriting rapidly	140	2.0
Ironing (with 5 tb iron)	144	2.06
Walking slowly (2.6 miles/hr)	200	2.86
Walking moderately fast (3.75 miles/hr)	300	4.28
Walking downstairs	364	5.20
Swimming	500	7.14
Running (5.3 miles/hr.)	570	8.14
Walking upstairs	1100	15.8
Walking very fast (5.3 miles/hr)	650	9.28

Table 24.3: Total calorie requirements for 24 hours

	Calories	
• ***Men***		
Shoe maker	2000-2400	(Sedentary work)
Carpenter or Mason	2700-3200	(Light work)
Farmer	3200-4000	(Moderate work)
Lumber man	4000 or more	(Heavy work)
• ***Women***		
House hold	2300-2900	
Seamstress (needle)	1800	
Seamstress (machine)	2300-2900	

Alternatively, using the data of ***Table 24.2*** calculation for the same carpenter will be:

8 hrs carpenter work at 240 C =	1920 C
8 hrs light work (sedentary) at 170 C	= 1360 C
8 hrs sleep 65 C/hr	= 520 C
SDA	= 96 C
Total	= 3896 C

The above two hypothetical cases, have about the same total caloric output.

In first case: We began with basal metabolic rate and added and subtracted additional energy factors + the SDA.

In the second case: The total caloric output per hour was tabulated + the SDA.

Metabolism in Children:

- The total metabolism in childhood is relatively much greater than, in adult life. There is, in the first place, the high BMR of childhood.
- The physical activity of children is usually greater, despite the fact that their period of sleep is longer than that of an adult.
- Their games and play involve tremendous amount of muscular exercise. The food intake, therefore, must cover the caloric needs in addition to the extra food required for growth.
- A child of 12 years consequently needs about the same amount of food as an adult, whereas an active boy of 16 years may require 3600 C or more per day.
- Caloric requirement of infants 0 to 1 year are determined on the weight basis.
  - Infants up to 2 months of age = 120 C/kg
  - Infants from 2 to 6 months = 110 C/kg
  - Infants from ½ to 1 year = 100 C/kg

Children: 1 to 10 years = 110 to 2200 C
Boys: 10 to 18 years = 2500 to 3000 C
Girls: 10 to 18 years = 2250 to 2300 C

Determination of Caloric requirements for a "Family": Caloric requirement of a family can be calculated from the formula:

Caloric requirement = "man value" of the family × energy required for each "man unit"

A ***'man unit'*** is defined as a normal man who has attained puberty and belongs to the age group of 15 to 45 years.

Man value: The *"man value"* of a family can be obtained by "adding the man units, of all the members which can be obtained with the help of the following table.

Table 24.4: Man value of different age groups

Age groups	*Man value*	*Age groups*	*Man value*
1-2 yrs	0.35	12 yrs.	0.90
3-4 yrs	0.42	13 yrs and above	1.0
5-6 yrs	0.50	Adult man and woman	1.0
7-8 yrs	0.60		
9-10 yrs	0.70	Pregnant woman	1.10
11 yrs	0.80	Lactating woman	1.30

Example: Let us consider a family consisting of an adult man, a pregnant wife, and four children of the age 2 yrs, 5 yrs, 7 yrs and 9 yrs.

∴" Man value" of the family
= 1.0 +1.10 + 0.35 + 0.50 + 0.60 + 0.70
= 4.25 man units.

If the energy requirements of a "man unit" is about 3000 C. Then caloric requirements of the family
= 3000 × 4.25,= 12,750 C.

☞ SALIENT POINTS TO REMEMBER

- Calorie value is defined as amount of heat energy obtained by burning 1.0 g of the food stuff completely in presence of O_2.
- The heat energy is a calorie (c). A calorie is defined as the amount of heat required to raise the temperature of 1.0 g of water by 1°C.
- Energy value of foods is expressed by "Kilo calorie" ('C').
- The Calorific values of carbohydrates, fats and proteins respectively are 4.0, 9.0 and 4.0 C/g.
- These three macronutrients supply energy to the body to meet the requirements of BMR, SDA and physical activity.

- Basal Metabolic Rate (BMR) is defined as the amount of heat given out by a subject who though awake is lying in a state of maximum physical and mental rest under comfortable conditions of temperature, pressure and humidity, 12 to 18 hours after meal (post-absorptive state).
- The normal BMR values-A healthy adult male has a BMR of about 40 C/sq.m/hour and an adult female about 37 C/sq.m/hr.
- Respiratory quotient (R.Q.) is the ratio of the volume of CO_2 produced by the volume of O_2 consumed, i.e. CO_2/O_2 during a given time.
- ***RQ is simply a ratio.***
- RQ of carbohydrate is 1, fats is about 0.7 and proteins 0.8. Normal RQ of a healthy adult on a mixed diet is 0.85.
- Specific dynamic action (SDA) is the extra heat produced by the body over and above the calculated calorific value of food stuffs.
- SDA is higher for proteins (30%), lower for carbohydrates (about 5 to 6%) and lowest for fats (about 4%).
- SDA of all together amounts to about 6% of the B.M.R.
- For calculation of caloric requirements one has to take into consideration:
  - Basal metabolic rate (1600 C/24 hr)
  - + SDA (96 C)
  - + energy supply for physical activity (most "variable") values taken from charts available.
  - + extra energy for periods of growth/and convalescence.
- Calorie requirements for a family can be calculated from the formula:
  Calorie requirement = "man value" of the family × energy required for each "man unit".
- A "man unit" is defined as a normal man who has attained puberty and belongs to the age group of 15 to 45 years.
- **"Man value** - The man value of a family can be obtained by adding the man units of all members which can be obtained from a table available.

PROTEIN FACTOR IN NUTRITION

The large amount of informations which are available on nutritive value of dietary proteins has been obtained mainly from experimental studies carried out on albino rats and to a limited extent studies carried out on the dogs, specially plasma proteins and Hb. The relatively few observations made on human volunteers support the view, that with occasional exceptions, the result of studies in these experimental animals may be generally applied to man.

Functions of Dietary Proteins: ***Proteins are primarily NOT meant for energy, their principal function is to synthesize tissue proteins of the body.*** Taken in excess, they may be utilized for the production of energy and may be converted to carbohydrates and fats.

Dietary Proteins and their Influence on Growth: Growth is manifested by formation of tissue proteins at a rate exceeding that of their degradation, i.e. + ve N-balance. Proteins in diet is much more critically concerned in growth and tissue repair than are carbohydrates and lipids. ***In this respect quality of proteins taken in diet is more important than the quantity consumed.*** One may take large amount of protein in the diet, but if it is not of good quality, i.e lacks essential amino acids, it will not be utilized for tissue protein synthesis and repair.

A. Quality of Proteins: Earlier stress was given more on how much proteins to be consumed but now with development of more satisfactory analytical methods for amino acids and accumulation of information on "essential; amino acids", it is now known that quality of proteins consumed is also of equal, rather more important than the quantity.

Quality of proteins can be discussed under the following heads.

- *Biological value of proteins*
- *Amino acid composition of the dietary proteins*
- *Availability of amino acids from foods*
- *Supplementary realtionship of amino acids*

1. Biological value: Food proteins differ considerably in the efficiency of their utilization for synthesis of body proteins.

Definition: Biological value is defined as that % of absorbed Nitrogen which is retained in the body.

Procedures:

There are several procedures which may be employed for evaluation of the biological value, i.e. quality of the protein.

a. ***Measurement of weight increase:*** Measurement of its influence on the weight increase of weanling animals. This can be expressed by ***protein efficiency ratio*** **(PER).**

Protein efficiency ratio (PER):

$$= \frac{\text{Weight increase (in gms)}}{\text{Gms of proteins consumed}}$$

b. ***On retention of abosrbed N_2:*** Determination of the biological value (BV) in terms of % of the absorbed N_2 retained by the organism. To estimate "biological value" (BV) of a protein:

- The animal is first kept on protein free diet for a couple of days and the faecal N_2 and urinary N_2 are estimated to obtain the amounts of the metabolic faecal N_2 and endogenous urinary N_2 respectively.
- Then the animal is fed with a measured amount of the test protein and the faecal and urinary N_2 are determined again.

Biological value (BV) is then calculated as follows:

$$\text{BV} = 100 \times \frac{\text{Food } N_2 - (\text{Faecal } N_2 - \text{Metabolic faecal } N_2) - (\text{Urinary } N_2 - \text{Endogenous Urinary } N_2)}{\text{Food } N_2 - (\text{Faecal } N_2 - \text{Metabolic Faecal } N_2)}$$

"Biological value" (BV) of some common proteins is given in ***Table 24.5.***

Table 24.5: Biological values (BV) of certain common food proteins

Animal protein	*BV*	*Vegetable protein*	*BV*
• Egg, whole	94	• Rice	86
• Milk (cow)	85	• Barley	71
• Milk powder	83	• Wheat	67
• Egg white	83	• Maize	60
• Fish	70 to 80	• Bengal gram	76
• Liver	77	• Green gram	51
• Pork	77	• Soya bean	64
• Beef	69	• Cashew nut	72
• Mutton	60	• Ground nut	54
		• Peas	56
		• Cotton seed	63

c. ***Net protein utilization (NPU):*** It is defined as % of food N_2 that is retained in the body. This depends on both:

- Content of essential amino acids and
- Digestibility and absorbability of the protein

$$\text{NPU} = \frac{\text{Digestibility coefficient} \times \text{Biological value}}{\text{Protein intake (Gm)}}$$

NPU values of some dietary proteins are as follows:

Dietary Proteins	*NPU*
• Egg Proteins	91
• Milk	75
• Meat	76
• Fish	72
• Liver	65
• Rice	57
• Maize	36
• Wheat	47
• Peas	45
• Ground nut	45
• Soybeans	54

d. Measurement of its influence on the rate of regain of body weight or of Liver protein by previously depleted animals.

e. Measurement of its influence on the rate of restoration of plasma proteins or Hb in animals previously depleted of these specific proteins (e.g. by plasmapheresis).

Classification of Quality of Proteins: Evaluated on the basis of above criteria, animal proteins generally are of "higher" quality ("first class" proteins/or ***'complete' proteins***) as compared to those of vegetable proteins (***'Incomplete' preoteins***)

- Whole egg and milk proteins specially lactalbumin rank highest in this respect and they contain the highest percentages of the "essential amino acids".
- Meat, fish, poultry and glandular tissues occupy next position in the scale. In the same class, are also yeast and soyabeans.

- Cereals, legumes (peas, beans, etc) and nuts are generally poor because they lack some essential amino acids and thus they are incomplete proteins and are of poor quality.

Gelatin:

- Commonly used in desserts and in preparation of ice cream. It does not occur naturally as such, but is prepared from collagen (cartilage, bone, tendon and skin) by boiling in water.
- The protein is palatable, tasty and easily digested and used in diets of children and invalids/convalescing patients.
- Though the protein is of animal origin, it is wholly ***an "inadequate protein", as it lacks essential amino acid tryptophan, and is also low in tyrosine and cystine.***

f. Chemical Score:

- Since egg proteins contain all essential amino acids in adequate amounts and possess the highest nutritive value, it has been assigned a chemical score of 100 (***reference protein***).
- Chemical scores of different proteins have been calculated in terms of egg proteins. It will depend on the essential amino acid most limiting in a particular dietary protein and thus it serves as an index of nutritive value of the particular protein.

Definition: The chemical score is defined as the ratio between the content of the most limiting amino acid in the test protein to the content of the same amino acid in egg protein expressed as a %.

Example:

- Milk protein: The limiting amino acid is S-containing amino acids.
- Chemical score = $\frac{3.4}{5.5} \times 100 = 65$
- Chemical score of Gelatin and Zein are 0 (zero). Chemical score of some of the common proteins are given below:

Proteins	*Chemical score*
• Egg proteins	100
• Milk Proteins	65
• Meat	70
• Fish	60
• Liver	66
• Rice	60
• Wheat	42
• Peas	42
• Bengal gram	44
• Soy bean	57
• Groundnut	44
• Gelatin	0
• Zein	0

2. Amino Acid Composition of Dietary Proteins: The role of essential amino acids has already been stressed. To be a 'complete' protein and of high biologic value the protein must have all the essential amino acids and ***they must be available to the organism together and simultaneously, so that they can be utilized for protein synthesis.*** It has been observed, ***if one of the essential amino acid is lacking and there is an interval of two hours or more, the amino acids are not utilized for protein synthesis.***

Proportionality Relationship of Essential Amino Acids: The biological value of protein is also ***related to proportionality relationship*** of its constituent essential amino acids. Studies in rats have shown that for optimal growth the following proportional relationship of E.A.A. is necessary taking tryptophan as unity.

• Tryptophan	1
• Threonine	2.5
• Isoleucine	2.5
• Methionine	3.0
• Phenylalanine	3.5
• Valine	3.5
• Leucine	4.0
• and Lysine	5.0

- There is evidence that above proportionality is also applicable approximately to human beings.
- Based on above, the following daily intake values in gm have been recommended tentatively for human beings, which is approximately double of the minimum requirement. This should provide an adequate excess from which cell can select the proper mixture for its specific protein synthesis.

	Minimal requirement	*Recommended daily intake*
• Tryptophan	0.25	0.5
• Threonine	0.5	1.0
• Isoleucine	0.7	1.4
• Valine	0.8	1.6
• Lysine	0.8	1.6
• Leucine	1.1	2.2
• Phenyl alanine	1.1	2.2
• Methionine	1.1	2.2

"Sparing" Action: Nonessential amino acids ***Tyrosine and cysteine can be synthesized in the body from essential amino acids phenylalanine and methionine respectively. Presence in diet of these two nonessential amino acids reduce the necessity of their corresponding essential amino acids ("Sparing" action).***

- On the other hand, if nonessential amino acids tyrosine and cysteine are not provided in diet, requirement of phenylalanine and methionine increases and the necessity for synthesis constitutes an additional excessive burden on the metabolic activities of the cells. This will be more under conditions of rapid growth, e.g. growing child, convalescing patient, pregnancy/and lactation.

3. Availability of Amino Acids of Foods: Digestibility of various proteins and the rates of release of amino acids may be affected by the way the foods are prepared before eating, e.g. heating during cooking-in some it may be beneficial and in some cases it may affect adversely.

Coefficient of Digestibility: Co-efficient of digestibility means that the amino acids are readily split off by the enzymes and are readily available for absorption.

Definition: It is the % of food N_2 that is absorbed from the alimentary canal after digestion.

For its determinations

- Animal is first kept on a protein free diet for a couple of days and its metabolic faecal N_2 is determined.
- Then the animal is fed with the test protein and its faecal N_2 is again estimated, while on the diet.

Calculation:

Digestibility co-efficient: This can be calculated as follows:

$$100 \times \frac{\text{Food } N_2 - (\text{Faecal } N_2 - \text{metabolic faecal } N_2)}{\text{Food } N_2}$$

Note:

- Usually vegetable proteins from cereals, legumes and seeds have lower digestibility co-efficient than what animal proteins have.
- Meat proteins have a high "co-efficient of digestibility". In this respect kidney is superior to other meats, liver is next and muscle meats third.

4. Supplementary Relationships of Amino Acids and time factor: This is a ***very important factor from nutritional point of view.*** As discussed above, most of vegetable proteins are ***"incomplete"*** proteins and of poor quality, lacking in one or the other of essential amino acids.

- ***A vegetable protein lacking a particular essential amino acid, if supplemented by another vegetable protein possessing that amino acid and taken simultaneously, the 'biological value' of each of these two low-quality proteins is enhanced*** and the constituent amino acids can be utilized for protein synthesis.

Some illustrative examples are given below:

- ***Wheat:*** An important dietary protein of Indians is deficient in lysine. All 'cereals' lack Lysine.
- ***Rice:*** Another staple food for Indians-not only lacks lysine, but also poor in threonine.
- ***Maize/corn:*** Lacks in tryptophan.

- *Legumes (peas and beans):* Usually deficient in methionine and also tryptophan.
- *Roots/tubers:* are generally deficient in methionine

Supplementary action is manifested as follows:

- ***The combination of wheat, low in lysine, but adequate in methionine, when taken together either with potatoes or peas, which is adequate in lysine but low in methionine, enhances the biological value of each of these low quality proteins*** to a considerable degree and the amino acids can be utilized for protein synthesis.
- Similar enhancement of the biological value of relatively low quality vegetable proteins is accomplished by the addition of high-quality animal proteins.

Time Factor: As stressed earlier, a protein molecule can be synthesized only if ***all the constituent 'essential' amino acids are available simultaneously and together in proper amounts.*** If an interval of one hour is allowed to elapse between ingestion of an "incomplete" amino acid mixtures and administration of the missing essential amino acid, the supplementary action is not seen, and the amino acids are not utilized for tissue protein synthesis resulting to 'Negative' N-balance.

B. Quantitative Aspect

- If the intake of protein is reduced gradually, urinary N-excretion also diminishes correspondingly and the organism may remain in N-equilibrium until a "critical intake" level above 0.25 to 0.33 gm/kg body weight is reached, below which the N-balance becomes negative. Continuation of such low protein diet for prolonged periods may endanger health and is harmful for body.
- What should be the "optimum quantity of protein to be consumed by an individual? This question has been discussed for years.
- Studies of various investigators have now established that ***an intake of about 1 gram of protein per kg of body weight is adequate to maintain N-equilibrium.*** In growing children, convalascent, and pregnancy and lactation, this must be increased considerably to permit growth of new tissues. In elderly persons, the proteins requirement is usually somewhat higher even though there is a somewhat lower calorie need. Negative N-balances are more common in this group. ***Hence it is recommended that elderly aged persons should consume more than 1 gm of "high-quality" proteins per kg of body weight daily.***

The "recommended daily allowance" (RDA) value for protein is given in the box.

RDA for proteins

Category	*Age in Years*	*Protein in gms*
• Men	18-35	70
	35-55	70
	55-75	70
• Women	18-35	58
	35-55	58
	55-75	58
• Pregnancy (2nd and 3rd trimesters)	-	+ 20
• Lactation	-	+ 40
• Infants	-	kg × 2.5 ± 0.5
• Children	1 to 3	32
	3 to 6	40
	6 to 9	52
• Boys	9 to 12	60
	12 to 15	75
	15 to 18	85
• Girls	9 to 12	55
	12 to 15	62
	15 to 18	58

The daily requirement of course will be influenced by the quality and biologic value of the proteins.

CONSEQUENCES OF PROTEINS DEFICIENCY

If the protein intake does not meet the immediate requirements, protein anabolism cannot be maintained at the required rate.

- In the child, growth is retarded and in the adult, weight is lost.
- Haemoglobin formation is impaired with consequent anaemia.
- Wound healing is delayed.
- If the deficiency is marked, excessive amount of fats may accumulate in Liver producing 'fatty liver', due to:
  - Choline deficiency, a consequence of methionine deficiency, and
  - Impaired 'apo-protein' synthesis, Lipoproteins formation suffers.
  - Fatty liver later on may lead to fibrosis (cirrhosis liver)
- Prolonged deficiency may result to inadequate synthesis of plasma proteins-specially albumin and fibrinogen.
- Fibrinogen deficiency, may lead to bleeding disorders.
- If the deficiency progresses to the point of significant decrease in plasma albumin concentration, oedema may develop, and also increased susceptibility to shock.
- Resistance to infections may be diminished as a result of impaired capacity for forming γ-globulins-antibodies (IgGs).
- In severe protein restrictions, certain hormones, protein in nature, such as those of anterior pituitary may not be synthesized in adequate amounts and endocrine abnormalities may appear, viz. amenorrhoea (gonadotropin deficiency).
- Since enzymes are proteins and must be synthesized in the body, the enzyme content of certain tissues (viz. liver cholinesterase, ornithine carbamoyl transferase (OCT), etc.) and enzymes in secretions (viz. pepsinogen in gastric juice, etc) falls in advanced deficiency stage. This may result in disturbances of function of organs affected.

ROLE OF CARBOHYDRATES IN DIET

- Glucose, fructose, galactose and to a minor degree, mannose, as well as those carbohydrates that yield them on digestion, are available to the body as energy producers. The pentoses in foods seem to be of limited value nutritionally. Ribose, deoxy-ribose required for nucleic acids synthesis, is obtained from HMP-Shunt. Moreover, pentoses form a very small fraction of the total carbohydrate intake of diet.
- Dietary polysaccharides or disaccharides cannot be utilized until digested to the monosaccharide stage. When introduced directly into blood stream, they act as foreign bodies and are excreted, chiefly by the kidneys.
- In as much as all biologically significant carbohydrates can be synthesized in the body, their ***main function in the diet is to provide readily utilizable source of energy for the maintenance of cell functions.***
- ***Requirement of carbohydrates in diet:*** Normally 55 to 65% of the total food calories should come from carbohydrates. ***A moderately active man requiring 3000 C/day, should take about 450 gm carbohydrates daily.*** But in India, poorer sections of the population derive more than 85% of the food calories from carbohydrates. ***Undue restriction of dietary carbohydrates influences both fat and protein metabolism adversely, even if the calorie intake is adequate.*** Fat mobilization from the depots and utilization are exaggerated, ***Ketogenesis is increased and ketosis may develop.*** The effect on protein metabolism is apparently of a specific nature, not shared by other substances e.g. fats, alcohol and not related to its calorigenic action. This is referred to as ***"protein sparing action of carbohydrates".***
- ***Protein sparing action of carbohydrates:*** Adequate amount of carbohydrate and fats in the diet may reduce the protein requirement. This may be due to:
  - Metabolic products of carbohydrates, e.g. oxalo-acetate (OAA), pyruvates (PA) and α-oxoglutarates provide the C-skeletons for the formation of non-essential amino acids through transamination,
  - Carbohydrates reduce the need for gluconeogenesis from amino acids, and,

- Both carbohydrates and fats are catabolized for energy and thus spare the proteins from being used for this purpose.
- *Action of Carbohydrates on Plasma lipids:* Replacement of a 'low' or moderate carbohydrate diet by a high carbohydrate diet may produce temporary rise in plasma TG and VLDL and temporary reduction in blood cholesterol. Substitution of starch by fructose or sucrose in the diet may also increase plasma TG by increasing lipogenesis from fructose.
- ***Relation with B-vitamins:*** With diets rich in carbohydrates ***the requirements for B-vitamins, particularly thiamine (vit B_1) increases*** because of their essential role in carbohydrate metabolism. Use of tubers, roots and sugars instead of cereals, as food sources for carbohydrates require supplementation with foods rich in B-vitamins as these foods are poorer than cereals in B-vitamin content.
- *Role of Cellulose:* Celluloses are polysaccharides found in plants. They are indigestible by human beings as there is ***no enzyme in our GI tract which can split β-1→4 linkage.*** But, cellulose in diet, contribute bulk to the intestinal contents, and therefore, in normal amounts promote intestinal motility, i.e. increases peristalsis ***("Roughage" action)*** and removes constipation. When present in excess, they may be irritating to intestinal mucous membrane, producing diarrhoea or a spastic type of constipation.
- *Excessive intake of carbohydrates in diet:* Ingestion of excessive amounts, specially in infants, may occasionally produce intestinal disturbances due to irritation induced by products of bacterial fermentation.

ROLE OF LIPIDS IN THE DIET

- A wide variety of lipids is provided in a balanced diet. In as much as, under normal circumstances, all components of biological significant lipids, with the exception of essential fatty acids, can be synthesized in the body from non-lipid prescursors. *The main function of dietary lipids, like that of carbohydrates, is to provide energy,* largely through oxidation of their constituent free fatty acids.
- The dietary lipids serve another indirect function, serving as ***"carriers of fat soluble vitamins (A,D,E & K)*** and provitamins like carotenes, which because of their solubility in fats, occur in nature mainly in association with these substances.
- Lipids my also exert a relatively minor ***"protein sparing effect"***, apart from their calorie contribution.
- *Requirements:* Neutral fats (TG), comprising the largest fraction of food lipids are quantitatively the most important of these substances. Under usual conditions ***fats provide 20 to 35% of the calories of the diet, i.e.*** 1 to 2 gm/kg of body weight in the average moderately active adult. Dietary fat has a ***high "satiety value",*** i. e. the ability to satisfy hunger.
- *Supply of polyunsaturated FA:* Food fats should contain adequate amounts of polyunsaturated FA to supply at least 1% of total calories in adult man and 4% of same in children. The nutritional significance of the polyunsaturated "EFA" have already been discussed (see chemistry of lipids). It is generally agreed that in man elevated plasma cholesterol levels of certain types may be lowered by
  - Restriction of fat intake and
  - Substitution of polyunsaturated FA for saturated FA.
- *Quality of fat:* Chain length and saturation of FA and MP of TG influence the nutritive quality of food fats. TG of short chain, medium chain, or polyunsaturated FA are more easily digested by ***Lipases*** in the intestine. While the TG of Caprylic acid (C_8) has a digestibility of more than 97%, that of palmitic acid (C_{16}) has a digestibility of about 70% only. Unsaturated TGs are also more readily absorbed than saturated ones. Oils of vegetable and seeds (e.g. sunflower oil, groundnut oil, soyabean oil, mustard oil) contain mainly unsaturated FA and are preferable.
- *Medium chain TG: has been used in treatment of chyluria and chylothorax as they are absorbed directly in portal blood.*

- ***Excess of fats in diet: An excessive high fat intake inhibits gastric secretion and motility, producing anorexia and gastric discomfort.*** Intestinal irritation and diarrhoea may result from excessive amounts of FA in the intestine. Excess of fats, particularly saturated fats, in the diet may reduce the gastric digestion of proteins, because fat digestion starts mainly in the intestine, thus preventing exposure of food proteins to pepsin. ***Excess fat intake can cause excessive production of ketone bodies, due to high FA oxidation and also can lead to Type 1 fatty liver.***
- Delay or failure of fat absorption may also reduce Ca^{++} absorption as calcium forms insoluble soaps with higher FA in intestine.
- Cotton seed oil contains a pigment ***"gossypol"*** which has ***anti-oxidant*** and ***antitryptic*** activity, diminishes appetite and interfere with protein digestion.

BALANCED DIET

Definition: A diet is said to be balanced one, when it includes proportionate quantities of food items ***selected from the different basic food groups*** so as to supply the essential nutrients in complete fulfilment of the requirements of the body.

Basis: A balanced diet should be based on:
- Locally available foods,
- Should be within the economic means of the people,
- Should fit with the local food habits,
- Diet should be easily digestible and palatable,
- Should contain enough roughage materials.

Such a diet containing the required quantities of the different essential nutrients would perform the basic functions of food.

Basic Food Groups: All essential nutrients including accessory food factors like vitamins and 'trace' elements required for the proper functioning of the body are distributed in varying quantities in different natural foods, constituting the ***"basic food groups"*** 'Basic food groups have

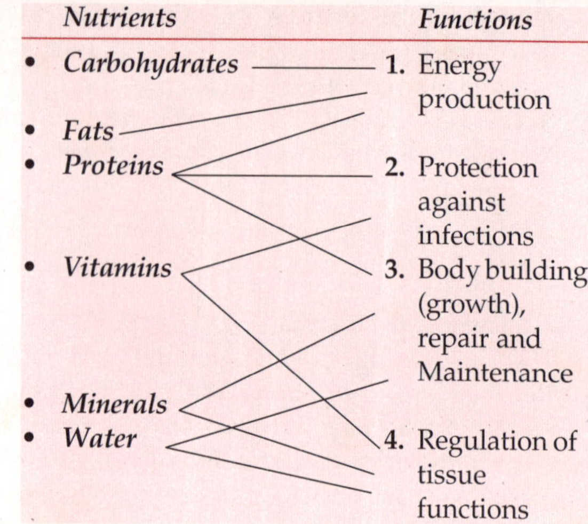

Fig. 24.2: Showing basic functions of foods (Nutrients)

been initially divided into seven, but now they have been put mainly into following ***4 groups:***

- ***Milk group*** including dairy products.
- ***Meat group*** including meat, fish, eggs and pulses/beans/nuts, etc.
- ***Green leafy vegetables and fruits*** group.
- ***Cereal groups*** including bread, rice, wheat, barley, etc.

A balanced diet should be an intelligent assortment of items from each of these four basic food groups so that different foods, rich in different nutrients can contribute to the total nutritive value of the diet.

How to plan a Balanced Diet?

- ***Age, Sex and Calorie Requirements:*** While planning diet for any individual, his/her age and sex, physical activity involved and special nutritional needs. viz. a growing child or a pregnant/lactating lady, if any, must be taken into account in determining the total calorie requirements and total daily requirement of nutrients.
- ***Selection of Nutrients from 'Basic Food Groups':*** The required quantities of food items are ***to be selected from the four basic food groups*** in such a way that their total nutritive values satisfy the

estimated requirements. The selection should be based on varieties of foods and if the requirements for calories and proteins are met, the vitamins and mineral requirements are automatically fulfilled.

- *Economic Status of the Individual:* In formulating balanced diet, it is imperative and necessary that the economic status of the individual is taken into account so that the diet is within the purchasing capacity of the individual.
- *High-Cost and Low –Cost diet:* For a rich person planning of a balanced diet does not pose any problem, because he can afford to purchase the foods recommended. In case of a person, belonging to low-income group, it poses the problem. Cheaper items have to be selected and at the same time care should be taken that nutritional and calorie requirements are fulfilled. ***A balanced diet formulated, loses relevance if it does not conform to purchasing capacity of the individual.***

Example of a Balanced Diet: A typical balanced diet (non-veg) for an adult man doing moderate work is shown in ***Table 24.6.*** Formation of any balanced diet must be followed by an approximate costing of the diet based on the local market values of the different commodities. ***The above diet provides about 2800 C and about 75gm proteins of high quality.***

Need For "Low Cost" Balanced Diet: Need for formulating 'low-cost' balanced diets is necessary to bring a compromise between the nutritive values and the cost. But now even the cheapest sources of nutrients like pulses, nuts, etc. have become costlier and as long as the diet is made a balanced one, the cost cannot be low. Hence the term 'Low-cost' diet should be replaced by ***'minimum cost' diet.*** An example of a "minimum cost" balanced diet for an adult male doing moderate work is given in ***Table 24.7.***

Such a diet will supply approx 2700 C and approximately 80 gm of vegetable proteins.

Table 24.6: Showing composition of a typical balanced diet for an adult male doing moderate work (non-veg)–*'high-cost' diet*

Food items (Nutrients)	*Quantity gm/day*
Cereals	475
Pulses	65
Green leafy vegetables	125
Other vegetables	75
Roots and Tubers	100
Fruits	30
Milk	100
Meat/fish	30
Fats and oils	40
Eggs	30
Sugars	40

Table 24.7: Shown the composition of a *"minimum cost"* balanced diet for an adult male doing moderate work

Food items (Nutrients)	*Quantity gm/day*
Cereals	285
Pulses	100
Green leafy vegetables	200
Potatoes	200
Colocasia	100
Ground nut (kernel)	50
Germinated Bengal Grams	50
Oils	35
Sugar	35

Note: Following to be noted:

- Costlier items like meat/fish/milk and eggs which are costlier, has been replaced by comparatively cheaper foods or vegetable origins. Their cost is less and nutritionally considered adequate.
- **Limitations:** With such a diet, based exclusively on vegetarian foods there will be a possibility of developing deficiency of vitamin B_{12} in future: ***The above can be prevented by taking small fishes once or twice a week or supplemented by an egg.*** As the requirement of vitamin B_{12} is very small and as the storage

capacity in liver very high, the chance of developing such a deficiency is rare.

Use of Certain Unconventional Food Items: Certain food items are discarded due to ignorance of their food values. Many of them are often found to be rich sources of proteins and calories and if consumed can effectively protect the body against nutritional disorders. Examples include: jack fruit seeds, pumpkin seeds, water-lilly seeds, water-melon seeds, etc. the kernel portions if suitably cooked can be good sources of calories and proteins. Similarly, small snails, oysters and crab meat are also delicious, highly nutritive and can be consumed. Various types of mushrooms, available in the rural areas are good sources of proteins and B vitamins and are extremely popular in developed countries.

Guidelines for Certain Dietary Food Stuffs

- *Nature of Lipids:* Avoid too much of fat in the diet. Saturated fats to be avoided and include oils having polyunsaturated fatty acids, use egg, meat, butter, ghee, cream, etc. in moderation, excess to be avoided.
- *Nature of carbohydrates:* Eat foods with complex carbohydrates like starches, e.g. cereals, whole grain breads, etc. than simple sugars.
- *Dietary fibres:* Vegetables, fruits, peas, beans and nuts should be included in the diet.
- *Avoid excess calorie:* Maintain ideal body weight according to height, obesity predisposes hypertension, diabetes mellitus and cardio-vascular diseases.
- *Variety of foods:* Should be taken to ensure an adequate intake of all essential nutrients. Choose food from basic food groups.
- Avoid too much of *salt.*
- If the individual drinks *alcohol,* it must be in a limited quantity. Heavy drinking is detrimental for health and can lead to fatty liver, cirrhosis of liver, and certain neurological disorders. *Alcohols are high in calorie value but low in nutrients.*

PROTEIN-ENERGY MALNUTRITION (PEM)

Synonym: Earlier used to be called as *"protein calories malnutrition" (PCM)*

What is Malnutrition ?

Malnutrition is a state arising from:

- An insufficient calorie intake causing under nutrition or inanition and/or
- Insufficient intake of one or more of the essential nutrients, specially proteins causing deficiency.

The above two are "primary" causes and responsible for Marasmus and Kwashiorkor respectively.

Other causes lead to "secondary" malnutrition:

- Due to inadequate absorption or utilization of essential nutrients (malabsorption syndrome) or
- Due to increases in their requirement, destruction or excretion generally secondary to diseases with special features superadded by the pre-existing disease.

Types: Protein-energy malnutrition (PEM) are mainly of **3 types:**

- *Marasmus*
- *Kwashiorkor*
- *Marasmic-Kwashiorkor*

The above are quite common diseases in children and often met with in India, Bangla Desh, SE Asian countries, West Africa and Arab countries. The two main types are discussed below and given in a tabular form to differentiate the two diseases *(Table 24.8)*

- *Marasmic-Kwashiorkor:* Symptoms of both Marasmus and Kwashiorkor are sometimes produced in a mixed way depending on the relative degrees of protein and calorie deficiencies. Marasmus and kwashiorkor may follow each other in some patients. Besides the above, symptoms of deficiencies of vitamins and minerals may also be found in these diseases, e.g. hypoprothrombinaemia (vitamin K-deficiency), pellagra (niacin deficiency), etc. and anaemia.

Table 24.8: Differentiation of marasmus from kwashiorkor

	Marasmus	*Kwashiorkor*
I.	Marasmus of primary or dietary origin is most common in tropics, results of starvation in small children.	Kwashiorkor is primarily due to diet very low in proteins.
II.	*Nature of Diet and calories:* Diet may be adequate in qualitative term but ***Insufficient in calories*** for the rapidly growing child. ***Calories become the most limiting factor.*** Infant survives on utilizing its own tissues	It is the result of ***a diet very low in proteins*** but provides enough calories to satisfy the need of the child. ***Proteins become the most limiting factor and not calorie.***
III.	*Causes:* • Exclusively breast fed infant of a malnourished mother. Milk supply is grossly reduced. • Prolonged breast feeding with inadequate supplementation of other foods. • Artificial feeds inadequate, less nutritive in proteins and calories. • Fear of diarrhoea, less feeding.	• Protein lack is quantitative and also qualitatively of low biological value. • Seen in artificially fed and weaned children. Occurs weeks or months after weanning. Proteins of low quality are fed, e.g. cereal grains, starchy foods and roots. No milk, eggs, etc.
IV.	*Predisposing factors:* • Premature babies • Local disease and/or • malformations of mouth and nose. interfere with adequate feeding.	Kwashiorkor seldom occurs as a consequence of an improper diet alone. In almost all cases an infectious disease acts as the precipitating factor. This may be: • Acute diarrhoea • A respiratory infection • Measles They add deterioration of diet, poorer utilization, and higher requirement.
V.	*Age:* Usually seen in infants less than one year	Seen in older children: In second/third year of life.
VI.	*Clinical features:* • Retarded growth, child is grossly emaciated, and underweight. Depleted of subcutaneous fats and muscles. • Infant is very hungry and cries continuously • ***Diarrhoea and vomiting.*** The infant may present frequent small dark green mucous Stools of ***"hunger diarrhoea".*** It aggravates the disease further. Vomiting is more common. • ***Skin and mucus membranes:*** skin is thin, attached to bone, flaccid and wrinkled. Bony prominences are marked. Mucous membranes of mouth are usually reddish. • ***Oedema:*** No oedema is present. • ***Hairs:*** Usually thin and lustreless Face: All the above features make up a typical • **Face** of marasmic child which has been Compared to a ***"little monkey".*** • ***Dehydration and electrolytes imbalances:***	• Retardation in growth and development has been described. Child is not emaciated like marasmus rather looks blown up due to oedema. • Apathy and anorexia are early manifestations. The child is less lively and refuses to eat. • Diarrhoea is almost always present. It becomes chronic and remittent. • ***Skin lesions*** although not always present are very characteristic, patches of hyperpigmentation, exfoliation, desquamation and ulceration are seen in skin of legs, buttocks and perineum. Unlike marasmus, some subcutaneous fats are present. • ***Pitting oedema*** is the main clinical characteristic on which the diagnosis is made. It is soft, painless. Usually first affects legs and then spreads to upper extremities and face. • Hairs usually dry and thin. Black hairs become brown or reddish-yellow and sometimes even white. Depigmented hairs alternate with more pigmented hairs, called as ***Flag sign.***
	May be present in both if complicated with excessive diarrhoea and vomiting.	

Contd...

Contd...

Marasmus	*Kwashiorkor*
VII. Haematological and Biochemical alterations:	
• ***Anaemia:*** Hb and haematocrit values are slightly reduced	• Some degree of anaemia is always found, it is mild to moderate. Type of anaemia varies,usually serum Fe and Cu are low.
• ***BMR*** Usually subnormal	• May be low
• ***Serum proteins:*** Total and differential and A:G ratio Total serum proteins and their fractions are reduced and but not to that extent as in kwashiorkor. Total serum protein usually ranges 5 to 6 gm% and albumin approx. 3.0 gm% A:G ratio: maintained	• Total serum proteins are always reduced. Albumin↓ ***Hypoalbuminaemia is a characteristic feature.*** α_1 α_2- globulins found to be relatively increased; β-globulins frequently decreased ↓. γ-globulins Variable, but usually high. A:G ratio: frequently reversed.
• ***Plasma Lipids:*** not much affected	• Unlike marasmus fall in plasma levels of cholesterol TG and β-lipoproteins seen.
• ***Fatty liver not common***	• ***fatty liver may be seen***
• ***Carbohydrate metabolism:*** Hypoglycaemia not a constant feature.	• Hypoglycaemia frequently found.
• ***Other electrolytes:*** not much altered.	• A marked K-depletion, primary at intracellular level is a constant and important alteration. Mg ↓ and Pi ↓ depletion also described.
• ***Serum enzymes*** also do not show much alterations.	• The serum activity of various enzymes, viz. Amylase, alkaline phosphatase, and others are frequently reduced.
VIII. ***Prognosis*** is good, unless severe complications Like dehydration and infections are present. Recover well with adequate dietary treatment. A complete and balanced diet adequate for his apparent or biological age but much higher in calories for normal child, 200 calories/kg or more may be required.	Not so good Even under the best conditions, the mortality of children admitted is still relatively high in the order of 10 to 20 percent.

Note: Histological , functional and metabolic alterations are less marked in marasmus than kwashiorkor. This is due to the fact that the child developing marasmus is forced in view of his very limited calorie intake to consume its own tissues.

Note: Protein energy malnutrition cases should be treated early with suitable diets and antibiotics and other ancillary measures, otherwise permanent stunting of growth, hepatic cirrhosis, permanent mental retardation, low IQ and even death may result.

DIET IN PREGNANCY AND LACTATION

Even though pregnancy and lactation are normal physiological processes, they increase considerably the nutritional requirements of the mother

- Due to nausea, vomiting and loss of appetite in early months of pregnancy, the food intake is generally reduced.
- Further, additional nutrients are required for the growth of the foetus.
  A baby weighing about 3.2 kg at birth, will contain about 500 gm of proteins, 30 gm of calcium and 0.4 gm of Fe and varying quantities of vitamins. This amount has to be supplied by the mother during whole of pregnancy.

- The increased nutritional requirements during lactation are due to the milk secreted by mother for feeding the baby.

COMPOSITION AND NUTRITIVE VALUE OF COMMON FOOD STUFFS

A. Nutritive Value of Milk: No other single food has as many nutritional virtues as that of milk. Milk supplies proteins of high biological value, easily digestibles fats, lactose (milk sugar) and calcium, phosphorus, vitamin A and B-vitamin in sufficient amounts. ***It is an ideal food for the infant,*** but it must be supplemented with other foods as the child grows. However, it is not a perfect food since **it lacks Fe, Cu and vitamin C.**

Chemistry:

- ***Proteins:*** **Chief proteins are:**
  - ***Caseinogen,***
  - ***Lactalbumin*** and
  - ***Lactglobulin.***

1. ***Caseinogen:*** Is a phosphoprotein (0.7% P) and carries Ca^{2+} bound with it, is more in amount in cow's milk (2.8%) as compared to human milk(0.5%). Boiling of milk increases digestibility of casein. Bovine caseins are more difficult to digest than human milk casein, as Bovine caseins form harder calcium paracaseinate during milk digestion due to higher Ca^{2+}: casein ratios. Caseinogen is insoluble at its isoelectric pH (pI = 4.6). Usual pH of fresh milk is 6.6 to 6.9.

$$\text{Casein} \xrightarrow{\text{Renin}} \underset{\text{(soluble)}}{\text{Paracasein}} \xrightarrow{Ca^{2+}} \underset{\text{Paracaseinate}}{\text{Insoluble}}$$

2. ***Lactalbumin and Lactglobulin:*** Have also very high biological values and both are good proteins. Lactalbumin is heat-coagulable and is most easily digested

Note: Milk proteins have sufficient amount of tryptophan and this compensates for the low Niacin content of milk.

- **Lipids:** Milk fats are in the form of very fine and stable emulsion and are the ***most palatable and digestible fats known.*** It differs from other fats in containing all saturated even carbon FA from butyric (C_4)to lignoceric acid (C_{24}) as well as a variety of unsaturated FA, viz. oleic acid, linoleic, linolenic and arachidonic acid. ***About 30 percent of FA in milk TG contains polyunsaturated fatty acids. Human milk differs from cow's milk*** in ***FA composition.*** Oleic acid predominates in both, 30 to 35% of total and FA C_{12} to C_{18} consists 80 to 90% of total. 10% of human milk FA are highly unsaturated (linoleic, linolenic, etc.) as opposed to 0.5% of cow's milk. Total fat content in human milk is 4.0 gm% as compared to cow's milk 5.0 gm%; other lipids include cholesterol and phsopholipids in small quantities. Boiling reduces the fat content of milk as some of the fat separates along with some of the coagulated ***lactalbumin*** as a floating layer of clotted cream.
- ***Carbohydrates:*** Principal carbohydrate present is the ***disaccharide 'Lactose' (milk sugar).*** Human milk contains 7.0 gm% as compared to cow's milk 5.0 gm%.
- ***Minerals:*** Milk is rich in mineral elements specially calcium, phosphorus, potassium, sodium, chloride and zinc. ***Milk is poor in iron and copper.*** Both humans and experimental animals develop a dietary anaemia, hypochromic microcytic type on an exclusive milk diet.

Calcium and phosphorus: About 120 mg Ca and 90 mg of P are present in 100 ml of cow's milk; the amounts are higher in buffalo's milk but much lower (Ca= 40 mg % and P = 30 mg %) in human milk. Calcium is present in combination with casein, as free Ca^{2+} and also as inorganic phosphates. Phosphorus is present as phosphoprotein casein, as inorganic phosphates and also non protein organic PO_4 esters. The ratio of Ca : P of milk facilitates the formation of soluble calcium phosphates in the intestine. Lactic acid produced by bacterial fermentation of lactose increases calcium absorption.

- ***Vitamins:*** Milk is a good source of vitamin A but it contains very little vitamin D, unless it is ***'fortified'*** and enriched by adding vitamin D or by irradiation with UV rays. α-Tocopherol content of human milk is about twice that of bovine milk. ***Vitamin C content of milk is very low*** and pasteurization destroys half of the original content. Milk has rather low concentrations of soluble B-vitamin group, but comparatively rich in riboflavine (B_2) and good in thiamine (B_1).

Human milk: Human milk differs markedly from cow's milk in a number of ways:

- The protein content of human milk is far lower.
- The lactose content of human milk is much higher.

	Cow's milk	*Human milk*
Caseinogen: Lactalbumin	3:1	1:2
Protein: non-protein N_2 ratio	11:1	3:1

Differentiation in composition of human milk and cow's milk is given in tabular from in ***Table 24.9.***

Table 24.9. Difference between the composition of human milk and cow's milk

	Human milk	*Cow's milk*
• Solids	12.5	13.5
• Water	87.5	87.0
• Proteins (gm %)	1.0 to 2.5 (1.5)	2.0 to 6.0 (4.0)
• Carbohydrates (gm%)	4.5 to 8.0 (7.0)	2.0 to 6.0 (5.0)
• Fats (gm%)	1.0 to 8.0 (4.0)	1.5 to 6.5 (5.0)
• Calcium (mg%)	40	120
• Phosphorus (mg%)	30	90
• Magnesium (mg %)	5	20
• Sodium (mg %)	15	50
• Potassium (mg %)	60	140
• Chloride (mg %)	40	110
• Vit A (μg%)	50	35
• Vit D (IU)	5.0	2.5
• Vit C (mg %)	4.5	2.0
• Vit B_1 (μg %)	15	45
• Riboflavin (μg %)	45	200
• Niacin (μg %)	180	80
• Vit. B_6 (μg %)	10	50
• Pantothenic acid (μg %)	200	350
• Calories/100 gm.	67	69

Humanisation of cow's Milk: Cow's milk, when fed to newborn babies has to be diluted with water to lower its protein content to that of human milk and lactose, glucose, maltose or sucrose has to be added to it to raise its sugar content to the level of human milk. This process is known as ***humanisation of cow's milk.***

Note: Bovine milk normally contains far less linoleic acid, α-tocopherol, vitamin C and niacin than those in human milk and hence humanised cow's milk will have still less of them due to the dilution.

Colostrum

- The secretion of the lactating mammary glands during the first few days of lactation (first 4 to 5 days) after parturition is called **colostrum.** It is thick, viscous yellow liquid and is **heat coagulable**. ***Heat coagulability is due to presence of increased amounts of globulins and lactalbumins.***
- Colostrum is richer than mature milk in proteins, vitamin A and D, α-tocopherols and calcium, but comparatively poorer than mature milk in casein, fats and lactose.
- ***Though it has less casein, but the total protein content is twice as much.*** The proteins have a high percentage of globulins and next is lactalbumins. Globulins which are the highest include some lactglobulins and ***various Igs (immunoglobulins)coming from the maternal blood. These immunoglobulins may be absorbed from the small intestine of newborns probably by 'pinocytosis' and confer temporary immunity.***
- A trypsin-like inhibitor present in colostrum may help to preserve the immunoglobulins in the alimentary canal of new borns by preventing hydrolysis.
- Colostrum also contains larger amounts of B-vitamins like thiamine, riboflavin and folic acid.

B. Nutritive Value of Egg: Egg is a delicious, palatable and enjoyable food item liked by adults as well as children. It can be taken in the diet in various forms and preparations. It is highly nutritive. From a nutritional stand point, the egg stands with dairy products and meat.

Composition of an Average Hen's Egg:

- It consists of approximately 30 percent yolk (yellow portion), 59 percent white and 11 percent shell.
- In the edible part there is 15 percent proteins, 10.5 percent fats and 1 percent ash.

I. *White part:* Is essentially a solution of proteins and salts.

***Proteins*:** Proteins of eggs are high quality proteins and are used as reference standard for assessing other proteins. The main proteins in white part are:

- ***Ovalbumin:*** A typical albumin
- ***Conalbumin:*** Another albumin
- ***Ovoglobulin:*** A globulin
- ***Ovo-mucoid:*** A glycoprotein

Note: The pale-yellow colour of egg white is partly due to riboflavin.

II. Yolk: It is more concentrated, containing only 51 percent of water. The chief constituents are proteins and fats. Also there is about 1 percent of mineral matters and vitamins.

1. ***Proteins:*** Proteins present in yolk are mainly two:
   - ***Vitellin*:** A phosphoprotein, resembeling caseinogen of milk.
   - ***Livetin*:** A globulin. Vitellin predominates and the ratio of Vitellin/Livetin = 3.6/1

The vitellin and lecithin present in yolk are associated as lipoprotein complex called Lecitho-vitellin.

2. ***Fats:*** Yolk contains nearly 30 percent of phospholipids-cephalin and lecithin mainly and to a small extent other phospholipids. ***Yolk is rich in cholesterol. An average hen's egg weighing 2 oz contains approximately 250 mg cholesterol.*** Fat present in egg-yolk is readily and thoroughly digested and absorbed. It contains appreciable amounts of polyunsaturated FA like linoleic acid.

3. ***Minerals*:** The yolk is well supplied with mineral matters, specially Ca, Fe and PO_4. ***It is very good source of Fe*** which is easily assimilable. Few foods supply as much available Fe as egg. It appears to be present practically all in inorganic forms. Much of the phosphates is present in phospholipids and vitellin.

4. ***Vitamins*:** The yolk is rich in vitamins A and D. Also in B-vitamins like thiamine, riboflavin but not in vitamin C. the other vitamins of B group and vitamin E are also present.

C. Other Basic Food Groups

1. ***Meat and Fish:*** Principal nutrient supplied is the proteins. Proteins of both meat and fish are of high biological value.

- Muscle meat excluding cartilages and bones, in itself is not a complete food as it is deficient in Ca and has high P content and this makes Ca : P ratio out of balance.
- Small fishes, though comparatively of cheaper cost are good sources of Ca and P because the whole fish is eaten.
- Fish and meat supplies adequate Fe but vitamin C, the fat soluble vitamins and certain B-vitamins are slightly deficient.

2. ***Pulses and Legumes:*** Pulses and legumes are commonly known as poor man's meat and are rich sources of protein. Now the pulses price has gone so high that it is not within the reach of poor men even.

- Chief protein is a globulin, called ***"Legumin"***. The protein content of dried pulses is from 20 to 25%, i.e. double that of cereals.
- They are rich sources of B-vitamins specially thiamine, riboflavin and niacin. Pulses and grams, if germinated, become rich sources of B-group vitamins and vitamin C as well.

Table 24.10: Shows the composition of different nutrients

	Water	*Proteins*	*Lipids*	*Carb*	*Calories*
	(in gm%)				*per 100 gm*
• *Whole egg*	73%	12.5	12.0	1.6	162
• *Yolk*	51%	16.0	33.0	2.1	381
• *White*	85%	11.5	trace (0.1)	1.4	51

Table 24.11: Shows vitamin contents of egg (fresh) per 100 gm of edible portion

Vit A	B_1	B_2	*Niacin*	*Vit. C*	*Vit D*
(I.U)	(mg)	(mg)	(mg)	(mg)	(I.U)
1000	0.15	0.40	0.1	0	60

3. ***Nuts:*** Nuts are characterized by a high fat and low carbohydrate content. The protein content is slightly lower than that of dried pulses.

4. ***Cereals:*** General composition of crude cereals (oats, wheat, barley, rice, rye, etc.) approximately protein 11 percent, carbohydrates 70 percent, minerals matter 2 percent, fats varying from 0.5 to 8 percent and water 11 percent.

a. ***Protein:*** Chief proteins of cereals are ***Glutelins*** and ***Gliadins***, usually they are not complete proteins as they may be deficient in certain amino acids. Some amounts of albumins and globulins are also present. Though protein content of cereals is not high, but in view of large quantities consumed per day, the total intake is good.

b. ***Carbohydrates***: Mainly in the form of starch, covered by a thin membrane of insoluble carbohydrate mainly cellulose, starch grains are insoluble and indigestible. Cooking by bursting the cellulose covering of the grains, renders, starch soluble and digestible.

c. ***Fats:*** Contain sufficient olein.

d. ***Minerals:*** Most abundant mineral constituents are Ca and PO_4, the latter is partly in the form of phytic acid (inositol hexaphosphate), which is not utilisable by humans and hinders the absorption of Ca ("anti calcifying effect"). The nutrition value of roller-milled white flour is considered less than the whole meal flour. There is great loss of vitamin E, and B-vitamins and mineral elements specially Ca, P and Fe. The quality and quantity of protein are slightly diminished.

5. ***Roots and Tubers:*** The most important tuber is potato, which is common food used daily. Sweet potatoes, colocasia, tapioca, carrots, etc. are other belonging to this group.

a. ***Carbohydrates:*** They are rich sources of carbohydrates and the most important substance present in starch. Main source of energy and gives 100 calories/100 gm, because of higher moisture content.

b. ***Proteins***: Only about half the total N_2 is present as protein chiefly as the globulin, ***"Tuberin"***. The remaining nitrogen is in the form of simple soluble nitrogenous compounds such as ***"Asparagine"***.

c. ***Minerals and Vitamins:*** Potatoes contain good quantities of vitamin C and Fe. Vitamin C content varies with the time of the year. Newly raised potatoes contain about 28 mg vitamin C per 100 gm, but on storage this amount gradually falls and the old potatoes contain less than 5 mg/100 gm. Carrots which are richest in sugar (10%) are valuable source of carotene, precursor of vitamin A.

6. ***Green Leafy Vegetables***: This is an important basic food group and includes fresh leafy vegetables of all kinds, e.g. spinach, amaranth, lettuce, cabbage, etc.

- Leafy vegetables ***are good sources of at least six essential nutrients.*** e.g. **carotene,** (Precursor for vitamin A), **B-vitamins like**-riboflavin **folic acid, vitamin C**, **Fe**, **Ca** and salts. The cost is quite cheap. If these nutrients, in similar quantities are to be obtained from alternate animal sources, the cost will be comparatively much higher. Excess of cabbage should be avoided as it is goitrogenic. Calorific value is rather small and are mostly due to sugar present.
- Cooking causes loss of B-vitamins and vitamin C, hence uncooked salads are, therefore more valuable. Cellulose present is not digested and absorbed, but add bulk to intestinal contents which stimulate peristalsis. ***Cellulose provides "roughage" value.***
- Green leafy vegetables are essentially ***protective foods*** due to their vitamin and mineral content, they prevent development of deficiency diseases.

7. ***Fruits:*** Fresh fruits are also ***essential Protective foods,*** although the energy value is twice that of green vegetables. This is due to sugars and starch. Proteins and fats usually amounting to less than 0.5 percent. Many fruits contain pentoses and pectins. Neither pentoses nor pectins are utilized by the body.

- They are good sources of B-vitamins, vitamin A and vitamin C.
- Fruits like orange, lemons and guava are good sources of vitamin C. ***Amla is the richest source of vitamin C.***

- Ripe yellow fruits, e.g. mango, or papaya contain carotene (precursor for vitamin A).
- Fruits are good 'alkalinisers' of blood and hence useful in pyrexia.
- ***Banana :*** Cheaper among the fruits and found plenty in our country. Ripe banana mainly contains carbohydrates and have definite energy value, contains starch as well as other sugars. It also has a higher protein content. Starch present in banana is said to be easily digested.

Table 24.12 shows nutritional value of some common food stuffs.

ROLE OF DIETARY FIBRES

Dietary fibres denote all plant cell wall components that cannot be digested by an animal's own digestive enzymes, e.g. ***cellulose, hemicellulose, pectins, gums, lignins and pentosans.*** Human beings cannot digest, but herbivores such as ruminants, can digest cellulose and that constitute the major source of energy for them.

Beneficial effects of high fibre diets:

- Helps in aiding water retention during passage of foods along the gut, and thereby producing larger, softer faeces.
- Help in increasing bulk of the faeces, which induces peristalsis ***("Roughage" action)*** and removes constipation. More insoluble fibres such as cellulose and lignin found in wheat bran helps in colonic function.
- More soluble fibres found in legumes and fruits, e.g. gums and pectins can lower blood cholesterol, probabaly:
  - By binding bile acids and
  - By binding dietary cholesterol thus preventing absorption.
- Soluble fibres also slow emptying of stomach and attenuate the post pradial rise in blood glucose, with consequent reduction in insulin secretion. This effect is beneficial to diabetic patients and to dieters because it reduce the rebound fall in blood glucose that stimulates appetite.

Clinical Importance

A fibre diet is associated with reduced incidence of:

- **Diverticulosis**
- **Cancer of colon**
- **Atherosclerosis and cardiovascular diseases**
- **Diabetes mellitus.**

Table 24.12: Shows nutritional value of some of common food stuffs

Items	*Calories*	*Proteins gm%*	*Carbohy-drates*	*Fats gm%*	*Fe mg%*	*Ca mg%*	*NaCl mg%*	*Vit A I.U*	*B_1 mg%*	*Riboflavine mg%*	*Niacin mg%*	*Vit C mg%*
• **Atta**	353	12.0	72.3	1.8	7.4	39	116	60	451	120	4.9	0
• **Rice (Raw, undermilled)**	349	7.1	79.0	0.4	2.8	11	88	0	198	53	1.8	0
• **Butter**	744	0.4	0	82.5	0	14	1764	2716	0	0	0	0
• **Cow's milk**	65	3.2	4.9	3.5	0	120	123	180	46	200	80	0
• **Buffalo's milk**	116	4.2	5.3	8.8	0.	21.2	–	162	–	–	–	–
• **Hen's Egg**	138	10.9	6.7	10.2	2.5	53	141	882	trace	353	0	0
• **Mutton (Goat) with bones**	155	14.8	0	10.9	1.8	123	141	28	49	219	5.3	0
• **Onions**	49	1.1	11.6	0	0.7	160	–	0	35	11	0.4	11
• **French beans**	14	1.1	2.5	0	0.7	46	–	120	71	46	0.4	11
• **Dal musoor**	346	26.1	60.1	0.7	2.1	134	88	250	444	–	1.4	0
• **Apple**	46	0.4	10.9	0.	1.4	8.8	–	trace	116	28	0.4	4
• **Banana**	102	1.1	24.0	0	0.4	7	282	trace	78	32	0.4	4

Effects of Cooking: Foods undergo considerable change in the process of cooking and preparation.

- Inedible portions are removed.
- Harmful bacteria and organisms are destroyed
- *Effect on raw meat:*
  - The chief difference between raw and cooked meat is that, the latter, even boiled, has less water, so that 4.0 gm of cooked meat has the nutritive value of approximately 5.0 gm of raw meat. The soluble portion is coagulated.
  - Some fats and extractives are lost, and collagen fibres are converted to gelatin, thus loosening the muscles fibres.
- *Effect on digestibility:* Cooking does not necessarily increase the digestibility, clinical practice, in fact, suggests that well-disintegrated raw or underdone meat is the most easily digested. But cooking, by breaking down connective fibres, makes meat easier to masticate and so assists digestion, it also increases the palatability of the meat. Overcooking, by causing shrinkage of coagulated proteins, decreases the digestibility.

Vegetables: Cooking usually increases both the water content and digestibility of vegetables. The chief effect of cooking is the loosening of the cellulose framework and liberation of starch grains (granules). Raw starch is practically indigestible.

Fats are little changed in the process of cooking

Taste and flavour: Cooking enhances the taste and flavour of food by the addition of seasoning and in dry cooking (like roasting and baking) by the formation of caramel from sugar and from partial decomposition products from fats and proteins. Many of these substances stimulates the secretion of digestive juices.

Loss of vitamins: Cooking involves loss in nearly all vitamins of foods, especially of soluble substances in boiling processes. Vitamin B_1 and C are specially liable to destruction when vegetables are cooked.

- *Effects of cooking on green vegetables:* may be summarized as follows:
- Vitamin A is unlikely to suffer damage.
- Water soluble B vitamins and vitamin C are likely to be lost by diffusion into the soaking or cooking water.
- Raw vegetables contain enzymes which destroy vitamins and become "active", if the vegetables are kept after bruising or cutting up.
- They act more rapidly if the temeprature is raised and are only themselves destroyed at about 80°C.
- It is therefore, better to cook vegetable by plunging them into boiling water or hot fat/oil rather than by raising to boil from cold. In the latter method; there may be considerable destruction of vitamins before the enzyme is destroyed.
- Water soluble vitamins are destroyed by prolonged heating and the vitamin content of cooked food diminishes if they are kept. These losses are reduced by adding salt or sugar before cooking.
- Vitamin B_1 and C are more stable in acid solution. Alkali, e.g. sodium bicarbonate hastens the destruction of vitamin B_1.

☞ SALIENT POINTS TO REMEMBER

- Proteins are primarily not meant for energy, their principal function is to synthesize tissue proteins of the body.
- Proteins are thus body building foods that supply essential amino acids. If required proteins (C-skeleton) can meet the body energy requirement (10-15 percent).
- Quality of proteins taken in the diet is more important than the quantity consumed.
- Several methods are available to assess the nutritive value of proteins. These include biological value (B.V.), protein efficiency ratio (PER), net protein utilization (NPU) and chemical score (C.S.).
- Presence of all essential aminoacids is mandatory for the protein to be utilized for tissue synthesis.
- If one of the essential amino acid is lacking and there is an interval of 2 hours or more, the

amino acids are not utilized for protein synthesis. Time factor is important.

- The combination of wheat, low in Lysine but adequate in methionine when taken together either with potatoes, or peas, which is adequate in Lysine but low in methionine enhances the biological value of each of these low quality vegetable proteins. This is called supplementary action of amino acids.
- The recommended dietary allowance (RDA) represent the quantities of nutrients to be provided daily in the diet for maintaining good health and physical efficiency.
- The RDA of protein is 1.0 gm/kg body weight per day.
- Carbohydrates are the major source of body "fuel" (energy) supplying about 55 to 65 percent of body calories.
- With diets rich in carbohydrates, the requirement for B-vitamins particularly thiamine (vit-B_1) increases.
- The nondigestible carbohydrates like cellulose, pectins, lignins, etc. are referred to as dietary "fibres".
- Adequate intake of fibres has "roughage value" and prevents constipation, improve glucose tolerance and reduces plasma cholesterol.
- A fibre diet is associated with reduced incidence of Diverticulosis, Cancer of colon, Diabetes mellitus, atherosclerosis and C.V. diseases.
- Lipids like carbohydrates is the concentrated source of energy. They also provide essential fatty acids (EFA), and fat soluble vitamins like A, D, K and E.
- Poly unsaturated fatty acids (PUFA) reduces the cholesterol level in blood.
- Medium chain TG has been used in treatment of chyluria and chylothorax as they are absorbed directly in portal blood.
- Excess fat intake with less carbohydrate intake can cause excessive production of ketonebodies due to high F.A. oxidation and can lead to Type 1 fatty liver.
- A diet is said to be a balanced one when it includes proportionate quantities of food items selected from the different basic food groups so as to supply the essential nutrients, viz proteins, fats, carbohydrates, minerals, vitamins and water, in complete fulfilment of the requirements of the body.
- Protein energy malnutrition (PEM), earlier called protein calorie matnutrition (PCM) is the most common nutritional disorder in the developing countries.
- PEM are mainly of 3 types:
  (i) Marasmus (ii) Kwashiorkor and (iii) Marasmic-Kwashiorkor
- Marasmus is primarily caused by calorie deficiency while Kwashiorkor is mainly due to inadequate protein intake.
- Milk is an ideal food but it lacks Fe, Cu and vitamin C.
- Milk proteins are high quality complete proteins. They are: Caseinogen (Phospho protein), Lactalbumin and Lactglobulin.
- Cow's milk diluted with water to lower its protein content and sugar (lactose, glucose, maltose/sucrose) is added to raise sugar content so that it simulates human milk. This is called as "humanisation of cow's milk".
- Colostrum is the thick, viscous yellow liquid, heat coagulable is secreted by the lactating mammary glands during the first few days of lactation (first 4 or 5 days) after parturition.
- Colostrum is richer than mature milk in proteins, vitamins A, D and E and Ca. Also contains Igs which absorbed by newborn baby gives temporary immunity.
- Egg is highly nutritive. White part of egg contains proteins, ovalbumin, conalbumin, ovoglobulin and ovomucoid.
- Yellow part of egg (yolk) contains vitellin (a phosphoprotein and livetin.
- The egg proteins are high quality proteins and are used as reference standard for assessing other proteins.
- Egg is very good source of Fe. Yolk of egg is rich in cholesterol.

MULTIPLE CHOICE QUESTIONS

Give one correct answer:

1. **Oxidation of which substance in the body yields the most calories per gram?**
   (a) Lipids (b) Carbohydrates
   (c) Proteins (d) Vitamins
   (e) Vegetable proteins
2. **Cellulose cannot be digested by the humans because of the inability to hydrolyze:**
   (a) α-amylopectins (b) α-amyloses
   (c) β-glycosidic bonds (d) Pectins
   (e) α - glycosidic bonds
3. **The RQ of a mixed diet is:**
   (a) 0.75 (b) 0.85
   (c) 1.0 (d) 0.95
   (e) 2.0
4. **The semi essential amino acid is:**
   (a) Glycine (b) Alanine
   (c) Serine (d) Arginine
   (e) Threonine
5. **Whole wheat is an excellent source of:**
   (a) Thiamine (b) Riboflavin
   (c) Niacin (d) Ascorbic acid
   (e) Lipoic acid
6. **Feeding of raw white of egg in the diet may result in deficiency of:**
   (a) Choline (b) Biotin
   (c) Pantothenic acid
   (d) Cyanocobalamine
   (e) Nicotinic acid
7. **The biological activity of vit E has been attributed in part to its action as:**
   (a) A reducing substance
   (b) An anticoagulant
   (c) A carrier in electron transport chain (ETC)
   (d) An antioxidant
   (e) An antidote to selenium poisoning
8. **Which of the following essential dietary factors is a precursor for a compound that can act as a carrier of "one carbon" moiety at different levels of oxidation?**
   (a) B_{12} (b) Folic acid
   (c) Methionine (d) Thiamine
   (e) Riboflavin
9. **Milk is notoriously deficient in which of the minerals?**
   (a) Ca (b) P
   (c) Fe (d) Na
   (e) K
10. **The intake of which food stuffs result in the greatest SDA:**
    (a) Proteins (b) Fats
    (c) Carbohydrates (d) Vitamins
    (e) Minerals
11. **Milk is notoriously deficient in which of the vitamins?**
    (a) Vitamin A (b) Vitamin B_1
    (c) Vitamin B_2 (d) Biotin
    (e) Ascorbic acid
12. **An important etiologic factor in kwashiorkor is:**
    (a) Dietary mineral deficiency
    (b) Dietary protein deficiency
    (c) Calorie deficiency
    (d) Mineral deficiency
    (e) Vitamin deficiency

ANSWERS

1. (a)	2. (c)	3. (b)
4. (d)	5. (a)	6. (b)
7. (d)	8. (b)	9. (c)
10. (a)	11. (e)	12. (b)

25 Water and Electrolyte Balance and Imbalance

DISTRIBUTION OF BODY WATER AND ELECTROLYTES

I. DISTRIBUTION OF BODY WATER

Total body water in an adult of 70 kg varies from 60 to 70% (36-49 litres) of total body weight, when expressed as percentage of ***"lean body mass"***, i.e. sum of the "fat-free tissue." The body water can be visualized to be distributed mainly in two "compartments", viz:

a. ***Intracellular fluid (ICF):*** The fluid present in the cells which is approximately 50% (35 L), and

b. ***Extracellular fluid (ECF):*** The fluid present outside the cells which constitutes approx 20% (14 L). The extracellular fluid (ECF) is considered to be present in the two compartments as follows:
   - ***Plasma:*** The fluid present in heart and blood vessels, approx, 5% (3L) and
   - ***Interstitial tissue fluid (ITF):*** 15% (11 L).

Distribution of body water is shown in ***Fig. 25.1.***

- ***"Transcellular" fluid:*** A variety of extracellular fluid collections formed by the "transport" or "secretory activity" of cells. *Examples are:*
  - Fluids found in salivary glands, pancreas, liver and biliary tract, skin, mucous membrane of respiratory and GI tracts; and
  - The fluids present in "spaces" within the eyes (aqueous humour), cerebrospinal fluid (CSF) in spinal canal and ventricles of brain, and that within the lumen of GI tract (mostly reabsorbed and not lost).

II. DISTRIBUTION OF ELECTROLYTES IN THE BODY

- ***Non-electrolytes:*** Such as glucose, urea, etc. do not dissociate in solution. While substances like NaCl, KCl in solution dissociate into sodium (Na^+), potassium (K^+) and chloride (Cl^-) ions, they are called as ***electrolytes.*** Water molecules completely surround these dissociated ions and prevent union of +vely charged particles with -vely charged ones.
- The + ve ions are called ***cations*** and -vely charged ions are called ***anions.***
- ***Law of electrical neutrality:*** Fluid in any body compartments will contain equal number of +vely charged and—vely charged ions.

Solutes in Body Fluids: Solutes in body fluids are mainly of *three* categories.

- ***"Organic" compounds of small molecular*** size like glucose, urea, uric acid, etc. They are ***"non-electrolytes"*** as they do not dissociate or ionize in solution. Since these substances diffuse relatively freely across cell membrane, they are not important in the distribution of water. If it is present in large quantities, however, they aid in retaining water and thus do influence total body water.
- ***"Organic" substances of large molecular size,*** mainly the ***proteins.*** Effect of protein fractions of the plasma and tissues is mainly on the

transfer of fluid from one compartment to another and **NOT** on the total body water.

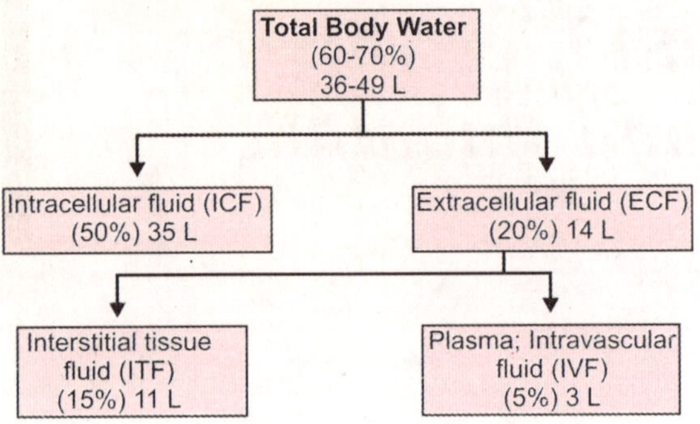

Fig. 25.1: Distribution of body water in an Adult of 70 kg

- ***Inorganic "Electrolytes":*** Because of the relatively large quantities of these materials in the body, they are by far the most important in distribution and retention of body water.

Electrolytes Composition of ECF: Both plasma (IVF) and tissue fluid (ISF) may be considered as ***one single compartment*** for all practical purposes as both resemble each other and both differ grossly from ICF

- Electrolytes composition of TF is similar to plasma except that Cl^- largely 'replaces' proteins as anion. Predominant cation is Na^+ ***(Table 25.1).***

Electrolytes Composition of ICF: ICF contains 195 mEq of cations and anions. Values of different electrolytes in ICF differs in different tissues. But chief cations are K^+ and then Mg^{++}. These are balanced by the chief anions PO_4^{--} and next by Pr^-.

- About two-thirds of K^+ within cells is ***"Proteinbound"***, while remaining one-third is 'free' which exchanges with ECF. Cl^-, HCO_3^- and Na^+ are present in intracellular fluid only in minimal amounts.
- ***Total electrolytes concentration is higher than that of the ECF (Table 25.2).***
- The phosphates of the cells are phosphoric esters of hexoses, certain phosphate, ATP and inorganic phosphates.

Table 25.1. Electrolytes of plasma and tissue fluid

Cations mEq/L			*Anions mEq/L*		
a. Plasma					
Na^+	=	143	Cl^-	=	103
K^+	=	5	HCO_3^-	=	27
Ca^{++}	=	5	HPO_4^{-2}	=	2
Mg^{++}	=	2	SO_4^{-2}	=	1
Total	=	**155**	$Proteins^-$	=	16
			Organic $acids^-$	=	6
			Total	=	**155**
b. Tissue fluid					
Na^+	=	145	Cl^-	=	116
K^+	=	5	HCO_3^-	=	27
Ca^{++}	=	3	HPO_4^{2-}	=	3
Mg^{++}	=	2	SO_4^{2-}	=	2
Total	=	**155**	$Proteins^-$	=	1
			Organic $acids^-$	=	6
			Total	=	**155**

Normal Fluid and Electrolytes Exchange in the Body: Under normal conditions in health, the relative volumes of water in above three compartments is kept constant ***(Fig. 25.2).***

Table 25.2: Electrolytes of ICF

Cations mEq/L			*Anions mEq/L*		
K^+	=	150	HPO_4^{-2}	=	110
Mg^{++}	=	40	Protein	=	50
Na^+	=	5	SO_4^{-2}	=	20
Total	=	**195**	HCO_3^-	=	10
			Cl^-	=	5
			Total	=	**195**

- Water can pass freely through the membrane which divide plasma from tissue fluid; and tissue fluid from intracellular fluid; ***but distribution of water is controlled by the osmotic pressure exerted by substances present in each compartment***, i.e. the electrolytes and protein molecules.
- Membrane separating ICF from tissue fluid is ***"Semi-permeable"*** called as ***"slow" membrane by Darrow***, and it allows only passage of water but not electrolytes and protein molecules in health.

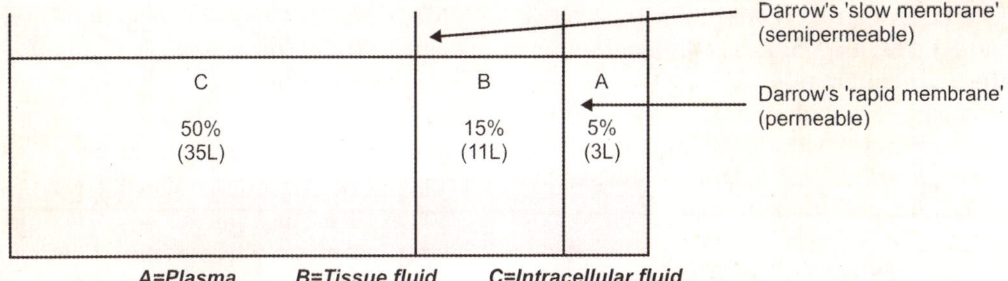

Fig. 25.2: Showing distribution of water in three compartments schematically

- Normally, there is osmotic equilibrium between these two compartments, but if this is disturbed, water is drawn from the compartment with lower osmotic pressure into that with higher osmotic pressure until equilibrium is restored. ***The osmotic imbalance between these two compartments results, in water being either sucked out of the cells (producing cellular dehydration) or water is drawn into the cells (producing cellular oedema) to restore the balance.***
- Membrane separating the vascular compartment from tissue fluid is more ***"permeable"***, called as ***"Rapid" membrane by Darrow,*** to water and electrolytes ***but not to protein molecules.***
- There is also fluid exchange taking place at the 'capillary beds'. The mechanism ***Starling hypothesis,*** provides for a continual circulation of fluid between the capillaries and the tissue spaces, a balance being maintained between the quantity of water filtered and that reabsorbed. ***Net filtration pressure that drives fluid out at the arterial end is 7 mmHg,*** (22 mmHg hydrostatic pressure—15 mmHg osmotic pressure), ***hydrostatic pressure being greater than osmotic pressure.*** On the other hand, ***at the venous end net absorption pressure which absorbs fluid is 8 mmHg,*** (15 mmHg osmotic pressure—7 mmHg hydrostatic pressure), ***osmotic pressure is greater than hydrosttic pressure*** (see chapter on Plasma Proteins).

Electrolytes Movements In and Out of Cells

- Much higher concentration of Na^+ and Cl^- in interstitial fluid and K^+ in intracellular fluid are accompanied by a differences in electrical potential. The resting skeletal muscle cells being ***about 90 mv -ve*** to the interstitial fluid. It is believed that the Lipid-protein membrane plays an important role in determining and maintaining these differences in concentration and potential.
- K^+ ions tend to diffuse out of and the Cl^- ions into the cells because of their concentration gradients, but this is almost exactly counterbalanced by a tendency to diffuse in the opposite direction due to the difference in electrical potential, i.e. the relative negativity on the inside of the cells tend to keep Cl^- out and K^+ in.
- ***In the case of Na^+, however, diffusion into the cells is favoured by both the concentration gradient and electrical potential. Cells do not allow accumulation of Na^+,*** hence under normal healthy conditions, there must be some mechanism for removing Na^+ from the cell, virtually as rapidly as it enters. Since this has to be accomplished in opposition to forces of concentration and electrical potential, it involves expenditure of energy, derived from cellular metabolism. **This process of "active transport" of Na^+ out of cells (Pumping out) is done by the *"Sodium Pump"*, which effectively extrudes Na^+ from the intracellular fluid.** This extrusion of Na^+ from

the cell is associated with splitting of ATP by **"Na^+-K^+ *ATP-ase*"** located at the inner surface of the cell membrane.

- The energy of hydrolysis of ATP is used by the transport mechanism for the coupled-exchange of Na^+ for K^+ ions between the intracellular and tissue fluids.

NORMAL WATER BALANCE

Body water is constantly exchanged with external environment.

1. Intake of Water: Water is normally absorbed into the body from the bowel (taken by mouth as water and beverages).

- Water also taken in cooked foods.
- *Metabolic water:* Formed from oxidation of food stuffs. Each gram of carbohydrates, fats and proteins yield 0.55 gm, 1.06 gm and 0.45 gm of water respectively on complete oxidation. In ml, on oxidation of 1 gm of carbohydrates, fats and proteins produces 0.56 ml, 1.07 ml, and 0.34 ml water respectively. ***In general 10 to 15 ml of water is produced per 100 calories of energy.***

2. Output of Water: Water is lost from the body constantly from various routes, they are as follows:

- ***Via kidney*** as urine: 1000 to 1500 ml in 24 hours.
- ***Via skin*** as "***insensible perspiration***": 600 to 800 ml of water in 24 hrs.
  N.B: Frank sweating is abnormal. ***Sweat is a "hypotonic" solution, 30 to 90 mEq/litre of NaCl are lost in sweating. In "insensible perspiration" there is no loss of salts, it is equivalent to distilled water.***
- ***Via lungs in the expired air:*** approximately 400 to 600 ml of water is lost in 24 hours.
- ***Via faeces:*** To a minor degree approximately 100 to 150 ml of water is lost in 24 hours from large intestine in faeces ***(Table 25.3).***

- **Normally in health,** the intake of water is more than the loss via skin, lungs and faeces and the surplus is excreted by the kidneys. Thus, **in health, the urinary volume largely depends on intake of water.**
- If the intake of water is low or excessive amounts are lost via extrarenal channels, the excretion of urine is diminished until only sufficient is excreted to eliminate the ***"waste products" (metabolic loads)*** of metabolism. Urinary volume may be reduced to 500-600 ml in 24 hours and this is called as ***minimum excretory*** volume. The exact quantity will depend on:
  - "Concentrating" power of the kidneys and
  - The quantity of "waste materials" required to be eliminated ***(solute load).***
- The loss through expired air (minimum 400 ml), by insensible perspiration through skin (minimum 600 ml), loss through faeces (minimum 100 ml) and the minimum excretory volume of kidney to eliminate waste products, i.e. 500 ml is called as ***obligatory losses (Approximately 1600 ml).*** This loss will continue as long as the individual is surviving.

Table 25.3: Average water intake and output in an adult

Intake		*Output*	
• Fluid by mouth as water and beverages	1000-1500 ml	• Urine (via kidney)	1000-1500 ml
• Water in food	700 ml	• Lungs	400 ml
• "Metabolic water"	400 ml	• Skin (insensible perspiration)	600 ml
		• Faeces	100 ml
Total	**2100-2600 ml**	**Total**	**2100-2600 ml**

NORMAL ELECTROLYTE BALANCE

- ***Though human systems consume fluids and food which vary markedly both in quality and quantity, electrolyte levels in subjects from any two widely located regions of the world are within narrow normal ranges.***
- The organs which are constantly regulating the electrolyte levels are the
  - **Intestine,** and
  - **The kidneys**, process is termed as the ***internal circulation of salts.***
- Principal ECF ions enter the lumen of GI tract and renal tubules and their near complete reabsorption regulate electrolyte levels.

a. GI Tract: About 8 litres of fluid of different electrolytes enter GI tract every day and are reabsorbed almost completely with fluid loss approximately 100 to 150 ml, and electrolyte loss of Na^+ around 10-30 mEq and of K^+ around 10 mEq ***(Table 25.4).***

b. Kidneys: ***Internal circulation of salts*** constantly occurring in kidneys is at a much faster rate than that observed in GI tract. In kidney a volume of plasma equal to ECF (12-15 L) is filtered and reabsorbed every 2 hours and about 25,000 mEq of Na^+ are filtered and reabsorbed every day ***(Table 25.5).***

- Na^+ is reabsorbed from the renal tubules in exchange with H^+ and NH^+_4 in proximal and distal tubules respectively by the following mechanisms.
  - ***H^+ exchange against bicarbonate (bicarbonate system).***
  - ***H^+ exchange against Na_2HPO_4 (phosphate system).***
  - ***Ammonia mechanism against NaCl. (Refer to chapter on acid base balance and imblance)***

REGULATORY MECHANISMS

In health, the volume and composition of various body fluid compartments are maintained within physiological limits even in the face of wide variations in intake of water and solutes.

- Osmolarity of ICF is determined mainly by its K^+ concentration, while that of ECF by Na^+ concentration. If the volumes of these compartments are to be maintained at constant levels, a mechanism must be provided for

Table 25.4: Electrolyte Composition of various secretions of GI tract

Secretions	*Volume ml/day*	*Electrolytes-mEq/L* Na^+	K^+	Cl^-	HCO^-_3
• **Saliva**	1500 ml	33	20	34	–
• **Gastric juice**	2500 ml	70	10	90	10
• **Bile**	500 ml	145	5	100	40
• **Pancreatic juice**	700 ml	145	5	70	115
• **Intestinal juice**	3000 ml	140	5	110	25
	8200 ml	533	45	404	190
Loss through faeces	**Fluid** — 100-150 ml				
	Na^+ — 10-30 mEq				
	K^+ — 10 mEq				

Table 25.5: Glomerular filtration and tubular reabsorption of water and Na^+

Substances	*Filtered per day*	*Excreted per day*	*Reabsorption*
• **Water**	180 L	IL	99.4%
• **Na^+**	180 × 140 mEq (25,000 mEq approx)	100 mEq	99.6%

adjustments in excretions of not only of water but also of Na^+ and K^+ in response to variations in amounts of each supplied to the organism. These adjustments are accomplished mainly by the kidneys. ***The kidneys respond promptly to deviations in osmolarity or individual ions concentration is ECF.***

- ***Homeostasis of body fluids,*** therefore involves mechanisms that
  - Responds to fluctuations in volume, as well as,
  - To changes in concentration of total solutes or of individual ions.
- Current concepts of the nature of the regulatory mechanisms include the existence of ***receptors*** sensitive to variations in:
  - Osmolar concentration (***osmoreceptors.***)
  - Individual ions ***(chemoreceptors)*** concentration in ECF,
  - To local or general variation in intravascular pressures (***baroreceptors***)
  - Plasma/or ECF volume (***volume receptors or stretch receptors***)
- The intrarenal mechanisms concerned with excretion of water and solutes may be influenced by stimuli initiated in these receptors either
  - By direct neural connections, or
  - Through the medium of "humoral factors", i.e. alterations in production and release of certain hormones, these are mainly two:
    - **Antidiuretic hormone (ADH) or Vasopressin.**
    - **Aldosterone,**

the former regulating the excretion of water and the latter Na^+ and K^+.

A. Thirst Mechanism (Neural Mechanism):

The intake of fluid is regulated by the mechanism of "thirst". ***A thirst centre is located in III ventricle,*** which regulates the amount of water, consumed as water or beverages. A deficient intake of water with continuing "obligatory losses" ***leads to concentration of body fluids with respect to solutes and a rise in osmotic pressure.*** This tends to draw water from ICF, ***the dehydration of the cells seem to be the main stimulus for thirst mechanisms*** through osmoreceptors as well as sensory nerves of mouth and pharynx (IX and X), which respond to dryness of the mouth and pharynx.

B. Antidiuretic Hormone (Vasopressin):

- A protein hormone; an octapeptide produced by the supraoptic nuclei in hypothalamus which exerts an antidiuretic effect. It affects renal tubules and provides for the facultative reabsorption of water from distal tubules, collecting tubules and parts of the loops of Henle.

C. Aldosterone:

Aldosterone, a steroid hormone, classified as mineralocorticoid, produced by Zona glomerulosa of adrenal cortex has the most important effect on mineral metabolism. ***The hormone increases the rate of tubular reabsorption of Na^+.*** The hormone has potent effect on the distal tubule, collecting tubule, and part of loop of Henle (accounts for 95% of all sodium reabsorption). ***Total lack of aldosterone can cause a loss of as much as 12.0 gm of sodium in 24 hours.*** Aldosterone also increases the reabsorption of Cl^- ions from the tubules, ***Na^+ reabsorption occurs at the expense of H^+ thus producing alkalosis.*** At the same time that aldosterone causes increased tubular reabsorption of Na^+, it also increases the loss of K^+ in the urine. (For Reninangiotensin system see chapter on Hormone).

D. Atrial Natriuretic Peptide (ANP):

For a number of years it has been known that if the GFR and aldosterone secretion rate are kept constant, an increase in intravascular volume (IVV) will result in natriuresis.

- Recently, a polypeptide of 152 aminoacids residues has been isolated from the cardiac atrium which has the following effects *in vivo:*
  - Increase in GFR ↑.
  - Increase in glomerular filtration fraction↑.
  - Causes natriuresis, diuresis and kaliuresis.
  - Decreases renin and aldosterone secretions, ↓, and

- Decreases blood pressure (antagonizes vasoconstriction) ↓.

Mechanism of action: Not clearly known. But it is postulated that ANP causes natriuresis ***by decreasing sodium reabsorption*** of the renal collecting duct. It is not yet certain what controls its release from the atrium, but it is proved that ANP is released in response to an increase in the IVV (intravascular volume).

ABNORMAL WATER AND ELECTROLYTE METABOLISM

Abnormalities can be of **two types:**

- **Dehydration:** Due to loss of water, or electrolytes or both and,
- **Water intoxication.**

I. DEHYDRATION

- Dehydration is a disturbance of water balance in which ***the output exceeds the intake,*** causing a reduction of body water below the normal level. Although the term implies loss of body fluid, the clinical state to which it refers is more than this; because, characteristically there is an accompanying disturbances of electrolytes.
- *Dehydration may be the result of:*
  - *Pure water depletion*
  - *Pure salt depletion or*
  - *Mixed type in which both water and salt depletion occurs.*
- **Marriott** called ***pure water depletion as "primary dehydration"***, and ***pure salt depletion as "secondary dehydration".***

  The following discussion will stress the two forms of depletion as separate entities in order to understand and emphasize certain basic pathophysiologic principles. However, it should be noted that most patients with dehydration have mixed type of depletion, with one or the other predominating.

A. PURE WATER DEPLETION (PRIMARY DEHYDRATION)

Definition: Pure water depletion occurs when water intake is stopped or water intake is inadequate and there is **no parallel loss of salt** in the secretions from the body.

Causes:

- When a patient is too weak or too ill to satisfy his/her water needs,
- In mental patients who refuse to drink,
- In cases of coma, dysphagia (difficulty in swallowing).
- In individuals lost in desert or shipwrecked.

Pathophysiology:

- Water depletion occurs almost always because of lack of intake, rather than because of losses from the body. When a person stops his intake of water, body water stores become depleted, because of the continuing ***"obligatory losses"*** and later on, supplemented by the ***continued excretion of "minimal volume" of urine required for excretion of "metabolic loads"***. Only source of water supply to the body in the complete absence of intake becomes the water obtained from oxidation of food staffs ("**metabolic water**").
- As obligatory water loss continues, the concentration of the electrolytes rises in the ECF, which becomes ***hypertonic (or hyperosmolar). Water flows from ICC to ECC to correct this imbalance*** and to maintain uniform osmotic pressure throughout the body. **Thus the volume of ECF is maintained almost to normal at the expense of ICF which is grossly reduced in volume** ***causing intracellular dehydration (Fig. 25.3).***

Clinical and Biochemical Findings:

- ***Thirst*** is the earliest ***symptom due to intracellular dehydration.*** Dehydration is shown by a dry tongue and 'pinched' facies.
- ***Oliguria:*** Hyperosmolarity stimulates the release of ADH, which causes reabsorption of water from kidney tubules, causing a gradual diminution of urine volume.
- A normal or slightly increased blood urea, a normal or slightly reduced plasma volume, may occur.
- There is usually no circulatory collapse or fall in BP seen as the plasma volume is maintained.

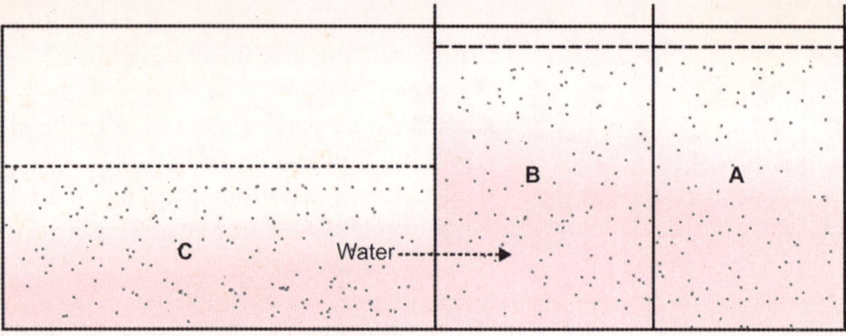

Fig. 25.3: Showing schematically distribution of water in three compartments in primary dehydration

- ***Urinary chlorides:*** It is important to note that in this type of dehydration ***urine will contain NaCl, rather it is to the higher side.***
- ***Death:*** Occurs when water loss amounts to approximately 15% of body weight (about 22% of total body water), which happens on about the 7th to 10th day of complete water deprivation, if not treated.

Estimation of Water Loss: **Marriott** divided states of water depletion into **three clinical phases** along with fluid deficit. ***(Table 25.6)***

B. PURE SALT DEPLETION

Definition: Pure salt depletion occurs when fluids of high Na^+ or Cl^- content are lost from the body and are **replaced by salt-deficient fluids** such as water by mouth or glucose solution IV.

Causes:

- Loss of Na^+ can occur by excessive sweating when only water is taken in as replacement.
- Another important means of sodium depletion is loss of GI fluids as in vomiting, diarrhoea, pancreatic/or biliary fistulae, cholera, and continous aspirations through intubation (suction).
- Urinary losses of Na^+ are perhaps not as common, but can occur in such clinical states as Addison's disease, diabetic acidosis, cerebral salt-wasting syndrome and certain instances of chronic renal disease. In these cases, loss of Na^+ may be aggravated by accompanying vomiting.
- Vigorous use of diuretics and low sodium or salt-free diets in the management of congestive heart failure may induce sodium depletion.

Pathophysiology:

- With sodium depletion, the ECF becomes ***hypotonic.*** The lowered osmotic pressure inhibits the release of ADH and the kidneys excrete water in an attempt to maintain normal extracellular Na^+ concentration. Because of the above, ***plasma and interstitial fluid volume are decreased.***
- Also the extracellular hypotonicity, allows water to flow into the cells where the concentration is greater, thus further reducing the volume of the ECF ***the cellular hydration is in contrast to cellular dehydration noted in pure water depletion.***
- The reduction of volume of the interstitial fluid exceeds that of the plasma. Probably because of two factors:
    - A higher osmotic pressure of plasma due to the proteins, and
    - Diminished filtration caused by decline of hydrostatic pressure within the circulation, a consequences of lowered plasma volume ***(Fig. 25.4).***

Table 25.6: Estimation of water loss in primary dehydration from clinical manifestations

Clinical phases	*Clinical features*	*Estimated deficit*
• *Early*	Thirst +	2% of body wt (approx 1.5 L)
• *Moderately severe* (72 to 96 hrs without water)	Thirst ++ Dry mouth pinched facies, oliguria, weakness, seriously ill early personality changes.	6% of Body wt (approx 4.2 L)
• *Very severe*	Above features + Diminution of physical and Mental capabilities, Hallucinations, and Delirium	7% to 14% of body wt (approx 5 to 10L)

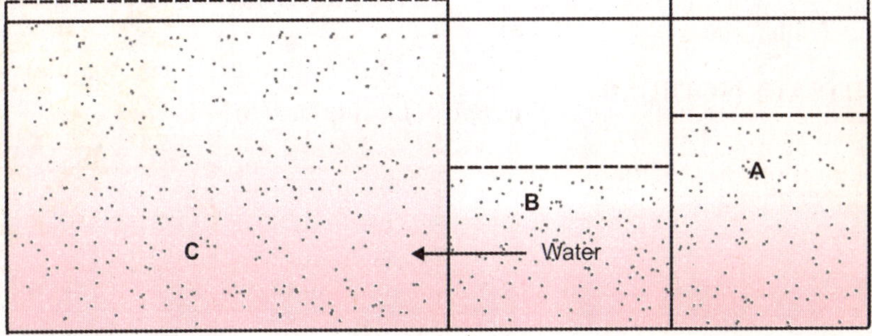

A = Plasma
B = Tissue fluid
C = Intracellular fluid

NB 1. Cellular hydration
2. Reduction in tissue fluid compartment more than plasma compartment

Fig. 25.4: Showing schematic distribution of water in three compartments in secondary dehydration

Clinical and Biochemical Features:

Clinical and biochemical findings mainly attributed to reduction in volume of ECF and sodium deficiency.

- Because of hypotonicity, ***Thirst is NOT a striking feature and absence of thirst is an important negative finding.***
- The patient appears apathetic and listless, mental changes are common and hallucinations, and confusions are common and sometimes delirious.
- Anorexia and nausea vomiting often aggravates the *"vicious cycle"* of sodium depletion. Thus

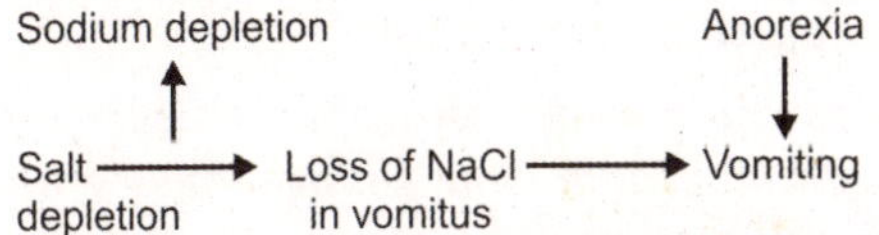

- *Cramps* are common and may occur in thigh, abdominal and respiratory muscles.
- Loss of interstitial fluid is manifested clinically by sunken eyes and inelastic skin.
- Reduced plasma volume leads to hemoconcentration. As a result of lowered blood volume there are decreased cardiac output, lowering of BP and a tendency to orthostatic fainting.
- Decreased glomerular filtration leads to N_2 retention with increase urea concentration.
- ***Urine analysis:*** Patients drinking freely maintain a nornal or slightly increased urinary volume, but ***there is no salt present in urine (except in Addison's disease).***
- *Death* is due to oligaemic shock.

Estimation of Loss of Fluids and Electrolytes:

Marriott divided states of water and salt depletion into ***three clinical phases*** alongwith fluid and salt deficit. ***(Table 25.7).***

Essential differences between two types of dehydration: Pure water depletion (primary

Table 25.7: Estimation of water and salt loss in secondary dehydration from clinical manifestations

Clinical phases	*Clinical features*	*Extimated deficit*
• *Early* (slight to moderate)	Lassitude, indifference/apathy, syncope, urine Cl^- = reduced	0.5 gm NaCl/kg = 4 L
• *Moderate to severe*	Above features + Nausea/vomiting, cramps, BP ↓ but > 90 mm Hg, urinary Cl^- =Absent	0.5 to 0.75 gm/kg (4.0-6.0 L)
• *Severe to very severe*	Above features + B.P. < 90 mm Hg, urinary Cl^- = absent	0.75 to 1.25 gm/kg (6.0-12.0 L)

dehydration) and pure salt depletion (secondary dehydration) are given in *Table 25.8.*

C. MIXED WATER AND SALT (SODIUM) DEPLETION

In clinical practice, depletion of both water and salt (sodium) is more common than depletion of either alone.

Definition: Mixed depletion occurs when there is loss of fluids containing high concentration of Na and Cl without a free intake of water.

Pathophysiology:

- Initially the ECF is *hypotonic. Later water loss outstrips the salt loss and ECF becomes hypertonic.*

Clinical and Biochemical Features: The clinical picture is a mixture of pure salt depletion and pure water depletion. The volume of fluid in both ECF and ICF is reduced. The patient appears dehydrated and complains of thirst. The BP may be lowered, blood urea is raised and there is hemoconcentration; urinary output is diminished and the excretion of salt is reduced.

Type of Fluids to Administer:

1. *For pure water depletion:* Water by mouth or per rectum or 5% Glucose by IV/SC or intraperitoneal routes depending on the case. **Note:** *Never give Isotonic Saline* which will increase hypertonicity.
2. *Pure sodium depletion:* Is corrected by isotonic saline solution.
3. *Mixed water and sodium depletion:* is treated with a mixture of saline and 5% Glucose, usually,
   - In the proportion 1:1 (half-normal saline)

     or
   - In 1 to 2 (one-third normal saline)

Urinary chloride level to be kept as a general guide:

- Normal saline to be given when chloride is absent from urine.
- Half normal saline when urinary chlorides are between 2.0 and 5.0 gm and
- Not more than one third normal saline for maintenance therapy, when urinary chloride excretion is greater than 5.0 gm per litre.

Estimation of Chloride Content of Urine: A rough estimate of chloride excretion can be obtained in bedside of patient by a simple test devised by **Fantus.**

Fantus's Test:

- Ten drops of urine are taken by a dropper/pipette into a clean test tube.
- Dropper/pipette is rinsed thoroughly in distilled water.
- One or two drops of 20% solution of potassium chromate is added as an indicator.
- The dropper/pipette is rinsed thoroughly again in distilled water.
- Take 2.9% solution of silver nitrate ($AgNO_3$) by the dropper/pipette and add drop by drop, the test tube being shaken after addition of each drop. *Count the drops.*

End Point: Is shown by a sharp colour change *from canary yellow to brown-brick red* due to formation of silver chromate

Result: The *number of drops of silver nitrate required to produce the change gives grams of sodium chloride per litre of urine.*

Table 25.8: Showing essential differences between pure water depletion (primary dehydration) and pure salt depletion (secondary dehydration)

Pure water depletion (Primary dehydration)	*Pure salt depletion (Secondary dehydration)*
• *Definition* Pure water depletion occurs when water intake stops or inadequate and there is no parallel loss of salt in the secretions.	Pure salt depletion occurs when the fluids of high Na^+ or Cl^- content are lost from the body and are replaced by salt deficient fluids such as water by mouth or glucose solution by IV
• *Causes* • Patient too weak or too ill to satisfy his water needs. • Mental patients. • Comatose patients • Patients with dysphagia • Individuals lost in desert or shipwrecked.	• Excessive sweating. • Loss of GI fluids: vomiting, diarrhoea, fistulae, continuous gastric suctions. • Urinary losses of Na^+: Addison's disease, • Diabetic acidosis, cerebral salt wasting syndrome, chronic renal disease. • Diuretics and low salt diet in congestive heart failure.
• *Nature of Dehydartion:* +++ Primary or simple, due to loss of ICF *(cellular dehydration)*	+++ Secondary or extracellular *due to loss of ECF*
• *Clinical features and findings:* • Thirst +++ (marked) • Lassitude + (slight) • Orthostatic fainting – Absent till date • Nausea and vomiting – Absent • Cramps—Absent • Pulse—Normal till late stage • BP— Normal till late	 • Absent • ++ to +++ (marked) • ++ to +++ (marked) • May be + to ++ • May be + to ++ • Rapid and thready • Fall in B P ++ to +++
• *Urinary Findings:* • Urine volume scanty (oliguria) • Sp. Gr. High • NaCl in urine Often + (usually to higher side)	 • Normal and colourless and increased volume • Usually low • Always absent except Addison's disease.
• *Biochemical findings:* • Tonicity of ECF — *Hypertonic* • Plasma volume — Normal till date • Haemo concentration — Not till late stage and slight • Blood viscosity — Normal till late • Plasma (Na^+) — Normal or slight increase in late stage • Blood urea + in late stage • Water absorption Rapid	 • *Hypotonic* • Decreased ++ to +++ • Increased ++ to +++ • Increased ++ to +++ • Decreased ++ to +++ • Usually increased ++ to +++ • Slow
• *Mode of death:* ? Due to rise in Os. Pr and cellular dehydration	• Oligaemic shock and peripheral circulatory failure.

Precautions:

- Same dropper/pipette should be used through out, as the whole test depends on the volume contained in the drops.
- Test should be repeated with distilled water instead of urine to ensure that potassium chromate solution is not contaminated with chlorides.

Interpretion:

- Urine normally contains 6.0 to 16.0 gm of NaCl per litre.
- Chloride may be regarded as absent if the colour changes with the first drop of $AgNO_3$. This may be normal finding in very dilute urine, which is unlikely to be encountered in dehydration.
- If urine of a sp. gr. 1020 or more contains less than 3.0 gm NaCl/litre, salt depletion is present.
- If the urine contains more than 5.0 gm/litre, chloride deficiency is unlikely unless the patient is suffering from Addison's dsease or saline is being given intravenously.

PATHOLOGICAL VARIATIONS OF WATER AND ELECTROLYTES

The variations seen pathologically in body fluid and electrolytes are not so simple as stated above. There may be ***three types of expansion:*** hypotonic, Isotonic, and hypertonic. Similarly, there may be ***three types of contraction:*** hypotonic, Isotonic and hypertonic. Salient features of these six types will be discussed briefly

1. *Hypotonic Expansion:* Accumulation of water without an equivalent amount of salt. It is occasionally encountered when copious quantities of salt free fluids viz. 5% glucose solution is given to persons with inadequate renal function. The accumulated water distributes osmotically among all the fluid compartments. The cells of CNS also share in this process, which may lead to convulsions and even death ***(water intoxication).***

Changes :

- Volume of ICF ↑
- Volume of ECF ↑
- Plasma $[Na^+]$ ↓, Haematocrit and plasma proteins↓
- Urinary excretion : Na^+↓ and H_2O↑(lower osmotic pressure inhibits A D H)

2. *Isotonic Expansion:* Accumulation of water and salt in isotonic amounts, i.e. accumulation of water with equivalent amount of salt. This expands the ECF, with no alteration of intracellular volume or composition. The water distributes between interstitial fluid (TF) and plasma, thereby lowering the concentration of plasma proteins and haematocrit. Clinically may manifest as palpable oedema of extremities or pulmonary oedema. Such a condition may arise as a serious complication of parenteral fluid therapy.

Changes :

- Volume of ICF —
- Volume of ECF ↓
- Plasma $[Na^+]$ —
- Haematocrit and plasma proteins↓
- Urinary excretion :
- Na^+↑
- H_2O↑

3. *Hypertonic Expansion:* Accumulation or retention of sodium leads to an increase in extracellular fluid volume (ECF). If somehow, this sodium is not accompanied by an equivalent amount of water, the resultant ECF becomes "hypertonic" and water is transferred from cells to ECF until osmotic equilibrium is attained. ***Thus ECF expands at the cost of cells, producing "Intracellular dehydration".*** If this state is allowed to continue, death may occur because CNS is damaged under such circumstances.

Changes :

- Volume of ICF ↓
ECF ↑
- Plasma $[Na^+]$ ↑
- Haematocrit and plasma proteins↓
- Urinary excretion : Na^+ ↑
H_2O ↑

4. *Hypotonic Contraction:* This results when salt is lost in excess from the body, unaccompanied by an equivalent amount of water, i.e. without simultaneous loss of equivalent amount of water. Excess water distributes itself in all the compartments. However, the serious aspects are those due to diminution in plasma volume. Such a condition can be seen in 'Adrenal cortical insufficiency'.

Changes :

- Volume of ICF ↑
  ECF ↓
- Plasma $[Na^+]$ ↓
- Haematocrit and plasma proteins↑
- Urinary excretion : Na^+↑, later ↓
  H_2O ↑

5. ***Isotonic Contraction:*** Most frequently encountered condition since there is no normal obligatory sodium loss from the body, isotonic contraction can occur by abnormal losses of Na^+ from the body, most commonly in one or more of the secretions of G.I. tract. These secretions are virtually isotonic with plasma.

The total daily production of these secretions is equal to 65% of the volume of entire ECF and continued loss of these secretions, if not treated, would soon be serious. As these fluids are all isotonic, their loss does not result in a change in ICF volume, and the entire loss must be from ECF, which contracts to an equivalent amount the water of interstitial fluid (TF) is drained, which results to dehydration, CV disturbances, oliguria and finally anuria. The patient may become unconscious and dies of circulatory collapse. Such a condition might arise in severe prolonged untreated diarrhoea.

Changes :

- Volume of ICF —
  ECF ↓
- Plasma $[Na^+]$ —
- Haematocrit and plasma proteins↑
- Urinary excretion : Na^+↓
  H_2O ↓

6. ***Hypertonic Contraction:*** The situation arises when there occurs excessive loss of water without simultaneous loss of Na^+. This results in contraction of both extracellular and intracellular compartments, such a condition is known as "hypertonic contraction" and it may arise in following conditions:
   - In patients with diabetes insipidus.
   - In persons who on account of debility are unable to feed themselves and remain unattended.
   - Those persons to whom water is unavailable, or
   - In persons who lose unusual amount of fluid in perspiration without getting it compensated.

Osmotic pressure of both compartments increases.

Changes :

- Volume of ICF ↓
  ECF ↓
- Plasma $[Na^+]$ ↑
- Haematocrit and plasma proteins↑
- Urinary excretion : Na^+↑
  H_2O ↓

Note: In practice, pure examples of these six situations are rarely encountered. Thus, although diarrhoea/or vomiting may produce *isotonic contraction,* the individual may fail to ingest water in sufficient quantity to meet the 'obligatory' water losses, thus converting the situation into *hypertonic contraction.*

Summary of the changes in six types is given in ***Table 25.9.***

Table 25.9: Showing changes in six types of contractions/expansions

Types	*Volume ICF*	*ECF*	*Plasma [Na^+]*	*Haematocrit and plasma proteins*	*Urinary excretion Na^+*	*H_2O*
• **Hypotonic Expansion**	↑	↑	↓	↓	↓	↑
• **Isotonic Expansion**	—	↑	—	↓	↑	↑
• **Hypertonic Expansion**	↓	↑	↑	↓	↑	↑
• **Hypotonic Contraction**	↑	↓	↓	↑	↑ late ↓	↑
• **Isotonic Contraction**	—	↓	—	↑	↓	↓
• **Hypertonic Contraction**	↓	↓	↑	↑	↑	↓

II. WATER INTOXICATION

This condition is caused by excess of water retention in the body and can occur due to the following causes:

- Renal failure
- Excessive administration of fluids parenterally.
- Hypersecretion of ADH following the administration of an anaesthesia for surgery, administration of narcotic drugs or in stress (including any surgery).
- Excess of aldosterone may lead to an overhydration of the body and subsequent water intoxication. (Conn's Syndrome).

Clinically: Headache, nausea, incoordination of movements, muscular weakness and delirium are the main symptoms of water intoxication.

Changes: PCV, Hb concentration and plasma proteins concentration are all decreased.

Plasma electrolytes are lowered

Urinary volume is usually increased and is of low sp. gr.

Treatment: Withholding fluids by mouth and administering 3 to 5 percent hypertonic saline IV.

☞ SALIENT POINTS TO REMEMBER

- Total body water in an adult of 70 kg varies from 60 to 70% (36 to 49 litres) of total body weight.
- It is distributed in cells, called intracellular fluid (ICF) constituting 50% (35L) and outside cells called extracellular fluid (ECF) constituting 20% (14 L).
- The daily water intake (by drinking, by water in food and metabolic water) and output (loss via urine, skin, lungs and faeces) maintain the body balance of water.
- Normally in health, the intake of water is more than loss via skin, lungs and faeces and the surplus is excreted in the urine.
- Thus, in health, the urinary volume largely depends on intake of water.
- If the intake of water is low or excessive amounts are lost via extra-renal channels, the excretion of urine is diminished until only sufficient is excreted to eliminate the "***Waste-products***" (metabolic load) which is approximately 500 to 600 ml. This is called "***minimum excretory volume***".

Electrolytes are distributed in the intracellular and extracellular fluids to maintain the osmotic equilibrium and water balance.

- Na^+ is the principal extracellular cation while K^+ is the main intracellular cation.
- As regards anions, Cl^- and HCO_3^- predominantly occur in the extra-cellular fluids while phosphates, proteins and organic acids are present in the I.C.F.
- Water and electrolyte balance are usually regulated together and this is under the control of hormones ADH (vasopressin) and aldosterone.
- Dehydration is a disturbance of water balance in which the output exceeds the intake, causing a reduction of body water below the normal level. There is also an accompanying disturbance of electrolytes.
- **Marriott** classified dehydration into following **three types:**
  - (i) Pure water depletion (Primary dehydration)
  - (ii) Pure salt depletion (secondary dehydration)
  - (iii) Mixed type in which both water and salt depletion occurs.
- Pure water depletion (primary dehydration) occurs when water intake is stopped or water intake is inadequate and there is no parallel loss of salt in the secretions from the body.
- Thirst is the earliest symptom due to intracellular dehydration.
- ECF becomes hypertonic (or hyper-osmolar) resulting to withdrawal of fluid from I.C.F. *leading to cellular dehydration.*
- Pure salt depletion (secondary dehydration) occurs when fluids of high Na^+ or Cl^- content are lost from the body and are replaced by salt-deficient fluids such as water by mouth or glucose solution by I.V.

- Thirst is conspicuously absent and is an important negative finding.
- ECF becomes hypotonic and cellular hydration is characteristic.
- Clinical manifestations in severe dehydration include increased pulse rate, low B.P. ↓, sunken eyeballs, decreased skin turgor, lethargy and coma.
- In clinical practice, mixed water and salt depletron seen more commonly. Mixed depletion occurs when there is loss of fluids containing high concentration of Na^+ and Cl^- without a free intake of water.
- Initially the ECF is hypotonic. Later water loss outstrips the salt loss and ECF becomes hypertonic.
- Pure water depletion should be treated by water given orally or 5% glucose I.V./S.C. *Never give isotonic saline which will increase hypertonicity of ECF.*
- Pure salt depletion is corrected by giving isotonic saline IV/SC
- Mixed water and salt depletion is treated with a mixture of saline and 5% glucose.

MULTIPLE CHOICE QUESTIONS

Give one correct answer:

1. **Predominant cation of plasma is Na^+ and it is balanced mainly by which of the anion?**
(a) HCO_3^- (b) Cl^-
(c) SO_4^{-2} (d) HPO_4^{-2}
(e) Organic acids
2. **Loss of water by insensible perspiration through the skin in 24 hours is:**
(a) 200 to 300 ml (b) 300 to 400 ml
(c) 400 to 500 ml (d) 600 to 800 ml
(e) 800 to 1000 ml
3. **Chief cation K^+ of ICF is mostly balanced by which of the following anions.**
(a) HPO_4^- (b) SO_4^-
(c) HCO_3^- (d) Cl^-
(e) Pr^-
4. **Minimum excretory volume to eliminate waste-products from the body in dehydration is:**
(a) 200 to 400 ml (b) 300 to 500 ml
(c) 500 to 600 ml (d) 600 to 700 ml
(e) Less than 200 ml
5. **In the arterial end of capillary loop, net filtration pressure which drives the fluid out is:**
(a) 5 mm Hg (b) 7 mm Hg
(c) 8 mm Hg (d) 9 mm Hg
(e) 10 mm Hg
6. **In primary dehydration, E.C.F. becomes:**
(a) Hypotonic (b) Hypertonic
(c) Isotonic (d) None of the above
7. **Net absorption pressure which draws fluid in at the venous end of capillary loop is:**
(a) 8 mm Hg (b) 9 mm Hg
(c) 10 mm Hg (d) 12 mm Hg
(e) 15 mm Hg
8. **Aldosterone is produced by**
(a) Zona glomerulosa
(b) Zona fasciculata
(c) Zone reticularis
(d) Zona glomerulosa + zona reticularis
(e) Zona reticulars + zone fasciculata
9. **Aldosterone increases**
(a) Excretion of Na^+
(b) Reabsorption of Na^+
(c) Reabsorption of K^+
(d) Excretion of water
(e) Excretion of Ca
10. **Urine normally contains NaCl in 24 hours urine:**
(a) 2 to 6 gm/litre
(b) 4 to 6 gm/litre
(c) 5 to 10 gm/litre
(d) 6 to 16 gm per litre
(e) 8 to 12 gm/litre

ANSWERS

1. (b)	2. (d)	3. (a)
4. (c)	5. (b)	6. (b)
7. (a)	8. (a)	9. (b)
10. (d)		

Acid-Base Balance and Imbalance

INTRODUCTION

Under normal conditions, the pH of ECF usually does not vary beyond the range 7.35 to 7.5 and is maintained approximately at 7.4, (pH of arterial blood is approximately 7.43 and venous blood is 7.4). ***Maintenance of this constant blood reaction is one of prime requisites of life*** and any material variation on either side, seriously disturbs the vital process and may lead to death. **pH < 7.3 leads to acidosis and pH>7.5 leads to alkalosis.**

- Large amounts of H^+ are continually contributed to these fluids from intracellular metabolic reactions, hence to maintain a constancy it is necessary and imperative that they are removed from the fluids effectively and promptly.
- The mechanisms of neutrality regulations are concerned, therefore, with maintaining a state of equilibrium between production, i.e. introduction H^+ ions and removal of the same.

ACID-BASE BALANCE IN NORMAL HEALTH

According to the modern concept of **Brönsted-Lowry:**

- An *acid* is defined as a substance, ion, molecule or particle, that yields H^+ ions (protons) in solution, and
- A *base* is anything that combines with H^+ ions (protons).

Accordingly, whereas H_2CO_3 is an acid, dissociating into H^+ and HCO_3^- ions, its anionic component HCO_3^- is a base.

Other examples are:

Acid		Base
HSO_4^-	⇔	$H^+ + SO_4^{2-}$
CH_3COOH	⇔	$H^+ + CH_3COO^-$
H_2PO_4	⇔	$H^+ + HPO_4^{2-}$

- $NaHCO_3$ acts as a base because it yields HCO_3^- ions, which can combine with H^+ ions.
- Water is a substance that can act either as acid or base.

H_2O **(Acid)** ⇔ $H^+ + OH^-$

$H^+ + H_2O$ **(Base)** ⇔ H_3O^+ **Hydroxonium ion (strong acid)**

- HCl is a strong acid by virtue of its extensive dissociation into H^+ and Cl^- ions, Cl^- ion is an extremely weak base, because it has very little capacity for combining firmly with H^+ ions. On the other hand, such anions as HCO_3^-, HPO_4^{2-}, $H_2PO_4^-$ and protein$^-$ are comparatively strong bases, because they have a relatively strong affinity for H^+ ions, forming weak acids (i.e. relatively slight dissociation).
- **The stronger the acid, the weaker the base,** which results from its dissociation and vice versa. Such pairs have been termed ***conjugate acid base pairs.*** Thus the conjugate base of the acid HCl is the Cl^- ions.

Several such pairs important in the body, arranged in order of descending strength of acid and hence of increasing strength of base are shown next page top.

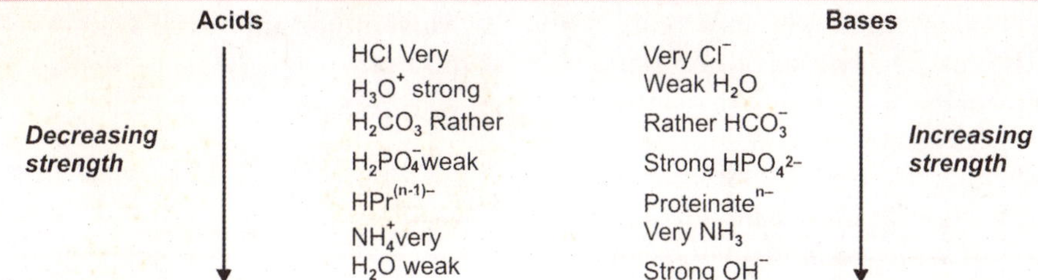

Note: It is to be noted that cations such as Na^+, K^+, Ca^{++}, Mg^{++} cannot donate or accept protons and so are neither acids nor bases. Such substances have been termed ***aprotes.*** All anions can accept usually protons and so are bases. Some can also act as acids at appropriate pHs.

BUFFERS

Definition: A buffer may be defined as a solution which resists the change in pH which might be expected to occur upon the addition of acid or base to the solution. ***Buffers consist of mixtures of weak acids and their corresponding salts,*** alternatively, weak bases and their salts. The former type is the more important and common in human body.

Mechanism of Action

Its action against added acid or base may be illustrated as follows: The sketchy diagram in box shows the weak acid HA and its completely ionized salt B^+A^-.

- ***Added H^+ ions,*** in the form of strong acid, combine with anions A^- (largely from the salt component of the buffer), to form the weakly dissociable HA, so that pH does not become as acid as it would in the absence of the buffer. The capacity to combine with added acid remains so long as there is a supply of the buffer salt in the medium.

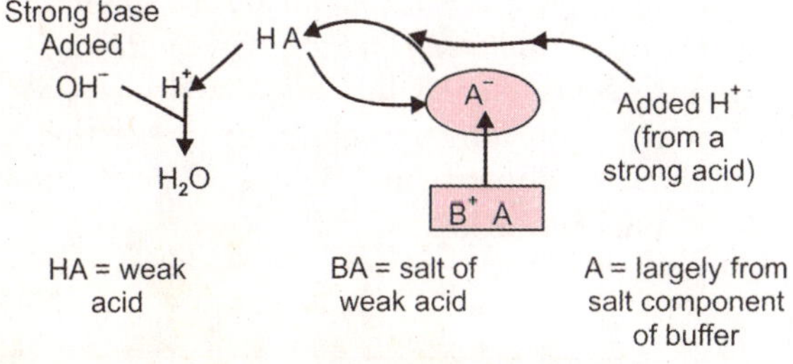

- ***Added OH^- ions,*** in the form of a strong base, combine with H^+ ions derived from the acid HA and form the weakly dissociable H_2O molecules. Hence pH does not become as alkaline as would happen in absence of the buffer. OH^- ions can be buffered as long as some of the acid HA remains to supply the H^+ ions.

Acids Produced in the Body

The following are the major sources of H^+ (protons) production in the human body.

- ***Carbonic Acid (H_2CO_3):*** It is the chief acid produced in the body in the course of oxidation in the cells. Approximately 300 litres of CO_2 are produced and eliminated daily in the body of an adult.
- ***Sulphuric Acid (H_2SO_4):*** A strong dissociable acid produced during oxidation of S-containing amino acids, e.g. cysteine/cystine and methionine.
- ***Phosphoric Acid (H_3PO_4):*** Products of metabolism of dietary phosphoproteins, nucleoproteins, phosphatides and hydrolysis of phospho-esters.
- ***Organic Acids:*** Abnormal production and ***accumulation of certain intermediary organic acids*** from oxidation of carbohydrates, fats and proteins, under certain circumstances, e.g. pyruvic acid, lactic acid, acetoacetic acid, β-OH-butyric acid, etc. Under ordinary conditions, PA/and LA and β-OH butyric acid are produced in quantities of about 80 to 120 millimoles daily, which may increase considerably under certain abnormal circumstances.
- ***Other sources:*** Certain medicines like NH_4Cl, mandelic acid, etc. may increase H^+ concentration of blood when administered in excess.

Both the H^+ ions and the anions produced by these acids must be disposed of, i.e. ultimately excreted from the body, in such a manner that their temporary sojourn in the EC fluids does not unduly affect the pH under normal health. ***The means whereby these ends are accomplished comprise the mechanism of regulation of acid-base balance.***

Mechanisms of Regulation of pH:

The mechanisms of regulation of blood pH involves the following factors.

1. *"Front-line" defence:* They are mainly
   - ***Buffer systems in the blood*** which restrict pH change in body fluids.
   - ***Respiratory mechanisms*** regulate excretion of CO_2 and hence, regulate H_2CO_3 concentration in EC fluid.

2. *"Second-line" defence:* This is achieved by kidneys. ***Renal mechanisms involve*** ultimate excretion of excess of acid or base and thus ultimate regulation of concentration of H^+ and HCO_3^- ions in ECF fluid.

3. *Dilution factor:* The acids introduced into and formed in the body are distributed throughout the ECF volume. Although this may not properly be regarded as a regulatory mechanism, entrance of a given amount of acid into a smaller volume of fluid, as in conditions of severe dehydration, results in relatively greater rise in H^+ ion concentration and decrease in effective buffer base.

Physiological Buffer Systems

The capacity of the EC fluids for transporting acids from the site of their formation (cells) to the site of their excretion (e.g. lungs and kidneys), without undue change in pH is dependent chiefly in the presence of efficient buffer systems in these fluids and in the erythrocytes.

Blood Buffers: Each of the buffer system consists of a mixture of a weak acid, HA, and its salt B.A., which give the mixture, the ability to resist change in the H^+ ion concentration and thus prevents any change of pH of the medium.

Most important buffer systems of blood are as follows:

1. *Plasma buffers:*

- $\frac{NaHCO_3}{H_2CO_3}$
- $\frac{Na_2HPO_4\ (Alk\text{-}PO_4)}{NaH_2PO_4\ (Acid\ PO_4)}$
- $\frac{Na\text{-}Pr}{HPr}$
- $\frac{Na\ Organic\ Acid}{H\ Organic\ Acid}$

2. *Buffers of RB Cells:*

- $\frac{K.HCO_3}{H_2CO_3}$
- $\frac{K_2HPO_4}{KH_2PO_4}$
- $\frac{K\ Hb}{H.\ Hb}$
- $\frac{K.\ Hb\ O_2}{H\ Hb.\ O_2}$
- $\frac{K\ Organic\ Acid}{H\ Organic\ Acid}$

In blood plasma: The bicarbonate buffer and plasma proteins and,

In erythrocytes: The bicarbonate buffers and Hb-system play the most significant and important role. These buffers act as the first line of defence. Whenever any acid alakali enters the blood stream, it is fixed up by these buffers and then disposed off by various ways.

A. ROLE OF DIFFERENT BUFFER SYSTEM

1. **Bicarbonate Buffer System:**

$$NaHCO_3/H_2CO_3 = [Salt]/[Acid]$$

- This consists of weak "Carbonic acid" (H_2CO_3) and its corresponding salt with strong base (HCO_3^-), $NaHCO_3$ (Sodium bicarbonate)
- **Normal ratio in blood** $\frac{NaHCO_3}{H_2CO_3} = \frac{20}{1}$
- This is the chief buffer of blood and constitutes the so called **alkali reserve.** ***Neutralization of strong and non-volatile acids entering the ECF is achieved by the bicarbonate buffer,*** Such acids, e.g. HCl, H_2SO_4, Lactic acid, etc. which are strong and non-volatile react with $NaHCO_3$ component. Thus, Lactic acid will be buffered as follows:

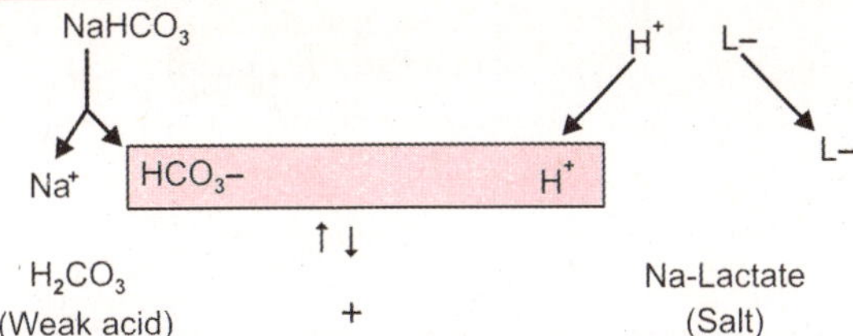

Inference

- ***A strong and nonvolatile acid is converted into weak (less dissociable) and volatile acid at the expense of $NaHCO_3$ (salt component of the buffer).***
- H_2CO_3 thus formed, as it is **volatile,** is eliminated through diffusion of CO_2 through alveoli of Lungs

Note: Proper lung functioning is important.

$$H_2CO_3 \xrightarrow[\text{Low } CO_2 \text{ tension}]{\boxed{CA}} H_2O + CO_2$$

CA = carbonic anhydrase

- Hence, ***bicarbonate buffer system sis directly linked up with respiration.***
- Similarly, when alkaline substance, e.g. NaOH enters the ECF, it reacts with the acid component, i.e. H_2CO_3 of the buffer system.

Alkali reserve: Is represented by the $NaHCO_3$ concentration in the blood has not yet combined with strong and non-volatile acid. Normally, all acids except carbonic acid reacts with bicarbonate to liberate CO_2.

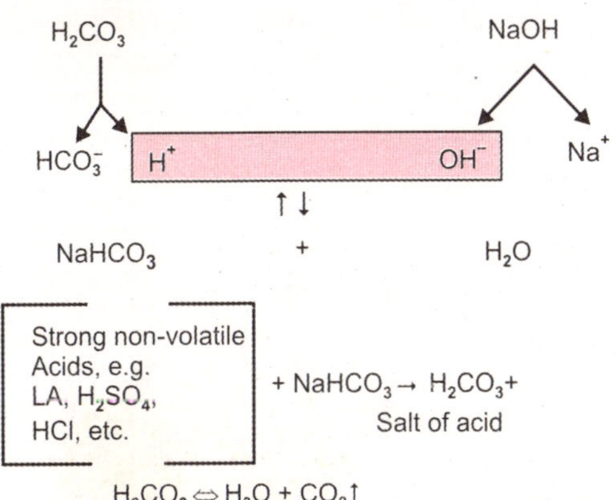

Advantages of bicarbonate buffer system: Bicarbonate buffer system is efficient as compared to other buffer systems.

- It *is present in very high concentration* than other buffer systems. (26 to28 millimole per litre)
- *It produces H_2CO_3,* which is a weak acid and volatile and CO_2 is exhaled out.
- Hence, ***it is a very good physiological buffer*** and acts as a front line defence.

Disadvantage: As a chemical buffer, it is rather weak, pKa is further away from the physiological pH.

2. Phosphate Buffer System:

Na_2HPO_4/NaH_2PO_4 = [Alk PO_4]/[Acid PO_4])

- ***Normal ratio in plasma is 4:1.*** This ratio is kept constant with the help of the kidneys. Thus, ***phosphate buffer system is directly linked up with the kidneys.***
- When a strong acid enters the blood, it is fixed up by alakaline PO_4 (Na_2 HPO_4) which is converted to acid PO_4 as follows:

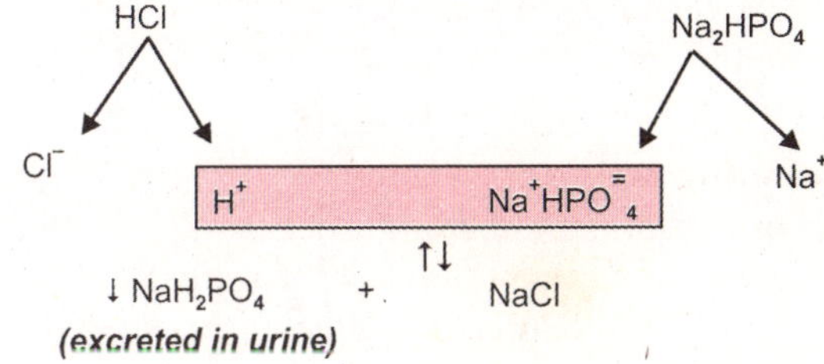

The acid PO_4 (NaH_2PO_4) thus produced is excreted by the kidneys, hence ***urine becomes more acidic.***

- When an alkali enters, it is buffered by the acid PO_4, which is converted to alkaline PO_4 and is excreted in urine, producing increased alkalinity of urine.

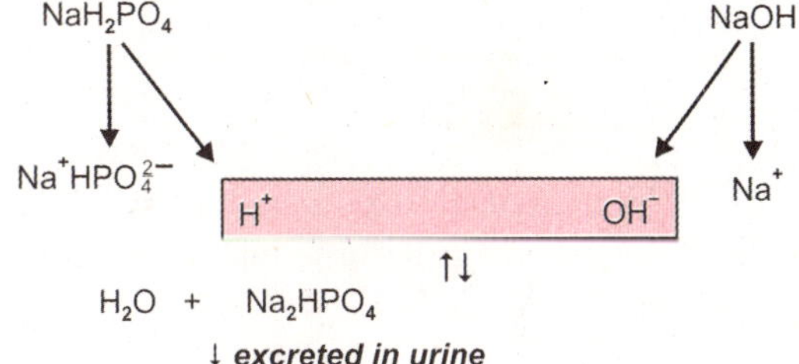

Thus, ***phosphates buffer system works in conjunction with the kidneys.*** A normal healthy kidney is necessary for proper functioning.

Advantage: As a chemical buffer it is very effective and better as pk_a approaches physiological pH

Disadvantage:

- Concentration in blood is low (1.0 millimole/litre),
- As a physiological buffer it is less efficient.

3. Protein Buffer System:

$$Na^+ Pr^- / H^+ Pr^- = [Salt]/[Acid]$$

Buffering capacity of plasma proteins is much less than Hb. The latter operates only in erythrocytes.

Example:

- One gm of Hb binds 0.183 mEq of H^+. On the other hand, one gm of plasma proteins binds 0.110 mEq of H^+, when titrated between pH 7.5 and 6.5.
- Hb of one litre of blood as buffer can bind 27.5 mEq of H^+. But plasma proteins present in one litre of blood can buffer 4.24 mEq of H^+ only between pH 7.5 and 6.5.

From the above examples, it is clear that ***Hb has more buffering capacity than plasma proteins.***

Buffering Action of Proteins

- ***In acidic medium, protein acts as a base,*** NH_2 group takes up H^+ ions from the medium forming NH_3^+ ***Proteins become +vely charged.***
- ***In alkaline medium, proteins act as an acid.*** Acidic COOH gr dissociates and gives H^+, forming COO^-.H^+ combines with OH^- to produce a molecule of water, ***proteins become –vely charged.***
- ***Na^+ Proteinate:*** Salt component can combine with strong acids and thus produces weak acid $H^+ Pr^-$.

$$\underset{\text{(strong acid)}}{Na^+Pr^- + \underset{\text{L.A.}}{H^+L}} \longrightarrow \underset{\text{(salt)}}{Na\,L} + \underset{\text{(weak acid)}}{H^+ Pr^-}$$

- Other factor that contributes to the removal of CO_2 is by formation of ***Carbamino-compounds,*** thus directly fixing CO_2.

$$PrNH_2 + CO_2 \Leftrightarrow PrNHCOOH$$

(Carbamino compound)

This reaction achieves the binding of CO_2 without passing through the carbonic acid stage.

4. Hemoglobin as a Buffering Agent:

- The buffering capacity of Hb, as of any protein, ***depends on the number of dissociable buffering groups,*** viz. acidic –COOH group, basic-NH_2 group, guanidino gr and most important is ***imidazole group,*** which varies with the pH of the medium.
- With the pH range of 7.0 to 7.8, ***most of the physiological buffering action of Hb is due to the "imidazole" group of amino acid "histidine".***
- **Imidazole contains two groups:**
  - Fe^{2+} containing group which is concerned with carriage of O_2, and
  - Imidazole N_2 group, which can give up and accept H^+ (proton) depending on the pH of the medium.

Thus, buffering capacity of Hb is due to the presence of "Imidazole" nitrogen group which remains dissociated in acidic medium and conjugate base forms.

- ***Oxygenated Hb is a stronger acid than deoxygenated Hb.*** On oxygenation, the imidazole N_2 group acts as acid and donates protons in the medium.

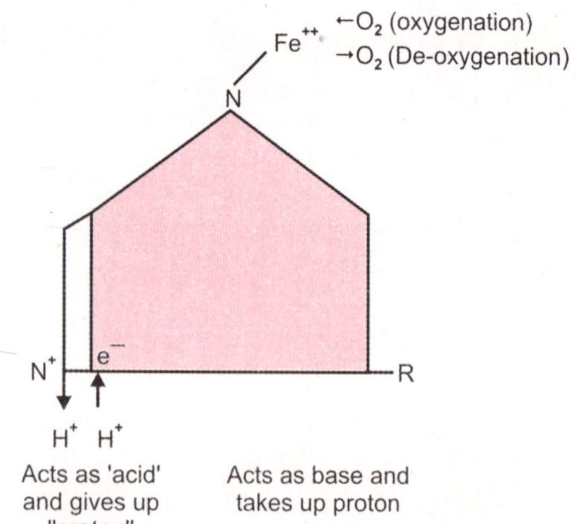

- ***Deoxygenated Hb is less acidic, less dissociable and imidazole N_2 group act as 'base'*** and takes up protons from the medium.
- ***Acidity of the medium favours delivery of O_2***
- ***Alkalinity of the medium favours oxygenation of Hb.***

Sequence of events that occur in lungs and tissues is shown schematically in Fig. 26.1.

In the lungs:

- The formation of oxy-Hb (Hb. O_2) from deoxygenated Hb (H. Hb), must release H^+ ions, which will react with HCO_3^- to form H_2CO_3.
- Because of low CO_2 tension in the lungs, the equilibrium then shifts towards the production of CO_2, which is continually eliminated in the expired air.

In tissues:

- Due to reduced O_2 tension, local acidity, and aided by CO_2 **Böhr effect,** Oxy-Hb (Hb.O_2) dissociates delivering O_2 to the cells and deoxygenated Hb (H.Hb) is formed.
- At the same time, CO_2 produced as a result of metabolism in the cells, is hydrated to form H_2CO_3, which ionizes to form H^+ and HCO_3^-.
- ***De-oxygenated Hb (H.Hb) acting as an anion, accepts the H^+ ions,*** forming so-called acid reduced Hb (H.Hb).
- Very little change in pH occurs because the newly arrived H^+ ions are buffered by formation of a very weak acid.

B. ROLE OF RESPIRATION IN ACID-BASE REGULATION

Participation of the respiratory mechanism, in the regulation of acid-base balance is dependent upon the following factors.

- The ***sensitivity of the respiratory centre (RC)*** in medulla oblongata to very slight changes in pH and pCO_2, and
- The ready diffusibility of CO_2 from the blood, across the pulmonary alveolar membrane, into the alveolar air.

  Hence, the lungs should be healthy so that diffusion of CO_2 takes place properly.
- ***An increase in blood pCO_2 ↑*** of only 1.5 mm Hg (0.2% increase in CO_2) results in 100% ***increase in pulmonary ventilation (stimulation of respiratory centre),*** which increases also with slight increases in H^+ ion concentration of the

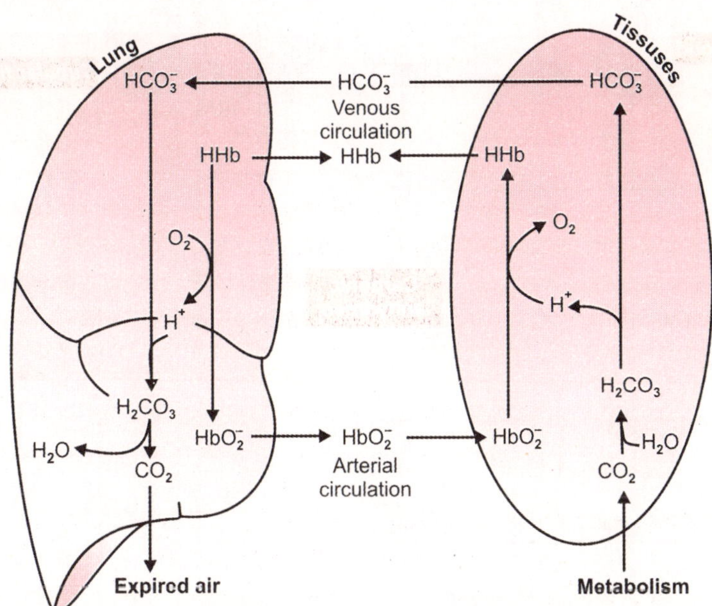

Fig. 26.1: Showing sequence of events that occur in lungs and tissues

blood (**acidosis**). The excess CO_2 is thereby promptly removed from the ECF in the expired air.

- *A decrease in blood* $pCO_2 \downarrow$ *or* H^+ *ion concentration (alkalosis), causes depression of respiratory centre,* with consequent slow and shallow respiration (hypoventilation) resulting to retention of CO_2 in the blood until the normal pCO_2 and pH are restored.

This respiratory mechanism, therefore, tends to maintain the normal B-H CO_3/H_2CO_3 ratio in the EC fluids.

C. RENAL MECHANISMS FOR REGULATION OF ACID-BASE BALANCE

Kidneys also affect acid-base equilibrium:

- *By providing for elimination of non-volatile acids,* viz. lactic acid, H_2SO_4 ketone bodies, etc. after being buffered with cations (principally Na^+) are first removed by glomerular filtration.
- *Body cannot afford to lose* Na^+ being extremely important. It is recovered as $NaHCO_3$ ("alkali reserve") in the renal tubules *by reabsorption in exchange of* H^+ *ions which are secreted.*

There are *Three mechanisms* by which the above is achieved:

- *Bicarbonate mechanism*
- *Phosphate mechanism*
- *Ammonia mechanism*

1. Bicarbonate Mechanism:

- Mobilization of H^+ ions for tubular secretion is accomplished by ionization of carbonic acid (H_2CO_3) which itself is formed from metabolic CO_2 and H_2O.
- This reaction $CO_2 + H_2O \Leftrightarrow H_2CO_3$ is catalyzed by the enzyme (Zn-containing enzyme) *carbonic anhydrase,* present in renal tubular epithelial cells.

Site: It operates in *proximal tubular epithelial cells.*

- The exchange of H^+ ions proceeds first against sodium bicarbonate.

Sequence of events that take place is shown in *Fig. 26.2.*

- Under normal conditions, the rate of H^+ secretion is about 3.50 millimoles per minute, and the rate of filtration of HCO_3^- ions is about

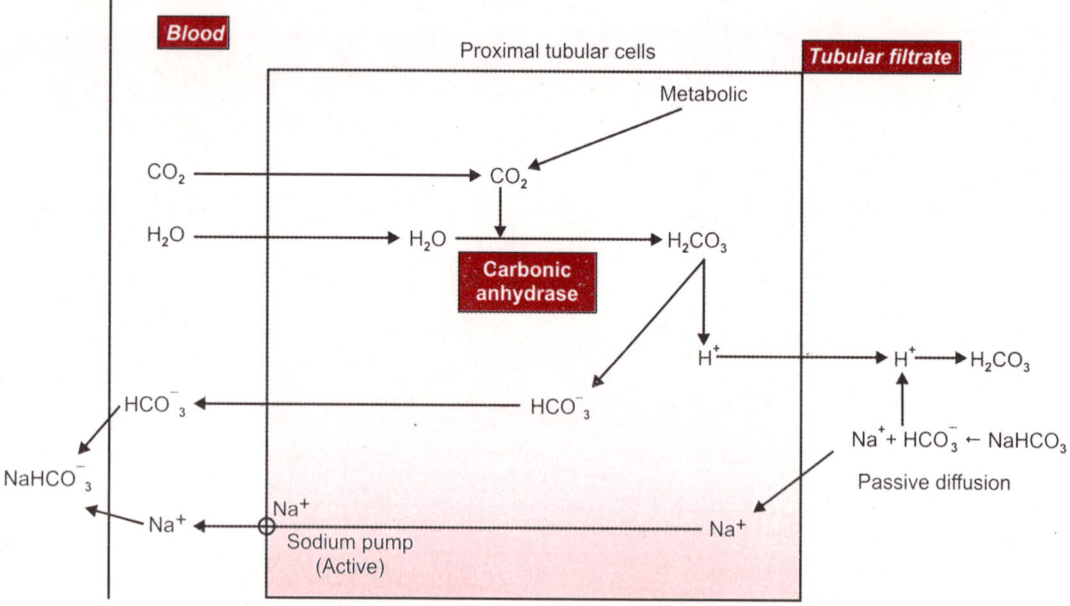

Fig. 26.2: Bicarbonate mechanism

3.49 millimoles per minute. Hence, all the HCO_3 ions are normally reabsorbed, while a slight excess of H^+ ions remains in the tubules to react with other substances and to be excreted in urine.

Above mechanism provides:

- *For complete reabsorption of all $NaHCO_3$.*
- *Reduction of H^+ ion load of plasma with little change in pH of urine.*

Note: *HCO_3^- moiety filtered is not that which is reabsorbed into the blood.*

Carbonic Anhydrase (CA): It in a Zn containing metalloenzyme. It specifically catalyzes of removal of CO_2 from H_2CO_3, however, the reaction is reversible. In the tissues, the formation of H_2CO_3 from CO_2 and H_2O is also accelerated by CA.

Source: The enzyme is present:

- *In RB cells,* associated with Hb; *never found in plasma,*
- Present in most of the tissues, where it catalyzes formation of H_2CO_3 from H_2O and metabolic CO_2.
- In *parietal cells of stomach,* where the enzyme is involved in secretion of HCl.
- In *renal tubular epithelial cells*-as stated above.

Recently, it has also been found in small quantities in muscles tissue, pancreas and spermatozoa.

Clinical Importance

In K deficiency, K^+ ions leave the cell. H^+ ions enter the cells producing intracellular acidosis. ECF becomes alkaline. More H^+ secretion from tubular epithelial cells and increased excretion of H^+, NaH_2PO_4 and NH_4Cl, ***increasing the titratable acidity. Though the ECF is alkaline, highly acidic urine is excreted.*** This condition is called as **paradoxic aciduria.** Such a situation may occur in:

- Patients treated for long with cortisone or corticotrophin (ACTH),
- Persons with hypercorticism (Cushing's syndrome), and
- Post-operative patients with K-free fluids, in whom depletion may occur due to continued loss in urine and GI fluids.

2. Phosphate Mechanisms:

- Both disodium hydrogen phosphate (Na_2HPO_4, alkaline PO_4) and monosodium dihydrogen PO_4 (NaH_2PO_4, acid phosphate) are present in the plasma.
- The pH of the urine is determined by the ratio of these two phosphates. In plasma, concentration of Na_2HPO_4 exceeds that NaH_2PO_4 and the ratio is maintained at 4:1 ***But in urine, the concentration of NaH_2PO_4 and the ratio becomes 9:1.***
- ***Glomerular filtrate of pH 7.4 is converted to a urine having pH- 6.0 or even as low ass 4.8.***
- After all the HCO_3^- has been reabsorbed by the mechanism stated above, H^+ secretion proceeds against Na_2HPO_4. The exchange of Na^+ ion for secreted H^+ ion changes Na_2HPO_4 to NaH_2PO_4 with consequent increase in acidity of urine, resulting in decrease in pH.
- ***Site:*** It operates in ***"distal tubule"*** of kidney ***(Fig. 26.3), see next page.***

3. Ammonia Mechanism:

A third mechanism operates in the ***distal renal tubule cells,*** for the elimination of H^+ ions and the conservation of Na^+, by production of NH_3 by the renal tubular epithelial cells.

Source of NH_3: NH_3 is produced by the hydrolysis of glutamine by the enzyme glutaminase which is present in these cells.

$$\text{Glutamine} \xrightarrow[\text{Glutaminase}]{H_2O} \text{Glutamic Acid} + NH_3$$

Mechanism: The NH_3 thus formed, forms NH^+_4 ions by combining with H^+ ions and NH^+_4 ions can exchange Na^+ ion from NaCl ***(Fig. 26.4).***

- The NH_3 production is greatly increased in metabolic acidosis and negligible in alkalosis.
- It is also observed that activity of renal *glutaminase* is enhanced in acidosis. The NH_3 mechanism is a valuable device for the conservation of fixed base.
- Under normal conditions, 30 to 50 mEq of H^+ ions are eliminated per day, by combination with NH_3 and about 10-30 mEq, as titratable acid, i.e. buffered with PO_4.

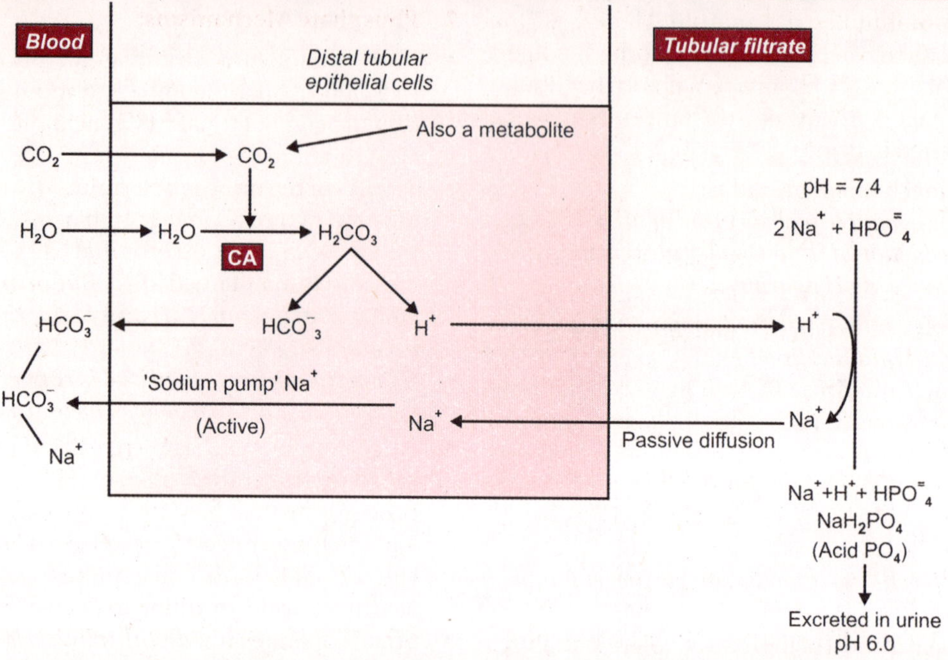

Fig. 26.3: Phosphate mechanism

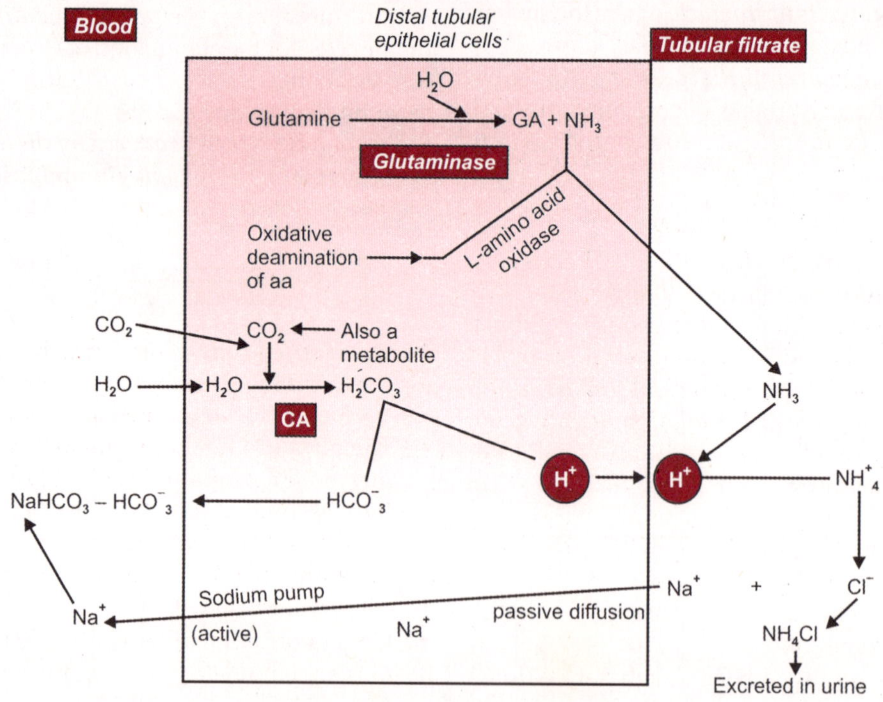

Fig. 26.4: Ammonia mechanism

ANION GAP

The "anion gap" is a mathematical approximation of the difference between the anions and cations routinely measured in serum.

Routine electrolyte measurements include Na^+, K^+, Cl^- and HCO_3^- (as total CO_2). The unmeasured cations, i.e., Ca^{++}, Mg^{++} average 7 mmol/L and the unmeasured anions, i.e. $PO_4^=$, $SO_4^=$, proteins⁻ and organic acids average 24 mmol/L.

If the Cl^- and the total CO_2 concentrations are summed and subtracted from the total of Na^+ and K^+ concentrations, the difference should be less than 17 mEq/L (mmol/L).

(a) ***If the anion gap exceeds 17 mmol/L this usually indicates significantly increased oncentrations of unmeasured anions.***

Causes:

- Uraemia with retention of "fixed" acids.
- Ketotic states, e.g. diabetes mellitus, alcoholism, starvation.
- Lactic acidosis, e.g. shock.
- Toxin ingestion, e.g. methanol, salicylate, ethylene glycol.
- Increased plasma proteins, e.g. in dehydration.

(b) ***An increased "anion gap" occurs occasionally in metabolic alkalosis.*** This is felt to be due to filtration of plasma proteins, resulting in loss of H^+ and consequent increase in the proteins net negative charge. In addition, plasma protein concentration may increase from the ECF deficit that occurs in metabolic alkalosis.

(c) ***Decreased anion gap less than 10 mMol/L can result from either:***

- An increase in the unmeasured cations, or
- A decrease in unmeasured anions.

1. ***An increase in unmeasured cations:*** This can be seen in:

- Lithium intoxication
- Hypermagnaesemia
- Multiple myeloma
- Polyclonal gammopathy and
- Polymyxin B therapy, since the drug is polycationic.

The reason for the decreased gap due to the presence of increased γ-globulins is the fact that these proteins may have net +ve charge at physiologic pH.

2. ***Decrease in unmeasured anions occurs in:***

- Hypoalbuminaemia and
- Hyponatraemia, with normal or increased EC fluid (e.g., SIADH). This is postulated to result from the selective renal excretion of unmeasured anions in this condition. Finally a spurious increase in measured Cl^- caused by Bromide intoxication can cause a spurious increase in the calculated gap.

Clinical Use

The "anion gap" is useful also for Quality control of laboratory results for Na^+, K^+, Cl^- and total CO_2. If an increased or decreased anion gap is calculated for a set of electrolytes from a healthy individual, this would indicate that one or more of the laboratory results are erroneous. Another possible explanation is that a mixed acid-base disturbance is present.

ACID BASE IMBALANCE

Acid Base imbalance can manifest as ***acidosis*** and ***alkalosis.***

A. *Acidosis* can be:

- ***Metabolic acidosis and***
- ***Respiratory acidosis.***

B. *Alkalosis* can be:

- ***Metabolic alkalosis*** and
- ***Respiratory alkalosis.***

All of the above may be in ***compensated*** phase and ***uncompensated*** phase.

A. ACIDOSIS

1. Metabolic Acidosis: Also called as ***primary alkali deficit.*** It is the commonest disturbance of acid-base balance observed clinically. It is ***caused when there is a reduction in the plasma*** HCO_3^- ↓ ***(B.*** HCO_3 ↓***) with either no or little change in the*** H_2CO_3 ***fraction.***

Mechanisms: If primary deficit of HCO_3^- occurs the ratio [HCO_3^-]/[H_2CO_3]=20/1, is **decreased,** i.e. pH is decreased resulting in metabolic acidosis (primary bicarbonate deficit).

1. ***Primary Compensatory Mechanism:*** The respiratory centre is stimulated by acidosis causing deep and rapid **(*Kausmaul*)** breathing. This increased ventilation will result in CO_2 loss and reduction in [H_2CO_3] ↓ (carbonic acid).
   - As a result, the ratio of [HCO_3^-]/[H_2CO_3] is restored towards 20:1, **as *levels of both in blood are reduced.***
   - However, ***increased ventilation causes reduction in pCO$_2$ ↓, which in turn depresses the respiratory centre.***
   - Thus, ***two opposing forces:***
     - acidosis stimulating respiratory centre and
     - Low pCO_2 depressing respiratory centre, are set against each other, and respiratory compensation is only partial.
   - During the early stages of alkali deficit, therefore, the organism is in a state of ***compensated acidosis,*** but as the condition progresses and the treatment is not instituted, the alkali deficit becomes more pronounced, the primary compensatory mechanism fails and the condition becomes one of ***uncompensated acidosis*** with an increase in H^+ ion concentration in blood.

2. ***Secondary Compensatory Mechanism is the Renal Mechanism:*** Renal mechanism attempt to correct the disturbance as follows:
   - By conserving cations
   - By increasing
     - NH_3 formation ↑
     - H^+ excretion compared to K^+ excretion in distal tubule
     - HCO_3^- reabsorption

Biochemical Characteristics

1. ***Uncompensated:*** **If uncompensated,** it is characterized biochemically in plasma or blood as follows
   - Disproportionate decrease in [HCO_3^-] ↓
   - Decrease in [H_2CO_3] ↓ and pCO_2 ↓
   - ***Decrease in total CO$_2$ content*** [HCO_3^-] + [H_2CO_3] ↓
   - Decrease in [HCO_3^-]: [H_2CO_3] ratio ↓
   - Decrease in pH ↓
2. ***Fully compensated :*** If fully compensated the CO_2 content is low, but the decrease in [HCO_3^-] and [H_2CO_3] is proportionate, the [HCO_3^-] : [H_2CO_3] ratio and pH remain within normal limits.

Urinary findings: The urinary NH_3 ↑ and titratable acidity ↑ are increased (if kidneys are functioning normally).

Causes of Metabolic Acidosis

I. ***Abnormal increase in "anions" other than HCO$_3^-$ ("acid-gain" acidosis) resulting from:***
- **Endogenous production of excessive acid ions** as occuring in:
  - *Diabetic acidosis,*
  - *Lactic acidosis,*
  - *Starvation,*
  - *High fever,*
  - *Violent exercise, and*
  - *Shock, haemorrhage and anoxia*
- ***Ingestion of acidifying salts: Dietary or iatrogenic:*** administration of excessive quantities of acids, e.g. acetyl salicylic acid, phosphoric acid, HCl, NH_4Cl and NH_4 NO_3, mandelic acid, etc.
- ***Renal insufficiency: Retention of acids normally produced:*** Acidosis is commonly obser-ved in the terminal stages of Nephritis, and destructive renal lesions such as polycystic kidneys, pyelonephritis, hydro and pyonephrosis, renal TB, etc.

Factors are:
- Decreased glomerular filtration with retention of 'acid' radicals,
- Decrease H^+-Na exchange,
- Decreased NH_3 formation,
- Nephritic acidosis is also contributed by the accumulation of certain organic acids.

II. Abnormal loss of HCO$_3^-$: Metabolic acidosis due to loss of base, may occur due to loss of excessive intestinal secretions, as in severe diarrhoeas, small bowel fistulaes, and/or severe biliary fistulaes.

2. **Respiratory Acidosis:** It is called as ***"primary [H$_2$CO$_3$] carbonic acid excess".***

- The underlying abnormality here is increase in $[H_2CO_3]$ ↑ in the blood, which follows decreased elimination of CO_2 (pCO_2↑) in the pulmonary alveoli. This may result from:
  - Breathing air containing abnormally high percent of CO_2, and
  - Conditions in which elimination of CO_2 through lungs is retarded.

Mechanism: If excretion of CO_2 through lungs is impaired (e.g. emphysema or depression of respiratory centre), more CO_2 will accumulate in blood, ***resulting in excess H_2CO_3 formation*** $[H_2CO_3]$ ↑. This results in lowering the ratio of $[HCO_3^-]$ / $[H_2CO_3]$, resulting lowering in pH ↓ and is described as ***"Respiratory acidosis" (carbonic acid excess).***

Compensatory mechanism: In this condition, the respiratory mechanism becomes secondary and renal mechanism becomes of prime importance.

1. ***Respiratory Mechanism:*** Increased stimulation to respiratory centre (RC) by the increased CO_2 tension (pCO_2 ↑) results in increased depth and rate of respiration with consequent increased ventilation. This mechanism becomes secondary in importance as the defect may be with the RC, its depression/or some pathology in the lungs. **As a result this compensatory mechanism becomes less effective.**
2. ***Renal Mechanism: Of prime importance More ions are reabsorbed from tubules*** in response to raised pCO_2 in blood and ratio of $[HCO_3^-]$ / $[H_2CO_3]$ is restored 20:1 as the levels of both in blood are increased.

Biochemical characteristics:

1. ***If uncompensated:*** It is characterized biochemically (plasma or blood) as follows:
   - Disproportionate increase in $[H_2CO_3]$ ↑ (pCO_2)↑
   - Increase in $[HCO_3^-]$ ↑
   - ***Increase in total CO_2 content*** ↑
   - Decrease in $[HCO_3^-]$: $[H_2CO_3]$ ratio ↓
   - Decrease in pH ↓.
2. ***If fully compensated:*** The CO_2-content is high, but the increase in $[HCO_3^-]$ and $[H_2CO_3]$ are proportionate, the $[HCO_3^-]$: $[H_2CO_3]$ ratio and pH remaining within normal limits.

Urinary findings: The urinary NH_3 ↑ and titratable acidity ↑ are increased (if kidneys are functioning normally)

Causes of respiratory acidosis:

I. ***Conditions in which there is depression or suppression of respiration:***

1. ***Damage to CNS:***
   - ***Brain damage:*** Trauma, inflammation, or compression and convulsive disorders.
   - ***Drug poisoning: like Morphine and Barbiturates.***
   - ***Excessive anaesthesia.***
   - ***Bulbar polio.***
2. ***Loss of "ventilatory functions" due to increased intrathoracic pressure or loss of elasticity.***
   - Tension cyst/and tension pneumothorax.
   - Pulmonary and mediastinal tumours.
   - Emphysema.
3. ***Effects of pain,*** e.g. Pleurisy

II. ***Conditions causing impairment of diffusion of CO_2 across alveolar membrane. (Reduced alveolorespiratory function):*** Reduction of respiratory surface:

- Emphysema,
- Pulmonary oedema, and congenital alveolar dysplasia (they also cause thickening of alveolar membrane or exudates).

III. ***Conditions in which there is an obstacle to the escape of CO_2 from the alveoli:***

- Obstruction to respiratory tract:
  - laryngeal obstruction,
  - asthma
- Rebreathing from a closed space.

IV. ***Conditions in which pulmonary blood flow is insufficient:***

- Certain congenital heart diseases
- Ayerza's disease.

For differentiation of metabolic and respiratory acidosis, refer to ***Table 26.1.***

Table 26.1: Differentiation of metabolic acidosis and respiratory acidosis

Metabolic acidosis	*Respiratory acidosis*
• Primary bicarbonate, HCO_3^- defict	• Primary carbonic acid H_2CO_3 excess
• $\frac{BHCO_3\downarrow}{H_2CO_3} = \frac{20}{1}\downarrow = pH\downarrow$	$\frac{BHCO_3}{H_2CO_3\uparrow} = \frac{20}{1}\downarrow = pH\downarrow$
• 1. *In uncompensated phase* • Disproportionate decrease in $[HCO_3^-]\downarrow$ • $[H_2CO_3]\downarrow$ • $p.CO_2\downarrow$ • **Total $CO_2\downarrow$ decreased** • Ratio $\downarrow$	• 1. *In uncompensated phase* • Disproportionate increase in $[H_2CO_3^-]\uparrow$ • $[HCO_3^-]\uparrow$ • $p.CO_2\uparrow$ • **Total $CO_2\uparrow$ increased** • Ratio $\downarrow$
2. *In fully compensated phase* Total CO_2 is low $\downarrow$, but the decrease in $[HCO_3^-]$ and $[H_2CO_3]$ is proportionate and ratio 20/1 and pH maintained	2. *In fully compensated phase* Total CO_2 content high $\uparrow$, but the increase in $[HCO_3^-]$ and $[H_2CO_3]$ is proportionate and ratio 20/1 and pH maintained
• *Compensatory mechanisms:* 1. **Primary:** Respiratory-low pH stimulates respiratory centre producing hyperventilation and decrease in $[H_2CO_3]\downarrow$ 2. *Secondary:* Renal • H^+—Na^+ exchange $\uparrow$ increased • HCO_3^- reabosrption $\uparrow$ increased • NH_3 formation $\uparrow$ increased	• *Compensatory mechanism:* 1. **Primary:** Renal-most important • Increase in H^+-Na^+ exchange • More HCO_3^- reabsorption • Increase NH_3 formation 2. *Secondary:* Respiratory partial Low pH and high CO_2 induce hyperventilation But CO_2 elimination is partial as the pathogenesis involves lung disorders/or depression of respiratory centre
3. *Urinary findings* • pH-acidic • Increase in excretion NH_4Cl and NaH_2PO_4 • Increase in titratable acidity	3. *Urinary findings* • pH-acidic • Increase in excretion of NH_4Cl and NaH_2PO_4 • Increase in titratable acidity
• *Causes* • Abnormal increase in anions other than HCO_3^- (acid gain acidosis) • Endogenous production of acid ions when excessive • Diabetic acidosis • Starvation • High fever • Violent exercise (LA) • Lactic acidosis due to other causes like shock and haemorrhage • Ingestion of acidifying salts • Renal insufficiency-Retention of acids normally produced • Abnormal loss of HCO_3^-, e.g. in severe diarrhoea, fistulae	• *Causes* • Conditions in which there is depression/or suppression of respiration • Damage to CNS • Brain damage (trauma, inflammation, compression), convulsion. • Drug poisoning like Morphine or Barbiturates • Excessive anaesthesia • Bulbar polio • Loss of "ventilatory functions" due to increased intrathoracic pressure or loss of elasticity, e.g. tension cyst, tension pneumothorax, pulmonary and mediastinal tumours, emphysema. • Effect of pain like pleurisy • Conditions causing impairment of diffusion of CO_2 across alveolar membrane—***"Reduced alveolar-respiratory function"*** Reduction of respiratory surface: Emphysema, pneumonia, pulmonary fibrosis, pulmonary oedema, etc. • Conditions in which there is 'obstruction' to escape of CO_2 from the alveoli; obstruction to respiratory tract, rebreathing from a closed space • Conditions in which pulmonary blood flow is Insufficient, e.g. certain congenital heart diseases, Ayerza's disease

B. ALKALOSIS

1. Metabolic Alkalosis: Also called as ***Primary alkali excess.*** This condition results from an absolute or relative increase in [HCO_3^-]. ***Primary alkali excess or increase in the " alkali reserve"*** is the most frequent cause of clinically observed alkalosis.

Mechanism:

- Excess of HCO_3^- accumulation (soluble alkali ingestion) cause an increase in the ratio of $[HCO_3]/[H_2CO_3^-]$ (i.e. pH is increased ↑) and it is known as ***"Metabolic alkalosis" ("bicarbonate excess").***
- ***The respiratory centre (RC) is inhibited by alkalosis*** causing shallow, irregular breathing. This reduced ventilation will result in CO_2 retention and increases in carbonic acid level $[H_2CO_3]$↑.
- The ratio of [HCO_3^-]/$[H_2CO_3]$ will be restored towards 20:1 as the levels of both in blood are increased.
- However, decreased ventilation raises pCO_2, which tends to stimulate the RC.

Again *opposing forces:*

- Alkalosis depressing, and
- Raised pCO_2 stimulating the RC are working simultaneously and the respiratory compensation is incomplete.

Renal Mechanism: It increases the excretions of:

- Cations ↑
- It also increases the excretion of HCO_3^- ↑ (replacing Cl^- in urine). Both are due to decreased H^+–Na^+ exchange.
- K^+ excretion increases in the distal tubules instead of H^+.
- There is reduced NH_3 ↓ formation and excretion of non-volatile acids, viz. lactic acid and keto-acids.

Following compensatory mechanisms operate:

- Decreased pulmonary respiration ↓
- Increased alkali excretion ↑
- Decreased acid excretion ↓
- Decreased NH_3 formation ↓
- Retention of acid metabolities

Urinary findings: Urinary acidity decreases ↓ and decreased NH_3 formation. Decrease in titratable acidity ↓.

Other Biochemical Changes and Clinical Manifestations:

Following biochemical and clinical manifestations accompany alkalosis:

- *Tetany:* In both types of alkalosis, respiratory/metabolic, tetany may occur due to decreased ionization of calcium salts in the EC fluid. ***The total serum calcium may remain within normal limits, but ionic calcium may dercrease to produce tetany.***
- *Hypokalemia:* Increased excretion of K^+ from distal tubules can produce K^+ depletion (decrease serum K^+ concentration–hypokalaemia)
- *Kidney damage:* Mainly degenerative changes in the tubules (nephrosis) occurs frequently with oliguria and N_2-retention.
- *Ketosis and Ketonuria:* Ketosis and Ketonuria may occur frequently in alkalosis, due to excessive vomiting because of inadequate carbohydrates intake.

Biochemical characteristics:

1. If ***uncompensated phase:*** It is characterized biochemically (plasma or blood) as follows:
   - Disproportionate increase in [HCO_3^-] ↑
   - Increase in $[H_2CO_3]$ ↑, pCO_2↑
   - ***Increase in total CO_2 content***
   - Increase in [HCO_3^-]:$[H_2CO_3]$ ratio ↑
   - Increase in pH ↑

2. ***If fully compensated:*** The CO_2 content is high, but the increase in [HCO_3^-]and $[H_2CO_3]$ are proportionate, and the [HCO_3^-]:$[H_2CO_3]$ ratio and pH remaining within normal limits.

Urinary findings: The urinary NH_3 ↓ and titratable acidity ↓, both are decreased (if kidneys are functioning normally).

Causes:

1. ***Excessive loss of HCl from stomach:*** The loss of excessive quantities of HCI from the stomach is encountered most frequently in individuals with following disorders:

- Pyloric obstruction and High intestinal obstruction
- Protracted gastric lavage without proper provision of acid replacement
- In infants with pylorospasm
- Sometimes in patients with generalized peritonitis.

As a result of the loss of Cl^- ions from the blood there is present in the body an excess of base, chiefly Na^+ and K^+, which is retained in the form of bicarbonate. ***In this way, a neutral salt (NaCl) is replaced by an alkaline salt (Na HCO_3)***

2. ***Alkali administration:*** Excessive intake of bases like $NaHCO_3$, Na and K acetates, lactates or citrates. **Lactates and citrates are converted into** HCO_3^- .

3. ***Potassium deficiency:*** Produces alkalosis (see above).

4. ***Roentgen ray, UV irradiation and Radium therapy:*** A decrease in the H^+ ion concentration of the blood plasma (i.e. increased pH) has been observed following deep X-ray therapy, radium therapy and prolonged exposure to UV rays. The mechanism is not clear. In some cases (radiation sickness), it may be due to excessive vomiting.

2. Respiratory Alkalosis: Also called as ***Primary H_2CO_3 deficit.*** This condition occurs when there is a decrease in $[H_2CO_3]$ ↓ fraction with no corresponding change in HCO_3^- in plasma.

Excessive quantities of CO_2 may be washed out of the body by hyperventilation.

Mechanism:

- Increased loss of CO_2 (due to hyperventilation), results in diminution of $[H_2CO_3]$ ↓
- The ratio of $[HCO_3^-]/[H_2CO_3]$ is increased ↑ (i.e. pH is increased) and is termed ***"respiratory alkalosis" (carbonic acid deficit)***
- In this condition, due to increased CO_2 loss, pCO_2 is low, which leads to less H^+–Na^+ exchange and less bicarbonate is reabsorbed (i.e. more HCO_3^- is excreted) by the renal, tubules and the ratio of $[HCO_3^-]/[H_2CO_3]$ returns towards normal i.e. 20:1, as levels of both in blood are decreased.
- ***Alkalosis and low p CO_2 depress respiratory centre and excretion of CO_2 is reduced.***

Compensatory mechanisms: In this condition, main compensatory mechanism is ***'renal'***

- Excretion of alkali in the form of HCO_3^-
- Decreased excretion of acid
- Decreased excretion of NH_3 in the urine
- Retention of Cl^- in the blood.

In view of the pathogenesis of this condition, the task of compensating for this defect falls on the kidneys. Other features are similar to metabolic alkalosis

Biochemical Characteristics:

1. ***If uncompensated:*** It is characterized biochemically (plasma or blood) as follows:
   - Disproportionate decrease in $[H_2CO_3]$↓ and pCO_2 ↓
   - Decrease in $[HCO_3^-]$ ↓
   - **Decrease in CO_2 content ↓**
   - Increase in $[HCO_3^-]:[H_2CO_3]$ ratio ↑
   - Increase in pH

2. ***If fully compensated:*** The CO_2 content is low, but the decrease in $[HCO_3^-]$ and $[H_2CO_3]$ is proportionate, the $[HCO_3^-]:[H_2CO_3]$ ratio and pH remaining within normal limits.

Urinary findings: The urinary NH_3 ↓ and titratable acidity ↓are both decreased (if kidneys are functioning normally).

Causes:

- ***Stimulation of Respiratory Centre (RC)***
  - ***In CNS diseases,*** e.g. meningitis, encephalitis–***alkalosis due to hyperventilation has been observed*** in some cases of meningitis/encephalitis, etc. manifesting hyperpnoea, over prolonged periods of time.
  - ***Salicylate poisoning:*** Large doses of salicylates, sometimes given in the treatment of acute rheumatic fever, produce stimulation of respiratory centre (RC) with consequent hyperventilation and tendency towards alkalosis.
  - ***Hyperpyrexia:*** Hyperventilation may occur as a result of the increased respiratory rate

associated with increase in body temperature.

- *Other causes:*
  - ***Hysteria:*** Hyperventilation during hysterical attacks.
  - ***Apprehensive blood donors:*** hyperventilation tetany with alkalosis has been observed in apprehensive and hyperexcitable donors.
  - ***High altitude effects:*** Hyperpnoea, occuring in untrained individulas ascending to high altitudes where the atmospheric O_2 tension is low (anoxic anoxaemia), commonly results in primary H_2CO_3 deficit and alkalosis.
  - ***Injudicious use of respirators***
  - Sometimes in ***hepatic coma.***

For differentiation of metabolic and respiratory alkalosis refer to ***Table 26.2 (see in next page).***

☞ SALIENT POINTS TO REMEMBER

- The normal pH of blood is maintained approximately at 7.4 (range 7.35 to 7.5). Maintenance of this constant blood reaction is of prime importance.
- Any material variation on either side seriously disturbs the vital process and may lead to death.
- The metabolism of body is accompanied by an over-all production of acids, viz carbonic acid, sulphuric acid, phosphoric acid and certain organic acids.
- The body has following lines of defence: (i) The first line of defence, viz. Buffer systems in blood and respiratory mechanisms, and (ii) second line of defence: Renal mechanisms.
- The above mechanisms regulate the acid-base balance and maintain the pH.
- Among the blood buffers, Bicarbonate buffer system is the most important *Physiological buffer*, with a ratio of HCO_3^- /H_2CO_3 as 20:1.
- When a strong and non-volatile acid is added, the $NaHCO_3$ component of the buffer system, reacts with the acid and forms salt and H_2CO_3 (weak and volatile acid).
- Due to low CO_2 tension in the lungs, H_2CO_3 breaks up to H_2O and CO_2, which is exhaled out. Thus, ***bicarbonate buffer system is directly linked up with respiration.***
- Phosphate buffer systems in the blood, in ratio of alkaline phosphate (Na_2 HPO_4)/to acid phosphate (NaH_2 PO_4) as 4:1.
- When a strong acid enters blood, it is buffered by Na_2HPO_4 which forms salt and acid phosphate (NaH_2PO_4) which is excreted in urine.
- ***In urine, NaH_2 PO_4 exceeds and ratio of NaH_2PO_4/Na_2HPO_4 becomes 9:1. Thus phosphate buffer system is directly linked with the kidneys.***
- Protein buffers and Hb also contribute to pH regulation.
- The respiratory system regulates concentration of carbonic acid (H_2CO_3) by controlling the elimination of CO_2 via lungs.
- The ranal mechanisms regulate pH of blood by excretion of H^+ and NH_4^+ ions and reabsorption of HCO_3^-. In the tubule, H^+ exchanges with Na^+ which is reabsorbed to blood.
- In proximal tubules, bicarbonate system operates and in the distal tubules, the phosphate system and amonia mechanisms operate.
- The acid-base disorders are classified as (i) acidosis-metabolic and respiratory and (ii) alkalosis-metabolic and respiratory respectively, due a rise or fall in blood pH.
- All of the above disorders may be in compensated phase and uncompensated phase.
- The metabolic disturbances, viz metabolic acidosis (primary alkali deficit) and metabolic alkalosis (Primary alkali excess) are associated with alterations in HCO_3^- concentration.
- The respiratory disorders, viz respiratory acidosis (primary carbonic acid excess) and respiratory alkalosis (Primary H_2CO_3 deficit) are due to changes in H_2CO_3 concentration.
- ***Biochemically the main differentiating feature between metabolic acidosis and respiratory acidosis is the total CO_2 content, which is decreased in former and increased in later.***
- ***Similarly the main differentiating feature biochemically between metabolic alkalosis and respiratory alkalosis is the total CO_2 content,*** which is increased in metabolic alkalosis and decreased in respiratory alkalosis.

Table 26.2: Differentiation of metabolic alkalosis and respiratory alkalosis

Metabolic alkalosis	*Respiratory alkalosis*
1. Primary bicarbonate HCO_3^- excess	1. Primary carbonic acid H_2CO_3 deficit
2. $\frac{BHCO_3 \uparrow}{H_2CO_3} = \frac{20}{1} \uparrow = pH \uparrow$	2. $\frac{BHCO_3}{H_2CO_3 \downarrow} = \frac{20}{1} \uparrow = pH \uparrow$
3. a. ***In uncompensated phase:*** Disproportionate increase • $[H_2CO_3] \uparrow$ • $[H_2CO_3] \uparrow$ or N • $p.CO_2 \uparrow$ or N • Ratio↑ • **Total $CO_2 \uparrow$ increased** • pH↑	3. a. ***In uncompensated phase:*** Disproportionate decrease • $[H_2CO_3] \downarrow$ • $[H_2CO_3] \downarrow$ or N • $p.CO_2 \downarrow$ or N • Ratio ↑ • **Total $CO_2 \downarrow$ decreased** • pH ↑
b. ***In fully compensated phase:*** Total CO_2 Is high ↑ but increase in $[HCO_3^-]$ and $[H_2CO_3]$ are proportionate and ratio 20/1 and pH maintained.	b. ***In fully compensated phase:*** Total CO_2 content is low ↓ decrease in $[HCO_3^-]$ and $[H_2CO_3]$ are proportionate and ratio 20/1 and pH maintained
4. ***Compensatory mechanisms:*** **a. Primary:** Respiratory Depression of RC and hypoventilation leading to retention of CO_2	4. ***Compensatory mechanisms:*** a. **Primary:** Renal • Decreased $H^+ \rightarrow Na^+$ exchange ↓ • Decreased excretion of acid ↓ • Increased excretion of HCO_3^- ↑ • Decreased excretion of NH_3 ↓ • K^+ excretion ↑ • Cl^- retention
b. ***Secondary:*** Renal • H^+–Na^+ exchange ↓ • NH_3 formation ↓ • Bicarbonate (HCO_3^-) reabsorption ↓ • K^+ excretion ↑ • Cl^- retention	**b.** ***Secondary:*** Respiratory–High pH and low pCO_2 produces hypoventilation and increase in H_2CO_3
c. ***Urinary findings*** • pH of urine alkaline • Decrease NH_3 ↓ • Decreased in titratable acidity ↓	c. ***Urinary findings*** • pH of urine-alkaline • Decrease in NH_3 ↓ • Decreased titratable acidity ↓
5. ***Other findings*** i. Low ionic Ca^{++} leading to tetany ii. K^+ depletion—leading to hypokalaemia iii. Ketosis and ketonuria may develop iv. Kidney damage-degenerative changes in tubules-leading to N_2-retention and oliguria may occur	 • Low ionic Ca^{++} leading to tetany • K^+ depletion—leading to hypokalaemia • Ketosis and ketonuria may develop • Kidney damage may occur leading to oliguria, N_2-retention.

6. ***Causes***
• Excessive loss of HCl
  • Protracted gastric lavage
  • Pyloric obstruction
  • High intestinal obstruction
  • Pylorospasm
• Alkali ingestion and alkali administration
• Excessive loss of K^+ leading to K^+ deficiency
• X-ray therapy, UV radiation and radiation therapy
	6. ***Causes***
	1. Stimulation of respiratory center (RC)
	• CNS disease meningitis, encephalitis, etc.
	• Salicylate poisoning
	• Hyperpyrexia.
	2. ***Other causes:***
	• Hysteria
	• Apprehensive blood donors
	• High altitude ascending
	• Injudicious use of respirator
	• Some cases of hepatic coma

MULTIPLE CHOICE QUESTIONS

Give one correct answer:

1. **The most important physiological buffer in the blood is:**
   (a) Phosphate buffer system
   (b) Haemoglobin buffer
   (c) Bicarbonate buffer system
   (d) Protein buffer system
   (e) Acetate buffer system
2. **The ratio of alkaline phosphate (Na_2HPO_4) to acid phosphate (NaH_2Po_4) in blood is:**
   (a) 2 : 1 (b) 4 : 1
   (c) 6 : 1 (d) 8 : 1
   (e) 10 : 1
3. **In which of the following enzyme, zinc constitutes an integral part of the enzyme:**
   (a) Cytochrome oxidase
   (b) Carbonic anhydrase
   (c) Xanthine oxidase
   (d) Trypsinogen
   (e) Pepsinogen
4. **If the pH of blood is 7.4, then the ratio of [HCO_3^-] and [H_2CO_3] is:**
   (a) 5 : 1 (b) 10 : 1
   (c) 15 : 1 (d) 20 : 1
   (e) 25 : 1
5. **All of the following are associated with metabolic alkalosis, *except:***
   (a) Ingestion of NH_4Cl
   (b) Loss of HCl
   (c) Pyloric obstruction
   (d) Prolonged steroid therapy
   (e) Diuretic thrapy
6. **All the following conditions can cause respiratory alkalosis, *except:***
   (a) Hysteria
   (b) Encephalitis
   (c) Salicylate poisoning
   (d) In apprehensive blood donors
   (e) Artificial ventilation
7. **Metabolic alkalosis associated with prolonged vomiting or gastric aspirations is due to loss of which of the following:**
   (a) Potassium ion
   (b) Sodium ion
   (c) Hydrogen ion
   (d) Chloride ion
   (e) None of the above
8. **Which of the following biochemical parameter is true in a case of Respiratory acidosis in uncompensated phase?**
   (a) Disproportionate increase in [H_2CO_3] ↑
   (b) Decrease in total CO_2 content ↓
   (c) Increase in ratio of [HCO_3^-]:[H_2CO_3]
   (d) Decrease in [HCO_3^-] ↓
   (e) None of the above
9. **Metabolic alkalosis is characterized by:**
   (a) Increase pCO_2 ↑
   (b) Elevated chloride level in serum
   (c) Hydrogen ion concentration in plasma ↑
   (d) Urinary pH near about 4.5
   (e) Low potassium level
10. **The ratio of acid phosphate (NaH_2PO_4) to alkaline phosphate (Na_2HPO_4) in urine is:**
    (a) 3 : 1 (b) 6 : 1
    (c) 9 : 1 (d) 12 : 1
    (e) 15 : 1

ANSWERS

1. (c)	2. (b)	3. (b)	4. (d)
5. (e)	6. (e)	7. (d)	8. (a)
9. (e)	10. (c)		

27 Renal Function Tests

INTRODUCTION

The body has a considerable factor of safety in renal as well as hepatic tissues. One healthy normal kidney can do the work of two, and if all other organs are functioning properly, less than a whole kidney can suffice. On the other hand, there are certain extrarenal factors which can interfere with kidney function, specially circulatory disturbances. Hence, methods that appraise the functional capacity of the kidney are very important. Such tests have been devised and are available, ***but it is stressed that no single test can measure all the kidney functions.*** Consequently, more than one test is indicated to assess the kidney function.

Preliminary Investigations to Renal Function Tests:

Assessment of renal function begins with the appreciation of:

- ***Patient's history:*** A proper history taking is important, particularly in respect of oliguria, polyuria, nocturia, ratio of frequency of urination in day time and night time. Appearance of oedema is important.
- ***Physical examination:*** This is followed by side room analysis of the urine specially for presence/or absence of albumin, and microscopic examination of urinary deposits specially for pus cells, RB cells and casts.
- ***Biochemical parameters:*** Certain biochemical parameters also help in assessing kidney function.

A step-wise increase in three nitrogenous constituents of blood is believed to reflect a deteriorating kidney function. Some authorities claim that ***serum uric acid normally rises first, followed by urea and finally increase in creatinine.*** By determining all the above three parameters a rough estimate of kidney function can be made. However, other causes of uric acid rise should be kept in mind.

Other biochemical parameters which help are determination of total plasma proteins, and albumin and globulins and total cholesterol. ***In nephrosis there is marked fall in albumin and rise in serum cholesterol level.***

PHYSIOLOGICAL ASPECT

Main functions of the kidneys are:

- To get rid the body of waste products of metabolism,
- To get rid of foreign and non-endogenous substances,
- To maintain salt and water balance, and
- To maintain acid-base balance of the body.

1. Glomerular Function: ***The glomeruli act as "filters"*** and the fluid which passes from the blood in the glomerular capillaries into Bowman's capsule ***is of the same composition of protein-free plasma.*** The effective filtration pressure which forces fluid through the filters is the result of:

- The blood pressure in the glomerular capillaries and
- The opposing osmotic pressure of plasma proteins, renal interstitial pressure and intratubular pressure. Thus,
  - Capillary pressure =75 mm Hg
  - Osmotic pressure of plasma proteins = 30 mm Hg

- Renal interstitial pressure = 10 mm Hg
- Renal intratubular pressure = 10 mm Hg

Hence, ***net effective filtration pressure***
= 75 – (30 + 10 +10)
= 25 mm Hg

Rate of filtration is influenced by:

- Variations in BP in glomerular capillary,
- Concentration of plasma proteins,
- Factors altering intratubular pressure, viz.
    - Rise with ureteral obstruction,
    - During osmotic diuresis.
- State of blood vessels.

If the efferent glomerular arteriole is constricted, the pressure in the glomerulus rises and the effective filtration pressure is increased. On the other hand, if the afferent glomerular arteriole is constricted, the filtration pressure is reduced.

The volume of glomerular filtrate formed depends on:

- The number of glomeruli functioning at a time,
- The volume of blood passing through the glomeruli per minute, and
- The effective glomerular filtration pressure.

Under normal circumstances, about 700 ml of plasma (contained in 1300 ml of blood or approximately 25% of entire cardiac output at rest) flow through the kidneys per minute and 120 ml of fluid are filtered into Bowman's capsule.

The volume of the filtrate is reduced in external conditions, such as ***dehydration***, ***oligaemic shock*** and ***cardiac failure*** which diminishes the volume of blood passing through the glomeruli, or lower the glomerular filtration pressure, and when there is constriction of the afferent glomerular arterioles or, changes in the glomeruli such as occur in glomerulonephritis. If the volume of glomerular filtrate is lowered below a certain point, the kidneys are unable to eliminate waste products which accumulate in blood.

2. Tubular Function: Whereas the glomerular cells act only as a passive semipermeable membrane, ***the tubular epithelial cells are a highly specialized tissue able to reabsorb selectively some substances and secrete others.*** About 170 litres of water are filtered through the glomeruli in 24 hours, and only 1.5 litre is excreted in the urine. Thus nearly 99% of the glomerular filtrate is reabsorbed in the tubules.

- ***Glucose*** is present in the glomerular filtrate in the same concentration as in the blood but practically none is excreted normally in health in detectable amount in urine and the tubules reabsorb about 170 gm/day. At an arterial plasma level of 100 mg/100 ml and a GFR of 120 ml/mt, approximately 120 mg of glucose are delivered in the glomerular filtrate in each minute. ***Maximum rate at which glucose can be reabsorbed is about 350 mg/mt (TmG), which is an 'active' process.***
- About 50 gm of ***urea*** are filtered through the glomeruli in 24 hours, but only 30 gm are excreted in the urine, ***this is a passive diffusion***.
- Certain substances foreign to the body, e.g. diodrast, para-amino hippuric acid (PAH) and phenol red are:
    - Filtered through the glomeruli and in addition, are
    - Secreted by the tubules.

  Thus the amount of these substances excreted per minute in the urine is greater than that filtered through the glomeruli per minute. At low blood levels, the tubular capacity for excreting these compounds is so great that the plasma passing through the kidneys is almost completely cleared of them
- Another group of substances, e.g. ***inulin, thiosulphate,* and *mannitol*** are eliminated exclusively by the glomeruli and are neither reabsorbed nor secreted by the tubules. Hence, amount of these substances excreted per minute in the urine is the same as the amount filtered through the glomeruli per minute, ***thus they give the glomerular filtration rate (GFR).***

RENAL FUNCTION TESTS

Classification

Based on the above functions, the renal function tests can be classified as follows:

I. *Tests based on Glomerular Filtration:*
- Urea clearance test.
- Endogenous creatinine clearance test.
- Inulin clearance test.

II. *Tests to measure Renal Plasma Flow (RPF):*
- Para-amino hippurate test (PAH)
- Filtration fraction

III. *Tests based on tubular function:*
- Concentration and dilution tests.
- 15 minute—PSP excretion test.
- Measurement of tubular secretory mass.

IV. *Certain Miscellaneous tests:* Which can determine size, shape, asymmetry, obstruction, tumour, infarct, etc.

I. GLOMERULAR FILTRATION TESTS

Three clearance tests are:
- ***Urea clearance,***
- ***Endogenous creatinine clearance,*** and
- ***Inulin clearance tests.***

These are used to examine for impairment of glomerular filtration.

What is meant by clearance test?

As a means of expressing quantitatively the rate of excretion of a given substance by the kidney, its "clearance" is frequently measured. This is ***defined as a volume of blood or plasma which contains the amount of the substances which is excreted in the urine in one minute,*** Or alternatively, the clearance of a substance may be defined as that volume of blood or plasma cleared of the amount of the substance found in one minute excretion of urine.

1. Urea Clearance Test: At present, the blood/plasma urea clearance test of Van Slyke is widely used. Blood urea clearance is an expression of the number of ml of blood/plasma, which are completely cleared of urea by the kidney per minute. As a matter of fact, the plasma is not completely cleared of urea. Only about 10 percent of the urea is removed. Consequently, 750 ml of plasma pass through the kidney per minute and 10 percent of the urea is removed, this is equivalent to completely clearing 75 ml of plasma per minute.

Maximum Clearance:

If the ***urine volume exceeds 2 ml/mt,*** the rate of urea elimination is at a maximum and is directly proportional to the concentration of urea in the blood. Thus, provided the blood urea remains unchanged, urea is excreted at the same rate whether the urinary output is 4 ml or 8 ml/mt. Volume of blood cleared of urea per minute can be calculated from the formula,

$$\frac{U \times V}{B}$$

Where,

U = Concentration of urea in urine (in mg/100 ml)

V = Volume of urine (in ml/mt)

B = The concentration of urea in blood (in mg/100 ml)

Substituting average values, the number of ml of blood cleared of urea per minute =

$$\frac{1000 \times 2.1}{28} = 75$$

A urea clearance of 75 does not mean that 75 ml of blood have passed through the kidneys in one minute and were completely cleared of urea. ***But it means that the amount of urea excreted in the urine in one minute is equal to the amount found in 75 ml of blood.*** The clearance which occurs when the urinary volume exceeds 2ml/mt is termed as ***Maximum urea clearance (Cm)*** and average normal value is 75.

$$\mathbf{Cm = 75\ ml\ (Normal\ range\ 75 \pm 10)}$$

Standard Clearance:

When the ***urinary volume is less than 2 ml/mt,*** the rate of urea elimination is reduced, because relatively more urea is reabsorbed in the tubules, and is proportional to the square root of the urinary volume. Such clearance is termed as ***standard clearance of urea (Cs)*** and average normal value is 54.

$$Cs = \frac{U \times \sqrt{V}}{B} = 54\text{ ml (Normal range} = 54 \pm 10)$$

Note: Provided no prerenal factors are temporarily reducing the clearance of urea, the volume of blood cleared of urea per minute is a index of renal function.

If a larger volume than normal is cleared/mt, renal function is satisfactory.

If a smaller volume is cleared, renal function is impaired.

Expression of Result as %: Sometimes the result of a urea clearance test is expressed as a per cent of the normal maximum or of the normal standard urea clearance depending on whether the urinary output is greater or lesser than 2 ml/mt.

Expressed as % of normal:

$$Cm = \frac{U \times V}{B} \times \frac{100}{75} \% = 1.33$$

$$Cs = \frac{U \times \sqrt{V}}{B} \times \frac{100}{54} \% = 1.85$$

Procedure: The test should be performed between breakfast and lunch, as excretion is more uniform during this time.

- The patient, who is kept at rest throughout the test, is given a light breakfast and 2 to 3 glasses of water.
- The bladder is emptied and the urine is discarded, the exact time of urination is noted.
- One hour later, urine is collected and a specimen of blood is withdrawn for determining urea content.
- A second specimen of urine is obtained at the end of another hour.

The volume of each specimen of urine is measured accurately and the concentration of urea in the specimen of blood and urine is determined.

The average value of the specimens of urine is used for assessing the quantity and urea content of urine.

Interpretation of the Test:

- Urea clearance of 70% or more of average normal function indicates that the kidneys are excreting satisfactorily.
- Values between 40 to 70% indicate mild impairment, between 20 to 40% moderate impairment and below 20% indicates severe impairment of renal function.
- ***In acute renal failure:*** The urea clearance Cm or Cs is lowered, usually less than half the normal and increases again with clinical improvement.
- ***In chronic nephritis:*** The urea clearance falls progressively and reaches a value half or less of the normal before the blood urea concentration begins to rise. With values below 20% of normal, prognosis is bad; the survival time rarely exceeds two years and death occurs within a year in more than 50% cases.
- ***Terminal uraemia:*** Is invariably found when the urea clearance falls to about 5% of the normal values.
- ***In Nephrotic syndrome:*** The urea clearance is usually normal until the onset of renal insufficiency sets in and produces the same changes as in chronic nephritis.

  In Benign hypertension: A normal urea clearance is usually maintained indefinitely except in few cases which assume a terminal malignant phase when it falls rapidly.

  Note: A very low protein diet can lead to low clearance value even in normal persons and in patients with mild renal disease.

2. Endogenous Creatinine Clearance Test:

At normal levels of creatinine, this metabolite is filtered at the glomerulus but neither secreted nor reabsorbed by the tubules. Hence, its clearance gives the GFR. This is a convenient method for estimation of GFR since:

- It is a normal metabolite in the body.
- It does not require the intravenous administration of any test material.
- Estimation of creatinine is simple.

Procedure of the Test:

- An accurate 24-hour urine specimen is collected ending at 7 AM and its total volume is measured.
- Collect a blood sample for serum creatinine determination.

- Estimate the serum and urinary creatinine concentration.

Result:

$$C\,cr = \frac{U \times V}{P}$$

Where,

U = Urine creatinine concentration in mg/dl
P = Serum creatinine in mg/dl.
V = Volume of urine in ml/mt.

Normal values for creatinine clearance varies from 95 to 105 ml/mt.

3. Inulin Clearance Test: Inulin, a homopolysaccharide, polymer of fructose is an ideal substance as:

- It is not metabolized in the body,
- Following IV administration, it is excreted entirely through glomerular filtration, being neither excreted nor reabsorbed by renal tubules.

Hence ***the number of ml of plasma which is cleared of inulin in one minute is equivalent to the volume of glomerular filtrate formed in one minute.***

Procedure of the Test:

- Preferably performed in the morning. Patient should be hospitalized overnight and kept reclining during the test.
- A light breakfast is given consisting of half glass milk, one slice of toast, can be given at 7.30 AM.
- At 8 AM 10 gm of inulin dissolved in 100 ml of saline, at body temperature, is injected IV at a rate of 10 ml per minute.
- One hour after (9 AM) the injection, the bladder is emptied and this urine is discarded.
- Note the time and collect urine one and two hours after. Volume of urine is measured and analyzed for inulin content.
- At the mid-point of each collection of urine, 30 and 90 minutes after the initial emptying of bladder, 10 to 15 ml of blood is withdrawn (in oxalated bottle), plasma is separated and analyzed for inulin concentration.

Calculation and Result: Values obtained of two samples of blood is averaged.

$$Cln = \frac{U \times V}{P}, \text{ where}$$

U = mg of inulin/100 of urine
V = ml of urine/mt
P = mg of inulin/100 ml of plasma (average of two samples)

Normal average: Inulin clearance in an adult (1.73 sq m) = 125 ml of plasma cleared of inulin/mt.

Range = 100 to 150 ml.

Note: Inulin clearance test is definitely superior for determination of GFR but requires tedious and intricate chemical procedure for determination.

4. Determination of ^{51} Cr-EDTA Clearance: Recently simplified single injection method for determination of ^{51} Cr-EDTA plasma clearance is widely used, for routine assessment of Glomerular filtration rate (GFR) in adults as well as in children. It is particularly convenient in children where it is not easy to collect 24 hour urine sample. It has been used for children younger than 1 year old.

II. TESTS FOR RENAL BLOOD FLOW

1. Measurement of Renal Plasma Flow (RPF):

- Para-amino hippurate (PAH) is filtered at the glomeruli and secreted by the tubules.
- At low blood concentration (2 mg or less/100 ml) of plasma, PAH is removed completely during a single circulation of the blood through the kidneys. Tubular capacity for excreting PAH of low blood levels is great.
- Thus, the amount of PAH in the urine becomes a measure for the value of plasma cleared of PAH in a unit time, i.e. PAH clearance at low blood levels meausres renal plasma flow (RPF).
- RPF (For a surface area of 1.73 sq. m) = 574 ml/mt.

2. Filtration Fraction (FF) : The filtration fraction (FF) is the fraction of plasma passing through the kidney which is filtered at the glomerulus, is obtained by dividing the Inulin clearance by the PAH clearance.

$$FF = \frac{C\ In}{C_{PAH}} = \frac{GFR}{RPF}$$

If we take, GFR = 125 and RPF = 574, then the

$$FF = \frac{125}{574} = 0.217\ (21.7\%)$$

Normal range = 0.16 to 0.21 in an adult.

Interpretations:

- The FF tends to be normal ***in early essential hypertension,*** but as the disease progresses, the decrease in RPF> than the decrease in the GFR. This produces an increase in FF.
- In the ***malignant phase of hypertension,*** these changes are much greater, consequently the FF rises considerably.
- ***In glomerulonephritis:*** The reverse situation prevails. In all stages of this disease, a progressive decrease in the FF is characteristic because of much greater decline in the glomerular filtration rate (GFR), than the renal plasma flow RPF.
- A rise in FF is also observed early ***in congestive cardiac failure.***

III. TESTS OF TUBULAR FUNCTION

A. Concentration Tests:

Principle: Based on the ability of the kidneys to concentrate urine, and based on measuring specific gravity of urine. They are ***simple bedside procedures, easy to carry out and extremely important.***

The tests are conducted either:

- Under conditions of restricted fluid intake, or
- By inhibiting diuresis by injection of ADH.

1. Fishberg Concentration Test: This test imposes less strenuous curtailment of fluid intake and may be completed in a shorter period of time. Most commonly used simple bedside concentration test.

Procedure:

- Patient is allowed no fluids from 8 PM until 10 AM next morning.
- The evening meal is given at 7 PM. It should be ***high protein*** and must have a ***fluid content of less than 200 ml***
- Urine passed in the night is discarded.
- Nothing by mouth next morning.
- Collect urine specimens next morning at 8 AM, 9 AM and 10 AM and determine the specific gravity of each.

Result and Interpretation:

- If tubular functioning is normal, the specific gravity of at least one of the specimens should be greater than 1.025, after appropriate correction made for temperature, albumin, and glucose.
- Impaired tubular function is shown by specific gravity of 1.020 or less and may be fixed at 1.010 in case of severe renal damage.

Note: A false result may be obtained, if the patient has:

- Congestive cardiac failure because elimination of oedema fluid in night will simulate inability to concentrate.
- Inability to concentrate is also characteristic of diabetes insipidus.

2. Lashmet and Newburg Concentration Test:

This test imposes:

- Severe fluid intake restriction over a period of 38 hours, and
- Involves the use of a special dry diet for one day.

3. Concentration Test with Posterior Pituitary Extract:

- The subcutaneous injection of 10 pressor units of posterior pituitary extract (0.5 ml of vasopressin injection) in a normal person will inhibit the diuresis produced the ingestion of 1600 ml of water in 15 minutes.
- The test has the advantage of short performance time, and minimizing the necessity of preparation of the patient.
- Posterior pituitary extract will also inhibit the diuresis seen in congestive heart failure

under active treatment as well as that of *diabetes insipidus,* allowing sufficient concentration to determine degree of tubular function in these conditions.

Interpretation: Under the condition of the test, individual with normal kidney function, excrete urine with specific gravity 1.020 or higher. Failure to concentrate to this degree indicates renal damage.

B. Water Dilution/Elimination Test:

Principle: The ability of the kidneys to eliminate water is tested by measuring the urinary output after ingesting a large volume of water.

Note: Water excretion is not only a renal function but also depends on extrarenal factors and prerenal deviation will reduce the ability of the kidneys to excrete urine.

Procedure:

- The patient remains in bed throughout the test because elimination of water is maximal in the horizontal position.
- On the day before the test, the patient has an evening meal but takes nothing by mouth after 8 PM.
- On the morning of the test, he empties his bladder at 8 AM which is discarded, and then drinks 1200 ml of water within half hour.
- The bladder is emptied at 9, 10, 11 and 12 noon and the volume and the specific gravity of the four specimens are measured.

Interpretations:

- If renal function is normal, more than 80% (1000 ml) of water is voided in 4 hours, the larger part being excreted in the first 2 hours. The ***specific gravity of atleast one specimen should be 1.003 or less.***
- If renal function is impaired, less than 80% (1000 ml) of water is excreted in 4 hours, and the ***specific gravity does not fall to 1.003 and remains fixed at 1.010 in cases of severe renal damage.***

C. Tests of Tubular Excretion and Reabsorption

Principle: The reserve function of secretion of foreign non-endogenous materials by the tubular epithelium is most conveniently tested for the use of certain dyes measuring their rate of excretion.

Phenol Sulphthalein (PSP) Excretion Test:

Use of PSP (Phenol red) to measure renal function was first introduced by **Rowntree** and **Geraghty** in 1912. Later on, **Smith** has shown that with the amount of dye employed, 94% excreted by tubular action and only 6% by glomerular filtration. Thus the test measures primarily tubular activity as well as being a measure of renal blood flow.

15-minute PSP Test: It has been shown, the test is reliable and sensitive if the amount of dye excreted in the first 15 minutes is taken as the criterion of renal function.

Test and Interpretation: When 1.0 ml of PSP (6 mg) is injected IV, normal kidneys will excrete 30 to 50% of the dye during the first 15 minutes.

- ***Excretion of less than 23% of the dye during this period regardless of the amount excreted in 2 hours indicates impaired renal function.***
- It is also used to determine the function of each kidney separately. Here, the appearances time as well as the rate of excretion of the dye is of importance. After IV injection, the normal appearance time of the dye at the tip of the catheters is 2 minutes or less and rate of excretion from each kidney is greater than 1 to 1.5% of the injected dye per ml. Increase in appearance time and decrease in excretion rate indicate impaired function.

IV. OTHER MISCELLANEOUS TESTS TO ASSESS RENAL FUNCTION

1. Intravenous Pyelography: When injected IV, certain radio-opaque organic compounds of iodine are excreted by the kidneys in sufficient concentrations to cast a shadow of the renal calyces, renal pelvis, ureters and the bladder on an X-ray film and gives lot of informations regarding size, shape, and functioning of the kidneys.

The most commonly used substances are:

- **Iodoxyl:** available as "Pyelectan", (Glaxo), Uropac (M & B), Uroselectan B, etc.
- **Diodone 30%:** more recently introduced, which gives better results. Available as Perabrodil (Bayer), Pyelosil (Glaxo), etc.

Indications: IV pyelography is widely used in the investigation of diseases of urinary tract and should be a routine procedure for investigation with patients:

- Of renal calculi,
- Repeated urinary infections,
- Renal pain and haematuria,
- Prostatic enlargement,
- Suspected tumours, and
- Congenital abnormalities.

By pyelography the relationship of the renal tract to calcified abdominal shadows and masses can be demonstrated. The excretion and concentration of Diodone may be used as a rough indication of renal function. If the calyces and pelvis of one kidney are outlined, while the other remains invisible, it can be assumed that the function of the invisible side is impaired.

Contraindications: IV Pyelography should not be done in patients with

- Acute nephritis
- Congestive cardiac failure,
- Severely impaired liver function,
- In frank uraemia,
- In hypersensitive patients and sensitivity to organic iodine compounds, sensitivity test should be done before injecting the drug.

2. Radio-active Renogram: ^{131}Labelled Hippuran is given IV and simultaneously the radioactivity from each kidney is recorded graphically in a stripchart recorder by electronic device. Hippuran-^{131}I is actively secreted by the kidney tubules and it is not concentrated in the liver.

Dose: 15 to 16 μci of Hippuran–^{131}I given IV slowly in single dose.

Interpretation: With the limitations and complexities of these interpretation of the results, the investigation is of great practical clinical use. The following information is obtained:

- Whether any major asymmetry in function between the two kidneys is present.
- A reasonable assessment of overall renal function, given by the ratio of bladder activity/heart activity in 10 minutes time.
- The presence of obstruction to urine flow in renal pelvis or ureters.

No other means exist for obtaining so much information in a short time about the differential functions of the kidneys.

3. Radio-active Scanning: A recent development is the renal scintiscan. This has the theoretical advantage over the renogram of being able to detect segmental lesions. In this technique, ^{203}Hg-labelled chlormerodrin or ^{197}Hg-labelled chlormerodrin is injected intravenously and a renal scan can be obtained by a scintillation counter over the lumbar regions.

Interpretations:

- Renal scanning is helpful for detection of abnormalities in size, shape and position of the kidneys.
- Renal tumours and renal infarcts are shown in scintiscan which may be missed in Pyelography.

☞ SALIENT POINTS TO REMEMBER

- The renal function is usually assessed by evaluating either the glomerular function by clearance tests or tubular function by urine concentration/dilution tests.
- The above is often guided by patient's history/examination, by urine examination for albumin and deposits and by blood analysis for urea and creatinine.
- The clearance is **defined** as the volume of the blood/plasma that would be completely cleared of a substance per minute.
- Urea clearance test and endogenous creatinine clearance are often used to assess renal function.
- The clearance which occurs when the urinary volume exceeds 2 ml/mt is termed as ***Maximum urea clearance*** (Cm). Cm = 75 ml (normal range 75 ± 10).

- When the urinary volume is less than 2 ml/mt, it is termed as ***standard clearance of urea*** (Cs). Cs = 54 ml (normal range = 54 ± 10).
- Normal values for endogenous creatinine clearance varies from 95 to 105 ml/mt.
- A decrease in the clearance tests is an indication of renal damage.
- Inulin clearance test represents GFR. It is superior to other clearance tests for GFR as it is excreted entirely through glomerular filtration, being neither excreted nor reabsorbed by renal tubules. It is not done in the laboratory routinely.
- Para-amino hippurate (PAH) clearance measures renal plasma flow (RPF).
- Inulin clearance is 125 ml/mt (Range 100 to 150 ml). PAH clearance C_{PAH} is 574 ml/mt.
- Filtration fraction (F.F.) is the fraction of plasma passing through the kidney which is filtered at the glomerulus, is obtained by dividing the Inulin clearance by the PAH clearance.

$$\text{F.F.} = \frac{C_{IN}}{C_{PAH}} = \frac{\text{GFR}}{\text{RPF}} = \frac{125}{574} \quad 0.217$$

Normal range = 0.16 to 0.21

- Water concentration/dilution tests are used to measure tubular function.
- Impairment in renal function is usually associated with elevated concentration of blood urea, serum creatinine, decrease in osmolality and specific gravity of urine by Fishberg concentration test

MULTIPLE CHOICE QUESTIONS

Give one correct answer:

1. **Normal maximum clearance of urea (Cm) in an adult averages about:**
   (a) 60 (b) 65
   (c) 75 (d) 85
   (e) 95
2. **In patients with renal failure all of the following are typically elevated in serum *except:***
   (a) Urea Nitrogen
   (b) Albumin
   (c) Phosphate
   (d) Creatinine
   (e) Uric acid
3. **Renal plasma flow (RPF) is measured by:**
   (a) Inulin clearance
   (b) Creatinine clearance
   (c) PSP excretion
   (d) Para amino hippurate clearance
   (e) Urine output
4. **To calculate the urea clearance, all of the following data are required *except:***
   (a) Blood urea level
   (b) Volume of urine in ml/minute
   (c) Urinary urea concentration
   (d) Patient's height and weight
   (e) Specific gravity of urine
5. **Normal renal plasma flow (RPF) in healthy adults averages about.**
   (a) 125 ml/mt (b) 250 ml/mt
   (c) 454 ml/mt (d) 574 ml/mt
   (e) 754 ml/mt
6. **Relationship between GFR and serum creatinine concentration is:**
   (a) Non-existent (b) Inverse
   (c) Direct (d) Indirect
   (e) None of the above
7. **Filtration fraction is obtained by dividing.**
   (a) PAH clearance by Inulin clearance
   (b) Urea clearance by PAH clearance
   (c) Creatinine clearance by PAH clearance
   (d) Inulin clearance by PAH clearance
   (e) Inulin clearance by urea clearance
8. **Which of the following renal function tests measures glomerular filtration rate (GFR)?**
   (a) Urea clearnace
   (b) Creatinine clearance
   (c) Inulin clearance
   (d) PAH clearance
   (e) PSP excretion

9. The Nephrotic syndrome includes all of the following *except:*
(a) Protein loss of 3 to 3.5 qm/24 hrs. or more in urine
(b) Low serum albumin level
(c) Dehydration
(d) Elevated serum cholesterol level
(e) Elevated levels of α_2 - globulin in serum

10. Of the following, the first laboratory evidence of chronic pyelonephritis is often:
(a) Loss of concentrating ability
(b) Decreased creatinine clearance
(c) Raised serum urea nitrogen level
(d) Raised serum uric acid level
(e) None of the above

ANSWERS

1. (c)	2. (b)	3. (d)
4. (e)	5. (d)	6. (b)
7. (d)	8. (c)	9. (c)
10. (a)		

28 Liver Function Tests

INTRODUCTION

Numerous **laboratory** investigations have been proposed in the assessment of liver diseases. From among these host of tests, the following battery of blood tests: Total bilirubin and VD Bergh test, total and differential proteins and A:G ratio and certain enzyme assays as aminotransferases, alkaline phosphatase and γ-GT have become widely known as ***"Standard Liver Function Tests" (LFTs).***

Urine tests for bilirubin and its metabolites and the prothrombin time (PT) and index (PI) are also often included under these heading; but tests such as turbidity/flocculation test, Icteric index, etc. are now becoming outdated. ***"Second generation"*** LFTs attempt to improve on this battery of tests and to gain a genuine measurement of liver function, i.e. quantitative assessment of functional hepatice mass. These include the capacity of the liver to eliminate exogenous compounds such as aminopyrine or caffeine or endogenous compounds such as bile acids which have gained much importance recently. However, such investigations are not yet routinely or widely used due to lack of facilities and are useful for reasearch purpose only. ***Hence in our discussion we will confine to "Standard LFTs" which are routinely done and possible in any standard laboratory***. It is ***stressed that with the advent of more sophisticated techniques for the diagnosis of liver diseases, particularly ultrasound and CT scanning together with percutaneous and endoscopic cholangiography and liver biopsies, routine use of standard LFTs being questioned now.***

FUNCTIONS OF THE LIVER

Liver is a versatile organ which is involved in metabolism and independently involved in many other biochemical functions. ***Regenerating power of liver cells is tremendous.*** Although details of the various functions performed by liver have been discussed under their respective places, a summary of these functions is given below in brief, so that students can easily group the tests of liver associating with its functions.

1. ***Metabolic Functions: Liver is the key organ and the principal site where the metabolism of carbohydrates, lipids, and proteins take place.***
   - Liver is the organ where NH_3 is converted to urea.
   - It is the principal organ where cholesterol is synthesized, and catabolized to form bile acids and bile salts.
   - Esterification of cholesterol takes place solely in liver.
   - In this organ absorbed monosacchrides other than glucose are converted to glucose, viz. galactose is converted to glucose.
   - Liver besides other organs can bring about catabolism and anabolism of nucleic acids.
   - Liver is also involved in metabolism of vitamins and minerals to certain extent.

2. ***Secretory function: Liver is responsible for the formation and secretion of bile in the intestine.*** Bile pigments-bilirubin formed from heme catabolism is conjugated in liver cells and secreated in the bile.

3. *Excretory function:* Certain exogenous dyes like BSP (bromsulphthalein) and Rose Bengal dye are exclusively excreted through liver cells.

4. *Synthesis of certain blood cogulation factors:* Liver cells are responsible for conversion of preprothrombin (inactive) to active prothrombin in the presence of vitamin K. It also produces other clotting factors V, VII and X. Fibrinogen involved in blood coagulation is also synthesized in liver.

5. *Synthesis of other proteins: Albumin is solely synthesized in liver* and also to some extent α and β globulins.

6. *Detoxication function and protective function:* Kupffer cells of liver remove foreign bodies from blood by phagocytosis. Liver cells can detoxicate drugs, hormones and convert them into less toxic substances for excretion.

7. *Storage function:* Liver stores glucose in the form of glycogen. It also stores Vit B_{12}, Vit A, etc.

8. *Miscellaneous functions:* Liver is involved in blood formation in embryo and in some abnormal states, it also forms blood in adult.

CLASSIFICATION OF LFTs

Tests used in the study of patients with liver and biliary tract diseases can be classified according to the specific functions of the liver involved.

I. *Tests based on abnormalities of pigment metabolism:*
   - Serum bilirubin and VD Bergh reaction
   - Icteric index (not done now)
   - Urine bilirubin
   - Urine and faecal urobilinogen

II. *Tests based on liver's part in carbohydrate metabolism*
   - Galactose tolerance test
   - Fructose tolerance test

III. *Tests based on changes in plasma proteins:*
   - Estimation of total plasma proteins, albumin and globulin and determination of A:G ratio.
   - Determination of plasma fibrinogen
   - Various Flocculation tests
   - Aminoacids in urine

IV. *Tests based on abnormalities of lipids:*
   - Determination of serum cholesterol and ester cholesterol and their ratio.
   - Determination of faecal fats

V. *Tests based on detoxicating function of liver:*
   - Hippuric acid synthesis test.

VI *Excretion of injected substances by the liver (Excretory function):*
   - Bromsulphthalein test (BSP retention test)
   - I^{131}-Rose bengal test

VII. *Formation of Prothrombin by liver:*
   - Determination of Prothrombin time and Index

VIII. *Tests based on amino acid catabolism:*
   - Determination of blood NH_3
   - Determiantion of glutamine in CS fluid (Indirect Liver Function Test)

IX. *Tests based on drug metabolism:*
   - MEGX Test
   - Antipyrine breath test

X. **Determination of serum Enzyme activities.**

All the liver function tests enumerated above will not be discussed, only the standard liver functions tests (LFTs), done in the laboratory routinely will be discussed. A few special tests, viz BSP test also will be considered

TESTS BASED ON ABNORMALITIES OF BILE PIGMENT METABOLISM

1. VD Bergh Reaction and Serum Bilirubin

Principle: Methods for detecting and estimating bilirubin in serum are based on the formation of a purple compound *"azo-bilirubin"* where bilirubin in serum is allowed to react with a freshly prepared, solution of VD Bergh's diazo reagent.

VD Bergh Reaction: Consists of two parts: Direct reaction and indirect reaction. The latter serves as the basis for a quantitative estimation of serum bilirubin (see below).

Ehrlich's diazo-reagent: This is freshly prepared before use. It **consists of two solutions:**

Solution A: Contains sulphanilic acid in conc HCl.

Solution B: Sodium nitrite in water. Fresh solutions is prepared by taking 10 ml of solution A+0.8 ml of solution B.

Procedure: Take 0.3 ml of serum into each of two small tubes. Add 0.3 ml of D.W. to one which serves as **"Control"** and 0.3 ml of freshly prepared diazoreagent into second **('test').** Mix both tubes and observe any colour change.

Basis of the reaction: Coupling of diazotized sulphanilic acid and bilirubin if present produces a ***"redish-purple" azo-compound.***

Responses: Three different responses may be observed:

- ***Immediate direct reaction:*** Immediate development of colour proceeding rapidly to a maximum.
- ***Delayed direct reaction:*** Colour only begins to appear after 5 to 30 minutes and develops slowly to a maximum.
- No direct reaction is obtained. Colour develops after addition of methanol **(*indirect reaction*).**

2. *Determination of Serum Bilirubin:* Indirect reaction is essentially a method for the quantitative estimation of serum bilirubin.

Principle: Serum is diluted with D.W. and methanol added in an amount insufficient to precipitiate the proteins, yet sufficient to permit all the bilirubin to react with the diazo-reagent.

N.B: Absolute methanol gives a clear solution than 95% ethanol.

Colour developed is compared with a standard solution of bilirubin similarly treated.

Note: Bilirubin is a costly chemical hence an artificial standard may be used.

Artificial Standard: It is a methyl red solution in glacial acetic acid of pH 4.6 to 4.7, which closely resembles the colour of azo-bilirubin.

Note: Before interpretation, students should know about 'Jaundice' and its causes.

JAUNDICE

In *jaundice* there is ***yellow colouration of conjunctivae, mucous membrane and skin*** due to increased bilirubin level. ***Jaundice is visible when serum bilirubin exceeds 2.4 mg/dl.***

Classification of Jaundice

1. Rolleston and McNee (1929), as modified by Maclagan, (1964): They classified jaundice ***in three groups:***

a. ***Haemolytic or pre-hepatic jaundice:*** In which there is increased breakdown of Hb, so that liver cells are unable to conjugate all the increased bilirubin formed hence unconjugated bilirubin increases.

Causes: Principally there are ***two categories:***

- ***Intrinsic:*** Abnormalities within the red blood cells by various haemoglobinopathies, hereditary spherocytosis, G-6-PD deficiency in red cells and favism.
- ***Extrinsic:*** Factors external to red blood cells, e.g. incompatible blood transfusion, Haemolytic disease of the newborn (HDN), autoimmune haemolytic anaemias, in malaria, etc.

b. ***Hepatocellular or hepatic jaundice:*** In which there is disease of the parenchymal cells of liver. This may be divided into **3 groups,** although there may be over-lappings.

- ***Conditions in which there is defective conjugation:*** There may be a reduction in the number of funtioning liver cells, e.g. in chronic hepatitis, in this all liver functions are impaired or there may be a specific defect in the conjugation process, e.g. in Gilbert's disease, Crigler-Najjar Syndrome, etc. In these the liver function is otherwise normal.
- ***Conditions such as viral hepatitis and toxic jaundice:*** In which there is extensive damage to liver cells, associated with considerable degree of intra-hepatic obstruction resulting in appreciable absorption of conjugated bilirubin.
- ***"Cholestatic" Jaundice:*** This ***occurs due to drugs, (drug-induced)*** such as chlorpromazine and some steroids in which there is mainly intrahepatic obstruction, liver function being essentially normal.

c. ***Obstrutive or post-hepatic jaundice:*** In which there is obstruction to the flow of bile in the extrahepatic ducts, e.g. due to gall stones, carcinoma of head of pancreas; enlarged lymph glands pressing on bile duct, etc.

II. Rich's classification of jaundice:

According to this classification jaundice is divided into mainly *two groups:*

a. Retention Jaundice: In which there is impaired removal of bilirubin from the blood, or excessive amount of bilirubin is produced and not cleared fully by liver cells. This group includes haemolytic jaundice and those conditions characterized by impaired conjugation of bilirubin.

b. Regurgitation jaundice: In which there is excess of conjugated bilirubin and it includes obstructive jaundice and those liver conditions in which there is considerable degree of intrahepatic obstruction (cholestasis).

Interpretations:

1. *VD Bergh reaction:* Correlation of different types of VD Bergh reaction is based on the fact how bilirubin reacts differently with the Diazo-reagent according to whether or not, it has been conjugated.

- Bilirubin formed from Hb and not passed through ***liver cells unconjugated bilirubin and it gives an indirect reaction.***
- On the other hand, bilirubin which has passed through liver cells and undergoes conjugation is called ***conjugated bilirubin and gives direct reaction.***
- *In haemolytic jaundice:* There is an increase in unconjugated bilirubin, hence indirect reaction is obtained, occasionally it may be a delayed direct reaction.
- *In obstructive jaundice:* Conjugated bilirubin is increased, hence an immediate direct reaction is obtained.
- *In hepatocellular jaundice:* Either or both may be present. In viral hepatitis: direct reaction is the rule, because it is associated with intrahepatic obstruction.
- An immediate direct reaction is also observed in *"cholestatic jaundice"*. In low-grade jaundice present in some cases of cirrhosis liver, results are variable, but an indirect reaction is usually seen.

An immediate direct reaction is obtained whether the obstruction is intrahepatic or extrahepatic. This does not, therefore, differentiate between an infectious hepatitis or toxic jaundice on one hand and post hepatic (obstructive jaundice) on the other. ***Hence a direct VD Bergh reaction is only of limited value.***

2. *Serum bilirubin:* It gives a ***measure of the intensity*** of jaundice. Higher values are found in obstructive jaundice than in haemolytic jaundice. Usefulness of quantitative estimation of serum bilirubin:

- *In subclinical jaundice:* Where the demonstration of small increases in serum bilirubin 1.0 to 3.0 mg/dl is of diagnostic value.
- *In Clinical jaundice:* Useful to follow the development and course of the jaundice.

3. Bile Pigments in Urine/Faeces (Bilirubinuria)

Principle: Most of the tests used for detection of bile pigments depend on the oxidation of bilirubin to differently coloured compounds such as biliverdin (green) and bilicyanin (blue).

Interpretations:

- ***Bilirubin is found in the urine in obstructive jaundice*** due to various causes and in "cholestasis". Conjugated bilirubin can pass through the glomerular filter.
- Bilirubin is not present in urine in most cases of haemolytic jaundice, as unconjugated bilirubin is carried in plasma attached to albumin, hence it cannot pass through the glomerular filter.
- ***Bilirubinuria is always accompanied with direct VD Bergh reaction.***

Note: Bilirubin in the urine may be detected even before clinical jaundice is noted.

Bile Pigments is Faeces

- Bilirubin is not normally present in faeces since bacteria in the intestine reduce it to urobilinogen.
- Some my be found if there is very rapid passage of materials along the intestine.

- Sometimes it is found in faeces of very young infants, if bacterial flora in the gut is not developed
- It is regularly found in faeces of patients who are being treated with gut sterilizing antibiotics such as neomycin.
- Biliverdin is found in meconium, the material excreted during the first day or two of life.

4. Urinary and Faecal Urobilinogen

a. ***Faecal Urobilinogen: Normal quantity of urobilinogen excreted in the faeces per day is from 50-250 mg.*** Since urobilinogen is formed in the intestine by the reduction of bilirubin, the amount of faecal urobilinogen depends primarily on the amount of bilirubin entering the intestine.

- Faecal urobilinogen is increased in haemolytic jaundice, in which ***dark clay-coloured faeces*** is passed.
- Faecal urobilinogen is decreased or absent if there is obstruction to the flow of bile ***in obstructive jaundice,*** in which ***clay-coloured faeces is passed.*** Complete degree of obstruction is found in tumors, whereas obstruction due to gall stones is intermittent. ***A complete absence of faecal urobilinogen is strongly suggestive of malignant obstruction.*** Thus, it may be useful in differentiating a non-malignant from a malignant obstruction.
- A decrease may also occur in extreme cases of diseases affecting hepatic parenchyma.

b. ***Urine Urobilinogen:*** Normally there are mere traces of urobilinogen in the urine. ***Average is 0.64 mg, maximum normal 4 mg/24 hours.***

- ***In obstructive jaundice:*** In case of complete obstruction, no urobilinogen is found in the urine. Since bilirubin is unable to get into the intestine to form it. ***The presence of bilirubin in the urine, without urobilinogen is strongly suggestive of obstructive jaundice either intrahepatic or post-hepatic.***
- ***In haemolytic jaundice:*** Increased production of bilirubin leads to increased production of urobilinogen which appears in urine in large amounts. **Thus, increased urobilinogen in urine and absence of bilirubin in urine are strongly suggestive of haemolytic jaundice.**

TESTS BASED ON LIVER'S PART IN CARBOHYDRATE METABOLISM

Basis: The tests are based on tolerance to various sugars since liver is involved in removal of these sugars by glycogenesis or in conversion of other monosaccharides to glucose.

1. Glucose Tolerance Test:

Not of much value in liver diseases. Although glucose tolerance is sometimes diminished, it is often dificult to separate the part played by the liver from other factors influencing glucose metabolism.

2. Galactose Tolerance Test:

Basis: The normal liver is able to convert galactose into glucose; but this function is impaired in intrahepatic diseases and the amount of blood galactose and galactose in urine is excessive.

Advantages of this test

- It is used primarily ***to detect liver cell injury.***
- ***It can be performed in presence of jaundice.***
- As it measures an intrinsic hepatic function, it may be used to distinguish obstructive and non-obstructive jaundice.

Note: In prolonged obstruction, if untreated, secondary involvement of liver leads to abnormality in the galactose tolerance.

Methods: This can be of ***two types:***

- ***Oral galactose tolerance test (Maclagan)*** and
- ***IV galactose tolerance test.***

a. ***Oral*** **Galactose Tolerance Test (Maclagan)**

The test is performed in the morning after a night's fast. A fasting blood sample is collected which serves as "control". 40 gm of galactose dissolved in a cup-full of water is given orally. Further blood samples are collected at ½ hourly intervals for two hours (similar to GTT).

Interpretations

- Normally or in obstructive jaundice 3 gm or less of galactose are excreted in the urine within 3 to 5 hours and the blood galactose returns to normal within one hour.
- In intrahepatic (Parenchymatous) jaundice: the excretion amounts to 4 to 5 gm or more during the first five hours.

Galactose index (Maclagan): It is obtained by adding the four blood galactose levels.

Interpretations:

- Upper limit of normal was taken as 160. In healthy medical students range varied from 0 to 110 and in hospital patients not suffering from liver disease the value ranged from 0 to 160.
- ***In liver diseases:*** Very high values are obtained. ***In infective and toxic hepatitis:*** values up to about 500 are seen, decreasing slowly as the clinical condition improves.
- ***In cirrhosis liver:*** Increased values may be obtained up to 500, depending on the severity of the disease.

b. ***IV galactose Tolerance Test (King):***

The test is performed in the morning after a night's fast. A fasting blood sample is collected which serves as "control". An IV injection of galactose, equivalent to 0.5 gm/kg body weight is given as a sterile 50% solution. Blood samples are collected after five minutes, ½ hour, 1 hour, 1 ½ hours, 2 hours and 2½ hours after IV injection and blood galactose level is estimated.

Interpretations:

- ***A normal response:*** Should have a curve beginning on the average at about 200 mg galactose/100 dl, falling steeply during the one hour and reaching a figure betwen 0 to 10 mg% by end of 2 hours.
- In most cases of ***Obstructive jaundice:*** Similar results are obtained, unless there is parenchymal damage.
- ***In parenchymatous diseases:*** With liver cell damage, the fall in blood galactose takes place more slowly. Normally no galactose is detected in 2½ hour sample, but in parenchymatous disease, value is greater than 20 mg/dl.

TESTS BASED ON CHANGES ON PLASMA PROTEINS

1. Determination of Total Plasma Proteins, Albumin and Globulin and A:G Ratio:

This yields most useful information in chronic liver diseases. ***Liver is the site of albumin synthesis and also possibly of some of alfa and beta globulins.***

Interpretations

- ***In Infectious hepatitis:*** Quantitative estimations of albumin and globulin may give normal results in the early stages. Qualitative changes may be present, in early stage rise in β-globulins and in later stages γ-globulins show rise.
- ***In obstructive jaundice:*** Normal values are the rule, as long as the obstructive jaundice is not associated with accompanying liver cell damage.
- ***In advanced parenchymal liver diseases and in cirrhosis liver:*** The albumin is grossly decreased and the globulins are often increased, so ***that A:G ratio is reversed, such a pattern is characteristically seen in cirrhosis liver.*** The albumin may fall below 2.5 gm% and may be a contributory factor in causing oedema in such cases. Fractionation of globulins, reveals that the increase is usually in the γ-globulin fraction, but in some cases there is a smaller increase in β–globulins.

Note:

- The severity of hypoalbuminaemia in chronic liver diseases is of diagnostic importance and may serve as a criterion of the degree of damage.
- A low serum albumin which fails to increase during treatment is usually a poor prognostic sign.

2. Estimation of plasma Fibrinogen: Fibrinogen is formed in the liver and likely to be affected if considerable liver damage is present.

- Normal value is 200-400 mg%.
- Values below 100 mg% have been reported in severe parenchymal liver damage. Such a situation is found in severe acute insufficiency such as may occur in:
  - ***Acute hepatic necrosis,***
  - ***Poisoning from carbontetrachloride,***
  - ***In advanced stages of liver cirrhosis.***

3. Flocculation Tests:

Principle: Flocculation tests depend on an alteration in the type of proteins present in the plasma. The alteration may be either quantitative or qualitative and most frequently involves one or more of the globulin fractions.

The flocculation tests are not done and have become obsolete.

4. Aminoacids in Urine (Aminoaciduria): The daily excretion of aminoacid nitrogen in normal healthy varies from 80 to 300 mg. Aminoaciduria found in severe liver diseases is of **"overflow" type**, ***with accompanying increase in plasma amino acids level.***

Clinical Importance

In severe liver diseases like acute yellow atrophy and some times in advanced cirrhosis of liver crystals of certain amino acids may be found in urinary deposits microscopically.

- *Tyrosine crystals*: Tyrosine crystallizes in sheaves or tufts of fine needles.
- *Leucine crystals:* Leucine has spherical shaped crystals, yellowish in colour, with radial and circular striations.

TESTS BASED ON ABNORMALITIES OF LIPIDS

- **Cholesterol-Cholesteryl Ester Ratio:**The liver plays an active and important role in the metabolism of cholesterol including its synthesis, esterification, oxidation and excretion.

Interpretations: Normal total blood cholesterol ranges from 150-250 mg/dl and approx. 60 to 70% of this is in esterified form.

- ***In obstructive jaundice: An increase in total blood cholesterol is common, but the ester fraction is also raised,*** so that per centage esterified does not change. It has been observed that the ratio of free and ester cholesterol is usually not changed unless accompanied by parenchymal damage.
- ***In parenchymatous liver diseases:*** There is either no rise or even ***decrease in total cholesterol and the ester fraction is always definitely reduced.*** The degree of reduction roughly parallels the degree of liver damage.
- ***In severe acute hepatic necrosis:*** The total serum cholesterol is usually low and may fall below 100 mg/dl, whilst there is marked reduction in the per centage present as esters.

TESTS BASED ON THE DETOXICATING FUNCTION OF THE LIVER

Hippuric Acid Test of Quick

Principle: Best known test for the detoxicating function of liver. Liver removes benzoic acid, administered as sodium benzoate, either orally, or IV, and combines with amino acid glycine to form hippuric acid. The amount of hippuric acid excreted in urine in a fixed time is determined. The test thus depends on *two factors:*

- ***The ability of liver cells to produce and provide sufficient glycine*** and
- ***The capacity of liver cells to conjugate it with the benzoic acid.***

For reliable result renal function must be normal. If there is any reason to suspect renal impairment, a urea clearance test should be done simultaneously.

Methods: Both oral and IV forms of the hippuric acid test are in use.

1. *Oral Hippuric Acid Test:* Dissolve 6.0 gm of sodium benzoate in approx 200 ml of water. The test may be started 3 hours after a light breakfast

of toast and tea. Food should not be given until late in the test. The patient empties the bladder, the urine being discarded. The patient is allowed to drink the sodium benzoate solution and **time is noted.** The bladder is again emptied 4 hrs later. Any urine passed during this 4 hours is kept and added to that passed at the end of 4 hours. The amount of hippuric acid excreted in this 4 hours period is estimated.

Interpretations:

- ***Normally,*** at least 3.0 gm of hippuric acid, expressed as Benzoic acid or 3.5 gm of sodium benzoate should be excreted in health.
- Smaller amounts are found when there is either acute or chronic liver damage. Amounts lower than 1.0 gm may be excreted by patients with infectious hepatitis.

2. ***IV Hippuric Acid Test:***

Indications: Normally oral test is preferred. An IV test is indicated:

- When there is impairment of absorption due to absorption defects.
- If there is accompanying nausea/vomiting.

Procedure: 1.77 gm of sodium benozate dissolved in 20 ml of DW as a sterile solution given IV. Shortly before the injection, the patient empties the bladder, which is discarded. The bladder is emptied after one hour and two hours after the injection.

Interpretations:

- In normal health, hippuric acid equivalent to at least 0.85 gm of sodium benzoate, or to 0.7 gm of benzoic acid should be excreted in the one hour, or equivalent to 1.15 gm of benzoic acid in the first two hours.
- Excretion of smaller amounts than above indicate the presence of liver damage.

TESTS BASED ON EXCRETORY FUNCTION OF LIVER

1. BSP Retention Test (Bromsulphthalein Test):

Principle:

1. The ability of the liver to excrete certain dyes, e.g. BSP is utilized in this test.
2. In normal healthy individual, a constant proportion (10 to 15% of the dye) is removed per minute.In hepatic damage and insufficiency, BSP removal is impaired by cellular failure, as damaged liver cells fail to conjugate the dye or due to decrease blood flow.
3. Removal of BSP by the liver ***involves conjugation of the dye as a mercaptide with the cysteine component of glutathione.*** The reaction of conjugation of BSP with glutathione is ***rate-limiting,*** and thus it exerts a controlling influence on the rate of removal of the dye.

Procedure: With the patient fasting, inject IV slowly, an amount of 5% BSP solution, which contains 5 mg of BSP/kg, body weight. Withdraw 5 to 10 ml of blood, 25 and 45 minutes after the injection and allow the specimens to clot. Separate the sera and estimate amount of the dye in each sample.

Interpretations:

- ***In normal*** healthy individual: Not more than 5% of the dye should remain in the blood at the end of 45 minutes. The bulk of the dye is removed in 25 minutes and less than 15% is left at the end of 25 minutes.
- ***In Parenchymatous Liver diseases:*** Removal proceeds more slowly. In advanced cirrhosis removal is very slow and 40 to 50% of the dye is retained in 45 minutes sample.

Contraindication: Since the dye is removed in bile after conjugation, this test can only be used in cases in which there is no obstruction to the flow of bile. Hence ***the test is of no value if obstruction of biliary tree exists (obstructive jaundice).***

Clinical Significance

- BSP-excretion test is a ***useful index of liver damage,*** particularly when the damage is diffuse and extensive.
- ***The test is most useful:***
  - ***In liver cell damage without jaundice***
  - ***In cirrhosis liver***
  - ***In chronic hepatitis.***

2. Rose-Bengal Dye Test: Rose Bengal is another dye which can be used to assess excretory function. 10 ml of a 1% solution of the dye is injected IV slowly.

Interpretation: Normally 50% or more of the dye disappears within 8 minutes.

I^{131} labelled Rose Bengal: I^{131} Rose Bengal has been used where isotope laboratory is present. I^{131} labelled Rose Bengal is administered IV. Then count is taken over the neck and abdomen. Initially, count is more in neck practically nil over abdomen. As the dye is excreted through liver, neck count goes down and count over abdomen increases.

Interpretation:

- ***In parenchymal liver diseases:*** High count in the neck persists and there is hardly rise in count over abdomen, as the dye is retained.

FORMATION OF PROTHROMBIN BY LIVER

1. *Determination Prothrombin Time:* ***Prothrombin is formed in the liver from inactive "pre-prothrombin" in presence of vitamin K. Prothrombin acitivity is measured as prothrombin time (PT).*** The term prothrombin time was given to time required for clotting to take place in citrated plasma to which optimum amounts of "thromboplastin" and Ca^{++} have been added. The "one-stage" technique introduced by Quick, the prothrombin time is related inversely to the concentration not only to prothrombin, but also of factors V, VII and X and it can be more sensitive to a lack of VII and X than to prothrombin alone. Inspite of above restriction, as it is simple and quick in performance, it is still much used.

Interpretations:

- ***Normal value*** Normal levels of prothrombin in control give prothrombin time of approx 14 seconds. (Range 10-16 Sec.) Results are alsways expressed as patient's prothrombin time in seconds to normal control value.
- ***In parenchymatous liver diseases:*** Depending on the degree of liver cells damage ***plasma prothrombin time may be increased from 22 to as much as 150 secs.***
- ***In obstructive jaundice:*** Due to absence of bile salts, there may be defective absorption of vitamin K,hence PT is increased, as prothrombin formation suffers.

Note:

- From above, ***it is observed that PT is increased both in obstructive jaundice and in diseases of liver cells damage. Hence PT cannot be used to differentiate between them.***
- ***However, if adequate vitamin K is administered parenterally, the PT returns rapidly to normal in uncomplicated obstructive jaundice, whereas in liver damage the response is less marked.***

Other Clinical Uses:

- PT is used mostly is controlling anticoagulant therapy.
- Determination of PT is also used to decide whether there is danger of bleeding at operation in biliary tract diseases.

2. ***Prothrombin index:*** Prothrombin activity is also sometimes expressed as ***"prothrombin index" in %***, which is the ratio of prothrombin time of the normal control to the patient's prothrombin time multiplied by 100. Thus

- $$\text{Prothrombin index} = \frac{\text{PT of normal control}}{\text{PT of patient}} \times 100$$

Normally index is 70 to 100%. The "critical level" below which bleeding may occur is not fixed one, but there is always a possibility of this occurring if prothrombin index is below 60%.

TESTS BASED ON AMINO ACID CATABOLISM

1. Determination of Blood NH_3: Nitrogen part of aminoacid is converted to NH_3 in the liver mainly by transamination and deamination (transdeamination) and it is converted to urea in liver only.

Interpretations:

- ***The normal range:*** Blood ammonia varies from 40 to 75 µg ammonia nitrogen per 100 ml of blood.
- ***In parenchymal liver diseases:*** The ability to remove NH_3 coming to liver from intestine

and other sources may be impaired. Increases in NH_3 can be found in more advanced cases of cirrhosis liver, particularly when there are associated neurological complications. In such cases blood levels may be over 200 μg/100 ml. Very high values may be obtained in hepatic coma.

2. Determination of Glutamine in CS Fluid (An Indirect Liver Function Test): Glutamine, the amide of glutamic acid, is formed by *glutamine synthetase* by glutamic acid and NH_3.Glutamine in CS fluid can be estimated by the method of **Whittaker (1955). The glutamine is hydrolyzed to glutamic acid and NH_3** by the action of dilute acid at 100 degree centigrade. A correction is made for a small amount of NH_3 produced from urea. No other substances present in CS fluid were found to form NH_3 under above conditions.

Interpretations: The normal range found to be 6.0 to 14.0 mg%.

- ***In infectious hepatitis:*** Found to range from 16to 28 mg%, but usually less than 30 mg%.
- ***In cirrhosis liver:*** The increase is more; depending on the severity. It varied from 22 to 36 mg% or more.
- ***In hepatic coma:*** Increase is very high, ranging from 30 to 60 mg% or more.
- In other types of coma, normal values are obtained.

Note: Some authorities put ***40 mg% as a critical level.*** Prognosis of the case is fatal if CS fluid glutamine level is more than 40 mg%, in case of cirrhosis liver and hepatic coma.

VALUE OF SERUM ENZYMES IN LIVER DISEASES

Quite a large number of enzyme estimations are available which are used to ascertain liver function. But most commonly and routinely employed in laboratories are two:

- *Serum transaminases (amino-transferases), and*
- *Serum alkaline phosphatase.*

a. Serum Transaminases (Aminotransferases)

Interpretations:

- Normal ranges for these enzymes are as follows: **SGOT (aspartate transaminase): 4 to 17 IU/L (7 to 35 units/ml)**

  SGPT (alanine transaminase): 3 to 15 IU/L (6 to 32 units/ml)
- Both these enzymes are found in most tissues, but the relative amounts vary. ***Heart muscles are richer in SGOT, whereas liver contains both but more of SGPT.***
- Increases in both transaminases are found in liver diseases, with SGPT much higher than SGOT.
- Their determination are of limited value in differential diagnosis of jaundice because of considerable overlapping.
- But their determination is of extreme use in ***assessing the severity and prognosis of parenchymal liver diseases*** specially acute infectious hepatitis and serum hepatitis. In these two conditions highest values, in thousand units are seen.
- Also useful in outbreak of infectious hepatitis (viral hepatitis), it is the most sensitive diagnostic index. ***The increase can be seen in prodromal stage, when jaundice has not appeared clinically.*** Such cases can be isolated and segregated from others, so that spread of the disease can be checked.
- Very high values are also obtained in toxic hepatitis, due to carbon tetrachloride poisoning. Increases are comparatively less in drug hepatitis (cholestatic) like chloropromazine.
- In obstructive jaundice (extrahepatic) also increases occur, but usually do not exceed 200 to 300 IU/L.

b. Serum Alkaline Phosphatase: Alkaline phosphatase enzyme is found in a number of organs, most plentiful in bones and liver, then in small intestine, kidney and placenta. ***Placental isoenzyme of alkaline phosphatase is heatstable.***

Table 28.1: Differentiation of three types of jaundice

	Haemolytic or prehepatic jaundice	*Hepatic or parenchymatous jaundice*	*Obstructive or posthepatic jaundice*
I. *Causes:*	Due to excessive haemolysis (a) Intrinsic: defects in RB cells (b) Extrinsic: causes external to RB cells	Disease of parenchymal cells of liver, viz. Viral hepatitis, toxic jaundice Cirrhosis liver-fibrosis	Due to obstruction of biliary Passage (a) Extrahepatic-gall stones, tumors, enlarged Lymph nodes, etc. (b) Intrahepatic cholestasis.
II. *Clinical findings:*			
(a) Degree of jaundice	Usually low +	Marked jaundice ++ to +++	Marked jaundice ++ to +++
(b) Faeces	Dark coloured	Variable, Usually pale	Clay coloured
III. **Biochemical findings:** Based on bile pigment metabolism:			
1. VD Bergh reaction	Indirect, may be delayed Positive	Biphasic	Direct
2. Type of bile pigment in circulation	Unconjugated bilirubin	Mixture of conjugated & unconjugated bilirubin	Conjugated bilirubin
3. Serum bilirubin	Usually low 3 to 5 mg%	High, up to 20 mg%	Very high, may be up to 50 mg%
4. Bile Pigments in urine:			
• Bilirubin	Not detected	Present	Present++
• Urobilinogen	Increased ++	May be increased + or normal	Decrease or Absent
5. Faecal Stercobilinogen	Increased ++	Decreased	Decreased or Absent
IV. *Steatorrhoea:*	Not present	Present	Present
V. *Other biochemical Features:*			
1. Prothrombin time (PT)	Normal	Increased	Increased, After parental vitamin K becomes normal
2. *Enzyme assays:*			
• Aminotransferase activity ALT (S-GPT)	Usually normal	Marked increase +++ to ++++ (goes in Thousand units). Usually 500 to 1500 IU/L or may be more	Increased to ++. Usually 100 to 300 IU/L Do not exceed 300 IU/L
• Alkaline Phosphatase (ALP)	Normal	Increased slightly(+) ***usually less than 30 KA Units %***	Marked increase 30 to 100 KA units%, ***more than 35 KA units % suggests obstructive jaundice.***

Interpretations:

- *Normal range:* For serum ALP as per King Armstrong method is 3 to 13 KA Units/100 ml (23 to 92 IU/L).
- ***It is used for many years in differential diagnosis of jaundice.*** It is increased in both infectious hepatitis (viral hepatitis) and post-hepatic jaundice (extra hepatic obstruction) but the rise is usually much greater in cases of obstructive jaundice. ***Dividing Line which has been suggested is 35 KA units/100 ml.*** A value higher than 35 KA units/100 ml is strongly suggestive of diagnosis of obstructive jaundice, in which very high figures even up to 200 units or more may be found. There is certain amount of over-lapping mostly in the range of 30 to 45 KA Units/100 ml.
- Very high values are occasionally found in certain liver diseases, e.g. xanthomatous biliary cirrhosis in which there is no extra hepatic obstruction.
- Higher values are also obtained in *space occupying lesions of liver, e.g.*
  - Abscess,
  - Primary carcinoma (hepatoma),
  - Metastatic carcinoma,
  - Infiltrative lesions like lymphoma,
  - Granuloma and amyloidosis.

A diagnostic triad suggested:

- ***High serum ALP,***
- ***Impaired BSP-retention*** and
- ***Normal/or almost normal serum bilirubin.***

- Serum ALP is found to be normal in haemolytic jaundice.

Mechanism of increase in ALP in liver diseases: Increase in the activity of ALP in liver diseases is not due to hepatic cell disruption, nor to a failure of clearance, but rather **to increased synthesis of hepatic ALP.** The stimulus for this increased synthesis in patients with liver diseases has been attributed to bile duct obstruction either extrahepatically by stones, tumors, strictures or intrahepatically *by infiltrative disorders or "space occupying lesions."*

Note:

- The relation of the aminotransferase to ALP level may provide better evidence than either test alone, as to whether or not the jaundice is cholestatic.
- **High ALP with low aminotransferase activity is usual in cholestasis and the converse occurs in non-cholestatic jaundice.** It is, however, stressed that there are several intrahepatic causes of cholestasis such as primary biliary cirrhosis, acute alcoholic hepatitis and sclerosing cholangitis in which laparotomy is in-appropriate, Hence even after a confident diagnosis of cholestatic jaundice based on the LFTs, further investigation to define the site of obstruction is imperative.

c. **Other enzymes:** Quite a large number of enzyme estimations have been evolved like serum 5'-nucleotidase, serum cholinesterases, serum ornithine carbamoyl transferase (OCT), serum leucine aminopeptidase (LAP), serum γ-glutamyl transferase (γ-GT), etc. but they are not done routinely in the laboratory. These enzyme estimations and their value will not be discussed here.

☞ SALIENT POINTS TO REMEMBER

- The liver function can be evaluated by the tests based on its various functions, viz. on its abnormalities of bile pigment metabolism (serum bilirubin, V.D Bergh reaction), serum enzymes (transaminases and alkaline Phosphatase), metabolic capability (Galactose tolerance test), pro-thrombin formation (Prothrombin time and index).
- Serum bilirubin (normal < 1 mg/dl) is derived mainly from hemedegradation and it is mostly 75 percent is in conjugated form.
- V.D. Bergh reaction is a simple and specific test to identify the nature of increased serum bilirubin.
- Conjugated bilirubin gives a direct +ve test while the unconjugated bilirubin gives indirect positive test.

- Serum enzymes namely ALT/and AST, ALP are routinely done in almost all laboratories for assessment of liver function. Increase in activity of these enzymes indicate an impairment of liver function.
- In viral hepatitis, serum ALT may show values more than thousand.
- Serum ALP > 35 KA units per 100 ml is indicative of obstructive jaundice.
- Jaundice is due to elevated serum bilirubin and is visible clinically when it is > 2 mg/dl.
- The three types of jaundice, viz. haemolytic, obstructive and parenchymatous can be differentially diagnosed by combination of biochemical tests.
- Increased unconjugated bilirubin ↑ and indirect V.D. Bergh test are indicative of haemolytic jaundice.
- Increased conjugated bilirubin ↑, and direct +ve V.D. Bergh test are suggestive of obstructive jaudice.
- Biphasic reaction seen in hepatic parenchymatous jaudice.
- Bilirubinuria is always accompanied with direct V.D. Bergh reaction.
- The presence of Bilirubin in urine without urobilinogen is strongly suggestive of obstructive jaundice either intrahepatic or post hepatic.
- A complete absence of faecal urobilinogen is strongly suggestive of malignant obstruction.
- Increased urobilinogen in urine and absence of bilirubin in urine are strongly suggestive of haemolytic jaudice.
- Impaired galactose tolerance test, diminished serum albumin and reverse A: G ratio, and prolonged prothrombin time, increased blood NH_3 level and C.S.F glutamine level are associated with liver malfunction.

MULTIPLE CHOICE QUESTIONS

Give one correct answer:

1. **In a case of jaundice, there is no trace of bile pigments in urine, the most probable diagnosis is:**
   (a) Infectious hepatitis
   (b) Obstructive jaundice
   (c) Serum hepatitis
   (d) Haemolytic jaundice
   (e) None of the above.
2. **Jaundice is clinically detected in sclerae when serum bilirubin concentration reaches above:**
   (a) 0.5 to 1 mg/100 ml
   (b) 1 to 2 mg/100 ml
   (c) 2 to 3 mg/100 ml
   (d) 3 to 4 mg/100 ml
   (e) >5 mg/100 ml.
3. **When jaundice results from hepatitis, the unconjugted fraction of total serum bilirubin is usually:**
   (a) At least 50% (b) Less than 50%
   (c) 50 to 85% (d) 85 to 90%
   (e) 90 to 100%.
4. **Patients with hepatocellular jaundice, as compared to those with purely obstructive jaundice, tend to have:**
   (a) Higher serum alkaline phosphatase, LDH and ALT activity
   (b) Higher serum alkaline phosphatase activity, lower LDH and ALT activity,
   (c) Lower serum alkaline phosphatase activity, LDH and ALT acitivity
   (d) Lower serum alkaline phosphatase activity, higher LDH and ALT activity
   (e) None of the above
5. **The slow moving fraction of LDH isoenzyme LD_5 (M_4) is typically elevated in patients with:**
   (a) Myocardial infarction
   (b) Cerebro vascular accident (stroke)
   (c) Pancreatitis
   (d) Hepatitis
   (e) In all of the above.
6. **Drugs can cause jaundice by all of the following mechanisms *except:***
   (a) By causing haemolysis
   (b) By selective toxic effects on kupffer cells of liver

(c) By causing intrahepatic cholestasis
(d) By competition with bilirubin for albumin binding site
(e) By direct toxic effect on hepatic cells.

7. Prothrombin time in obstructive jaundice:
(a) Normal
(b) Decreases
(c) Becomes normal after vit K injection
(d) Increases after vit K injection
(e) None of the above.

8. Prothrombin time in parenchymal disease of the liver:
(a) Normal
(b) Decreases
(c) Increases
(d) Becomes normal after parenteral vit K injection
(e) None of the above.

9. Increased unconjugated bilirubin is found in all of the following *except:*
(a) Hemolytic anemia
(b) Crigglar Najjar syndrome
(c) Gilbert's syndrome
(d) Dubin Johnson syndrome
(e) Physiological jaundice in infants.

10. In the liver, a substantial proportion of the activity of the following enzyme is membrane bound
(a) Aspartate Aminotransferase
(b) Alanine Aminotransferase
(c) Lactate dehydrogenase
(d) Alkaline phosphatase
(e) Ornithine Transcarbamoylase.

ANSWERS

1. (d)	2. (c)	3. (b)
4. (d)	5. (d)	6. (b)
7. (c)	8. (c)	9. (d)
10. (d)		

29 Mechanism of Action of Drugs

When a drug is administered it produces an effect which can be seen or measured in most cases, e.g. effect of adrenaline or atropine. In most of the cases the mechanism of drug action or how the effect is produced is known and it may be conveniently grouped into the following categories:

I. PHYSICAL ACTION

The mechanism of action of some drugs can be explained on the basis of the simple physical property of drugs.

- *Osmotic Effect:* Magnesium sulphate and sodium sulphate when administered orally are not absorbed from intestine and exerts an osmotic effect and act as purgative. Similarly, if Mannitol is given intravenously being a non-threshold substance is excreted by the kidney acts as a diuretic.
- *Adsorptive Property:* Activated charcoal is used as an ingredient of universal antidote as it can adsorb poisons.
- *Emollients:* Fixed oils, vaseline are used for preventing the cracking of skin.
- *Demulscents:* Syrups, honey, glycerine are used for cough because of this property.
- *Radioactivity:* Radioisotopes are used because of selective localisation for diagnostic and therapeutic uses, e.g. I^{131}.
- *Radio opacity:* Organic iodine compounds are used as diagnostic agents for intravenous pyelography or angiography.
- *Color:* Fluorescein, a dye is used locally in the eye to see for corneal ulcers.

II. CHEMICAL ACTIONS

Some drugs react chemically extracellularly to produce effects.

- *Antacids:* Aluminium hydroxide and magnesium trisilicate can be used orally to reduce gastric acidity. Sodium bicarbonate can be used intravenously to counteract acidosis in cases of diabetic ketoacidosis.
- *Oxidizing agents:* Potassium permanganate can be used to oxidise alkaloids in cases of poisoning. Iodine is used as a germicidal agent because of its oxidising property.
- *Chelating agents:* Calcium acetate, dimercaprol, penicillamine are used in metallic poisoning because those form non-ionisable complex with metallic ions in the body.

III. ENZYMES

Almost all biological reactions are carried out under the catalytic influence of enzymes; hence enzymes form a very important target of drug action. The drugs may inhibit selectively the enzymes, such inhibitions may be competitive or non-competitive. (Refer for details the chapter on "Chemistry of enzymes").

(a) *Competitive (Equilibrium Type):* The drug competes with normal substrate or coenzyme, so that a new equilibrium is achieved in the presence of the drug.

* Contributed by Dr SK Gupta, MBBS, MD (Pharmacology), Ex Professor and Head of Pharmacology, Armed Forces of Medical College, Pune 411 040.

- Physostigmine and Neostigmine compete with acetylcholine for *"choline esterase"*.
- Sulphonamides compete with PABA (Para amino benzoic acid) for bacterial *"folate synthetase"*.
- Allopurinol competes with hypoxanthine for *"Xanthine oxidase"* which reduces uric acid formation.
- Carbidopa and methyldopa competes with levodopa for *"dopadecarboxylase"*.

A non-equilibrium type of enzyme inhibition can also occur with drugs which react with the same catalytic site of the enzyme but either form strong covalent bonds or have such high affinity for the enzyme that the normal substrate is not able to displace the inhibitor. For example, organophosphates react covalently with the esteratic site of the enzyme cholinesterase. Methotrexate has 50000 times higher affinity for *"dehydrofolate reductase"* than the normal substrate dihydrofolic acid (DHFA).

(b) ***Non-competitive inhibition:*** The inhibitor reacts with an adjacent site and not with the catalytic site but alters the enzyme in such a way that it looses its catalytic property.

Examples are:

Drugs	*Enzymes*
• Aspirin	- Cyclo-oxygenase
• Acetazolamide	- Carbonic anhydrase
• Disulfiram	- Aldehyde dehydrogenase
• Digoxin	- Na^+/K^+ – ATP ase
• Theophylline	- Phosphodiesterase
• Propyl thiouracil	- Peroxidase in thyroid.

IV. ACTION THROUGH RECEPTORS

A large number of drugs act through specific macromolecular components of the cell which regulate critical functions like enzyme activity, permeability, structural features, template functions, etc. These macromolecules or the sites on them which bind and interact with the drug are called receptors.

Receptor is defined as a binding site with functional correlate(s). Receptors are situated on the surface or inside the effector cell, and specific agonists combine with them to initiate the characteristic response.

- ***Agonist:*** It activates a receptor to produce an effect. It has affinity and intrinsic activity.
- ***Antagonist:*** It prevents the action of an agonist on a receptor but does not have any effect of its own. It has affinity but no intrinsic activity.
- ***Ligand:*** It is a molecule which attaches selectively to particular receptors or sites. The term only indicates affinity without regard to functional change: agonists and competitive antagonists are both ligands of the same receptor.

Many drugs act upon physiological receptors which mediate responses to transmitters, hormones, autacoids and other endogenous mediators, e.g. cholinergic, adrenergic, histaminergic and other receptors. In addition now some truly drug receptors have been described for which there are no known physiological ligands, e.g. benzodiazepine receptors, cardiac glycoside receptor, thiazide receptor.

Action effect sequence: ***"Drug action"*** and ***"Drug effect"*** are often loosely used inter-changeably, but are not synonymous.

- ***Drug action:*** It is the initial combination of the drug with its receptor resulting in a conformational change in the latter (in case of agonist) or prevention of conformational change through exclusion of the agonist (in case of antagonists).
- ***Drug effect:*** It is the ultimate change in biological function brought about as a consequence of drug action, through a series of intermediate steps.

Function of receptors: Receptors subserve two essential functions, viz. recognition of the specific ligand molecule and transduction of the signal into a response. Accordingly, the ***receptor molecule*** has a ***ligand binding domain*** and ***an effector domain (Fig. 29.1)*** which undergoes a functional conformational change.

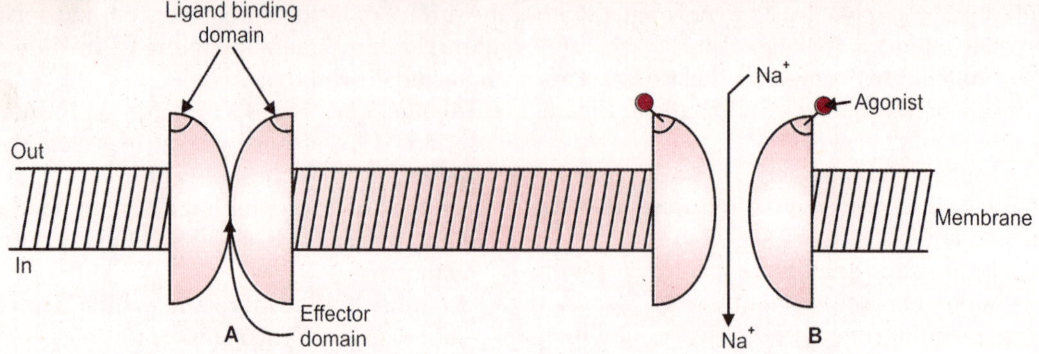

Fig. 29.1: Diagrammatic representation of direct receptor mediated operation of membrane ion channel

A. Normally the channel is closed

B. When two molecules of agonists (say acetyl choline) bind to the effector domain, the channel opens up and Na^+ enter the cell causing depolarization

Transducer Mechanisms (Signalling mechanisms)

Four basic mechanisms of transmembrane signalling are well understood and shown in *Fig. 29.2.*

Four Mechanisms are described below:

1. G-Protein coupled receptors: These are a family of cellmembrane receptors which are linked to the effector (enzyme/channel/carrier protein) through one or more GTP activated proteins (G-Proteins) for response effectuation.

There are three major effector pathways through which G-protein coupled receptors function.

(a) ***Adenylyl cyclase:*** cAMP pathway: Activation of adenylyl cyclase (AC) results in intracellular accumulation of second messenger cAMP which functions almost exclusively through cAMP - dependant protein kinase (PK_A). The PK_A phosphorylates and alters the function of many enzymes, ion channels, carriers, and structural proteins to manifest as increased contractility (heart), relaxation (smooth muscles), glycogenolysis, lipolysis, inhibition of secretion/mediator release, modulation of junctional transmission, hormone synthesis, etc. The reverse occurs when AC is inhibited through inhibitory G-Protein.

(b) ***Phospholipase C; IP_3-DAG Pathway:*** Activation of Phospholipase C (PLc) hydrolyses the membrane phospholipid ***"Phosphatidyl inositol 4, 5 bi-phosphate" (PIP_2)*** to generate the second messenger ***"inositol 1, 4, 5 triphosphate" (IP_3)*** and ***diacyl glycerol (DAG).*** IP_3 mobilises Ca^{++} from intracellular organellar depots and DAG enhances Protein Kinase C (PKc) activation by Ca^{++}. Cytosolic Ca^{++} (third messenger in this setting) is a regulator through calmodulin (CAM), PKc and other effectors-mediates/modulates contraction, secretion/transmitter release, neuronal excitability, intracellular movements, membrane function, metabolism, cell proliferation, etc. Like AC, PLc can also be inhibited through inhibitory G-Protein when opposite responses would be expected.

(c) ***Channel regulation:*** The activated G-Proteins can also open or close ionic channels specific for Ca^{++}, K^+ or Na^+ and bring about hyperpolarisation/depolarisation/changes in intracellular Ca^{++}; e.g., ***Gs opens Ca^{++} channels in myocardium and skeletal muscle as well as close neuronal Ca^{++} channels***. Physiological responses like changes in ionotropy chronotropy, transmitter release, neuronal activity and smooth muscle relaxation follow. Receptors found to regulate ionic channels through G-Proteins are given below.

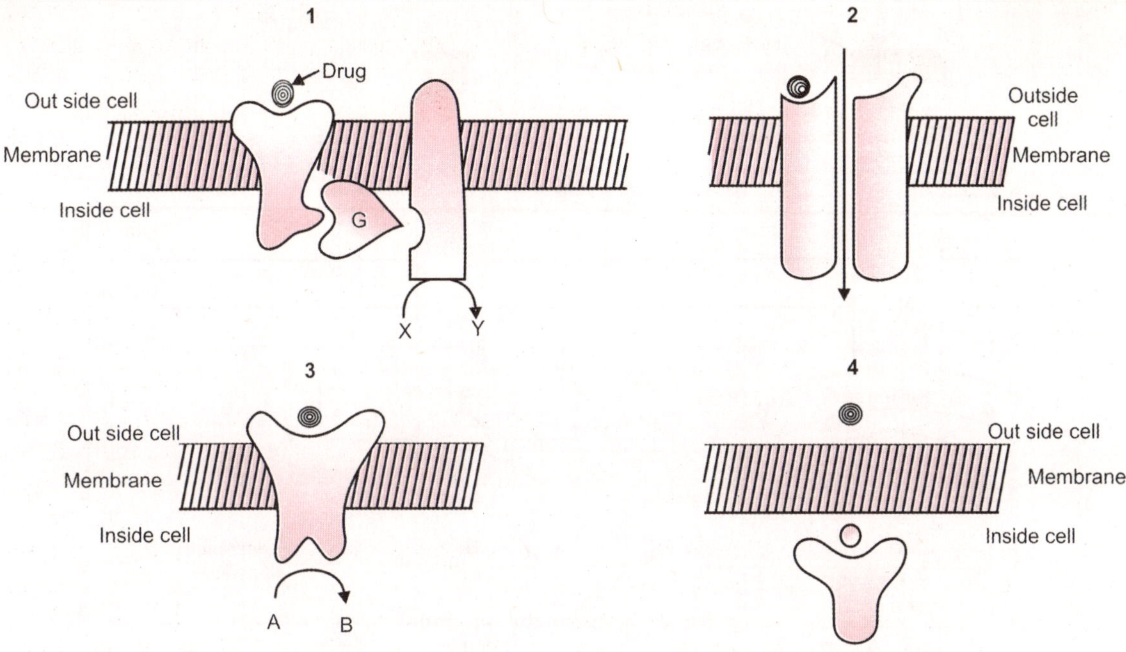

Fig. 29.2: Showing four basic mechanisms of transmembrane signalling

Key:
1. The signal binds to a cell surface receptor linked to an effector enzyme by a G-Protein.
2. The signal binds to and directly regulates the opening of an ion channel.
3. The signal binds to the extracellular domain of a transmembrane protein, thereby activating an enzymatic activity of its cytoplasmic domain.
4. A lipid soluble chemical signal crosses the plasma membrane and acts on an intracellular receptor (which may be an enzyme or a regulator of gene transcription).

Ca^{++} ↑	Ca^{++} ↓	K^+ ↑
• Adrenergic β-receptors (Heart, skeletal muscle)	• Dopamine D_2 • GABA-B • Opioid K • Adenosine A_1 • Somatostatin	• Adrenergic α_1-receptors • Muscarine M_2 • Dopamine-D_2 • 5-HT_{1A} • GABA-B • Opioid-μ, δ

2. Receptors with intrinsic ion channels: These cell surface receptors enclose ion selective channels (for Na^+, K^+, Ca^{++} or Cl^-) within their molecules. Agonist binding opens the channel and causes depolarisation/hyperpolarisation/changes in cytosolic ionic composition, depending on the ion that flows through. The nicotinic cholinergic, GABA-A, Glycine (inhibitory) excitatory aminoacids and 5-HT_3 receptors fall in this category.

Thus, in these receptors, agonists directly operate ion channels, without the intervention of any coupling protein or second messenger. The onset and offset of responses through this class of receptors is the fastest.

3. Enzymatic receptors: This class of receptors themselves are enzymatic proteins. The agonist binding site and the catalytic site lie respectively on the outer and innerface of the plasma membrane. These two domains are interconnected through a single transmembrane stretch of peptide chain.

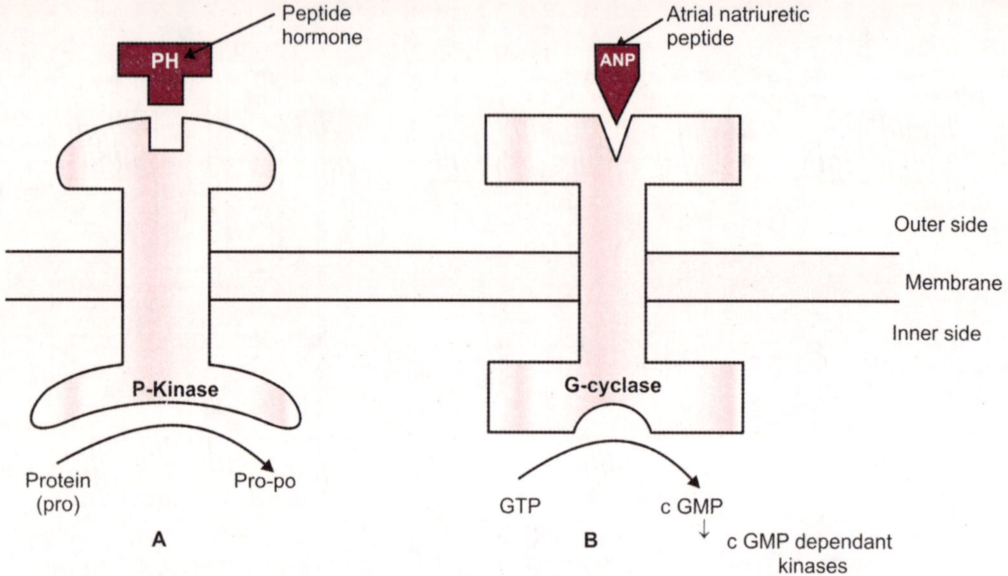

Fig. 29.3: Enzymatic receptors

A. In case of peptide hormones (pH) and some cytokinase use tyrosine protein kinase (in case of insulin, epidermal growth factor, certain interleukins) and the intracellular events are triggered by phosphorylation of relevant proteins. In addition, the receptors itself gets auto-phosphorylated on tyrosine residues which promotes association of several receptor molecules → organising the complex signalling mechanism. A common feature of this class of receptors is that their activation and association also promotes receptor internalisation and down regulation.

B. ***The enzyme can also be guanylyl cyclase (GC) as in the case of atrial natriuretic peptide (ANP):*** Agonist activation of the receptor generates cGMP as the second messenger in the cytosol which inturn activates cGMP-dependant protein kinase and modulates cellular activity.

Some peptide hormones and some cytokines utilise this class of receptors.

4. Receptors regulating gene expression (Transcription factors): In contrast to the above three classes of receptors, these are intracellular (cytoplasmic or nuclear) soluble proteins which respond to lipid soluble chemical messengers that penetrate the cell. The receptor-protein (specific for each hormone/regulator) is inherently capable of binding to specific genes but is kept inhibited till the hormone binds near its carboxy terminus and exposes the DNA binding regulatory segment located in the middle of the molecule. Attachment of the receptor protein to the genes facilitates their expression so that specific messenger RNA is synthesized on the template of the gene. This messenger RNA moves to the ribosomes and directs synthesis of specific proteins which regulate the activity of the target cells. All steroidal hormones (glucocorticoids, mineralocorticoids, androgens, oestrogens, progesterone), thyroxines, Vit-D and Vit A function in this manner. This transduction mechanism is then slowed in its course of action.

Biochemistry of AIDS

INTRODUCTION

The acquired immunodeficiency syndrome (AIDS) was recognized in the United States in 1981 with a sudden outbreak of opportunistic infections, *Pneumocystis carinii* pneumonia, and Kaposi's sarcoma (KS). On the basis of the epidemiologic features, association with the loss of $CD4^+$ lymphocytes and immunosuppression, and likely infectious etiology, a new human retrovirus was pursued as a causal agent. The field of retrovirology had opened just a decade earlier with the description of *reverse transcriptase* (RT) and with the discovery of human T cell leukemia/lymphoma virus type I and type II (HTLV-1 and HTLV-II), the first two known human retroviruses, in 1979 and 1981 (reported in 1980 and 1982, respectively). ***By 1984, the detection, isolation, and propagation of the human immunodeficiency virus type 1 (HIV-1), the third human retrovirus, had led to the development of a diagnostic test, an increasingly detailed understanding of the molecular biology of this virus, and, most important, the beginning of rational antiviral therapy.*** Human immunodeficiency virus (HIV) is the most significant emerging pathogen. Since recognition in 1981 HIV has produced a world wide epidemic.

DISCOVERY OF HIV

The first indication that AIDS could be caused by a retrovirus came in 1983 when **Barre-Sinoussi** and coworkers at the Pasteur Institute recovered a *reverse transcriptase* containing virus from the lymph node of a man with persistent lymphadenopathy syndrome (LAS). However further studies in 1983 by **Luc Montagnier** and co workers indicated that this human retrovirus although similar to HTLV in infecting $CD4^+$ lymphocytes but instead of propagating in cell culture as does HTLV, ***it killed $CD4^+$ cells***. **Robert Gallo** and his team in 1984 reported characterization of another human retrovirus distinct from HTLV that they called HTLV III. **JA Levy** and coworkers in the year 1984 reported identification of retrovirus from AIDS patient in San Francisco and named it as AIDS associated retrovirus (ARV). **Rabson and his colleagues** in the year 1985 found that the proteins and the genome of the AIDS virus were distinct from HTLV. For all these reasons, in 1986 the International Committee on Taxonomy of Viruses recommended giving the AIDS virus a separate name, the Human Immunodeficiency Virus (HIV).

RETROVIRAL BACKGROUND

Retroviruses constitute a large and diverse family of **enveloped RNA viruses** that use as a replication strategy the transcription of virion RNA into linear double-stranded DNA with subsequent integration into the host genome. The characteristic enzyme used for this process, an ***RNA-dependent*** *DNA polymerase* that reverses the flow of genetic information, is known as ***reverse transcriptase***. The unique lifestyle of the retrovirus involves two forms, a ***DNA provirus*** and ***an RNA-containing infectious virion***. The basic structure,

*Contributed by Lt Col AK Sahni, MD, DNBm PhD and Lt Col RM Gupta, MD, DNB, Associate Professors, Department of Microbiology, Armed Forces Medical College, Pune 411 040.

genetic organization, and life cycle of HIV-1 are similar to those of most retroviruses, but with some additional features.

As RNA viruses, retroviruses have the survival advantage of great genetic diversity. As viruses with a DNA intermediate in their replication cycle, they also have the advantage of latency, as do many DNA viruses, but even more so because the DNA provirus is integrated into the chromosomal DNA. As a $CD4^+$ T-cell-and macrophage-tropic virus, HIV has the advantage of reducing the effectiveness of host immune attacks. Retroviruses are typically 100 nm in diameter and contain two single strands of RNA, which permits recombination between the strands. ***The typical genome is 10-kilo bases (Kb) in size*** and ***contains three major structural genes***, namely, **gag, pol,** and **env** HIV-1 also contains several additional genes; similar "extra" genes-first described in HTLV-1 are essential to viral replication. These complicated genomes are characteristic of human retroviruses. Although sharing T-cell tropism, genomic complexity, and functional similarities, the four known human retroviruses-HIV-1 and 2 and HTLV-I and II and related animal viruses belong to two different groups.

Retroviruses have been classified by a number of different biologic features, and at present, ***infectious retroviruses are grouped into at least seven genera. The human retroviruses include lentiviruses (HIV-1 and 2), onc viruses (HTLV-I and II), and human endogenous virus (HERV-K).***

STRUCTURE AND MOLECULAR FEATURES OF HIV

VIRION STRUCTURE

HIV-1 virion ***(Fig. 30.1)***, according to electron microscopic observation, has a **cone shaped core** or **capsid** which consists of:

a. The major capsid protein p24;
b. The nucleocapsid protein, p7/p9;
c. The diploid single stranded RNA genome; and
d. The three viral enzymes, protease, reverse transcriptase and *integrase.*

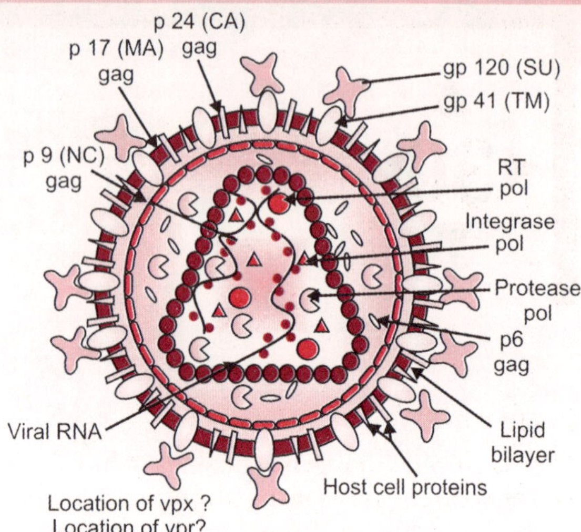

Fig. 30.1: Schematic diagram of HIV virion

Reverse transcriptase is the hallmark of a retrovirus and is capable of transcribing its genomic RNA into double stranded DNA. This DNA copy of the retroviral genome is called a **"provirus"**. After integration into the host genome, the provirus serves as a template for cellular *DNA-dependent RNA polymerases* to generate new viral RNA genomes as well as shorter subgenomic messenger RNAs. The unspliced and singly spliced viral RNAs are translated into the protein components of the viral core and the envelope proteins and the multispliced viral RNAs into the small accessory/regulatory proteins. **Surrounding the capsid lies the matrix constituted by myristylated p17 gag protein**, which is located underneath the virion envelope. The matrix protein is involved in the early stages of the viral replication cycle and plays a part in the formation and transport of the preintegra-tion DNA complex into the nucleus of the host cell. The **virion envelope** consists of a lipid bilayer membrane, derived from the host cell. Like all retroviruses, an envelope consisting of viral glycoproteins embedded in a host cell derived lipid bilayer surrounds HIV-1. ***The virus surface is constituted by 72 knob containing trimers and tetramers.*** The **envelope glycoproteins are synthesized as gp160** precursor in the rough endoplasmic reticulum. Aspargine linked, high mannose sugar chains are added to gp 160, which is then assembled into oligomers. These are then transported to the Golgi apparatus where cellular proteases cleave gp 160 into the external surface (SU) envelope protein or gp 120 and transmembrane (TM) protein or gp 41. These proteins are transported to the cell surface, where part of the central and N-terminal portion of the gp 41 is also expressed on the outside of the virion. The gp 41 glycoprotein has an ectodomain that is largely responsible for trimerization. Most of the surface exposed elements of the mature oligomeric envelope glycoprotein complex are located in gp 120. Selected, well-exposed, carbohydrates on the gp 120 glycoprotein are modified in the Golgi by the addition of complex sugars. The gp 120 and gp 41 are maintained in the assembled trimer by noncovalent, labile interactions between the gp 41 ectodomain and discontinuous structures composed of N- and C-terminal gp 120 sequences. ***For entry of the virus in the target host cell, the viral envelope fuses with the plasma membrane of the cell by a process mediated by the viral envelope glycoproteins.***

GENOME

The ***size of HIV-1 genome is about 9.8 kb*** with open reading frames coding for several viral gene products which are **flanked on each end by long terminal repeat (LTR) sequences *(Fig. 30.2)*. The three major genes are gag, pol and env.**

- The **gag gene codes** for the gag precursor protein p55, which is **cleaved by viral protease to generate p24, p17, p9 and p6 gag proteins.**
- The **pol gene** codes for the pol precursor, which is cloven into ***reverse transcriptase (RT), protease (PR),*** and ***integrase (IN)***. Protease processes the gag and pol polyproteins. Integrase is involved in the integration of the proviral DNA, generated from the viral RNA genome by reverse transcriptase into the host cell chromosomal DNA.
- The **env gene** codes for the envelope precursor gp 160, which is cloven into gp 120 and gp 41. Gene products of other spliced mRNA make up various viral regulatory and accessory proteins.
- **The tat gene** codes for the transactivating protein. **Tat**, which along with certain cellular proteins, interacts with a region in the RNA loop formed at the 3′ LTR region called **Tat responsive element (TAR)**. ***Tat is involved in the upregulation of HIV replication.***
- **The rev gene:** produces **Rev** (regulator of viral protein expression). Rev interacts with a cis acting RNA loop structure called the **Rev responsive element or RRE**. The Rev protein promotes the export from the nucleus of the unspliced or singly spliced viral RNAs that act, respectively, as genomic RNA/template for the translation of gag/pol proteins and template for envelope proteins. ***In the absence of Rev, no structural proteins are made.***

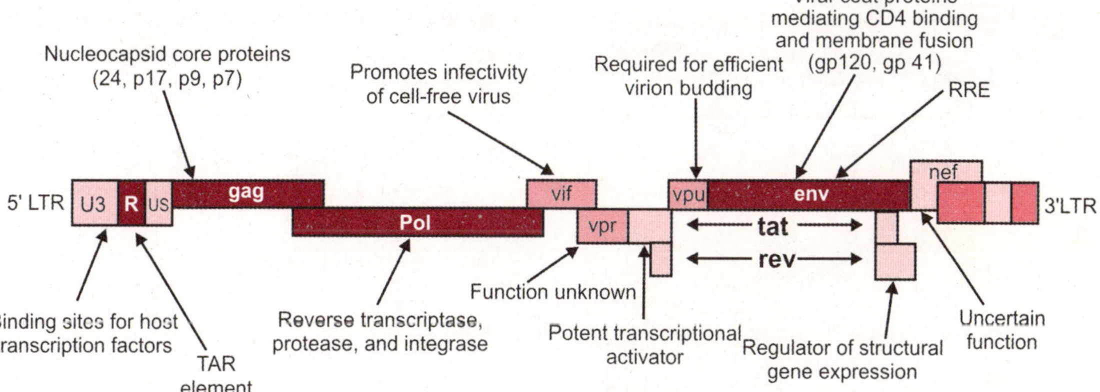

Fig. 30.2: Schematic diagram of HIV genome

- **The Nef gene:** Another viral gene product, Nef, coded by the *nef* gene, appears to have a variety of potential functions, including downregulation of viral expression. It appears that the Nef mRNA represents the majority of the earliest mRNA species following integration.

  However, most studies have indicated a pleiotropic function of Nef and that it is not always associated with downregulation of replication. **Tat, Rev, and Nef** are not incorporated into virion particles but are first viral components produced from multiply spliced viral mRNA.

  The **other accessory viral gene** products are **Vif, Vpr** and **Vpu**.
- **Vif** is reported to increase virus infectivity and cell-to-cell transmission. ***It helps in proviral DNA synthesis*** and might play a role in virion assembly.
- **Vpr** ***helps in virus replication.***
- **Vpu**, whose expression appears to be regulated by Vpr, ***helps in release of the virus.***

VIRUS LIFE CYCLE

The life cycle of HIV-1 can be considered in **two distinct phases** *(Fig. 30.3)*.

The **initial** early events occur within a short time and include viral attachment, entry, reverse transcription, entry into the nucleus, and integration of the double-stranded DNA (the provirus).

The **second phase** occurs over the lifetime of the infected cell as viral and cellular proteins regulate the production of viral proteins and new infectious virions.

HIV is an RNA virus whose hallmark is the reverse transcription of its genomic RNA to DNA by the enzyme reverse transcriptase. The replication cycle of HIV begins with the high-affinity binding of the gp120 protein via a portion of its V1 region near the N terminus to its receptor on the host cell surface, the CD4 molecule.

The CD4 molecule is a 55-kDa protein found predominantly on a subset of T lymphocytes that are responsible for helper or inducer function in the immune system. It is also expressed on the surface of monocytes/macrophages and dendritic/Langerhans cells. In order for HIV-1 to fuse to and enter its target cell, it must also bind to one of a group of co-receptors.

The **two major co-receptors** for **HIV-1** are **CCR5** and **CXCR4**. ***Both receptors belong to the family of seven-transmembrane-domain G***

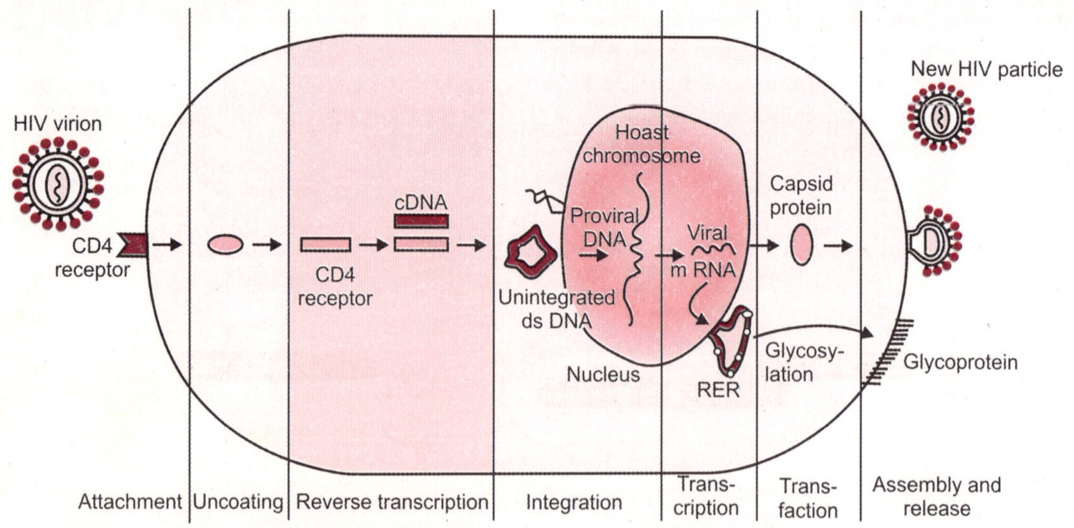

Fig. 30.3: Schematic diagram of HIV life cycle

protein-coupled cellular receptors, and the use of one or the other or both receptors by the virus for entry into the cell is an important determinant of the cellular tropism of the virus (see below for details). Following binding, the conformation of the viral envelope changes dramatically, and fusion with the host cell membrane occurs in a coiled-spring fashion via the newly exposed gp41 molecule; the ***HIV genomic RNA is uncoated and internalized into the target cell. The reverse transcriptase enzyme, which is contained in the infecting virion, then catalyzes the reverse transcription of the genomic RNA into double-stranded DNA.*** The DNA translocates to the nucleus, where it is integrated randomly into the host cell chromosomes through the action of another virally encoded enzyme, *integrase*. This provirus may remain transcriptionally inactive (latent), or it may manifest varying levels of gene expression, up to active production of virus.

Cellular activation plays an important role in the life cycle of HIV and is critical to the pathogenesis of HIV disease. Following initial binding and internalization of virions into the target cell, incompletely reverse-transcribed DNA intermediates are labile in quiescent cells and will not integrate efficiently into the host cell genome unless cellular activation occurs shortly after infection. Furthermore, some degree of activation of the host cell is required for the initiation of transcription of the integrated proviral DNA into either genomic RNA or mRNA. In this regard, activation of HIV expression from the latent state depends on the interaction of a number of cellular and viral factors. Following transcription, HIV mRNA is translated into proteins that undergo modification through glycosylation, myristylation, phosphorylation, and cleavage. The viral particle is formed by the assembly of HIV proteins, enzymes, and genomic RNA at the plasma membrane of the cells. Budding of the progeny virion occurs through the host cell membrane, where the core acquires its external envelope. The virally encoded protease then catalyzes the cleavage of the gag-pol precursor to yield the mature virion. ***Each point in the life cycle of HIV is a real or potential target for therapeutic intervention.***

MODES OF TRANSMISSION

The transmission of a virus can be greatly influenced by the amount of infectious virus in a body fluid and the extent of contact with that body fluid. Epidemiological studies conducted during 1981 and 1982 first indicated that the major routes of transmission of AIDS were intimate sexual contact and contaminated blood. Moreover, it became evident that transfusion recipients and hemophiliacs could contract the virus from blood or blood products and mothers could transfer the causative agent to newborn infants. ***These three principal means of transmission • blood, •sexual contact and • mother-to-child-have not changed. The other modes of transmission of the virus are by • sharing of the needles by the intravenous drug users and by • needle stick injuries.***

Blood and Blood Products

All blood samples of HIV sero-positive individual contain circulating infectious virus whether the individual is asymptomatic or has AIDS. HIV is readily found during acute (primary) infection. Subsequently, within weeks, the level of free virus detected in the blood is markedly reduced. The total amount of infectious free virus present in the blood of asymptomatic individuals averages 100 IP (infectious particles) per ml. In the years before the screening of blood, HIV present in blood and blood products such as factors VIII and IX could infect transfusion recipients and hemophiliacs. ***The potential risk of infection of transfusion recipients depends on the virus load and appears to be greatest as an infected individual (as donor) advances to disease.*** In hemophiliacs, this transmission could be caused only by free virus and was associated with receipt of many vials of unheated clotting factors.

The Transmission of HIV by Genital Fluids

The transmission of HIV by genital fluids most probably occurs through virus-infected cells since these can be present in larger numbers than free virus in the body fluids. Moreover, recent studies suggest that these infected cells transfer HIV to epithelial cells best when present in seminal fluid, because cell-to-cell contact is increased most probably via factors in semen. The presence of different levels of infected cells in the genital fluids probably explains the variations in virus transmission among sexual partners. **The amount of virus in genital fluids is important for sexual transmission.** Generally, 10 to 30% of seminal and vaginal fluid specimens have shown the presence of free infectious virus and/or virus-infected cells. The finding of HIV in the bowel mucosa itself provides another reason, besides abrasions, for the high risk of transmission associated with anogenital contact.

Transmission from Mother to Child

Mother to child transmission of HIV includes transmission during pregnancy, during delivery, and through breast-feeding. HIV-1 is transmitted to the fetus or infant by 13 to 48% of infected mothers. Data from various countries suggest that as many as 15% of babies' breast fed by HIV infected mothers may become infected through breast-feeding.

Transmission by Needle Stick Injury

The chances of transmission of HIV from infected individual by needle stick injury are only 0.03-0.3%.

NATURAL HISTORY OF HIV INFECTION

According to CDC classification AIDS case definition includes all HIV-infected persons who have less than 200 $CD4^+$ T-lymphocytes/µl, or a $CD4^+$ T-lymphocyte percentage of total lymphocytes of less than 14. This includes the addition of three clinical conditions pulmonary tuberculosis, recurrent pneumonia, and invasive cervical cancer and retains the 23 clinical conditions in the AIDS surveillance case definition published in 1987. HIV infected individuals are classified as asymptomatic (A), symptomatic (B), and AIDS cases representing AIDS indicator conditions (C) depending on their CD4 counts and associated symptoms. ***$CD4^+$ counts are divisible into three categories (1) > 500/µl, (2) 200-499/µl and (3) < 200/µl.***

Classically the natural history of HIV infection *(Fig. 30.4)* can be divided into **three distinct stages**,

- *acute primary infection syndrome,*
- *asymptomatic latent state* and
- *symptomatic HIV infection, AIDS.*
- **Acute primary infection syndrome** *can be asymptomatic*, or it may be associated with influenza like illness with fevers, malaise, diarrhea and neurological symptoms such as headache. This illness usually lasts **2 to 3 weeks, with full recovery.**
- **Asymptomatic infection** refers to the asymptomatic carrier state that follows initial infection. *It typically lasts for many years, with a gradual decline in the number of circulating $CD4^+$ T cells.* In a minority of cases, infection does not proceed beyond this asymptomatic phase and CD4 counts remain stable.
- **Symptomatic HIV infection and AIDS**, *typically occurs about 10 to 12 years after initial HIV-1 infection.* The stage is **defined by more serious AIDS-defining illnesses and/or by a decline in the circulating CD4 count to below 200 cells/mml.** Examples of AIDS-defining illnesses include infections like, *Pneumocystis carinii pneumonia, Mycobacterial tuberculosis, esophageal candidiasis, toxoplasmosis of the brain, CMV retinitis and cancers: cervical cancer, Kaposi's sarcoma, various B-cell lymphomas linked to EBV, HIV-related encephalopathy, HIV-related wasting syndrome, lymphoid interstitial pneumonia.*

The **pathogenesis of HIV-1 infection** *(Fig. 30.5)* reflects a complex interplay between virus replication, virus-induced lymphocyte killing, and the immune response of the host. **HIV-1 replication and virus load are the driving forces behind viral pathogenesis**. This has been convincingly demonstrated by several studies. Studies have shown that among persons with

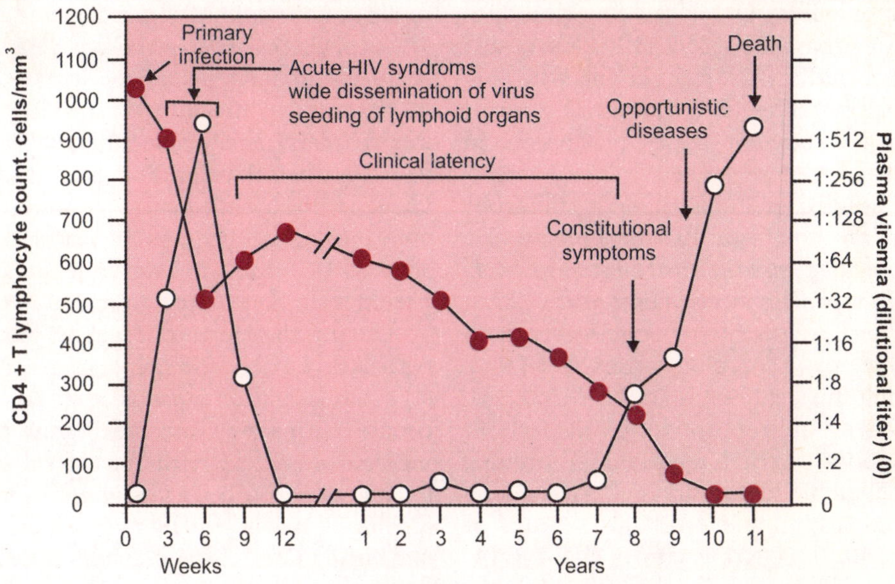

Fig. 30.4: Natural history of HIV infection
(*Adapted from* Pantaleo G Graziosi C Fauci AS: New concepts in the immunopathogenesis of human immunodeficiency virus infection. N Engl J Med 1993, 328: 327-335)

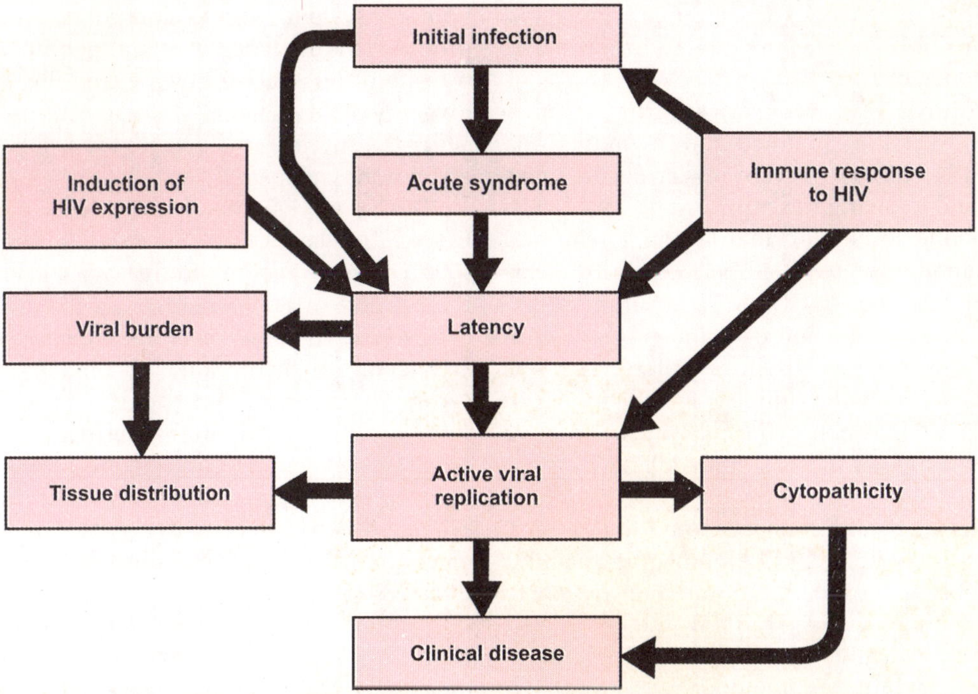

Initial infection
Acute syndrome
Immune response to HIV
Induction of HIV expression
Latency
Viral burden
Tissue distribution
Active viral replication
Cytopathicity
Clinical disease

Fig. 30.5: Pathogenesis of HIV infection and interaction of multiple factors (*Adapted from* Fauci AS: Multifactorial nature of human immunodeficiency virus disease: Iimplications for therapy. Science1993, 12, 262[5136]: 1011-8)

equivalent baseline $CD4^+$ T cell counts, individuals with high baseline plasma HIV-1 RNA loads died more rapidly than individuals with low baseline plasma HIV-1 RNA loads. This initial set point is indicative of disease progression in the patient.

In the natural course of infection, a primary or acute viral infection results within a few weeks. ***During the acute phase the viral doubling time is 10 hrs and the peak of viremia occurs at 21 days after infection*** the virus thus replicates to very high levels and there is a sharp decline in the $CD4^+$ T cells. During this acute phase of HIV infection, there is active viral replication, particularly in $CD4^+$ lymphocytes, and a marked HIV viremia. This peripheral blood viremia is at least as high as 50,000-copies/ml and often in the range of 1,000,000 to 10,000,000 copies/ml of HIV-1 RNA. ***High titers of cytopathic HIV are detectable in the blood*** so that ***the p24 antigen test is usually (but not always) positive,*** while HIV antibody tests (such as enzyme immunoassay) are often negative in the first three weeks. The viremia is greater in persons whose primary HIV infection is symptomatic.

Within a few weeks, a specific immune response to HIV is mounted, and viral replication is greatly reduced thereby lowering the virus load, and allowing the number of $CD4^+$ T cells to rebound to near-normal levels. A temporal association was identified between the appearance of virus specific $CD8^+$ CTL in the peripheral blood and the decline of primary viremia in acutely infected patients. In several studies it was established that the initial burst of viremia in acute HIV-1 infection is controlled by the immune system primarily by the Cytotoxic T cell responses. The neutralizing antibodies seem to appear later during the infection, at about 8 to 10 weeks.

Thereafter, the $CD4^+$ T lymphocytes rebound in number after primary HIV infection, but not to pre-infection levels. The HIV infection then becomes clinically "latent". Though no clinical signs and symptoms are apparent, the immune system primarily deteriorates through depletion of $CD4^+$ lymphocytes. The virus continues to replicate in lymphoid organs, despite a low level or lack of viremia. HIV can be found trapped extracellularly, in the follicular dendritic cell network of germinal centers in lymphoid tissues or intracellularly, as either latent or replicating virus in mononuclear cells. The **period of clinical latency** with HIV infection, when infected persons appear in good health, **can be variable—from as short as 18 months to over 15 years. This latent period lasts, on average, from 8 to 10 years.**

During the chronic infection phase HIV-1 replicates at a rate of 180 generations per year, for a period of ten or more years. The viral load continues to slowly but inexorably increase in most patients. The ***HIV RNA levels rise by roughly 0.1 log 10 per year. It has been estimated that roughly 10 billion viral particles are produced and one billion $CD4^+$ T lymphocytes are killed each day.*** Owing to the highly error prone reverse transcription, this leads to rapid emergence of genetic variants (quasispecies), that eventually escape all means of controls excised by the body's immune system. **Nowak and colleagues** have proposed the existence of an **"antigenic diversity threshold"**, in which the ever-expanding genetic diversity of HIV-1 eventually exhausts the capacity of the immune system to respond, resulting in an immune collapse.

The hallmarks of emergence of HIV infection from clinical latency, are a marked decline in the CD4 lymphocyte count and an increase in viremia. Replication of HIV increases as the infection progresses. There is loss of normal lymph node architecture as the immune system fails. Before serologic and immunologic markers for HIV infection became available, **clinical criteria established emergence from latency by development of generalized lymphadenopathy.** This condition, described by the term **persistent generalized lymphadenopathy (PGL),** is not life threatening.

Another phase of HIV infection described clinically, but no longer commonly diagnosed in practice, is the condition known as **AIDS-related complex (ARC),** which is not necessarily preceded by PGL. ARC lacks only the opportunistic infections and neoplasms, which define AIDS. ARC patients usually show ***symptoms of fatigue, weight loss, and night sweats, along with superficial fungal infections of the mouth (oral thrush) and fingernails and toenails*** (onychomycosis). It is uncommon for HIV-infected persons to die at the stage of ARC. The staging of HIV disease progression through the use of CD4 lymphocyte counts and plasma HIV-1 RNA levels has made use of the terms PGL and ARC obsolete.

The **stage of clinical disease**, AIDS, is reached years after initial infection is marked by the **appearance of one or more of the typical opportunistic infections or neoplasms** diagnostic of AIDS by definitional criteria. The progression to clinical AIDS is also marked by the appearance of syncytia-forming (SI) variants of HIV in about half of HIV-infected patients. These SI viral variants, derived from non-syncytia-forming (NSI) variants, have greater $CD4^+$ cell tropism and are associated with more rapid $CD4^+$ cell decline. The SI variants typically arise in association with a peripheral blood CD4 lymphocyte count between 400 and 500/microliter, prior to the onset of clinical AIDS. Appearance of the SI phenotype of HIV also serves as a marker for progression to AIDS that is independent of $CD4^+$ cell counts.

IMMUNOLOGICAL RESPONSE IN HIV

HIV-1, as most other viruses, **induces a strong immunological response during infection.** In many other viral infections the combined action of host humoral and cellular immune responses clears the virus from the body after a primary replication state of the virus. In HIV-1 infection also, the concentration of the virus in the blood decreases after a primary state of rapid replication and virus production, but some virus remains in the body. The number of lymphocytes carrying the proviral DNA is low in the blood, but higher amounts of infected cells and virus particles may be seen in the lymph nodes and spleen. ***This suggests that during clinical latency, HIV accumulates in the lymphoid organs and replicates actively despite a low viral burden and low to absent viral replication in Peripheral blood mononuclear cells (PBMCs). Therefore, a state of true microbiological latency does not exist during the course of HIV infection.***

Following initial exposure to HIV, the generation of cellular immune responses against HIV may take a while to develop, therefore neutralizing antibodies against free virus are important to dampen initial viral spread. Subsequently, generation of ***HIV-specific T-helper lymphocytes (THL)*** *and* ***Cytotoxic T Lymphocyte (CTL)*** responses becomes important in removing HIV-infected cells from the host and in controlling further activation and spread of the virus once established in the host. ***Thus, both arms of the immune system are important in the immunological control of HIV infection.***

Humoral immunity involves neutralizing antibodies directed at various epitopes on the viral surface. Cellular responses, particularly the CTLs, are targeted at the epitopes present on an HIV infected host cell. HIV specific THLs and generation of various cytokines trigger the CTL response. The HIV specific THLs are recruited when $CD4^+$ cells are activated. Antigen presenting cells (APCs) such as dendritic cells and macrophages engulf the infecting virus, break it down into smaller epitopes and present this to the CD_4^+ cells, thus activating it. However, in most cases of HIV infection, the rapid loss of HIV-specific THLs and functional abnormalities in a variety of other immune cells ultimately lead to the establishment of chronic infection with high viral load, which, if untreated over time, results in further progressive loss of immune function. Moreover, the neutralizing antibodies have a limited ability to bind to gp 120, as it is heavily glycosylated.

The peripheral blood does not accurately reflect the actual state of HIV disease, particularly early in the clinical course of HIV infection. Viral replication in lymphoid organs takes place despite a vigorous production of antibodies against most viral proteins, as well as a cellular response involving both cytotoxic and natural killer cells. ***Eventually the persistent***

replication of the virus leads to the breakdown of the immune system, immune deficiency and the death of the host, usually due to opportunistic infection.

There are several mechanisms, which might explain the persistence of the virus and escape from the immune clearance. • ***The virus might enter a quiescent state of replication,*** where provirus expression and antigen production are down regulated, so that no antigenic viral proteins are expressed and become inaccessible to the immunological clearance. • ***The virus may also replicate in tissues where it escapes the immune system.*** Also, • ***if the virus destroys all CD_4^+ T cells that carry specificity's needed for virus neutralization*** or specific killing of infected cells, or stops expression of neutralization epitopes, it would be able to continue replication in the body. • A fourth and perhaps most likely mechanism for escape, ***is the generation of viral variants during replication, with point mutation in antigenic sites.*** Such point mutants cannot be recognized by previously generated immunity as a result the virus escapes neutralization and killing, leading to persistent infection and replication. Ten billion new HIV virions, with a half-life in plasma of only 6 hrs are produced each day. This results from a relatively short virus life cycle (the time from virion binding to the cell to the release of progeny) of approximately 1,2 days.

DIAGNOSIS OF HIV INFECTION

The diagnosis of HIV infection depends upon the demonstration of antibodies to HIV and/or the direct detection of HIV or one of its components.

- The **standard screening test for HIV infection** is the **ELISA**, also referred to as an **enzyme immunoassay (EIA)**. This solid-phase assay is an extremely **good screening** test with a **sensitivity of > 99.5%**. Most diagnostic laboratories use a commercial EIA kit that contains antigens from both HIV-1 and HIV-2 and thus are able to detect either. These kits use both natural and recombinant antigens and are continuously updated to increase their sensitivity to newly discovered species, such as group O viruses. ***EIA tests are generally scored as • positive*** (highly reactive), • ***negative*** (nonreactive), or • ***indeterminate*** (partially reactive). While the EIA is an extremely sensitive test, **it is not optimal with regard to specificity**. This is particularly true in studies of low-risk individuals, such as volunteer blood donors. In this latter population, only 10% of EIA-positive individuals are subsequently confirmed to have HIV infection. Among the factors associated with false-positive EIA tests are antibodies to class II antigens, autoantibodies, hepatic disease, recent influenza vaccination, and acute viral infections. For these reasons, anyone suspected of having HIV infection based upon a positive or inconclusive EIA rsult must have the result confirmed with a more specific assay.
- The ***most commonly used confirmatory test is the western blot.*** This assay takes advantage of the fact that ***multiple HIV antigens of different, well-characterized molecular weights elicit the production of specific antibodies.*** These antigens can be separated on the basis of molecular weight, and antibodies to each component can be detected as discrete bands on the western blot. A negative western blot is one in which no bands are present at molecular weights corresponding to HIV gene products. In a patient with a positive or indeterminate EIA and a negative western blot, one can conclude with certainty that the EIA reactivity was a false positive. On the other hand, a ***western blot demonstrating antibodies to products of all three of the major genes of HIV (gag, pol, and env) is conclusive evidence of infection with HIV.*** By definition, western blot patterns of reactivity that do not fall into the positive or negative categories are considered "indeterminate". **There are two possible explanations for an indeterminate western blot result.**
- The most likely explanation in a low-risk individual is that the patient being tested has antibodies that cross-react with one of the

proteins of HIV. The most common patterns of cross-reactivity are antibodies that react with p24 and/or p55.

- The least likely explanation in this setting is that the individual is infected with HIV and is in the process of mounting a classic antibody response. *In either instance,* the *western blot should be repeated in 1 month to determine whether or not the indeterminate pattern is a pattern in evolution.*

In addition, **one may attempt to confirm a diagnosis of HIV infection with the p24 antigen capture assay** or one of the tests for HIV RNA. While the western blot is an excellent confirmatory test for HIV infection in patients with a positive or indeterminate EIA, it is a poor screening test. Among individuals with a negative EIA and PCR for HIV, 20 to 30% may show one or more bands on western blot. While these bands are usually faint and represent cross-reactivity, their presence creates a situation in which other diagnostic modalities **[such as DNA PCR, RNA PCR, the (b) DNA assay, or p24 antigen capture]** must be employed to ensure that the bands do not indicate early HIV infection.

A *variety of laboratory tests are available for the direct detection of HIV or its components.* These tests may be of considerable help in making a diagnosis of HIV infection when the western blot results are indeterminate. In addition, the tests detecting levels of HIV RNA can be used to determine prognosis and to assess the response to antiretroviral therapies. The simplest of the direct detection tests is the *p24 antigen capture assay*. This is an EIA-type assay in which the solid phase consists of antibodies to the p24 antigen of HIV. *It detects the viral protein p24 in the blood of HIV-infected individuals where it exists either as free antigen or complexed to anti-p24 antibodies.* Overall, approximately 30% of individuals with untreated HIV infection have detectable levels of free p24 antigen. This increases to about 50% when samples are treated with a weak acid to dissociate antigen-antibody complexes. Throughout the course of HIV infection, an equilibrium exists between p24 antigen and anti-p24 antibodies. *During the first few weeks of infection, before an immune response develops, there is a brisk rise in p24 antigen levels. After the development of anti-p24 antibodies, these levels decline.* Late in the course of infection, when circulating levels of virus are high, p24 antigen levels also increase, particularly when detected by techniques involving dissociation of antigen-antibody complexes. *This assay has its greatest use as a screening test for HIV infection in patients suspected of having the acute HIV syndrome, as high levels of p24 antigen are present prior to the development of antibodies.* In addition, it is currently routinely used along with the HIV EIA assay to screen blood donors in the United States for evidence of HIV infection. *Its utility as an assay is decreasing with the increased use of the reverse transcriptase PCR (RT-PCR) and bDNA technique for direct detection of HIV RNA.*

The ability to measure and monitor levels of HIV RNA in the plasma of patients with HIV infection has been of extraordinary value in furthering our understanding of the pathogenesis of HIV infection and in providing a diagnostic tool in settings where measurements of anti-HIV antibodies may be misleading, such as in acute infection and neonatal infection. **Two assays are predominantly used** for this purpose. They are the **• RT-PCR (Amplicor) and the • bDNA (Quantiplex).** It should be pointed out that the *only test approved by the FDA at this time for the measurement of HIV RNA levels is the RT-PCR test.* While this approval is limited to the use of the test for determining prognosis, it is the general consensus that these tests as well as the bDNA test are also of value for monitoring the effects of therapy and in making a diagnosis of HIV infection. *In addition to these two commercially available tests, the DNA PCR is also employed by research laboratories for making a diagnosis of HIV infection by amplifying HIV proviral DNA from peripheral blood mononuclear cells.* The commercially available RNA detection tests have a sensitivity of 40 to 50 copies of HIV RNA per milliliter of plasma, while the DNA PCR tests can detect proviral DNA at a frequency of one copy per 10,000 to 100,000 cells. Thus, **these tests are extremely sensitive.** One frequent consequence of a high degree of sensitivity is some loss of specificity, and false-positive results have been reported with each of these techniques. For this reason, ***a positive EIA with a confirmatory western blot remains the "gold standard" for a diagnosis of HIV infection,*** and the interpretation of other test results must be done with this in mind.

In the **RT-PCR technique,** following DNAase treatment, a cDNA copy is made of all RNA species present in plasma. Insofar as HIV is an RNA virus, this will result in the production of DNA copies of the HIV genome in amounts proportional to the amount of HIV RNA present in plasma. This proviral DNA is then amplified and characterized using standard PCR techniques, employing primer pairs that can distinguish genomic cDNA from messenger cDNA. The bDNA assay involves the use of solid-phase nucleic acid capture system and signal amplification through successive nucleic acid hybridizations to detect small quantities of HIV RNA. Both tests can achieve a tenfold increase in sensitivity to 40 to 50 copies of HIV RNA per milliliter with a preconcentration step in which plasma undergoes ultracentrifugation to pellet the viral particles. ***In addition to being a diagnostic and prognostic tool, RT-PCR is also useful for amplifying defined areas of the HIV genome for sequence analysis and has become an important technique for studies of sequence diversity and microbial resistance to antiretroviral agents. In patients with a positive or indeterminate EIA test and an indeterminate western blot, and in patients in whom serologic testing may be unreliable (such as patients with hypogammaglobulinemia or advanced HIV disease), these tests provide valuable tools for making a diagnosis of HIV infection. They should only be used for diagnosis when standard serologic testing has failed to provide a definitive result.***

ANTIRETROVIRAL THERAPY (ART)

There has been reduction in number of new AIDS cases in the developed countries with the advent of ***Highly Active Anti-Retroviral Therapy [HAART].*** When potent combination therapy is administered effectively, the levels of RNA in plasma and infected cells in lymphoid tissue clear rapidly. Virtually all the compounds that are currently used, or under advanced clinical trial, for the treatment of HIV infections, belong to one of the following classes:

- ***Nucleoside/nucleotide reverse transcriptase inhibitors (NRTIs):*** i.e. zidovudine (AZT), didanosine (ddI), zalcitabine (ddC), stavudine (d4T), lamivudine (3TC), abacavir (ABC), emtricitabine [(-) FTC], tenofovir (PMPA) disoproxil fumarate;
- ***Non-nucleoside reverse transcriptase inhibitros (NNRTIs):*** i.e. nevirapine, delavirdine, efavirenz, emivirine (MKC-442); and
- ***Protease inhibitors (PIs):*** i.e. saquinavir, ritonavir, indinavir, nelfinavir, amprenavir, and lopinavir.

In addition to the reverse transcriptase and protease step, various other events in the HIV replicative cycle are potential targets for chemotherapeutic intervention:

- ***Viral adsorption, through binding to the viral envelope glycoprotein gp120*** (polysulfates, polysulfonates, polyoxometalates, zintevir, negatively charged albumins, cosalane analogues);
- ***Viral entry, through blockade of the viral coreceptors CXCR4 and CCR5*** [bicyclams (i.e. AMD3100), polyphemusins (T22), TAK-779, MIP-1 alpha LD78 beta isoform];
- ***Virus-cell fusion, through binding to the viral glycoprotein gp41*** [T-20 (DP-178), T-1249 (DP-107), siamycins, betulinic acid derivatives];
- ***Viral assembly and disassembly, through NCp7 zinc finger-targeted agents*** [2,2′-dithiobisbenzamides (DIBAs), azadicarbonamide (ADA) and NCp7 peptide mimics];
- ***Proviral DNA integration, through integrase inhibitors such*** as L-chicoric acid and diketo acids (i.e. L-731, 988);
- ***Viral mRNA transcription, through inhibitors of the transcription (transactivation) process***

(fluoroquinolone K-12, Streptomyces product EM2487, temacrazine, CGP64222).

Also, in recent years new NRTIs, NNRTIs and PIs have been developed that possess respectively improved metabolic characteristics. Although, a multitude of anti-HIV agents are being pursued actively, it has not been possible to eradicate HIV completely in an infected individual. The viral suppression is inadequate (failure to reduce viral copy number to less than 50 copies/ml) and unsustainable. Over a period of time expansion of resistant variants takes place and these viral populations overtake the immune system leading eventually to AIDS. According to the guidelines laid down, ***it is advised to administer a multi drug regimen consisting of non-nucleoside reverse transcriptase inhibitors, nucleoside reverse transcriptase inhibitors and protease inhibitors to avoid faster emergence of resistant viruses.*** The use of existing therapies in the developing world, where more than two thirds of the total HIV infection prevails, is limited owing to their high cost. Apart from the high cost and emergence of resistant mutants, another limiting factor is low patient compliance owing to the cumbersome drug regimens and side effects.

HIV VACCINE

Identifying the epitopes of HIV that are most critical in establishing infection or, conversely, which epitopes should be targeted for the development of cell-mediated and humoral immune responses to control HIV, is a major concern in vaccine development. **HIV vaccine can be either preventive vaccine**, which can be given to healthy individuals who are HIV negative, or it can be a **therapeutic vaccine,** which can be given to people who are already ill with the goal of curing them or improving their health:

The **goals for an HIV vaccine** should include

- Protection against HIV infection, i.e. against all routes of transmission, against intravenous transmission only, against mucosal transmission only;
- protection against progression to disease i.e., reduction of the viral load;
- reduction of transmission, i.e. vaccines likely to have lower viral load or lower transmission rate.

An Ideal HIV Vaccine

The ideal characteristic of an AIDS vaccine would include:

- Efficacy in preventing transmission by the mucosal and parenteral route
- Excellent safety profile
- Single dose administration
- Long lived effect resulting in protection many years after vaccination
- Low cost
- Stability under field conditions
- Ease of transportation and administration and
- Ability to induce protection against infection with diverse viral isolates preventing the need for many isolate specific vaccines.

Although the overall strategy is to achieve sterilizing immunity, a more realistic goal is to develop a vaccine, which could control viral replication, delay the onset of the disease and to reduce viral transmission. Modeling studies have revealed that even a partially efficacious vaccine would still have a major medical and socio-economic impact particularly in the developing countries.

Barriers to HIV Vaccine Development

Obstacles to the development of an effective HIV vaccine include factors related to the biology of HIV-1 infection and practical realities of developing and testing an AIDS vaccine are as follows:

- ***Sequence variation:*** The rapid replication of HIV-1 *in vivo* produces 10^{10} new virions/day which facilitates rapid generation of sequence variants. Because a significant proportion of HIV specific neutralizing antibodies and CTL are subtype specific, this sequence diversity has fostered efforts to induce broadly reactive immune responses or to utilize multivalent HIV vaccine.
- ***Protective immunity:*** Another fundamental barrier is the lack of information regarding the type of immune response that may protect

against HIV infection. CTL responses may be important to induce vaccine mediated protective immunity. HIV vaccine should be able to induce both HIV specific CTL and neutralizing antibody responses.

- *Latency:* Like other retroviruses, HIV integrates into the host genome where it can remain in a latent form that does not express HIV structural proteins and is thus less likely to be eliminated by the host cellular and humoral immune responses.
- *Transmission:* HIV-1 is predominantly transmitted by mucosal route. Yet our knowledge of the event occurring during mucosal infection and immune responses responsible for defending against mucosal infection are quite limited. In addition, HIV transmission may occur by both cell free and cell associated virus particles. Cell associated virus is thought to be resistant to neutralizing antibodies and will not be recognized by the host CTL responses, unless there is a fortuitous match between the HLA molecules between the host and the donor.

HIV Vaccine Concepts

Several different HIV vaccine concepts have been used in the animal model to elicit HIV specific immune response as follows:

- *Recombinant subunit vaccine:* A vaccine produced by genetic engineering simulating a part of the outer surface envelope or other part of HIV. gp 120 is the most well studied candidate HIV-1 vaccine. **VaxGen**, a San Francisco-based company, initiated the first phase III-efficacy trial of an HIV vaccine in 1998 *using its gp 120-subunit vaccine known as AIDS VAX.*
- *Synthetic peptide vaccines:* Synthetic peptides of HIV are small epitopes of HIV proteins. Peptide based approaches offer the advantage of targeting specific epitopes that lie within the conserved area of the virus. Synthetic peptides can be linked to lipid molecules (e.g., lipopeptides) to facilitate induction of cellular immune responses such as CTLs. Finally *the peptide can be combined as a multipeptide vaccine in a strategy to include diverse subtypes so as to increase the breadth of the vaccine induced response.*
- *Virus like particles (VLP) and pseudovirions:* These are non-infectious particles resembling HIV that has one or more HIV proteins. Pseudovirions are replication incompetent viruses produced in mammalian cell cultures that contain all the viral proteins required for viral assembly, but do not contain the RNA genome, thus making it non-infectious. For example, core particles of hepatitis B virus have been engineered and evaluated preclinically to present HIV antigens.
- *Live vector vaccine: A live bacteria or a virus that is harmless to humans and is used to transport a gene that makes HIV proteins.* These include live attenuated bacterial vectors such as • **Bacille Calmette-Guerin (BCG)** and • **Salmonella**. These vectors are safe and can establish infection via a mucosal route and can elicit strong mucosal immune responses.
- *Whole killed or inactivated vaccine:* In this, the entire virus particle is presented to the immune system but it cannot infect or replicate and thus safer.
- *Live-attenuated vaccines:* Live attenuated virus vaccines have been successfully used to protect against a great number of diseases including polio and measles. *Nef*-deleted strains of simian immunodeficiency viruses (SIV) have shown promising immune protection from challenge with infectious SIV. Safety is a serious concern with this vaccine as the chances of reverting back to a more virulent HIV strain is quite high.
- *DNA immunization (Naked DNA or nucleic acid vaccine):* One of the newest technologies for vaccine design offer significant advantages in ease of manufacturing. Pieces of HIV DNA are incorporated into harmless plasmid DNA from bacteria. These bacterial plasmids that have been genetically engineered to contain viral genes are injected into the muscle or skin.

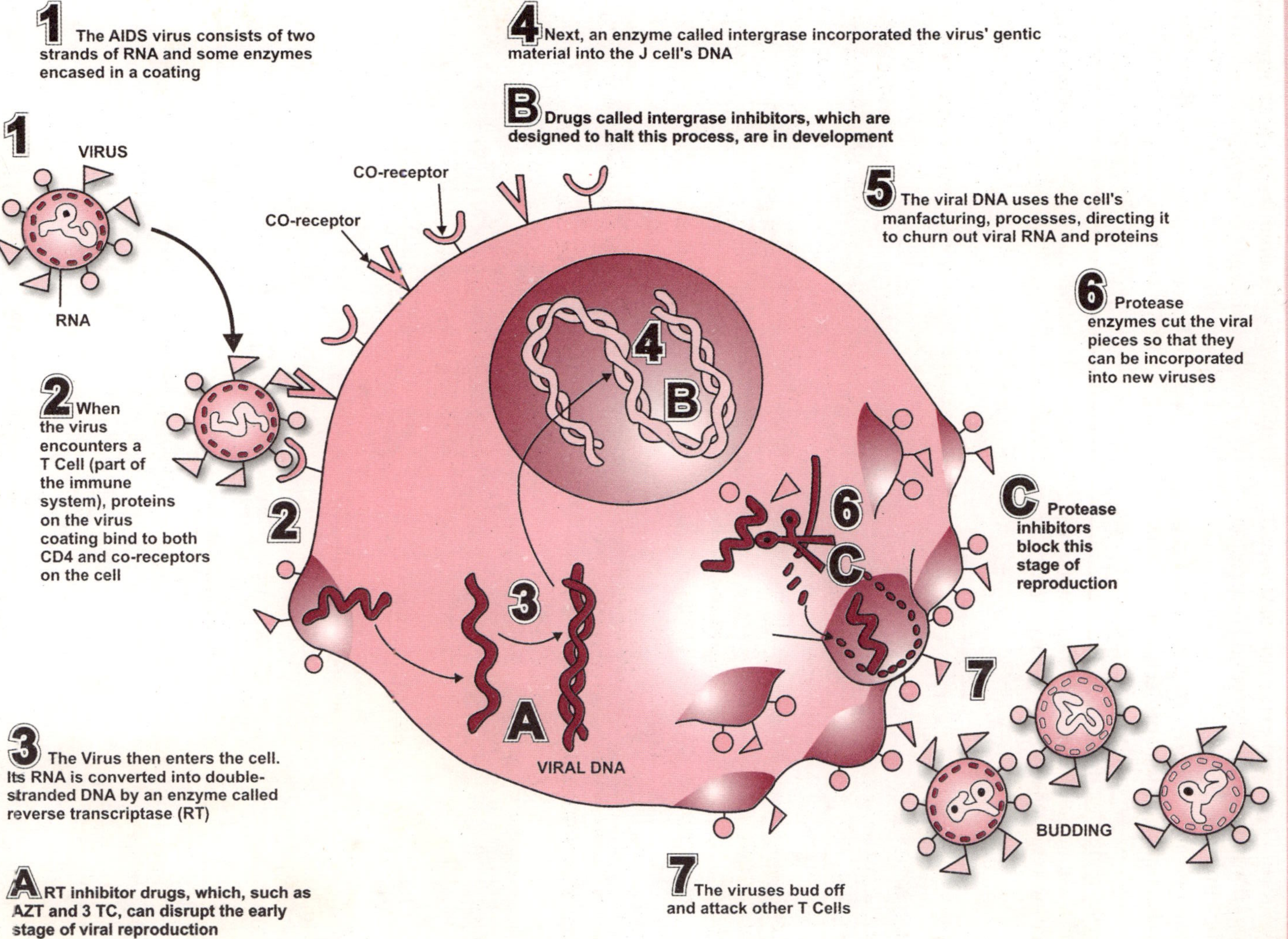

Fig. 30.6: Diagrammatic representation of life cycle of AIDS virus and possible methods to stop the disease

HIV DNA vaccines have been developed using HIV antigen from the *env* and core region of the virus.

- ***Prime boost protocols/combination vaccines:*** Recognizing that protection from HIV may require a broad spectrum of immune responses including humoral, cellular and mucosal immunity, scientists have designed **combination regimens** in attempts to **elicit such broad-spectrum immunity**. Prime boost refers to a vaccination regimen involving a primary vaccination with one vaccine generating CMI response followed by a boost with another vaccine, often a subunit protein to elicit humoral response. Combination vaccine approaches elicit the most potent immune responses in non-human primates and in humans.

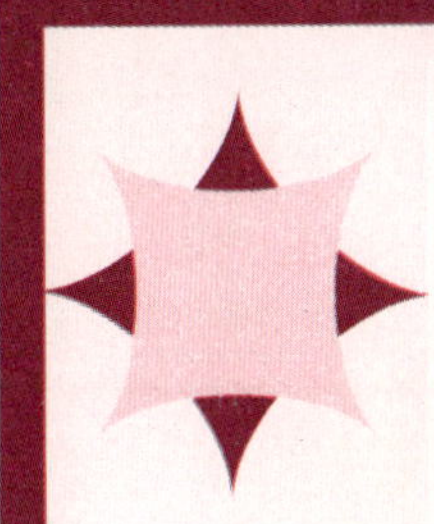

References

1. Baron DN: *A Short Textbook of Chemical Pathology*; 4th edn, 1982.
2. Bell GH, Davidson JN and Scarborough: *Textbook of Physiology and Biochemistry,* E and S Livingstone, 1965.
3. Bloom SR and Polak JM: *Gut Hormones*, 2nd edn, Churchill Livingstone, 1981.
4. Bondy PK and Rosenberg LE: *Duncan's Disease of Metabolism*, 7th edn, WB Saunders, Philadelphia, LOndon, 1974.
5. Bowen HJA: *Trace Elements in Biochemistry*, Academic Press, New York, 1966.
6. Brewer HB and Bronzert TJ: *Human Plasma Lipoproteins,* Fractions No-1, 1977.
7. Cantarow A and Schepartz B: Biochemistry, 4th edn, WB Saunders, Philadelphia, London, 1970 (reprint).
8. Conn EE and Stumpf PK: *Outlines of Biochemistry,* 2nd edn, Wiley Eastern, NEw Delhi, 1969.
9. Coodley EL: *Diagnostic Enzymology*, Lea and Febiger, Philadelphia, 1970.
10 Davidson JN: *Biochemistry of Nucleic Acids*, 5 th edn, Willey, New York, 1965
11. Daven Port HW: *ABC of Acid-base Chemistry*, 6th edn, university of Chicago Press, 1974.
12. De Luca HF and Schnoes HK: Vitamin D: *Recent Advances*, Ann Rev Biochem, 1983.
13. Dixon M and Webb EC: *Enzymes*, 2nd edn, Academic Press, New York, 1964.
14. Fersht A: *Enzymes Structure and Mechanism*, 2nd edn, Freeman, 1985.
15. Frisell WR: Acid-Base *Chemistry in Medicine*, Macmillan, New york, 1968.
16. Fruton JS and Simmonds SS: *General Biochemistry*, 2nd edn, John Wiley and Sons, New York, 1965
17. Ganong WF: *Review of Medical Physiology*, 6th edn. Lange Medical Publications, 1973.
18. Goldberger, *Emanuel: A Primer of Water, Electrolytes and Acid-Base Syndromes*, 4th edn, Lea and Febiger, Philadelphia, 1971.
19. Goodhart RS and Maurice E shils: *Modern Nutrition in Health and Disease,* 5th edn, Lea and Febiger, 1973.
20. Gopalan C and Rao, Nara Singa BS: *Dietary Allowances for Indians*, Indian Council of Medicl Research, New Delhi, 1980.
21. Halkerston lan DK: *Biochemistry,* 2nd edn. John Wiley and Sons, 1990.
22. Hoffman WS: *The Biochemistry of Clinical Medicine*, 4th edn, Year Book Medical Publishers, Chicago, 1970.
23. Harper HA: *Review of Physiological Chemistry*, 17th edn, Lange Medical Publication, 1979.
24. Hobbs JR: Immunoglobulins in Clinical Chemistry, *Advances in Clinical Chemistry*, 1971.
25. Heftman E (Ed): *Chromatography*, 3rd edn, Reinhold, 1975.
26. Hsia DY: *Inborn Errors of Metabolism*, 2nd edn, Year Book Medical Publications, Chicago, 1970.

27. King EJ: *Practical Clinical Enxymology,* D Von Nostrand, London, 1965.
28. Kleiner IS and Orten JM: *Biochemistry*, 7th edn, CV Mosby, St Louis,1966.
29. Khan RH and Lands WEM: Prostaglandins and cyclic AMP, Academic Press, New York, 1973.
30. Kornberg A: *DNA Replication*, Freeman, 1980.
31. Krishna Swamy K: Selemum in Human Health, *ICMR Bulletin*, 1990.
32. Lands WEM: *The biosynthesis and metabolism of prostaglandins*, Ann Rev Physiol, 1979.
33. Latner AL: Cantarow and Trumper: *Clinical Biochemistry*, 7th edn. Saunders, Philadelphia, 1975.
34. Lehninger AL: *Biochemistry*, 2nd edn, (Reprint) kalyani Publishers, Ludhiana, New Delhi, 1984
35. Mazur A and Harrow B: *Textbook of Biochemistry*, 10th edn. Saunders, Philadelphia, 1971.
36. Moncada S (Ed): Prostacyclin, thromboxane and leukotrienes, *Brit Med Bull*, 1983.
37. Mc Gilvery RW: *Biochemistry-A Functional Approach*, 3rd edn. Saunders, Philadelphia, 1983.
38. Murray: *Harpers Biochemistry*, Harper and Row, 1990.
39. Orten JM and Neuhaus W: *Human Biochemistry*, 10th edn. CV Mosby, BI Publications Ltd, New Delhi.
40. Prasad AS: *Trace Elements and Iron in Human Metabolism* Plenum Press, 1978.
41. Putman FW Ed: *The Plasma Proteins: Structure, Function and Genetic Control*, 2nd edn, Academic Press, New York, 1977.
42. Rawn JD: *Biochemistry*, Neil Patterson Publishers, Burlington, North Carolina, 1989.
43. *Samson Wright's Applied Physiology:* The English Language Book Society and Oxford University Press, London, 12th edn, 1971.
44. Smith LC: Plasma Lipoproteins: Structure and metabolism. *Ann Rev Biochem*, 1978.
45. Smith EL, Hill RL, Lehman IR, Lefkwitz RZ, Handler P and White A: *Priniciples of Biochemistry*, 7th edn. McGraw-Hill International, 1983.
46. Stryer L: *Biochemistry*, 3rd edn. WH Freeman, 1975
47. Sunderman FW and Sunderman FW Jr: *Serum proteins and the Dysproteinaemias*, Pitman Medical Publication, Philadelphia, 1964.
48. Suttie John W: *Introduction to Biochemistry*, Holt Rinehart and Winston, New York, 1977.
49. Thompson G: Plasma lipoproteins and their disorders, *Medicine*, 3rd series, 1978.
50. Thompson RHS and Wotton IDP: *Biochemical Disorders in Human Diseases*, 3rd edn. J and Churchill Ltd, London 1970.
51. Thorpe WB, Bray HG and James HP: *Biochemistry for Medical Students*, 9th edn, Churchill, London, 1970.
52. Underwood EJ: *Trace Elements in Human and Animal Nutrition*, 4th edn, Acdemic Press, New York, 1977.
53. Varley H: *Practical Clinical Biochemistry*, William Heinemann Medical Books Ltd. London, 1969.
54. Wasserman RH (Ed): *Calcium Binding Proteins and Calcium Function*, Elsevier, 1977.
55. Weisberg HF: *Water, Electrolytes and Acid-Base balance*, 2nd edn, William and Wilkins, Baltimore 1962.
56. West ES, Todd WR, Mason HS and Van Bruggen JT: *Textbook of biochemistry*, Macmillan, New York, 1966.
57. Wilkinson JH (Ed): *Principles and Practice of Diagnostic Enzymology*, Edward Arnold, London,1976.
58. Williams RH: *Textbook of endocrinology*, WB Saunders, Philadelphia, Indian Reprin,1970.
59. Yudkin M and offord K: *Comprehensive Biochemistry*, Longman (England), 1973.
60. Zubay Geoffrey: *Biochemistry*; 2nd Edn, Maxwell Macmillan (International edn), 1989.

Index

A

B

C

D

G

H

I

J

K

L

M

N

O

P

Q

R

S

T

U

V

W

X

Z